WO 100

WO 100

Essential Surgical Practice

Basic Surgical Training

Essential Surgical Practice

Basic Surgical Training

FOURTH EDITION

Edited by

Sir Alfred Cuschieri FRSE, MD (Malta), MD ((Liverpool), ChM (Liverpool), FRCSEd, FRCSEng, FRCSGlas, FRCSI
Professor of Surgery & Honorary Consultant Surgeon, Department of Surgery & Molecular Oncology, University of Dundee; Honorary Consultant Surgeon, Tayside University Hospitals NHS Trust

Robert J. C. Steele MD FRCS
Professor of Surgical Oncology & Honorary Consultant Surgeon, Department of Surgery & Molecular Oncology, University of Dundee; Honorary Consultant Surgeon, Tayside University Hospitals NHS Trst

Abdool Rahim Moossa MD FRCS FACS
Professor & Chairman, Department of Surgery, University of California, San Diego, Medical Center

A member of the Hodder Headline Group
LONDON
Co-published in the United States of America by
Oxford University Press Inc., New York

First published in Great Britain in 2000 by Butterworth Heinemann

This impression published in Great Britain in 2001 by
Arnold, a member of the Hodder Headline Group,
338 Euston Road, London NW1 3BH

First published 1982
Second Edition 1988
Third Edition 1995

http://www.arnoldpublishers.com

Distributed in the United States of America by
Oxford University Press Inc.,
198 Madison Avenue, New York, NY10016
Oxford is a registered trademark of Oxford University Press

Whilst the advice and information in this book are believed to be true and
accurate at the date of going to press, neither the author[s] nor the publisher
can accept any legal responsibility or liability for any errors or omissions
that may be made. In particular (but without limiting the generality of the
preceding disclaimer) every effort has been made to check drug dosages;
however it is still possible that errors have been missed. Furthermore,
dosage schedules are constantly being revised and new side-effects
recognized. For these reasons the reader is strongly urged to consult the
drug companies' printed instructions before administering any of the drugs
recommended in this book.

British Library Cataloguing in Publication Data
A catalogue record for this book is available from the British Library

Library of Congress Cataloging-in-Publication Data
A catalog record for this book is available from the Library of Congress

ISBN 0 340 80683 4 (hardback)
ISBN 0 340 80686 9 (International Students Edition)

1 2 3 4 5 6 7 8 9 10

Produced and typeset by Gray Publishing, Tunbridge Wells, Kent
Printed and bound in Great Britain

Contents

List of contributors

Jeff W. Allen MD
Instructor in Surgery, University of Louisville,
Louisville

John Camilleri-Brennan MD FRCS (Glasgow)
Surgical Research Fellow, Ninewells Hospital, Tayside
University Hospitals NHS Trust

Derek J. Byrne MD, FRCS
Consultant Urologist, Ninewells Hospital, Tayside
University Hospitals NHS Trust

Sir Alfred Cuschieri FRSE, MD (Malta), MD
(Liverpool), ChM (Liverpool), FRCSEd, FRCSEng,
FRCSGlas, FRCSI
Professor of Surgery and Honorary Consultant
Surgeon, Department of Surgery and Molecular
Oncology, University of Dundee; Honorary
Consultant Surgeon, Tayside University Hospitals
NHS Trust

Sandra Engelhardt MD
Clinical Instructor of Surgery, University of
California, San Diego, Medical Center

Pamela R. Ferguson LLB, PhD, DipLP
Solicitor and Senior Lecturer, Department of Law,
University of Dundee

Douglas Gentleman BSc (Hons), MB, ChB (Hons),
FRCS (Glasgow), FRCS (England)
Honorary Consultant Neurosurgeon, Ninewells
Hospital, Tayside University Hospitals NHS Trust;
Consultant, Centre for Brain Injury Rehabilitation,
Royal Victoria Hospital, Dundee

Ian S. Grant MD, FRCA, FRCS
Director and Consultant Anaesthetist, Intensive Care
Unit, Western General Hospitals NHS Trust
Edinburgh

Gareth Griffiths MB, ChB, MD, FRCS
Consultant Surgeon, Ninewells Hospital, Tayside
University Hospitals NHS Trust

John F. Hansbrough MD
Director, Regional Burn Center, Professor of
Surgery, University of California, San Diego,
Medical Center

Iain S. Henderson MB, FRCP, ChB
Consultant Physician, Ninewells Hospital, Tayside
University Hospitals NHS Trust

Graeme Houston MD, FRCP, FRCR
Consultant Radiologist, Ninewells Hospital, Tayside
University Hospitals NHS Trust

David B. Hoyt MD, FACS
Associate Professor of Surgery, Chief Division of
Trauma, The Monroe E. Trout Professor of Surgery,
University of California, San Diego, Medical Center

Michael C. Jones BSc (Hons), MD (Hons), FRCP
(Edin), FRCP (Glas)
Consultant Physician, Ninewells Hospital, Tayside
University Hospitals NHS Trust

Roland T. Jung MA, MD (Cantab), FRCP (Edin),
FRCP (London)
Consultant Physician, Director of Research and
Development, Tayside NHS Consortium, Diabetes
and Endocrinology, The Diabetes Centre, Ninewells
Hospital, Tayside University Hospitals NHS Trust;
Honorary Professor in Medicine, University of
Dundee

Murray Lough FRCGP
Assistant Director of Postgraduate Medical Education,
University of Glasgow

Ellon McGregor MB, ChB, MRCP
Consultant Physician, Ninewells Hospital, Tayside
University Hospitals NHS Trust

Andrew Mikulaschek MD
Clinical Instructor of Surgery, University of
California, San Diego, Medical Center

A. R. Moossa MD
Professor and Chairman, Department of Surgery,
University of California, San Diego, Medical Center

Stephen Palmer PhD
Centre for Health Economics, University of York

Christopher R. Pennington BSc, MD, FRCP,
FRCPE
Consultant Physician and Gastroenterologist, Ninewells
Hospital, Tayside University Hospitals NHS Trust;
Honorary Professor in Medicine, University of
Dundee

Martijn Poeze MD
Algemene Heelkunde, Academisch Ziekenhuis,
Maastricht

Graham Ramsay MD, FRCS
Surgeon, Algemene Heelkunde, Academisch
Ziekenhuis, Maastricht

Ian C. Reid MB, ChB, BMedBiol, PhD, MRCPsych
Professor of Psychiatry and Consultant Psychiatrist,
Department of Psychiatry, University of Dundee

Ian W. Ricketts BSc Elec Eng, PhD Computing
Professor in Assistive Systems and Healthcare
Computing, Department of Applied Computing,
University of Dundee

Iian Rubinfeld MD
Clinical Instructor of Surgery, University of
California, San Diego, Medical Center

Mark Sculpher PhD
Centre for Health Economics, University of York

R. J. C. Steele MD, FRCS
Professor of Surgical Oncology and Honorary
Consultant Surgeon, Department of Surgery and
Molecular Oncology, University of Dundee;
Honorary Consultant Surgeon, Tayside University
Hospitals NHS Trust

A. M. Stewart MRCPsych, FDSRCPS
Consultant In Liaison and General Adult Psychiatry,
Royal Dundee Liff Hospital

Peter Arno Stonebridge ChM, MB, ChB,
FRCS (Ed)
Consultant Surgeon, Ninewells Hospital, Tayside
University Hospitals NHS Trust

Alan Struthers MB, ChB (Hons), BSc (Hons), MD,
FRCP, FRCP(Ed), MRCP, FESC, DCH
Professor and Consultant Physician in Clinical
Pharmacology, Dept. Of Clinical Pharmacology,
University of Dundee

Alastair M. Thompson MD, FRCSEd (Gen)
Senior Lecturer and Honorary Consultant
Surgeon, Department of Surgery and Molecular
Oncology, University of Dundee; Honorary
Consultant Surgeon, Tayside University Hospitals
NHS Trust

C. Wallis MD, FRCA
Consultant Anaesthetist, Western General Hospitals
NHS Trust, Edinburgh

Robert J. Winchell MD FACS
Associate Professor of Clinical Surgery, University of
California, San Diego, Medical Center

Preface

It is now 18 years since the first edition of *Essential Surgical Practice* was published. During this time life, surgical practice and surgical training have all changed greatly. Largely for these reasons, the editors of the Fourth Edition, in association with the publishers, decided on a radical change in format and presentation. At the same time we also wanted to pave the way for expectations regarding surgical practice in the new millennium.

Within the United Kingdom, the most significant changes in surgical training date from the Calman Report. The period of surgical training is now shorter and has two distinct phases: basic training and higher surgical training within a recognized surgical specialty, with an exit examination towards the end of the training period. The basic format adopted reflects this fundamental change and the Fourth Edition thus consists of two volumes. The first volume caters for the needs of the junior trainee undertaking his or her basic training in 'the generality of surgery' up to the MRCS/AFRCS examination. The second volume is intended for the higher surgical trainee in General Surgery, including Vascular Surgery, Breast and Endocrine Surgery as these are currently grouped with this surgical specialty, although the situation may change in the future.

The format adopted in this edition is also different from the previous editions in its use of topic-related modules incorporating allied sections with the emphasis on management of patients with the various surgical disorders. The account, especially in Volume I, is thus patient orientated rather than disease orientated. Several new topics have been included for the first time in an effort to enhance the totality of patient care and management covered, and because of the increasing importance of the Internet in continued medical education and professional development, a section on its use is included in one of the modules. In many ways, the format adopted for the Fourth Edition is that in common usage in distance learning.

In Volume II, the intention has been to cover in detail all the necessary material for higher surgical training in General Surgery. Other sections are addressed from the viewpoint of what the general surgeon should know about disease processes and conditions managed by other surgical specialists; that is, core information as distinct from specialist knowledge. This required an exercise of refined judgement from us as editors and from all the contributors, but we are confident that we have achieved the right balance.

The production of a new edition is always a labour of love and this has been no exception. The task has been exacting, but at the same time highly educational to us. Disraeli's remark that 'the best way to learn a subject is to write a book about it' is indeed true. The task would have been impossible without the support we received from our publishers, especially Dr. G. Smaldon, who has consistently cajoled and prodded us to finish the job, and from all our authors, to whom we owe an immense debt for the excellence of their contributions. As we move into the new millennium, we hope that *Essential Surgical Practice* will continue to provide assistance to surgical trainees world-wide and that they will find within its pages encouragement to acquire knowledge, skill and compassion, which are the cornerstones of surgical practice.

A. Cuschieri
R.J. Steele
A.R. Moossa

Surgical biology and pathological examination

'The world can only be grasped by action, not by contemplation ... the hand is the cutting edge of the mind' – Jacob Bronowski 1908–1974

Section 1.1 • Wound healing and repair

In earlier times the wound was assessed somewhat indirectly by studies of the breaking strength and collagen content. Today we look beyond these parameters to the behaviour of the individual cells in the wound since these are the prime movers in the healing process. Uneventful healing is dependent on their health and, in turn, this is determined by their microenvironment and a whole host of growth factors supplemented by growth-promoting and chemotactic substances produced primarily by platelets, lymphocyte cells and macrophages.

The elements of healing

Three distinct processes contribute to the process of wound healing.

Epithelialization
This is the process by which the surface covering of the wound is restored by a combination of cell migration and multiplication. The stimulus for epithelial repair is unknown. The loss of contact between cells undoubtedly plays a part. When an area is denuded of epithelium, the marginal cells divide and migrate across the bare area. The activity ceases when epithelial contact is re-established. There is also evidence that the loss of the epithelial cover is associated with a fall in the level of a local inhibitory hormone or chalone that is synthesized by the epithelial cells. Epithelialization proceeds most rapidly in a most highly oxygenated environment.

Contraction
This is the process by which the edges of an open wound gradually close together. It is a form of tissue migration that involves the entire thickness of the skin and subcutaneous tissues. It therefore proceeds most readily in areas where the skin is loose, such as the buttocks and the back of the neck. Contraction is due to forces exerted by specialized fibroblasts in the wound.

These cells have contractile elements in their cytoplasm and are known as myofibroblasts. The process of contraction is physiological and must be distinguished from the pathological process of scar contracture or cicatrization that causes distortion and limitation of movement.

Connective tissue formation
This is the process by which the main body of the wound is united. It plays a fundamental role in all but the most superficial injuries, and the strength of the wound following surgery is dependent on it. Connective tissue formation is the most important element of the three components, and many studies of wound healing are simply an examination of this component in isolation.

Types of healing

Although the elements of tissue repair are the same, open and closed wounds heal rather differently. When a surgical incision is closed with sutures or clips and heals without complication, it is said to heal by first intention. Union takes place by a combination of epithelialization and connective tissue formation. When an open wound is allowed to close naturally, union is accomplished by a combination of all three: wound contraction, connective tissue formation and epithelialization. This is known as healing by second intention or by granulation. These wounds heal from the bottom by abundant vascular connective tissue that has a granular appearance, hence the name.

Prior to the development of connective tissue, the closed wound is much more susceptible to infection than the open wound. For this reason, a heavily contaminated wound is often only partially closed. The deeper layers are secured but the subcutaneous tissues and the skin are left open. Once healing is established and granulation tissue has formed, the wound may be closed without fear of invasive infection developing. The technique is called delayed primary closure or secondary suture, and this type of healing is known as healing by third intention.

Phases of healing

In deeper wounds, the strength recovery is often an important attribute. Studies in the 1920s demonstrated that this occurred in the phasic manner typical of many biological processes. In the first few days, the wound has no recordable strength. Following this, strength increases rapidly. Finally, after a few weeks, the process slows down and further increases in strength occur gradually. These features of strength recovery correlate well with observed changes in the wound, and healing is often considered as a three-phase event.

During the first few days, when the wound has no strength, little seems to be happening and this is called the lag phase. However, there is intense enzymic and leucocytic activity with breakdown and removal of devitalized tissue. A better term is the preparation phase, as the foundations for repair are being laid. During the next few weeks the scene is dominated by the proliferation of cells and capillaries. Neutrophils and macrophages are prominent and fibroblasts lay down collagen in increasing amounts. In an open wound, this vascular fibrocellular tissue is recognized as granulation tissue. This is the phase of proliferation or fibroplasia. After a variable number of weeks, these wound activities slow down. Fibroblasts and capillaries are less in evidence but strength increases progressively. This third phase is the one of maturation or differentiation that lasts for several months.

The organ of repair

During the phase of proliferation the new tissue in the wound can be thought of as a repair organ (Figure 1.1).

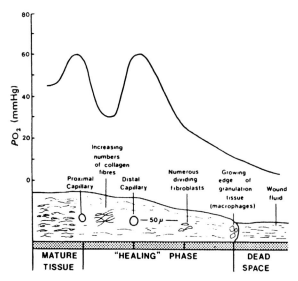

Figure 1.1 Profile of a healing wound. It is a delicate system of cells and capillaries. New tissue grows from the 'vital' edge towards the central dead space. Direct measurements of P_{O_2} in this granulation tissue shows a steady fall from the normal mature tissue level of around 45 mmHg to anoxic levels in the centre of the wound. Macrophages have a lower oxygen requirement than fibroblasts and are found at the free edge of the growing tissue. (After Silver, 1980.)

Its delicate stroma and extensive capillary network provide both physical and nutritional support for its component cells. The function of this organ is connective tissue formation. The fibroblast is the key cell synthesizing collagen and intercellular ground substance. Its activities, together with those of the support macrophages, are dependent on a readily available supply of oxygen. As a result, cells and capillaries develop together as a unit and grow until the wound is filled. This new vascular connective tissue is most obvious in open wounds but it is also present between the edges of a healing, closed, incised wound. As time passes, the fibroblasts and the capillaries become much less prominent and a mature fibrous scar remains.

Wound strength

The recovery of strength has obvious clinical significance and has proved to be one of the most useful indications of the progress of repair. Early studies of wound-breaking strength showed that the apparently well-healed wound was still remarkably weak. Skin and scar tissue are complex viscoelastic materials that cannot be fully characterized unless tensile strength and extension (stretch) are recorded simultaneously. Plotted together, they describe a curve (load–extension) that reflects the ability of the scar to resist rupture (energy absorption) (see Figure 1.2a–c). The findings are remarkably uniform, demonstrating only a 50–70% recovery of strength by the end of 6 months. It appears that total recovery is rarely achieved. Such low recordings need not cause alarm, for the absolute values are more than enough to meet the stresses imposed by everyday life.

Wound histology

Light microscopy shows a characteristic sequence of events (Figure 1.3). As time elapses after wounding, specific cell populations appear on the scene. Neutrophils predominate in the first day and monocytes peak about 24 h later. By 5–6 days, fibroblasts are found in large numbers and their presence is synchronous with the establishment of a microcirculation. Collagen is readily identified in increasing amounts after the fourth day.

A characteristic sequence of enzyme changes is also seen (Figure 1.4). When identified histochemically, these can be used to calculate the age of the wound in hours. Collagen is responsible for most of the strength of the wound, and scar weakness is associated with physical changes in the collagen. When the wound is examined by polarized light, normal collagen stands out as a clearly birefringent material. However, the wound scar does not exhibit this property during the first 6 months of healing. This lack of birefringence indicates a failure of organization at the molecular and small fibril level. Physical factors, e.g. fibre shape and weave, are important in determining the mechanical properties of skin and scar. These are best displayed by scanning electron microscopy. In unwounded skin, the collagen fibrils lie in well-organized bundles (Figure

(a)

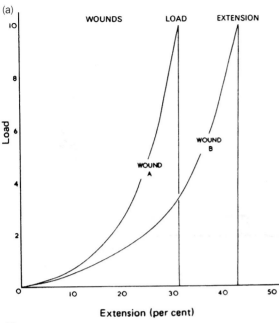

(b)

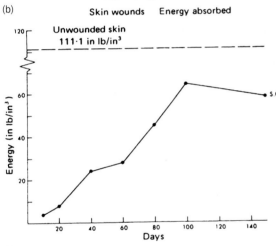

(c)

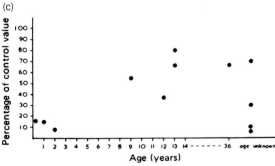

Figure 1.2 (a) Load–extension curves for wounds, which break under the same load but differ in the degree of extension. Wound A is less pliable than wound B and is therefore easily ruptured. The ability to resist rupture (energy absorption) is measured by the area under the curve. (b) The ability of a wound to resist rupture expressed as its energy absorption. There is only a 50% recovery by 150 days. (From Forrester *et al.*, *J Surg Res* 1969; **9**: 207–212, with permission.) (c) The tensile strength of human skin wounds expressed as a percentage of intact skin. In the first 2-year period, skin wounds are less than 20% of control value and even at 13 years there is still a marked weakness. (From Douglas *et al.*, *Br J Surg* 1969; **56**: 219–222, with permission.)

HISTOLOGICAL EVENTS

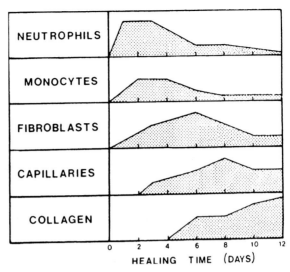

Figure 1.3 Characteristic sequence of events in the first few days of wound healing. Neutrophils and monocytes appear first. Collagen appears following the development of a functioning fibroblast–capillary system.

1.5). In sutured wounds, the collagen fibrils lie in a relatively haphazard manner (Figure 1.6). As time passes, the collagen fibrils in the wound coalesce to form large irregular masses (Figure 1.7), remodelling being minimal. As yet there is no evidence that the normal architectural network is ever restored.

Wound biochemistry

Of all the soft-tissue constituents of the body, only collagen has sufficient strength of its own to be responsible for the observed mechanical properties of unwounded tissue and firmly healed scar. The total amount of collagen rises rapidly in a healing wound and normal levels are usually attained within a few weeks. However, strength continues to increase long after the collagen content has returned to normal. Clearly, the quality of the collagen in the wound alters as time goes by.

Studies using radioactive tracer techniques have clarified the situation (Figure 1.8). The amount of collagen in the wound stabilizes after a few weeks but the rate of collagen synthesis and lysis remains high for considerably longer. This balance of synthesis and lysis may explain several healing defects. In keloid and hypertrophic scars, overproduction of collagen seems to be due to a relatively low rate of lysis. In scurvy, it is the synthesis of collagen that fails, and the wound weakens under the continued lytic process.

Collagen forms 30% of the total protein content of most animals. The collagen molecule is a rigid rod 300 nm long and 1.5 nm wide. Each molecule is composed of three polypeptide chains bound in a left-handed helix. The molecule itself is twisted the opposite way into a right-handed superhelix. The polypeptide chains of collagen are themselves remarkable.

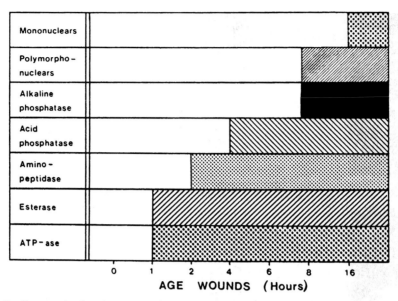

	0	1	2	4	6	8	16

Mononuclears, Polymorpho-nuclears, Alkaline phosphatase, Acid phosphatase, Amino-peptidase, Esterase, ATP-ase

AGE WOUNDS (Hours)

Figure 1.4 Schematic diagram showing the histochemical estimation of age of antemortem skin wounds. (From Rawkallio, *J Forensic Sci* 1972; **1:** 3–16, with permission.)

Over half of the molecule is composed of the three amino acids glycine, proline and hydroxyproline. Both the carboxyl-end and the amino-terminal of the molecule are non-helical and the entire structure is held together by hydrogen bonds. These bonds are relatively weak and the bulk of the strength of mature collagen is attributed to strong intermolecular and intramolecular covalent bonds. The individual amino acids are assembled in the endoplasmic reticulum of the fibroblast (Figure 1.9), beginning at the amino-terminal and proceeding towards the carboxyl-end. A unique feature in the synthesis is that neither hydroxyproline nor hydroxylysine is incorporated directly into the collagen molecule. Instead, a proline-rich collagen precursor (protocollagen) is formed. Hydroxylation then proceeds under the influence of protocollagen hydroxylase. Requirements of the enzyme are oxygen, α-ketoglutarate, ferrous iron and ascorbic acid. Each of these may interfere with collagen metabolism but the only one of practical importance is ascorbic acid, deficiency of which delays collagen synthesis. The incompletely synthesized collagen cannot be excreted from the fibroblasts and distends their endoplasmic reticulum in a characteristic way (Figure 1.10). Several different genes direct synthesis and 13 distinct types of collagen have been identified in vertebrate tissues. Type I characterizes mature bone and skin. Type II is found in hyaline cartilage and type

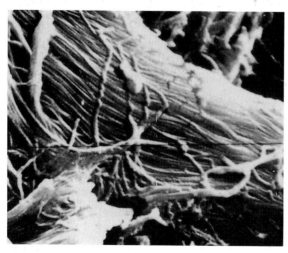

Figure 1.5 Scanning electron micrograph of part of a normal collagen fibre showing that it is made up of bundles of cross-banded fibrils (× 9000). (From Forrester *et al., Nature* 1969; **221:** 373–374, with permission.)

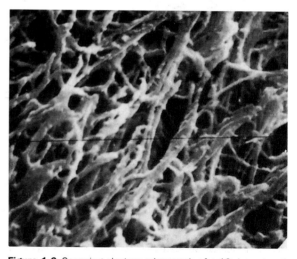

Figure 1.6 Scanning electron micrograph of a 10-day sutured wound showing the randomly orientated collagen fibrils. They show little tendency to aggregate. Cross-banding is not apparent (× 9000). (From Forrester *et al., Nature* 1969; **221:** 373–374, with permission.)

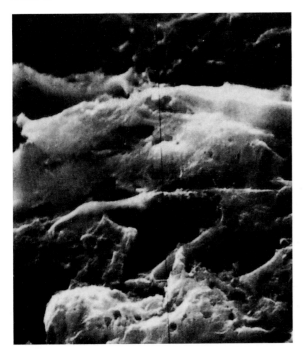

Figure 1.7 Scanning electron micrograph of a representative portion of a 100-day wound. The collagen fibrils have aggregated to form large collagen masses but normal fibre architecture has not been restored (× 3150). (From Forrester *et al., Nature* 1969; **221:** 373–374, with permission.)

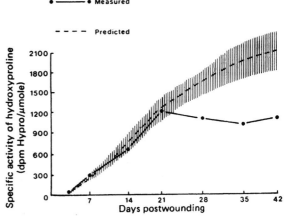

Figure 1.8 Comparison of scar collagen accumulation predicted from its rate of synthesis with that actually measured. Total collagen does not increase after 3 weeks, even though it continues to be synthesized and deposited at a rapid rate. Collagen is now being removed as quickly as it is formed (collagenolysis). The difference between the curves represents scar collagen turnover. (From Madden and Peacock, *J Ann Surg* 1971; **174:** 511–520, with permission.)

III in cardiovascular structures, infant skin and the granulation tissue of healing skin wounds. Types IV and V are associated with basement membranes, and the others with a variety of tissues including cartilage and certain tumours. The significance of these different forms of collagen is not yet clear but their existence does help to explain why cutaneous scar tissue behaves in a different way from the surrounding dermis. Scar collagen contains both types I and III and differs in its degree of hydroxylation of lysine and glycosylation of hydroxylysine. The cross-linking pattern is also different.

All connective tissues contain varying amounts of ground substance. This amorphous matrix between the cells and fibres contains protein–glycosaminoglycan complexes called proteoglycans. The fibroblast synthesizes collagen, glycosaminoglycans and fibronectin. The latter component of the matrix is a large glycoprotein with important influences on both intercellular adhesion and cell to matrix adhesion. The functions of the proteoglycans and fibronectin are incompletely understood, but they appear to play a part in the organization

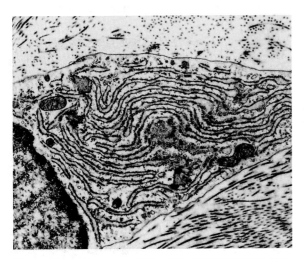

Figure 1.9 Electron micrograph of a normal fibroblast. Note the characteristic well-developed endoplasmic reticulum. The lining ribosomes, which are responsible for its rough appearance, are the active site of collagen synthesis. New collagen fibrils are rapidly excreted and are seen here surrounding the cell (× 9000). (Courtesy of Professor Russell Ross, Seattle.)

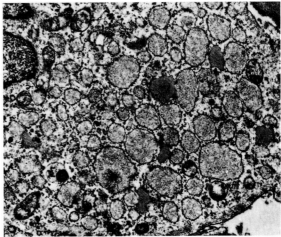

Figure 1.10 Electron micrograph of part of a scorbutic fibroblast. Note the typical distended endoplasmic reticulum. There is no sign of collagen but it will appear within 24 h of providing ascorbic acid (× 9000). (Courtesy of Professor Russell Ross, Seattle.)

and precipitation of collagen fibres. The ground substance has, in addition, important effects on the mechanical properties of mature tissue. The wound is a fibre–gel–fluid system and the mechanical properties of this complex material differ significantly from those of fibrous tissue alone.

Factors affecting healing

A number of factors influence the rate of wound healing. However, some have unpredictable effects. Thus, jaundice and uraemia adversely affect wound healing in animals but not in humans. The important factors influencing healing in clinical practice are: age, nutrition, vascular supply, sepsis, oxygen and wound dressing.

Age

Healing proceeds more rapidly in the young provided they are well nourished. The increased vigour of repair may explain why hypertrophic scars and keloids are more common in early life.

Nutrition

To a certain extent, wounds do not heal well in the debilitated and malnourished. However, several studies have documented the biological priority of healing wounds. Thus, patients have to be very severely protein depleted before healing is impaired. Ascorbic acid is required for the synthesis and maintenance of collagen. Following injury, body stores are rapidly depleted and a scorbutic state may be induced. When this happens, collagen synthesis is impaired with delayed healing. In older wounds where collagen turnover is still active, scars have been known to reopen. Healing is also delayed by zinc deficiency.

Vascularity

Wounds heal well in areas such as the face where the blood supply is good and vice versa. The most striking examples are found in ischaemic vascular disease of the lower limb. Both wound healing and the overall metabolic response to trauma are optimal when the environmental temperature is raised to 30°C. The combination of increased blood flow and warmth following sympathectomy has been shown to improve healing in patients with peripheral vascular disease.

A minimal inflammatory stimulus is required for healing to progress normally. If anti-inflammatory drugs, e.g. cortisone, are administered in the first few days after wounding, healing is likely to be delayed. Once healing is established, cortisone does not appear to interfere with the healing process. In practice, wounds do heal in patients receiving long-term steroid therapy but the process is slow and more susceptible to complications.

Sepsis

Local infection is perhaps the most important cause of delayed wound healing and dehiscence. Collagen synthesis is depressed and collagenolysis increased, thereby enhancing the softening of the wound edges

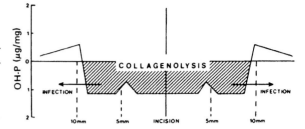

Figure 1.11 The chemically active zone of an incised wound extends for at least 5 mm on either side of the wound. Collagen lysis is prominent in the first week and is more marked when infection is present. (After Adamsons *et al.*, *Surg Gynec Obstet* 1966; **123**: 515–521.) The zero line is the concentration in normal abdominal wall..

(Figure 1.11). This adversely affects the strength of the repair and makes cutting out of the sutures more likely.

Oxygen

Oxygen is crucial for wound healing. Direct examination of the granulation tissue growing into a wound chamber shows a number of regular features. The partial pressure of oxygen (P_{O_2}) falls steadily from the normal mature tissue level of around 45 mmHg (6.0 kPa) to levels close to zero in the centre of the wound. Fibroblastic activity is maximal up to 50–80 μm away from the nearest normally perfused capillary. At this point, P_{O_2} levels between 10 and 20 mmHg (1.3–2.6 kPa) are regularly recorded. Macrophages have lower oxygen requirements than fibroblasts and are found at the free edge of the growing granulation tissue. Even in these areas of very low oxygen tension, they are still able to ingest bacteria but there is uncertainty about their ability to kill the ingested organisms. Increased oxygen uptake is invariably associated with bactericidal activity since the process is mediated by the peroxidase system.

The delivery of nutrient oxygen to the wound is impaired by a number of local factors, such as tissue trauma and tight suturing techniques. More serious problems arise when wound capillary perfusion is impaired by systemic disorders. By far the most serious of these is the capillary shutdown associated with hypovolaemia. The wound, together with the splanchnic and cutaneous circulation is the first to shut down in an attempt to maintain circulation to the vital organs. Similar effects are observed in states of increased blood viscosity and cardiopulmonary decompensation. Finally, there is evidence that increasing the oxygen supply to a wound induces greater collagen production (Figure 1.12), although it does not appear to affect the overall rate of healing.

Wound dressings

The undisturbed wound heals best and dressings may therefore impair healing, especially of open wounds, by damaging the delicate new cells and capillaries on the wound surface. These wounds have to be packed with non-adherent materials that permit surface oxygenation and do not encourage bacterial overgrowth.

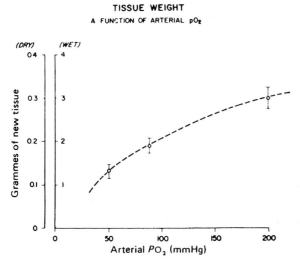

Figure 1.12 The amount of new tissue formed in a wound is considerably greater when arterial P_{O_2} is increased by changing the ambient oxygen from 14–20% to 45% for 25 days. (From Hunt, *Trauma* 1970; **10**: 1001–1009, with permission.)

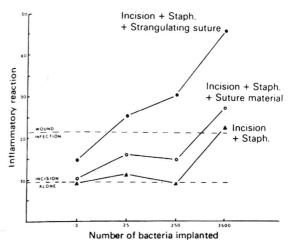

Figure 1.14 The presence of extraneous material in a wound enhances the likelihood of infection developing. The presence of one tied silk suture doubles the chance of a contaminated wound becoming infected. (After Howe, *Surg Gynec Obstet* 1966; **123**: 507–514.)

Wound failure

Although healing is a unified response to injury, failures tend to present in three quite distinct ways. Acute failures are wound infection and dehiscence. Chronic failure is the condition of pathological fibrosis resulting from the overproduction of scar tissue (hypertrophic scar, keloid).

Acute failures

Wound infection

This is the most common and troublesome disorder of wound healing. A primarily closed wound has no resistance at all to bacteria swabbed on its surface during the first 6 h (Figure 1.13). After this time, it becomes increasingly difficult to infect the wound, until at 5 days it is as resistant as the surrounding skin. Thus, an

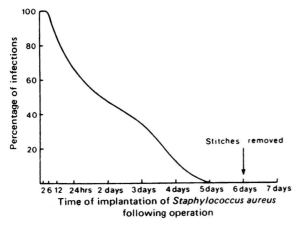

Figure 1.13 Vulnerability of a healing incised wound to surface contamination with micro-organisms. During the first 6 h it has no resistance. Thereafter, it becomes increasingly resistant to invasion, and by 5 days it is as resistant as normal skin. (After DuMortier, *Surg Gynec Obstet* 1933; **56**: 762–766.)

occlusive dressing is advisable only during the first few days unless there is an obvious nearby source of contamination, e.g. colostomy. **The main source of wound infection is endogenous from the patient's own bacteria at the time of surgery [see Modules 5, 18, Vol. I]**.

Factors predisposing to wound infection include:

- local trauma from excessive retraction, extensive electrocoagulation, defective haemostasis
- the presence of foreign material: the presence of a single piece of sterile silk suture material doubles the chance of a contaminated wound becoming infected (Figure 1.14)
- diminished perfusion.

Wound dehiscence

This is always a catastrophe. At least, the patient requires a second operation and hospital stay is prolonged. In other situations, particularly cardiac and vascular, it may prove fatal. In a high proportion of cases, wound infection precedes and determines the result [see Module 18, Vol. I].

Wound fibrosis

This abnormally contracting tissue is often a late consequence of injury or inflammatory disease and features a whole range of chronic fibrotic processes, from simple adhesions in peritoneum and tendon sheaths to interstitial fibrosis. Other troublesome examples are benign oesophageal stricture, mitral stenosis and hepatic cirrhosis. In primary closed wounds pathological fibrosis results in either a hypertrophied scar or keloid. Wound scarring is also increased in wounds that become infected before they heal. Attempts have been made to control this pathological fibrosis by specific antifibrotic treatment of the scar (β-aminopropionitrile, penicillamine, steroids, zinc) and non-specific methods aimed at diminishing the inflammatory process that precedes fibroblast activation.

The present methods of managing hypertrophic scars and keloids are imprecise and rely on compression, surgical excision and judicious use of corticosteroids (triamcinolone).

Section 1.2 • Blood and haemostasis

Although the cardinal function of blood and an effective circulation is the provision of adequate tissue perfusion for the supply of oxygen and for export of waste products, the cellular component and the plasma fraction of blood subserve several other functions, some of which involve the participation of the monocyte–macrophage system.

Blood groups and histocompatibility antigens

Blood groups

The most important is the ABO system. The surface antigens A and B are coupled to ceramide, a lipid component of the cell membrane of the erythrocyte. Both are derived from substance H as a result of the activity of two specific transferases coded by the respective allelic genes A and B on chromosome 9. Blood group O individuals do not possess either of these transferase enzymes and thus carry the H substance unchanged. Antibodies to antigen A or B are present in the plasma when the respective antigen is absent from the red cells. Thus, group A have anti-B, group B have anti-A, group O have both anti-A and anti-B, and group AB do not have any. Although group O individuals are often referred to as 'universal donors', they should always be screened for anti-A and anti-B before their blood is administered to group A and B patients. These natural antibodies, which belong to the immunoglobulin M (IgM) class, are haemolysins and are thought to arise as a result of immunization by gut bacterial antigens closely allied in composition to the A and B antigens. The characteristics of the ABO blood group system are outlined in Table 1.1.

Of the other blood-group systems (Rhesus, Kelly, Duffy and Kidd), the most clinically relevant is the Rhesus (Rh) system. This is inherited by a single complex gene on chromosome 1, which gives various combinations of C or c, D or d, and E or e. An Rh-negative mother (genotype = dd) will be immunized by her fetus if this is Rh positive (genotype = DD), usually as a result of placental bleeding during delivery of the firstborn, with the production of anti-D haemolysins. During subsequent pregnancies, these IgG anti-D antibodies cross the placenta and cause haemolytic disease of the newborn if the fetus is Rh positive. This disease has been virtually eliminated as a result of treatment of the mother with preformed anti-D IgG at the time of birth of her first baby to haemolyse any Rh-positive cells from the baby that reach the maternal circulation.

Leucocyte and platelet antigens

Antigens on the surface of leucocytes and platelets may be cell specific or present on other cells of the body. The latter are known as shared antigens and the most important group in this category is the human leucocyte antigen (HLA) system. It is also referred to as the major histocompatibility complex (MHC) and provides the mechanism by which the immune system recognizes self. These antigens belong to two classes (I and II) and are of great importance in organ transplantation.

Erythropoiesis and function of the erythrocyte

Erythropoiesis

Normal physiological function is dependent on the maintenance of a constant mass of circulating red blood cells (approx. 309×10^9 dl), the primary function of which is the supply of oxygen and removal of CO_2 essential for cellular respiration, continued viability and metabolic activity.

The circulating red cell mass is controlled by balanced replacement of erythrocyte loss due to senescence (normal life span of 120 days) with production (erythropoiesis) in the bone marrow and liver (fetus). Effete erythrocytes are removed by the monocyte–macrophage system, predominantly in the spleen. Marrow hyperplasia and increased activity are encountered in all conditions associated with abnormal red cell destruction, i.e. haemolytic anaemias.

Erythrocytes originate from a pluripotential cell via the common haemopoietic progenitor (spleen colony-forming unit, CFU-S). Under the influence of erythropoietin, some of these CFU-S differentiate into several erythroid colony-forming units (CFU-E), which then differentiate further and mature into red blood corpuscles (Figure 1.15). Erythropoiesis is predominantly regulated by the oxygen tension in the renal blood, which regulates the release of proerythropoietin that is then activated to erythropoietin in the plasma. Low renal oxygen tension leads to increased release of erythropoietic factor by the kidneys and thus enhanced erythropoiesis. Recombinant erythropoietin is now available and is used predominantly in the treatment of anaemia associated with chronic renal disease. In addition to erythropoietin, several other growth factors, hormones (growth, thyroid, insulin, androgens), vita-

Table 1.1 ABO blood groups

Phenotype (group)	Genotype	Erythrocyte antigens	Antibodies	Incidence (%)
O	OO	H	Anti-A, anti-B	47
A	AA/AO	A	Anti-B	42
B	BB/BO	B	Anti-A	9
AB	AB	AB	None	3

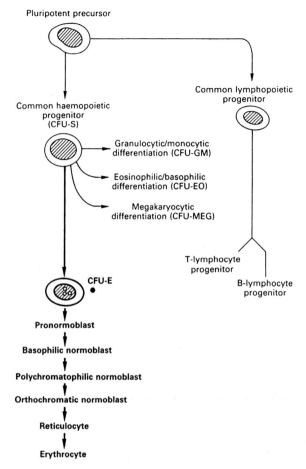

Figure 1.15 Schematic representation of normal erythropoiesis.

mins (B_6, B_{12}), folate, iron and inhibitors (T-lymphocyte factors) are involved in this multistage process. The earliest microscopically recognizable erythrocyte precursor in the bone marrow is the pronormoblast (rubriblast, proerythroblast).

Red cell function

The major fuel supply to the erythrocyte is glucose that is metabolized largely through anaerobic glycolysis (Embden–Meyerhof pathway) and, to a much lesser extent, via the pentose phosphate pathway. Anaerobic glycolysis yields ATP (to meet cellular energy requirements), NADH and 2,3-diphosphoglycerate (2,3-DPG), which influences the affinity of haemoglobin (Hb) for oxygen. The pentose phosphate pathway produces NADPH. The NADH/NADPH system is necessary to protect against oxidative damage to the Hb.

The main function of the erythrocyte is the transport of oxygen and CO_2. Haemoglobin is essential for the carriage of oxygen, as this is only slightly soluble in water. For this reason at normal atmospheric pressure, only a very small amount of oxygen (approximately 3.0 ml/l) is in solution in the plasma. Thus, the bulk of the oxygen requirement (250 ml of O_2/min at rest) is carried by the erythrocytes. The haemoglobin mole-

cule consists of two α- and two β-chains with each chain being folded over a haem group. This configuration enables the binding of four molecules of oxygen (one per chain). Thus, oxyhaemoglobin is represented as $Hb(O_2)_4$. At normal atmospheric pressure, the partial pressure of inspired air in the alveoli normally exceeds 100 mmHg (13.3 kPa), whereas the partial pressure in the pulmonary arterial blood reaching the alveolar capillary network is much lower (40 mmHg; 5.3 kPa). This pressure gradient permits rapid diffusion across the alveolocapillary membrane to the plasma for uptake by the Hb in the erythrocytes. This results in 95% saturation of the Hb with oxygen. The partial pressure of oxygen in the blood (Po_2) and thus the amount of oxygen in solution in the plasma can be increased by oxygen therapy and especially by hyperbaric therapy without affecting the amount of oxygen carried by Hb (because this is fully saturated). Hence, breathing pure oxygen instead of air (which contains only 21% oxygen) can raise the arterial Po_2 to 600 mmHg (80 kPa), increasing the amount of oxygen in solution accordingly. Much higher partial pressures of oxygen in the arterial blood are obtained by hyperbaric therapy.

At the blood–tissue interface, oxyhaemoglobin releases oxygen (dissociates) as a result of complex changes in its chemical and structural configuration. Primarily, the extent of dissociation (and conversely the percentage saturation) of Hb is dependent on the Po_2 in the interstitial fluid. This is outlined by the sigmoid oxyhaemoglobin dissociation curve (Figure 1.16). This dissociation curve can be shifted to the left (Figure 1.16), reflecting an increased affinity of Hb for oxygen. This is deleterious as oxygen is less readily released to the tissues. A shift to the left can be brought about by:

- low Pco_2 (hyperventilation)
- high pH (alkalosis)

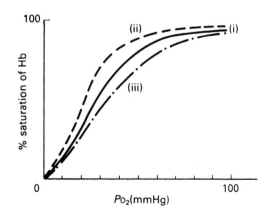

Figure 1.16 Oxyhaemoglobin dissociation curves: (i) normal curve; (ii) dissociation curve shifted to the left reflecting an increased affinity of Hb for oxygen, which is deleterious as oxygen is less readily available to the tissues; (iii) shift to the right implies decreased affinity of Hb for oxygen and thus increased delivery of oxygen to the tissues. It is encountered as a physiological compensatory mechanism in pyrexia, acidosis and hypercapnia. The relation between shifts of the oxyhaemoglobin and pH changes is known as the Bohr effect.

- hypothermia
- reduced content of 2,3-DPG (stored blood).

By contrast, a shift to the right implies decreased affinity of Hb for oxygen and thus increased delivery of oxygen to the tissues. It is encountered as a physiological compensatory mechanism in pyrexia from any cause, acidosis and hypercapnia. The relation between shifts in the oxyhaemoglobin and pH changes is known as the Bohr effect.

Simultaneously with the release of oxygen to the tissues, CO_2 diffuses into the erythrocytes. Thus, the essential ongoing first reaction at the blood–tissue interface is:

$$Hb(O_2)_4^- + H_2O + CO_2 \leftrightarrow Hb^- + H_2CO_3 + 4O_2$$

This reaction is catalysed by the enzyme carbonic anhydrase. Within the physiological pH range, most of the carbonic acid, H_2CO_3, dissociates:

$$H_2CO_3 \leftrightarrow H^+ + HCO_3^-$$

The reduced Hb^- takes up the liberated H^+ to form HHb (isohydric exchange) and the HCO_3^- diffuses out of the cell in exchange for Cl^- (chloride shift). By this process, the pH of venous blood is not significantly altered despite carriage of CO_2. These reactions are reversed at the alveolar capillary membrane in the lungs with the release and escape of CO_2 into the alveolar air and oxygenation of the reduced haemoglobin.

Abnormal haemoglobins

Abnormal affinity for oxygen, increased red cell aggregation or haemolytic episodes can be caused by a varied of disorders of haemoglobin (congenital and acquired). These include hereditary genetic coding disorders characterized by either qualitative (haemoglobinopathies, e.g. HbSS in sickle cell disease) or quantitative changes, e.g. reduction or absence (thalassaemia) of the globin polypeptide chains. In addition, there are abnormal non-functioning derivatives of haemoglobin. The latter are often acquired and include methaemoglobin (drug induced, e.g. sulfonamides, severe acute pancreatitis), sulfhaemoglobin (drug induced) and carboxyhaemoglobin (CO poisoning, smoking).

Monocyte–macrophage system

Also known as the reticuloendothelial system, this consists of the circulating monocytes and fixed macrophages in lymph nodes, spleen, lungs and the liver, which is the largest component [see Module 11, Vol. I]. It is now generally believed that the fixed tissue macrophages are derived from the circulating monocytes. The main functions of the monocyte–macrophage system are as follows:

- **phagocytosis and degradation** by lysosomal enzymes of particulate matter and bacteria. In this respect, the Kupffer cells and the macrophages in the lung filter bacteria from the blood stream
- **removal of senescent red blood cells**, especially in the spleen and, to a lesser extent, in the liver
- **antigen presentation**: in lymphoid tissue macrophages ingest and break down large antigens into soluble fragments, which are then presented on the surface to B-cells and MHC class II-bearing T-cells. Specialized antigen-presenting macrophages in the lymphoid follicles have dendritic processes that capture immune complexes, retain the antigen from these complexes for long periods and present it to numerous B-lymphocytes, including memory cells. Antigen presentation to T-cells in the paracortical areas of lymph nodes is performed by a different type of macrophage, possibly derived from the dendritic Langerhans cells of the skin
- **storage of iron** involving intracellular binding to apoferritin
- **synthesis of** coagulant factors (e.g. fibrinogen), proteinases (e.g. α_2-macroglobulin), cytokines (interleukin-1; IL-1), lymphokines (e.g. as colony stimulating factors that regulate proliferation and differentiation of granulocytes, macrophage precursors and erythropoiesis), erythropoietin, etc.

The monocyte–macrophage system is implicated in various hereditary storage disorders resulting from specific enzyme deficiencies, e.g. various mucopolysaccharidoses and several lipidoses, the most common of which is Gaucher's disease.

Function of plasma proteins

The plasma proteins are largely responsible for the oncotic pressure that is crucial to the exchange of fluid across the capillary membrane. In addition, they have other important functions. These include blood clotting, anticoagulation and inhibition of fibrinolysis, transport, buffering of acid metabolites, acute phase response and defence against microbial invasion through the complement–antibody response assisted by the immune cellular response.

Oncotic pressure

The plasma proteins, particularly the albumin fraction, are responsible for maintenance of the circulating blood volume. The effect is mediated by the oncotic pressure that they exert. This reverses the fluid flux from the interstitial space to the intravascular compartment at the venular end of the capillary where the effective oncotic pressure of the plasma proteins exceeds the capillary hydrostatic pressure. This delicately balanced mechanism is disturbed if the plasma protein level is decreased (hypoalbuminaemia) or the hydrostatic pressure in the capillary bed is elevated through congestion (e.g. right heart failure, circulatory overload, varicose veins) or the permeability of the capillary membrane is increased (sepsis, inflammation).

Table 1.2 Natural plasma inhibitors

- Antithrombin III (heparin cofactor)
- Heparin cofactor II
- α_2-macroglobulin
- α_1-antitrypsin
- α_2-antiplasmin (α_2-plasmin inhibitor)
- C1-inactivator (C1-esterase inhibitor)
- Extrinsic pathway inhibitor
- Activated protein C inhibitor

All of these events result in expansion of the interstitial fluid compartment with oedema formation.

The normal bidirectional flow of fluid across the capillary membrane also supports the exchange of nutrients and waste products between the capillary blood and the interstitial fluid. The actual exchange is, however, independent of net flow and is governed by the movement of solutes along concentration gradients.

Anticoagulation

A substantial percentage of the globulin fraction of the plasma proteins (*c.* 20%) is made up of agents that inhibit the activity of activated clotting factors and fibrinolytic enzymes (Table 1.2). Essentially, these are antiproteinases and some have other specific physiological roles. As a group they limit and localize thrombosis, fibrinolysis and inflammatory reactions. Hereditary deficiency states may result in recurrent thrombosis [see Module 20, Vol. I], bleeding tendency (α_2-antiplasmin, plasminogen activator inhibitor I), pulmonary emphysema (α_1-antitrypsin) or hereditary angioneurotic oedema (C1 inactivator).

Transport

The plasma proteins act as an efficient transport system for a variety of endogenous and exogenous substances: hormones, bilirubin, iron (transferrin), copper (caeruloplasmin), vitamins (retinol binding protein), drugs, etc. In some instances binding also serves to reduce the innate toxicity of material (e.g. binding of unconjugated bilirubin to albumin). In general, when a substance is bound to the plasma proteins, it is inactive. Thus, release from the bound state is necessary for the physiological effect of the hormones on target organs.

Buffer action

Plasma proteins, like all other body proteins, have a high content of weakly acidic and basic groups and thereby contribute to the general buffering mechanism of blood. CO_2 generated by cellular respiration dissolves in the aqueous component of tissue fluid and blood to form carbonic acid (H_2CO_3), which readily dissociates at the normal blood pH range to hydrogen ions (H^+) and bicarbonate (HCO_3^-). Thus, carriage of CO_2 by the venous blood tends to lower pH by increasing the H^+ concentration. In the physiological healthy state, however, the pH of venous blood is only marginally lower than that of arterial blood. This is in part due to the buffer base supplied by plasma phosphates and plasma proteins. However, oxyhaemoglobin–haemoglobin provides the main buffering of H^+ generated by CO_2 carriage through the process of isohydric exchange [see Module 13, Vol. I].

Defence against microbial infection: complement system, immunoglobulins and acute phase reactants

Complement system

Similarly to blood coagulation, the complement system consists of a series of enzyme proteins, which acts on each other in a sequential manner to produce molecular fragments and complexes, which subserve important functions in the host's defence against invading microbes. Thus, coating of bacteria with C3b facilitates their adherence to phagocytes that have cell surface receptors for this component. Small peptide complement fragments (C3a and C5a) have specific biological activity and either trigger the release of preformed mediators from mast cells and basophils (histamine, tryptase, chemotactic factors for polymorphs and eosinophils and platelet activating factor) or activate phospholipase, which releases arachidonic acid from the phospholipids of the cell membrane of the mast cells. The arachidonic acid is then converted to leukotrienes (lipo-oxygenase pathway) or to prostaglandins and thromboxanes (cyclo-oxygenase route). Leukotrienes induce vasodilatation, bronchoconstriction and chemotaxis, whereas prostaglandins and thromboxanes cause platelet aggregation and vasodilatation. Collectively, these agents provide the final common motor pathway for the acute inflammatory response (vasodilatation, exudation of plasma proteins and accumulation of polymorphs). Finally, complement by the formation of the membrane attack complexes (MAC), consisting of several complement components (C5b, C6–C9) on the surface of the invading organism, increases the permeability of its cell membrane. Thereafter, water and electrolytes enter the cell attracted by osmotic forces in such quantities as to induce cell disruption and lysis.

The complement system is activated by two mechanisms: the alternative and the classical pathways. Some micro-organisms can bind the C3 cleaving (convertase) enzyme directly to their surface polysaccharide molecules and protect it from inhibition. The activated enzyme (C3bBb) then generates large amounts of C3b cleavage products from C3 that are deposited on the surface of the organisms. This direct activation occurring in the absence of antibody constitutes the alternative pathway of complement activation. By contrast, the classical pathway is initiated by binding of antibody to the surface antigens of the invading organism. This binds to and activates the C1q component of complement, setting off a multistep cascade reaction involving several complement components and leading to the formation of an activated enzyme (C4b2b) that has C3 convertase activity. Thus, the two pathways converge at the cleavage of the C3 component, which is pivotal to the complement system.

Antibodies

The body has a vast army of B-lymphocytes bearing different antibodies with specific recognition sites for all possible foreign antigenic material. Thus, when an organism gains access, lymphocytes with the appropriate surface antibody dock with the antigen and thereafter proliferate to form a clone of plasma cells programmed to produce large amounts of the required antibody needed to eliminate the invading organism. This process of proliferation of a specific line of B-lymphocytes is known as clonal selection and forms the basis of the acquired immune response. This encounter with a specific pathogen is permanently coded in some of these lymphocytes, which persist as memory cells. When compared with the primary response described above, these cells are capable of mounting a more rapid and vigorous antibody response (higher antibody titres) in the event of a second encounter with the same pathogen (secondary response).

Acute phase reactants

This is a collective term for a group of plasma proteins, the concentration of which rises dramatically in acute inflammation and trauma (Table 1.3). The group includes a wide range of proteins, which normally subserve specific physiological functions: ferritin, fibrinogen, C-reactive protein, caeruloplasmin, α_1-antitrypsin, α_2-macroglobulin, C9, haptoglobin, etc. The most clinically useful in the context of acute illness is C-reactive protein, which is synthesized and secreted by the liver. Endotoxin (during an infection) stimulates the release of IL-1 from the Kupffer cells, which leads to enhanced hepatic synthesis of the protein. In turn, C-reactive protein binds to some bacteria and thereby activates complement. Hence, it performs a useful opsonizing effect, i.e. encourages adherence to phagocytes. In surgical practice, circulating levels of C-reactive protein are often used as an index of severity of the illness, e.g. acute pancreatitis.

Haemostasis

In health, perfusion of tissues and organs is dependent on vascular patency, adequate perfusion pressure, normal

Table 1.3 Disorders inducing a major acute-phase response

- Bacterial infections
- Rheumatic disease: rheumatoid arthritis, seronegative spondarthritis
- Vasculitis
- Crohn's disease
- Trauma including burns and surgery
- Malignancy

Table 1.4 Mechanisms responsible for preventing intravascular coagulation in the healthy state

- Blood flow
- Naturally occurring plasma inhibitors
- Heparin sulfate–antithrombin III mechanism
- Protein C–thrombomodulin–protein S mechanism
- Fibrinolysis
- Endothelial prostacyclin
- Hepatic clearance of activated factors

blood rheology and interacting physiological mechanisms that prevent intravascular coagulation. At the same time, the body can mount a rapid co-ordinated response aimed at achieving efficient haemostasis in the event of vascular injury. Disorders of the mechanisms responsible for maintaining the fluid nature of blood result in the hypercoaguable state with a tendency to recurrent thrombosis. By contrast, defects in the haemostatic mechanism are manifested by bleeding, which may be spontaneous or occasioned by trivial injury.

Physiological control mechanisms against intravascular coagulation

These are outlined in Table 1.4. An adequate blood flow is crucial to the prevention of intravascular thrombosis as it dilutes and clears activated coagulants away from the site of the injury. In clinical practice this is well exemplified by venous thrombosis, where the combination of a hypercoaguable state and venous stasis is required to initiate this pathological event.

In addition to the plasma protein inhibitors described previously, two important mechanisms play a key role in the prevention of intravascular coagulation. These are the heparin sulfate–antithrombin-III (AT-III) mechanism and the protein C pathway. AT-III is a protease inhibitor synthesized and secreted by the liver. Native AT-III neutralizes the activity of thrombin and other clotting factors rather slowly but becomes a rapid and potent inhibitor in the presence of mucopolysaccharides such as heparin sulfate elaborated by the vascular endothelium. The physiological role of the heparin sulfate–AT-III mechanism is therefore to neutralize activated clotting factors on the vascular endothelial surface. Protein C is a vitamin K-dependent serine protease synthesized and secreted by the liver as a zymogen which, together with protein S (also synthesized by the liver) and a vascular endothelial protein (thrombomodulin), provides a major naturally occurring anticoagulant system. When thrombin is generated intravascularly it binds to thrombomodulin on the cell surface of the vascular endothelium. This complex activates protein C, which then forms a complex with protein S on the surface of both vascular endothelium and platelets. This protein C–S complex inactivates factor Va and factor VIIIa and plasminogen activator inhibitor. Thus, in addition to abrogating clotting on these surfaces, the protein C pathway stimulates fibrinolysis. The extrinsic pathway inhibitor (EPI) is a low-molecular-weight plasma protein that stops coagulation initiated by the factor VIIa–tissue factor complex.

Other vascular endothelial defences against thrombosis include the secretion of tissue plasminogen activator (promotes fibrinolysis) and the elaboration of prostacyclin, which is a potent vasodilator and inhibitor of platelet adhesion.

The haemostatic response

The haemostatic response, which prevents exsanguination after vascular injury, has two components:

- **primary response**: vasoconstriction and formation of platelet plug
- **secondary response (haemostasis)**: formation of a fibrin seal that ensures continued haemostasis until healing of the vascular injury is complete.

Primary response

The factors that initiate and maintain the vasoconstriction are not known, although platelet factors such as thromboxane A_2 (TXA_2, a potent vasoconstrictor) and substances released from the endothelium are probably involved. Contrary to former belief, serotonin does not mediate the initial vasoconstrictor response.

The formation of the platelet plug involves three interrelated stages: platelet adhesion, the release reaction and platelet aggregation. Platelet adhesion to the vascular endothelium and adjacent perivascular connective tissue (predominantly collagen) is the initial event and appears to be receptor mediated (von Willibrand factor; vWf). Congenital absence of this factor (von Willibrand's disease) results in a prolonged bleeding time with a normal clotting time. Following adherence to collagen, the platelets change shape from flat discs to spheres with polypoidal projections and actively secrete a number of factors from their α-granules (release reaction). These include adenosine diphosphate (ADP), β-thromboglobulin (β-TG), platelet factor-4 (PF4), platelet-derived growth factor (PDGF) and vWf. ADP is largely responsible for the platelet aggregation and this is augmented by TXA_2 derived from arachidonic acid (released from platelet membrane phospholipids) via the cyclo-oxygenase pathway. The actual aggregation (binding of platelets to each other) requires the presence of fibrinogen that binds to specific surface receptors on several platelets, thereby linking them together. Patients with congenital absence of fibrinogen (afibrinogenemia) or absence of the specific platelet receptors for fibrinogen (Glanzman's thrombasthenia) have prolonged bleeding times due to defective platelet aggregation. Several of the clotting factors synthesized by megakaryocytes (fibrinogen, factor V, etc.) are stored in platelets from which they are liberated during the release reaction, thus contributing to the coagulation cascade. In addition, activated platelets provide a procoagulant factor (PF3), which enhances the activation of prothrombin to thrombin by factor Xa.

Secondary response (blood coagulation)

The essence of blood coagulation is a chain reaction or cascade of proenzyme to enzyme conversions, with each enzyme activating the next proenzyme down the line until thrombin acts on fibrinogen to produce fibrin monomer, which then polymerizes to the stable fibrin. The various clotting factors are shown in Table 1.5.

By convention, two pathways of blood coagulation are recognized: extrinsic and intrinsic. Both lead to the activation of factor X (Xa) and thereafter follow the same cascade reaction (Figure 1.17). This division is, however, somewhat arbitrary as the two systems con-

Table 1.5 Coagulation factors

Designation	Synonym
I	Fibrinogen
II	Prothrombin
III	Tissue thromboplastin
IV	Calcium ion
V	Proaccelerin, labile factor
VII	Serum prothrombin conversion accelerator
VIII	Antihaemophilic factor
VWf	von Willebrand factor
IX	Christmas factor
X	Stuart–Prower factor
XI	Plasma thromboplastin antecedent
XII	Hageman factor
XIII	Fibrin stabilizing factor
Prekallikrein	Fletcher factor
HMW kininogen	Contact activation factor

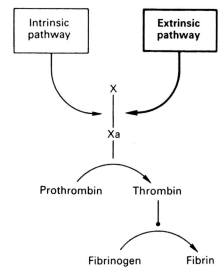

Figure 1.17 The two pathways of blood coagulation: extrinsic and intrinsic. Both lead to the activation of factor X (Xa) and thereafter follow the same cascade reaction.

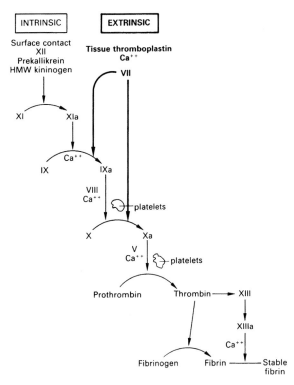

Figure 1.18 Simplified system of the blood coagulation cascade.

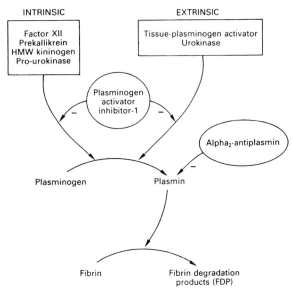

Figure 1.19 The fibrinolytic system.

verge at other levels (e.g. factor IX). However, the distinction is of practical value as, while the prothrombin time reflects the activity of both pathways, the partial thromboplastin time measures the activity of the intrinsic system only. The extrinsic system is initiated by exposure of blood to injured tissue via the release of tissue thromboplastin (i.e. tissue factor that is extrinsic to the blood). By contrast, the intrinsic pathway is triggered by contact of Hageman factor with a foreign surface and no extrinsic component is needed for the coagulation process. A simplified system of the blood coagulation cascade is shown in Figure 1.18.

Formation of a stable fibrin clot
Thrombin cleaves four fibrinopeptides from fibrinogen with the formation, of fibrin polymer, which polymerizes spontaneously to form fibrin. The stabilization of this to yield the insoluble fibrin requires the action of XIIIa (activated by thrombin) and calcium ions.

Fibrinolysis
The lysis of fibrin by plasmin is an important physiological mechanism which guards against occlusion of blood vessels and is important in tissue repair. Following haemorrhage due to vascular injury, fibrinolysis is temporarily switched off. Premature activation will result in renewed bleeding and this mechanism may be responsible for recurrent bleeding from gastrointestinal ulceration. Abnormal fibrinolysis is associated with severe bleeding disorders and is involved in tumour spread. There are both intrinsic (factor XII, prekallik-

rein, high-molecular-weight kininogen and pro-urokinase) and extrinsic activators (tissue-plasminogen activator, urokinase) of plasminogen. Inhibition is achieved by the activities of plasminogen activator inhibitor-1 (PAI-1 produced by endothelial cells, hepatocytes and fibroblasts) and α_2-plasmin inhibitor (Figure 1.19).

Section 1.3 · Surgical immunology

Normally, the immune response is directed against the antigenic characteristics of micro-organisms and, to a much lesser extent, cancer cells. A breakdown in the immune system can take two forms: (i) a lack of appropriate response to a pathogen; or (ii) a reaction by the immune system against host antigens causing disease or rejection. In order to understand these processes, it is necessary to describe the components of the immune system.

Major histocompatibility complex

The MHC is central to the immunological identity. The MHC consists of a series of antigens expressed on nucleated cells. Thus, red blood cells do not have these antigens but instead have the blood group isoantigens (A, B).

The MHC was first identified on leucocytes, where it is known as the HLA system, the genes for which are located on the short arm of chromosome 6. The MHC gene region encodes for three groups of antigens: class I, class II and class III. The HLA system is made up of class I and II antigens. The function of class III gene product is not clear. There are three class I loci (A, B, C) and three class II loci (DR, DQ, DP) on the chromosome. Thus, this system is highly polymorphic, there being at least 20 alleles in A, 40 in B, eight in C,

16 in DR, three in DQ and six in DP. The inheritance of MHC genes is Mendelian and the expression codominant, so each individual expresses two alleles at each of the loci.

Class I antigens are expressed on all nucleated cells, whereas class II antigens are found on cells involved in the immune response. Both classes are involved in immune recognition, the molecules forming a binding site for processed antigen to be identified by the T-cell receptor (see below).

The reason for the diversity of the MHC system is not completely understood but like all genetic diversity it appears to have a survival advantage, e.g. it enables different individuals to mount different responses to invading micro-organisms, i.e. virulent agents are lethal to some but not to other individuals. The MHC is associated with certain disorders often with an underlying autoimmune basis, e.g. ankylosing spondylitis, which is 20 times more common in individuals possessing HLA B27 and juvenile insulin-dependent diabetes.

In addition to the MHC, there are numerous other tissue antigens collectively referred to as the minor histocompatibility antigens. The loci for these are widely distributed within the genome. They may be the major source of organ allograft rejection in patients matched at the MHC.

Cellular components of the immune system

Phagocytes

Phagocytes are found in the blood stream (neutrophils and monocytes) and in the tissues as part of the monocyte–macrophage (reticuloendothelial) system as tissue macrophages, Kupffer cells in the liver, microglia in the brain, mesangial cells in the kidneys and dendritic cells in the skin. Phagocytes of the monocyte type are responsible for processing antigens, pathogens and other particles. After alteration of the phagocytosed material by intracellular lysosomes, the phagocytes present the foreign material or antigens to the lymphocytes, which then initiate the immune response. This process is called antigen presentation and any cell undertaking this function is termed an antigen-presenting cell (APC). The interaction among the antigen, the APC and the lymphocyte leads to the release of chemical messengers called cytokines. In turn, these cytokines enhance the ability of macrophages and other competent cells to recognize and assimilate further antigenic material. Neutrophils do not act as APCs. Instead, they completely degrade the phagocytosed material.

The ability of phagocytes to take up pathogenic material is dependent on surface receptors that can recognize activated complement (C3 system) and the Fc fragment of immunoglobulin (see below), both acting as opsonins, i.e. they coat the invading antigen. The density of these receptors on the cell surface determines the level of phagocytosis and the activity of their intracellular lysosomal enzymes.

The processed antigenic fragments become com-plexed with class II MHC antigens and migrate to the surface of the APC. Here the combined processed foreign antigen/class II complex becomes exposed for antigen recognition by the immune system. Most antigen recognition requires the combination of foreign antigen with self-MHC for T-cell activation, but there are exceptions. Thus, MHC alloantigens, e.g. tissue antigens of an organ graft, can be recognized more directly by specific T-cells, presumably because these alloantigens resemble the type of modification to self-MHC normally produced by combination with a foreign antigen.

The most active APCs appear to be the tissue macrophages that originate from blood monocytes and continue to recirculate carrying processed antigen from the periphery to the regional lymph nodes, where they initiate the immune response. In addition, the Kupffer cells lining the sinusoids of the liver act as APCs and present processed antigen to the circulating T-cells.

Lymphocytes

Lymphocytes form 20% of the white cell population and are of two kinds: T- and B-cells. The functional classification of lymphocytes depends on the detection of cell-surface markers that are identified using specific monoclonal antibodies. These cell-surface markers are termed clusters of differentiation (CD) and have been defined by international agreement. Some of these markers are specific adhesion molecules, e.g. CD54, which is intercellular adhesion molecule-1 (ICAM-1).

T-lymphocytes
T-cells differentiate in the thymus (at least in the fetus) and carry a number of important functions:

- regulation of the level of the immune response
- cytotoxic activity against bacteria
- assistance to B-cells in the destruction of virally infected cells
- initiation of cytotoxic activity of other immune effector cells.

All T-cells carry a receptor (Figure 1.20) that recognizes antigens and MHC molecules. This receptor is related to immunoglobulin and is associated with the CD3 molecule that is thus used as a pan T-cell marker. Both CD3 and the T-cell receptor are members of the immunoglobulin superfamily, as are CD4 and CD6. The T-cell receptor/CD3 complex is essential for the functioning of the immune system. Activated (but not resting) T-cells also carry class II MHC molecules and have receptors for the cytokine IL-2.

There are two main types of T-lymphocyte (helper and suppressor), which are differentiated by their surface markers and function. T-helper cells are characterized by the surface receptor CD4, the ligand of which is part of the MHC class II complex on the APC. Processed antigen is expressed with the MHC class II molecule to the T-cell receptor/CD3 complex on the cell, thereby initiating the immune recognition and response. This response involves the T-helper

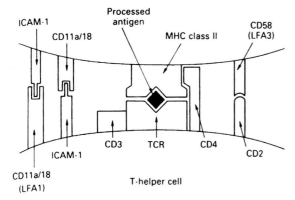

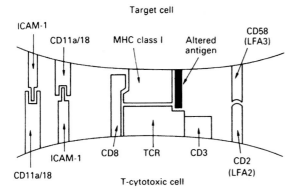

Figure 1.20 Cellular interactions involving the major histocompatibility complex (MHC) and the T-cell receptor (TCR). Processed antigen is presented to the TCR on the T-helper cell by the antigen-presenting cell (APC) together with MHC class II, whereas altered (e.g. viral) cellular antigen is presented to the T-cytotoxic cell with MHC class I. These interactions are also dependent on CD4 and CD8, respectively, and aided by a number of adhesion molecules.

lymphocyte producing several cytokines, particularly IL-2, which are involved in the maturation of T-cytotoxic lymphocytes, B-lymphocytes and various other functions of the immune system.

Cytotoxic T-lymphocytes express the surface receptor CD8, which recognizes class I MHC molecules (expressed in all nucleated cells). When foreign antigen, e.g. from virally infected or tumour cells, is expressed together with MHC class I molecule, this is recognized by the T-cell receptor/CD3 complex on the cytotoxic T-cell. This then releases various proteases that puncture the cell membrane, destroying the abnormal cell.

The T-lymphocytes with suppressor function form an ill-defined group that also expresses the CD8 marker. There is no doubt that suppressor activity exists but the existence of specific T-suppressor cells remains unconfirmed.

B-lymphocytes
B-Lymphocytes develop in the bone marrow and fetal liver. Activated B-cells proliferate and mature under the influence of T-cells. They ultimately differentiate into plasma cells that are characterized by an expanded cytoplasm, a large endoplasmic reticulum and a synthetic system entirely concerned with antibody pro-

duction. The characteristic surface marker of B-lymphocytes is an immunoglobulin. In addition, B-cells have receptors (C1, C2 and receptor for the Fc fragment of antibody). B-cells produce antibodies (immunoglobulins) in the presence of foreign antigens with the help of antigen-specific T-cells. Immunoglobulin is the B-cell equivalent of the T-cell receptor.

Null cells are a distinct group of leucocytes that exhibit neither T-cell nor B-cell characteristics. They carry a mixture of surface markers including CD16 and CD56. In appearance they are large, granular lymphocytes. The presence of receptor for the Fc portion of immunoglobulin G (IgG) allows null cells to mediate antibody-dependent cellular cytotoxicity (ADCC). Some cytotoxic T-cells also express the Fc receptor and are thus capable of ADCC (see below).

Natural killer (NK) lymphocytes are able to recognize antigenic determinants on the surface of some tumour and virally infected cells and destroy these without the assistance of antibody, although they are also capable of ADCC. The direct cytotoxic activity is not MHC restricted. NK cells express receptors for γ-interferon and IL-2. They are thought to serve a surveillance role with activity against circulating tumour cells, especially those of lymphoid origin. There is also some evidence that reduced NK activity correlates with tumour dissemination and with postoperative infective complications. Most NK function is undertaken by large granular lymphocytes.

NK cells do not have any cytotoxic activity against solid tumours. However, they can be transformed into lymphokine-activated killer (LAK) cells by incubation with IL-2. LAK cells are cytotoxic against various tumour cell lines. This form of immunotherapy (infusion of *ex vivo* produced LAK cells from a patient's NK cells) has been demonstrated to show some activity against certain human solid tumours, particularly melanoma and renal carcinoma, but its excessive toxicity has limited its usage and acceptance. Both NK and LAK cells are capable of ADCC.

Cytokines
These are water-soluble, low-molecular-weight peptides that act on or are produced by lymphocytes. They are grouped as follows:

- **interleukins:** IL-1 to IL-13
- **interferons:** α-interferon, β-interferon, γ-interferon
- **colony-stimulating factors:** macrophage-colony stimulating factor (M-CSF), granulocyte–macrophage-colony stimulating factor (GM-CSF), granulocyte-colony stimulating factor (G-CTF).

Cytokines subserve several functions. In the first instance, some members are involved in the initiation of the inflammatory process. Others promote cell recruitment to the damaged area during the process of repair. Some cytokines are able to act more specifically, e.g. macrophage-stimulating factor enhances the ability of macrophages to ingest micro-organisms. An important function of cytokines is to provide a short-range

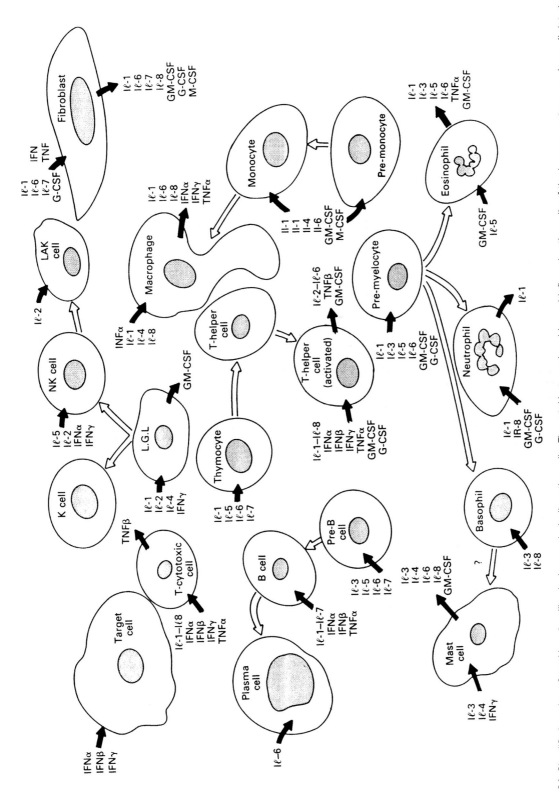

Figure 1.21 Simplified version of cytokine signalling by immunologically active cells. The cytokines produced by and influencing the cells of the immune system are shown. Il, interleukin; IFN, interferon; TNF, tumour necrosis factor; GM-CSF/G-CSF/M-CSF, granulocyte/macrophage, granulocyte and monocyte/macrophage-colony stimulating factors; LGL, large granular lymphocyte; K, killer; NK, natural killer; LAK, lymphokine-activated killer.

messenger system of communication between cells of the immune response, hence the name interleukins. The cytokine signalling is extremely complex and a simplified version is shown in Figure 1.21.

IL-1 is produced by macrophages and, to a lesser extent, by lymphocytes and fibroblasts. It acts as a short-range messenger in combination with antigen to cause T-cells to release IL-2 and probably express the IL-2 receptor (IL-2R). IL-1 also acts as a circulating humoral agent and induces the liver to manufacture acute-phase reactive proteins and the hypothalamus to raise the body temperature. It also stimulates B-cells and induces the macrophages to release prostaglandin E_2 and tumour necrosis factor (TNF). IL-1 is responsible for certain symptoms, including arthralgia and myalgia. It also causes weight loss and tissue destruction in certain disorders. The production of IL-1 can be reduced or suppressed by aspirin, indomethacin, corticosteroids and antimalarial agents.

IL-2 is produced by T-cells. It acts as a T-cell growth factor causing clonal proliferation in response to an antigen. Most T-cell subsets will proliferate in the presence of IL-2, the extent depending on the density of the IL-2 receptor, the level of expression of which requires restimulation and further exposure to antigen. IL-2 levels are reduced by immunosuppressive agents, e.g. cyclosporin and corticosteroids. The effect of corticosteroids is probably secondary to suppression of IL-1 production. IL-2 receptors are also found on B-cells, monocytes and null cells.

IL-3 is produced mainly by T-helper cells and mast cells, which produce histamine. It acts as a colony-stimulating factor on all haemopoietic cells. Its presence is obligatory for the development of mast cells.

IL-4 is produced by T-helper cells, for which it acts as an autocrine growth factor. It also stimulates B-cells to proliferate. Activity appears to extend to most haemopoietic cells. IL-4 is of crucial importance in the induction of several immunoglobulins.

IL-5 is produced mainly by T-cells and induces proliferation of both B-cells and eosinophils. It is thus involved in type I allergic reactions. IL-5 acts in synergy with IL-2 in the induction of LAK activity in peripheral blood lymphocytes but is inactive in this respect on its own.

IL-6 is an inflammatory cytokine produced by macrophages, fibroblasts, mast cells and T-cells. It acts on a variety of targets in the immune and haemopoietic systems. Many of the activities thought to be due to IL-1 are actually secondary to the induction of IL-6. It is also a B-cell growth factor, being involved in the production of plasma cells. IL-6 stimulates malignant myeloma cells.

IL-7 is produced by fibroblasts and stromal cells. It stimulates the growth of early lymphoid cells, especially those of the B-lineage.

IL-8 is an inflammatory cytokine produced by stromal cells, endothelium and gastrointestinal mucosal cells. It stimulates neutrophil infiltration.

IL-10 is derived from T-cells and inhibits the production of cytokines from monocytes and macrophages.

Interferons are produced by leucocytes (α-interferon), fibroblasts (β-interferon) and antigen-activated lymphocytes (γ-interferon). The overall role of interferons is to synergize with other cytokines, but α- and β-interferons also enhance class I MHC antigens expression, whereas γ-interferon enhances class II expression. All act as antiviral agents and together with IL-2 augment NK cell cytotoxicity against certain target tumour cells.

TNF is derived from macrophages and lymphocytes and kills tumour cells in some animal systems but not in humans. TNF exists in two forms, α and β. Cachectin is related to TNF and is possibly the same substance. High levels of TNF are accompanied by wasting of both adipose tissue and muscle and are responsible, together with other cytokines/factors, for wasting syndromes. Thus, prolonged infusion of TNF alone in humans does not result in cachexia. Most of the current interest in TNF relates to its role as one of the mediators of multiple organ failure, although monoclonal antibodies against TNF and endotoxin have proved ineffective against the systemic inflammatory response syndrome (SIRS) **[see Module 19, Vol. I]**.

The colony-stimulating factors are manufactured by several cells, including stromal cells, fibroblasts, endothelium and lymphocytes. GM-CSF promotes the growth of granulocyte and monocyte progenitor cells. It has proved useful in aiding the recovery of the bone marrow from cytotoxic chemotherapy and radiotherapy (bone marrow rescue). G-CSF acts in a similar fashion on granulocytes and M-CSF stimulates cells of the monocyte–macrophage lineage.

Immunoglobulins

Immunoglobulins (antibodies) are classified on a structural basis into types and classes: IgG (four classes), IgA (two classes), IgM, IgD and IgE, and are either membrane bound (surface) or secreted. Each has a non-antigen binding Fc fragment and an antigen-binding Fab moiety. All immunoglobulins are constructed of two identical light and two identical heavy chains cross-linked by disulfide bonds (Figure 1.22). The N-terminal domains are formed from one heavy and one light chain that serves as the antigen-binding site (paratope) reacting with a specific part of the antigen molecule (epitope). The structure of these domains varies with the different antibodies (variable domain), with the antigenic determinant for each being termed the idiotype. The remaining part of the molecule (Fc fragment and part of the Fab moiety) is constant within classes of immunoglobulin and this antigenic determinant is referred to as the isotype.

The specificity of an antibody for an antigen is dependent on the variable region, which is coded for by gene segments named V, D and J. Variability is consequent on a process of mutation and genetic

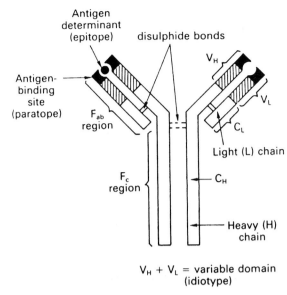

$$V_H + V_L = \text{variable domain (idiotype)}$$

Figure 1.22 Structure of immunoglobulin of the IgG type. This is formed from two heavy chains and two light chains linked together by disulfide bonds. Both heavy and light chains have constant (C_H and C_L) and variable (V_H and V_L) regions. The C_H/C_L region is termed the isotype and the V_H/V_L region, which contains the binding site (paratope), is termed the idiotype.

rearrangements within these gene segments in the B-cell. By these mechanisms, each individual has an enormous heterogeneity of antibody molecules; in fact, more than could be contained in the genome. Membrane-bound immunoglobulin is found on the surface of the B-cells, where it functions as a cell receptor. This immunoglobulin has the same antigenic-binding characteristics as the immunoglobulin that may be produced by cells originating from this lineage.

Each B-cell can produce only one idiotype. Thus, effective antibody production against a specific antigen results from clonal expansion and maturation of individual B-cells into plasma cells. A particular cell can, however, change the Fc portion and hence the class of antibody without changing the characteristics of the antigen-binding site. This is because the genes coding the C and V regions are separate and fragments are only spliced as proteins. This explains why the primary response to an antigen may be mainly IgM, whereas the secondary response is mostly composed of the more avidly binding IgG.

The constant areas of the immunoglobulin molecule are concerned with the interaction between the antibody and the receptor on the cell surface. Many of the effector functions are mediated via the Fc receptors on the cell surface and this permits a variety of functions, e.g. the receptor for the Fc fragment of IgG enables macrophages to phagocytose antigenic particles coated with the antibody, or kill an invading organism (ADCC). Similarly, receptors for IgA located on the deep side of epithelial cells facilitate the transfer of the antibody across the cell to be discharged in the secretions. IgE receptors found on mast cells are involved in the release of inflammatory mediators and lymphokines on contact of these cells with specific antigen, and thus initiate the inflammatory response. Antibodies thus subserve two functions:

- they bind with antigens via the variable domain
- they connect with the host's defence effector system through the constant domain.

Immunoglobulin G

This is the most abundant immunoglobulin and it constitutes the major antibody produced during a secondary response. It has the ability to cross the placenta into the fetus and is reinforced by colostral IgG during neonatal life. IgG diffuses readily into the extravascular spaces and thus its predominant role is to neutralize bacterial toxins and bind micro-organisms when it activates complement (classical pathway), thereby inducing chemotaxis and phagocytosis. IgG coating sensitizes the target cells to destruction by killer lymphocytes.

Immunoglobulin A

IgA is found in the secretions of exposed mucosal surfaces, e.g. saliva, nasal mucosa, tears, gastrointestinal tract, bronchial and genitourinary epithelium, as a dimer that is stabilized by a protein synthesized by the epithelial cells (secretory component). The purpose of this mechanism is the prevention of bacterial adherence to the exposed mucosal cells and hence invasion.

Immunoglobulin M

These star-shaped antibodies are also known as macroglobulins because of their high molecular weight. These antibodies induce agglutination and cytolysis. IgM antibodies are the first isotype to appear during the course of an infection and are largely confined to the intravascular compartment. Hence, their primary role is thought to be the containment of bacteraemia.

Immunoglobulin D

IgD is nearly all bound to the surface of some of the circulating lymphocytes. It is probably involved in the control of lymphocyte proliferation and suppression and may be involved in establishing tolerance to certain antigens, although its exact function remains unknown. Some consider it to be an evolutionary relic.

Immunoglobulin E

Only a small subpopulation of plasma cells synthesizes IgE and these are mainly confined to mucosal surfaces. Plasma levels of IgE are normally low but levels rise considerably during parasitic infestations. These antibodies, by coating the parasites, sensitize them to destruction by eosinophils. IgE is also associated with the defence of mucosal surfaces in association with mast cells. Encounter with a foreign antigen induces degranulation of the mast cells with the liberation of vasoactive amines, e.g. histamine, causing increased capillary permeability and exudation of plasma factors into the area. It is the mechanism involved in allergic reactions such as extrinsic asthma and hay fever.

Autoimmune disease

Several mechanisms exist to limit the possibility that the immune mechanism may react and damage the host's tissues. In the first instance, clones of T-cells that express self-recognizing receptors are destroyed in the thymus in early life, a process known as clonal deletion. Secondly, self-reacting clones are functionally suppressed. This is termed clonal anergy. T-cells are crucial in immune regulation. Thus, it is often possible to detect self-reacting B-cell clones but in the absence of specifically reacting T-helper cells (deleted in the thymus) they are unable to proliferate. In addition, other suppressor mechanisms specifically involving T-cytotoxic cells appear to limit the host response to self.

None the less, these protective mechanisms may fail. Fortunately, although many individuals appear to suffer a breakdown in tolerance towards their own antigenic make-up, only a few develop autoimmune disease. Individuals who develop autoimmune disease show an alteration in the T-helper/cytotoxic ratio in their peripheral blood because the suppressor mechanism has failed. Sometimes there are alterations in the target organs, e.g. thyroid and pancreas, when cells from these organs express class II MHC antigens that are not found in normal individuals. This abnormal expression can be induced by infection, normal physiological triggering, e.g. lactation, or by the action of interferons and TNF-α. In this situation, class II MHC expression is invariably associated with lymphocytic infiltration, which explains the histological appearance of Hashimoto's thyroiditis [see **Disorders of the Thyroid, Vol. II**].

Autoimmune disorders are classified as:

- **organ specific**: primary thyrotoxicosis (Graves' disease), Hashimoto's thyroiditis, Addison's disease, type I diabetes mellitus and pernicious anaemia (megaloblastic anaemia, atrophic gastritis and achlorhydria)
- **non-organ specific**: rheumatoid arthritis, systemic lupus erythematosus, chronic active hepatitis and primary biliary cirrhosis.

Autoantibodies can be detected in the serum of patients with these disorders, e.g. IgG autoantibody to TSH in Graves' disease, IgM autoantibody (rheumatoid factor, RF) to the patient's own IgG in rheumatoid arthritis, and antibodies to double-stranded DNA (anti-nuclear factor, ANF) in systemic lupus erythematosus.

The organ damage is induced by the cytotoxicity of macrophages, NK cells and B-cells primed with the respective autoantibody, as well as cytotoxic T-lymphocytes.

The inflammatory response

The inflammatory response can be acute, subacute or chronic. The clinical histology (especially the cellular response) varies accordingly, with neutrophils predominating in acute inflammations and lymphocytes and macrophages in chronic and subacute inflammations. Some conditions are primarily chronic in nature, while others begin as acute but progress to a chronic stage, especially if treatment is suboptimal. Alternatively, acute episodes of inflammation may subside for a time (remissions) with reactivation of the inflammatory process and renewed symptoms and signs (relapses) during the natural history of the disease. This is exemplified by inflammatory bowel disease.

Although in clinical practice infection by micro-organisms is the most important cause of inflammation, this may be caused by non-infectious putative agents: chemical agents, antigen–antibody complexes, trauma, etc. Indeed, traumatic inflammation is an essential part of the healing/repair process and accounts for the changes of the 'lag phase' of healing described earlier in this module.

Acute inflammatory response

The well-recognized features of acute inflammation are pain, swelling, erythema and heat. All of these manifestations are due to the release of chemical mediators. The response varies with the nature of the putative agent. The inflammatory response related to infection is best considered as a mechanism that allows the rapid accumulation of immunologically competent cells and phagocytes to destroy the invading micro-organisms. In this respect, the host's response depends on a number of factors, including the type of organism and the infecting dose, previous exposure and the site of invasion.

Complement fragments C3a, C5a and bacterial endotoxin activate neutrophils, rendering them adherent to the vascular endothelium. Endotoxin also stimulates macrophages to produce and release IL-1 and TNF, itself a potent neutrophil activator. Both cytokines increase the adhesiveness of endothelium for neutrophils. Various products of arachidonic acid metabolism, including platelet activating factor, leukotriene B4, the peptidoleukotrienes C4, D4 E4 and TXA$_2$, are also involved in the inflammatory response.

The first stage in the acute inflammatory response consists of the migration of neutrophils through the vascular endothelium to the inflammatory source. This involves adherence to the endothelium. The activated neutrophils leave the central column of blood cells of the flowing blood and tumble on the activated endothelial lining before they stick (a phenomenon known as rolling). The binding itself is mediated by two adhesion molecules, L-selectin (leucocyte adhesion molecule 1; LAM-1) and E-selectin (endothelium leucocyte adhesion molecule 1; ELAM-1). This is followed by the binding of other molecules known as β$_2$-integrins on the neutrophils with intercellular adhesion molecules 1 and 2 on the vascular endothelium (ICAM-1 and ICAM-2).

The fully activated extravasated neutrophils produce elastase and free radicals or species, e.g. superoxide ions and hydrogen peroxide designed to destroy the invader but which can also damage the host's own tissues. This mechanism, with the production of highly destructive reactive species, can be disadvantageous to the host, as in the ischaemia reperfusion injury and in certain specific infections such as tuberculosis and leprosy. It may also be involved in SIRS.

Immunocompromised patients

The patient with immune deficiency is unable to mount an appropriate defence against invading organisms and is thus liable to serious infections and, moreover, may show minimal signs in the presence of severe disease. The risk is determined by the severity of the immune deficiency and, in the clinical context, this is more important than the underlying cause. Low-risk patients are more susceptible to infections by organisms that are known to be pathogenic to immunologically competent individuals. Patients with moderate immune deficiency are additionally susceptible to infections by organisms that are normally considered to be harmless commensals. Malnourished patients, patients on steroid therapy and organ transplant recipients belong in this moderate-risk group. In patients within the high-risk group (severely immunocompromised), the risk of fatal infections with both pathogenic and commensal organisms is so high that these patients may require isolation and the use of prophylactic antibiotics.

Minor degrees of immune deficiency are very common in surgical practice and are frequently overlooked. Some of the factors often encountered in surgical practice include:

- **age**: neonates, infants and advanced age
- **metabolic factors**: chronic renal and liver disease
- **drugs**: antibiotics, non-steroidal anti-inflammatory drugs (NSAIDs), steroids, gastric antisecretory drugs, tobacco
- **specific disorders**: diabetes mellitus, advanced malignancy, collagen disorders, rheumatoid arthritis, cystic fibrosis
- **malnutrition**
- **surgical procedures**: intravenous cannulae, bladder catheterization, endotracheal intubation, nasogastric intubation, abdominal drains.

Aside from cystic fibrosis, congenital disorders causing immune deficiency are rare and include congenital neutropenia, deficiencies in antibody production and cell-mediated immunity.

Serious immunosuppression

The causes include drug-induced bone marrow failure from cytotoxic chemotherapy, total body irradiation and graft-versus-host disease. A severe degree of immunosuppression results from total body irradiation (1000 Gy), normally used to treat residual leukaemia. This therapy destroys most immunocompetent lymphocytes and there is a decrease in the granulocytes and monocytes, leading to impaired reticulo-endothelial activity and antibody formation. Furthermore, radiation also causes chromosomal damage so that the immunoglobulin structure may be altered and less effective. Severe infections per se can cause a fall in the neutrophil count in addition to a defect in neutrophil function, detected as toxic granulation in the circulating neutrophils.

The risk of infection is proportional to the level and duration of the neutropenia and is compounded by the anaemia and thrombocytopenia that accompany bone marrow failure. Organisms that commonly cause infections in these patients include pyogenic and endogenous enteric bacteria. The patient is also at risk from exogenous enteric pathogens, e.g. *Pseudomonas*, *Klebsiella* spp., *Serratia*, *Actinobacter* and endogenous *Candida* spp. and airborne *Aspergillus*.

The management of these patients is primarily directed to the prevention of infection until the severely immunocompromised state recovers or is reversed by bone marrow rescue or transplantation. Measures used to achieve this objective include strict personal hygiene, use of prophylactic antibiotics including gut decontamination, protective isolation in rooms with a laminar flow system, and controls over food and visitors.

Mucosal barriers

The skin clearly has a major role in protection as a physical barrier against invading micro-organisms, but it is also immunologically active, as exemplified by its resident large numbers of antigen-presenting dendritic cells. The protective skin barrier is breached by extensive trauma including burns in normal individuals. Immunocompromised individuals are prone to significant infections even after mild skin injuries. Pressure sores (decubitus ulcers) are important sources of infection, common organisms being *Staphylococcus aureus* and *epidermidis*. In compromised patients, colonization with *Pseudomonas* and *Candida* is common in moist skin areas and enteric organisms are prevalent on the perianal skin.

The gastrointestinal tract also acts as a barrier and harbours immunologically competent cells. The mucosa of the normal gastrointestinal tract is protected by both mucin and secreted IgA, which prevent the adherence of pathogens. Some pathogens are capable of destroying the mucin protection and, in the event of mucin deficiency, certain normal enteric organisms are capable of attacking the intestinal mucosa. In a similar fashion gastric acid acts as a strong barrier to infection, but in the event of gastric haemorrhage, gastric neoplasm and the use of gastric antisecretory drugs, e.g. H_2 receptor blockers and proton pump inhibitors, this acid barrier is lost or its efficacy reduced. Normally, commensal organisms with the gastrointestinal tract (the gut microflora) adhere to the mucosa. Invading micro-organisms have to compete for binding sites and available nutrients. This phenomenon is termed colonization resistance. If a patient is prescribed a broad-spectrum antibiotic, especially if this is poorly absorbed, the commensal gut microflora is reduced by a factor of 10^3–10^5. This allows an organism that is resistant to the antibiotic used to become established and cause a clinical infection, e.g. *Clostridium difficile* pseudomembraneous colitis [see **Gastrointestinal Disorders, Vol. II**]. Even minor trauma to the mucosal surface, e.g. following endoscopy, can prevent adherence of commensal organisms.

Aside from immune mechanisms, the integrity of the gastrointestinal barrier is dependent on physical continuity of the mucosal lining, adequate blood supply and luminal supply of calories and specific amino acids such as glutamine. There is also evidence that the permeability is increased in severe cholestatic jaundice. The pathological significance of lost or impaired barrier function is the translocation of pathogenic Gram-negative bacteria and/or endotoxins into the portal blood stream. If the Kupffer cell barrier function is overwhelmed, systemic bacteraemia and endotoxinaemia ensue. Thus, significant translocation of bacteria and endotoxin may be encountered:

- after major trauma including major surgery
- in severe sepsis
- in patients on prolonged parenteral feeding
- in patients with intestinal ischaemia
- in patients with severe cholestatic jaundice and liver failure.

A similar pathological mechanism has been implicated in SIRS, which results in multiorgan failure. The widespread damage to the endothelium is now thought to be the result of systemic activation/trafficking of systemic neutrophils. Previously endotoxin/TNF was held to be primarily responsible, but other substances including cell-wall aminophospholipids may be involved in the widespread activation and endothelial damage [see **Module 19, Vol. I**]. In an attempt to reduce this usually fatal condition, selective decontamination of the digestive tract (SDD) has been advocated for critically ill patients within intensive care units. This involves the application of antibiotic and antifungal pastes to the oral cavity and pharynx, and oral administration of non-absorbable antibiotics. At least one trial has shown benefit in patients on ventilatory support, although the practice of SDD is still not in widespread usage.

Colonization resistance is also important in the respiratory tract, but only in the upper respiratory passages. In normal individuals, inhaled micro-organisms are rapidly cleared by alveolar macrophages, although this function is impaired in patients with even mild changes in immune function. When an endotracheal tube has been in place for a few days, there is severe mucosal damage, allowing colonization with enterobacteria. Flow of urine is the major factor preventing infection in the urinary tract.

Trauma

Trauma, including surgery, is associated with a multi-factorial non-specific immune depression that involves the cell-mediated rather than the humoral response. This is demonstrated by reduced delayed-type sensitivity on skin testing to recall antigens, e.g. *Candida* and tuberculin. Changes in lymphocyte function that have been documented after trauma and surgery include a decrease in the CD4/CD8 ratio, decreased IL-2 production from T-lymphocytes (CD4$^+$ T-helper cells), reduced NK activity and reduced generation of LAK cells from peripheral lymphocytes. Monocytes are also affected, with the most notable change being reduced class II MHC expression. Indeed, persistent depression of class II MHC expression is associated with a poor prognosis after major trauma. Perioperative blood transfusion adds to the immune depression after surgery and has been shown to be associated with an increased incidence of postoperative infection. Recombinant cytokines and other immunological agents may have a place in patients undergoing major surgery for cancer and in patients sustaining major trauma. Thus, low-dose IL-2 prevents the fall in NK activity and LAK cell generation after surgery. The clinical efficacy of these agents in these situations, however, remains to be confirmed by prospective studies.

Nutrition

Severe malnutrition has profound effects on the immune system but these are largely confined to the cell-mediated response. All of the commonly measured tests of cell-mediated immunity are depressed. Thus, there is a generalized lymphopenia with marked depletion of the CD4$^+$ T-helper cells, impaired IL-2 production, reduced lymphocyte proliferative response to mitogens, reduced NK activity and generalized atrophy of the lymphoid organs. As with severe trauma, the delayed-type sensitivity to recall antigens is severely impaired and in extreme cases the patient fails to react (anergy). There are no significant changes in the humoral immunity and the B-cells and immuno-globulin production are not impaired.

Section 1.4 • Pathological techniques

Perhaps the most important requirement is the establishment of good communication between the surgeon and the pathologist in terms of the provision of the relevant clinical information, correctly obtained biopsy specimens and the need or otherwise for its fixation prior to dispatch to the pathology department. In some situations special laboratory techniques are required in the handling of certain specimens. These necessitate prior consultation with the pathologist to ensure that the laboratory is set up for the correct handling of the specimen when it arrives. The pathologist can only report on the material received. This may not always be representative of the disease process. In this respect, the surgeon must have the necessary experience and knowledge of surgical pathology to be able to obtain the appropriate biopsy of the lesion in any given situation.

Tissue harvest: biopsy techniques

Tissue diagnosis by the examination of biopsy material, histology, is the final arbiter in establishing the nature of the disease process. The alternative, which is applicable to certain situations and may indeed complement histology, is cytology. This attempts to characterize the cell yield obtained as normal, hyperplastic or neoplastic. The accuracy of both techniques depends on three factors: the skill in obtaining the right representative material, adequate processing and staining of the specimen, and the interpretative skill of the histopathologist or cytologist.

Biopsy

By definition, this involves the removal of a piece of tissue for the examination of the histological architecture and cellular details. It can be open (obtained during surgery), endoscopic or closed (percutaneous). The latter two are always partial, whereas open biopsy can be incisional or excisional (total).

Percutaneous closed biopsy

This involves the targeted removal of a needle core of tissue from the suspected site. When this is deeply situated it can be performed 'blind' as in percutaneous liver biopsy, or under visual control (guided biopsy) by X-ray techniques (fluoroscopy, computed tomography; CT), ultrasound or laparoscopy **[see Module 21, Vol. I]**. The type of biopsy needle varies with the nature of the tissue involved, e.g. Abrahams needle for pleural biopsy or Menghini needle for liver biopsy, although the most commonly used implement for soft-tissue biopsy (including liver) nowadays is the Tru-cut needle. Automatic, spring-loaded modifications of this needle, e.g. Biopty device (Figure 1.23), are used for guided needle-core biopsy. With the advent of Tru-cut needle systems, the use of high-speed drill biopsy has become largely confined to bone.

Open biopsy

Open biopsy can be incisional or excisional. Incisional biopsy entails the removal of a wedge of the lesion with adjacent normal margin, whereas in excisional biopsy the entire lesion is excised with surrounding rim of normal tissue. In practice, all small lesions should be excised *in toto*. Incisional biopsy is used for large lesions prior to treatment.

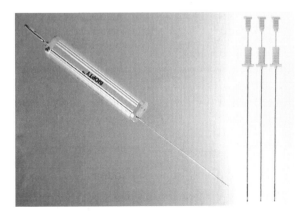

Figure 1.23 Biopsy device: a mechanized form of Tru-cut needle-core biopsy.

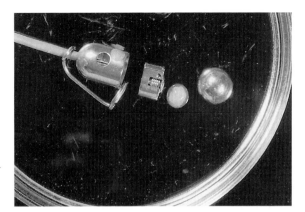

Figure 1.24 Opened Crosby capsule with jejunal mucosal biopsy specimen in Petri dish.

Endoscopic biopsy

This is now the most commonly performed tissue-sampling procedure. The technique is used in association with both rigid and flexible endoscopy with a variety of biopsy forceps, which have cutting cup-shaped jaws. As the specimens obtained are small, interpretation may be difficult and multiple biopsies are desirable. Endoscopic biopsy is often accompanied by brush cytology, especially for upper gastrointestinal tract lesions, and the combined use of the two techniques enhances the overall diagnostic yield. For inaccessible regions such as the small intestine, special techniques are used. This involves the swallowing of a suction biopsy capsule on a lead (e.g. Crosby capsule). When the desired location as determined by X-rays is reached, suction is applied and the cutting knife situated at the outlet of the capsule activated, thereby enclosing the desired portion of tissue, after which the capsule is retrieved (Figure 1.24).

Rules governing tissue biopsy

The objective is the harvest of a tissue sample with its tissue architecture preserved and which is representative of the underlying pathological process. This may, on occasion, prove problematic and there is a number of practical difficulties with the various techniques that may limit the usefulness of the histological interpretation. In general, however, certain guidelines may be followed.

- The larger the lesion the greater the number of biopsies needed for adequate evaluation: multiple biopsies overcome the problem of heterogeneity.
- Biopsies should not be taken from the central crater of ulcerated lesions because this region usually consists largely of necrotic tissue. A wedge peripheral slice that includes the adjacent normal margin is likely to be more informative.
- Whenever safe, the biopsy should include the whole thickness of the lesion so that the pathologist can establish the relationship with the surrounding tissue. This is especially important in providing information on the depth of the lesion: used in the staging of some tumours, e.g. malignant melanoma.

■ Large, deeply situated masses are often surrounded by a pronounced peripheral tissue reaction that can form a thick layer simulating a 'capsule'. It is important for the surgeon to ensure that the biopsy wedge transgresses the capsule to include a representative portion of the lesion itself.

■ When electrocautery is used to obtain the wedge biopsy, the surgeon should use a cutting current and the biopsy should be larger to ensure that there is sufficient tissue within the wedge that is suitable for histological interpretation.

■ The tissue should be handled gently with minimal grasping of the wedge to avoid crushing damage and distortion of the histological features.

■ Vascular lesions should be biopsied with extreme care and biopsy should not be attempted unless the surgeon is able to deal with any resulting haemorrhage. These lesions should be excised *in toto* if considered necessary on clinical or pathological grounds.

■ Special considerations apply with regard to the biopsy of lymph nodes. This procedure should be considered only after a detailed examination of the patient and the non-invasive appropriate tests have been carried out. The following must precede all lymph-node biopsies: search for a primary tumour, exclusion of infectious disease, documentation of the generalized or localized nature of the lymphadenopathy and, in the case of cervical lymphadenopathy, a full ear, nose and throat (ENT) examination. Whenever possible, lymph nodes should be biopsied intact with the removal of a single node or a group of nodes. When this is not possible because of fixation and matting, a good wedge that includes the capsule and surrounding stroma of the mass is obtained. All lymph-node biopsies should be sent fresh to the pathology department, as they often require special immunohistochemical staining and electron microscopy.

■ Orientation is essential when the surgeon requires information on resection margins and staging. This has to be performed by the surgeon at the time of excision using easily identifiable markers (e.g. sutures of different materials or lengths), as it may be impossible for the pathologist to orientate the specimen after it has been excised.

■ Special considerations apply to liver tumours.

Cytology

In terms of the techniques used, cytology may be exfoliative, brush, imprint or aspiration. The latter is obtained by aspiration of fluid or solid masses using a fine-gauge needle and, for this reason, it is commonly referred to as fine needle aspiration cytology or FNA. It is used most commonly by surgeons for the diagnosis of fluid collections (ascites, pleural effusion, etc.), breast lumps and other subcutaneous lesions, thyroid swellings and prostatic enlargement, although it is applicable to a

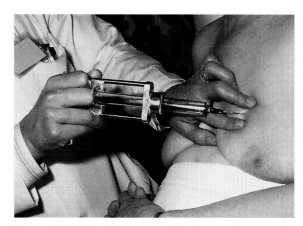

Figure 1.25 Aspiration gun used for fine needle aspiration cytology. It allows the surgeon to fix the lump with the left hand while aspirating the lump in several directions with the right hand.

wide variety of conditions and is used routinely by chest physicians for the diagnosis of pulmonary lesions. For breast lesions, a special aspiration gun is often used (Figure 1.25). This enables the surgeon to fix the lump with the left hand while the lesion is aspirated in several directions by the right hand. Deep-seated lesions within the abdomen (e.g. hilar tumours and renal lesions) can also be subjected to FNA under CT or ultrasound control [see Module 21, Vol. I].

Brush cytology is employed in endoscopic work. A special brush, introduced through the operating channel of the endoscope, is used and brushings are obtained from the entire surface of the lesion. Some of the superficial cells of the lesions are caught amongst the bristles and are then transferred to a glass slide. In China, 'blind' brush cytology is used for screening for oesophageal cancer. The patient swallows a small abrasive balloon tied to a piece of string. Once in the stomach, this is pulled up and slide smears are prepared.

Although valuable, imprint cytology is infrequently used by surgeons. One technique entails the application of a sterile glass microscope slide to the cut surface of the tissue, e.g. lymph node. The surface cells become adherent to the glass slide, which is then processed in the usual way and subjected to cytological examination. Another method, scrape cytology, produces a consistently better cell yield. The edge of one end of a glass slide is used to scrape the surface of the tissue and the resulting 'scoop' on the upper surface of the glass edge is then transferred to a second glass slide before a squash preparation is made. Imprint cytology, especially when combined with labelled monoclonal antibody to tumour surface antigens, is a very sensitive method for the detection of secondary deposits in lymph nodes. Perhaps a more surgically useful application of imprint cytology is in checking whether the resection margins contain or are free of tumour. In this respect, it is superior to frozen section but necessitates the availability of immediate reporting by a skilled cytologist.

Irrespective of the technique used, cytology smears are made on glass slides (both fresh and fixed in carbowax) for staining prior to examination by the cytologist. The stains most commonly used are the Giemsa and the Papanicolaou, but it is important to stress that many of the special stains used in histopathology can be used for the evaluation of cytological material, e.g. stains for glycogen, melanin and mucin. Indeed, it is now possible to determine the oestrogen receptor status of a breast cancer by immunoperoxidase staining of the fine needle aspirate using special antibodies.

Cytological diagnosis is based on the cellular characteristics (nuclear size, chromatin architecture, nucleoli, etc.) and the degree of cohesion of the cells (reduced in cancer aspirates) (Figure 1.26). There are several disadvantages to the existing practice whereby the surgeon obtains the fine needle aspirate of a solid lump and then sends the smears to the cytological department for examination. The most important of these is the high incidence of unsatisfactory samples (smears containing stroma only). This necessitates a repeat of the procedure on a separate occasion. There are several ways in which this problem can be overcome. In some countries such as Sweden, the cytologist takes the FNA. In the UK, the preferred option is immediate reporting by the cytologist. This entails the provision of a small laboratory near the clinic. The surgeon hands the fine needle aspirate to the technician, who prepares the smears and stains one with a special haematology stain, 'Diff Quik'. This enables the cytologist to give a definite answer within 5 min. Moreover, if the specimen obtained is unsatisfactory, the procedure is repeated immediately.

Basic handling of specimens

Fixation

The first consideration relates to fixation of the tissue. Although most specimens should be fixed as soon as possible after removal, there are certain situations where maximum information is better obtained by the examination of unfixed (fresh) tissue. The usual fixative is 10% buffered formalin and this is suitable for most specimens. However, certain tissues are better fixed in alternative solutions, e.g. Bouin's solution for testicular biopsies and peripheral nerves, chromate solutions for chromaffinomas and glutaraldehyde for tissues to be submitted for electron microscopy. The most important practical consideration relating to the fixation of tissue is the use of a suitably sized container that can accommodate at least 10 times the volume of fixative relative to the specimen. Furthermore, the specimen must be totally immersed in the fixative and the pot accurately labelled.

Certain tissue specimens are best sent fresh to the pathology department for a variety of reasons, e.g. preparation of dabs or smears, culture, enzyme histochemistry and electron microscopy. There must be minimum delay between obtaining the tissue and its arrival at the laboratory and the staff there must be given prior warning and subsequently informed when the specimen is on its way.

Request form

Every specimen must be labelled correctly and accompanied by a completed and signed request form. The information on the request form must correspond to that on the label of the specimen jar. The form must contain details of the following: patient identification, unit and consultant in charge, nature of specimen, date, previous histopathology report numbers (if any), clinical features, operative findings and presumptive

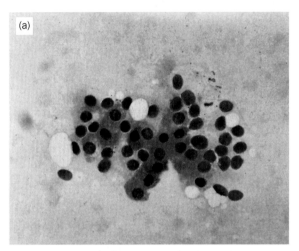

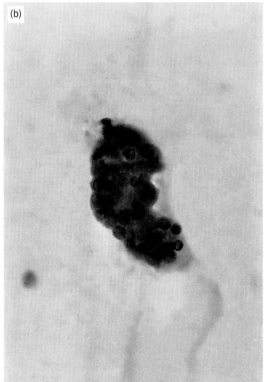

Figure 1.26 (a) Benign cytological aspirate from a fibroadenoma. (b) Malignant aspirate from an invasive breast cancer.

diagnosis. If the specimen is considered to be infectious, this should be clearly stated on the form. In addition, most hospitals use hazard stickers for this purpose. In this event, the specimen is usually left in the fixative for a longer period before being examined and cut up in a class I safety cabinet. Culture swabs may be taken from the fresh specimen by the surgeon before fixation and sent to the microbiological department.

Cut-up

All specimens are measured and their macroscopic features described. Solid organs are weighed. Biopsy material is put through for processing intact. The rest are cut up and representative pieces of the tissue processed.

Specimens of organs are best left uncut (solid) or unopened (hollow) and simply immersed in the fixative solution, providing they arrive at the pathology department on the same day. The pathologist can then cut or open the specimen, clean it if necessary and thereafter, in the case of hollow organs, pin it out on a cork board. The material is then immersed in fresh fixative for representative blocks to be taken on the following day. This ensures good preservation of the interior of the specimen or mucosal lining, avoids distortion and permits better histological evaluation. One exasperated pathologist, upset by the persistent habit of surgeons in opening the specimens, was known to reiterate, 'surgeons should get out of the habit of opening their bowels in theatre'.

The removal of pieces of fresh tissue for any purpose, e.g. estimation of oestrogen receptors or research, is best undertaken by the pathologist, who can ensure that the correct pieces are given while retaining sufficient material to enable a firm histological diagnosis. Gross specimens, if considered to be of special interest, are photographed before blocks are taken for processing and histological analysis.

Tissue processing, cutting and staining

Processing and embedding

The aim of tissue processing is to embed the fixed tissue in a supporting medium that will permit the subsequent cutting of histological sections without deformation or damage of the tissue. In practice, paraffin wax is the most satisfactory routine embedding medium. The actual steps involved after fixation include:

- dehydration to remove the fixative and the tissue water by alcohol and acetone
- clearing of the tissue by substances, which are miscible with the dehydrating agents and the embedding medium, i.e. xylene or toluene
- embedding in hot wax.

Nowadays, the dehydration and clearing of the fixed tissue are conducted by the automatic tissue processor.

Cutting and staining

Sections are cut on a microtome and are then mounted on glass slides before staining. The routine stain used is haematoxylin and eosin (H&E), and this provides

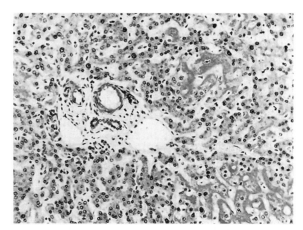

Figure 1.27 Liver stained by Congo red to demonstrate deposition of amyloid.

enough details of cellular and tissue architecture to enable the vast majority of routine histopathological diagnoses to be made. However, there are situations where special stains including histochemical staining (Figures 1.27 and 1.28) are needed to identify specific tissue components or cellular inclusions.

Reporting

Laboratories do vary, but usually a report should be available to the clinician within 2–3 days. If an urgent report is required, the pathologist can give the specimen priority and examine it before the rest, thus enabling issue of an early report. This practice, which is in widespread usage, must not be abused, as this would render impossible the organization of a priority service by the pathologist. The request for urgent paraffin must be clearly indicated on the form and telephone or 'bleep' details of the contact doctor included.

Although routine reports are issued within 24–48 h, this is not always possible for a variety of reasons. Some tissues require longer to fix (infectious) or process (fatty tissue, breast) or require special treatment, e.g. decalcification, before processing (bone). Further material may need to be examined and deeper levels cut or special staining or electron microscopy carried out before a firm pathological diagnosis can be reached. Finally, difficulties may be encountered with pathological interpretation that may require consultation and, in some cases, outside specialist opinion. However, in these situations, it is usually possible for the pathologist to issue an interim report.

Frozen section

In this technique, the fresh tissue is frozen (−25°C) using solid CO_2 or liquid nitrogen and then sectioned in a special cabinet (cryostat) containing a microtome. The cut frozen sections are stained, usually with H&E, for immediate reporting to the surgeon. It is an exacting technique that requires the services of an

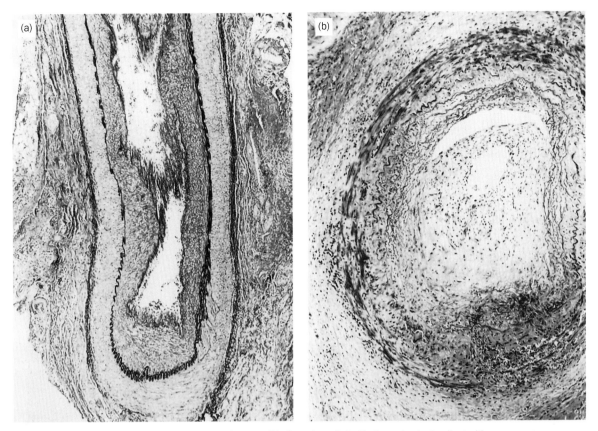

Figure 1.28 Elastica red yellow stain: (a) normal artery; (b) disruption of elastic tissue in giant cell arteritis.

experienced histopathologist, as the interpretation is more difficult than that experienced with fixed paraffin sections. Furthermore, there is some pressure on the pathologist to provide the information needed in a short time interval. In all cases it is essential that the pathologist be briefed with the details of the clinical features and the nature of the biopsy taken. If all of these conditions are fulfilled, the accuracy of frozen section reporting is high, with low false-positive (0.2%) and false-negative (0.6%) results.

Frozen section is used for three purposes during surgery:

- to establish the nature of suspect lesions: is it benign or malignant?
- to ensure disease-free margins in resections for malignancy
- to establish whether the biopsy obtained in a difficult case contains sufficient material for a diagnosis to be established with subsequent paraffin histology.

Although the pathologist is able to give a definite diagnosis in the majority of cases, there are instances when this is not possible and the diagnosis has to be deferred until permanent sections are examined. In this situation, the surgeon, after ensuring that the pathologist has received adequate tissue, may opt to terminate the procedure and postpone definite surgical

treatment until the result of the paraffin histology is available.

All frozen sections in patients undergoing elective surgery should be booked with the pathology department prior to the operation. There is no doubt that the frozen section service is abused by surgeons and a large number (50% in one reported audit) is unnecessary. **The most important guideline to the surgeon in deciding the need or otherwise for a frozen section is whether the findings of this process influence the nature of the procedure carried out at that time.**

Handling of special specimens

Breast screening

Breast-screening programmes are based on mammography performed in screening units or mobile vans. If an abnormality is detected on the initial screen, the woman is called for more detailed mammography and clinical examination. Some of these individuals are found to have palpable breast lumps. Others have impalpable lesions, which appear on the mammographic films as 'areas of disordered architecture', 'microcalcification' or 'localized densities', or a combination of these. These lesions require preoperative localization by special techniques (most commonly by the Mammolock needle inserted by the radiologist) immediately prior to excision biopsy performed under general anaesthesia [see Disorders of the Breast, Vol. II].

The specimen with the localizing needle is X-rayed in the pathology department using a Faxitron machine. These specimen films are compared with the pre-operative mammographic films to determine whether the lesion has been removed. If the abnormality is not identified, the surgeon is informed and more tissue is removed and the process repeated until X-ray confirmation of excision of the lesion is obtained. In practice, most lesions are identified on the first biopsy (Figure 1.29).

The circumference of the specimen is then marked with dye. Following inspection and palpation, the

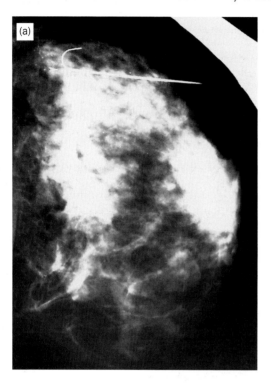

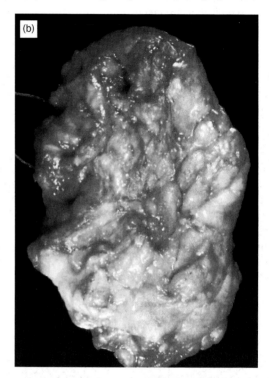

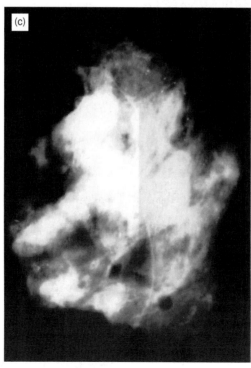

Figure 1.29 (a) Localizing mammogram with Mammalock needle; (b) excisional biopsy of above lesion; (c) radiograph of the same specimen.

specimen is cut in serial coronal slices to a predetermined thickness (5.0 mm) on a special board. The tissue slices are then placed in sequence on an X-ray film, which is then exposed to determine the exact location and extent of the lesion (Figure 1.30). Blocks of tissue are taken from the slices containing the X-ray abnormalities and are labelled to match with the slices from which they are taken. Particular attention is paid to the resection margins. The blocks are then fixed in formalin and processed for routine paraffin histology.

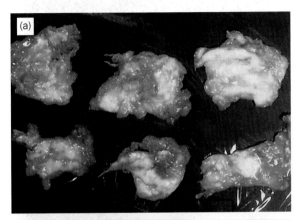

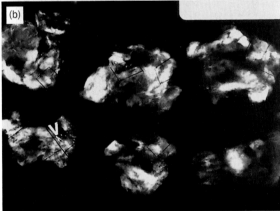

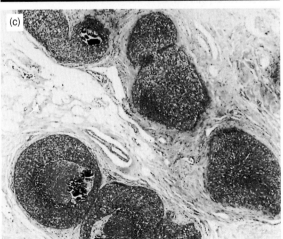

Figure 1.30 (a) Slices of the specimen; (b) radiograph of the same with arrow depicting microcalcification in one of the slices; (c) histology of the lesion from this slice (ductal carcinoma *in situ*).

Approximately 50% of the subclinical lesions identified by screening are benign (sclerosing adenosis, duct ectasia, etc.) and the rest malignant. Non-invasive cancer (ductal carcinoma *in situ*, lobular carcinoma *in situ*) is more commonly found than invasive cancer in these screening biopsies. Compared with the naturally presenting disease, a greater incidence of tubular and cribriform invasive cancer is found by breast screening.

Lymph nodes

Ideally, these should be received fresh and are handled by the pathologist in a safety cabinet. The node is bisected and dabs (imprint cytological smears) are made on glass slides. These are stained with Giemsa and Lieshman stains. Thereafter, the following procedure is followed.

▪ Representative cross-sections of the nodes are fixed in formalin for paraffin embedding and routine H&E staining.
▪ Another piece is fixed in formalin but is embedded in resin to enable cutting of semithin sections (1–2 μm) which give better morphological details of lymphoid cells (Figure 1.31).
▪ Small cubes (2.0 mm^3) are fixed in glutaraldehyde for electron microscopy.
▪ A piece is snap frozen (−70°C) for enzyme and immunohistochemistry. The latter is important for the identification of T- and B-cells using specific monoclonal antibodies.
▪ A small piece is kept in the refrigerator at 4°C for microbiological examination should this be desirable: the infective nature of the lesion may not have been appreciated at the time of the biopsy. In this situation, culture of the retained fresh lymph node may furnish valuable confirmatory evidence for the establishment of a definite diagnosis.

Small intestinal biopsy

The specimen is removed from the capsule and dabs made on to glass slides, which are then stained with

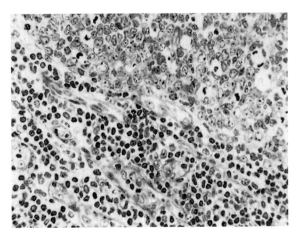

Figure 1.31 Semithin section showing greater cellular detail of the lymph node.

Giemsa or toluidine blue in the search for *Giardia lamblia*. The specimen is then placed in a Petri dish containing isotonic saline and examined under the dissecting microscope to assess the villous architecture. The orientation of these small specimens before embedding is important for accurate histological interpretation. If enzyme histochemistry is desired a portion is kept deep frozen.

Skin biopsies

Most skin biopsies are fixed in formalin as the purpose of the biopsy is usually to exclude malignancy or confirm the exact diagnosis of benign lesions. However, when certain skin disorders are suspected, e.g. chronic autoimmune vesiculobullous disorders, all forms of lupus erythematosus, leucocytoclastic vasculitis, etc., the skin biopsies are sent fresh. These are processed in a special manner. The skin ellipse is divided longitudinally and one half is frozen for direct immunofluorescent examination to detect IgA, IgG, IgM and C3. The other half is fixed in formalin for routine paraffin blocks and H&E staining.

Muscle biopsies

The specimen should be received fresh so that special procedures can be carried out and the correct orientation obtained. The specimen is divided into three portions. Small blocks are fixed in glutaraldehyde for electron microscopy. A representative cross-section is snap frozen for diagnostic enzyme histochemical studies. These include staining with Gomori trichrome, PAS with and without diastase, ATPase at various pH, NADH diaphorase, non-specific esterase and SR19. A myophosphorylase is performed if glycogen deficiency is suspected. The remainder is left to relax on a piece of cardboard for 10 min before being cut in longitudinal and transverse blocks for fixation in formalin, paraffin embedding and routine H&E staining.

Enzyme histochemistry

As enzyme activity is partially or totally lost when tissue is fixed and processed in paraffin blocks, enzyme histochemistry is usually performed on fresh-frozen material. These techniques are not employed routinely but are indicated in certain specific circumstances, the most important of which are:

- myopathies: where a specimen of skeletal muscle is stained for the following enzymes involved in normal muscle metabolism and contraction: ATPase (which differentiates type I from type II fibres; Figure 1.32), phosphorylase, cytochrome oxidase, phosphofructokinase and aldolase
- malabsorption: for the diagnosis of alactasia, a jejunal biopsy is examined for lactase and sucrase deficiency, whereas in suspected gluten enteropathy, the jejunal biopsy may be stained for acid and alkaline phosphatase

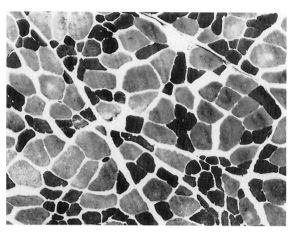

Figure 1.32 Muscle biopsy stained with ATPase showing type I and type II fibres.

- diagnosis of Hirshsprung's disease: rectal biopsy is stained by the acetylcholinesterase method for the identification of nerves and ganglia
- detection of acid phosphatase in metastatic prostatic cancer
- detection of alkaline phosphatase in vascular endothelial tumours.

Immunohistochemistry

This is a technique by which specific antibodies are utilized to detect cellular or tissue constituents. Direct techniques involve the application of the specific antibody to the tissue. As the antibody is labelled (by conjungation with a marker), the presence and site of the antigen–antibody reaction can be determined (Figure 1.33). These direct methods are, however, insensitive. They have been largely superseded by indirect (sandwich) immunohistochemical techniques that are much cleaner and more sensitive. The indirect method employs two antibodies. The primary antibody (for the detection of the desired antigen) is unlabelled and is applied to the tissue. The second tracer antibody raised in a different animal species against the primary antibody is labelled. When applied to the section it will bind to the primary antibody and the resulting complex (tracer antibody + primary antibody + antigen) is detected by the marker on the tracer antibody. The most sensitive indirect method is the avidin–biotin complex technique, where use is made of the fact that avidin (derived from egg white) binds with high affinity four molecules of biotin (a water-soluble vitamin). The labelled biotin is conjugated to the tracer antibody (biotinylated). The first stage consists of the application of the mouse primary monoclonal antibody to the tissue for binding to the target antigen. In the second stage, the labelled biotinylated anti-mouse tracer antibody is added. This binds to the primary antibody. Finally, the addition of avidin-labelled biotin complex results in the formation of the avidin–biotin complex binding the entire conglomerate by strong molecular bridging (Figure 1.33b). This technique has been modified with

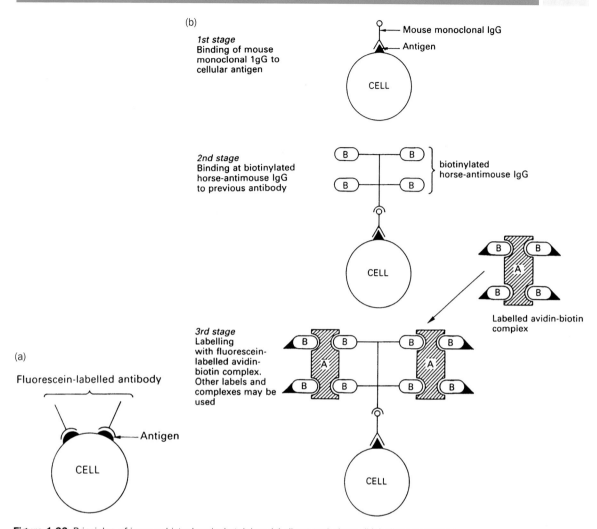

Figure 1.33 Principles of immunohistochemical staining: (a) direct technique; (b) indirect technique.

the substitution of avidin with streptavidin (protein component of *Streptomyces avidinii*), which is less prone to non-specific attachment to tissue lectins.

The most common markers or labels used as conjugates with the tracer antibodies are enzymes (horseradish peroxidase, calf intestinal phosphatase, glucose oxidase), since these can be readily identified by specific colour reactions with chromogenic substrates. Other markers include colloidal metals (gold, silver, silver-enhanced gold, ferritin), radioisotopes and fluorescent labels. Radiolabels are used for quantitative immunocytochemistry and autoradiography.

The most important significant advance to contribute to the widespread routine use of immunohistochemistry was the development of the hybridoma technique for the production of monoclonal antibodies. It consists of the fusion of a normal plasma cell or transformed B-lymphocyte with a neoplastic myeloma cell. The resulting hybridoma cells are immortal and during *in vitro* cell culture can produce large quantities of a variety of antibodies when exposed to antigen. By careful subculture the clone producing

the desired antibody that is specific to the antigen in question and which does not react with any other molecules is isolated. The resulting pure antibody is referred to as monoclonal (derived from one clone of cells) to distinguish it from polyclonal antibody, i.e. by several clones of plasma cells, as happens when a host animal is immunized with a purified specific antigen.

In general, the fixation of tissue does not destroy the antigens of interest to diagnostic histopathology and thus immunohistochemistry can be used on fixed tissues. There are, however, some exceptions. The important ones include lymphoid cell-surface antigens, cell membrane or nuclear receptors, hormones and neuropeptides. These are best detected on freeze-dried specimens or frozen sections.

In practice, immunohistochemistry is important in the following situations.

Typing of lymphoid tumours with the use of antibodies that recognize specific surface antigens on leucocytes. These are referred to by the CD system and are used to classify lymphomas into

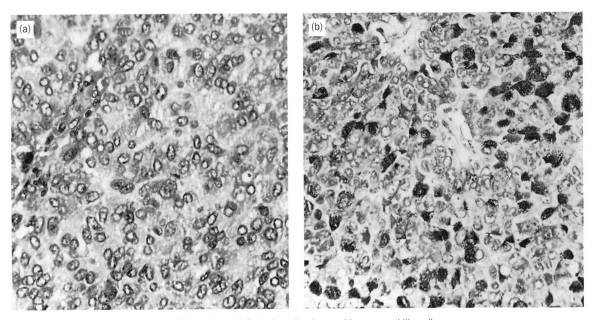

Figure 1.34 Carcinoid tumour: (a) H&E staining; (b) Grimelius showing positive argyrophilic cells.

B-cell origin (CD45R), T-cell origin (CD3), Hodgkin's (CD30, CD15) and histiocytic lymphomas (CD68).

- **Identification of specific tumours:** (i) germ-cell tumours by placental alkaline phosphatase (seminomas, dysgerminoma), α-fetoprotein (non-seminomatous germ-cell tumours, embryonal carcinoma), human chorionic gonadotrophin (malignant teratoma trophoblastic), human placental lactogen (HCG-positive germ-cell tumours); (ii) carcinoid tumours by Singh (argentaffin) and Grimelius (argyrophil) (Figure 1.34); (iii) prostatic tumours by prostate specific antigen (Figure 1.35), prostatic acid phosphatase; (iv) melanoma by S100, HMB45 and vimentin; (v) thyroid tumours by thyroglobulin for thyroid epithelial lesions and calcitonin for medullary carcinoma; (vi) vascular tumours by endothelial markers – factor VIII (CD34); and (vii) early lymph-node metastatic deposits (Figure 1.36).

- **Soft-tissue tumours:** in these tumours, immunohistochemistry is used to identify specific intermediate filaments such as vimentin, actin and desmin. The latter is found in skeletal and smooth-muscle cells (normal and neoplastic). Actin identifies myoepithelial cell origin.

- **Anaplastic tumours:** some tumours are so anaplastic that ordinary histological examination cannot even identify the tissue of origin of the tumour: epithelial, soft tissue or lymphoma. This problem can be resolved by immunohistochemical staining with a panel of monoclonal antibodies. The first step in the solution to this problem is the differentiation of the tissue of origin: epithelial, lymphoid or mesenchymal. Epithelial origin is identified by a panel of antibodies to cytokeratins, epithelial membrane antigen and CEA, lymphomatous origin by leucocyte common antigen, mesenchymal origin by vimentin and desmin (Table 1.6).

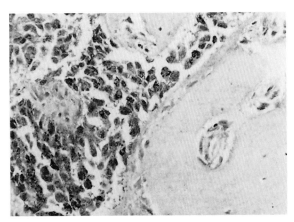

Figure 1.35 Bone biopsy. Positive staining of the tumour cells for prostate-specific antigen.

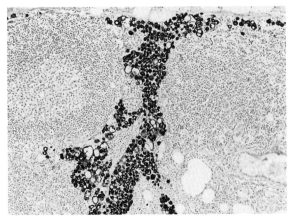

Figure 1.36 Lymph node stained to reveal cytokeratin positive cells (metastatic breast carcinoma).

Table 1.6 Immunohistochemical characterization of anaplastic tumours

Antibody against	Nature of tumour
Cytokeratins	Epithelial
Epithelial membrane antigen	Epithelial
Leucocyte common antigen	Lymphoid
Vimentin	Mesenchymal, lymphoid
Desmin	Muscle
Actin	Myoepithelial
Neuron-specific enolase	Neuroendocrine, neuronal
S100	Melanocyte, nerve sheath
Factor VIII	Endothelial
CD34 (QB end)	Endothelial

Immunofluorescent techniques

Fluorochromes (fluorescein isothiocyanate isomer I, tetramethyl rhodamine isothiocyanate isomer R) are used as labels for the tracer antibody. A fluorochrome absorbs radiation in the ultraviolet or visible light range. As it is bound irreversibly to the antibody, the site of the antigen–antibody complex is visible by fluorescence even at the subcellular level, e.g. mitochondria, microsomes and muscle fibres. This technique is often used in flow cytometry (see below).

The main routine indications for immunofluorescent staining are skin and renal biopsies. In the former they serve to outline the patterns of immunoglobulin distribution in systemic lupus erythematosus, bullous disorders and the vasculitides. In renal biopsies immunofluorescent techniques are used to localize immunoglobulins, complement and fibrin within the glomerular basement membrane, mesangium and vessel walls. Various renal disorders exhibit different specific distribution of these substances (Figure 1.37).

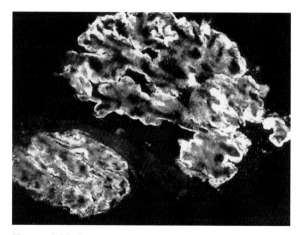

Figure 1.37 Renal biopsy: fluorescent staining of frozen section specimen showing positive IgG in membrano-proliferative glomerulonephritis type I.

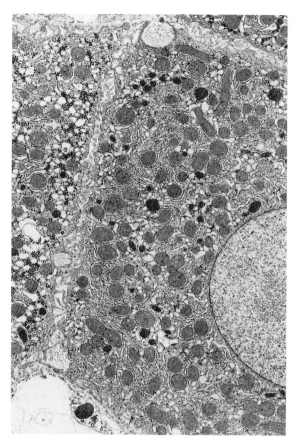

Figure 1.38 Transmission electron microscopy: liver hepatocyte.

Electron microscopy

Electron microscopy uses an electron beam produced by an electron gun. There are two types of instrument: transmission and scanning electron microscopes (SEM), although modern versions of the former have a scanning capability. Special fixatives (e.g. osmium tetroxide, glutaraldehyde), embedding media (e.g. epoxy resin) and stains (e.g. lead citrate, uranyl acetate) are used for electron microscopy.

Transmission electron microscopy

The principle is similar to that of light microscopy. However, instead of visible light a high-velocity homogeneous beam of electrons is focused on the specimen that is thin enough to transmit at least 50% of the incident electrons. The transmitted beam then enters the imaging system composed of a series of lenses, which together produce the final, highly magnified image of the specimen (Figure 1.38). Modern instruments can achieve a resolution of 0.14 nm.

Scanning electron microscopy

When an electron beam hits a specimen, some electrons are transmitted or back scattered, whereas other interact with the atoms of the specimen to produce secondary electrons (low energy), X-rays and visible light (cathode luminescence). The secondary

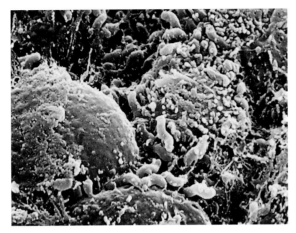

Figure 1.39 Scanning electron microscopy: *Helicobacter pylori* in gastric mucosa.

electrons are used to form three-dimensional images of the surface architecture of the specimen when the instrument is in the emissive mode (Figure 1.39). In the X-ray mode, the SEM can be used to provide a chemical analysis of the specimen.

Diagnostic use of electron microscopy

In routine practice, electron microscopy is employed for the following procedures:

- interpretation of renal biopsy material: for the identification of immune complex deposits in basement membranes and mesangium (Figure 1.40)
- tumour diagnosis: electron microscopy is used to differentiate an anaplastic carcinoma from a lymphoma, in the identification of neurosecretory granules in APUD tumours (e.g. carcinoids, medullary carcinoma of thyroid), and identification of melanosomes in suspected melanomas and in the differentiation of spindle cell tumours and lymphomas. Even with histochemistry, spindle cell tumours can be difficult to interpret. In these

tumours, electron microscopy can help to differentiate epithelial (spindle cell carcinoma) from smooth-muscle or fibroblastic tumours. Although electron microscopy can be used to identify the cell origin of lymphomas, this is better achieved nowadays with immunohistochemistry.

- diagnosis of inborn errors of metabolism
- diagnosis of viral and other infections
- skin disorders: electron microscopy is useful in the diagnosis of viral disorders, skin infiltration by T-cell lymphomas, classification of epidermolysis bullosa, histocytosis X, etc.
- identification of amyloid.

Quantitative techniques

Histometry and stereology

The techniques of histometry provide quantitative measurements of histological preparations such as volume proportions, surface area, particle/tissue component numbers and particle dimensions. The techniques involve the use of purpose-designed glass covers, which incorporate parallel lines (straight or sinusoidal) or spatially related dots (e.g. outlining equilateral triangles) on the mounted specimens. The number of particles, cells, etc., under study that is crossed by the lines or superimposed by the dots is counted (point counting). Histometric techniques have a number of applications:

- measurement of certain histological changes: cellularity, staining intensity and grading of tumours
- examination of three-dimensional features from the two-dimensional planes using geometrical procedures (stereology), e.g. number of cells per volume, surface area per volume
- valid comparisons of histological studies from different centres because the results can be standardized.

Flow cytometry

This technology is in established usage for the following:

- rapid measurement of the biological properties of cells or subcellular organelles
- physical separation of desired subpopulations of cells based on these measured properties
- objective measurements of cellular features, including tumour cell DNA analysis (e.g. ploidy)
- cell-cycle analysis.

Flow cytometry is applicable to blood, bone marrow, malignant effusions, lymphoid tissues and cell suspensions from solid tumours, although the latter are more difficult to prepare and require extensive mechanical or enzymic disaggregation. The flow-cytometric work published during the 1990s has led to a better understanding of the behaviour and classification of many tumours. The main application of flow cytometry has been in the study of solid tumours and cellular immune response to tumours and organ allografts. Flow-cyto-

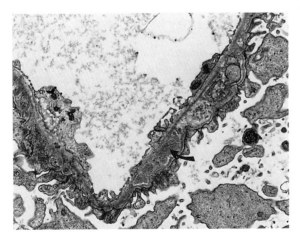

Figure 1.40 Renal biopsy: deposits in the basement membrane (arrowed) in membranous glomerulonephritis.

metric examination of tumours can support the diagnosis when morphological examination is equivocal and has provided useful data in the study of borderline lesions. In addition, the ploidy status of a tumour can provide useful prognostic information, which is independent of stage and grade. It has been used to monitor responses to chemotherapy and to evaluate tumour recurrence after successful treatment.

The principle of flow cytometry entails the passage of a single column of cells in suspension through a transparent chamber. The cell column is irradiated by a beam of laser light that is scattered at various angles depending on the characteristics of the cells and their inclusions. The scattered light is detected and converted to electronic signals, which are digitized and stored by an on-line computer that is able to generate the required information in histogram form, e.g. cell size, viability and cell granules. Specific stains are used according to the intended investigation. For tumour ploidy and proliferative activity a DNA fluorochrome (propidium iodide) is used to stain nuclear suspensions obtained from the tumour. The flow-cytometric profile of normal cells consists of a predominant peak in the diploid (2N) region and a much smaller peak in the tetraploid region (4N). The former corresponds to cells in the G0–G1 phase (resting) and the latter to the G2–M phase (post-DNA synthesis/mitosis) of the cell cycle. Tumour cells exhibit additional (abnormal) aneuploid peaks with nuclei containing abnormal amounts of DNA relative to the diploid state. The degree of aneuploidy is defined by the DNA index, which is the ratio of the DNA content of the G0–G1 aneuploid peak/DNA content of the G0–G1 diploid peak. For most tumours, this is greater than 1.0 (hyperdiploid) and, much less commonly, lower than 1.0 (hypodiploid).

Flow cytometry is also used to provide data on the cell-cycle kinetics of tumours. With the aid of specific computer programs and specialized techniques (bromodeoxyuridine uptake, Ki-67 monoclonal antibody), the relative proportions of cells in the G0–G1, S1 and G2–M phases can be calculated. In general, DNA aneuploidy and elevated proportions of cells in the S phase (synthesizing DNA) indicate aggressive tumours with a poor prognosis.

Autoradiography

In autoradiography a radioactive label (β-emitting isotope) such as tritium (^{3}H) or ^{125}I is introduced into the tissue either by injecting an animal or following *in vitro* incubation of tissue or cells. The labelled tissue is then opposed to a special water-soaked film (Kodak AR 10 stripping film) or dipped in special photographic emulsions (Eastman-Kodak, Ilford). The autoradiographic process results from the activation of the emulsion by the β-radiation from the radioisotope as it decays. The resulting image reproduces in great detail the distribution of the radioactive label within the section.

Autoradiography is rarely used for routine purposes but is an extremely useful tool in biological research, including studies involving *in situ* hybridization for the detection of DNA and RNA sequences with radiolabelled probes.

Hybridization techniques

In the production of cellular polypeptides, the genetic instructions contained in the double-stranded DNA genome are copied on to the single-stranded messenger RNA (mRNA) by a process known as transcription, with the DNA acting as the template. The message encoded in the mRNA is then used in the process of translation to form the specific polypeptides. The detection of abnormal DNA or mRNA can be achieved in the laboratory in two ways. The first consists of immobilization by heating of preparations of the DNA or RNA on inert supporting membranes (nitrocellulose or Nylon), followed by the addition of specific labelled (radioactive or chromogenic) nucleic acid probes (produced by recombinant biotechnology) which then hybridize with the specific sequences. In the case of DNA, denaturation by alkali is essential to convert the molecule into a single strand prior to the application of the specific probe. Examples of filter hybridization (or blotting techniques) are dot-blot hybridization for measuring specific amounts of DNA or RNA extracted from tissues, Southern blotting for the detection of DNA fragments produced by digestion using special enzymes called restriction endonucleases, Northern blotting for the determination of the molecular size of specific mRNAs and Western blotting for the detection and sizing of specific polypeptides.

The second technique involves the demonstration of the abnormal DNA and RNA in the tissues (formalin fixed or fresh) and is known as *in situ* hybridization. The process is essentially similar to that involved in the blotting techniques. The cellular DNA is first denatured by heat or alkali, specific labelled nucleic acid probes are applied in the presence of formamide and 1.2 M NaCl and the specimen is then incubated for several hours. Non-specific staining is minimized by using the smallest amount of labelled probe possible and an excess of unlabelled non-competing DNA or RNA to block non-specific binding sites.

Although *in situ* hybridization is likely to play an increasing role in histopathology in the future, at present its use is restricted to research institutions and major centres. Currently, it is employed in the detection of viral colonization (e.g. cytomegalovirus, human papillomavirus, Epstein–Barr virus), examination of genomic material in hereditary disorders and clonal derivation of lymphomas.

Guide to further reading

Bancroft, J. D. and Stevens, A., eds (1990). *Theory and Practice of Histological Techniques*, Churchill Livingstone, Edinburgh.

Jaun, R. (1989). *Ackerman's Surgical Pathology*, CV Mosby, St Louis, MO.

Roitt, I. M. (1997). *Essential Immunology*, Blackwell Scientific Publications, Oxford.

Surgical craft and technology

1 • Categories of operation

2 • Surgical exposure

3 • Dissection and fascial planes

4 • Tissue approximation

5 • Arrest of haemorrhage

6 • Surgical technology

'The hand of the beginner is heavy' – Moynihan

Surgeons require (i) knowledge of the disease processes that they manage; (ii) cognitive skills that underline clinical judgement and decision making; and (iii) the necessary level of psychomotor skills to ensure technical operative competence. All of these components of surgical practice are important but the level of technical competence distinguishes the master surgeon from the average. In the end, surgical competence depends on the ability of the individual. In psychomotor research, ability is defined as 'the adaptive capacity, trait, attribute or aptitude that an individual brings to a given task', whereas skill is the result of a specific combination of abilities (reinforced by practice and training) that an individual brings to a given task. Ability is innate and determines the ultimate level of skill that an individual will attain with practice and experience. Performance relates to the overall efficiency with which a complex activity such as a surgical operation is executed. Competence is reached when an individual can perform a task safely, to an acceptable standard and within an acceptable time frame, i.e. the individual can perform the operation expeditiously and with good patient outcome. Proficiency indicates that competence is consistent and has reached

the 'expert level' as a result of experience and reinforcement by a sustained caseload. This is the level that every surgical trainee must aspire to as an independent consultant. The achievement of this objective is not easy. Aside from the necessary attributes, it demands a real commitment to refine the technical skills, constant exposure to operative surgery and subspecialization within a defined field of operative surgery, e.g. gastrointestinal or vascular.

Until recently, operative training was based exclusively on the apprenticeship system. This entails graded exposure to operative work depending on progress as assessed by the consultant. The trainee graduated from second to first assistant, to performing minor operations under supervision by more senior surgeons, followed by exposure to major surgery initially as first assistant, then as principal surgeon under supervision until competence to perform certain operations unsupervised is reached. Competence is, of course, speciality and procedure related. Increasingly, the apprenticeship system is being supplemented by training of component operative generic skills, e.g. suturing and anastomosis, in purpose-designed skills laboratories or units. This has assumed greater importance since the period of surgical training was reduced.

Section 2.1 • Categories of operation

Operations can be classified by various criteria:

- total operative insult to the patient
- risk of infection by the procedure
- urgency of treatment
- remedial
- ablative or functional
- prophylactic
- validated.

Total operative insult

An operation, however expeditiously performed, inflicts injury to the patient and can really be defined

as a controlled assault on a patient with a therapeutic intent. The total operative trauma has two components: (i) the trauma of the exposure needed to reach the operative site; and (ii) the trauma of the procedure itself (procedural trauma). There is no correlation between the access trauma and the procedure trauma. Indeed, with some operations, the access trauma accounts for the major part of the total operative insult, e.g. vagotomy or cardiomyotomy. The ratio of access:procedure trauma of specific operations determines the benefit obtained by using the laparoscopic approach instead of open access by laparotomy. Benefit is likely only if this ratio is high [see Module 21, Vol. I].

The extent of the total operative insult is used to classify operations into minor, medium and major, and it determines the rate of recovery of the patient from the intervention. The surgical trauma is responsible for the catabolic response [see Module 4, Vol. I] and, together with general anaesthesia, for the non-specific immunosuppression. There is an established correlation between the severity of the catabolic response and the extent of the injury. Although there is a relation between magnitude of the operation and the perioperative risks, it is important to stress that other factors are involved, chief amongst which is the preoperative state of the patient [see Modules 15, 16 Vol. I].

Major operations require intensive or high-dependency care for this and other reasons, including cardio-vascular and respiratory care and support. Patients undergoing medium operations require intensive or high-dependency postoperative care only if their preoperative condition is compromised by comorbid disease [see Module 3, Vol. I]. Recovery from major operations includes a period of intensive or high-dependency care, followed by a stay in a surgical ward, discharge and convalescence before return to full activity or work. Convalescence is referred to in North America as the period of short-term disability (PSD). There is a wide variation in the PSD following a major operation, as many factors operate in the individual case: personality type, social class, motivation, general health before the operation, type of health-care provision (private or national), employment, etc.

Minor operations pose no immediate risk but none the less can be attended by complications. As the overall risk is minor, most of these patients are treated in day-case or ambulatory care surgical units [see Module 16, Vol. I].

Risk of infection

The majority of infections complicating surgical procedures are endogenous from the patient's own resident microflora. With good modern theatre practice, the risk of airborne infection is low and can be ignored except in prosthetic implant surgery and in the immuno-compromised patient. The use of microenvironment modules and biological isolators is an established practice in joint-replacement surgery and in patients at risk from opportunistic infections.

It is customary to classify surgical procedures into three categories depending on their infectivity risk. **Clean** operations do not involve bowel and are conducted in the absence of sepsis. Ideally, these operations should carry a negligible infection rate. **Potentially infected (clean-contaminated)** procedures include all elective operations on hollow viscera, which usually, or on occasions, harbour pathogenic organisms, e.g. the biliary tract and the gastrointestinal tract. The postoperative infection rate in this group is due largely to endogenous infection and can be substantially minimized by appropriate antibiotic prophylaxis and careful surgery designed to avoid spillage of the intraluminal contents with contamination of the peritoneal cavity and wound. Procedures carried out for or in the pre-

sence of sepsis are referred to as **infected operations**. The surgical principles governing the management of infected cases include treatment of the underlying pathology, efficient peritoneal toilet that entails complete evacuation of pus and culture of infected material. In addition, there is clear evidence for the value of two procedures in the management of severe intra-abdominal sepsis:

- peritoneal lavage with isotonic saline solution to which antibiotics may be added (tetracycline, cephalosporins)
- delayed closure of the abdominal wall: this usually refers to delayed closure of the skin and subcutaneous tissue layers on the premise that wound infection is likely. The musculoaponeurotic layer is closed with 1/0 monofilament absorbable material such as polydioxanone (PDS), and the wound then packed with gauze soaked in proflavine emulsion. The skin is closed 4–7 days later once granulation tissue has formed.

In situations where gross sepsis is encountered and recurrent intra-abdominal sepsis or abscess formation is considered likely, the entire laparotomy wound is left unsutured and the infected region of the peritoneal cavity and the wound are packed. Evisceration is prevented either by application of an Opsite dressing (Figure 2.1) or by a prosthetic mesh (prolene or polyester) fitted with a zip (or the two halves are sutured). The edge of each half is sutured to the edges of the skin wound. Irrespective of the method used, the peritoneal cavity is opened under sedation and the packing renewed at intervals of 1–2 days, when the wound and

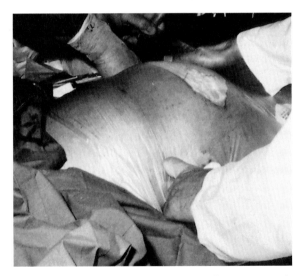

Figure 2.1 Non-closure of the abdominal wall in severe sepsis (anteriror coeliotomy, marsupuliazation). The patient had pancreatic necrosis with peripancreatic abscess formation. After resection of the pancreatic sequestrum, evacuation of the abscess and saline lavage, the space between the transverse colon and the stomach extending between the pancreatic bed and the parietes is packed with proflavine emulsion gauze. Evisceration is prevented by the application of an Opsite dressing.

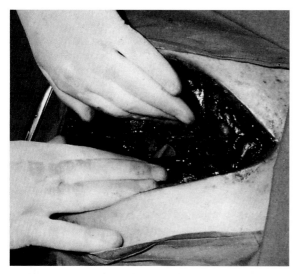

Figure 2.2 Renewal of the pack and toilet of the cavity is performed every 24–48 h under intravenous sedation in the operating theatre until sepsis is eliminated and healing is well under way.

the affected region are inspected and any necessary toilet and debridement carried out. In these severely septic patients, the antibiotic regimen must be based on the results of the bacteriological culture and sensitivity tests, and advice from the hospital microbiologist sought. Usually, the infection is a mixed one with both Gram-negative aerobes and anaerobes. Extra precautions are instituted in the operating theatre during and immediately after completion of infected cases to prevent the spread of infection. The theatre is thoroughly cleaned and the floor mopped with antiseptic solution before its further use.

Clean operations should precede potentially infected procedures in elective surgical lists. Infected cases are performed last, or preferably in a separate theatre reserved for these cases.

Urgency of treatment

Patients may require surgical treatment for the following reasons.

■ They have chronic symptoms attributable to a diagnosed surgical disorder but have no acute manifestations or immediate life-threatening complications. In this instance, the operation is conducted on an elective basis. This category (elective operations) carries the lowest risk as there is time for detailed assessment and the patient is fully prepared physically, mentally and prophylactically for the planned operation [see Module 16, Vol. I]. The underlying condition may, of course be serious, e.g. cancer. In this situation, careful treatment planning on a multidisciplinary basis is essential in the individual case. In some instances chemotherapy or radiation therapy or both (chemoirradiation) is undertaken before the operation itself.

■ Patients develop a life-threatening condition from trauma or because of an acute complication of an underlying benign or malignant disorder. These patients require emergency operation after adequate resuscitation (if needed). For all non-cardiac operations, the single most important risk factor is an emergency intervention. Thus, all emergency operations carry a definite risk of death but this varies with the nature, extent and severity of the underlying pathology, the cardiorespiratory reserve and age of the patient. Some surgical disorders are treated most commonly as an emergency because the involved organ does not usually present with chronic symptoms, e.g. acute appendicitis or acute Meckel's diverticulitis.

Emergency laparoscopy is nowadays increasingly used primarily to establish the diagnosis of acute right lower abdominal pain, but also to deal with conditions such as acute appendicitis and perforated ulcer. Overall, the benefit from interventional emergency laparoscopy (as opposed to diagnostic) is marginal, although it can be substantial in the individual case. Thus, in patients with a perforated duodenal ulcer, if the laparoscopy confirms that the perforation is well sealed, all that is needed is peritoneal lavage of the right paracolic gutter and pelvis and, perhaps, the insertion of a drain. Hence, laparotomy is avoided and this is undoubtedly beneficial in elderly patients and those with compromised cardiorespiratory function. It has to be stressed that the recovery of a patient from localized peritonitis caused, for example, by appendicitis, is determined by the severity of the peritoneal infection and is unlikely to be materially influenced by whether the appendix is removed through a grid-iron incision or by the laparoscopic approach. The argument that laparoscopic appendectomy is not justified because it does not reduce the hospital stay is illogical. Once the diagnosis of acute appendicitis is established by laparoscopy, the choice between open and laparoscopic appendectomy depends on the surgeon's preference and expertise. There have been 12 randomized trials comparing open with laparoscopic appendectomy. All have shown equivalent morbidity. The benefits for the laparoscopic approach registered by the majority of these studies are improved diagnosis of other causes of peritonitis (appendix inflamed secondarily as a result of disease elsewhere, e.g. perforated diverticulitis) and earlier return to school and games in children. Laparoscopic examination and treatment of intestinal obstruction are both ill-advised as all the published experience indicates inadequate diagnosis and treatment with increased morbidity compared to open surgery [see Module 17, Vol. I].

■ Some patients have signs and symptoms that suggest an impending major complication. These patients are usually in hospital on conservative management or medical therapy with frequent observations and assessment of physical signs. Lack of progress with conservative management is an indication for

urgent (planned or scheduled) intervention. In many instances, this decision is taken in consultation with the gastroenterologist and anaesthetist. A typical example is the acute exacerbation of ulcerative colitis with megacolon that does not settle with high steroid therapy [see Hepatobiliary Pancreatic Surgery and Gastrointestinal Surgery, Vol. II].

Remedial

This term is reserved for operations on patients designed to correct:

1. an iatrogenic complication
2. persistent adverse symptoms that occur as a consequence of an operation that was otherwise successful in curing the patient of the disease or symptoms
3. deformity and restoration of the patient's body image.

By and large, these are specialized operations conducted by expert surgeons and the interest of the patients is best served by referral to tertiary referral centres. The repair of bile-duct strictures following iatrogenic injury to the common bile duct during cholecystectomy is a case in point. The general surgeon should not attempt correction and is well advised to refer the patient to a hepatobiliary centre. There is good evidence that the best results in patients with bile duct strictures are obtained when the first corrective operation is conducted by a hepatobiliary surgeon experienced in dealing with this pathology [see Hepatobiliary Pancreatic Surgery, Vol. II].

Remedial surgery for persistent disabling symptoms is usually encountered in patients after surgery on the upper gastrointestinal tract, e.g. vagotomy, gastric resections and antireflux surgery. These patients are very difficult to treat because they often have a multiplicity of symptoms, although on careful history taking, one is always able to determine the dominant symptom. Remedial surgery is aimed primarily at correcting this. In general, remedial surgery for adverse gastrointestinal symptoms results in amelioration rather than cure, although the gain from surgery may be substantial, e.g. a patient with small stomach syndrome or severe dumping can eat, or a patient with severe intractable diarrhoea can lead a reasonable social life. The management of these patients entails careful selection, choice of the appropriate operation and expert dietetic management. Again, management in a tertiary referral centre gives the best results [see Gastrointestinal Surgery, Vol. II].

Surgery to deal with deformity is usually conducted after ablative operations for cancer, e.g. breast reconstruction after mastectomy, although primary reconstruction at the time of mastectomy is undertaken more frequently nowadays. Scar revision, usually following surgery on the face, neck and exposed extremities, is undertaken by plastic and reconstructive surgeons.

Ablative or functional

Operations can also be classified as ablative or functional.

In the course of an ablative operation, the surgeon removes a block of tissue (surgical specimen). Such operations can be minor, e.g. removal of a subcutaneous swelling, moderate, e.g. cholecystectomy and partial thyroidectomy, or major, e.g. curative resections for cancer. It is axiomatic that all resected specimens must be submitted for histological examination.

By contrast, functional operations are designed to correct a pathophysiological defect or abnormality, e.g. cervicodorsal sympathectomy for hyperhidrosis, cardiomyotomy for achalasia and fundoplication for pathological gastro-oesophageal reflux. As previously indicated, functional operations are best conducted through the minimal access approach as the access trauma (laparotomy or thoracotomy) constitutes the major component of the operative traumatic insult to the patient.

Prophylactic

These operations are only undertaken in patients at risk to prevent the development of serious disease, usually cancer, and thus increase life expectancy in the individual patient. Examples include prophylactic proctocolectomy in patients with familial polyposis coli and in patients with long-standing total ulcerative colitis on a surveillance programme. It is likely, with advances in molecular genetics and the identification of genes responsible for hereditary cancer, that more prophylactic operations including mastectomy will be undertaken in the future.

To a large extent, bariatric surgery (surgery for morbid obesity) has a prophylactic intent as the weight loss not only improves the quality of life of the patient (immediate effect) but will reduce the risk of heart disease and disabling osteoarthritis/spondylosis, and increase the life expectancy and quality of life of these patients [see Module 3, Vol. I].

Validated versus non-validated

Validated operations are those in established practice, the efficacy and outcome of which are known from past long-term usage or clinical studies. Non-validated operations are new procedures that have not been evaluated in terms of their efficacy and safety. The fact that an operation is carried out by the minimal access approach does not necessarily mean that it is a non-validated operation. Thus, for example, laparoscopic cholecystectomy, even when it was introduced, was a validated operation as the nature of the operation was unchanged from traditional open cholecystectomy. By contrast, laparoscopic hernia repair, when first introduced, was not a validated operation because both the anatomical approach and the nature of the repair differed from the traditional anterior inguinal canal approach. Subsequent clinical trials have established the merits and disadvantages of the laparoscopic approach.

It takes some time (years) to validate a new operation or interventional procedure. **Heneage Ogilvie said of gastric operations, 'every gastric operation is good … until it is found out'.** In the ideal situation, new operations or interventions should initially be conducted in a few selected centres with strict external audit of the results. This preliminary assessment determines efficacy and safety, the documentation of which is essential before dissemination to other centres (after adequate training of staff) **[see Module 20, Vol. I]**.

There is a learning curve for a new operation or intervention during which the surgeon's ability to perform the operation improves to the level of proficiency needed to obtain consistent good results with minimum morbidity. The problem is to ensure that surgeons go through this learning curve without inflicting morbidity on the patients. This can only be achieved by preceptorship training, by which is meant assistance by an approved expert until proficiency is reached. This approach ensures operative training with minimum morbidity and mortality.

Within the UK, the Safety and Efficacy Register of New Interventional Procedures (SERNIP) was set up by the Medical Royal Colleges for new operations and interventions in 1993. SERNIP's role is to act as an intelligence centre to co-ordinate the experiences of doctors, developing new techniques and advising on the need for further research. SERNIP does not attempt to evaluate 'effectiveness' in general use (it does not audit), nor does it adjudicate on economic issues (cost–benefit). The Advisory Committee of SERNIP is made up of experts nominated by the Royal Colleges who allocate procedures to one of four categories:

- safety and efficacy established, procedure may be used
- sufficiently close to a procedure of established safety and efficacy to give no reasonable grounds for questioning safety and/or efficacy; procedure may be used
- safety and/or efficacy not yet established; procedure requires a fully controlled evaluation and may be used only as part of systemic research consisting of a randomized, controlled trial and advising the Standing Group of Health Technology accordingly
- safety and/or efficacy shown to be unsatisfactory; procedure should not be used.

Section 2.2 • Surgical exposure

The adequate exposure of the anatomical site of the operation is crucial to the efficient and safe execution of the procedure. Until recently, maximal exposure with a large enough incision was considered axiomatic. The advent of minimal access surgery (MAS) would, at first glance, appear to have changed this surgical principle, but in fact it has not.

The surgical exposure needed depends on the operation and the build of the patient. In practice, the options are:

- open surgical exposure
- laparoscopic exposure with or without positive pressure pneumoperitoneum
- combined exposure or laparoscopically assisted operations
- thoracoscopic approach
- video-assisted thoracic surgery.

Open surgical exposure

Abdomen
Laparotomy or exposure of the peritoneal cavity is derived from the Greek *laparos*, meaning flank.

General considerations
Certain general considerations should be taken into account. In the first instance, the length of the incision depends on the thickness of the subcutaneous fat, which becomes a real problem in the morbidly obese. These patients require large incisions and the subcutaneous fat should be split by distraction of the wound edges rather than cut, as this causes less bleeding from the large subcutaneous veins embedded in the fat (difficult to control by electrocoagulation). Secondly, females have a more commodious intraperitoneal space (including pelvis) than males who, especially when young and muscular, have tightly packed organs. The thicker musculoaponeurotic layer in males adds to the exposure problems and necessitates more strenuous retraction. In general, males have a deeper upper abdomen and, for this reason, access to the subdiaphragmatic space is more difficult. This becomes a real problem in males with chronic obstructive airways disease (COAD) and a barrel chest.

In addition to obesity, the type of build of the patient (asthenic, hypersthenic) is also important in the correct choice of incision. Thus, in patients with hypersthenic build and a long narrow subcostal angle, an upper transverse/oblique incision gives a very limited approach to the supracolic compartment. These patients are better served by a midline approach.

Incisions
Abdominal incisions may be longitudinal (midline, paramedian), transverse, oblique or a combination. Transverse incisions heal more successfully and are less painful than longitudinal but, to provide equal access, they need to be longer. The paramedian longitudinal approach is a poor choice of incision. It used to be popular because of its trap-door design: the rectus muscle is interposed between the incisions on the anterior and posterior rectus sheath when the wound is closed. The medial mobilization of the rectus muscle from the anterior and posterior rectus sheath inevitably devitalizes sections of this muscle close to the tendinous intersections and, for this reason, results in partial atrophy of the muscle. If a longitudinal approach is

preferred, the midline incision through the linea alba is a better proposition. The midline incision is advised when the diagnosis is not clear (exploratory laparotomy).

Both oblique and transverse abdominal incisions are muscle cutting to a greater or lesser extent but do not usually cause denervation problems, contrary to the longitudinal muscle-cutting rectus incision. The exception is the right subcostal (oblique) incision used commonly for open cholecystectomy, where damage/division of the right subcostal nerve is almost inevitable and may cause subsequent neuralgic type pain. The grid-iron incision (transverse or oblique) centred over McBurney's point (junction of the outer with the middle third of a line joining the anterior–superior iliac spine and umbilicus) is a muscle-splitting incision used routinely for open appendectomy. It may cause damage to the ileo-inguinal nerve and thus weaken the musculoaponeurotic components of the inguinal canal, thereby predisposing to subsequent formation of an inguinal hernia on the ipsilateral side.

The bilateral subcostal incision used for wide exposure of the supracolic compartment of the abdomen is an example of a combination incision. Often, a third midline component is added between the two subcostal incisions and this combination (which may split the lower sternum) is referred to as the Mercedes incision. Other types of combination incision include the trap-door variety, where one component is at right angles to the other. In the USA, a large curved transverse incision in the upper abdomen, which crosses the entire epigastric region, is often referred to as the 'sabre slash'.

Mini-laparotomy
The extent or size of a mini-laparotomy has never been defined and, to a large extent, the term is relative, i.e. the incision is smaller than the standard approach. On average, however, mini-laparotomy incisions are 7.0 cm in length. In practice, mini-laparotomy is used either as the only access for an operation, e.g. mini-cholecystectomy or as part of laparoscopic-assisted surgery (see below).

Wound protection
In principle, wound protection is a sensible practice designed to prevent contamination by bacteria and thus wound infection and, in cancer patients, to reduce the incidence of implantation of exfoliated viable tumour cells and the subsequent development of tumour implantation deposits.

As almost all of wound infections are endogenous in origin, protection of the operative wound from gross contamination is practised by some, either as plastic drapes or with antiseptic-soaked swabs (e.g. chlorhexidine). The disadvantage of plastic drapes is that their removal cannot be achieved without some contamination of the wound. To date, there has not been any firm evidence that the use of wound protectors significantly reduces the incidence of postoperative

wound infection, which depends on (i) bacterial count of the wound edges at the end of the operation; and (ii) surgical technique (surgeon factor).

The exact incidence of tumour deposits in the wound following open surgery for cancer is not known. Current estimates are based on a large retrospective report on patients undergoing resections for colorectal cancer. This showed an incidence of 0.6% at 12 months, rising to 1% over the subsequent few years. Tumour deposits are related to the implantation of viable exfoliated tumour cells (spontaneous or induced by surgical manipulations). Lavage cytology studies have shown that gastrointestinal tumours (stomach, colon) that have reached the serosa, pancreatic and ovarian cancer shed viable cancer cells spontaneously in 30–40% (in the absence of obvious peritoneal deposits). With the advent of MAS, concern arose from early reports of an increased incidence of tumour deposits in the access port wounds (port site deposits). In fact, the median reported incidence of port site deposits after laparoscopic surgery for potentially curative cancer is 1.5%, and again it appears to be surgeon related. Correct surgical technique based on oncological principles, selection of cases and wound protection during delivery of the specimen are crucial in the prevention of wound deposits **[see Module 21, Vol. I]**.

Closure of abdominal incisions
Abdominal incisions are nowadays closed in a single layer (mass closure) in preference to layered closure, which has been popular in the past. Mass closure is quicker and gives consistently good results. Strong monofilament (1/0 gauge), as opposed to braided suture material, is preferred for closure of abdominal wounds for two reasons: (i) improved tissue slide; and (ii) less bacterial adherence. The monofilament material may be non-absorbable, e.g. prolene, or biodegradable, e.g. PDS. Contrary to popular belief, nylon is biodegradable, as is silk. The use of large tension sutures to relieve tension on the suture line is favoured by some, especially when closure of the abdomen is difficult or prolonged postoperative ileus is predicted. Tension sutures should be tied loosely as otherwise they devascularize the wound.

Chest
The chest can be opened by (i) posterolateral thoracotomy, (ii) prone thoracotomy – favoured in children, (iii) anterolateral thoracotomy or (iv) median sternotomy.

Posterolateral thoracotomy
This is the classical open access approach to the right or left chest cavity. The patient is placed on his or her side with the table split underneath the lower chest to widen the intercostal spaces. Appropriate supports for the arm, back and neck of the patient are essential. The incision is oblique and follows the line of the sixth rib. It should skirt a distance of 2.0 cm below the inferior

angle of the scapula to avoid scapular adhesion after the operation. Posterolateral thoracotomy gives an excellent access but is accompanied by a high incidence of post-thoracotomy deafferentation pain. The right thoracic approach is favoured by most surgeons for subtotal oesophagectomy.

Correct positioning of the patient in a stable secure position is the responsibility of the surgeon. A double-lumen endotracheal tube (Carlen's or equivalent) is used to block and collapse the lung on the operating side (single-lung anaesthesia). In prolonged operations, this collapse is held partially responsible for some of the postoperative chest complications. Periodic reinflation for a few minutes intermittently during the course of the operation is practised by some to improve the cardiovascular condition of the patient during surgery and to reduce the risk of postoperative pulmonary collapse. Some patients are found at operation to be intolerant of single-lung anaesthesia, despite adequate lung volume estimates (spirometry) before the operation. In these cases, the surgeon has to operate with an inflated lung, using gentle compression to obtain the relevant access.

Anterolateral thoracotomy

The patient is in the supine position and the chest wall is open anteriorly on one or other side, usually along the fifth or sixth rib. A mini-anterolateral thoracotomy is used in video-assisted thoracoscopic surgery, e.g. lobar resection, pneumonectomy and Belsey mark IV procedure for reflux and hiatus hernia.

Median sternotomy

This provides access to the heart, great vessels and the trachea (central mediastinum) and to both sides of the chest. The skin incision is midline and the sternum is split by means of an electrical oscillating saw. Median sternotomy is the approach used for open cardiac surgery in combination with cardiopulmonary bypass (CPB), systemic hypothermia and cardioplegic arrest. The CPB systems use either a bubble or membrane oxygenator with roller or centrifugal pumps that provide a non-pulsatile flow. A heat exchanger is incorporated in the system for cooling and rewarming the patient. All CBP systems cause activation of the fibrinolytic and complement systems, and damage the blood cellular components. None the less, CBB systems are quite safe for a period of up to 4–6 h of use. Hypothermia (25–30°C) is used in most cases to decrease the patient's metabolic rate and tissue oxygen demands. Further selective cooling of the heart is achieved by topical cold solution within the pericardial sac and/or by infusion of cold (4°C) cardioplegia crystalloid solution into the coronary circulation.

Laparoscopic exposure

Positive-pressure pneumoperitoneum

In laparoscopic MAS, the standard exposure is through the creation of a positive-pressure pneumoperitoneum by an inert gas, traditionally CO_2. Other gases may be used, such as nitrous oxide, and this is preferred when laparoscopy is carried out for diagnostic purposes under local anaesthesia, as it appears to induce less pain.

The surgical exposure of the operative field by a positive-pressure pneumoperitoneum (10–12 mmHg) is undoubtedly better than that achieved by open surgery, particularly for relatively inaccessible areas such as the subdiaphragmatic space and pelvis. Therefore, the surgical principle of maximal exposure of the relevant anatomy is not compromised. Indeed, the anatomy with the standard laparoscopes is magnified approximately two times. **However, the positive-pressure pneumoperitoneal laparoscopic approach has some drawbacks: (i) the laparoscope–charged couple device (CCD) camera provides a tunnel view without any peripheral vision of the rest of the abdominal cavity; (ii) the CO_2, which is kept at a set pressure by the automatic insufflator, creates convection currents that may be responsible for the spread of exfoliative tumour cells or bacteria; and (iii) the raised intra-abdominal pressure has adverse respiratory, cardiovascular, hormonal and metabolic effects.** Although with good anaesthesia these can be tolerated by fit patients, the same cannot be said for patients with cardio-respiratory compromise. There is a clear correlation between the incidence and severity of adverse cardiovascular and respiratory complications and the level of positive pressure used for insufflation of the peritoneal cavity. Thus, the operative principle is to use the minimum pressure that gives adequate exposure. In children, this should rarely exceed 6.0 mmHg [see Module 21, Vol. I].

Gasless laparoscopy

Gasless laparoscopy is still evolving in terms of the technology needed to elevate the anterior abdominal wall and thus create the necessary workspace. Its development is aimed at the abolition or reduction of the positive-pressure pneumoperitoneum. The initial techniques consisted of either insertion of slings through the anterior abdominal wall around the midline and surrounding the falciform, or metal 'hooks' of varying shapes. Both are fixed to a chain that is then attached to an overlying gantry once sufficient lift is achieved (Figure 2.3). The anterior wall sling is simple and very useful. It permits conduct of a standard laparoscopic procedure (e.g. cholecystectomy, antireflux surgery) with the intra-abdominal pressure set at 4.0 mmHg. There is now good evidence from randomized studies that abdominal wall-lift devices (completely gasless or low pressure-pneumoperitoneum) substantially reduce adverse cardiovascular, hormonal and metabolic changes, accelerate recovery from anaesthesia without the problems of CO_2 narcosis and are accompanied by less postoperative pain.

However, the current generation of abdominal wall-lift devices has two major disadvantages: (i) tenting effect with reduced exposure; and

(ii) trauma to the parietal peritoneum of the anterior abdominal wall. The space created by these lift devices is a conical space with the apex at the point of elevation by the retracting device, compared with the ovoid workspace created by positive-pressure pneumoperitoneum. It is thus difficult to undertake complex operations with the gasless approach and the risk of iatrogenic injury during the dissection may be increased. The second problem concerns the sustained compression/ischaemic trauma by the retractor on the parietal peritoneum of the anterior abdominal wall, especially during long procedures. This will encourage adhesion formation and, possibly, tumour implantation in operations for cancer.

The second generation of abdominal wall-lift devices are in the early stages of clinical evaluation and attempt to reduce these problems by (i) providing extraperitoneal elevation; and (ii) minimizing the tenting effect. One example is the LaparoTensor (Figure 2.4), which is based on the insertion of two curvilinear needles in the subcutaneous plane of the anterior abdominal wall over the operative field. When inserted, the needles enclose a large circle open at one end. The butts of the needles projecting at one end beyond the skin are clamped together and to the lifting device. The shape of the needles has been designed by mathematical modelling of the abdominal wall (Figure 2.4) to provide a better work space (the apex of the cone is widened), although this is still not as commodious as that provided by positive-pressure pneumoperitoneum **[see Module 21, Vol. I]**.

Extraperitoneal and retroperitoneal exposure

In this situation, there is no natural cavity, but one is created by finger and balloon distention of the loose areolar tissue surrounding an organ or anatomical region. Once the space is created, CO_2 insufflation through the optical port maintains the exposure. This approach is used for endoscopic adrenal surgery (as an alternative to the laparoscopic approach), lumbar sympathectomy, extraperitoneal inguinal hernia repair, pelvic node dissection for tumour staging of urological and pelvic tumours, etc. There is some evidence that the risk of CO_2 embolism is higher during retroperitoneal endoscopic than laparoscopic (intraperitoneal) surgery.

Combined exposure: laparoscopically assisted

There is no precise definition of laparoscopically assisted surgical operations. The endoscopic purist would regard an operation as laparoscopically assisted when the entire dissection is completed laparoscopically, and a mini-laparotomy is used at the end of the operation to deliver the specimen and perform the reconstruction of the gut, e.g. laparoscopic partial gastrectomy, laparoscopic right hemicolectomy and laparoscopic left colectomy or anterior resection. The ratio of the endoscopic to the external component of the operation can be varied and, in some instances, the combined approach is used to reduce the size of the abdominal incision for an open intervention. A pertinent example of this situation is anterior resection when, for whatever reason, the laparoscopic approach is contraindicated. In this situation, preliminary mobilization of the splenic flexure and adjacent transverse colon will permit an 'open' anterior resection through a transverse suprapubic (Pfannenstiel) or a lower midline incision. This combination provides 'the best of both options'.

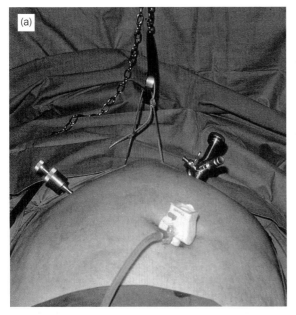
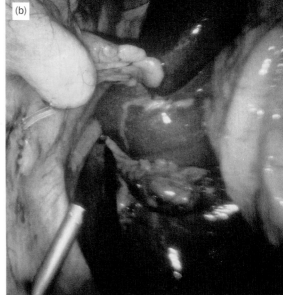

Figure 2.3 Anterior round ligament sling for low-pressure pneumoperitoneum: (a) external; (b) internal view during laparoscopic cholecystectomy with a pressure of 4.0 mmHg.

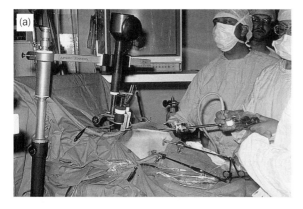

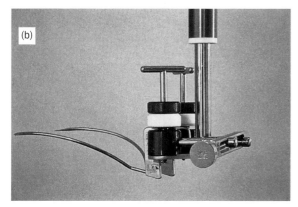

Figure 2.4 (a) LaparoTensor in use; (b) the subcutaneous needles provide a more uniform lift than intraperitoneal lift devices.

There is no evidence that laparoscopically assisted operations are safer than the totally laparoscopic intervention in terms of the risk of iatrogenic injuries. The adoption of the combined approach, however, reduces the operating time and results in a better functional reconstruction of the gastrointestinal tract. This is particularly the case after partial gastrectomy.

Thoracoscopic and video-assisted thoracic approach

The advantages of avoiding a large thoracotomy include accelerated recovery, especially in patients with compromised cardiorespiratory reserve and less pain. The instruments and equipment used are similar to those used in laparoscopic surgery. There are several techniques for safe endoscopic access to the pleural cavity and the procedures can be carried out with (i) single-lung anaesthesia (endobronchial occlusion by a double-lumen tube); or (ii) bilateral ventilation, when intrapleural CO_2 at a pressure of 6–8 mmHg is used to compress the lung. This level of positive intrathoracic pressure is well tolerated by most but not all patients [see Module 21, Vol. I].

Thoracoscopic approach

The complete thoracoscopic approach is now the standard treatment in many centres for pulmonary wedge biopsies, mediastinal node biopsy, for treating patients with spontaneous pneumothorax, for sympathetic denervation, mobilization of the intrathoracic oesophagus, for pulmonary segmentectomies and assessment/management of chest injuries. The approach can be anterior, posterolateral or posterior depending on the procedure and preference of the surgeon. The prone posterior approach (Figure 2.5) is particularly useful for sympathetic denervation (cervicodorsal ganglionectomy and splanchnicectomy), for mediastinal node biopsy and for mobilization of the intrathoracic oesophagus. The telescope port is placed 2.5 cm below and in line with the inferior angle of the scapula with the elbows suspended along the edges of the operating table.

Video–assisted thoracoscopic approach

In this instance, a 5.0 cm mini-thoracotomy (equivalent to mini-laparotomy) is made at the start of the procedure. Its exact location depends on the nature of the operation being performed. Video-assisted thoracoscopic approach is used for major interventions such as Belsey mark IV fundoplication, pulmonary lobectomies, pneumopnectomy and coronary artery bypass surgery.

Section 2.3 • Dissection and fascial planes

'There is no such thing as a surgical postoperative complication – all are enacted on the operating table.'

General principles

The above is a quotation from a master Liverpool surgeon. It is correct in so far as technical complications are concerned, but ignores the systemic complica-

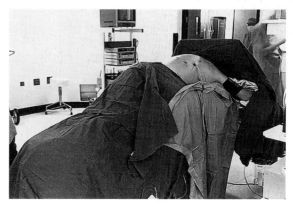

Figure 2.5 Prone posterior thoracoscopic approach. This allows access to both pleural cavities without changing the position of the patient. In addition, simple procedures can be carried out without single-lung anaesthesia.

tions that may complicate surgical intervention. None the less, it stresses, by exaggeration, the importance of technical execution (task quality) to the clinical outcome. Whatever the complexity of the pathological anatomy and density of adhesions, the operation progressed at a steady pace and the tissue planes seemed to open up as he dissected. When watched, he appeared to be slow but, in fact, the operations were completed fairly quickly. When once asked to explain his technique, his reply was 'this is how I have always done it'. On reflection, the operative work of this individual and other master surgeons has the following characteristics:

- immediate grasp in three dimensions of the abnormal anatomy of the case (spatial perception)
- appreciation of tissue planes
- economy of movements with purposeful manipulations
- operative choreography
- upper- limb co-ordination and manual dexterity
- gentle but firm touch
- strict adherence to the sequential steps of an operation.

This surgeon had reached the stage when he rarely committed any execution errors. He had developed these skills over many years to an extent that his brain was conditioned to execute 'macro-operative programmes'. He operated on autopilot and, for this reason, could not specify the components of his surgical operative skill. These are the skills that every surgical trainee should strive by constant effort to improve and hone his or her operative manipulations. Some of these skills are worth considering in some detail.

Touch

The essence of good dissection is the application of the right amount of stretch on the tissue with the assisting hand before division/suture, etc., of the tissue with the active hand. The correct amount of stretch on the tissue (without trauma) is entirely dependent on the tactile force feedback that the surgeon has developed from the innate level with which he or she was born. It is the level of appreciation by the surgeon of this sensory feedback to the hand that distinguishes the surgeon with the gentle touch from the rough one. Research into psychomotor skills has shown that left-handed are by nature more gentle than right-handed individuals, although the latter are more precise and commit fewer errors. A gentle touch must be accompanied by accuracy and decisive manipulations by the active hand. Tentative active manipulations, e.g. scratching with the scissors or inadequate needle passage, should be avoided.

Identification of tissue planes

Normal tissue planes are made up of condensations of areolar tissue and are relatively avascular, permitting separation with ease and without significant blood loss if the surgeon proceeds in the correct plane. Otherwise, bleeding, difficulty and resistance to separation are encountered. These are indications that the dissection has deviated to the incorrect plane. These normal fascial planes are altered by previous surgery and inflammation: the fibrotic component is increased and this is most dense close to the visceral side, becoming less so as the parieties and retroperitoneum are reached. The transition between the dense fibrous layers and the outer areolar tissue forms a distinctive 'white line'. This indicates the correct plane of dissection.

Economy of movement

All movements made by the surgeon in performing tasks are deliberate and purposeful, and achieve the desired objective. Unproductive movements not only waste time but also increase the risk of error. Another aspect of this skill requires that a step of an operation be completed before proceeding to the next. Thus, flitting from one step to another is counterproductive to the progress of an operation.

Choreography

Each operation is made up of a number of steps which, in turn, are composed of a series of sequential tasks. Choreography implies a co-ordinated performance of the various component tasks of a step such that the execution of one task facilitates the performance of the subsequent one. In this fashion, the step is executed smoothly and efficiently. Errors are of two kinds: intrastep (execution) or interstep (procedural). An intrastep or execution error means that the task is executed poorly, e.g. a needle swivels during passage through the tissue, or scissors cut the wrong layer. By contrast, a procedural or interstep error indicates missing a step or the wrong order of steps, e.g. failure to clamp or coagulate an arteriole before dividing it. In essence, choreography signifies that a surgeon has an orderly checklist of the steps of an operation in mind and, in executing the procedure, he or she follows this rigidly.

Types of dissection

Surgical dissection can be either blunt, i.e. the tissue planes are teased apart, or sharp, when a cutting device is used.

Blunt dissection

When used judiciously, blunt dissection is effective and safe. It requires the presence of loose areolar tissue that allows easy separation as a shear force is applied by hand or using a gauze swab or a pledget (peanut) held in a forceps (or long, secure grasper in endoscopic surgery). It relies for its safety on tactile feedback to the surgeon's hand and, unless this is refined, excessive shear force can be inadvertently applied so that tissues are torn and vessels avulsed. Blunt dissection is very useful in anatomically crowded areas or when the correct anatomy cannot be identified, especially if important structures, the integrity of which must be preserved, are known to be present within the block of tissue.

Sharp dissection

Sharp dissection, which involves division of tissue and separation of tissue planes, is carried out by mechanical (scissors, scalpel) or energized equipment (HF electrosurgery, ultrasonic devices, etc.). Irrespective of the equipment used, sharp dissection is a two-handed procedure that involves the application of the correct amount of tension by the assisting hand (often with atraumatic dissecting forceps, but sometimes directly with the hand over a gauze swab), while the division/separation is effected by the active hand. Clean separation and cleavage is as much dependent on the 'cutting instrument' as on the amount of stretch applied to the tissue.

HF electrosurgery is the most commonly used form of energized sharp dissection but, during the 1990s, vibrating (ultrasonic) equipment, water-jet and laser devices have been introduced both in open and in endoscopic surgery. The physical principles governing the safe use of these forms of energized dissection are discussed in the section of this module on 'Technology'.

Adhesions

Adhesions result from previous inflammation or operative interventions within serous cavities. The reported incidence of adhesions after open general abdominal operations ranges from 67 to 93%, although there is great variation in the formation of adhesions between individuals. Adhesions are also much less common after laparoscopic surgery. The adverse consequences of adhesions are shown in Table 2.1.

The division of adhesions is an integral part of abdominal surgery. Adhesiolysis may be necessary to obtain exposure or because the adhesions are responsible for the primary pathology, i.e. mechanical small bowel obstruction [see **Gastrointestinal Surgery, Vol. II**].

Adhesiolysis

Aside from causing symptoms and intestinal obstruction, adhesions influence the surgical access used and the level of technical difficulty of an operation, whether this is open or endoscopic. **Undoubtedly, adhesions increase the morbidity from iatrogenic injury in laparoscopic surgery, especially during the creation of the pneumoperitoneum,** when adherent bowel can be impaled by the **Veress needle or, worse, by the optical trocar cannula**. There are now safe techniques for the creation of pneumoperitoneum in patients with adhesions from previous surgery [see **Module 21, Vol. I**]. In open surgery, the technique for safe adhesiolysis relies on:

- establishing the anatomy of the adhesions
- putting the adhesions on the stretch (usually with the flat of the assisting hand over a swab), to identify the white line. This marks the insertion of the adhesion, which is completely avascular and can thus be divided by scissors without bleeding
- separating adhesions over a wide front; otherwise, the surgeon 'digs himself into a deep hole', with poor exposure and risk of damage to bowel loops.

Adhesions must not be separated by energized dissection and should not be clamped and divided between ligatures. This obscures the tissue planes and promotes further adhesions.

Section 2.4 • Tissue approximation

Accurate tissue approximation is essential for operative repair of defects and execution of safe anastomosis. Aside from gentle handling of tissues and careful dissection, the approximation must be achieved without tension and without compromise of the integrity of the blood supply essential to the healing process. The approximation itself can be performed by:

- sutures
- staples or clips
- glues.

Approximation by suturing

Approximation of edges involved in the anastomoses of hollow viscera, closure of wounds and repair of defects by interrupted or continuous suturing is an acquired craft based on established surgical principles.

The key principles involved are:

- preservation of the blood supply
- approximation of the edges without tension. This applies equally to repair of hernias and to intestinal anastomoses that should 'sit' rather than 'stand'
- meticulous technique with attention to detail and execution in the same way every time
- correct suture spacing and suture bites. It should be remembered that wounds heal despite sutures, which tend to devascularize the wound edges. Thus, especially in gastrointestinal anastomosis, the balance between creating a seal and devascularization is fine. In this respect, crowding the

Table 2.1 Complications of adhesions

- Intestinal obstruction
- Difficult reoperative surgery
- Chronic pain
- Infertility
- Increased health-care costs

anastomotic line with too many sutures predisposes to failure of the anastomosis. As a general rule, the space between the individual sutures should approximate to the size of the individual suture bites
- selection of the correct suture materials.

Continuous and interrupted suturing

Although in some instances either continuous or interrupted suturing can be used with equally good results, this is not always the case and certain specific anastomoses require the use of one and not the other of these two techniques. Continuous suturing is quicker than interrupted suturing and results in a more leakproof and haemostatic join. Hence, it is the technique deployed in vascular anastomoses. The 'purse-string' effect inherent to continuous suturing is minimized by correct suture spacing (the greater the distance between suture bites, the more pronounced the purse-string effect) and by the use of separate sutures for the posterior and anterior suture walls of the anastomosis. Even so, such an anastomosis cannot enlarge and this is an important consideration in children, where an anastomosis has to allow for growth. Continuous suturing is inadvisable in the anastomosis of small tubular structures and is difficult in deep cavity work.

Interrupted suturing is slower but allows more accurate suture placement. It is the technique used routinely in microsurgical work. Although less waterproof than the continuous technique, interrupted suturing is preferred by most surgeons for oesophageal, small bowel and colonic/rectal anastomoses. The sutures are placed on the back wall of the anastomosis before they are tied and the procedure is then repeated for the anterior wall. This technique ensures correct suture placement and precise coaptation of the edges. Interrupted suturing is less likely to devascularize gastrointestinal anastomoses. This is an important consideration in high-risk areas such as oesophageal and colonic anastomoses. Both interrupted suturing and stapling (see below) are accompanied by a higher incidence of postoperative suture line bleeding from anastomoses involving the stomach, particularly gastrojejunostomy.

Ligatures and suture materials

Ligatures, as opposed to sutures, are lengths of biocompatible thread used to tie structures such as blood vessels. The vast majority of sutures used in surgery nowadays is atraumatic, i.e. the needle is attached to the material either by swaging or crimping. In swaging, the rear of the needle is flattened and then folded over as a tunnel to hold the suture. Crimping, which is used for larger needles, entails drilling a canal at the rear of the needle (by laser) to accommodate the thread, which is then crimped in place. Crimping provides a more secure join between thread and needle. Swaging is used for fine atraumatic and detachable sutures (controlled-release or pop-off), where the attachment is intentionally set to a minimum strength, so that after passage through the tissue the needle can be easily pulled off. Controlled-release atraumatic sutures are invaluable for interrupted suturing in deep cavity work. They should not be used for continuous suturing.

The attachment of the thread to the needle by either technique creates a problem because the diameter of the needle at the junction is always larger than the suture. In practice, this ratio averages 2:1 for large and 3:1 for small sutures. The adverse effect of this step is that the suture lies loosely in the tissue, as the tunnel made by the needle is at least twice the size of the suture. Atraumatic sutures made from expanded polytetrafluoroethylene (ePTFE; Gortex) provide an exception to this, since the compressible sponge-like nature of this material results in a ratio of 1:0.8, i.e. the suture fits snugly in the tissues, improving the seal.

All materials used, whether natural or synthetic, meet certain mechanical, biological and handling requirements.

The important **mechanical** characteristics are tensile strength, yield point, elasticity and breaking strength retention (BSR). A high tensile (breaking) strength is always a good attribute because it permits the use of a finer suture. In terms of the bulk of the suture material in contact with the tissue, a 2/0 suture has a circumference that is double that of the 3/0 equivalent; hence, the inflammatory response is higher and the risk of infection greater. The tensile strength is also important in relation to knotting, since the strength of a perfect knot is, at most, only 50% of the tensile strength of untied ligature or suture material from which it is made. The BSR is an important mechanical characteristic. It is a reflection of the rate and extent of biodegradability of the suture following immersion in fluids (*in vitro* BSR) or implantation in animal tissues (*in vivo* BSR). When a suture is subjected to progressive distraction in a tensiometer, a certain point is reached when the material starts to deform and stretch permanently before it breaks if the distraction force is continued beyond this yield point. Young's modulus of elasticity (which is measured from the start of the distraction force to the yield point) is an expression of the resistance to elongation of the suture before it breaks. The higher the modulus, the less elastic the suture. A measure of elasticity is a good attribute as it enables the material to undergo elastic deformation when tied, thereby increasing knot security. By contrast, excessive elasticity is a nuisance as the material lengthens and distorts (crinkles) during knotting. The ideal combination is a suture with a high tensile strength, good BSR and a low to medium modulus of elasticity.

The **biological** characteristics depend on the composition, structure and surface charge of the material. They include biodegradability, reactivity (extent of inflammatory reaction), tissue incorporation (tissue growth into the interstitial microstructure of the material), effects of infection and site-specific adverse effects, e.g. deposition of calcium on non-absorbable

Table 2.2 Size of suture/ligature material: empirical gauge versus metric systems

Empirical gauge	Metric size (mm)
10/0	0.02
9/0	0.03
8/0	0.05
7/0	0.07
6/0	0.1
5/0	0.15
4/0	0.20
3/0	0.25
2/0	0.35
0	0.4
1	0.45
2	0.55

material in the urinary tract, and calcium bilirubinate in the biliary tract.

The **surgical/handling** characteristics relate to the ease of handling, slide through the tissue, knot run-down and knot security. The friction coefficient of a suture determines the ease of slide through the tissue, the knot run-down and the resistance to knot slip. Monofilament sutures slide more easily through tissues (and are thus less traumatic) than their braided equivalents. In the case of synthetic sutures, this disadvantage of braided sutures is largely, but not completely, overcome by coating the braid with a lubricant copolymer such as polybutylene. A low-friction suture exhibits excellent tissue slide and good knot run-down at the expense of an increased tendency to spilling. Thus, knots fashioned from these sutures require several throws (minimum of five) as opposed to the traditional three. The visibility of a suture is an important yet overlooked property. Only a limited range of dyes is approved for dyeing sutures and ligatures (violet, black, shades of blue–green). The visibility of a suture helps considerably in the execution of correct suturing and is an important characteristic in laparoscopic work, where blue–green is the most appropriate. Transparent (undyed) biodegradable monofilament sutures are difficult to use, especially in the smaller gauges, but are preferred by plastic surgeons for subcuticular closure as the dyed sutures may lead to tattooing when the dye leaches out as the material degrades.

Traditionally, the size (diameter) of sutures and ligatures is expressed by the empirical gauge system. The equivalent metric size (diameter in tenths of a millimetre) is shown in Table 2.2. The gauge range used in general surgery is from 1 to 5/0 (0.45–0.15 mm).

Natural materials
These include catgut (plain, chromic, alcohol packaged, dry), silk, linen, cotton and collagen. From a physical standpoint, they can be considered as twines of fibrous polymers. As a group, they have excellent handling characteristics and knotting properties. However, they excite a prominent inflammatory response within the tissues and, moreover, are easily colonized by bacteria, which invade the interstices of the twine and are then less susceptible to antibiotics.

All of the natural materials (including silk) are biodegraded by proteolytic digestion. The degradation is rapid with catgut and slow with silk and cotton. Another property of the natural materials is that they absorb water (tissue fluid) and thus swell following implantation. This swelling increases the knot security and is probably the reason why black silk and catgut are still popular with some surgeons.

The BSR of plain catgut (now derived from bovine intestine) is poor, and this material loses 50% of its tensile strength within a few days of implantation. Chromic catgut has twice the BSR of plain catgut and is thus preferable. Chromic catgut is an ideal material for external slip-knots and endoloops used in MAS for three reasons: (i) its stiffness (when dry); (ii) its rough twine texture, which resists reverse slipping; and (iii) because it swells following implantation, thus adding to the security of the slip-knot [see Module 21, Vol. I].

Synthetic non-absorbable materials
These **hydrocarbon polymers** are all derived from coal and oil. They are hydrophobic and therefore do not swell following implantation. Although generally regarded as non-biodegradable, some, such as polyamide (nylon), degrade in the tissues slowly with time. The group characteristics include flexibility, high tensile strength, resistance to creep and relative inertness. The main disadvantage of these hydrocarbon polymers in the monofilament form is their poor knot-retaining quality, with a tendency to knot spilling. The development of multifilamentous copolymers (by braiding of multifilaments or by looping from a single filament) has solved this problem.

Polypropylene (Olefin) is marketed as Prolene (Ethicon) and Surgipro (USSC). It is a monofilament material with a low friction coefficient (slides well through the tissues), excites a minimal tissue reaction and handles better than nylon. It is, however, elastic and can fracture. Knots tend to spill unless tied and drawn properly. Five throws are recommended for security. Polypropylene is used extensively in general surgery (e.g. mass closure of the abdomen) and for vascular anastomoses. Subcutaneous knots must be buried as otherwise localized tenderness/sinus formation may occur.

Polyamide (nylon) is available as monofilament (Dermalon, Ethilon, Monosot) and braided (Nuralon). Polyamide combines strength and elasticity but is slowly biodegradable, retaining two-thirds of its strength for up to 6 months. In the monofilament form, it is a difficult material to handle and does not tie well, with a tendency for the knot to spill. Despite this, it is popular with many surgeons for mass closure of laparotomy wounds. The braided form (Nuralon) handles and

Table 2.3 Synthetic absorbable suture materials

Monofilament	Braided
PDS (polydioxanone)	Braided polydioxanone
Maxon (polyglyconate)	Dexon (coated polyglycolic acid)
Monocryl (polyglecaprone)	Vicryl (coated polyglactin)
Biosyn (glycomer)	Polysorb (coated lactomer*copolymer)

ties well and is used extensively for single-layer gastrointestinal anastomoses by many surgeons.

Polyester (Dacron) is the strongest of the nonabsorbable polymers and has the best mechanical and handling properties. It knots and handles very well. Polyester is available as the uncoated braid (Mersilene) and as a braided suture coated with polytetrafluoroethylene (Ethibond, Surgidac).

Expanded polytetrafluoroethylene (ePTFE, Gortex) is an excellent suture and excites the least inflammatory reaction of all biomaterials used in surgical practice. Its microporous structure allows tissue ingrowth. ePTFE handles extremely well, although the knots tend to spill unless locked tightly. A minimum of four throws is recommended for knot security.

Synthetic absorbable materials
These are much less reactive than catgut, i.e. cause less inflammatory reaction after implantation. They are degraded slowly by hydrolysis rather than proteolytic digestion and exhibit a BSR of several weeks. The degradation by hydrolysis is important as this process releases hydrogen ions, thereby lowering the pH in the vicinity of the wound. This is thought to reduce bacterial colonization and infection. Synthetic absorbable suture materials can be monofilament or braided. The latter are available as coated and uncoated braids (Table 2.3).

Needles
Surgical needles are essentially penetrating devices designed to pass sutures through tissue with minimum trauma. As mentioned previously, most sutures are nowadays attached to the needle by crimping or swaging (atraumatic sutures) and the French eyelet needle is rarely used. The important characteristics of surgical needles are shape, size, tip and configuration of the shaft (body).

Shape
Needles can be straight, curved, compound curved and customized. The large, straight Keith needle is still popular for hand suturing and small, straight needles are used by some surgeons for laparoscopic suturing. The straight needle is not ideal for suturing, however, because it does not allow the smooth wrist-scooping movement. In addition, the straight needle results in a 'cutting' effect as the tissue is stretched on the shaft when the needle is picked and pulled out at the exit

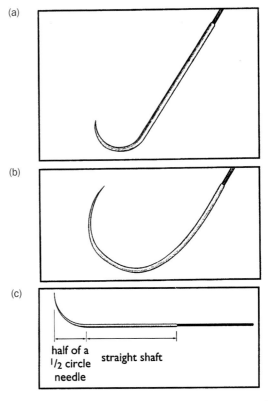

(a)

(b)

(c)

half of a
1/2 circle   straight shaft
needle

Figure 2.6 Examples of compound curved needles: (a) J-shaped; (b) fishhook; (c) endoski needles.

point. Curved needles do not have these problems. They are based on various sections of a circle (1/8, 1/4, 3/8, 1/2 and 5/8). The most commonly used curved needles in general surgery are the 1/2 and 3/8-circle configuration. The half-circle needle is ideal for end-to-side anastomosis, whereas the 3/8 circle is better for tissue plane approximation and end-to-end anastomosis. The compound curved needles have different profiles at the tip and body and are exemplified by the J-shaped needle, fishhook needle and the endoski needle used in MAS (Figure 2.6).

Size
This relates to the length and diameter of the needle. The length chosen is dictated by the distance between the entry and exit bites and by the length of the needle that needs to emerge from the exit point so that it can be picked up by the needle driver without damage to the tip. The gauge (diameter) chosen depends on the resistance of the tissue and its texture. In atraumatic sutures, the needle is always thicker than the suture and the ratio of the two is seldom below 2:1. The ratios of needle to suture diameters for atraumatic sutures used in general surgery are shown in Table 2.4.

Tip
The sharpness of the tip and the tapering ratio determine the penetrating characteristics of the needle. The tapering ratio describes the extent of the taper from the maximal cross-section of the shaft (shoulder) to the

Table 2.4 Atraumatic suture sizes and needle:suture ratios used in general surgery

USP size	Needle diameter (mm)	Suture diameter (mm)	Needle:suture ratio
6/0	0.3	0.1	2.7:1
5/0	0.4	0.15	2.7:1
4/0	0.5	0.2	2.5:1
3/0	0.65	0.25	2.6:1
2/0	0.75	0.34	2.2:1
0	0.9	0.4	2.2:1
1	1.1	0.47	2.3:1
2	1.4	0.57	2.4:1

needle tip and is calculated from:

$$\text{Tapering ratio} = \frac{\text{Distance between shoulder and tip}}{\text{Diameter of the shaft}}$$

The longer the taper, the more the needle penetrates atraumatically. Sharp needles with a long tapering ratio are use for suturing delicate tissues or those softened by inflammatory oedema. Sharp needles, however, increase the possibility of injury to the surgeons and operating staff. This is an important consideration in infected cases. Closure of the abdominal wound with blunt needles is advisable in these cases.

The tip of the needle is either conical, with a round cross-section (tapered), or cutting, where the shape is pyramidal and the cross-section triangular, with either a cutting inside edge (conventional), a cutting outside edge (reverse cutting) or both cutting outside and inner edges (cutting tip). Cutting needles are used for penetrating tough tissues, e.g. skin and cornea.

Body
The shaft or body of the needle is the longest section and extends from the shoulder to the join with the suture. Its cross-sectional shape determines: (i) the extent of trauma to the tissues during needle passage; and (ii) security of hold by the jaws of the needle driver (preventing deflection and swivel). The least traumatic configuration is the round-bodied needle, which should always be used for suturing delicate tissue, but this needle offers the least secure grip. The oval needle is fairly atraumatic and provides a better grip with fewer tendencies to swivel. It is preferable to the round-bodied variety in laparoscopic work. Various other shaft shapes are available for specialized work: ribbed, flattened hexagonal, triangular, etc.

Approximation by clips and staples

Edge approximation by clips
Clips are often used instead of sutures to close skin wounds, for skin grafts and to attach prosthetic mesh in hernia repair. Clips used for this purpose are made of titanium alloys that are fully biocompatible and virtually non-reactive. The advantages of skin closure with clips include speed of application, good coaptation, minimal disturbance of the blood supply to the edges (constant occlusive force) and ease of removal. There are many clip applicators (disposable and reusable) but essentially they fall into two types: side and end applicators. The side applicators (Figure 2.7) are ideal for skin closures. They are used extensively in:

- head and neck surgery
- skin closure after peripheral vascular surgery
- skin grafting.

End-clip applicators deliver a clip at the end of the instrument and are ideal for the attachment of prosthetic mesh during hernia repair since they permit precise application. They are used extensively in laparoscopic hernia repair. The morbidity following use of clips for this purpose is related to the risk of nerve entrapment by the clip, especially during laparoscopic hernia repair. For this reason, in both transabdominal

DIRECTIONS FOR USE:

1
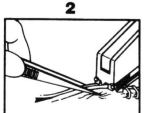
Evert skin edges.

2
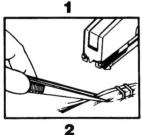
Position the stapler over the centre of the everted skin edges. Close by squeezing the handles together.

3
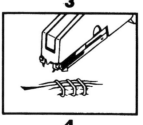
Alternately, the skin stapler can be precocked to enable more precise placement of the staples. Simply squeeze the handles until the points of the staple are visible and the trigger is in the precocked position. The staple then can be placed exactly where desired and implanted by completing the squeeze.

4
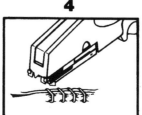
Release the trigger to achieve staple release.

Figure 2.7 Disposable side-clip applicator for skin closure.

preperitoneal repair (TAPP) and extraperitoneal repair, clips are being used less frequently and only at the superior margin of the prosthetic mesh. The important factor in the prevention of recurrence is not the fixation but the size of the mesh, which must be large enough to overlap the defect by a significant margin.

Anastomosis by stapling

Anastomotic staplers are mechanical devices that enable the performance of anastomosis of hollow organs (side to side, end to end and end to side) by a single-layer technique using a treble row of evenly spaced titanium staples that join the approximated organs from the mucosal aspect while a central blade cuts out an opening inside the staple lines. In circular staplers, the blade is circular and cuts out a 'doughnut' inside the circular staple line, whereas in linear staplers, the straight blades cut in a linear fashion the opposing walls of the two organs between the two rows of staples.

There is no doubt that staplers have been a significant technological advance since their introduction (first in Russia and Hungary) and their subsequent development as fully loaded, disposable but multifire instruments in North America in the 1980s and 1990s.

The advantages of staplers, especially in surgical gastroenterology, include:

▪ the ability to perform safe anastomoses in surgically inaccessible or difficult areas. This is best exemplified in colorectal surgery, where staplers have undoubtedly increased the number of sphincter-saving low anterior resections for cancer without compromising adequate distal margins

▪ uniform surgical results: the overall performance of low rectal and oesophageal anastomosis (effectiveness) has improved as stapling has evened out surgical skill in the execution of these difficult anastomoses

▪ compared with hand suturing, anastomotic stapling is considerably quicker to execute

▪ less risk of contamination

▪ avoidance of the need for occluding clamps.

The widespread use of staplers has not been an unmixed blessing. In the first instance, they have encouraged some surgeons to abandon hand-sutured anastomosis in all situations, thus being a disincentive to the acquisition and maintenance of suturing skills. Secondly, there are situations where the use of staplers not only represents an unnecessary additional cost, but also may enhance morbidity by an increased risk of postoperative suture-line bleeding. This is best exemplified by gastroenterostomy, where bleeding, usually from the gastric side of the staple line, is attributed to the prominent vascular supply of this organ. Finally, although stapler failure is uncommon, the integrity of the stapled anastomosis is dependent on the correct technique, which includes the correct size of stapler and staples, adequate preparation of the two anastomotic ends and anastomosis without tension. Some consider that stenosis is more common after stapled than hand-sutured anastomosis. With stainless-

steel staples, corrosion and leaching of iron and other constituents of steel has been documented experimentally, although this problem has been solved with the use of titanium staples. Both types of staple produce confusing artefacts on subsequent magnetic resonance imaging. Hand suturing and stapling techniques are not mutually exclusive and, indeed, should be regarded as complementary since the vast majority of stapling techniques require some hand suturing for optimal results.

Underlying mechanism of tissue approximation by staples

Within the cartridge of the instrument, the staples are U-shaped. When fired the staples grip the outer layers and assume the characteristic B-configuration that is essential for inverted coaptation of the edges without impairment of the capillary and nutrient blood flow to the anastomosis. This process works only if the surfaces of the two organs are in apposition throughout the intended anastomotic site. If extraneous tissue, e.g. fat, lies anywhere in between the stapling ring, the fixation of the tissue at this point is defective and the anastomosis will leak. Thus, adequate preparation of the two ends is essential. As an additional precaution, the integrity of stapled low rectal anastomosis is tested by insufflation of air through the anus after submerging the anastomosis in isotonic saline. The selection of the correct cartridge deploying the appropriate size of staples (2.4–4.8 mm) is crucial for the execution of a safe anastomosis. The smallest staples should be restricted for the closure of blood vessels.

Types of stapling device

From the functional standpoint, staplers are either occlusive non-cutting or anastomotic cutting (linear or circular). Occlusive staplers (Figure 2.8) approximate the two walls of an organ without cutting it and are used extensively to close the stapler insertion site after a linear stapled anastomosis and in bariatric surgery. Although circular staplers from different companies vary in detail, they are essentially of the same basic design. Circular staplers (Figure 2.9) have a detachable anvil that is inserted in one of the hollow organs and this is then closed tightly around the stem by a purse-

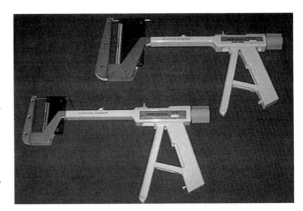

Figure 2.8 Occlusive disposable stapler: the device approximates and staples the two walls of an organ without cutting it.

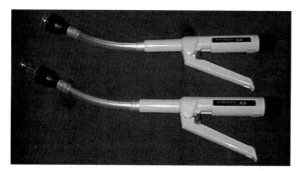

Figure 2.9 Circular cutting stapler used for oesophageal and colorectal anastomoses. The anvil is detachable.

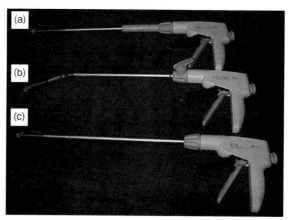

Figure 2.12 Endoscopic linear stapler; (a) occlusive stapler; (b) linear cutting anastomotic stapler with deflecting head; (c) linear cutting anastomotic stapler.

string suture. The rest of the instrument is composed of the cartridge (containing staggered rows of staples), a docking mechanism (for the stem of the anvil), advancement mechanism for approximation of the two organs and a firing mechanism, which drives both the staples and the circular blade.

Linear staplers (Figure 2.10) consist of two docking limbs, one of which carries the cartridge containing the staplers and the other the knife mechanism. Most modern linear staplers are multifires, i.e. the cartridge can be replaced for multiple applications (up to six times). In most instances, the stapling length is fixed

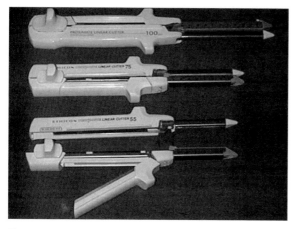

Figure 2.10 Linear cutting stapler. The instrument has two docking limbs, one of which carries the cartridge containing the staplers and the other the knife mechanism. Most modern linear staplers are multifires, i.e. the cartridge can be replaced for multiple applications (up to six times).

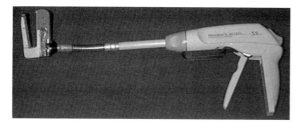

Figure 2.11 Linear occlusive stapler with adjustable stapling head.

(e.g. 30 mm, 60 mm). Thus, if a long side–side anastomosis is needed (e.g. creation of an ileal pouch), sequential application of the linear stapler along the intended anastomosis is necessary. This is an entirely safe and well-validated technique. Some of the newer staplers permit adjustment of the stapling length (Figure 2.11).

In some situations, both linear and circular staplers are used (double stapling). This is usually the case in low anterior resection where, in the first instance, the rectum is stapled and transected by a linear cutting stapler and the stapled transected proximal colon is then anastomosed to the rectal stump by a circular stapler. This entails insertion of the anvil of the circular stapler through the antimesentric taenia of the proximal colon and insertion of the stapler fitted with a perforating plastic trocar through the anus. The plastic trocar is made to perforate the closed rectal stump by the approximating mechanism. The plastic trocar is then removed and the two parts of the instrument are docked and approximated before the instrument is fired.

Both occlusive and anastomotic staplers have been developed for MAS (Figure 2.12). Some are powered and others have a deflecting staple head that facilitates precise application through the laparoscopic ports (Figure 2.12). Others have adjustable anastomotic lengths (Figure 2.13).

Long steerable flexible staplers are currently being developed for oesophageal and colonic anastomosis following open or endoscopic resection.

Approximation by biocompatible glues (sealants)

There has been a resurgence in the use of glues during the past few years. The search continues for biocompatible glue that would allow completely suture-free anastomoses. No currently available products are suitable for this purpose, although some are used to reinforce sutured or stapled anastomoses, and skin closure with medical-grade cyanoacrylte adhesives is possible. Glues fall into two main categories:

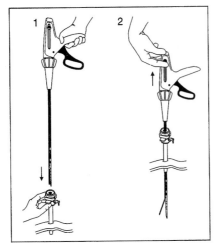

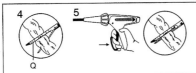

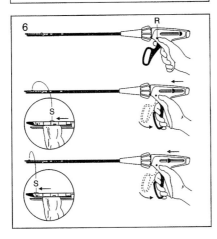

Figure 2.13 The newer generation of endoscopic cutting anastomotic stapler with adjustable anastomotic length.

- biological: these include fibrin-based glues (Tisseal, Scottish, Beriplast, etc.), Thrombin, Avitene (collagen sealant), Surgicel, Spongostan, and collagen-based sealant systems incorporating fibrin components (Tacocomb), as well as other polymers. Surgicel is one of the most frequently used products in general surgery. It is a sterile, absorbable, knitted fabric prepared by the controlled oxidation of regenerated cellulose. In addition to its local haemostatic action, Surgicel is bactericidal *in vitro*
- synthetic: polymer protein-based sealants, synthetic hydrogel (Focal Seal) and medical-grade cyanoacrylite adhesives.

Fibrin glues

These are more efficacious than the other varieties of biological sealant. In the classical formulation, fibrin glues consist of two components: fibrinogen and thrombin plus calcium, with additives that vary with

the preparation. When mixed at the point of application, the concentration of fibrinogen and thrombin influences the rate of polymerization of fibrinogen to fibrin and the strength of the final product. Some contain an antiproteinase (aprotinin), which is added with the intention of prolonging the integrity of the fibrin clot (ultimately dissolved by fibrinolysis) and increasing its adherence to the tissue. The two solutions have to be made up prior to use from the freeze-dried materials and then drawn into separate syringes that are connected to the applicator system. In essence, this consists of a Y-connection leading to a long double-lumen tube (one for each solution), with the two lumens joining at the tip where mixing of the two solutions occur, i.e. at the point of application.

Tachocomb is a new formulation of fibrin glue designed to avoid the need for making up the solutions of the procoagulant factors before use. It consists of a sponge-like membrane of equine collagen that is coated on one surface with the fibrinogen and thrombin plus calcium. The sheet is applied to the surface and then gently pressed with a saline-soaked swab until it adheres to the tissue. Tachocomb undergoes complete dissolution (phagocytosed by leucocytes and monocytes) within 6 weeks. Early clinical trials with this product have been promising but the reported experience is limited. FibFix is another formulation that is still being evaluated experimentally. It is a single-syringe formulation of fibrin glue that allows precise control of coagulation through light activation process.

The main disadvantage of all fibrin glues is the possibility of transmission of viral disease. Although all products are heat treated to destroy known viruses, there is the remote possibility of transmission of as-yet unidentified viruses. In some products, the thrombin is of bovine origin. This is a cause of some concern in view of the possibility of contamination with the bovine spongiform encephalopathy virus, and thus the risk of new variant Creutzfeldt-Jakob disease (CJD).

The established uses of fibrin sealants are:

- control of bleeding: cardiac bypass surgery, liver surgery and hepatic cryosurgery
- sealing of cerebrospinal fluid leaks in neurosurgery
- closure of pulmonary air leaks
- sealing of vascular grafts and catheter cannulation sites
- reinforcement of difficult gastrointestinal anastomoses.

The potential uses of fibrin glues include: (i) to attach skin flaps to the chest wall after mastectomy and thus reduce seroma formation; and (ii) as drug delivery systems (high-dose controlled release chemotherapy).

Section 2.5 • Arrest of haemorrhage

The ability to arrest haemorrhage is an essential component of surgical skill. Haemorrhage can arise spontaneously as a result of disease or from blunt and penetrating trauma, or may be encountered during the course of an operation.

The techniques for effective control of bleeding fall into three categories:

- endoscopic: injection, thermal and photocoagulation, banding
- radiological: embolization of bleeding vessels
- surgical: techniques deployed during open and MAS.

Endoscopic and radiological techniques are covered elsewhere [see Module 21, Vol. I].

Control of surgical bleeding

Types of bleeding

Bleeding may be encountered during surgery or as a result of trauma (primary bleeding), within 24–48 h after operation (reactionary bleeding) or be delayed for several days to weeks (secondary bleeding). Reactionary bleeding from small blood vessels within raw surfaces, minor capsular lacerations (liver, spleen) or from anastomotic suture or staple lines occurs as a result of the rise in the blood pressure after surgery. Reactionary bleeding is a special problem in laparoscopic surgery as small vessels compressed by the positive pressure pneumoperitoneum may bleed following desufflation. Thus, careful haemostasis is essential throughout these procedures. A more serious cause of reactionary bleeding arises from a slipped ligature or clip used to secure an artery. Secondary bleeding is due to infection and is always a major problem. It is best exemplified by bleeding from infected vascular grafts, often requiring removal of the infected graft and some form of non-anatomical bypass through a non-infected region [see Vascular Section, Vol. II]. Internal (concealed) bleeding is defined as haemorrhage within closed body compartments or serous cavities with no visible external losses, and manifests externally as hypovolaemic shock.

Bleeding during surgery

'Bloody surgery is bloody bad.'

The primary objective is the execution of operative interventions in a bloodless field or with minimal blood loss. The advantages from this are several, the most important being reduced blood-transfusion requirements, improved healing, maintenance of normal function of organ and systems, and reduction of infective complications. In many instances, bleeding during surgery is best prevented by careful dissection techniques. This is especially important in MAS, where control of bleeding is more difficult than in open surgery and is a common indication for conversion.

The following surgical methods are used for the control of haemorrhage.

- Packing: adequate packing of major or uncontrollable bleeding has saved many lives. During open surgery, when substantial bleeding is encountered in a deep cavity or inaccessible region, the first measure should be the application of compression by packs. This provides immediate control, allows the surgeon to obtain the necessary instruments and sutures and enables him or her to define the appropriate strategy. In addition, it gives the anaesthetist the opportunity to restore an adequate blood volume. In some situations, such as in major liver injuries, packing is the correct treatment and is preferable to hepatic resections, which carry a prohibitive mortality in this situation. Once bleeding is controlled by packs, the abdomen is closed and packs are removed or replaced 24–48 h later.

  Packing is not possible in MAS but control by compression can be achieved by grasping adjacent tissue with an atraumatic grasper and applying this over the bleeding area. An additional port is inserted to enable application of suction and irrigation. As the assistant maintains soft-tissue compression, the surgeon approaches the bleeding area with a coagulating forceps or clip applicator in the dominant hand and suction irrigation in the assisting hand. If bleeding cannot be controlled within a few minutes, the case should be converted to the open approach, in which event soft-tissue compression is maintained while the abdomen is being opened.

- Vascular control (proximal and distal) to the operative field is a wise precaution for dissection of lesions adjacent to or adherent to major blood vessels. This entails insertion of vascular sling around the vessels at the limits of the operative field, so that vascular clamps can be readily applied in the event of haemorrhage.

- During partial resection of solid organs (liver, spleen and kidneys), temporary occlusion of the inflow vessels is undertaken, e.g. Pringle manoeuvre during hepatic resection and management of bleeding hepatic lacerations. A careful note must be kept of the period of 'warm ischaemia' of the organ in question. The duration of warm ischaemia that the organ can tolerate should not be exceeded (45 min for the liver) unless the organ is cooled locally.

- Surface oozing over a wide area is best controlled by spray coagulation using the Argon beam system (see below).

Surgical vascular control and haemostasis

Vessels can be secured before division by a variety of techniques:

- thermal coaptation and sealing by energized systems: electrocoagulation, photocoagulation, ultrasonic sealing
- ligature and clipping
- transfixation
- vascular suturing or stapling
- application of fibrin glue.

The appropriate technique used depends on the size and the exact location. Energized coagulation by electrocoagulation, photocoagulation or ultrasonic systems (see below) is perfectly safe for vessels (arteries and veins) up to 2.0 mm in diameter but is not secure for larger vessels. Clips and simple ligatures (preferably with synthetic braided absorbable materials) are used for vessels between 2.0 and 3.0 mm in diameter. The correct application of clips, which must encompass the vessel totally and be applied at right angles to the long axis of the vessel, is crucial for safe vascular control by this technique, which is useful in deep cavity work and during laparoscopic surgery. The vessel should be divided at some distance (a few millimetres) from the clip or ligature, as the splayed-out cuff is the determining factor in preventing slippage by the force exerted by the systemic blood pressure. Overtightening of a ligature should be avoided as this will result in weakening of the vessel wall by the cheese-wire-cutting effect. This is especially the case in the less pliant atherosclerotic arteries of older patients. The mechanism of closure of the lumen of an artery is a complex physical process but involves gradual reduction of the lumen (by infolding of the walls) such that blood flow ceases when the walls of the vessel collapse. When studied, the force needed to achieve this in blood vessels subjected to normal blood pressure is very small (approximately 5–7 N).

Larger arteries (3.0–4.0 mm) are more securely controlled by either transfixion or double ligature, especially if the artery arises directly from the aorta (e.g. inferior mesenteric). Vessels greater than 4.0 mm are best secured by vascular clamps on either side of the proposed section. The proximal end is then sutured by 4/0 prolene before the clamp is released. The distal end can be ligated as this will come out with the specimen. Vascular control of these large vessels by suture provides maximum security and also avoids narrowing and distortion of the parent vessel. This is especially important in securing large

veins, e.g. the splenic vein at the junction with the portal vein. An alternative technique for securing large blood vessels is by vascular staplers. These are very commonly used for securing the pulmonary arteries and veins during lung resections. **Whether a vascular suture or a stapling is used to secure large vessels, it is important that 'flush' control is achieved such that the parent vessel is not constricted or a blind out-pouch is left. Either situation may result in thrombosis of the parent vessel** (Figure 2.14).

Section 2.6 · Surgical technology

General considerations

Surgical intervention is becoming increasingly dependent on high-technology devices. **This introduces new variables affecting the performance and outcome of an intervention, including malfunction of the equipment and misuse by the surgeon. The risk of errors for any particular procedure increases as the technology used becomes more complex. In addition, the technology itself is a potential source of hazard to both the staff and the patient.**

Important considerations that relate to high-technology equipment used in surgical treatment include proper maintenance and training of the surgeons in safe and efficient usage. In this respect, it is essential that the surgeon understands the physics underlying the function of a particular device. **Irrespective of its nature, all energized equipment that delivers energy to the patient is potentially harmful.**

The power-density level reached during surgery with conventional instruments (scissors, scalpel) is a function of the sharpness of the instrument and the force applied by the surgeon. Power density is the amount of energy (mechanical, electrical, ultrasonic, photonic) applied per cm^2 surface area of tissue and determines the effect, i.e. cutting or coagulation. In other words, the tissue effect depends on the power (W) and the surface area of

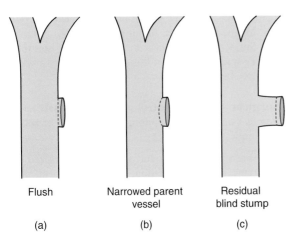

Figure 2.14 Vascular suture or a stapling of a tributary: (a) correct 'flush' control; (b) faulty because parent vessel is constricted; and (c) faulty because a blind out-pouch is left. Both (b) and (c) predispose to thrombosis of the parent vessel.

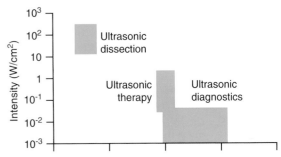

Figure 2.15 Energy levels of the various technologies used in dissection and ablation in surgery. (Reproduced from Muller and Fritzsch, *Endosc Surg Allied Technol* 1994; **2:** 205–210.)

contact, i.e. the effect of the same amount of energy will depend on the contact area between the instrument or probe tip and the tissue. The energy levels of the various technologies used in dissection and ablation in surgery are shown in Figure 2.15.

The visual-display technology (telescopes, camera, monitors, etc.) used in MAS is covered elsewhere [see Module 21, Vol. I].

High-frequency electrosurgery

The underlying principle involves the passage of an electric current through the tissue by means of a potential difference (voltage). The resultant flow of electrons excites the tissue molecules, notably water, creating heat energy, which causes water evaporation

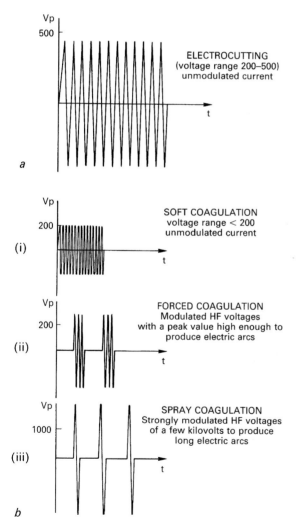

a

b

Figure 2.16 Characteristics of the applied currents in HF electrosurgery. (a) Unmodulated continuous sine wave in the voltage range 200–500 for **electrocutting**. (b) (i) Unmodulated current with a voltage output below 200 volts for **soft coagulation**. This voltage does not generate electric arcs; (ii) modulated HF voltages with a peak value high enough to produce electric arcs for **forced coagulation**; (iii) strongly modulated HF voltages of a few kilovolts to produce long electric arcs for **spray coagulation**.

and tissue coagulation. High-frequency (HF) currents (greater than 100 000 Hz) are used to minimize the risk of electrical shocks. The characteristic of the applied current can be varied from sine wave to modulated, to favour cutting or coagulation, respectively (Figure 2.16). HF electrosurgery can be monopolar, bipolar or quasipolar.

Monopolar high-frequency electrosurgery

Here, the current escapes from the electrode tip, dissipates into the receptive tissue and exits through the grounding pad (patient neutral electrode; Figure 2.17). The neutral grounding pad should have a large, even surface and is applied to the patient's upper thigh, covering a large area of clean, hairless skin to ensure a low current density. **Special efforts should be made to ensure that the patient's skin does not come in contact with metal components of the operating table, chucks and restraining devices, and damp clothing.** The connecting cables to the neutral and active electrode (appliance use by the surgeon) must be in perfect condition with respect to their insulation and connector plugs.

The potential hazards of HF electrosurgery include unwanted discharge and absorption of low-frequency currents (shocks), HF current burns (to patient and staff), sparking to unwanted areas (collateral damage) and capacitive coupling (applies to MAS) [see Module 21, Vol. I]. Electrical current leakage can also cause malfunction of pacemakers and monitors. The monopolar HF unit must not be operated in the vicinity of an electrocardiogram electrode (minimum distance of 15 cm).

Modern electrosurgical generators, such as produced by ValleyLab and Erbe, are smart devices in that they incorporate a microprocessor with sensor electronics that provides the necessary feedback from the electrode–tissue interface to the computer inside the generator. Used correctly, these smart generators adjust the power output to the lowest level necessary to achieve the effect. In addition, the strict limitation to the purposeful voltage range (200–500 Vp) preserves the integrity of the electrodes and increases the safety margin.

Electrocutting
HF monopolar electrocutting is achieved by the use of a continuous sine-wave (unmodulated) current (Figure 2.18) of sufficient voltage (200–500 V) to produce electric arcs at the tip of the active electrode. These arcs cause an immediate vaporization of tissue in contact with the electrode, creating a series of 'cellular mini-explosions' that collectively result in cleavage. If the voltage drops below 200 V, tissue cutting cannot be achieved since the electric arcs are not generated. Conversely, if the voltage rises above 500 V, the electric arcs produced are so intense that the tissue is carbonized and the electrode may be damaged. Within the safe operating range, the depth of coagulation of

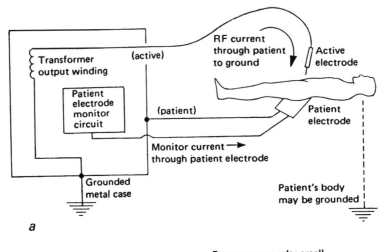

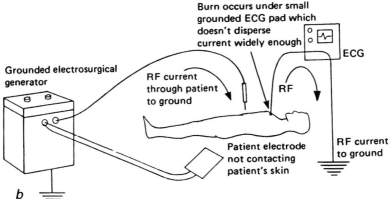

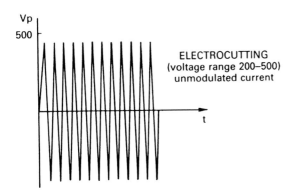

Figure 2.17 Sequence of events leading to a thermoelectric burn of the patient following faulty application of the indifferent electrode of a diathermy generator using the conventional earthing system. (a) Correct application of the indifferent (patient's) electrode; (b) faulty application of the patient's electrode.

the cut edges increases with increasing voltage and intensity of the electric arcs. In practice, the depth of coagulation during electrocutting is determined by the setting of the HF output power and the degree of modulation of the current (blend or mix). It is also influenced by three other factors:

- thickness of the cutting electrode
- rate and depth of cutting
- impedance of the generator.

With a conventional HF unit having an impedance of 250 Ω, fluctuations in the current or output voltage and intensity of the electric arcs are produced by variations in the depth and rate of cutting. This may lead to carbonization of the tissue along the cut edges, particularly at the beginning and end of the cut. This problem is obviated by smart HF generators that incorporate microprocessor-controlled automatic circuits with sensory electronics referred to previously.

Electrocoagulation
When an HF-modulated alternating electric current is applied specifically for heating living tissue, the temperature rise is proportional to the specific electrical resistance of the tissue, the duration of current flow and the square of the root-mean-square of the electrical current density. Largely because of the irregular current density distribution in the tissue, the temperature rises at different rates in various zones within the tissue. As the current density is largest in the zone of contact

Figure 2.18 Characteristics of the applied currents in HF electrosurgery. Unmodulated continuous sine wave in the voltage range 200–500 V for **electrocutting**.

between the tissue and the electrode, the maximum temperature is reached there, with the temperature decreasing proportionately with the distance from the contact area. On this phenomenon depends the safe deployment of monopolar electrocoagulation, since the further away the tissue from the contact area, the less likely the damage.

Once the temperature of the tissue near the contact surface has reached the boiling point, a layer of vapour forms between the tissue and the electrode, which impedes current flow. Thereafter, the sequence of changes depends on the peak voltage. If this is less than 200 V, the coagulation process slows down until the tissue next to the electrode has dried out, when current flow ceases. If the current is not switched off, the coagulum becomes adherent to the electrode. When this happens, removal of the electrode will dislodge the coagulum and precipitate renewed bleeding. If the peak voltage exceeds 200 V, once the tissue next to the contact area has dried out, electric arcs are produced that carbonize and puncture the coagulum, thereby causing the coagulation process to continue unabated until the generator is switched off or the dried-up coagulum becomes so thick that it resists further puncture by the electric arcs.

There are three coagulation modes that can be used:

- soft
- forced
- spray.

Soft coagulation is the safest for both open and laparoscopic surgery. As the peak voltage is less than 200 V, no electric arcs are generated between the electrode and the tissue. It results in desiccation of the tissue with shrinkage and no charring.

Forced coagulation deploys high peak voltages (>500 V) to generate electric arcs to achieve deep coagulation. This may be needed in vascular areas but the risk of collateral damage is substantially higher. Forced coagulation should never be used in close proximity to important structures such as the bile duct or ureter.

Spray coagulation is a non-contact mode where long electric arcs are intentionally generated by strongly modulated HF voltages (a few kilovolts) to surface coagulate raw and bleeding areas or to achieve haemostasis from inaccessible vessels. Spray coagulation is used in urology during transurethral resection of the prostate.

Ion plasma beam coagulation

This is a modification of monopolar HF electrocoagulation. It utilizes a plasma of ions of an inert gas (most commonly argon) to deliver the electrical current and is directed as a focused beam to the desired target. The argon gas beamer works with certain specific generators (Erbe, ValleyLab), which are capable of providing a spray coagulating current. The electrical arcs from this current produce a conductive channel of argon ions (the plasma) in the centre of the gas cone. It thus pro-

vides non-contact coagulation with minimal charring and depth of tissue necrosis under the coagulum. The argon ion plasma appears as a blue lightning flame that darts to other wet areas of the tissue surface once the incident zone has been desiccated, hence the limited depth of coagulation. Other advantages of the system include the displacement of blood by the gas spray, thereby permitting a more direct application of current to the bleeding area, and cooling around the coagulating zone by the outer layers of the gas, thereby minimizing lateral thermal damage. There is an optional setting of the gas flow in litres in relation to the generator power output, i.e. the greater the power the greater the gas flow required. When operating on vascular organs such as the liver, spleen and kidneys, the argon flow rate must not exceed 10.0 l/min because of the risk of gas embolism.

The delivery handpiece (disposable or reusable, flexible or rigid) essentially consists of a tube containing the energizing copper-wire or tungsten-wire electrode (Figure 2.19). Ion plasma coagulation can be used in open surgery, MAS and interventional flexible endoscopy to control bleeding from surface lesions, and is especially useful in arresting haemorrhage from large

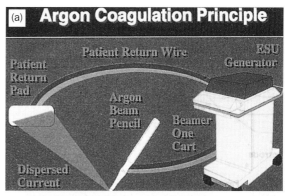

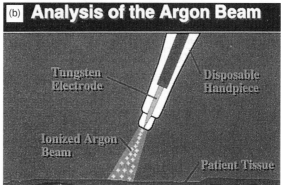

Figure 2.19 (a) The argon gas beamer works with certain specific monopolar generators, which are capable of providing a spray coagulating current. A ground pad is essential for the return current and the patient must be insulated from any metal component or wet surface. (b) The electric arcs from this current produce a conductive channel of ionized argon gas in the centre of the gas cone resulting in non-contact precise coagulation with minimal charring and depth of tissue necrosis underneath the coagulum.

oozing surfaces, during liver resections and partial splenectomy or nephrectomy. During laparoscopic and thoracoscopic surgery, one of the ports must be kept open during deployment of ion plasma coagulation, to avoid a dangerous rise in the intra-abdominal and intrathoracic pressures, respectively.

Bipolar electrocoagulation

Some dedicated bipolar generators operate only with bipolar probes, while others are capable of operating in both the monopolar and bipolar modes. In bipolar electrocoagulation, the current crosses between the two prongs of the electrode and returns to the generator without flowing through the patient. Thus, a patient ground (neutral) pad is not required and bipolar electrocoagulation is undoubtedly safer than the monopolar variety. Heating of the tissue in bipolar electrocoagulation is confined to the area between the two ends of the probe and thus collateral thermal damage is not possible. When using bipolar electrocoagulation, the minimum power necessary is used and every precaution must be taken to avoid contact between the active electrode and metal instruments. The tips of the bipolar electrode must be kept clean, as fouling with encrusted coagulum impairs the coagulation efficiency.

Although bipolar generators do not require a neutral patient ground pad, combined machines, which incorporate monopolar and bipolar circuits, do, and the safeguards described previously with regard to the safe application of the neutral ground pad must be strictly adhered to.

Quasi-bipolar electrocutting

This is designed to achieve electrocutting without the unmodulated current passing through the patient. Although standard monopolar/bipolar generators are used, specially designed cutting probes, which incorporate active (cutting) and return elements, are employed to apply the unmodulated current (Figure 2.20). The system is not, strictly speaking, bipolar and some current leakage to the patient is possible, especially if the return component of the electrode is fouled by charred tissue debris. A neutral ground pad is thus advisable.

Chemical composition of electrosurgical smoke

Electrosurgical smoke contains charred debris, cell-sized fragments, breathable aerosols and various complex

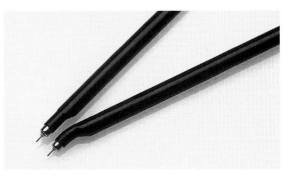

Figure 2.20 Bipolar electrocutting knife. The cutting needle can be retracted inside the instrument and the 'return' electrode.

organic molecules. Electrosurgical smoke used to be considered sterile but this has been questioned, particularly in relation to viral agents. The same applies to the smoke (plume) caused by lasers. At least 21 toxic or carcinogenic compounds have been positively identified in electrosurgical smoke (Table 2.5). The use of smoke-evacuation devices and safety precautions against inhalation by theatre staff has been recommended. In endoscopic surgery, compounds produced by the high-temperature pyrolysis of protein and fat are absorbed into the systemic circulation of the patient and lead to an increased level of carboxyhaemoglobin and methaemoglobin in patients after prolonged laparoscopic operations. *In vitro* studies have shown that high concentrations of electrosurgical smoke are cytotoxic and low (sublethal) concentrations stimulate white cells and the vascular endothelium.

Ultrasonic dissection

Ultrasound waves are mechanical waves that are not audible by the human ear, i.e. have a frequency above 20 000 cycles/s (20 kHz; 1 cycle/s = 1 Hz) and propagate in matter but not in air (hence the need for acoustic coupling by conductive gel during contact diagnostic ultrasound). Ultrasonic dissectors impart a higher power density than mechanical non-energized dissection but utilize less energy than HF electrosurgery or laser surgery. As a result of this, they cause less heating of tissue with reduced penetration.

The ultrasonic frequency range used for surgical dissection ranges between 20 and 60 kHz. The tissue

Table 2.5 Chemicals identified in electrosurgical smoke

Hydrocarbons	Nitriles	Amines	Aldehydes	Miscellaneous
2,3-Dihydroindene	3-Butenenitrile	Pyrrole	3-Methyl propanol	2-Methyl furan
1 Decene	Benzonitrile	6-Methyl indole	3-Methyl butenal	5-Dimethyl furan
1 Undecene	2-Propylene nitrile	Indole	Furfural	Hexadecanoic acid
Ethynyl benzene			Benzaldehyde	4-Methyl phenol
Ethyl benzene				
Toluene				

effects (separation, cutting, coagulation) are due to the high power density (around 100 W/s) compared with diagnostic ultrasound which, because of the low power density (0.01 W/s), has no discernible effect.

Basic design of ultrasonic dissectors

All ultrasonic dissectors, irrespective of make, consist of (i) an electrical generator; (ii) a piezoelectric transducer; and (iii) the dissection instrument (disposable or non-disposable). The transducer and dissection instrument is incorporated in the handpiece, which is connected to the generator by an electrical cable. The generator supplies the electrical energy to the system.

Piezoelectric transducers

These are ferroelectric ceramic crystals that vibrate (expand and contract rapidly), thereby producing ultrasound waves when energized by an electric current. The vibration frequency (Hz) varies with the extent of polarization of the crystals. By contrast, when piezoceramic crystals are compressed, they generate an electrical current, i.e. convert mechanical into electrical energy. It is this latter effect that is used in many household and car appliances, e.g. ignition systems. The former effect, conversion of electrical to mechanical (ultrasound) energy, is used in both diagnostic ultrasound and ultrasonic dissection.

The vibrations generated by the piezoelectric transducer are conducted by a metal rod, the length, diameter and shape of which influence the conducting efficiency to the tip of the instrument. A number of silicon rings fixed at specific vibration nodal points (Figure 2.21) prevents the rod from touching the outer protective sheath. Alternatively, the rod is covered in a Teflon sheath. An efficient system transmits most of the vibration energy to the tip of the instrument (hook knife, shears, ball, etc.) with little heating of the shaft of the instrument.

Low-power ultrasonic dissectors

These operate at a frequency of around 25 kHz and the handpiece, consisting of the transducer and free (unsheathed) rod, is non-disposable. The system allows irrigation and suction during activation, and handpieces for both open and laparoscopic surgery are available (Figures 2.22 and 2.23). Low-power ultrasonic dissectors are the safest form of energized dissection. They do not coagulate or cut, but only cleave cells with a high water content by a process called cavitation: the intracellular water, when subjected to the pressure waves, vaporizes, forming vacuoles, which then

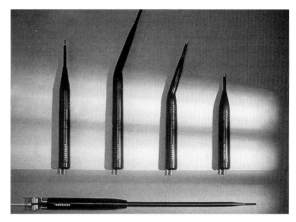

Figure 2.22 Selector probes (Spembley Medical) for low-power ultrasonic dissection; top for open surgery, bottom for laparoscopic surgery.

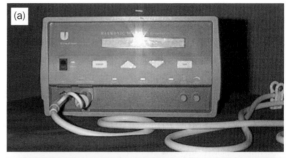

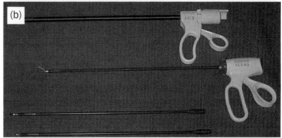

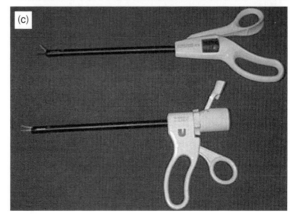

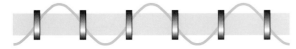

Figure 2.21 A number of silicon rings fixed at specific nodal points prevents the vibrating rod from touching the outer protective sheath of the handpiece of the ultrasonic dissector.

Figure 2.23 High-power ultrasonic dissection system (Ethicon). (a) Generator; (b) transducer and hand pieces for endoscopic surgery; (c) hand pieces for open surgery.

resonate with the vibrating rod, leading to implosion of the cell. These low-power ultrasonic dissectors cannot cut fibrous organized structures (arteries, veins, ureters, etc.) and impart very little, if any, collateral damage. They are used extensively for hepatic resections, where they cleave the hepatic parenchyma, exposing the intra-hepatic ducts and vessels for clipping or ligation.

High-power ultrasonic dissectors
High-power ultrasonic dissectors have become very popular for both laparoscopic and open surgical interventions in view of their efficiency in effective coagulation and cutting, thus reducing the instrument traffic and the duration of the procedure. Instead of smoke, they produce mist that can obscure the view in laparoscopic work, especially when the sprayback fouls the lens of the telescope.

These devices operate at a frequency of 55.5 kHz and thus deliver a very high vibrational energy to the tissue such that significant heating (as much as 120°C at the instrument tip), deformation and friction effects occur at the instrument–tissue interface. Cutting is mainly due to 'tissue sawing' (high-speed frictional deformation) coupled with linear compression of the tissue (by the surgeon). Although very efficient, these high-power ultrasonic dissectors can cause collateral tissue damage, especially when the generator is used at maximum power. Animal experiments have demonstrated significant damage (on subsequent histology) to the walls of the aorta, bile duct, etc., after high-power ultrasonic dissection in the vicinity of these structures. Each generator has five power levels (power levels 1–5). Although the vibration frequency is unaltered, the excursion at the tip of the instrument varies from 50 μm at power setting 1 to 100 μm at power level 5 (Figure 2.23). Collateral damage to vital structures is diminished by operating at a maximum power setting of 3. The trade-off is slower cutting, but safety is increased. For coagulation, the power setting should be minimal (level 1) and pressure is applied gently to coapt the vessel walls and create a seal over a wide area before cutting it.

Lasers

Laser is an acronym for 'light amplification by stimulated emission of radiation' and essentially consists of a beam of highly collimated (waves are in synchrony) monochromatic light (of a single wavelength). Visible light is the relatively small range of wavelengths of the electromagnetic spectrum (380–700 nm) that can be detected by the human eye (Figure 2.24). Electromagnetic radiation of wavelengths below (ultraviolet, X-rays and γ-rays) or above (infrared, microwaves and radiowaves) this range is invisible.

Laser beams can be generated of wavelengths that cover the entire visible portion of the electromagnetic spectrum (380–700 nm) as well as the ultraviolet and infrared regions (Figure 2.24).

Production of laser beams
The three components of a laser device are: the lasing medium, a power source often referred to as pump source and a resonator or optical cavity (Figure 2.25).

The lasing medium may be solid (crystals, e.g. ruby, semiconductor diodes, e.g. Gallium arsenide), gas (CO_2, helium, argon, metal vapours) or liquid (usually organic dyes in suitable solvents, e.g. rhodamine 6G in methanol). The lasing medium is energized by the pump source (electric current or light) inside the resonator. This is essentially a vacuum tube with a mirror at either end, one being totally reflective, i.e. bounces back all incident photons (light particles), and the other partially reflective. i.e. lets some photons through, and thus provides the exit point of the laser beam.

Within the resonator, the atoms of the lasing medium are excited from their resting or ground state to a higher energy level by absorption of the electrical or light energy from the power source. When the lasing medium has been excited sufficiently, a stage is reached when more of its atoms are at the upper energy level than at the ground state. This population inversion of the molecules of the lasing medium is essential for the lasing action to begin. Then, some of the excited atoms return spontaneously to the ground state, releasing this extra energy as photons of light of a wavelength characteristic of the lasing medium used (spontaneous emission of radiation). These photons interact with other excited atoms, which then return to the ground state, releasing more photons (stimulated emission of radiation). The net result is the production of waves of the same wavelength (monochromatic) travelling in the same direction and in phase with one another (spatially

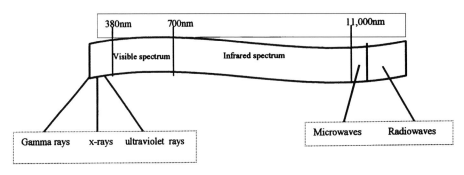

Figure 2.24 Electromagnetic spectrum.

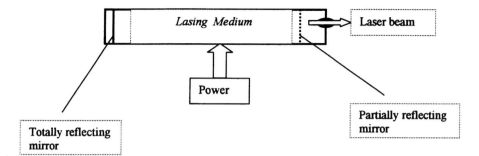

Figure 2.25 Components of laser devices: the lasing medium, a power source often referred to as pump source and a resonator or an optical cavity.

coherent). These photons are reflected backwards and forwards between the two mirrors, causing further stimulated emission of radiation from other excited molecules of the lasing medium. The partially reflective mirror allows some of this radiation to escape from the resonator, forming the laser beam.

Properties of laser beams

Most lasers produce collimated light; that is, the beam is parallel with minimal divergence with distance. This property enables high irradiance of tissue (power per unit area irradiated or power density). The semiconductor diode-array lasers are an exception as the light output from these solid-state devices is poorly collimated and requires focusing by suitable optics. The second property is being monochromatic (single or very narrow lines at characteristic wavelengths). Therapeutically, this enables the choice of laser for a given effect, coagulation, cutting or activation of specific chemicals. The third property of laser beams is spatial coherence of the component waves (in phase), although this is reduced to some extent when laser light is transmitted through an optical fibre and is rapidly lost as the light penetrates the tissue.

Classification

Lasers can emit light continuously (continuous-wave lasers) or in the form of discrete multiple pulses of higher energy around 1 ms (pulsed lasers). Both types can be Q-switched. Essentially, this consists of a very fast shutter in the resonator cavity between the lasing medium and partially reflecting mirror. When the shutter is closed, there is a tremendous build-up of light energy in the chamber, which is released as a giant high-energy pulse when the shutter is open (Figure 2.26).

The majority of medical lasers operate at specific wavelengths depending on the lasing medium. Thus, if a different wavelength is needed, another laser system has to be used. This has been the main limitation of lasers in medical therapy. A tunable laser, i.e. one that enables the clinician to select different output wavelength beams for a wide range of specific applications, does not currently exist, although the dye lasers and the more recent solid state diode-array lasers are tunable over a narrow range. Diode-array lasers will probably replace all other types in view of their portability and because they are largely maintenance free.

From the safety aspects (potential damage to the eye and skin), lasers are classified as 1, 2, 3A, 3B and 4, with class 1 being safe and 4 the most hazardous, requiring strict safety procedures. The vast majority of medical lasers falls into class 4 because of the power needed. For this reason, laser safety management is mandatory within the National Health Service.

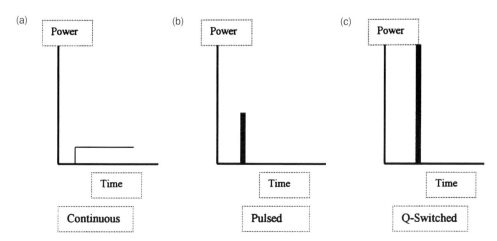

Figure 2.26 Schematic representation of power output of (a) continuous-wave lasers; (b) pulsed lasers; (c) Q-switched lasers. The latter releases a giant high-energy pulse when the shutter is open.

Table 2.6 Examples of medical lasers in current usage

Laser type	Wavelength (γ) (nm)	Output power	Beam output	Class 1–4	Beam transport
Helium/neon	630 (red)	0.5–10 mW	C W	1, 2, 3A, 3B	Fibreoptic or mirrors
Argon ion	490–510 (blue–green)	3–10 W	CW and		
Q-switched	4	Fibreoptic			
Nd:YAG	1060 (infrared)	70 W	CW and pulsed	4	Fibreoptic
Carbon dioxide	10 600	5–30 W	C W and		
Q-switched	4	Mirrors			
Dye lasers	<400 to >700	15 J	Pulsed	4	Fibreoptic
Excimer	200 (ultraviolet)	0.1 J	Pulsed	4	Direct
KTP	532	15 W	Q-switched	4	Fibreoptic
Diomed–diode array laser	730			4	Fibreoptic

CW, continuous wave; W, Watt; J, Joule (Watt-second).

Laser safety management

This involves:

- **a laser protection adviser**: a physicist certified for competence in laser radiation protection
- provision of **local rules** for each specific application of a laser. These address the nature of hazards, training, user's responsibilities, methods of safe working, personal protective equipment, especially eyewear, etc.
- **a laser protection supervisor** who ensures that the local rules are implemented and is usually the clinician responsible for the use of the laser
- **a laser controlled area**: the operating environment of the laser. The occupancy and activity of all persons in this area are subject to control and supervision to prevent exposure to radiation in excess of the maximum permissible exposure (MPE). This is the level of laser radiation to which the eye and the skin may be exposed without suffering adverse effects. The MPE varies with the wavelength of the radiation, the pulse duration or exposure time and, for lasers operating in the 400–1400 nm range, the size of the retinal image. The distance at which the radiation exposure from the laser equals the corneal MPE is defined as the nominal ocular hazard distance (NOHD). This is taken into account when specifying the boundaries of the laser controlled area. Warning signs are provided at every entrance to the laser controlled areas that medical lasers that fall within class 3B or 4 should only be operated by **authorized users** and a register kept of all authorized users for each laser installation.

Examples of medical lasers and their characteristics are shown in Table 2.6.

Medical applications of lasers

Lasers are used to achieve: (i) therapeutic effects, (ii) stimulation of healing, (iii) diagnosis, and (iv) optical alignment.

Therapeutic effects

These are achieved by the deposition of laser energy at a radiant exposure of 10^5–10^7 J m^{-2} and may be

(i) photochemical, (ii) photothermal, (iii) photoablative, or (iv) photomechanical.

- **Photochemical effect**: in clinical practice, this is referred to as photodynamic therapy (PDT). The basis for the treatment is the prior administration of a photosensitizer, e.g. haematoporphyrin derivative (HpD, Photophrin II) or various chlorin compounds, to the patient. The photosensitizer is taken up and retained by the tumour or dysplastic tissue. If this is irradiated by the appropriate laser light (630 in the case of HpD), the light interacts with the photosensitizer (photochemical reaction), leading to the production of highly toxic reactive species such as singlet oxygen with necrosis of the tumour. The actual destruction is far more complex and involves both a direct cytotoxic effect on the tumour cells and destruction of the tumour circulation. With HpD, the major factor in the necrosis of the tumour is destruction of its blood supply. The problem with PDT centres on the prolonged time it takes for the body to clear the photosensitizer. This may vary from several days to weeks (depending on the photosensitizer used). During this time, the patient has to avoid exposure to sunlight because of the risk of a major burn. PDT has been used in palliation, e.g. inoperable oesophageal and bronchial carcinomas, in the ablation of mucosal cancer of the gastrointestinal tract and urinary bladder, and in the destruction of Barrett's mucosa in association with medical (proton–pump inhibitors) or surgical treatment of the acid reflux. Following this treatment, regeneration with squamous epithelium may occur in some but not all cases.
- **Photothermal effects**: these are used to obtain photocoagulation, cutting and ablation by vaporization. Some 90% of the CO_2 laser radiation is totally absorbed by tissue water within a depth of 0.2 mm. This laser is therefore ideal for surgical cutting and for vaporization of tissues. Argon laser penetrates more deeply before absorption (0.5 mm) and Nd:YAG (neodymium:yttrium aluminium garnet) 2 mm. The argon laser is used extensively in

ophthalmology and in photocoagulation because of the high absorption of the blue–green light by haemoglobin and melanin. However, for endoscopic control of bleeding the Nd:YAG laser produces more effective coagulation and shrinkage of blood vessels in view of its greater penetration. The addition of a sapphire tip at the end of the conducting fibre or sculptured fibre tips enable contact mode laser delivery, permitting more precise endoscopic application with less smoke than the free beam mode. Interstitial laser hyperthermia produced by implantation of fibres conducting laser light into the tumour is an established modality of *in situ* ablation of tumours in solid organs such as the liver. The pulsed dye laser is the most effective laser for the treatment of port wine stains and has replaced the argon laser for this purpose.

- **Photoablative effects**: ultraviolet light is highly absorbed in tissue. Excimer lasers (argon fluoride, xenon chloride), which output in the ultraviolet range are used in ophthalmology for controlled precise ablation, e.g. band keratoplasy and to refashion the corneal curvature for refractive correction. Experimentally, excimer lasers have been used to remove atherosclerotic plaques from peripheral blood vessels.
- **Photomechanical effects**: these require giant pulse laser energy with power densities of around 10^{16} W m^{-2}, such as that produced by Q-switched Nd:YAG laser. These pulses generate localized shock waves and are used in ophthalmology for capsulotomy and iridotomy. Intraluminal stone fragmentation (e.g. impacted ductal calculi) is achieved by creating these shock waves with the end of the optical fibre touching the stones. Other lasers used for intraluminal lithotripsy are the Holmium:YAG (2100 nm) and pulsed dye laser systems (504 nm).

Stimulation of healing
Low-power laser energy (10–100 mW) produced by helium–neon (HeNe), gallium arsenide (GaAs), etc., emitting at the red end of the spectrum or near infrared region, has been shown to stimulate healing and is used in soft-tissue trauma, wound healing and relief of chronic pain due to musculoskeletal disorders.

Diagnosis
The photochemical effect can be used in the early diagnosis of severe dysplasia and *in situ* cancer of mucosal tumours accessible by endoscopy (gastrointestinal tract, bronchus and urinary bladder). For this purpose, the naturally occurring substance α-amino-levulenic acid (ALA) is administered intravenously or by mouth. ALA is itself not a photosensitizer, but following administration it is converted into protoporphyrin ix (Ppix) which fluoresces bright pink when irradiated with violet light (410 nm). The dose given and the power density of the light used are minimal, thereby a photoablative effect is not achieved. The procedure is known as fluorescent endoscopy and has the potential

for increasing the earlier detection of severe dysplasia and *in situ* cancer. Initial experience with fluorescent endoscopy using ALA has demonstrated a much higher detection of *in situ* cancer of the oesophagus, bronchus and urinary bladder compared with ordinary white-light endoscopy. Other photosensitizers can be used for fluorescent endoscopy but ALA is the ideal substance for this purpose because it is rapidly cleared from the body (within 24 h) and is thus free of the problem of delayed cutaneous sensitivity to sunlight.

Laser Doppler velocimeters incorporating low-power HeNe or diode lasers (up to 2 mW) are in routine use to measure skin blood flow, blood pressure and oxygen saturation (pulse oximeters) during surgery and in high-dependency and intensive care units.

Optical alignment
Low-power lasers emitting in the red are used routinely in optical alignment systems for patient positioning in radiotherapy and also as a light-guide for invisible lasers (Nd:YAG) during photocoagulation.

Cryosurgery

Cryosurgery is a long-established modality for tissue destruction by rapid freezing followed by slow thawing. It has been used in the treatment of skin, head and neck, prostate and liver tumours (primary and secondary cancer). Recent technological developments include laparoscopic probes that enable cryoablation through the laparoscopic approach. The advantage of this is twofold.

(i) The procedure can be repeated several times: this is particularly important in the management of patients with secondary hepatic tumours.
(ii) There is experimental evidence that cryosurgery, carried out through the laparoscopic approach with positive pressure pneumoperitoneum, results in a greater immediate tumour cell kill. This is probably related to the reduced liver perfusion consequent on the reduction of the portal blood flow by the positive intra-abdominal pressure.

Basis of cryoablation
Rapid cooling of cells to below −40°C results in supercooling and the formation of intracellular ice crystals that disrupt cell membranes and intracellular organelles. In addition, osmotic damage occurs with rapid freezing and slow thawing. During the freezing stage, blood flow ceases completely in the iceball and, when scanned by the contact ultrasound probe, the lesion does not transmit ultrasound waves. These are reflected from the surface of the iceball, giving a characteristic hyperechoic white margin overlying an area of acoustic shadowing (Figure 2.27). As the lesion thaws, blood flow returns for several hours. During this period, fixed tumour antigens, intracellular enzymes, etc., leak into the circulation. The escape of the fixed tumour antigens is thought to initiate an immunological response, although its significance in humans remains uncertain. The serum

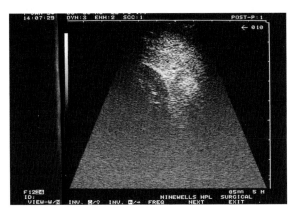

Figure 2.27 Ultrasound appearance of hepatic iceball during laparoscopic cryotherapy. The ultrasound waves are reflected from the surface of the iceball, giving a characteristic hyperechoic white margin overlying an area of acoustic shadowing.

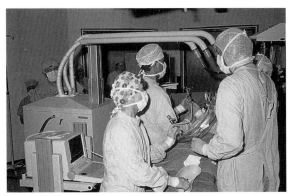

Figure 2.29 Modern cryosurgical unit with gantry that accepts up to three cryoprobes simultaneously (Spembly Medical).

lactic dehydrogenase level correlates most closely with the extent of cryodestruction on the day after cryosurgery, but transaminases and carcinoembryonic antigens (in the case of secondary deposits from colorectal cancer) are elevated for several days. The revascularization accounts for the 'systemic stress' syndrome after hepatic cryosurgery and limits the extent of freezing possible during any one session (to approximately 12 cm^3). During this period there is a degree of disseminated intravascular coagulation with a fall in platelets, which is maximal between the second and third postoperative day. For this reason, when large volumes of liver are frozen, haematological support is necessary. The revascularization of the cryolesion is only temporary and is invariably followed by occlusion of the blood vessels. The haemorrhagic necrosis becomes encapsulated and undergoes liquefaction over a period of several weeks. Eventually, the lesion shrinks down to a scar.

Modern equipment for cryosurgery of tumours

Although many cooling systems are available, the appropriate coolant used in cryosurgery for *in situ* ablation is liquid nitrogen as this has a boiling temperature of −190°C. All modern cryosurgical machines used for cryoablation of tumours use implantable rather than surface probes. These are shaped like blunt needles and those for laparoscopic use are 2.0 mm and 3.0 mm in diameter. They produce pear-shaped iceballs measuring 4–6 cm in diameter (Figure 2.28). More

than one probe can be inserted into big lesions simultaneously such that the two iceballs merge to encompass the tumour. The objective is to create an iceball that is larger than the lesion by at least 1.0 cm. Modern cryosurgery machines have a gantry into which the cryoprobes dock (Figure 2.29). The cryosurgery process is monitored with ultrasound and thermocouples placed at the periphery of the lesion.

Freezing regimens

Currently, there are two schools of thought. Some practise repeated freeze–thaw cycles, on the basis that the first freeze–thaw cycle alters the thermal conductivity and thus a larger frozen volume is achieved with the second freeze. Other surgeons practise a single freeze, usually of about 20 min duration, on the grounds that there is no material evidence that multiple-freeze cycle regime produces a larger iceball than a single freeze of the same duration. In addition, the procedure is shorter.

Treatment options

Currently, hepatic cryosurgery is limited to patients who are considered inoperable either because the hepatic reserve is compromised by cirrhosis (primary liver tumours) or because the disease is bilateral and extensive (secondary deposits). However, in the latter instance, cryosurgery may be used in conjunction with resection of a liver lobe. As previously indicated, laparoscopic cryosurgery is preferable to open cryosurgery as it permits repeated application at intervals of 6–8 weeks. Repeated cryotherapy combined with systemic chemotherapy (Raltidrex of high-dose 5-FU) is being investigated in phase II trials.

Radiofrequency thermal ablation

In situ thermal ablation of inoperable hepatic tumours is an alternative to cryosurgery since tumour cells are susceptible to temperatures over 45°C. Experimentally, there is a documented synergistic tumour cell kill between hyperthermia and chemotherapy or radiotherapy. Thermal ablation can be achieved by interstitial

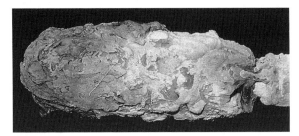

Figure 2.28 Iceball formed by a 2.0 mm laparoscopic needle cryoprobe.

laser hyperthermia, high-intensity focused ultrasound and RF current. Interstitial laser hyperthermia requires expensive technology and costly maintenance. High-intensity focused ultrasound is still at the experimental stage.

Mechanism of action

RF localized heating is currently the most feasible and cost-effective means of achieving targeted precise thermal ablation and is in established use in cardiology (e.g. treatment of arrythmias) and neurosurgery. During RF *in situ* tissue thermal ablation, the HF alternating electric current (200 000–500 000 Hz) flows from the non-insulated tip of an electrode into the tissue. This current flow induces ionic agitation within the tissue surrounding the electrode, resulting in frictional heating, which is quite different from electrocautery, where the current heats the probe. As a result, a localized ellipsoid lesion centred round the non-insulated tip of the probe forms. The thermal lesion is hyperechoic and its generation and size can thus be monitored by ultrasound scanning. The heat generated in the lesion depends on the current intensity (I) and its duration (T) and is described by I^2T. Although current intensity has a much greater effect on lesion volume, a minimum duration of application is needed to achieve the maximum lesion size. During application, heat is continuously generated and lost (by tissue conduction, by convection by the circulating blood and by shunting of RF current along low-resistance electrical paths) until equilibrium, determining the size of the thermal lesion, is reached. Tissue heating decreases rapidly with distance from the tip of the probe ($1/r^4$).

Modern equipment for radiofrequency *in situ* ablation of tumours

The long axis of the ellipsoid thermal lesion is approximately twice the length of the bare tip and its diameter approximates to two-thirds of the long axis. This has meant that until recently the largest thermal lesion that could be achieved *in vivo* by RF thermal ablation was approximately 2.5–3.0 cm and this limited its efficacy. Technological developments in recent years have led to (i) a new generation of microprocessor-controlled RF generators (Figure 2.30), and (ii) multielectrode probes that permit the insertion of an array of single electrodes

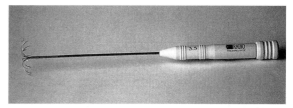

Figure 2.31 Multielectrode probe that permits the insertion of an array of electrodes conducting RF current into the lesion following a single puncture.

conducting RF current into the lesion following a single puncture (Figure 2.31). This configuration enables the creation of thermal lesions of up to 4.0 cm in diameter. The new RF generators provide information on the resistance of the tissue surrounding the probe, the temperature of the electrode tip, the RF current intensity passing from electrode and the RF voltage producing the current. Thus, the control on the size of the lesion is much more precise. A neutral ground pad (electrode) is essential as current travels through the patient. Cooling of the electrode during use improves ablative power (Figure 2.30).

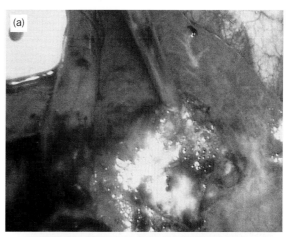

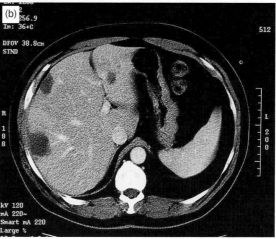

Figure 2.32 (a) Laparoscopic RF ablation of secondary hepatic tumour; (b) appearance of thermally ablated lesion 1 week after treatment: the lesion has a necrotic fluid centre with surrounding fibrosis.

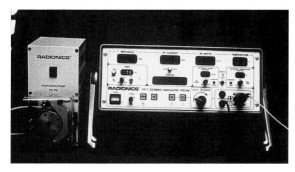

Figure 2.30 New generation of microprocessor-controlled RF generators with cooling of the electrode during use. This increases the thermal ablative zone.

RF ablation has been mostly used in the treatment of secondary hepatic tumours. It can be applied percutaneously under ultrasound or computed tomographic guidance. The laparoscopic approach with contact ultrasound scanning provides a more precise and controlled approach (Figure 2.32).

Guide to further reading

Becker, J. M., Dayton, M. T., Fazio, V. W., *et al.* (1996). Prevention of postoperative abdominal adhesions by a sodium hyaluronate-based bioresorbable membrane: a prospective randomized double-blind multicentre study. *J Am Coll Surg* **183**: 297–306.

Cuschieri, A. and Hanna, G. B. (1997). Surgical competence, training and privileges, in *Laparoscopic Surgery* (M. Hobsley, T. Treasure and J. Northover, eds), Arnold, London, pp. 21–41.

Cuschieri, A., Wilson, R. G., Sunderland, G., *et al.* (1997). Training initiative list scheme (TILS) for minimal access therapy: the MATTUS experience. *J R Coll Surg Edin* **42**: 295–302.

Guidelines for perioperative cardiovascular evaluation for noncardiac surgery (1996). Report of the American College of Cardiology/American Heart Association Task Force on Practical Guidelines. *Circulation* **93**: 1278–1317.

Hensman, C., Baty, D., Willis, R. G. and Cuschieri, A. (1998). Chemical composition of smoke produced by high-frequency electrosurgery in a closed gaseous environment. *Surg Endosc* **12**: 1017–1019.

Muller, W. and Fritzsch, G. (1994). Mechanicotechnical basis of surgery using invasive ultrasound energy. *Endosc Surg Allied Technol* **2**: 205–210.

Risk assessment in surgery

1 • Risk factors

2 • Preoperative assessment

3 • Risk-assessment scoring systems

'Mistakes are always initial' – Cesare Pavese

Risk assessment is a fundamental component of surgical practice. It is important for two main reasons. Firstly, the appropriate selection of patients for surgery depends on the balance between the benefit likely to be derived from the surgical procedure and the risk posed by that procedure. Thus, a patient considered to be fit for resection of a partially obstructing carcinoma of the colon might not be advised to undergo cholecystectomy for minimally symptomatic gallstones. Secondly, an assessment of risk will guide the surgeon and the anaesthetist as to the degree of supportive care that will be necessary in the postoperative period, and sometimes in the immediate preoperative phase. There is, however, a third reason for having an accurate measure of risk. Increasingly, surgeons are expected to submit their results to public scrutiny, and unless outcomes are adjusted for risks, which are outside the surgeon's control, publication of morbidity and mortality rates may provide extremely misleading information.

Risk assessment can be carried out at various levels. At its most subjective, the surgeon's 'gut feeling' can be a reasonable predictor of outcome, but this is highly dependent on the individual's experience. Most commonly, patients will have a careful history and physical examination, and they will then be required to undergo a series of investigations that will vary according to age, state of health as determined by the history and examination, and the severity of the surgical intervention. At the most objective end of the scale, a 'risk assessment score' can be calculated from a number of parameters that have been chosen arbitrarily, tested retrospectively and then validated prospectively. There are many different disease-specific risk-assessment scores, and a smaller number of generic scoring systems.

This module consists of three sections. In the first, the important risk factors are covered. In the second, methods of preoperative assessment are considered, and the third section describes some of the commonly used risk-scoring systems.

Section 3.1 • Risk factors

Risk factors relate to age, comorbid disease, the nature of the operation, the surgeon and the patient's medication:

- age
- cardiovascular disease
- respiratory disease and smoking
- gastrointestinal: malnutrition, adhesions, jaundice
- renal disease
- haematological conditions
- obesity
- diabetes mellitus
- surgeon, operative severity and emergency surgery
- drugs.

Age

Patients over 60 years of age are at increased risk of serious complications following surgery as a result of limited mobility, frequent presence of intercurrent disease and diminished reserve of cardiac, respiratory or renal function, which restricts the ability to cope with the stress of surgery or postoperative complications. This increased risk is dependent more on the physiological state of the patient than the chronological age and no one should be denied an operation on the basis of age alone. Elderly patients therefore require careful preoperative evaluation to assess their cardiac, respiratory and renal functions. Intravenous fluid and blood transfusion must be administered cautiously and with adequate monitoring as elderly patients are more likely to develop cardiac failure as a result of circulatory overload. Elderly patients also require smaller doses of narcotic analgesics or sedatives, as these are likely to precipitate confusion, both as a result of a direct action on the central nervous system (CNS) and from resulting hypoxia from respiratory depression.

Wound infection rates tend to be higher in elderly patients but this may be due to the fact that such patients require more time in hospital after a given operation and therefore wound infections are more likely to be recorded.

Postoperative stroke occurs in 1% of patients above the age 65 years and in 3% of those above 80 years. There does not appear to be an increased incidence of postoperative stroke in patients with a history of old stroke or in those with a symptomatic carotid bruit. However, a recent stroke (within 2–3 months of the operation) is thought to increase the risk of a recurrent episode. As the autoregulation of the cerebral circulation becomes impaired with age, extremes of hypotension and hypertension must be avoided throughout the perioperative period.

Cardiovascular disease

Overall, myocardial infarction and congestive heart failure are the most common causes of perioperative death in patients undergoing non-cardiac surgery. The Committee of Perioperative Cardiovascular Evaluation for Non-cardiac Surgery (American College of Cardiology and American Heart Association Task Force) identifies major, intermediate and minor clinical predictors of increased perioperative cardiovascular risks (Table 3.1) for myocardial infarction, congestive heart failure and death. Recent myocardial infarction is defined by the American College of Cardiology as greater than 7 days but less than or equal to 30 days. When present, major predictors (Table 3.1) necessitate intensive management and delay or cancellation unless the condition

requires emergency surgery to save life. The intermediate predictors (Table 3.1) enhance the risk of perioperative cardiac complications and require careful assessment by objective testing of the patient's cardiac performance. It should be noted that a history of myocardial infarction (more than 30 days) or pathological Q wave on the electrocardiogram (ECG) is considered as an intermediate risk factor, compared with a recent MI which is listed as a major predictor. Minor predictors (Table 3.1) are recognized markers for cardiovascular disease that have not been proven independently to increase perioperative risk.

In practice, these guidelines translate into the following management pathway.

▪ Major predictors present: surgery cancelled unless condition is immediately life threatening. Intensive cardiological management takes priority. Some may require myocardial revascularization (when the stress of elective non-cardiac surgery is likely to exceed the stress of daily life) in the first instance.

▪ Intermediate predictors: objective performance of cardiac status (e.g. echocardiography, stress ECG) undertaken, on which is based the individual risk that should influence the decision to go ahead with surgery.

▪ Minor predictors: surgery can proceed with adequate monitoring and postoperative support.

Although moderate hypertension is not an independent risk factor, its presence is often an indictor of coexisting coronary artery disease (CAD) and intraoperative fluctuations of the blood pressure in hypertensive patients are associated with myocardial ischaemic episodes. Furthermore, patients with preoperative hypertension are more likely to develop hypotension during surgery than normotensive patients, especially when blood volume is decreased. Thus, hypertension should be controlled prior to elective surgery. The exact details of any antihypertensive therapy that the patient is taking must be recorded, so that the anaesthetist can avoid adverse drug interactions and hypotensive episodes. Dysrhythmias are also important and patients with heart rates of less than 40 beats/min in the presence of a normal or increased supraventricular rate should have a pacemaker inserted preoperatively, even as an emergency. Likewise, patients with Stokes–Adams attacks have a great risk of developing complete heart block during anaesthesia and should also be paced preoperatively.

While most experts agree that pulmonary hypertension (associated with congenital heart disease, corrected or uncorrected) increases the risk of non-cardiac surgery, there have been no reported studies that quantitate the risk; however, it does appear that these patients do not tolerate intraoperative and postoperative hypoxia as well as normal individuals. Antibiotic prophylaxis against bacterial endocarditis in these patients when undergoing non-cardiac surgery is essential.

Table 3.1 Clinical predictors of increased perioperative cardiovascular risk (myocardial infarction, congestive heart failure, death)

Major
- **Unstable coronary syndromes**
  (i) Recent myocardial infarction with evidence of important ischaemic risk by clinical symptoms or non-invasive study
  (ii) Unstable or severe angina (Canadian class III/IV)
- **Decompensated congestive heart failure**
- **Significant arrhythmias**
  (i) High-grade atrioventricular block
  (ii) Symptomatic ventricular arrhythmias in the presence of underlying heart disease
  (iii) Supraventricular arrhythmias with uncontrolled ventricular rate
- **Severe valvular disease**

Intermediate
- **Mild angina pectoris (Canadian class I/II)**
- **Prior myocardial infarction by history or pathological Q waves**
- **Compensated or prior congestive heart failure**
- **Diabetes mellitus**

Minor
- ? Advanced age
- ? Abnormal ECG (left ventricular hypertrophy, left bundle branch block, ST-T abnormalities)
- ? Rhythm other than sinus (e.g. atrial fibrillation)
- ? Low functional capacity (inability to climb one flight of stairs)
- ? History of stroke
- ? Uncontrolled systemic hypertension

Respiratory disease and smoking

The incidence of respiratory disease in surgical patients varies with the population and in Western countries this ranges from 25 to 50%. The presence of either obstructive or restrictive pulmonary disease increases the risk of postoperative pulmonary complications and carries an adverse effect on the cardiovascular system. Thus, hypoxaemia, hypercapnia, acidosis and the increased work of breathing can cause further deterioration in patients with compromised cardiac function. Chronic obstructive airways disease is followed by a higher incidence of postoperative pulmonary complications than is restrictive airway disease. In patients with significant pulmonary disease, estimation of functional capacity (spirometry and blood gas analysis) form part of the preoperative evaluation. Wherever possible, surgery in patients with acute respiratory infections should be postponed until 2 weeks after the resolution of the infection. The timing of elective surgery in patients with chronic respiratory disease should coincide with remission and after a period of intensive physiotherapy and appropriate treatment with antibiotics and bronchodilators. Postoperative problems, particularly chest infections and segmental or lobar collapse, are exceedingly common in patients with chronic bronchitis and in heavy smokers.

Smoking increases the risk of surgery and anaesthesia as a result of its adverse effects on the cardiovascular and respiratory systems. Carbon monoxide and nicotine are responsible for the immediate cardiovascular effects. Consequent on the formation of carboxyhaemoglobin, carbon monoxide reduces the amount of haemoglobin available for combination with oxygen and alters the oxygen dissociation curve such that the affinity of haemoglobin for oxygen is enhanced. It also has a weak negative inotropic action on the heart. Nicotine causes an increase in heart rate and blood pressure; thus, it enhances the demand of the myocardium for oxygen while carbon monoxide decreases the supply. Elimination of both carbon monoxide and nicotine with improvement in the cardiovascular fitness is complete following a 12–24 h abstention from smoking.

There is a sixfold increase in the postoperative respiratory morbidity in patients who smoke more than 10 cigarettes per day. The responsible factors include small airways disease, hypersecretion of a thick viscid mucus and impairment of tracheobronchial clearance. Smoking also depresses the immune system. It induces reduction in immunoglobulin levels, natural killer cell activity, neutrophil chemotaxis and pulmonary alveolar macrophage activity.

It is therefore recommended that smokers should abstain from smoking for about 3 months prior to surgery, as this will result in an improvement in pulmonary function, a reduction in the likelihood of postoperative respiratory morbidity and the return towards a normal immune response. Those who find it impossible to stop smoking for this period will derive some benefit in terms of improved cardiovascular function from a short period of abstinence (12–24 h before their operation). This applies particularly to patients with ischaemic heart disease.

Gastrointestinal

Malnutrition

The patient with malnutrition, as a result of either impaired gastrointestinal function or inadequate diet, is at increased risk of morbidity associated with surgery. However, assessment of nutritional status can be difficult and is covered in detail elsewhere [see Module 8, Vol. I]. In essence, it is important to obtain an accurate history and probably the most vital piece of information is the amount of weight loss. There is evidence that loss of 15–20% of body weight is likely to be associated with impairment of physiological function and increased postoperative complications.

Physical examination should be directed towards determining body stores of fat and protein. Inspection of the temporalis, spinatus and interosseous muscles is a good indication of muscle wasting and the presence of oedema is suggestive of protein (kwashiorkor-like) malnutrition. Contrary to popular belief, the level of plasma albumin is not a particularly good index of malnutrition. Albumin is most useful as a negative acute-phase reactant and in a patient who is metabolically stressed, usually by sepsis, a low serum albumin can be expected. Thus, in the patient who is suspected of malnutrition and has a low plasma albumin, a focus of sepsis should be sought.

In the past it has been common practice for patients suspected of malnutrition to undergo a period of supplemental parenteral nutrition prior to surgery, but recent prospective studies have failed to demonstrate any benefit from this approach. Nevertheless, as a general guideline, body weight loss of 15–20% below the patient's ideal weight, accompanied by clinical evidence of muscle weakness and wasting, is still a reasonable indication for nutritional repletion before undertaking surgery. If possible, this should be carried out using the enteral route, although in patients with severe gastrointestinal malfunction parenteral nutrition may be required.

Adhesions

Another important gastrointestinal problem, which may affect the outcome of surgery, is the presence of intra-abdominal adhesions. The problem of adhesions is dealt with elsewhere [see Module 17, Vol. I]. In the preoperative assessment of a patient undergoing surgery, the possibility of encountering adhesions must be borne in mind, both in terms of obtaining access to the abdominal cavity and in terms of estimating the length of the procedure. Previous laparoscopy is unlikely to be associated with significant adhesions but **in the patient who has undergone a laparotomy there is a high likelihood of small and sometimes large bowel being adherent to the deep surface of the**

wound. Thus, when a laparotomy is to be performed in a patient who has already undergone major open intra-abdominal surgery, great care must be exercised to identify adherent loops of bowel and to avoid damaging them. This is best achieved by obtaining access to the abdominal cavity by extending the incision beyond the extent of the previous scar. When multiple dense adhesions are found within the abdominal cavity, great care should be exercised in separating out loops of bowel as **multiple accidental enterotomies lead to a significant risk of postoperative intestinal fistulation.**

Jaundice

The patient with jaundice is also at significant risk of postoperative complications, particularly sepsis, disorders of clotting, renal failure, liver failure, and fluid and electrolyte abnormalities. In addition, the conjugation and metabolism of drugs and anaesthetic agents are impaired because of hepatocyte malfunction.

Contrary to popular belief, there is no evidence to support the view that wound healing is impaired in the presence of jaundice. Wound-healing problems are usually confined to patients who have jaundice as a result of underlying malignancy and are the result of the disease and its association with poor nutrition. The nutritional deficits in jaundice patients are variable and parenteral nutrition should only be used very selectively because of the risk of infection. A high intake of carbohydrate is essential and amino acid solutions containing aromatic amino acids should be used sparingly as these may precipitate encephalopathy in susceptible patients. The oral route for nutritional supplementation should be used whenever possible.

Infective complications are usually due to the fact that most patients with jaundice undergoing surgery have an obstructed biliary tree and the bile in these patients may be infected by aerobic Gram-negative organisms. Coagulation disorders are usually due to a prolonged prothrombin time resulting from a deficiency of vitamin K-dependent factors consequent on the malabsorption of this vitamin that occurs in cholestatic jaundice [see Hepatobiliary and Pancreatic Surgery, Vol. II]. A more serious bleeding disorder may arise in the severely jaundiced patient, who may develop a consumptive coagulopathy from disseminated intravascular coagulation due to the presence of circulating endotoxin. This serious haematological complication requires careful monitoring of fibrinogen levels, fibrinogen degradation products and platelet counts. It may improve with control of infection but often requires specific treatment with fresh-frozen plasma alone or in combination with heparin. Under normal circumstances, however, the patient with jaundice who is about to undergo surgery merely requires an intramuscular injection of phytomenadione (10–20 mg). This will reverse the multifactorial clotting deficiency within 1–3 days. With severe hepatic disease, the prothrombin time may remain abnormally prolonged despite this treatment and in this case adminis-

tration of fresh-frozen plasma is necessary to cover the perioperative period.

The association between postoperative renal failure and severe conjugated hyperbilirubinaemia (the hepatorenal syndrome) is well known, although the precise mechanism is poorly understood. A reduced glomerular filtration is present and even in the absence of infection, endotoxaemia is frequently present. This is due to absorption of endotoxin produced by the intestinal microflora, which is usually bound by bile salts, which are absent in obstructive jaundice. Irrespective of the exact cause of the renal damage, there is now good evidence that adequate hydration and preoperative induction of a natriuresis or diuresis reduces the incidence of renal failure after surgical intervention in jaundiced patients. It is therefore current routine practice to administer intravenous fluids for 12–24 h before surgery and this is followed by an osmotic diuretic (Mannitol) or a loop diuretic (Frusemide) administered intravenously at the time of induction of anaesthesia.

All patients undergoing surgery should be catheterized and the urine output measured hourly. Further administration of diuretics is indicated if urine output falls consistently below 40 ml/h (despite adequate hydration and a normovolaemia) during operation and thereafter. Preoperative administration of oral chenodeoxycholic acid, commencing a few days before surgery, is practised in some centres and one clinical trial has shown a reduction in the incidence of renal failure, although a second trial with ursodeoxycholic acid did not report any benefit. More recently, the administration of oral lactulose has been shown to reduce the incidence of renal failure in jaundiced patients undergoing surgical treatment, but this has not yet been confirmed by other studies.

Renal

It is very important to obtain an assessment of renal function prior to surgery. The patient with renal failure may require dialysis and it is particularly important to establish the potassium levels as both hypokalaemia and hyperkalaemia increase the risk of cardiac dysrhythmias. Renal failure is commonly associated with heart disease and complicates its management. Correction of prerenal failure is particularly important in the emergency situation. For the management of fluid and electrolyte imbalance [see Module 7, Vol. I].

Haematological conditions

Anaemia

The patient with profound anaemia should have this corrected preoperatively as the reduced oxygen-carrying capacity of the blood will put undue strain on the cardiovascular system and exacerbate myocardial ischaemia or precipitate heart failure. In patients with iron-deficient anaemia, this should ideally be corrected by means of oral iron therapy if there is sufficient time to achieve this. Alternatively, the patient may require a blood transfusion, but this should be performed at least

1 week prior to surgery for elective conditions to allow for haemodynamic stabilization. It must be emphasized, however, that correction of mild anaemia is neither necessary nor desirable before surgical intervention. Most patients in this category have adjusted to the reduced haemoglobin load and the associated haemodilution may be beneficial in ensuring adequate tissue perfusion in the perioperative period. Indeed, controlled haemodilution down to a packed cell volume of 30–35% has been reported to reduce morbidity.

Polycythaemia, thrombocytosis and other conditions that increase blood viscosity may enhance the risk of thromboembolism or haemorrhage or both. Sickle cell disease, which is common in certain African ethnic groups, must be recognized before surgery. The condition can occur as the homozygous state (SS), resulting in the full-blown disease with attacks of sickle cell crises and haemolytic anaemia, or as the heterozygous condition (sickle cell trait). This rarely causes problems and is associated with a normal lifespan. Although the abnormal Hb S is soluble when oxygenated, it polymerizes and crystallizes out when it loses oxygen. As a result of this conformational change, the red cells become elongated, sickle shaped and rigid, leading to increased blood viscosity and an abnormal rheological state. The rigid cells block the microcirculation to various organs, inducing episodes of pain and infarction (joints, small bones of the hands and feet, spleen, etc.). Attacks of vaso-occlusive crises are precipitated by dehydration, infection, hypoxaemia (during surgery and anaesthesia), severe physical exertion, childbirth and high-altitude flying. Repeated attacks of splenic infarction can lead to an increased susceptibility to infection by *Streptococcus pneumoniae*. If sickle cell disease is suspected, the patient must be screened using the dithionite solubility test, and special precautions taken if surgery and general anaesthesia are required (adequate hydration, avoidance of hypoxaemic episodes, oxygen therapy).

In patients with a suspected bleeding disorder, a full coagulation screen must be carried out. The management of hereditary and acquired bleeding disorders is covered in Module 20, Vol. I.

Diabetes mellitus

Patients with diabetes mellitus require special management, which is discussed elsewhere [see Module 20, Vol. I]. The most important feature in the management of the diabetic patient is to avoid dehydration. Patients with diabetes mellitus have a much higher incidence of coronary artery disease (CAD) and, when present, myocardial ischaemia is more likely to be silent than in the general population.

Obesity

Obese patients have an increased risk of respiratory complications, deep vein thrombosis, wound infection and wound dehiscence [see Module 9, Vol. I]. In addition, they have a higher incidence of intercurrent disease and have restricted mobility. The technical difficulty of the operative procedure is also increased, making the risk of iatrogenic injury during surgery more likely. Whenever possible, controlled weight reduction is recommended before elective surgical treatment. **Morbidly obese patients are at risk of postoperative pulmonary failure and a significant percentage suffers from sleep apnoea.** Thus, all morbidly obese patients require intensive care following both elective and emergency surgery.

Drugs

Many patients coming to surgery are on drug therapy. Some drugs should be continued right up to the time of operation. These include antihypertensive agents and steroids. Other drugs must be discontinued for 2 weeks before general anaesthesia. These include:

- **monoamine oxidase inhibitors** (MAOI), which cause accumulation of noradrenaline in nerve terminals, leading to severe hypertension, pyrexia and convulsions when administered with vasopressors and narcotics
- **tricyclic antidepressants**, which block the uptake of noradrenaline into nerve terminals and have anticholinergic properties. These potentiate the actions of noradrenaline and atropine-like drugs
- **fenfluramine**, which interacts with halogenated anaesthetics, inducing dysrhythmias, and lithium, which prolongs the action of neuromuscular blocking agents
- **phenothiazine,** which may induce tremor and restlessness during intravenous induction with barbiturates.

Oral contraceptives pose the specific risk of postoperative deep-vein thrombosis. In women using the combined (oestrogen plus progesterone) pill, this risk is double that of non-users. This is related to a reduction in the activity of antithrombin III induced by the additive affect of the contraceptive and general anaesthesia. This enhanced risk is not seen with the progesterone-only pill, which need not be stopped over the time of elective surgery. Oestrogen-containing contraceptives should be discontinued 4 weeks before major elective surgery and alternative contraceptive arrangements made. In the emergency situation, prophylactic low-dose heparin should be used. There is no evidence that hormone-replacement therapy in postmenopausal patients increases the risk of postoperative venous thromboembolism.

Patients on warfarin are at risk of haemorrhagic complications. These patients should have the warfarin discontinued at least 3 days prior to surgery. If anticoagulation is considered vital, the warfarin should be converted to a low-molecular weight-heparin. This can be continued up to 12 h before operation and recommenced about 12 h postoperatively.

Operative severity and operating surgeon

The magnitude of the operation is an important risk factor. Operations are usually classified as minor, moderate, major or major+:

- **minor**: local anaesthetic procedures, uncomplicated groin hernia repairs, uncomplicated varicose vein operations
- **moderate**: appendicectomy, cholecystectomy, mastectomy, transurethral resection of prostate
- **major**: any laparotomy, bowel resection, cholecystectomy with choledochotomy, peripheral vascular procedure or major amputation
- **major+**: any aortic procedure, abdominoperineal resection, pancreatic or liver resection, oesophagectomy, total gastrectomy.

These classifications are used in the operative severity score of the POSSUM Scoring system (see below).

There have been several studies comparing cardiac complications in elective versus emergency operations and a recent review of the literature concluded that cardiac complications are two to five times more likely to occur with emergency surgical procedures than with elective operations. Thus, emergency surgery is itself an important risk factor.

It is also an important, if unpalatable fact, that the individual surgeon is a significant risk factor. It is now generally recognized that the outcome of similar operations can vary widely according to the skill of the operating surgeon and it is important for all surgeons to be aware of their own results and to ensure that they conform to a reasonable standard. In the future, training must ensure that all surgery is carried out to an acceptable standard.

Section 3.2 • Preoperative assessment

Preoperative assessment is an essential aspect of surgical care as the ultimate outcome will be largely dependent on measures taken as a result of the assessment of operative risks and fitness for general anaesthesia. Adequate preoperative care consists of the following:

- assessment of operative risks; appropriate selection of patient
- assessment of fitness for general anaesthesia and surgery
- adequate explanation to the patient of the nature of the operative procedure, so that fully informed consent can be obtained
- correction of nutritional, blood volume, fluid and electrolyte deficiencies
- institution of prophylactic measures against common postoperative complications [see Module 18, Vol. I]
- general preparation of the patient for surgery
- estimation of the amount of blood required to cover the operation
- assessment of the likely postoperative course and probable need for high-dependency or intensive care after the operation.

There is some truth in the statement that the beneficial effects of a surgical operation are inversely proportional to its magnitude. This emphasizes the need for careful patient selection that involves balancing the relative benefits from a given surgical procedure against the known risks and complications of the treatment. This decision is taken against the background knowledge regarding the natural history of the untreated disease from which the patient is suffering. Whereas the decision to operate may be straightforward, as in the emergency treatment of life-threatening disorders, it is often more difficult for planned elective procedures. Nowhere is this decision more difficult than in the use of prophylactic operations for latent or symptomless disease.

Extreme attitudes are always wrong and such statements as 'the patient has to earn the operation' are expressions of rigid views borne of an unaudited experience and testify to an inadequate appreciation of human suffering. Moreover, the careful selection of patients for surgery should not entail the rejection of patients for surgical treatment because of the presence of risk factors that could adversely affect the overall results of a given personal series. The prime consideration must always be the welfare of the patient and patient selection is exclusively concerned with the decision regarding the best form of treatment for a particular patient in the light of individual and personal circumstances (age and current disease, mental attitude and overall risks). This must of course include the patient's own expressed wishes.

Good selection of patients for surgery also entails an early decision that the medical or conservative management has failed since, other risk factors being equal, the overall operative mortality is lower for procedures undertaken under elective conditions. Thus, for example, the mortality following colectomy for ulcerative colitis is highest when this is performed as an emergency because of colonic perforation, intermediate when undertaken urgently for toxic megacolon and lowest when the procedure is performed electively because of failure of medical treatment.

Another aspect of patient selection is referral for specialized treatment. This concerns both interspecialty and intraspecialty tertiary referrals. The latter include patients with iatrogenic injuries (e.g. bile duct strictures), major hepatic surgery patients with severe and persistent symptoms after gastric surgery, bleeding oesophageal varices and major reconstructive procedures on the gastrointestinal tract. These situations require special expertise and back-up facilities, as the optimal results of remedial surgery are obtained at the first attempt at correction; the surgeon who does not have the necessary expertise should not 'have a go'.

History

When assessing a patient for surgery a full history must be taken, but particular attention must be paid to the following:

- cardiac and vascular disease, including deep vein thrombosis. Recent myocardial infarction is a significant risk factor
- respiratory disease and smoking habits
- other medical disorders, particularly hypertension, diabetes, bleeding diatheses and previous stroke
- detailed account of all drugs being taken
- alcohol intake
- previous experience of anaesthetics, especially intractable vomiting, volatile agents used and specific anaesthetic complications, such as suxamethonium, apnoea and malignant hyperpyrexia.

Physical examination

Again, a full physical examination must be carried out, but the following are particularly important:

- cardiovascular system
- respiratory system
- nutritional status
- mental state
- abnormalities of the jaw and neck
- presence of dentures.

Investigations

Investigation can be divided into routine preoperative investigations and special investigations.

Routine investigations

When carrying out routine preoperative investigations, it is important to ensure that adequate information is obtained, but not at the expense of carrying out large numbers of unnecessary investigations. For this reason it is useful to think of these investigations as mandatory, discretionary or unnecessary in terms of the type of operation or the status of the patient. In general, the standard routine investigations are haemoglobin level, urea and electrolytes with creatinine, liver function tests, sickle cell screening, chest X-ray, ECG, neck X-ray and thoracic inlet X-ray. Each of these will be considered in turn.

Haemoglobin
Mandatory:

- history of/or anticipated blood loss, e.g. menorrhagia or major surgery
- cardiorespiratory disease
- adult female patients.

Discretionary:

- all patients not in the mandatory or unnecessary categories.

Unnecessary:

- healthy male patients
- children having minor surgery.

Urea and electrolytes plus creatinine
Mandatory:

- diuretics
- major urological intestinal or renal surgery
- hypertension
- cardiac failure
- renal failure.

Discretionary:

- elderly patients undergoing major surgery.

Unnecessary:

- most patients having minor procedures.

Liver function tests
Mandatory:

- liver disease
- unexplained fever after recent general anaesthetic
- alcoholism
- any previous hepatitis.

Unnecessary:

- all patients not in the mandatory category.

Sickle-cell screening
Mandatory:

- status not known in Afro-Caribbeans.

Unnecessary:

- status known (card carried or in notes).

Chest X-ray
Mandatory:

- heart failure
- pulmonary disease with localizing chest signs
- malignancy.

Discretionary:

- heavy smokers
- hypertension.

Unnecessary:

- angina
- uncomplicated asthma
- chronic obstructive airways disease where a recent chest X-ray has been performed.

Electrocardiogram
Mandatory:

- hypertension
- arrhythmias
- ischaemic heart disease.

major surgery in the elderly (over 60 years).

Discretionary:

any of the categories in the mandatory column with fairly recent ECG.

Unnecessary:

all other patients.

Neck X-ray
Mandatory:

rheumatoid arthritis with neck symptoms.

Unnecessary:

cervical spondylosis

all other patients.

Thoracic inlet X-ray
Mandatory:

thyroid enlargement.

Unnecessary:

all other patients.

Special investigations
Pulmonary function tests and blood gas analyses are advisable in patients with respiratory disease that limits function and in patients undergoing thoracotomy. Forced expiratory volume in one second (FEV_1) and forced vital capacity (FVC) are good indices of obstructive and restrictive airways disease and can easily be measured by means of a Vitallograph. A coagulation screen should always be carried out when a bleeding diatheses is suspected or when a patient is taking anticoagulants. A cardiological opinion and tests of cardiac function (24-h ECG monitoring for ST depression, stress ECG, echocardiography, thallium scanning, etc.) are needed in patients with intermediate predictors of risk for perioperative cardiac morbidity. The exact assessment for estimation of risk in the individual patient is left to the cardiologist.

Section 3.3 • Risk-assessment scoring systems

For the majority of patients, assessment of risk is based largely on clinical assessment. In essence, this is a judgement based on history and examination of the clinical, physiological and nutritional state of the patient. If carried out by an experienced clinician, this overall assessment is probably as reliable as any complex scoring system. Usually, the clinical assessment is supplemented by taking into consideration the influence of individual factors (variables), which are known to have a documented adverse effect on outcome, e.g. old age, respiratory disease, cardiac disease and renal impairment. This type of additional assessment of risk is known as univariate, as the individual risk factors are considered one at a time. By contrast, multivariate (multifactorial) assessments provide a cumulative account (score) made up of the collective contributions of various data (clinical and laboratory), which reflect the overall risk and therefore the likely outcome. Some of these are generic, i.e. they can be used across a wide range of disease states, and others refer to specific disease processes.

Generic scoring systems

ASA
The term ASA refers to the scoring system devised by the American Society of Anaesthesiologists. This provides a measure of the preoperative physical status of the patient and is described in Table 3.2. Initially, the system was introduced to describe and select patients for clinical trials but it has now been adopted for routine clinical use. It has the advantage of simplicity but as it does not employ specific parameters, grading of the patient relies on a certain degree of subjectivity.

APACHE
Assessment of outcome is an important consideration in patients requiring intensive care treatment, for several reasons. Firstly, intensive care is an extremely costly resource. The cost–benefit ratio cannot therefore be ignored and it is generally agreed that intensive care is inappropriate when the probability of survival is negligible. Within any hospital, the facilities for intensive care treatment are finite and often limited. If a selective policy is not adopted, the available resource becomes readily exhausted and salvageable patients who become acutely ill and require intensive care support may be denied this treatment. Thus, a policy of admitting inappropriate patients to the intensive care unit, aside from being wasteful, is actually counterproductive.

Table 3.2 Physical status scale of the American Society of Anaesthesiologists (ASA)

Class	Physical status
1	A normally healthy individual: no organic, physiological, biochemical or psychiatric disturbance
2	A patient with mild to moderate systemic disease: this may or may not be related to the disorder requiring surgical treatment, e.g. diabetes mellitus, hypertension
3	A patient with severe systemic disease that is not incapacitating, e.g. heart disease with limited exercise tolerance, uncontrolled hypertension or diabetes
4	A patient with incapacitating systemic disease that is a constant threat to life with or without surgery, e.g. congestive cardiac failure, severe and persistent angina
5	A moribund patient who is not expected to live and where surgery is performed as a last resort, e.g. ruptured aortic aneurysm
E	A patient who requires an emergency operation

There has therefore been considerable clinical research into techniques and methods that afford reliable and precise estimates for outcome. The method that has been most validated and is now widely accepted is the APACHE (Acute Physiology and Chronic Health Evaluation) system. It measures the severity of the acute disease by quantifying the degree of abnormality of multiphysiological variables. The APACHE system gives a score, which is the sum total of:

- acute physiological score (APS)
- age points
- chronic health points.

The maximum possible score with a revised APACHE system (APACHE II) is 71. In practice, no patient has ever exceeded 55 and scores in excess of 35 are associated with a mortality exceeding 85% (Table 3.3).

Acute physiological score
The original APACHE I system had 34 potential physiological variables, making up the APS. As this was found to be impracticable, the infrequently measured and redundant variables have been dropped in the revised APACHE II, so that the APS is now made up from 12 variables (Table 3.3). The weighting system is based on a scale of 0 (normal range) to 4 (high or low abnormal). In practice, the APS is assessed on these variables over a 24-h period, when the most deranged physiological value for each parameter for that day is used to calculate the score, e.g. the lowest blood-pressure recording, lowest pH and highest respiratory rate.

Age points
Chronological age is an independent variable in its own right and, for this reason, points are assigned to the age in years as follows: 44 and below (0), 45–54 (2), 55–64 (3), 65–74 (5), 75 and over (6).

Chronic health points
As outcome is also adversely influenced by previous history of severe organ or system disorders and immunodeficiency states, points are allocated for these chronic health problems. The organ insufficiency and/or immunocompromised state must have been present before the current severe illness. The risk of death is higher when acutely ill patients with these previous chronic health problems require emergency surgical or non-operative treatment and when they undergo elective surgical operations and are electively admitted to the intensive care unit directly from the recovery room. For this reason, five points are awarded to non-operative or emergency postoperative patients as opposed to two points for elective postoperative patients with the same chronic health problems.

Mortality and APACHE II scores in patients treated in intensive care units
The relationship of the APACHE II system with mortality in patients admitted to the intensive care units is illustrated in Figure 3.1. There is a clear-cut inverse correlation between APACHE scores and survival; when this exceeds 29, the mortality increases sharply and above 35 the chances of survival are so small as to be negligible. Within a given APACHE score range, the overall risk of hospital death varies in accordance with the underlying aetiology of the acute disease. Thus, in the score range 10–19, intensive care unit patients with gastrointestinal bleeding or septic shock have a mortality of 27–30%, as distinct from 13% in patients with congestive cardiac failure.

POSSUM
While the APACHE II system is ideal for predicting mortality in the intensive care unit, it is not so useful for the prediction of mortality and morbidity across the general surgical spectrum. The reasons for this are that it requires 24 h of observation and the analysis of a large number of variables. For this reason, a simple scoring system for general surgical patients whose main use would be in surgical audit was developed. To start with, 62 factors were assessed by a multivariate discriminant retrospective analysis to reduce the number of variables. Of these, 35 factors were then assessed prospectively to produce a system that has been termed POSSUM (Physiological and Operative Severity Score for the Enumeration of Mortality and Morbidity). This is divided into two sections: the physiological score, to be scored at the time of surgery, and the operative severity score. These are detailed in Tables 3.4 and 3.5.

Thus, POSSUM requires scores from 12 physiological and six operative severity variables to estimate the risk of postoperative morbidity or mortality. For morbidity, the equation is:

$$\ln [R/(1 - R)] = -5.91 + (0.16 \times \text{physiological score}) + (0.19 \times \text{operative severity score})$$

For mortality, the risk equation is:

$$\ln [R/(1 - R)] = -7.04 + (0.13 \times \text{physiological score}) + (0.16 \times \text{operative severity score}).$$

Prospective studies have shown POSSUM to be highly accurate in predicting both morbidity and mortality.

Disease-specific scoring systems

Over the years many scoring systems for different disease states or forms of trauma have been developed. In order to provide a representative example, the commonly used scoring systems for cirrhosis of the liver, pancreatitis, head injury, general trauma and tumour prognosis are described below.

Cirrhosis of the liver
In cirrhosis of the liver, the prognosis is largely dependent on liver function. This is particularly important in assessing the risk of surgical procedures on patients with cirrhosis. The most important factors are as follows:

Table 3.3 The APACHE II Severity of Disease Classification System

Physiological variable	High abnormal range				0	Low abnormal range			
	+4	+3	+2	+1		+1	+2	+3	+4
Temperature; rectal (°C)	≥ 41	39–40.9		38.5–38.9	36–38.4	34–35.9	32–33.9	30–31.9	≤ 29.9
Mean arterial pressure (mmHg)	≥ 160	130–159	110–129		70–109		50–69		≤ 49
Heart rate (ventricular response)	≥ 180	140–179	110–139		70–109		55–69	40–54	≤ 39
Respiratory rate (non-ventilated or ventilated)	≥ 50	35–49		25–34	12–24	10–11	6–9		≤ 5
Oxygenation: $A\text{-}aDo_2$ or Pa,o_2 (mmHg)									
a) $Fi,o_2 \geq 0.5$ record $A\text{-}aDo_2$	≥ 500	350–499	200–349		< 200				
b) $Fi,o_2 < 0.5$ record only Pa,o_2					$Po_2 > 70$	Po_2 61–70		Po_2 55–60	$Po_2 < 55$
Arterial pH	≥ 7.7	7.6–7.69		7.5–7.59	7.33–7.49		7.25–7.32	7.15–7.24	< 7.15
Serum sodium (mmol/l)	≥ 180	160–179	155–159	150–154	130–149		120–129	111–119	≤ 110
Serum potassium (mmol/l)	≥ 7	6–6.9		5.5–5.9	3.5–5.4	3–3.4	2.5–2.9		< 2.5
Serum creatinine (mg/100 ml) (double point score for acute renal failure)	≥ 3.5	2–3.4	1.5–1.9		0.6–1.4		< 0.6		
Haematocrit (%)	≥ 60		50–59.9	46–49.9	30–45.9		20–29.9		< 20
White blood count (total/mm³) (in 1000s)	≥ 40		20–39.9	15–19.9	3–14.9		1–2.9		< 1
Glasgow Coma Score (GCS) Score = 15 minus actual GCS									
(A) Total Acute Physiology Score (APS): sum of the 12 individual variable points	≥ 52	41–51.9	32–40.9		22–31.9		18–21.9	15–17.9	< 15

Serum HCO_2 (venous; mmol/l) (not preferred, use if no ABG)

Table 3.3 *Continued.*

(B) Age points: assign points to age as follows:

Age (years)	Points
≤ 44	0
45–54	2
55–64	3
65–74	5
≥ 75	6

(C) Chronic health points

If the patient has a history of severe organ system insufficiency or is immunocompromised assign points as follows:

(a) for non-operative or emergency postoperative patients: five points or

(b) for elective postoperative patients: two points

Definitions

Organ insufficiency or immunocompromised state must have been evident **prior** to this hospital admission and conform to the following criteria:

Liver	Biopsy-proven cirrhosis and documented portal hypertension: episodes of past upper GI bleeding attributed to portal hypertension; or prior episodes of hepatic failure/encephalopathy/coma
Cardiovascular	New York Heart Association Class IV
Respiratory	Chronic restrictive, obstructive, or vascular disease resulting in severe exercise restriction, i.e. unable to climb stairs or perform household duties; or documented chronic hypoxia, hypertension (> 40 mmHg) or respirator dependency
Renal	Receiving chronic dialysis
Immunocompromised	The patient has received therapy that suppresses resistance to infection, e.g. immunosuppression, chemotherapy, radiation, long-term or recent high-dose steroids, or has a disease that is sufficiently advanced to suppress resistance to infection, e.g. leukaemia, lymphoma, AIDS

APACHE II Score

Sum of (A) + (B) + (C)

(A) APS points . . . .

(B) Age points . . . .

(C) Chronic health points . . . .

Total APACHE II . . . .

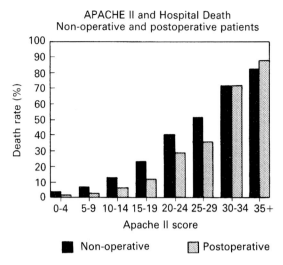

Figure 3.1 Relationship between APACHE II scores and hospital mortality ($n = 5815$). (From: Knaus *et al. Crit Care Med* 1985; **13:** 818–829.)

- size of the liver: large livers have a better prognosis than small, shrunken organs
- jaundice is a poor prognostic sign unless the diagnosis is primary biliary cirrhosis
- ascites: this is a poor prognostic sign
- albumin: low albumin is a poor prognostic sign
- hypoprothrombinemia: if persistent, this is a poor prognostic sign
- portosystemic encephalopathy: this is a poor prognostic sign
- alcoholic history: if a patient abstains from further alcohol intake the prognosis is better than cirrhosis of unknown origin (cryptogenic).

These factors, however, only give a rough impression of prognosis and, for this reason, various grading systems have been devised. The most widely used is that of Child, modified by Pugh (Table 3.6). Grade A indicates a good prognosis, grade B a moderate prognosis and grade C a poor prognosis. An alternative classification is that of the Paul Brousse Hospital devised by Bismuth (Table 3.7).

Table 3.4 POSSUM: Physiological score (to be scored at the time of surgery)

			Score	
	1	2	4	8
Age (years)	< 60	61–70	> 71	
Cardiac signs	No failure	Diuretic, digoxin, antianginal or hypertensive therapy	Peripheral oedema; warfarin therapy	Raised jugular venous pressure
Chest radiograph			Borderline cardiomegaly	Cardiomegaly
Respiratory history	No dyspnoea	Dyspnoea on exertion	Limiting dyspnoea (one flight)	Dyspnoea at rest (rate > 30/min)
Chest radiograph		Mild COAD	Moderate COAD	Fibrosis of consolidation
Blood pressure (systolic) (mmHg)	110–130	131–170	> 171	–
		100–109	90–99	< 89
Pulse (beats/min)	50–80	81–100	101–120	> 121
		40–49		< 39
Glasgow coma score	15	12–14	9–11	< 8
Haemoglobin (g/100 ml)	3–16	11.5–12.9	16.1–17.0	10.0–11.4
		17.1–18.0	< 9.9	> 18.1
White cell count ($\times 10^{12}$/1)	4–10	10.1–20.0	> 20.1	
		3.1–4.0	< 3.0	
Urea (mmol/1)	< 7.5	7.6–10.0	10.1–15.0	> 15.1
Sodium (mmol/1)	> 136	131–135	126–130	< 125
Potassium (mmol/1)	3.5–5.0	3.2–3.4	2.9–3.1	< 2.8
		5.1–5.3	5.4–5.9	> 6.0
Electrocardiogram	Normal		Atrial fibrillation (rate 60–90)	Any other abnormal rhythm or > 5 ectopics/min Q waves or ST/T wave changes

COAD, chronic obstructive airways disease.

Table 3.5 POSSUM: Operative severity score

	Score			
	1	2	4	8
Operative severity[a]	Minor	Moderate	Major	Major+
Multiple procedures	1		2	> 2
Total blood loss (ml)	< 100	101–500	501–999	> 1000
Peritoneal soiling or blood	None	Minor (serous fluid)	Local pus	Free bowel content, pus
Presence of malignancy	None	Primary only	Nodal metastases	Distant metastases
Mode of surgery	Elective		Emergency resuscitation of > 2 h possible[b]	Emergency (surgery < 2 h needed)

Definitions of surgical procedures with regard to severity are guidelines; not all procedures are listed and the closest should be selected.
[a]Surgery of moderate severity includes appendicetomy, cholecystectomy, mastectomy, transurethral resection of prostate; major surgery includes any laparotomy, bowel resection, cholecystectomy with choledochotomy, peripheral vascular procedure or major amputation; major+ surgery includes any aortic procedure, abdominoperineal resection, pancreatic or liver resection, oesophagogastrectomy; [b]resuscitation is possible, even if this period is not actually utilized.

Acute pancreatitis

In acute pancreatitis the diagnosis is confirmed by a rise in the serum amylase (greater than 1000 IU/l). The level of the amylase is not prognostic, although a very high amylase level may indicate a gallstone aetiology. It is important to have some index of prognosis, not only for comparative studies of different treatment regimes, but also to provide an indication of whether or not high-dependency or intensive care is indicated and whether or not early endoscopic retrograde cholangiopancreatography (ERCP) in patients with gallstone disease is appropriate. For this reason, scoring systems have been developed using largely biochemical parameters. The most widely used systems are the Ranson and Glasgow criteria, which are given in Table 3.8.

Scoring system for the assessment of head injury

One of the most frequent problems encountered by the clinician is to decide whether a patient is responding normally and fully aware of his or her surroundings. This problem is equalled by the difficulty in conveying to his or her colleagues exactly what is meant by the descriptive terms used in the account of the patient's

Table 3.7 Paul Brousse Hospital classification of severity of chronic liver disease

Parameter	Number of criteria
Albuminaemia < 3.0 g/100 ml	1
Hyperbilirubinaemia > 30 mol/l	1
Encephalopathy	1
Clinical ascites	1
Coagulation factor II and V 40–60%	1
Coagulation factor II and V < 40%	2

A, none of the criteria; B, one or two criteria; C, three or more criteria.

Table 3.8 Prognostic grading systems for acute pancreatitis

Ranson	Glasgow/Imrie
At admission/diagnosis Age > 55 years WBC > 16 000/mm³ Blood glucose > 10 mmol/l AST > 250 SF units/dl LDH > 350 IU/l	**Within 48 h** Age > 55 years WBC > 15 000/mm³ Blood glucose > 10 mmol/l (not diabetic) Serum albumin < 32 g/l Blood urea > 16 mmol/l (no response to i.v. fluids) LDH > 600 IU/l Pao₂ < 60 mmHg AST/ALT > 100 IU/l Serum calcium < 2.0 mmol/l
Within 48 h Haematocrit fall > 10% Blood urea nitrogen rise > 5 mg/dl Serum calcium < 2.0 mmol/l Pao₂ < 60 mmHg Base deficit > 4 mEq/l Estimated fluid sequestration > 61	

Three or more positive criteria in either system predicts a severe attack of acute pancreatitis.

WBC, white blood cells; LDH, lactate dehydrogenase; AST, aspartate aminotransferase; ALT, alanine aminotransferase.

Table 3.6 Pugh modification of Child's classification system for assessing severity of hepatic dysfunction in cirrhosis

	Points awarded for abnormality		
	1	2	3
Encephalopathy	None	1–2	34
Ascites	Absent	Slight	Moderate
Albumin(g/l)	35	28–35	<28
Prothrombin time (s prolonged)	14	4–6	6+
Bilirubin (mmol/l)	15–30	30–45	45+
Bilirubin patients in primary biliary cirrhosis	15–60	60–150	150+

Grade A, 5–6 points; grade B, 7–9 points; grade C, 10+ points.

Table 3.9 The Glasgow Coma Scale

Eye opening		
Spontaneous	4	
To speech	3	E
To pain	2	
Nil	1	
Best motor response		
Obeys	6	
Localizes	5	
Withdraws (flexion)	4	M
Abnormal flexion	3	
Extensor response	2	
Nil	1	
Verbal response		
Orientated	5	
Confused conversation	4	
Inappropriate words	3	V
Incomprehensible sounds	2	
Nil	1	

Coma score: (responsiveness sum = 3–15 (E + M + V)).

condition. Terms such as 'semiconscious', 'semico-matose' and 'stuporose' have vastly different meanings to different people and so it is important to be as precise as possible regarding the clinical findings. Fully conscious implies being fully aware of and interacting in an appropriate fashion to one's environment. The patient may, however, have an organic mental state which, although allowing him or her to be conscious, impairs the intellect, personality or memory. If the patient is not fully conscious, the clinician must be able to describe the degree of consciousness.

The Glasgow Coma Scale (Table 3.9) uses eye opening, best motor response and verbal response to assess the level of consciousness. This has the advantage of providing an objective means of assessing level of consciousness which is highly reproducible. It can therefore be used to monitor a patient's progress and its use has now extended beyond the assessment of head injury. It is also used as part of other scoring systems, e.g. POSSUM.

Injury severity score

In trauma patients the extent of injury and the proba-bility of survival can be defined using the injury severity scoring system (ISS). Points are assigned to major organ systems depending on the type and severity of injury, i.e. minor = 1, moderate = 2, severe but not life threatening = 3, life threatening but survival probable = 4, and survival not probable = 5. Fatal cardiovascular CNS or burn injuries are allocated a score of 6. The three highest scores are then squared and summated. Scores of around 25–40 are associated with a 50% mortality, depending on the patient's age.

Prognostic scoring systems in cancer

There have been many attempts at producing prognostic indices for various types of cancer, but probably the most accurate system remains the pathological TNM system [see Module 15, Vol. I]. This involves combining primary tumour characteristics (size and/or invasion through organ of origin and/or involvement of adjacent organs, lymph-node status in terms of tumour involvement and the presence of absence of distant metastases). Various other approaches have been attempted, however, e.g. in breast cancer, a prognostic index combining tumour size, nodal status, oestrogen receptor status and histological tumour differentiation has been developed. In addition, there has been a huge amount of work looking at other prognostic factors in various tumours and the recent exponential growth of knowledge in the area of molecular oncology has provided many further candidates to enhance this process. It has to be said, however, that simple pathological grading still remains the most useful and most widely used system.

Guide to further reading

Copeland, G. P., Jones, D. and Walters, M. (1991). POSSUM: a scoring system for surgical audit. *Br J Surg* **78**: 356–360.

Guidelines for Perioperative Cardiovascular Evaluation for Noncardiac Surgery (1996). *Circulation* **93**: 1278–1317.

Knaus, W. A., Draper, E. A., Wagner, D. P. and Zimmerman, J. E. (1985). APACHE II: a severity of disease classification system. *Crit Care Med* **13**: 818–829.

Mangano, D. T. (1990). Perioperative cardiac morbidity. *Anesthesiology* **72**: 153–184.

MODULE 4
The injured patient

1 • General considerations

2 • Metabolic response to trauma

3 • Prehospital care and transport

4 • Assessment of the injured patient

5 • Management of the burns victim

'Extreme remedies are most appropriate for extreme diseases' – Hippocrates, c. 460–377 BC

This module deals with the general aspects of modern care of the injured patient, including the management of the burns victim. The surgical treatment of specific injuries (neck, chest, abdominal, genitourinary and vascular) is covered in Volume II [Trauma, Vol. II].

Section 4.1 • General considerations

Trauma remains one of the leading causes of death and disability throughout the world. In the USA, it is the largest cause of death in the population 44 years old and younger, more than all other causes of death combined for this age group. It is exceeded only by atherosclerosis and cancer as the major cause of death in all age groups. Approximately 60 million people are injured annually; 30 million require medical treatment and 3.6 million require hospitalization. On average, 150 000 people per year die from trauma-related causes and almost half a million people sustain injuries leading to permanent disability. Motor vehicle accidents remain the single most common cause of trauma-related mortality (32%), followed by gunshot wounds (22%) and falls (9%). Trauma-related monetary costs in the USA are greater than $400 billion annually, when one considers the need for acute and chronic care and the loss of productive life. Arguably, it is the single most costly health-care problem today in the USA, and possibly the world.

If the number of fatalities due to trauma is plotted as a function of time after injury, three peaks appear. The **first peak**, which consists of approximately 50% of all trauma-related deaths, contains those patients who die instantaneously or very soon after injury. These fatalities are generally due to an injury or a combination of injuries considered to be lethal, such as a brainstem laceration or a ruptured heart. Few of these patients will be saved by health-care systems, as they die from injury before reaching the hospital. In general, survival from these injuries will be increased by prevention; either by the development of devices that prevent injury or the introduction of laws that limit behaviour that may result in injury. The **second peak**, which contains approximately 30% of trauma fatalities, occurs within hours of injury and is usually due to severe haemorrhage. Considerable reduction in the number of people dying during this period can occur if there is rapid transport from the scene of the accident to a hospital fully staffed and equipped to care for victims suffering severe injuries. The development of a 'systems' approach to trauma care has resulted in a significant reduction in the mortality of patients dying within hours of injury. **A trauma system operates within a geographical region (i.e. city, county, state) and provides for rapid transport of victims of major trauma to specified hospitals within that region**. These specific hospitals are called trauma centres because they have concentrated resources and expertise to treat severely injured patients immediately and effectively. The integration of prehospital care, rapid transport and immediate surgical treatment within a trauma system has been demonstrated to reduce preventable deaths due to trauma from 20–30% to 2–9%. In general, further development of trauma systems, organized protocols for care of predictable injuries and expanding the availability of these systems to rural areas will result in the reduction of mortality during this period.

The **third peak** in trauma deaths occurs days to weeks after injury and is usually due to infection and multiple organ failure. The development of trauma systems has changed the epidemiology of death in this peak in regions where trauma care is more developed. The availability of early rapid transport and early, aggressive in-hospital care has improved early resuscitation and changed the character of the third traditional peak following injury into three smaller peaks. Occurring within the first week following injury, inability to control intracranial hypertension following severe head injury now accounts for a significant portion of late mortality.

Sepsis and accompanying multiple organ failure have diminished as a result of better, more aggressive resuscitation and early care. They now account for approximately 5% of overall mortality and only 30% of late mortality in an organized system of care. Fatal pulmonary embolus accounts for a significant portion of the late mortality peak as well. Continued understanding of the epidemiology of death and immunosuppression in this third peak will refocus our attention on care and research strategies to deal with this changing pattern during acute care.

The scope of the problem should not be limited to mortality. Morbidity accounts for the majority of efforts provided by both the acute care team and the rehabilitation team. In essence, society's efforts will have to parallel the peaks in mortality and morbidity following injury to make an impact on the problem. Prevention aimed at aetiologies of injury and better protection against injury will reduce the first peak, ongoing development of trauma systems will deal with the second peak, and better understanding of late death along with focused research towards those problems identified will impact the third peak.

Preventive strategies in communities are starting to have an effect. States with mandatory helmet laws for bicycle and motorcycle riders have reported fewer fatal head injuries since the laws have been in effect. The adverse effects of alcohol on driving are disseminated through the media and stiffer laws and penalties have been instituted for offenders. Mandatory seatbelt use in automobiles has contributed to the lowest highway motor vehicle fatality rate in 20 years. Car and truck manufacturers are studying the dynamics of crash mechanisms more closely and are building safer vehicles with more safety devices for occupant protection. However, these measures, although steps in the right direction, are not enough to decrease significantly the overall impact and cost of trauma.

Biomechanics of injury

As with most diseases in medicine, injuries incurred from trauma have predictable patterns based on the mechanism. Understanding how these mechanisms cause injury will help the surgeon to anticipate the patient's needs upon arrival at the trauma centre which, in turn, will hopefully translate into lower overall morbidity and mortality.

Traumatic injuries occur when a transfer of energy takes place between the environment and the patient. The energy can originate from mechanical, electric, thermal or chemical forces within the environment and usually results in a physiological imbalance or a structural change in the patient, causing an alteration of normal homeostatic function.

In discussing mechanisms of trauma, the most common type of energy causing injury is the energy associated with movement called kinetic energy, whether it is the movement of a car, a baseball bat or a bullet. Kinetic energy is a function of the mass and velocity of a given object and is described mathematically as one-half of the mass of the object times its velocity squared, or:

$$KE = M/2 \times V^2.$$

For purposes of discussion, weight and speed can be substituted for mass and velocity, respectively. Using this equation, one can see that, since velocity is squared, the speed of an object, rather than its weight, has a much greater impact on the overall energy produced. This is most easily illustrated by examining firearm ballistics (see later in this Module). The energy produced from a heavy bullet fired from a low-velocity gun is significantly less than that of a lighter bullet fired from a high-velocity rifle.

Injury occurs when the kinetic energy is imparted to the trauma patient. The term used to describe this phenomenon is the 'impact force', which is determined by several factors including the rate of onset of the energy, duration and direction of application, and its magnitude (proportional to the weight and speed of the object and the area of application). The resultant physical deformities of the victim's body produced by the impact force are known collectively as 'strain'. Strain can be further classified as 'tensile' strain, in which the force is acting along the longitudinal axis of a particular structure, causing stretching or compression, and 'shear' strain, in which the force is acting perpendicular to the longitudinal axis of a particular structure, causing shearing or tearing.

As the force strikes the body, the tissues will react to the energy transfer. A phenomenon called cavitation occurs, in which tissue impacted by an outside force will move away from the point of impact. If considered on a cellular level, energy is being transmitted to the cells as movement which, in turn, causes these cells to collide into neighbouring cells, much like what happens when playing billiards when a rack of billiard balls is struck by the cue ball.

Two types of cavity can be created, depending on the nature of the impact force. Temporary cavities are created when the surface and structural tissues of the body are stretched but the overall shape of the body is maintained. This is most often seen in blunt trauma where the effects of cavitation may be apparent, i.e. broken bones or soft tissue disruption, but no distinct cavity is identified afterwards owing to the overall elasticity (described below) of the tissues. A permanent cavity is created along the lines of an impact force that causes tearing or compression of the tissues, leaving a permanent deformity of the affected tissues that can be identified later. This is most easily demonstrated with penetrating trauma, where the site of contact of the knife or bullet to the body is readily seen.

Various factors related to the victim will also determine the amount of injury sustained. Body tissues have properties known as elasticity and viscosity that are important in determining the amount of damage sustained. The elasticity of a tissue is its tendency to regain its original shape after being deformed by an outside force. The viscosity of a tissue is its tendency to resist change of shape while in motion. When the applied impact force deforms a specific body structure beyond the limits of either its elasticity or viscosity, the cohesiveness of the tissue is lost and disruption of the structure occurs. Examples of these types of injury are punctures, lacerations, abrasions, or contusions to the skin or soft tissues, fractures of bones, and parenchymal disruptions of solid organ viscera.

Several other factors will also influence the extent of injury sustained during a traumatic event. The amount of damage sustained by the tissues is directly proportional to the rate of application of the energy to the tissue, called the rate of energy loading. Essentially, applying a force more rapidly increases the likelihood of overcoming the shear strain tolerance and tensile strength of the tissue, and thereby causes more damage than when applied at a slower rate. This also emphasizes the importance of velocity to the amount of energy produced. Another important factor is the surface area over which the force is applied. The same force applied over a small surface area will cause greater damage than when applied over a larger surface area. The reason is that, with the larger surface area, the energy is more widely and evenly distributed over the impact area, imparting less energy per unit surface area. If the energy is more spread out, there is less likelihood that the tensile strength and the shear strain tolerance of the tissues will be overcome and, thus, permanent damage is less likely. If that same amount of force is applied to a smaller surface area at the same rate of load, the chances are greater that the tensile strength and the shear strain tolerance of the tissues will be overcome and damage to the tissues will be sustained. This is best illustrated when considering knife wounds. Although these are low-velocity penetrating wounds, they penetrate because the energy is concentrated at the point or edge of the knife as it comes into contact with the victim, thereby disrupting the tissues.

Blunt trauma

Blunt trauma occurs when two objects come into contact with one another and one object changes speed more quickly than the other object. The energy imparted is distributed over a wider surface area compared with penetrating mechanisms and the forces involved during the impact create both shear and tensile strain, creating a temporary cavity. Injury results when the energy imparted by the force of impact exceeds the tensile strength and shear strain tolerance of the tissue. Examples include falls, automobile and motorcycle accidents, pedestrians struck by automobiles, blunt assaults and most sport-related injuries. Blunt trauma is the most common type of injury in the USA, with motor vehicle accidents and pedestrians struck by cars being the two most common mechanisms.

Motor vehicle accidents

Several factors influence the severity and pattern of injuries sustained in a motor vehicle accident. The size of the car is important in that injury frequency is higher in smaller cars. The position of the occupant within the car at the time of impact will also determine the severity and type of injuries sustained. This is related to the occupant's risk of hitting the wheel and steering column, windscreen or side windows, or any supporting structure such as the A pillar (between the windscreen and side window) of the car. The occupant's body habitus is an important determinant of injury severity. Studies have shown that obese individuals have a lower incidence of facial and closed head injuries. It is postulated that the obese torso acts like an intrinsic airbag, absorbing the impact force of the crash. The use and type of restraint device have also been shown to affect significantly injury severity. Finally, the type of accident, described below, greatly affects the type of injury patterns seen.

At the time immediately preceding a motor vehicle accident, the occupants of the car and the car itself are travelling at the same rate of speed. In general, an accident occurs when the vehicle strikes another object in the environment, i.e. another vehicle or a stationary object such as a telegraph pole. This results in a rapid deceleration of the vehicle and its occupants in which three collisions are occurring.

- **The first collision is the vehicle striking the object in the environment. Although the vehicle stops, the occupant is still moving forwards inside the car.**
- **The second collision occurs when the restraint devices or the interior of the car stop the occupant's forward movement.**
- **The third collision occurs when the forward movement of the occupant's internal organs are stopped, usually by a cavity wall, another organ, or ligaments, fascia, vessels or muscle.**

Each of these collisions causes a different type of injury. However, these injuries can be predicted based on the force vector (i.e. direction of the force of the accident) as it is applied to the vehicle.

Frontal impact
Frontal impact occurs when the vehicle is abruptly stopped from moving forwards. This rapid deceleration causes an unrestrained victim to follow one of two paths within the car: down-and-under or up-and-over. The down-and-under path causes the victim to move downwards on to the seat and forwards into the steering column or dashboard. Lower extremity injuries are common with this type of motion. The foot can twist on a pedal or floorboard, causing ankle dislocation or fracture. The knees usually take the brunt of the force as they hit the dashboard. If the tibia strikes first, the femur can override the tibial plateau, causing a dislocation of the knee joint and possible proximal tibial fracture. As the popliteal artery is fixed at this point,

stretching or avulsion can occur, which may result in an ischaemic lower leg. If the femoral condyles strike the dashboard first, the femur must absorb the impact and may fracture. Alternatively, the pelvis may continue in a forward motion causing the femoral head to override the acetabulum, resulting in a posterior hip dislocation and possible acetabular fracture. After impact of the lower extremities, the upper body may rotate forwards, with the abdomen or thorax striking the steering column or dashboard and resulting in intra-abdominal or intrathoracic injuries.

In the up-and-over path, the occupant is launched from his or her seat over the dashboard or steering column. The head and face become the lead point of the body, striking the windscreen or windscreen frame. The chest or abdomen then strikes the steering column, potentially resulting in both compression and shear type internal injuries. Compression injuries occur as the body is forced against the car structure, causing disruption to the solid abdominal organs such as the liver, spleen, kidneys and pancreas, which are relatively inelastic. This mechanism is responsible for cardiac contusions as well as rupture of abdominal hollow organs. Shear injuries can also occur, where the internal organs are torn from their normal anatomical support structures by their forward momentum. Again, the solid organs are most vulnerable and this can result in vascular injuries as the vascular pedicles are stretched. This mechanism is also responsible for aortic disruption, where the heart continues its forward motion while the distal aortic arch is relatively fixed to the spine at the ligamentum arteriosum.

Lateral impact

In a lateral impact collision, the vehicle is struck from the side, displacing it laterally. This causes injuries through a number of mechanisms. First, the lateral aspect of the car being forced into the passenger compartment strikes the victim, causing lateral compression-type injuries. The ribs on the side of impact are commonly fractured and flail chest and pulmonary contusions can occur. Solid organs such as the spleen, liver or kidneys are vulnerable to injury, depending on whether the occupant was struck on the right or left side of the body. Other bony injuries include clavicle fractures on the side of impact as well as pelvis and femur fractures. With the lateral compression mechanism, sometimes the femoral head can be forced into the acetabulum, causing an acetabular fracture. Extremity fractures on the side of impact are not uncommon. Head, scalp and facial injuries occur as the side window or doorpost is forced inwards. These injuries can range from a simple scalp laceration to a severe closed head injury with skull fractures, cerebral contusions and intracranial haematomas.

A second type of injury occurs if the patient is wearing restraining belts. As the car is displaced laterally, the victim is pulled away from the impact point and the initial centre of gravity. As the body is displaced laterally, the head tends to continue to move in the original direction of travel until pulled in the direction of impact by the neck. This causes both rotation and lateral flexion injuries to the cervical spine. A similar mechanism is also responsible for thoracic aortic disruptions from lateral impact collisions, as the fixed thoracic aorta is pulled away from the relatively mobile heart and aortic arch.

Finally, the occupants are also subject to injury from secondary collisions where an occupant is struck by another occupant, such as the head of occupant A being forced into the shoulder of occupant B. This potentially causes injuries to both occupants.

Rollover and ejection

Rollover or ejection-type motor vehicle accidents are particularly worrisome because of the potential for high-energy transfer to the victim and resultant severe injuries. During a rollover, the vehicle is undergoing multiple impacts in rapid succession, occurring at different impact angles in relation to the victim. The victim's body and internal organs are then undergoing these same impacts with the potential for each impact to cause tissue injury. No set injury pattern has been identified for this injury mechanism, as almost any type is possible.

Ejection also implies a high-energy transfer to the victim in that the rapid deceleration or change of direction imparted by the collision is enough to force the occupant through the window or roof of the vehicle. This can result in severe head, neck, facial and torso injuries. The victim is then subject to additional deceleration forces when coming into contact with the ground. Again, it is impossible to predict injuries with this mechanism. **Victims of both ejection and rollover-type mechanisms should be taken to the nearest trauma centre after stabilization and assumed to have life-threatening injuries until proven otherwise**.

Pedestrian struck

Children, intoxicated adults and the elderly are the most common victims of being struck by moving vehicles. This particular mechanism of injury is associated with a high degree of energy transfer to an unprotected victim. These patients should be considered to have multisystem trauma and transported to the nearest trauma centre for evaluation.

There are three distinct impact moments when a pedestrian is struck by a moving vehicle. The first impact occurs as the bumper of the vehicle strikes the lower extremities of the victim, potentially fracturing the tibia, fibula or distal femur. As the legs are displaced out from underneath the pelvis and torso, the second impact occurs in which the torso rolls up on to the bonnet of the vehicle. The proximal femurs, pelvis, abdomen and thorax potentially can be injured, resulting in fractures to the femur, pelvis, spine and ribs and significant intra-abdominal and intrathoracic organ damage. At this point during the accident, the victim's head, neck and face are also vulnerable as they may strike the hood or windscreen of the car, causing serious damage to the skull, brain, facial bones and cervical spine. The third impact occurs as the victim falls away from the car, sometimes propelled a significant distance through the air, depending on how quickly the car was moving at initial contact, striking the ground. In general, the victim lands on one side of the body, causing additional injury to the extremities, thorax and abdomen coming into contact with the ground. Head and spinal injuries are also common with this type of impact.

Children, by virtue of being smaller, are usually struck anatomically higher than adults, resulting in relatively fewer lower leg and more femur, pelvic and torso injuries. Moreover, as a child's mass is less than that of an adult, the child may not be thrown clear of the vehicle and may be dragged by the front end of the vehicle for a considerable distance. The child victim also may fall underneath the car where almost any type of injury can occur, including being run over by the tyres. As with an adult victim, significant closed head injury and an unstable spine must be assumed and appropriate care given until proven otherwise.

Depending on the age of the victim, different types of injury pattern are sustained. When an adult realizes that he or she is about to be struck by a vehicle, an attempt is made to turn away from the vehicle in an effort to protect himself or herself. The injuries sustained are along the lateral or posterior aspect of the body. By comparison, a child will face the oncoming vehicle with resultant anterior injuries. The pattern of injury will also depend on the type of vehicle that strikes the victim. Passenger cars produce mostly lower extremity and pelvis injuries, while light trucks and vans cause a higher incidence of abdominal and thoracic injuries.

Penetrating trauma

Penetrating trauma causes injury by separating and crushing the tissues along the path of the penetrating object. Both temporary and permanent cavities are formed, in which the energy transmitted by the penetrating object is concentrated on a relatively small area. As the force of the missile is imparted to the surrounding tissues, a temporary cavity is formed where the tissue expands away from the pathway of the missile in both the frontal and lateral directions. When the force of this energy exceeds the tensile strength and shear stress tolerance of the tissues, tissue disruption occurs.

Weapon types

Penetrating trauma is categorized by the energy level imparted by the source of injury and is usually discussed in terms of low-, medium- and high-energy weapons. Knife or ice-pick wounds are generally considered to be low-energy mechanisms, whereas handguns and rifles are considered medium- and high-energy mechanisms. However, when discussing ballistics and wounding potential, some authors may

consider the less powerful handguns as low-energy as well.

Hand-driven weapons such as knives or ice picks produce damage only with their sharp points or cutting edge. Because of the low energy imparted to the surrounding tissue, there is relatively little secondary damage caused by temporary cavitation. Injuries can be roughly predicted based on a description of the weapon (size and length) and the site of entrance of the wound. Additional information helpful to determining potential injuries includes the gender of the attacker. Men tend to hold the knife with the blade originating from the thumb side of the hand and thrust upwards, whereas women tend to hold the knife with the blade originating from the little finger side of the hand and thrust downwards. In general, men are able to generate more force than women, owing to their increased strength and mass. Military training in hand-to-hand combat techniques teaches that to cause more damage once penetration has occurred, the attacker should move the blade from side to side or up and down while it is inside the victim in order to create more damage to surrounding organs and tissues. These types of injury should always be suspected when encountering a knife or similar type wound, regardless of the size of the entry point. Evaluation of knife wounds should always include a complete visual inspection of the victim in order to determine whether there are additional points of entry or associated injuries incurred from falling or attempts to flee the attack.

As mentioned above, guns can be described as low-, medium- or high-energy weapons. This is determined by the muzzle velocity of the projectile as it leaves the barrel of the gun (Table 4.1). Low-energy weapons are those with muzzle velocities of less than 1100 feet/s. Medium-velocity weapons have muzzle velocities between 1100 and 2000 feet/s and high-energy weapons have velocities of greater than 2000 or 2500 feet/s, depending on the author's particular bias. Higher velocity weapons tend to cause more tissue destruction because of the larger temporary cavity formed and the effects of fragmentation.

Table 4.1 Weight of projectile, muzzle velocity and approximate maximum kinetic energy of frequently used firearms

Description (calibre)	Projectile weight (g)	Muzzle velocity (feet/s)	KE (feet/lb $\times 10^2$)
Pistols			
0.22 short	29	1000	0.5
0.38 special	158	870	1.8
9 mm Luger	125	1150	2.6
0.45	250	860	2.8
0.357 magnum	158	1430	5.0
0.44 magnum	240	1470	8.1
Rifles			
0.22 long	40	1150	0.8
5.56 mm M-16	55	3250	9.1
Winchester	170	2200	12.8

Bullets come in a variety of configurations and cause damage through a variety of mechanisms. Common shapes of bullets include round-nose, wadcutter and semi-wadcutter. The wadcutter design are bullets with a flattened nose for target shooting, whereas the semi-wadcutters have a tapered nose with a sharp shoulder midway back on the bullet and are designed primarily for target shooting with semi-automatic handguns. Bullets can be pure lead, partially or fully jacketed. Jacketed refers to a hard copper or copper alloy covering the lead that will prevent fouling of the rifled barrel. Partially jacketed bullets have the soft lead exposed at the nose and are referred to as soft points. Soft points that have their tip hollowed out are referred to as hollow points. Both the soft and hollow points will expand when striking tissue, causing more tumbling and a wider impact zone, leading to more tissue destruction.

Handguns are usually considered low- to medium-energy weapons and are available in a wide variety of shapes and sizes. Their wounding potential is dependent on multiple factors. The calibre of a gun refers to the internal diameter of the barrel and is usually measured in fractions of an inch (e.g. .38 or .45) or in millimetres (e.g. 9 mm). The larger the calibre, the larger the missile that is fired. The bullet is held within a brass casing with gunpowder. When the firing pin or hammer of the gun falls on the primer of the bullet, it ignites the gunpowder, producing an explosion that propels the bullet out of the gun. Magnum loads have a larger amount of gunpowder than standard loads for a given calibre of gun. The amount of gunpowder within the cartridge is one of the main determinants of the velocity and, therefore, the kinetic energy produced by the projectile.

Revolvers are handguns in which the bullets, numbering anywhere from five to eight depending on the calibre and size of the gun, are held in a rotating cylinder. Single-action revolvers require manual cocking of the hammer, which is then released when the trigger is pulled. Double-action revolvers are so-called because the action of pulling the trigger will both cock the hammer and then cause its release. Semi-automatic and automatic handguns contain their bullets within a magazine. When a bullet is fired from the gun, the spent casing is ejected and a new round is automatically chambered. Semi-automatic weapons will fire one bullet each time the trigger is pulled. Fully automatic weapons fire continuously as long as the trigger is depressed and US law forbids their sale and use by the general public. Unfortunately, many semi-automatic weapons can be easily converted to fully automatic.

Rifles and derivations thereof, including assault weapons and carbines, are high-energy weapons. As with handguns, a variety of configurations exists, including single shot, magazine-fed lever, bolt or slide action, and gas-operated semi-automatic and automatic. They typically fire smaller bullets than some of the larger handguns, but the muzzle velocity attained can be two to three times greater and result in significantly more damage. Depending on the size of the bullet and the amount of gunpowder in the bullet, handguns rarely achieve muzzle velocities exceeding 1500 feet/s. In contrast, rifles can exceed 3000 feet/s muzzle velocities and, since velocity is more important than mass in the generation of kinetic energy, it is easy to see why an injury from a rifle can be devastating.

Shotgun calibre is measured in gauge; the lower the gauge number, the wider the internal diameter of the gun. The bullets for shotguns range from single lead slugs with rifling grooves on the side to improve accuracy, to numerous steel or lead pellets. These pellets are close together at the muzzle but rapidly spread out as the distance from the gun increases. In order to keep tighter groupings of the pellets, shotguns use chokes that help to keep the pellets from too rapid a dispersion when shooting at more distant targets. At close range they are highly destructive, but they cause less significant injury as the range increases. Close-range wounds should be inspected for embedded shotgun shell wadding or part of the shell, as these are potential sources of infection if not debrided.

Ballistics

Ballistics refers to the behaviour of the projectile from initial take-off to complete stop. For trauma surgeons, the two most important aspects of ballistics are external ballistics, which refers to the flight of the projectile from gun to victim, and terminal ballistics, which refers to projectile activity after it has struck the victim. Wounding potential is a clinical application of terminal ballistics and is dependent on the bullet's weight, shape and impact velocity, the stability of the bullet in the tissues, the resistance to the bullet exerted by the tissues as the bullet passes through (referred to as drag) and a combination of shape and velocity of the bullet and the viscosity and elastic properties of the tissue (referred to as the coefficient of drag).

In the majority of civilian shootings, the assailant and victim are usually separated by less than 10 m. At that distance, impact velocity is approximately the same as initial muzzle velocity (the speed of the bullet as it leaves the barrel of the gun). At greater distances, however, several factors can affect the external ballistics of the bullet. The ballistic coefficient is used to describe a bullet's ability to overcome air resistance during flight; the lower the number, the greater the velocity lost during its flight and the smaller amount of kinetic energy available for tissue destruction at impact. Other factors refer to bullet instability during flight. These include yaw, which is the bullet's deviation from the longitudinal axis of flight; precession, which is a circular motion of the nose of the bullet perpendicular to the longitudinal axis of flight; and nutation, which is similar to precession except that a rosette pattern is made by the nose of the bullet. Yaw can lead to tumbling of the bullet after it impacts the body of the victim, causing increased tissue damage. Nutation increases the chances that the bullet will strike the victim at an angle to its true longitudinal axis of flight.

This increases the surface impact area and can lead to greater tissue destruction.

Bullets cause damage by a number of mechanisms. Direct injury is caused by the bullet or fragments cutting through the tissues and the transfer of heat. This type of injury mechanism predominates with the lower velocity handguns that cause relatively small temporary cavities. However, if the bullet hits a vital structure such as the heart, brain or a major blood vessel, death can result. Indirect injury is caused by the creation of the temporary cavity owing to the transfer of the kinetic energy from the bullet to the surrounding tissues through high-displacement shear waves. These shear waves compress and accelerate the tissue away from the point of impact. Studies of high-velocity bullets shot through 10% gelatin blocks have demonstrated that the temporary cavity created is approximately 10–20 times the diameter of the bullet. Finally, the elastic and viscosity properties of the body tissue struck will also determine the amount of damage sustained. Relatively elastic tissue, such as muscle, will sustain less injury than denser, less elastic tissue, such as the spleen or liver.

Fragmentation has been identified as a major cause of tissue destruction and occurs when the bullet breaks up after striking the victim and the resulting pieces create their own paths through the tissue. Alternatively, other parts of the body, such as teeth or bone fragments, can become missiles, causing damage to surrounding tissue.

Section 4.2 • Metabolic response to trauma

Metabolism is the complex system of interrelated biochemical reactions and physiological responses required to maintain life. These reactions and responses involve almost every physiological and homeostatic process in some way. Traumatic injury is one of the many nonspecific stimuli that trigger a set of metabolic changes known as the **stress response**. **The stress response is the body's damage control system, intended to maintain homeostasis on a cellular as well as a systemic level, and to provide substrate for repair of injury**. The stress response involves a set of hormonal and inflammatory signals that produces a hyperdynamic and hypermetabolic state. Hyperglycaemia and mobilization of additional energy substrate from muscle and fat stores occur in order to fuel vital body functions, and to support hepatic protein synthesis. An inflammatory cascade mediated by cytokines serves to mobilize the immunological response needed to promote haemostasis, wound healing and control of infection. The stress response is an adaptive process that generally works quite well at maintaining homeostasis, yet some of its mediators and effects are locally or systemically harmful. **Systemic inflammatory response syndrome (SIRS) is a label used to describe the pathological extension of the stress response**. An understanding of the components of the stress response, and the harmful effects of sustained triggering of the response, is essential in guiding the care of the injured patient.

Specific changes in the stress response

Severity and type of injury are important determinants of the intensity and character of the stress response. The timing of the response is variable, and depends on these factors as well. Resolution, if possible, requires removal of secondary insults (e.g. ischaemia, infection, haemodynamic instability, hypoxia) and ongoing trauma (e.g. compartment syndrome). The general physiological response has been characterized as an 'ebb and flow' phenomenon. The early, or ebb phase is characterized by a hypovolaemic state and regional hypoperfusion. Often, physiological variables such as heart rate, cardiac output, oxygen consumption, urine output and blood pressure are all somewhat depressed. Lactic acidosis resulting from anaerobic metabolism may exist as well and may be evidenced by an increase in the base deficit noted on the arterial blood gas analysis, corresponding to an under-resuscitated state. During this time the inflammatory and hormonal mediators begin to accumulate and the entire response may be in a pattern of holding and build-up.

As the patient stabilizes and sources of ongoing injury are removed, a **hyperdynamic state** develops. This is the flow phase of the metabolic response, which can take as long as 12–24 h to achieve. The hyperdynamic state is characterized by increased cardiac output and oxygen delivery, tachycardia, fever and restoration of normal haemodynamic parameters. Volume status returns to baseline and urine output increases slightly. Anaerobic metabolism will diminish, allowing lactate to clear and the base deficit to normalize. **During this hyperdynamic state, carbohydrate, protein and fat metabolism are significantly altered**. Hyperglycaemia, protein catabolism and lipolysis are prominent features of the response. The underlying purpose of these changes is the mobilization of energy and substrate for survival and wound healing. Muscle protein can be rapidly mobilized for creation of glucose, which is the primary energy substrate of the body. The amino acids can be used for creation of acute-phase proteins, which aid in mediating the stress response and healing.

Fluid and electrolyte conservation

Decreases in fluid volume from haemorrhage lead to multiple signals directed at restoring circulating volume. Aortic and carotid body pressure receptors and atrial stretch receptors signal the brain of decreases in their respective inputs. The changes in atrial pressure also lead to decreased levels of atrial natriuretic peptide (ANP). In addition, sensory afferent fibres trigger a direct neurally mediated response at the level of the central nervous system (CNS). These inputs are mediated through the hypothalamus and lead to the release of antidiuretic hormone (ADH) from the posterior pituitary. Increased levels of ADH and decreased levels of ANP lead to the conservation of sodium and free water at the level of the renal tubule. The same changes in circulating volume lead to increased levels of aldosterone, mediated by the renin–angiotensin system. This increase in aldosterone contributes to the conservation of sodium and relative wasting of potassium and hydrogen ions in the renal tubule. These changes in fluid and electrolyte handling, and subsequent retention of sodium and water, usually persist despite removal of the initiating trauma and adequate resuscitation. The intensity of the response, and hence the degree of sodium and water retention, is a reflection of the severity of the systemic insult.

Hypermetabolism

The hyperdynamic state is not without cost. At a cellular level, the process requires a great deal of energy in the form of adenosine triphosphate (ATP) and NADH. The basal metabolic rate (BMR) is a global measure of the energy expenditure of an individual, and normal BMR can be predicted based on age, gender and body size. BMR can be measured using continuous monitoring of respiratory gas exchange, focusing on oxygen consumption and carbon dioxide production. **In general, oxygen consumption in litres per unit time multiplied by 4.8 estimates the BMR in kilocalories per unit time**. Metabolic rate is markedly increased in the postinjury patient. Severely injured patients may have a BMR that is 1.5 times normal and severe burns patients may have as much as double the predicted BMR.

Alterations in glucose metabolism

Hyperglycaemia is typical in the postinjury state, and has led to the phrase 'diabetes of stress'. This effect is also proportional to the type and severity of injury. Initially, during the ebb phase, hyperglycaemia and hypo-insulinaemia are present. Later, insulin levels rise to normal but hyperglycaemia persists. Glucagon, adrenaline (epinephrine), noradrenaline, vasopressin and angiotensin II are secreted in the stress response and all promote glucose mobilization and production. This mobilization of glucose is accomplished in the liver by promotion of glycogenolysis, cessation of glycogenesis and increased gluconeogenesis. These signals are also responsible for muscle catabolism to facilitate this increase in gluconeogenesis. Lactate production is increased because of anaerobic metabolism, with the lactate recovered in the liver through the Cori cycle creating more glucose.

Usual physiological controls on hyperglycaemia are lost in the stressed state. Exogenous glucose and insulin no longer suppress hepatic synthesis of glucose. Hepatic lipolysis also continues, contributing to increased glucose levels. At the same time that glucose production is increased, glucose disposal is kept relatively fixed, owing to peripheral insulin resistance. Under normal circumstances, insulin functions to promote muscular glucose uptake and anabolism, and it is maximally effective at a mere 2% of receptor activation. The stress response is characterized by peripheral insulin resistance, in which normal or supranormal levels of insulin fail to control hyperglycaemia. The primary site of this resistance is in the skeletal muscle, thus preserving glucose for hepatic use, and as the primary energy source for the heart and brain.

Alterations in protein metabolism

Following injury, a catabolic state exists; a time when muscle breakdown exceeds production. The usual protective effects of the fasting state are absent and high protein mobilization occurs despite a lack of protein input. Exogenous nutrition high in protein can help to attenuate this response, but will not prevent it. Skeletal muscle serves as the primary reserve pool of amino acids that are mobilized for gluconeogenesis. As gluconeogenesis increases in response to stress, there is a fivefold increase in the rate of transport of amino acids from the periphery to the liver. Phenylalanine is not a substrate for gluconeogenesis, and its serum level increases disproportionately. Branched-chain amino acids are utilized directly for energy and substituted into the Krebs cycle. Alanine and glutamine are mobilized preferentially, making up half of the amino acids mobilized, although they make up little more than 10% of the body's total amino acids. Alanine is important for gluconeogenesis in the liver because it can be directly converted to pyruvate for use in the Krebs cycle. Glutamine serves two unique purposes in the stressed state. It is utilized by gut enterocytes as their primary energy source, and it is also utilized in the kidney for ammonia generation, in order to assist with acid secretion. In addition, glutamine is used by fibroblasts, endothelial cells and cells of the immune system. Despite their systemic importance, metabolic pathways for glutamine and alanine favour excretion as urea and ammonia, which tends to increase their rate of mobilization from muscle stores.

Alterations in fat metabolism

The stressed postinjury state favours lipolysis. This effect is not attenuated by exogenous nutritional sources and is thought to be perpetuated by continued high sympathetic tone and catecholamine levels. Mobilization and oxidation of free fatty acids are promoted and accelerated, with systemic levels rising in proportion to injury severity. Exogenous fat may even be burned as fuel. Ketosis seldom complicates this hypermetabolic state, unlike starvation and other syndromes where fatty acids are relied on for energy. High levels of free fatty acids may promote pathways of prostenoid production with resultant immuno-suppressive effects owing to increased levels of prostaglandin E_2. It is thought that limiting fat intake to 2 g/kg body weight/day may help to avoid this immunosuppressive effect. In addition, modification of the specific fatty acid composition of dietary fat may be of value in modifying the response of the immune system.

Immunological and inflammatory alterations

The immune response following injury is complex and only superficially understood. It begins with local tissue damage, in which damaged cells release chemical signals that trigger local inflammation. These signals function as autocrine, paracrine and eventually endocrine mediators of the inflammatory response. Capillary leak results in interstitial oedema and leucocyte infiltration follows through these breaks in the capillary endothelium. Local production of free oxygen radicals and lysozymes by polymorphonucleocytes results in ongoing tissue damage. **The leucocyte-produced cytokines involved in mediating inflammation include interleukin-1 (IL-1), IL-2, tumour necrosis factor-α (TNF-α) and interferon-γ (IFN-γ)**. If the local insult is significant enough, the cytokine mediators eventually spill into the central circulation and act to propagate the systemic inflammatory response. From an immunological perspective, this results in leucocyte demargination and mobilization of leucocytes from the bone marrow and splenic reserves. The resultant leucocytosis is biased towards immature cell types, also referred to as 'left shift' of the differential count.

Alterations in oxygen utilization and transport

Oxygen and energy metabolism are both altered following injury. In healthy, normal adults, oxygen delivery (V_{O_2}) exceeds oxygen consumption (D_{O_2}) by a ratio of approximately 5:1. This reserve is diminished in the stressed state, owing to decreases in delivery and increased rate of consumption. Haemoglobin levels can be low from haemorrhage, oxygenation can be low from airway or thoracic injury, and cardiac function may be diminished because of direct trauma or other myocardial depressant effects. Local factors such as tissue oedema, and microcirculatory alterations including capillary plugging and shunting may all contribute to difficulties with getting oxygen to the cell. Hypermetabolic changes induced by the stress response lead to an increased demand for oxygen at the cellular level. At the mitochondrial level there is an uncoupling of the normal process of oxidative phosphorylation, which is believed to occur at the cytochrome on the inner mitochondria membrane. Oxidative phosphorylation is the key process in energy metabolism in which the mitochondrion produces the high-energy phosphate bonds of ATP, the key energy source for most metabolic processes. This can lead to a reliance on anaerobic pathways, despite adequate oxygen delivery.

Mediators of the stress response to injury

Injury can trigger the immune and hypermetabolic responses in multiple ways. Pain, fear, anxiety and agitation act to initiate the stress response. Changes in circulating volume trigger hormonally mediated volume conservation. Trauma causes direct tissue damage, with resultant release of inflammatory mediators. Haemorrhagic shock or vascular injury may cause ischaemia, leading to cellular damage. Subsequent reperfusion often exacerbates the cellular injury, and hence the inflammatory response, and allows systemic distribution of inflammatory mediators. Infective sources, such as gastrointestinal perforation or aspiration, also promote an inflammatory response.

The stress response has two control arms, the neurohormonal arm and the inflammatory arm. The neurohormonal arm is composed of the neural reflex arcs associated with volume restoration and the catecholamine-mediated 'fight or flight' response. Afferent pathways signal the brain, resulting in the release of noradrenaline from peripheral nerves and stimulation of the adrenal medulla, which releases adrenaline. Another hypothalamically mediated response is the release of cortisol. The afferent signal received in the hypothalamus causes the release of cortisol releasing hormone (CRH), which signals the anterior pituitary gland to release adrenocorticotropic hormone (ACTH). ACTH travels via the bloodstream to the adrenal glands and causes them to release cortisol and other glucocorticoids.

The inflammatory arm of the stress response is mediated by cytokines, which are messenger compounds released by cells as a result of trauma, infection, ischaemia or shock. These messengers act at both a local level and a systemic level. Through complex activation pathways, the resultant inflammatory humoral cascades that follow can involve the complement system, eicosanoids and platelet-activating factor. Because the signals are greatly amplified, and feed back into one another at many levels, the inflammatory arm is capable of perpetuating the entire stress response long after the initial insult has been removed.

Minor wounds may have a limited pain response and limited tissue damage, resulting in minimal activation of either arm of stress response activation. Massive crush, as a counter example, could have significant hormonal activation due to pain, fear and stress, as well as a massive inflammatory response based on extensive tissue destruction, ischaemia/reperfusion, vascular injury and wound contamination. Under such circumstances, the intensity and prolonged activation of the stress response may lead to major morbidity or mortality.

Hormonal mediators

Glucagon, cortisol and catecholamines are the primary hormonal mediators of the stress response. Infusion of these three hormones serves as a laboratory model of the stress response. The early phase of trauma is characterized by a catecholamine surge. Persistent elevation in levels can be detected long after the initial event and correlate with injury severity. These levels slowly approach normal as the patient's condition normalizes, often days later. The catecholamines serve a vasopressor function, causing vasoconstriction, tachycardia and anxiety at the CNS level. They also act to increase lactate production in peripheral tissues, often despite adequate energy substrate.

Catecholamines are important in promoting hepatic glycolysis, gluconeogenesis, peripheral lipolysis and muscle catabolism. The degree of hypermetabolism is directly related to catecholamine levels.

Cortisol and glucagon levels are also elevated in the stress response. Cortisol and other glucocorticoids are released from the adrenal gland in response to hypothalamic–pituitary signalling. They function to increase serum glucose levels by promoting gluconeogenesis and glycogenolysis, and to increase intravascular amino acid levels. Glucagon is released from the alpha cells of the islets of Langerhans in the pancreas, and serves as an anti-insulin hormone. It, too, promotes gluconeogenesis and glycogenolysis, although it is less important in inducing catabolism.

Several other hormones are involved in the stress response, but to a lesser degree. Thyroid hormones are unchanged or slightly reduced during the stress response. Growth hormone levels are unchanged during the stress state but exogenous administration may have therapeutic potential (see below). Insulin serves as an anabolic hormone, leading to increased glycogen production, increased glucose utilization at the cellular level, increased amino acid incorporation into protein and increased assimilation of free fatty acids into fat. These effects are opposite to those induced by the stress response. Insulin may be protective as a regulator of the stress response, decreasing the potential for damage from the unopposed effects of other stress hormones.

Cytokine mediators
Cytokines are peptide compounds, first produced at the site of injury. They play an important role in the initiation and promotion of the stress response. Cytokines are intercellular messengers, produced primarily by reticuloendothelial cells, a category composed of macrophages, lymphocytes, monocytes and hepatic Kupffer cells. Cytokines can act locally in an autocrine or paracrine fashion, and act systemically to promote release of other cytokines and inflammatory mediators, or to prime distant immune-competent cells.

Cytokines are present in almost undetectable levels in the healthy state, yet rapid propagation of the inflammatory response leads to high serum levels very quickly. A cascade develops in which cytokines amplify and diversify production of other cytokines and inflammatory factors. The system responds even more rapidly after priming by previous trauma or other triggers. Although serum levels may fall rapidly for some mediators, their effects may continue for some time. This behaviour is thought to be related to unmeasured and unrecognized secondary mediators produced by the initial cascade, which serve to perpetuate the response. The major cytokines identified as components of the inflammatory response are:

- TNF-α
- IL-1
- IL-2
- IL-6
- IFN-γ
- colony stimulating factors.

TNF-α, sometimes referred to as cachectin, is one of the main cytokines responsible for the stress response. TNF-α is produced most often by macrophages, but can also be manufactured by lymphocytes and Kupffer cells. Release of TNF-α from macrophages is stimulated primarily by endotoxin, although trauma is also a trigger for its release. TNF-α is responsible for many of the systemic effects that are the hallmarks of the inflammatory response, including fever, anorexia, tachypnoea and tachycardia. Higher levels of TNF-α are associated with hypotension, organ failure and death. TNF-α is responsible for neutrophil release from the bone marrow, neutrophil margination and activation, as well as release of oxidants, superoxide, lysozyme and arachidonic acid metabolites from leucocytes. Fever is achieved by direct action on the suprachiasmatic nucleus of the hypothalamus. Other effects on the hypothalamic–pituitary axis include stimulation of ACTH and cortisol production, an area of crossover with the neurohumoral control system.

TNF-α is chemotactic for neutrophils and helps to promote bacterial killing. TNF-α is also responsible for increased vascular permeability, procoagulant effects, fibroblast proliferation and local inflammation necessary for wound healing. Effects on metabolism include promotion of proteolysis, skeletal muscle wasting, catabolism, negative nitrogen balance and increased hepatic uptake of amino acids. It is this array of metabolic effects that led to its other name – cachectin. In the presence of TNF-α, the liver shifts to production of acute-phase proteins. Lipoprotein lipase activity is diminished and plasma levels of triglycerides and free fatty acids rise. Finally, TNF-α leads to the production of several other cytokines, expanding and sustaining the response.

IL-1 works in a variety of ways, many of which are similar to the actions of TNF-α. IL-1 is usually released from tissue macrophages and blood monocytes and is active when bound to cell membranes. Even small doses can cause fever by the same pathway as TNF-α. This effect is so prominent that IL-1 has been referred to as endogenous pyrogen. IL-1 stimulates the release of IL-2 and IL-6 and helps to shift the liver to production of acute-phase proteins. Like TNF-α, IL-1 causes neutrophilia resulting from bone marrow release and is chemotactic to neutrophils. Also like TNF-α, it causes increased endothelial permeability and catabolism, and acts as a procoagulant. IL-1 is associated with anaemia and low levels of zinc and iron, all thought to be protective in the presence of microbial infection.

Less is known about the functions of IL-2 and IL-6, both of which are stimulated by IL-1. IL-2 is produced by T-lymphocytes, and it exists only at very low levels in health, possibly owing to the presence of serum suppressive factors. It functions to stimulate cell-mediated immunity by enhancing cytotoxic T-cell function. The usual rise in levels of IL-2 in situations of physiological stress is suppressed in trauma and burns patients, and the degree of suppression correlates with mortality. Prostaglandin E_2 is one of the possible serum suppressive agents.

In contrast, IL-6 is increased in trauma and burns patients. IL-6 is released from fibroblasts and activated B-lymphocytes and promotes fibroblast, B-cell and hepatocyte proliferation. It is also thought to play a major role in shifting hepatic synthesis to acute-phase proteins. Unlike many other cytokines with brief appearances in the serum, IL-6 often peaks at 1 week after the initial insult. Levels of IL-6 correlate with injury severity or endotoxin levels. Deleterious effects of IL-6 have not yet been described.

IFN-γ is produced by helper T-cells and some macrophages. It serves as a priming agent for macrophage function. IFN-γ increases production of other cytokines, such as TNF-α, thus promoting the cascade. Beyond these functions, specific roles for IFN-γ are poorly described.

Colony stimulating factors are newly associated with the cytokines of the stress response. These are glycoproteins such as erythropoietin, granulocyte colony stimulating factor and granulocyte–macrophage colony stimulating factor. In traumatic wounds they function by promoting wound healing, increasing leucocyte response and decreasing bacterial counts.

Other inflammatory mediators

There are several other mediators of the stress response, which are currently less well understood but under increasing investigation. The **leukotrienes** are a family of chemical products of the lipoxygenase pathway of arachidonic acid metabolism. They are produced in vascular tissue and lung parenchyma by macrophages, mast cells and neutrophils. Leukotrienes serve as chemoattractants and smooth-muscle vasoconstrictors, and serve to accentuate local tissue ischaemia in the inflammatory state. **Prostenoids** are another family of products of arachidonic acid metabolism, but stem from the cyclooxygenase pathway. Examples of this group include prostacyclin, which serves as a vasodilator, and thromboxane A_2, which causes vasoconstriction, increases platelet aggregation and promotes neutrophil margination.

Another prostenoid, prostaglandin E_2, is involved in several important functions. The febrile response induced by IL-1 is thought to be mediated by prostaglandin E_2 in the hypothalamus. This is the point at which non-steroidal anti-inflammatory drugs (NSAIDs) and aspirin, which are inhibitors of prostenoid synthesis, inhibit the development of fever. Prostaglandin E_2 is thought to be immunosuppressive, through the mechanism of decreasing IL-2 levels.

Other agents involved in the inflammatory response to injury include **oxygen radicals** and **bacterial endotoxin**. Oxygen radicals, including superoxide, hydrogen peroxide and lipid peroxides, are often produced during reperfusion after ischaemia, or are byproducts of neutrophil function. Oxygen radicals have a number of toxic effects, causing damage to cell membranes, increasing cell permeability, initiating local inflammation, disrupting interstitial matrix, impairing macrophage phagocytosis, causing alteration in cell DNA and stimulating arachidonic acid metabolism. Endotoxin plays a role in postinjury sepsis, even without overt bacterial infection. The gut is often implicated as the source. Disruption of gut mucosal integrity owing to regional hypoperfusion and inadequate enterocyte substrate potentially leads to the release of bacteria or endotoxin into the systemic circulation. The systemic effects of endotoxin are dramatic. Endotoxin is a potent stimulator of inflammation through the release of arachidonic acid metabolites, oxidants and cytokines (especially TNF-α).

Specific organ system changes

Owing to its central role in metabolism, the liver undergoes major changes in response to injury. Blood flow is diminished in the shock state as a result of splanchnic vasoconstriction, a response designed to protect cardiac and CNS blood flow. Although blood and oxygen are in short supply, the liver is even more highly active. Gluconeogenesis and recycling of lactate through the Cori cycle are increased dramatically. Ureagenesis must continue at a high level to clear nitrogen byproducts, which are the result of increased protein catabolism. The liver also serves to clear aromatic amino acids, which can serve as false neurotransmitters. Hepatic protein synthesis is shifted away from albumin and towards acute-phase proteins. IL-6 is considered the primary mediator in this shift in production.

Although not yet fully understood, the acute-phase proteins produced in the liver serve a protective function during the inflammatory response. C-reactive protein serves as a free radical scavenger and an opsonin. Fibrinogen is essential for haemostasis and assists in wound healing. Ceruloplasmin functions as an oxygen scavenger and transports protein. The antiproteases produced as acute-phase proteins serve to reduce tissue damage caused by proteases released by dead or dying cells.

Under the stress of these severe metabolic demands, the liver becomes gradually overwhelmed and diverted from daily activities. Cholestasis and steatosis develop as fat metabolism becomes of secondary importance. If the stress on the hepatocytes is too great, frank hepatic failure may result. Because of the crucial role of liver function, hepatic failure under these circumstances is associated with high mortality.

Lung function is significantly affected by the inflammatory response, and the lung is often the first organ to show signs of failure. As metabolism increases, carbon dioxide production increases, necessitating an increase in minute ventilation. Alveolar metabolism increases to clear circulating vasoactive agents. In addition to these increased functional demands, the lung is particularly vulnerable to the secondary effects of the inflammatory process. The lung contains a large number of macrophages and other immune-competent cells. As systemic inflammation develops and the immunological system is primed, lung macrophages are stimulated to release inflammatory mediators locally, causing alveolar damage and further promoting local inflammation. This sequence of events can lead to a self-perpetuating inflammatory process resulting in the adult respiratory distress syndrome (ARDS).

Kidney function is also strongly affected by the stress response, and some degree of renal dysfunction is extremely common under circumstances of prolonged stress. In the early stages of the stress response, preservation of intravascular volume is the priority. Oliguria results both from the direct effects of hypovolaemia, and also as a result of increased levels of aldosterone and ADH. As the stress response develops, the kidney is called upon to increase clearance of metabolic byproducts in order to keep up with increased production. The higher solute load requires higher renal blood flow, which may not be available. Azotaemia develops if the increased urea production that results from ongoing protein metabolism surpasses the ability of the kidney to excrete. In addition, circulating factors such as inflammatory mediators and cytokines, or nephrotoxins such as intravenous contrast and various pharmacological agents, may cause direct damage to renal cells. Heavily increased metabolic load under circumstances of poor perfusion and exposure to nephrotoxins can lead to acute tubular necrosis and severe renal dysfunction. Fortunately, there are very effective means of renal replacement therapy available in the intensive care unit (ICU). Renal failure is a contributing factor to postinjury mortality, but rarely the primary cause. Acute renal failure, which develops under severe physiological stress, is usually reversible. Renal function usually returns after several weeks if the patient survives.

Gut function and mucosal integrity are altered following injury. As blood flow is redirected to vital organs, splanchnic blood flow is diminished and the gut often becomes relatively, or frankly, ischaemic. Splanchnic vasculature also may be injured by systemic low flow states, endotoxaemia, deposition of inflammatory mediators and complement, and reperfusion injury. This chronic ischaemic insult rarely causes frank necrosis, but is likely to produce a number of adverse sequelae.

The gut mucosal barrier serves to protect the body from the mass of potentially pathogenic bacteria normally resident in the gut lumen. Barrier function is metabolically demanding and depends on rapid enterocyte replacement, local IgA production, mucous production and active peristalsis. Maintenance of barrier function is dependent on splanchnic blood flow, blood oxygenation and enteral nutrition. As inflammation persists, the demands of the enterocyte cannot be met and mucosal integrity is compromised. Loss of the mucosal barrier may lead to clinically important bacterial translocation, where enteric bacteria enter the systemic circulation. Although established in laboratory animal models, human evidence of this phenomenon is lacking. It is postulated that endotoxin is able to translocate without physical translocation of bacteria, leading to excessive propagation of the inflammatory response without frank bacteraemia. Experience in several patient groups strongly suggests that measures that promote maintenance of enterocyte function lead to a decrease in the incidence of systemic consequences of unchecked inflammation.

The CNS is also heavily involved in the response to injury. Anxiety, pain and even 'ICU psychosis' can lead to ongoing stimulation of the neurohumoral arm of the stress response. Hypothalamic and pituitary-mediated feedback pathways result in ongoing catecholamine release. Chronically elevated catecholamine levels contribute to ongoing hypermetabolism, promoting catabolism, release of inflammatory mediators and increasing predisposition to serious infections. Cortical function may deteriorate as a result of regional ischaemia, or the accumulation of metabolic byproducts and pharmacological agents that cannot be cleared owing to impaired liver and kidney function. Global CNS function usually returns to baseline as the other organ systems return to normal function.

Modification of the stress response

Enteral nutrition

Early nutritional support of the injured patient has become a standard of trauma care. Even small amounts of glucose in maintenance fluids may attenuate the catabolic effects of the inflammatory state. Although catabolism is not completely eliminated, full nutritional support is essential to promote wound healing, prevent infectious complications, maintain lean body mass, provide substrate for the liver to prevent mobilization of muscle mass and maintain gut mucosal integrity. Enteral nutrition is by far the preferred route of feeding, with parenteral nutrition reserved for circumstances in which enteral feeding is impossible or impractical. Enteral feeding is less expensive, does not require central access, is more physiological and serves a trophic function in the gut by increasing the production of maintenance gut hormones.

The goal of nutritional support is the provision of adequate metabolic substrate and the preservation of normal gut mucosal function. The specific requirements of an individual patient are difficult to predict with accuracy. General formulae will provide a rough estimate, but care must be taken to ensure that the nutritional regimen is appropriate to the circumstances. Therefore, nutritional support should be monitored as objectively as possible, with sequential measurement of physiological markers in order to establish adequacy of feeding and to avoid overfeeding.

Nutritional modification

Beyond the general benefits of enteral feeding, there is a growing body of evidence that the immune response can be altered by specific nutritional supplements. One such substance is glutamine. Glutamine is the primary energy source for enterocytes and is also a component in the production of glutathione, an endogenous anti-oxidant. Critical illness results in severe glutamine depletion. Although glutamine is difficult to include in formulations of amino acids for parenteral nutrition, it is easily included in enteral formulae, and is possibly more effective when delivered intraluminally. Supplementation of glutamine improves muscle protein synthesis, improves nitrogen balance, maintains lean body mass and attenuates fluid accumulation in the inflammatory state. All of these effects are of potential benefit to the critically ill patient, and in some studies glutamine supplementation has been associated with decreased length of hospital stay.

Another amino acid, arginine, is thought to have an immunomodulatory function, including augmentation of macrophage activity and natural killer cell activity. In healthy adults, this amino acid is rarely required as a supplement owing to sufficient endogenous production. However, when arginine is provided as a supplement to physiologically stressed patients, it improves nitrogen balance, wound healing, immune function and maintenance of lean body mass.

Manipulation of lipids in nutritional support is also promising as a possible method of immunomodulation. Diets rich in ω-6 fatty acids are thought to be immunosuppressive and proinflammatory, favouring production of the more damaging eicosanoid species. Alterations in dietary lipid composition can effect changes in subsequent metabolic pathways. Short-chain fatty acids may be enterotrophic. Medium-chain triglycerides, ω-3 fatty acids and 'structured' lipids are beneficial in improving nitrogen balance, decreasing infection rates and possibly increasing survival.

Pharmacological modification

Since many cytokines have been associated with deleterious systemic effects, the blockade of cytokine production, or of specific cytokine receptors, has the potential to control the stress response. A number of specific cytokine blockade strategies has been attempted. Antibody to TNF-α has been used successfully to blunt the inflammatory response, but has resulted in increased mortality in some clinical trials. Other cytokine-specific antibodies are being studied, both alone and in combination with other approaches selectively to block negative pathways. To date, there has been no clear success with these techniques in clinical practice.

Cyclooxygenase inhibition using non-steroidal anti-inflammatory compounds has the potential to inhibit the deleterious effects of inflammation and has met with limited success in certain circumstances. Local and regional anaesthetic techniques have been found to be beneficial in limiting the inflammatory response to surgical trauma. Early and effective analgesia in injured patients may similarly be beneficial.

As research in immunology develops, a better understanding of the role of various compounds may lead to more effective manipulation of the inflammatory response. The primary difficulty lies in blocking only the damaging aspects of the response without impeding the essential functions of the same inflammatory mediators.

Several hormonal interventions are promising in modifying the stress response. Growth factors administered topically on burn wounds or systemically have been beneficial in injured patients, leading to accelerated wound healing and resultant decrease in inflammatory stimulus. Systemic administration of growth hormone has been shown to improve nitrogen balance, attenuate catabolism and stimulate protein synthesis. The use of insulin to control hyperglycaemia and promote anabolism is also beneficial in a broader sense. It was once thought that both hyperglycaemia and exogenous insulin should be avoided in the injured patient, so glucose was withheld despite its potential metabolic benefits. Although control of hyperglycaemia is important, especially in the head-injured patient, the use of insulin for control of hyperglycaemia may directly attenuate catabolism, in addition to facilitating adequate nutrition. Owing to the relatively insulin-resistant state present after stress, a high dose of insulin may be required, and the dose should be titrated to clinical effect.

Conclusion

The body's response to injury is a complex process, with the goal of maintenance of homeostasis. Beginning with immediate postinjury survival, and then continuing through the inflammatory response, wound healing and fighting infections, the body must adapt and adjust constantly. Mechanisms that are adaptive for survival, especially in the absence of medical intervention, may be beneficial in the short term and harmful in the long term. The majority of late trauma deaths is the result of sepsis and multisystem organ failure, which are largely the results of these negative effects. As understanding of the entire process improves, it may be possible to select only the positive aspects of the response and suppress the negative aspects. Carefully targeted modification of the metabolic responses to initial injury may be the key to preventing these deaths.

Section 4.3 • Prehospital care and transport

Prehospital response

The prehospital response describes the systematic approach to the delivery of prehospital care to the acutely injured patient. The intention is to provide the injured patient access to the trauma system and aid in the overall management by initiating evaluation and treatment by trained personnel at the scene of the accident. This system, referred to as emergency medical services (EMS), is usually organized on a local governmental level and works within a medical system that will supervise and evaluate its activities and performance.

The 'golden hour' after a traumatic event is the optimum period in which proper evaluation and treatment will provide the best outcome for the trauma patient. The major goals of an EMS system are to provide:

- rapid access by well-equipped vehicles
- appropriate field management by trained personnel
- rapid transport to an appropriate hospital while providing good care *en route*.

These goals are realized through the rapid assessment of the patient and the situation causing the traumatic event, appropriate airway management, field control of haemorrhage, stabilization of fractures and initiation of volume replacement while *en route* to a hospital equipped to manage rapidly and effectively the potential injuries sustained by the patient.

In order to achieve these goals, the EMS system is organized into three distinct phases:

- the prospective phase
- the immediate phase
- the retrospective phase.

Each phase plays an integral part in maintaining the standards required for appropriate patient care.

The prospective phase occurs before the EMS service has been established within a community and is then maintained through consideration of what will be required before patient contact is made. It should establish an adequate and a consistent source of funding to ensure that the entire system is maintained. It also includes the initial training and continuing education of relevant personnel, purchasing and equipping of vehicles, as well as restocking of supplies before each emergency call, adequate and appropriate staffing of units, and development, updating and approval of treatment protocols.

The immediate phase takes place after the ambulance leaves the station and while patient care is being provided. It is initiated when access to the system is made, usually through a 999 or 911 call (or similar emergency call system). Upon arrival at the scene, the emergency medical technicians (EMTs) should evaluate the situation that caused the incident, determine the number of patients involved and ascertain whether additional equipment or personnel are needed. The patient is then assessed and treatment started with the use of established guidelines and treatment protocols. Care is continued while *en route* to the hospital and hospital personnel are notified prior to arrival. Information provided to the hospital should be succinct and to the point. The algorithm MIVT (mechanism, identified injuries, vital signs, treatment rendered) is a useful way to convey vital information.

The retrospective phase consists of a review of every call after it has been completed to assure that proper medical care was provided. This phase is designed primarily for quality control and assurance within the EMS system and is also used to help to develop a continuing education programme.

The components that go into the make-up of an EMS system consist of the personnel involved, the equipment required to carry out the specified duties, and defined guidelines and treatment protocols within which the EMTs provide care to the accident victim. The medical director of the EMS service plays a vital role in the long-term planning and day to day running of the service. This person is usually a physician who has been appointed by the political entity responsible for the development and maintenance of the EMS service and is approved by the appropriate medical body that oversees the medical management. The medical director should have the authority to make any and all decisions affecting medical care in the prehospital arena. As such, this person should have knowledge and demonstrated ability in the planning and operation of prehospital EMS systems, experience in the prehospital provisions of emergency care for acutely ill or injured patients, experience in training and ongoing education of EMS personnel, and knowledge and experience in the application of medical control to an EMS system. This person should also be knowledgeable in the administrative and legislative processes that affect the system.

The EMTs are responsible for field assessment, treatment and transport of the trauma victim. There are three different levels of EMT based on the amount and type of training. Basic EMTs have completed a standardized 110-h course and have passed both a written and practical examination. They are able to perform basic life-support skills including cardiopulmonary resuscitation, splinting and bandaging, extrication, emergency childbirth techniques, MAST trouser application and simple airway management. Intermediate EMTs have completed the training, and demonstrated proficiency in all of the basic EMT requirements. In addition, they have undergone an additional 150–200 h of training with emphasis on knowledge in assessment and physiology in resuscitation, and evaluation and management of the critically injured trauma patient. Additional skills acquired include the application and use of intravenous (i.v.) fluid therapy and endotracheal tube placement. Paramedic EMTs are trained in all the skills taught to Intermediate EMTs and have additional training in the use of specific drugs that may be useful in the field, such as adrenaline, insulin, glucose, naloxone, morphine, valium, sodium bicarbonate, calcium and frusemide. Finally, nurses can be employed as EMT instructors and quality-control auditors. In some areas nurses have also taken part in field operations with EMTs; however, they require additional instruction similar to that undergone by EMTs in order to do so safely.

The equipment used in prehospital care has been listed in the American College of Surgeons (ACS) Committee on Trauma document entitled 'Essential Equipment List for Ambulances'. The most current version was published in 1994. Most of the equipment and supplies listed are universally accepted and readers are referred to the ACS document for additional details.

In order to evaluate and manage patients adequately in the field, treatment protocols should be established for almost all medical conditions likely to be encountered. Treatment protocols are the overall steps in patient care management taken by EMTs with every patient contact. Each protocol consists of specific standing orders, which the EMTs initiate in order to evaluate and stabilize the trauma patient. It is important to realize that evaluation and emergency management is the primary emphasis when designing these protocols. Obtaining accurate diagnoses in the prehospital setting is difficult and is better accomplished at the hospital, where definitive care can be provided.

Access and triage

The first step in access to trauma care is recognition that an injury has taken place. This can be a problem in rural areas, where recognition that an accident has occurred may be delayed by the lower population density. Steps taken to try to improve access in both urban and rural areas include the use of a universal emergency telephone number, and the deployment of emergency access phones along main roads that provide for communication to emergency medical services and access to the nearest trauma system. The recent increase in the number of cellular phones used by the general public may also help to alleviate this problem. Public safety programmes and educational programmes in school are used to educate the public on how properly to access and use these systems.

Once recognition of an injury has taken place and after providing initial stabilization, the EMS personnel must then decide what level of care the injured patient will require for optimal outcome. Trauma patients can be divided into three different groups, based on the extent of their injuries: those that are rapidly fatal, those that are potentially fatal and those that are not fatal. The first group consists of patients who have sustained mortal injuries and expire within the first 10–15 min after the incident. They represent approximately 5% of all patients sustaining trauma. Prehospital care is unlikely to benefit these patients. The third group consists of patients whose injuries are minor and will not cause a threat to life if treatment is delayed. These injuries are usually confined to the soft tissues or isolated extremity fractures and represent about 80% of all trauma patients. The remaining second group, approximately 7–15% of all trauma patients, consists of patients who have sustained potentially fatal injuries, and it is this group of patients who will benefit most from established prehospital and trauma systems. Studies have shown that when these patients are taken to designated trauma centres, the numbers of potentially salvageable deaths and cases of unacceptable care are significantly reduced. Field triage techniques are used to help to identify these patients.

Triage is the sorting and classification of casualties and determination of the priority of need and proper place of treatment. The purpose is to be selective because there is a finite amount of resource available for the care of patients within a given medical system.

Field triage systems use physiological, anatomical and mechanism of injury data to make decisions that determine how a patient will be subsequently treated. These data are used in the field to determine whether the patient has a possibility of having sustained a serious or potentially life-threatening injury and, if so, what hospital resources are going to be required in order to diagnose and treat those injuries adequately. The field triage system in use by a trauma system should be reviewed periodically for cases of under-triage and over-triage. **Under-triage** occurs when a patient is not felt to have a serious injury but actually does and results in potentially preventable morbidity and mortality. **Over-triage** occurs when a patient is felt to have sustained a serious injury but actually has not and can result in overutilization of finite material, financial and human resources.

The information gathered in the field is combined and quantified using triage scoring systems, which help the field personnel to quantify the severity of injury and aid in making a decision as to whether the trauma victim requires the resources of a trauma centre. The first trauma triage tools reported in the literature used physiological parameters in their assessment of trauma victims. Physiological criteria include measurements of basic body function parameters such as heart rate, blood pressure, respiratory rate and effort, level of consciousness and temperature. Currently, the Revised Trauma Score is the most widely used field system (Table 4.2). It assumes that the physiological reflections of the blood pressure, respiratory rate and head injury as measured by the Glasgow Coma Score (GCS) (Table 4.3) can be used together mathematically to assess injury severity and predict which patients are in need of the most developed care.

Anatomic criteria are used in determining the potential for serious or life-threatening injury. This includes, but is not limited to: penetrating injury to the head, neck, torso or proximal extremity, two or more proximal long bone fractures, pelvic fracture, flail chest, amputation proximal to the wrist or ankle, limb paralysis, greater than 10% total body surface area (TBSA) burn or inhalation injury.

Table 4.2 Revised trauma score components

Glasgow Coma Scale	Systolic blood pressure (mmHg)	Respiratory rate	Coded value
13–15	> 89	10–29	4
9–12	76–89	> 29	3
6–8	50–75	6–9	2
4–5	1–49	1–5	1
3	0	0	0

Table 4.3 Glasgow Coma Score

Eye opening	
Spontaneous	4
To voice	3
To pain	2
None	1
Verbal response	
Orientated	5
Confused	4
Inappropriate words	3
Incomprehensible	2
None	1
Motor response	
Obeys command	6
Localizes pain	5
Withdraws (pain)	4
Flexion (pain)	3
Extension (pain)	2
None	1
Total	3–15

Mechanism of injury criteria help to predict the likelihood of injury by estimating the amount and direction of force applied to the body. Mechanisms of injury felt to have a high potential for major trauma include falls of more than 5 m, motor vehicle accidents with a fatality at the scene, passenger ejection, prolonged extrication (> 20 min), or major intrusion of the passenger compartment, pedestrians struck by a motor vehicle, motorcycle accidents at a speed of more than 20 mph, or any penetrating injuries to the head, neck, torso or proximal extremities. When used as a triage criterion by itself, mechanism of injury results in a high over-triage rate. However, when combined with other triage components, it improves the sensitivity and specificity of the triage process.

Other criteria used in triage decisions include the patient's age, associated medical conditions, environmental conditions, paramedic judgement and length of time to transport to the nearest trauma centre. Elderly patients, patients with chronic diseases and patients exposed to environmental extremes have been shown to be at increased risk for morbidity and mortality following trauma. In addition, studies have shown that haemodynamic and respiratory dysfunction, as well as mortality, are increased with increasing transport times. Finally, studies have shown that EMS field personnel judgement can be as accurate or more so than the available triage scoring methods commonly in use.

Perhaps the best triage system is one that employs a combination of the above-mentioned criteria. Mechanism of injury, anatomic region and type of injury, pre-existing illnesses and paramedic judgement provide additional information that, when combined with physiological data, help to determine whether a patient requires transport to a designated trauma centre. The ACS Field Triage System described in the Resources for Optimal Care of the Injured

Patient uses all of the above-mentioned criteria as a decision scheme in deciding whether a patient requires trauma centre level of care. It is widely used throughout the USA and represents the state-of-the-art in field triage decision schemes. Perhaps the best that can be accomplished with present methodology is for each trauma system to define its own criteria for major trauma and decide which of the present field triage scoring schemes will provide the lowest rates of under-triage and over-triage.

Basic life support

Once the injured patient is assessed and stabilized, the patient is transported to the nearest trauma centre for definitive care. The level of training of the EMS responders and the capabilities of the transporting unit can vary. The needs of the injured patient should be anticipated and the appropriate unit dispatched to the accident scene.

Currently, almost all prehospital EMTs have completed a 110-h course on basic life-saving measures (BLS) and have passed both a written and practical examination. The skills acquired are aimed at providing stabilization of the injured patient, namely, that airway, breathing and circulation are assessed and aided, and measures are taken to prevent any further injury during transport. The skills required at this level include the use of oral or nasal airways and bag–valve mask, cardio-pulmonary resuscitation, extrication, immobilization, splinting and bandaging, control of external haemorrhage, emergency childbirth and application of pneumatic antishock garments. Oral or nasal airways and the bag–valve mask are devices used to assist in airway gas exchange. Extrication, immobilization, control of external haemorrhage, and splinting and bandaging techniques are used to prevent further injury to the patient while the initial assessment and transport are taking place.

Basic cardiopulmonary resuscitation is an important circulatory assisting manoeuvre used on patients who do not have a measurable blood pressure. However, airway control and adequate ventilation must be assured for cardiac massage to be effective. Pneumatic antishock garments are also aimed at assisting circulation; however, the use of this device has become more limited in scope following studies showing minimal effects on blood pressure and potentially significant complications. Both of these skills are often ineffective in the severely injured patient and, while they should always be tried when indicated, their use should not delay transport.

Advanced life support

Advanced life support (ALS) is provided by paramedics who have had additional training beyond that required for BLS. Since airway compromise, haemorrhage and head injuries are responsible for the majority of early deaths due to trauma, the ALS provider is taught to recognize these problems and the necessary skills to stabilize the patient. These skills include airway maintenance and field intubation and, in many centres, pleural decompression and obtaining a surgical airway. Intravenous access and volume resuscitation are also taught, in addition to application of the pneumatic antishock garment. ALS providers are also instructed on the use of various medications and have advanced cardiac support skills as well. Finally, they are knowledgeable on the use of invasive monitors.

Methods of transport

Ground versus air transport

The principle is to move the trauma patient to the receiving hospital as quickly and as safely as possible. Since outcome is directly related to time to definitive care, the quickest mode of transport that assures patient safety should be chosen. However, choosing the best mode of transport can be dependent on the distance, geography, weather and patient status, as well as the availability and skills of the transport personnel and the equipment that are likely to be needed during transport.

Several options are available at major trauma centres, including ground transport, helicopter and fixed-wing air transport. There are conflicting data in the literature as to which transport modality provides the best patient outcome, probably because of the lack of controlling for patient injury acuity and resuscitative techniques provided during transport. However, there are several salient points that can be made. When transport is needed in the local urban setting, helicopter transport offers no advantage over an organized ground transportation system, and the increased cost of using helicopters in this manner is probably not justified.

The main benefit of air transport, in terms of patient survival, is its use for long-distance transport. This benefit can be realized up to an 800-mile radius from the trauma centre when fixed-wing air transport systems are used. However, air transport is subject to unique complications found specifically when a patient is taken up to high altitudes. These include expansion of gases within body cavities such as the thorax or abdomen, as well as potential spaces such as tissues with gas gangrene or penetrating eye injuries. This phenomenon can also occur with equipment such as air splints used for limb stabilization and endotracheal cuff balloons. When used in an air transport setting, these devices must be periodically checked to prevent tissue ischaemia from compression. The available working space within most air transport vehicles is significantly less than that found in ground transport vehicles. As such, specific protocols should be devised that address situations in which the patient becomes unstable, and the air flight crew should be trained in advanced life-support skills.

Interhospital transfer

Hospital categorization as a designated trauma centre, as defined by the ACS, is divided into four levels. While all four levels are maximally committed to the care of the trauma victim, the distinction between them is the availability of resources and personnel capable of caring for the acutely injured patient. Level III and IV designation is reserved for those small suburban or rural communities that do not have the resources to be a level I or II trauma centre. Part of the planning for the care of the injured at a level III or IV centre should include arrangements made for the transfer of the severely injured to a centre with a higher level of resource availability when needed.

Many trauma victims who live in rural communities do not have immediate access to a designated trauma centre or regional trauma system. Previous studies have shown that these patients are at an increased risk of death. Some of the factors that have been implicated in contributing to potentially avoidable mortality in this situation include failure to recognize the severity of the injury, lack of adequate resuscitative measures, and delay in or lack of necessary treatment procedures for stabilization. It is imperative that the initial treating physician is able to recognize that the trauma victim may have injuries that require diagnostic or therapeutic modalities beyond the scope of the initial receiving hospital. If this situation is identified, then transfer of the patient to a 'higher level of care' is appropriate.

Interhospital transfers should occur from one facility to another that will provide the additional resources needed. However, one must recognize that the period of transport is one of potential instability for the patient and the risks of transport must be balanced against the benefits of a higher level of care. Risk to the patient can be minimized with the use of proper equipment, personnel and planning. In addition to the medical aspects of interhospital transfer, physicians must comply with certain federal and local legal regulations. Failure to do so has serious ramifications for the transferring hospital, as well as for the individual physician.

Criteria for transfer

Identification of a trauma victim who may benefit from transfer to a designated trauma centre is based on specific criteria. A number of factors must be examined when making this decision, including patient status and recognition of possible injuries and comorbid factors as well as the personnel and equipment resources necessary for optimal patient care.

The physiological criteria that identify a patient as a 'major trauma victim' in the field can also be applied when deciding whether the patient may benefit from interhospital transfer. Upon arrival at the emergency department, the central nervous, cardiovascular and respiratory systems need to be objectively assessed. This can be done using the field triage scoring tools described above. Derangements in the patient's physiological status should be identified and, to the best of the physician's and initial receiving hospital's ability, stabilized prior to transport. Ongoing deterioration of the patient's status despite resuscitation attempts may benefit from urgent transfer but needs to be managed on a case-by-case basis.

Specific types of injuries, when suspected or diagnosed, may be best treated at designated trauma centres. These include injuries that will require prompt attention by surgical subspecialty services. Examples are significant CNS injuries such as depressed or open skull fractures, penetrating injuries, injuries resulting in coma or lateralizing signs, or spinal cord injuries. Major chest injuries including suspected aortic dissection, flail chest or cardiac injuries, as well as pelvic ring disruption accompanied by evidence of shock or ongoing blood loss, open fracture, or evidence of pelvic visceral organ injury should be considered for transfer. In addition, patients with known or suspected multiple system injuries, severe facial injuries, significant burns, and combined head, abdomen, chest or pelvic injuries, and patients who require microvascular reconstruction should be considered.

Finally, individual physician assessment plays a key role in the transfer of the injured patient. The initial care physician should know what resources are available at that particular hospital. This physician should also be able to recognize serious potential injuries based on mechanism of injury or significant comorbid factors. If the initial care physician feels that the patient requires transfer for optimal care of the injuries based on any part of this general assessment, the physician should institute transfer to the nearest trauma centre.

Methods of transfer

Transfer of the trauma victim must be organized in a way that minimizes the risk to the patient during the transfer process. This requires establishing transfer protocols at the EMS and institutional levels prior to transport. It also includes the planning that is necessary after the decision for transfer is made in individual cases with respect to the type of equipment, mode of transport and personnel necessary to maximize patient safety.

Transfer agreements are established protocols between hospitals that ensure rapid and efficient passage of pertinent patient information prior to the actual transfer. This should include patient identification, history and physical examination findings, diagnostic and therapeutic procedures performed and their results, and the initial impression and a clear identification of the referring and receiving physician. This information then allows the trauma surgeon at the receiving hospital to suggest possible diagnostic or therapeutic manoeuvres that may be required prior to transfer, such as intubation, insertion of a nasogastric tube, Foley catheter or thoracostomy tube. It also allows for mobilization of resources, such as an ICU bed or operating room, at the receiving hospital in anticipation of possible injuries. The physicians involved should also discuss the mode of transportation, accompanying personnel and equipment that may be needed for optimal transfer. Discussion should include who will assume medical control of the patient during transport. Full documentation including a summary of care from the referring hospital and copies of all studies should accompany the patient to the receiving hospital.

Transport modality

The mode of transportation will depend on the availability of a particular mode, distance, geography, weather, patient status, the skills of the transport personnel and the equipment that is likely to be needed during transport. This should be discussed between the referring and receiving physicians with each transfer. Knowledge of transporting agencies in the area and their availability should be ascertained as soon as the need for transport is recognized.

The patient should have appropriate monitoring of physiological indices, including invasive monitoring, during the transport period. This includes monitoring of respiratory rate, cardiac rhythm and blood pressure, intracranial pressure, central venous or pulmonary artery pressure. If the patient is intubated, end-tidal CO_2 should be monitored and the transport ventilator should have alarms to indicate disconnection and high airway pressures. The other additional equipment necessary for safe transport is that needed for effective advanced cardiac life support/advanced trauma life support interventions and has been outlined in a number of publications.

The transport team should consist of two people in addition to the vehicle operator, one of whom should have requisite training in advanced airway management, intravenous therapy, cardiac dysrhythmia recognition and treatment, and advanced trauma life support. If the transporting personnel do not have the necessary training or skills, a nurse or physician should accompany the patient during transport to ensure optimal care.

Section 4.4 • Assessment of the injured patient

Prehospital phase

Care of the injured patient begins in the prehospital setting with a tightly integrated emergency medical response system designed to provide immediate access to life-saving medical care. In most locations, this involves a first-response team of paramedics who provide basic life-support measures, splinting and spine stabilization within minutes of a traumatic event. Often, these prehospital personnel can also perform advanced procedures including intravenous access, maintenance of the airway and intubation, pleural decompression and cricothyroidotomy. The patient is stabilized and rapidly transported to a trauma centre, where resuscitation is continued and injuries are identified and treated expeditiously.

Hospital phase

The transfer of patient care from prehospital to in-hospital teams should occur in an organized fashion with a report that rapidly details the mechanism of injury, the patient's vital signs and obvious injuries, and interventions provided by prehospital providers. The report becomes the formal mechanism by which transfer of care occurs. Assessment and treatment then follow a logical sequence based on clinical judgement and the principles of the Advanced Trauma Life Support programme developed by the ACS Committee on Trauma. A team approach involving physicians, nurses, technicians and trained paramedical personnel allows resuscitation to occur while ongoing evaluation is conducted.

The team must have a captain responsible for organizing the team efforts and performing the primary survey. He or she should rapidly determine the nature of diagnostic tests or interventions required by the patient, and the order in which those activities should be performed. Various tasks can be accomplished simultaneously by team members, all of which should be co-ordinated by the team leader.

Primary survey

Airway

During the primary survey in the resuscitation suite, life-threatening conditions are identified and management is begun simultaneously. The injured patient's potentially most life-threatening problem is loss of the airway; therefore, this is the first priority of the trauma team. The patient who answers when questioned has an adequate, protected airway. **The patient who is unconscious or who demonstrates respiratory insufficiency is at risk for aspiration, hypoxia and hypercarbia, and requires definitive airway control.**

The airway should be cleared of blood, vomitus and foreign bodies. During this time, any interventions require an awareness of the possibility of cervical spine fracture; therefore, hyperextension and hyperflexion of the neck must be avoided. Suctioning, oropharyngeal airways and the use of bag–mask devices may be all that is required to restore oxygenation. **If there continues to be evidence of respiratory insufficiency after these manoeuvres, or if the patient remains unable to protect the airway, definitive airway control with endotracheal intubation or cricothyroidotomy is necessary.** These measures ensure control of gas exchange, protection from aspiration and the ability to hyperventilate to assist in the management of intracranial pressure in patients with closed head injury.

Breathing

After establishing a patent, controlled airway, the next priority is to ensure that adequate gas exchange is occurring. Injuries that can compromise breathing include:

- **compression of the pulmonary parenchyma by blood, air, or visceral herniation**
- **flail chest from multiple rib fractures**
- **pulmonary contusion**
- **airway obstruction**
- **pneumonitis from aspiration.**

If ventilation is compromised owing to pneumothorax or massive haemothorax, an early decision regarding pleural drainage must be made. During the initial evaluation, the examiner should note crepitus, absence of breath sounds and inadequate ventilation suggesting one of these possibilities. In the absence of breath sounds on one side, particularly with mediastinal deviation or dullness to percussion, pleural drainage should be established. Radiography to document the pathology is not indicated, particularly in patients who are hypotensive. Chest tubes should be placed in the anterior axillary line, in the inframammary groove at the fifth interspace. Flail chest, contusion and aspiration, although rarely immediately life-threatening, often cause progressive ventilatory failure. When patients with these conditions develop evidence of ventilatory insufficiency, such as the use of accessory muscles to breathe, progressive hypoxaemia or hypercapnoea, they benefit from endotracheal intubation.

Circulation

The next priority is estimation of the patient's circulatory status. Blood pressure, pulse, skin perfusion, urine output, mental status and central venous pressure are clinically useful indicators of haemodynamic condition. During the primary survey, assessment is limited to the first three parameters. The goal is to determine whether the patient is in shock and, if so, the magnitude of the shock (Table 4.4).

Shock in a trauma patient initially must be assumed to be due to hypovolaemia and is therefore treated with volume expansion. The insertion of one or two large-bore intravenous lines in the upper extremities during the prehospital phase can facilitate resuscitation. Placement of such lines,

Table 4.4 Classification of shock in adults based on initial presentation (for a 70-kg man)

	Class I	Cl.ass II	Class III	Class IV
Blood loss (ml)	≤ 750	750–1500	1500–2000	≥ 2000
Blood loss (% blood volume)	≤ 15	15–30	30–40	≥ 40
Pulse rate	< 100	> 100	> 120	> 140
Blood pressure	Normal	Normal	↓	↓
Pulse pressure	Normal or ↑	↓	↓	↓
Capillary refill	Normal	Delayed	Delayed	Delayed

however, must not delay transport of the patient. In the past, standard care of the hypotensive patient in the field dictated volume resuscitation and use of the pneumatic antishock garment (MAST). Recent data have raised questions about both therapies.

A large, prospective, randomized trial found that in an urban setting with predominantly penetrating trauma, use of the MAST offered no survival benefit and actually increased mortality in patients with thoracic trauma. The study suggested that MAST might benefit patients with a systolic blood pressure of less than 50 mmHg, a finding that was confirmed by a second study. The MAST may also be beneficial in the haemodynamic stabilization of patients with severe pelvic fractures, owing to its ability to enhance the tamponade of retroperitoneal haematomas

The controversy regarding **field stabilization** versus the **scoop and run** philosophy can be addressed pragmatically. Patients who are close to a trauma centre should be rapidly taken there. Transport should not be delayed by attempts at intravenous access. In contrast, patients who are far from trauma centres or who require prolonged extrication benefit from obtaining intravenous access in the field.

During the primary survey, resuscitation should begin as soon as the extent of hypovolaemia is appreciated. At least two large-bore intravenous lines should be started, if this was not done during the prehospital phase. Rapid infusion of 1–2 litres of Ringer's lactate promptly re-establishes and maintains normal blood pressure in patients who do not have ongoing bleeding. If the initial infusion of 2 litres of Ringer's lactate fails to restore blood pressure, blood must be given in addition to crystalloid. Type O, Rh-negative blood is the appropriate blood product for a severely hypotensive patient. If the patient's blood type is known, un-cross-matched, type-specific blood can be used as soon as it is obtained from the blood bank. It is the blood product of choice until cross-matched blood becomes available.

Ongoing fluid requirements indicate significant bleeding and necessitate immediate measures to identify and control the source of haemorrhage. A decision must be made as to whether there is cavitary (intra-thoracic or intra-abdominal) or non-cavitary (external bleeding and fractures) haemorrhage. Sources of external bleeding should be controlled with direct pressure. Splinting of extremity fractures will reduce blood loss at fracture sites. Significant intrathoracic or intra-abdominal bleeding should be suspected in all hypotensive patients, even though many will have only a non-cavitary source of haemorrhage. Potential sources of bleeding should be investigated with chest radiographs and objective evaluation of the abdomen. Unstable patients should undergo diagnostic peritoneal lavage (DPL). Further assessment of the stable patient's abdomen can be performed during the secondary survey.

Improvements in prehospital care have resulted in the more frequent transport of patients in extremis to trauma centres. Rapid assessment of these patients is required to decide who will benefit from aggressive resuscitative efforts. If initial examination reveals an absence of peripheral pulses, it must be determined whether the patient has a cardiac rhythm. Lack of a rhythm is synonymous with death. Those patients still maintaining electrical activity may have electromechanical disassociation (EMD) secondary to cardiac tamponade or exsanguinating haemorrhage. In such cases, external cardiac massage and volume replacement should be initiated while preparations are made for resuscitative thoracotomy. If cardiac tamponade is suspected owing to hypotension and distended neck veins with an appropriately placed wound, confirmation of the diagnosis through a subxyphoid window, followed by immediate thoracotomy, is indicated. Likewise, patients with EMD secondary to hypovolaemia may benefit from aortic cross-clamping via thoracotomy with concomitant volume resuscitation and attempt to control the source of their exsanguinating haemorrhage.

The routine use of thoracotomy in all patients suffering traumatic cardiac arrest cannot be justified. A meta-analysis of reports concerning the outcome of resuscitative thoracotomy for trauma found an overall survival rate of 11%. There were no survivors among patients without signs of life at the scene of injury. There were no neurologically intact survivors among those patients arriving at the hospital without signs of life. (In these studies, signs of life were defined as pupillary reactivity, agonal respirations or cardiac electrical activity.) **Considering these findings, it seems justifiable to perform resuscitative thoracotomy only on penetrating trauma patients with signs of life at the scene and loss of vital signs within 5 min of hospital arrival. In blunt trauma patients, only those with signs of life upon arrival at the resuscitation area should undergo thoracotomy**. Patients who meet these strict criteria and undergo resuscitative thoracotomy have the highest potential for functional survival.

Brain resuscitation
A brief neurological examination utilizing the components of the GCS (Table 4.3), a determination of pupillary size and reactivity, and an assessment of lateralizing signs complete the primary survey. Establishment of an airway and initiation of mild hyperventilation to an arterial carbon dioxide tension (Pa,CO_2) of 30–35 mmHg are the first line of therapy for patients with severe closed head injury. Resuscitation of circulating blood volume to maintain cerebral perfusion pressure is also of obvious importance. Maintenance of adequate oxygenation and avoidance of hypotension are paramount in minimizing secondary injury to the traumatized brain. **Patients with a GCS of 8 or less or lateralizing signs are very likely to have an intracranial mass lesion requiring prompt surgical intervention**. For this reason, such patients should receive a computed tomographic (CT) scan of the head as soon as possible.

In summary, the primary survey is directed at airway, breathing and circulation management, initial neurological assessment and brain resuscitation. None of the aspects of initial assessment is forgiving of delay in diagnosis; therefore, it is vital that resuscitation and evaluation occur aggressively and simultaneously.

Secondary survey

The secondary survey is a comprehensive assessment directed at identification of suspected and unsuspected injuries. If possible, a history should be obtained. This begins with the prehospital provider's report and should include the mechanism of injury, the patient's vital signs and treatments given during transport. Knowledge of the mechanism of injury can help the physician to judge those areas of the body that may have sustained the greatest energy transfer so that subsequent investigations can be directed appropriately. The patient's past medical history, including allergies, medications, known past illness and the time of the last meal, should also be determined.

Assuming sufficient team size, many components of the secondary survey, such as detailed physical examination, blood drawing and radiography, can be performed simultaneously. For the purposes of description, these activities, including the physical examination, will be broken down into their basic components. As the secondary survey progresses, more specialized tests or therapy may be needed as directed by clinical findings. Throughout the evaluation, the patient must be reassessed continually to monitor the response to ongoing resuscitative efforts. The unstable patient should have a rapid assessment to identify sources of haemorrhage and then be taken to the operating room immediately. The completely stable patient should undergo a thorough physical examination as well as appropriate radiographic and biochemical testing before proceeding to the treatment phase.

All trauma patients should have an arterial blood gas drawn and basic radiographs obtained. The blood gas will help to assess the acid–base status and adequacy of respiration. The specimen also should be sent for type, screening and haematocrit determination. Additional blood can be held in case a toxicology screen or other biochemical investigation is deemed necessary. Basic radiographic evaluation should include chest and anteroposterior X-ray, lateral and odontoid view cervical spine films. A swimmer's view is obtained if the lateral view does not visualize the junction of the seventh cervical and first thoracic vertebral bodies. The need for these X-rays in penetrating trauma should be based on clinical assessment. Penetrating wounds should be marked with metallic clips prior to filming to assist in anatomical localization.

A complete physical examination is performed from head to toe, looking for any evidence of injury. The head is palpated for haematomas, lacerations and fractures. Scalp lacerations can result in significant blood loss and should be rapidly closed with a running suture

to provide haemostasis. The eyes are evaluated for pupillary reactivity and visual acuity. The ears are checked for haemotympanum or otorrhoea and the nose is assessed for epistaxis or rhinorrhoea. Any of these findings may be indicative of a basilar skull fracture. The mouth is examined for retropharyngeal haematomas and aspirated foreign bodies. The facial bones should be palpated to identify step-offs or crepitus associated with facial fractures. Cranial nerve function should be examined and recorded.

While axial immobilization is maintained, the cervical collar is removed and the neck is evaluated for venous distention or tracheal deviation, and palpated for tenderness or bony step-offs. Penetrating injuries should be assessed for platysma penetration but should not be probed. Skin abrasions on the neck associated with the use of a shoulder harness should alert the examiner to the possibility of a blunt carotid injury and should prompt further evaluation with carotid ultrasound.

Inspection of the chest will identify penetrating or sucking chest wounds or the paradoxical movement of a flail chest. Palpation will reveal crepitus and rib or sternal pain, indicating possible fractures. Auscultation can help to identify pneumothorax and haemothorax. Distant heart sounds in conjunction with distended neck veins may indicate cardiac tamponade and should prompt further evaluation. The chest radiograph obtained during the secondary survey will aid in the diagnosis of these entities, as well as pulmonary contusion, aspiration and blunt aortic injury.

All patients with thoracic trauma documented by history or physical examination should have an electrocardiogram (ECG) performed during the secondary survey as well as continuous cardiac monitoring throughout their resuscitation. **Patients with ECG changes may have blunt cardiac injury and should be monitored with telemetry for at least 24 h**. If there are any signs of cardiac failure, invasive monitoring and echocardiography are indicated to delineate further any cardiac dysfunction.

Patients with rapid deceleration injuries are at risk for transection of the thoracic aorta. **Suspicion of this injury should be raised by an anteroposterior radiograph demonstrating a mediastinum more than 8 cm wide, loss of the normal aortic contour, apical capping of the lung, or tracheal or nasogastric tube deviation**. Patients with an appropriate mechanism of injury and an abnormal mediastinum on chest X-ray should undergo a definitive study to rule out aortic disruption. Arch aortography is considered the gold standard for evaluation of the thoracic aorta. Spiral CT and transoesophageal echocardiography have also been used successfully at some centres, but currently cannot be considered as standard care.

Suspicion of a ruptured hemidiaphragm should be raised when the chest radiograph demonstrates failure of resolution of a suspected haemothorax after tube thoracostomy, or the

presence of the nasogastric tube or bowel gas above the normal plane of the diaphragm. Patients with diaphragmatic injury should undergo prompt laparotomy for repair of the defect.

Penetrating chest wounds are managed according to the presumed trajectory of the missile based on physical examination. Wounds confined to one hemithorax are treated with tube thoracostomy, with anticipated re-expansion of the lung. Further evaluation is necessary if the trajectory crosses the mediastinum, potentially including bronchoscopy, oesophagoscopy, aortography and echocardiography.

The abdominal examination helps to determine whether there is injury significant enough to warrant surgical intervention. Inspection of the abdomen for bruising or abrasions may suggest underlying organ injury. Auscultation is generally not helpful unless bowel sounds are absent, thereby raising the suspicion of significant visceral injury. In unstable patients, it is necessary to determine rapidly whether there is signifi-cant intraperitoneal bleeding. **DPL accomplishes this goal safely and quickly, and should be the diagnostic test of choice in circumstances in which time is critical**. DPL is considered grossly positive if more than 10 ml of blood is aspirated upon insertion of the catheter into the peritoneum. If less blood is aspirated, 1 litre of normal saline is infused into the peritoneum and subsequently drained. The fluid is sent for microscopic analysis. A red blood cell count of more than 100 000 for blunt trauma is considered positive and warrants eventual laparotomy. A haemo-dynamically unstable patient with a microscopically positive DPL is likely to have a source of bleeding elsewhere and needs further evaluation. For example, such a patient who also has a pelvic fracture may have uncontrolled retroperitoneal bleeding and may benefit from early angiography and therapeutic embolization prior to laparotomy.

Haemodynamically stable patients also require objec-tive evaluation of the abdomen. A CT scan of the abdo-men is most commonly used for this purpose, although DPL can also be employed. In some centres, focused abdominal ultrasound is used as a screening tool to identify fluid within the peritoneum, pleural space or pericardium. Identification of free fluid in the abdomen requires abdominal CT scan to quantify the fluid's vol-ume and identify its source. Indications for laparotomy following evaluation of blunt trauma patients with ultrasound or CT are not well established. Management should be based on objective findings and the patient's clinical status. **It must be remembered that neither ultrasound nor CT is 100% sensitive, and serial examination of the patient's abdomen in the setting of a negative test is mandatory**.

Abdominal gunshot wounds require explora-tory laparotomy because 90–95% of patients will have intra-abdominal injury. Abdominal stab wounds can be managed using a policy of selective exploration, as intraperitoneal injury is less common than in patients sustaining abdominal gunshot wounds.

First, the stab wound must be assessed for fascial pene-tration using local wound exploration. When penetra-tion is present, DPL is indicated. Criteria mandating laparotomy are controversial, varying from a red blood cell count of 1000 to 100 000. Most centres favour using a lower cell count, which maximizes the test's sensitivity for visceral injury. Stab wounds to the back and flank can be evaluated using DPL and intravenous urogram in conjunction with serial abdominal examinations. Similarly, abdominal and pelvic CT scan also can be used to investigate these wounds.

The presence of pubic or iliac crest pain, pelvic instability or perineal haematomas should raise the suspicion of a major pelvic fracture and prompt a pelvic radiograph. If blood is present at the urethral meatus or a pelvic fracture is documented, a cystourethrogram should be performed. Rectal examination should be performed prior to the placement of a Foley catheter to determine the presence of blood and to assess the possibility of prostatic injury. In posterior urethral injury, the prostate may not be palpable owing to its being separated from the urethra. If there is no blood at the meatus or evidence of urethral injury, a Foley catheter should be inserted to decompress the bladder and monitor urine output. The presence of haematuria should suggest retroperitoneal injury. Patients with pelvic fracture and haem-positive stool should undergo further evaluation. Those with rectal injuries will require diverting colostomy.

Maintaining axial spine alignment, a detailed examination of the back of the chest and abdomen should be made by turning the patient on the side. Direct palpation of the thoracic and lumber spine should be performed and other entrance or exit wounds noted. Radiographs of the spine are indicated if tenderness to palpation, bony abnormalities or neurological deficits are found.

The extremities should be assessed for tenderness, ecchymosis, crepitus, skin integrity, and the presence of peripheral pulses and neurological deficit. Evaluation for vascular injury should include inspection and palpation of all extremities for the presence of pulses, bruits and expanding haematomas. Abnormalities should prompt angiographic appraisal.

Neurological examination should include complete motor and sensory evaluation, including assessment of rectal tone and bulbocavernosus and anal wink reflexes, as well as continued re-evaluation of the patient's level of consciousness, pupillary size and GCS assessment.

Monitoring

During the initial resuscitation, an awareness of the adequacy of treatment for hypovolaemic shock, respiratory distress and intracranial hypertension is essential. Constant ECG monitoring is indicated in all patients with significant injury. A Foley catheter is mandatory for assessing urinary output. An arterial line is useful to document fluctuations in blood pressure as well as adequacy of gas exchange. A central venous pressure monitor is helpful in following trends in volume resuscitation. Although often impractical in the resuscitation suite, a pulmonary artery catheter may be a useful adjunct in patients with significant underlying cardiopulmonary or renal disease. Patients with significant head injury should undergo placement of an intracranial pressure-monitoring device. The use of any combination of these monitors allows one to assess the effect of volume resuscitation on physiological end-points such as blood pressure, central venous pressure, urinary output, arterial pH, base deficit and intracranial pressure. Minute-to-minute assessment of the patient's physiological responses to interventions will help to guide further therapy.

Where to resuscitate

Most patients with major trauma, either blunt or penetrating, will be well served by evaluation in a dedicated trauma resuscitation suite. Direct admission to the operating room where surgical management can be effected rapidly may benefit a minority of patients with injuries requiring immediate attention (between 5 and 10% of major trauma casualties). The indications for operating room resuscitation in the present author's institution include:

- systolic blood pressure < 100 mmHg after penetrating injury to the neck, chest or abdomen
- blunt abdominal trauma and systolic blood pressure < 100 mmHg despite prehospital administration of 2 litres of crystalloid
- amputation above the knee or elbow
- complex wounds with hypotension
- paramedic judgement.

Treatment of patients requiring immediate surgery is facilitated by receiving them in an operating room staffed by a full team including the anaesthetist, surgeon, surgical technician and nursing staff. The roles and responsibilities of trauma team members are essentially the same whether the patient is resuscitated in the operating room or in the resuscitation area.

In summary, early hospital care, or the resuscitation phase, should follow an ordered set of priorities that include a primary survey, with assessment of airway, breathing, circulation, neurological disability and complete exposure of the patient to assess all injuries. Simultaneous with the resuscitative effort, life-threatening problems identified during the primary survey are treated, shock management is initiated, the cervical spine is stabilized and external haemorrhage is controlled. The secondary survey then includes a complete evaluation of the head, neck, chest, abdomen, pelvis, rectum, extremities and nervous system. Laboratory and radiological investigations should be selected and performed in priority order. Whether the patient should be resuscitated in the operating room or in the emergency department should be determined prior to arrival at the hospital based on the patient's overall condition and severity of injury, and resources available at the trauma centre.

Operative phase

Surgical procedures are directed at arresting haemorrhage, controlling enteric contamination, removing devitalized tissue, repairing injured soft tissues and stabilizing fractures. The distinction between the resuscitative and operative phases can be artificial, especially in the most critically injured patients. For example, control of the airway and support of the circulation may occur in conjunction with resuscitative thoracotomy and laparotomy in patients who suffer cardiopulmonary arrest after penetrating trauma. Likewise, simultaneous operations by multiple teams are often necessary in patients who suffer polysystem injury. Co-ordination of surgery by several teams decreases operative time and minimizes the need for repeated trips to the operating room.

The importance of early and expeditious operation in trauma patients cannot be overstated. Lack of recognition of the need for operation and delay in surgical management continue to be leading causes of morbidity and preventable death due to trauma. In addition, early operation for many injuries, such as stabilization of fractures, has been shown to decrease morbidity, as well as the cost and duration of hospitalization.

Intensive-care phase

Improvements in transport, resuscitation and operative management of many injuries have reduced early mortality and increasingly shifted the burden of support to the postinjury/postoperative arena. Patients who have suffered severe injuries with or without operation will require a period of intense observation and care. Invasive monitoring of cardiac function, intracranial pressure, and arterial and venous pressure is common. Particular attention is paid to fluid and electrolyte balance, and haematological and coagulation parameters. Careful observation allows for early recognition of problems and early institution of therapy. Changes in the status of the patient warrant careful evaluation. As in the early hospital phase, delays in recognition or management of problems can lead to disastrous complications and death.

Rehabilitation phase

Rehabilitation is the process by which biological and psychosocial functions are restored sufficiently to allow an injured person to enjoy maximum autonomy. The objective is to return the patient to the level of function that existed prior to the injury. Rehabilitation requires a team approach that often draws on the skills of the neurosurgeon, orthopaedic surgeon, plastic surgeon, occupational therapist, physiotherapist and social worker. Involvement of the rehabilitation team early in the patient's course can facilitate later efforts directed at placement of the patient in a setting appropriate for his or her level of function.

Summary

Initial management and evaluation of trauma patients begin in the field and extend to the trauma centre. Primary assessment involves simultaneous evaluation of airway, ventilation, circulation and the potential for significant head injury. Once initial evaluation and initiation of resuscitation are complete, a formal secondary survey should be conducted, followed by definitive care. Ongoing reassessment throughout this time allows for continual evaluation of adequacy of resuscitation and definitive treatment. Changes in the treatment plan should be based on the patient's clinical status. The ultimate goal is to return the patient to the pre-injury level of function.

Section 4.5 • Management of the burns victim

Millions of individuals throughout the world are hospitalized for the treatment of burns each year, and thousands die. The burn injury can be one of the most serious and devastating forms of trauma. The daily cost of modern care for burns victims is very high. The economic loss is also staggering and must be measured not only in terms of costs of treatment but in the permanent loss of many productive years of life. This loss is magnified by the fact that 50% of major burns occur during the formative and productive years.

Destruction of the skin by heat results in severe local and systemic physiological alterations. Management of the burns victim requires understanding of the pathophysiology, diagnosis and treatment not only of the local skin injury, but also of the derangements that occur in the haemodynamic, metabolic, nutritional, immunological and psychological homeostatic mechanisms. Proper patient care demands that the burn wound, the accompanying systemic changes and the alterations produced by treatment be conceptually viewed as dynamic, interrelated processes, not as isolated phenomena.

Even when treatment may be successful, the burns victim may require a recovery period extending over months or years, even with successful treatment. The evaluation and treatment of diverse physiological changes over a prolonged time requires a co-ordinated team of health professionals. Indeed, recognition of the need to develop highly specialized teams and burn-care facilities has been the major advance in the management of burns in the last quarter of the twentieth century.

Final success or failure of treatment of the burns victim is difficult to measure. Survival or death is today not always an adequate yardstick. Death of the victim with a nearly total body surface injury, hands and face burned beyond recognition, and so deep as to preclude fully functional reconstruction and rehabilitation, may not be considered failure. Similarly, survival without consideration of the functional and social rehabilitation of the victim should not be the only measure of success. The burns teams must treat the patient as a whole person when measuring success or failure, not how they understand and treat the burn, but how they understand, treat and rehabilitate the burned person.

Evaluation of the burns victim

The first essential step in treating a burns victim is to treat immediate life-threatening problems, including airway management and shock. The next step is to determine the severity of the injury and then to decide the level of expertise necessary to care for the patient. A careful history and physical examination specifically modified for the burns victim must be rapidly performed.

The ultimate determinants of the severity of the burn injury are the extent of tissue destroyed and whether the victim in a particular state of health can withstand the injury. The guidelines used to evaluate the burn severity are the victim's age, the extent of the burn, the depth of the injury, the area of the body involved, whether an associated inhalation injury occurred at the time of burning, and the presence of comorbid factors in addition to the burn injury that will affect the treatment or eventual outcome.

Age

Burn injuries incurred at the extremes of age carry greater morbidity and mortality. The age of the patient determines the natural thickness of the skin and also dictates the amount of stress that the victim can withstand. A good guideline is that burns in people under the age of 3 years or over the age of 60 years tend to be more severe. For example, a patient 80 years of age with 20% TBSA deep burns may have a non-survivable injury, while the same burns in a younger patient would be well tolerated.

Extent of burn

The extent of the burn surface involved can be determined by careful observation and should be recorded graphically. This is important not only for diagnosis and treatment but also for prognosis and statistics. It is customary to record the extent of injury in terms of percentage of body surface involved. Only areas of partial- and full-thickness burn are included in this assessment, since first-degree burns do not have appreciable morbidity. A rough estimate of the extent of burn can be made by using the rule of nines (Figure 4.1), but more detailed assessment requires careful mapping of the areas of burn injury on a specialized charting form. Children require modification of the rule of nines because the child's head is proportionally larger, and the legs smaller, compared to the adult.

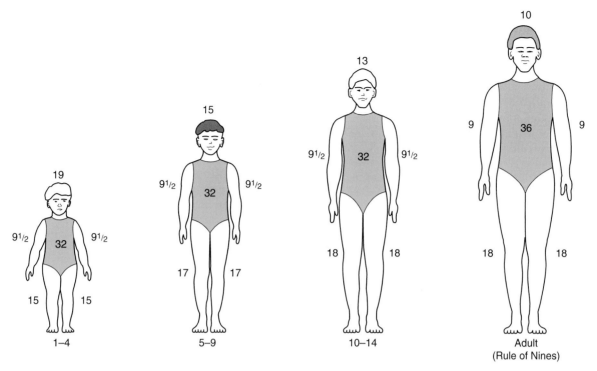

Figure 4.1 The 'Rule of Nines' is used to determine the total body surface area (TBSA) of injury. Only areas of partial- and full-thickness injury are included in the estimate. Compared with an adult, the head of a child is relatively large in per cent surface area and the lower extremities are relatively small.

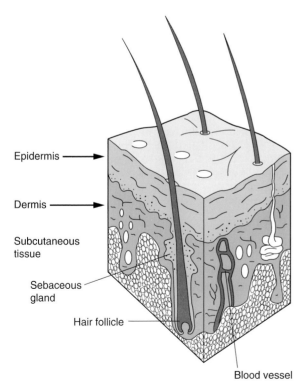

Figure 4.2 The skin is now recognized as a complex organ. The epidermal layer is protective, while the dermal layer contains organelles including hair follicles, nerve endings, sebaceous and sweat glands. Partial-thickness burns can re-epithelialize from basal cells that line the hair follicle shafts.

Depth of burn

Since the volume of tissue destroyed is ultimately important, both the depth and the extent of injury must be evaluated. The skin is viewed as a complex organ, with many structures and functions (Figure 4.2). Unfortunately, the depth of the burn may be difficult to assess accurately. Although many elaborate tests have been proposed to evaluate depth of the burn, none has proven to be totally reliable. Depth of the injury may be non-uniform throughout the burn's extent and the depth may progress with time. Scald burns, other than those due to immersion, tend to be more superficial than burns produced by exposure to flames or contact with hot objects. Chemical and electrical burns tend to be deep even though they may appear superficial at the time of initial evaluation. Erythema of the wound, blanching of the tissues and thin watery blisters are associated with superficial burns, while thick-walled blisters and a pale, poorly or non-blanching wound bed or a dry, leathery eschar are associated with deeper burns. However, appearance may be deceptive, as will be discussed later under 'Pathophysiology'.

Sensation may be unreliable for determining burn depth. Even full-thickness burns have pressure sensation because the pressure receptors, Paccinian corpuscles, are located beneath the dermis. Pin prick is absent in deep burns, and it can also be absent in burns of moderate depth. Therefore, it is not a good predictor of full-thickness injury as has often been reported.

For the initial treatment of the burns victim, it is only necessary to separate those injuries that are deeper and will require hospitalization and specialized care. The full extent of the injury will reveal itself between 4 and 14 days after the thermal insult.

Location

The location of the burn injury is important. Burns to the face and neck, hands, feet, perineum and genitalia carry specific problems in their treatment, reconstruction and eventual rehabilitation. These areas are considered primary areas. Significant burns of the primary areas become major by location, regardless of the total body extent or depth of the injury.

Inhalation injury

The associated inhalation of noxious gases and smoke that cause pulmonary damage increased the mortality in the McIndoe Regional Burns Unit from 13.9% to 58%. In a study of patients with TBSA burns greater than 80%, inhalation injury was found in two out of 19 survivors (11%) versus six out of 13 non-survivors (46%). Thus, suspicion of inhalation should be determined on initial evaluation. Victims injured in a closed space with the presence of heavy smoke are likely to have inhaled significant smoke. Similarly, patients who present with singed nasal vibrissae, conjunctivitis, pharyngeal oedema, carbonaceous sputum, bronchorrhoea, hoarseness or stridor should be suspected of having inhalation injury.

Comorbid factors

Associated trauma at the time of burning increases the severity of the burn. In addition, existing disease states prior to the thermal event can help to determine the treatment and outcome. Cardiovascular, respiratory, renal or metabolic diseases can complicate care and increase mortality. Seizure disorders and alcohol or drug misuse tend to predispose patients to burn and complicate their treatment. The presence of pre-admission hypovolaemia or shock has also been identified as a risk factor. In patients with burns greater than 80% TBSA, preadmission under-resuscitation was found in zero out of 19 survivors and in four of 13 non-sur-

vivors (31%), stressing the need for prompt transportation of the patient to a qualified burns centre.

Categorization

Using the above criteria, burns can be categorized conveniently for determination of severity. The classification adopted by the American Burn Association is presented in Table 4.5. Additional useful information prior to the initiation of treatment includes the history of the victim's immunizations, especially against tetanus, history of known allergies and the social circumstances surrounding the burn. Suicide or homicide attempts, child abuse and inability of the victim to care for himself or herself may all influence the initial evaluation of the burns victim and assist in determining the level of expertise necessary for proper treatment and follow-up.

Pathophysiology of the local burn injury

Within the limits of biological variability, human skin will tolerate temperatures up to 40°C for brief periods. Temperatures above this level result in progressively increased tissue destruction that is worsened by increased time of exposure. Three concentric zones of significant thermal injury were described by Jackson (Figure 4.3). In the centre of the injury at the point of contact with the heat, cells are immediately destroyed by coagulation. Next, there is a zone of injured cells which might under ideal circumstances survive, but usually progress to tissue death over 24–48 h. This zone has been labelled the zone of stasis. Finally, there is a volume of tissue known as the zone of hyperaemia, which has been minimally injured and may recover over a period of 7 days.

Clinically, the amount of tissue destroyed or injured determines the treatment plan. Therefore, the depth of the burn injury is important (Table 4.5). Burns may not be uniform in depth, and in any given area the depth will vary depending on the thermal energy transferred to the skin, the blood supply, thermal conductivity and evaporative water loss from this skin. The **first-degree burn** is characterized by erythema and discomfort

Table 4.5 Classification of thermal burns

	Major burn	Moderate burn	Minor burn
Partial-thickness size	> 25% adults	10–25% adults	< 15% adults
	> 20% children	10–20% children	< 10% children
Full-thickness size	> 10%	2–10%	< 2%
Significant burns of hands, feet, face, perineum, genitalia	Yes	No	No
Inhalation injury	Major burn if present	No	No
Comorbid factors	Poor risk patients	Relatively good risk patient	Not present
Associated injury	Major burn if present	Not present	Not present
Treatment facility	Specialized burn care facility	General hospital with designated team	Frequently managed as outpatient

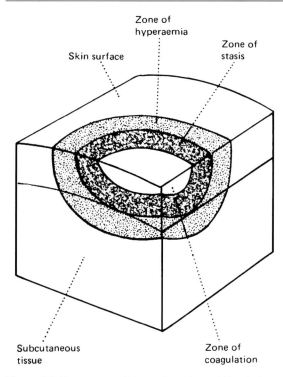

Figure 4.3 Three zones within a primary burn. (After Jackson, 1953.)

decreases to 50% of normal, cell death occurs. The response of the cells involved in burns is neither uniform nor static. The blood supply and local environment of the wound will help to determine the cellular response. Additional trauma, oedema, decreased vascular supply or microbial invasion will further injure or destroy cells that survive the initial thermal insult.

In addition to cell damage, there are both immediate and delayed vascular and cellular inflammatory responses at the burned site. Accumulation of fluid in the burn wound is a prominent feature of thermal injury. The fluid and electrolyte shifts within the wound are related to the type and severity of the injury. This appears to be secondary to a series of mediators released following the thermal insult. These mediators include vasoactive amines, prostaglandins, thromboxanes, leukotrienes, free oxygen radicals and cytokines such as IL-1, IL-2 and IL-6. Thermal injury produces immediate spasm of venules, vasoconstriction of arterioles and dilatation of capillaries. Capillaries and venules become permeable in the burned area allowing leakage of fluid, electrolytes and proteins. The immediate response is followed within 6 h by a delayed response with venular dilatation and further increased capillary permeability. The most rapid fluid loss occurs during the first 12 h postburn and is accompanied by cell margination and emigration, as seen in inflammation from other causes. Another cause of loss of fluid into the burn wound (besides capillary permeability) is the breakdown of the cell membrane by the thermal injury that injures the transmembrane sodium pump. This produces increased intracellular sodium and water and an efflux of potassium.

A typical local cellular response accompanies the fluid response. Neutrophils emigrate from vessels into the tissues and are attracted by chemotactic factors such as IL-6 to the site of the injury. Monocytes migrate into the area and tissue macrophages differentiate in the area as needed for repair. Wound macrophages influence healing by releasing numerous substances such as angiogenesis factors and various mitogenic and chemotactic growth factors.

Systemic response to local injury

As the above events are occurring at the local site of burning, systemic changes also take place. The functions of all organ systems are eventually altered owing to the effects of a major burn. Some of the changes are related to burning itself, and some are in response to the stress of injury.

Cardiovascular response
Among the most immediate and severe changes are those in the heart and blood vessels. A precipitate drop in cardiac output of up to 50% is frequently seen in major burns. Although this response was originally thought to be due to a poorly defined myocardial depressant factor, it now appears to be secondary to changes in the interstitium in the wound and adjacent

only. Within a few days the outer injured cells peel off the totally healed skin with no scarring. The **second-degree burn** is best divided into two subcategories: superficial partial-thickness and deep partial-thickness. The **superficial partial-thickness injury** is characterized by blisters. Removal or breaking of the blisters results in weeping from the burn surface. Since the basal layers of the skin are not destroyed in this injury, regeneration is prompt and these burns usually heal in 10–17 days in the absence of infection. The **deep partial-thickness burn** is more severe, with many areas of marginally viable tissue. This skin will only survive and heal under the most optimal conditions. The **third-degree** or **full-thickness burn** contains totally destroyed skin. Whereas the more superficial injuries are characterized by increased vascularity, this is an avascular injury. Coagulation necrosis of the cells, thrombosis of vessels, and accumulation of fluids and cellular infiltrate in the margins of the wound characterize the injury. This burn cannot heal itself. Total-thickness skin loss can be restored only by ingrowth from the margins of the wound or by application of skin grafts from non-burned portions of the body. Finally, **fourth-degree injuries** involve death or injury to subcutaneous tissues such as fat, fascia, muscle or bone.

Cytological damage occurs as protein is denatured by rising temperatures. Many of the changes are reversible. Only at temperatures in excess of 45°C does denaturation exceed the ability of the cell to repair the damage. At this temperature, thermolabile enzyme systems are blocked and when the enzymic activity unburned tissue and also to circulating hormones. Release of osmotically active cellular elements and transcapillary migration of plasma proteins produce increased interstitial oncotic pressure. When this osmotic gradient forms across an injured basement membrane, massive oedema can occur. As blood volume and plasma volume fall, further decreases in cardiac output occur until levels as low as 20% of normal are reached. A direct toxic effect of the burn or burn byproducts may cause myocardial failure. More recently, enormous elevations in catecholamines, vasopressin and angiotensin II have been documented in the acute shock period (Figures 4.4 and 4.5). These hormones may decrease cardiac function by increasing afterload and limiting venous return to the heart, and they may also cause coronary vasoconstriction, resulting in myocardial ischaemia. The initial cardiac effect appears to be self-limited, and cardiac output returns towards normal within 36–48 h.

The fluid shifts in the local burn area are accompanied by total body fluid shifts in the larger injuries. Nearly total body capillary permeability occurs in patients with greater than 30% body surface area burns. The fluid–electrolyte–protein loss renders Starling's hypothesis ineffective and the fluid enters a functional third space. This represents an overall haemodynamic defect. Fully 60% of the extracellular fluid volume may be lost in a major burn through capillary permeability, the intracellular fluid shifting into the heat-injured cells, and evaporation following destruction of the skin barrier. Most of the loss occurs within the first 8–12 h, but additional fluid losses continue internally for at least 48 h after injury. Added to these losses specific for the burn injury is the obligatory fluid loss by respiration and urine. The fluid loss to the outside and to the internal functional third space results in haemodynamic instability or burn shock. The understanding of burn shock was necessary before adequate resuscitation techniques could be devised.

Besides the fluid portion of the vascular system, the systemic cellular elements also have a predictable response. Progressive anaemia occurs beyond that pre-

dicted in response to direct erythrocyte destruction by heat. Erythrocyte survival is decreased and the normal hypoxic stimulus for haemopoiesis appears to malfunction. Red cell trapping by the reticuloendothelial system and losses through capillary permeability and thrombus formation further diminish the red cell mass. Platelet changes postburn are biphasic. An initial thrombocytopenia may be severe and is followed by prolonged thrombocytosis, accompanied by hypofibrinogenaemia and a brief state of diffuse intravascular coagulopathy. Neutrophils are affected by burn injury and this affects the systemic host defences. Phagocytic capacity and microbial killing are decreased although, curiously, an increase in neutrophil intracellular oxidant content is found.

Renal response

Renal function is altered in the burns victim as in any trauma victim. The posterior pituitary releases high levels of ADH (arginine vasopressin) for several days (Figure 4.5), causing maximal reabsorption of water in the renal tubules. Maximum sodium reabsorption occurs simultaneously because of aldosterone release from the adrenals. This combination results in excretion of a small amount of concentrated urine containing a decreased sodium concentration.

The injured cells in the burn wound release increased amounts of myoglobin, haemoglobin and toxic products, which are presented to the kidney. If adequate glomerular filtration rate (GFR) is not maintained, or if renal ischaemia occurs, these products cannot be effectively removed and acute tubular necrosis ensues. This is the basis of renal failure, which was previously a common accompaniment of burn shock. Myoglobin is the most injurious of these agents; significant myoglobinuria usually requires extensive muscle injury, most commonly occurring with high-voltage electrical transmission injury. **Absorption of myoglobin into the circulation is greatly increased if a subfascial compartment syndrome occurs and persists without relief by escharotomy and/or fasciotomy.**

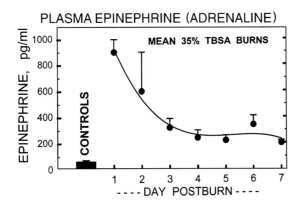

Figure 4.4 Plasma adrenaline levels are markedly elevated in patients with major burns. This hormone causes tachycardia and vasoconstriction, and contributes to the hypermetabolic response.

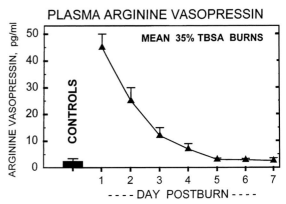

Figure 4.5 Plasma arginine vasopressin levels are enormously elevated in patients with major burns. This hormone is an intense vasoconstrictor.

If volume losses are replaced by a similar fluid and volume to that being lost, renal blood flow is maintained. This results in an adequate GFR and urine volume. Since urine volume reflects solute load and GFR, decreased renal function is almost inevitably a result of inadequate fluid and electrolyte replacement. Urine flow rates of 30–50 ml/h in adults and 1 ml/kg/h in children are adequate for the kidneys to remove toxic breakdown products and maintain function during the period of haemodynamic instability.

Pulmonary response

The pulmonary system may be exposed to a hypoxic environment in a fire and this may be aggravated by inhalation of noxious stimuli, primarily smoke particles but also gases, at the time of injury. The hypoxia is a stimulus for release of injurious free oxygen radicals as well as arachidonic acid metabolites. Although the heat is usually dissipated before it can cause a pulmonary burn, it causes damage to the upper airway leading to oedema and obstruction. As the burns victim becomes oedematous and the cardiac output falls, the vascular space contracts, leading to a ventilation–perfusion imbalance. This leads to inadequate peripheral perfusion and lactic acidosis. The prolonged poor perfusion results in cell damage and microthrombosis in the capillaries.

To effect the resuscitation, large volumes of salt-containing fluid are given, resulting in a weight gain of 15–20%, making the chest wall heavy and hard to move. This excursion may be further limited by an unyielding, leathery burn eschar encasing the anterior thorax. Unless severe smoke inhalation occurs, there does not appear to be altered permeability in the lungs, so lung water is not usually increased. However, excessive amounts of resuscitation fluids can result in pulmonary oedema and worsen outcome. The level of the diaphragm may be elevated by a reflex gastrointestinal ileus, further decreasing intrathoracic volume.

Burns victims frequently exhibit hyperventilation. Ventilation is about twice normal, with minute volumes up to 14 litres at a ventilatory rate of 20 breaths/min. This is due to increased oxygen demands and increased carbon dioxide production, as the body enters the hypermetabolic phase, and to a ventilation–perfusion imbalance. In addition, patients with burns of 40% TBSA or more may develop restrictive disease with a mild to moderate decrease in lung volume, a decreased vital capacity and an increase in pulmonary resistance.

Gastrointestinal response

The initial response of the gastrointestinal tract to a major burn is a reflex ileus due to splanchnic vasoconstriction. Acute gastric dilatation, vomiting and aspiration can occur. As soon as the ileus resolves, which is usually within 2–4 days, it has been the custom to initiate enteral alimentation. However, experience in the past decade has shown that enteral feedings can be initiated immediately upon admission, with close sur-veillance of the gastric residual volumes by frequent aspiration of the nasogastric tube. Early nutrition delivered to the gastrointestinal tract can help to minimize the ileus. Prokinetic agents such as metoclopramide also aid the acceptance of feeding, as does placement of the feeding tube distal to the pylorus. Aggressive nutritional support delivers the markedly increased calorie requirements of the burns patient, and decreases the incidence of potential gastrointestinal complications. In the past, gastroduodenal mucosal ulceration was a frequent occurrence in the burns victim. This may not always be clinically evident. The ulcerations may not be due to true hyperacidity, but may relate to ischaemia of the gastric mucosa. Gastrin does not appear to be increased in the burns patient. However, the ulcerations seem to be due to a relative hyperacidity, and during the first 72 h postburn, patients seem to have a higher basal acid output than later in their burn course. **When enteral feeding is early and continuous, gastro-duodenal ulcerations are virtually eliminated.** This may be due to neutralization of gastric acid, but may also be attributed to direct nourishment of the gastrointestinal mucosa.

Liver function is altered following thermal injury. These changes are probably due to decreased splanchnic circulation and hypoxia, and the effects of toxic waste products. Liver biopsies have shown cloudy swelling and evidence of glycogenolysis as early as 3 h after injury. Overfeeding will lead to hepatic steatosis and should be avoided.

Musculoskeletal response

Direct injury to the fascia, tendon, muscle and outer cortex of bone can occur at the time of burning. Localized or generalized osteoporosis and demineralization may result from the burn per se or be secondary to prolonged immobilization. New periosteal bone growth, myositis ossificans and heterotopic bone formation have all been reported in burns victims.

Neuroendocrine response

Adrenaline and noradrenaline are released in high amounts following thermal trauma. This would appear to be a protective mechanism, since the mortality is higher in burns victims who cannot sustain this increased response. However, catecholamine-medicated hypermetabolism, tachycardia and hyperdynamic cardiac activity may also lead to postburn cardiac dysfunction and death. To study this further, six severely burned patients were treated with intravenous propranolol in an attempt to decrease myocardial oxygen requirements, with apparent success. The adrenal cortex also responds with increased secretion of 17-hydroxycorticosteroids. These corticosteroids remain elevated as in a standard stress reaction until the patient is healed. Mineralocorticoids, specifically aldosterone, increase to conserve the decreasing sodium ion to the third space at the time of injury. This helps to prevent hypovolaemia by conserving sodium ions.

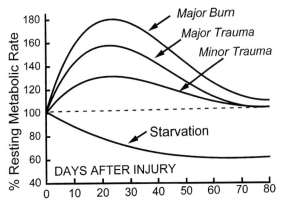

Figure 4.6 The metabolic rate is markedly elevated in burns patients, more so than in comparison groups of traumatized, non-burned individuals. The elevated metabolism can extend well into the rehabilitative period.

Metabolic–nutritional response

The metabolic rate of the burns victim is greatly accelerated (Figure 4.6). Oxygen consumption is increased and nitrogen losses are magnified. Associated with this hypermetabolic response are protein catabolism, ureagenesis, lipolysis and increased gluconeogenesis (Figure 4.7). As the water-holding lipid in the skin is destroyed, evaporative water losses increase at tremendous energy expense. The resultant body cooling results in shivering, thus adding to energy demands. However, these mechanisms do not totally explain the hypermetabolism, and warming the environment or prevention of evaporative water losses by impermeable dressings do

not eliminate it. Excision of the burned tissue and immediate wound closure do not minimize the hypermetabolism (Figure 4.8).

The hypermetabolic state following burn injury results in profound catabolism with decreased glucagon:insulin ratios and extreme intracellular cation alterations. Muscle breakdown weakens the skeletal muscles, including the muscles required for ventilation. The negative nitrogen balance accompanying hypermetabolism can result in nitrogen requirements of up to 20 g of nitrogen per square metre of TBSA burn per day during the first month after the burn. This nitrogen need results from both increased protein catabolism and decreased protein synthesis.

Counter-regulatory hormones, glucagon, cortisol and catecholamines are elevated in patients with burns and are believed to play a major role in mediating the catabolic response to injury. These endocrine mediators, working with various inflammatory mediators released from the burn wound, appear to be responsible for the various metabolic responses that occur after a major burn. Cytokines such as TNF and IL-1 also appear to play a role in the catabolic response to burns.

Monitoring of the hypermetabolic state and determination of caloric needs in the burns patient have been problematic. The calculation of nitrogen balance by measuring nitrogen intake (easy) and nitrogen output (difficult) is fraught with errors. More recently, continuous metabolic monitoring by equipment that measures oxygen consumption and carbon dioxide production appears to yield more reproducible results

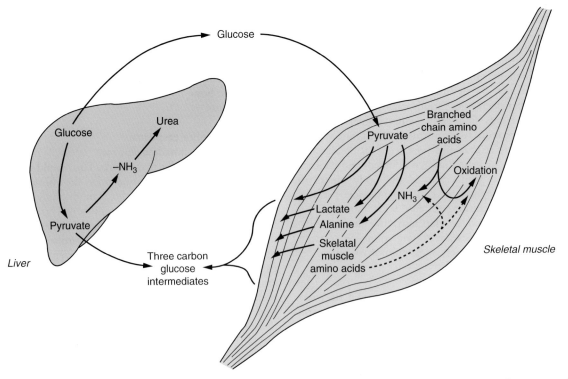

Figure 4.7 The catabolic response to injury results in breakdown of muscle protein and shunting of three carbon fragments to the liver for gluconeogenesis. This response is only partially blunted by aggressive feeding.

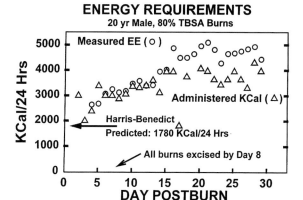

Figure 4.8 Continuous daily metabolic expenditures were measured by a metabolic monitor in this 20-year-old male who sustained mostly full-thickness flame burns over 80% of his body. Even though all burns were excised by day 8 postburn, and in spite of aggressive enteral nutritional support, the metabolic rate continued to climb and remained elevated. This patient's metabolic rate rose to 250% compared with baseline levels calculated by the Harris–Benedict equation. EE, energy expenditure.

(Figure 4.8). However, this equipment is only useful in patients who are connected to ventilators.

There was hope that the metabolic rate could be lessened by early wound excision and closure, but intense metabolic monitoring of burns patients indicates that the hypermetabolic state continues and can even increase after wound closure, as shown in Figure 4.8.

Immune response

The systemic immune responses are altered by burn injury. Defects have been identified in both the cellular and humoral immunological defence mechanisms. Impaired cellular immunity is suggested by an overall lymphopenia with a relative increase in T-suppressor cells, a decrease in IL-2 and delayed rejection of allograft skin. The decreased number of lymphocytes is further altered by a decreased responsiveness of peripheral blood lymphocytes to T-cell mitogens. An increase also occurs in immunosuppressive substances in burn sera that participate in the generation of suppressor T-cells. Potential lymphocyte suppressor substances identified are arachidonic acid metabolites, interferons, bacterial endotoxin, cutaneous 'burn toxin', denatured protein, metabolic hormones (corticosteroids), neutrophil products, vasoactive amines (histamine), serotonin, serum proteins (immunoglobulins), immune complexes, α-globulins, complement and antibiotics (parenteral and topical). Humoral defects such as depression of the immunoglobulins and complement titres have been documented. Isolation of an immunosuppressive peptide from burns victims' serum has shed light on immune system abnormalities.

There are other changes in host defences following thermal injury. Some aspects of the inflammatory reaction are depressed; neutrophil chemotaxis is inhibited and phagocytosis is less than optimal. In addition, once phagocytosis occurs, intracellular killing of microorgan-

isms is diminished. However, neutrophil intracellular accumulation of oxidant intermediates, such as superoxide anion and hydrogen peroxide, increases. The increased production of oxidant species has been implicated in tissue injury by extravasated neutrophils, leading to progression of the local burn injury, acute lung injury and multiple organ failure. The inflammatory responses may be more important in determining outcome from burns than alterations in T-cell and humoral immunity.

Psychiatric response

Victims respond to the psychological stresses attendant with major trauma in individualized patterns. These patterns may be more dependent on the patient's preburn personality than on a specific response to the burn injury. Situational depression is a uniform response, but true psychosis is unusual. Temporary toxic psychotic symptoms can accompany the other physiological alterations such as shock, hypoxia, water imbalance, electrolyte disturbance and sepsis. Iatrogenic factors such as inadequate relief of pain and anxiety, injudicious use of drugs and sleep deprivation can all trigger various responses of the psyche.

The above responses can be expected from any major burn. Other local and systemic alterations are seen as complications occur. These will be discussed in the section on 'Complications'.

Emergency department treatment

The initial treatment of the burns victim is contingent upon proper evaluation and the understanding of the local and systemic pathophysiological alterations. The same attention to cardiorespiratory function, haemorrhage and associated injures given to any trauma patient must be directed to the burns victim.

The emergency department treatment will depend on the category of burn. Minor burns can be treated in an ambulatory setting. For these patients, the treatment consists of tetanus prophylaxis and analgesia. In patients who have had effective tetanus immunization within the past 10 years, a tetanus toxoid booster should be administered. In patents not previously immunized against tetanus, human antitetanus immune globulin should be given for passive protection and standard active immunization begun. In the minor burn wound, true burn wound sepsis is rare. It has long been the custom that penicillin is necessary in the early burn period for avoiding infection from virulent β-haemolytic *Streptococcus*. However, careful studies have shown that prophylactic treatment with penicillin or other antibiotics does not alter the clinical course in major or minor burns. Topical antibacterials are unnecessary for burns of limited size. The wound needs only to be cleaned with a bland soap and carefully dressed. In smaller wounds, the decision as to whether or not to debride blisters is a matter of individual preference. The wound can be easily dressed by applying a non-adhering gauze next to the wound followed by a bulky absorptive dressing. The parts should be immobilized in a safe functional position and the injured extremity elevated if possible. The wound then must be inspected at 24 h and periodically until healing occurs. The minor burn will usually be a superficial partial-thickness injury and thus be quite painful. Therefore, a consideration of analgesia completes the initial treatment.

Moderate and major burns require hospitalization. Therefore, the emergency department treatment is not definitive. It is important that the initial emergent care does not complicate later definitive treatment. Immediate treatment of the impending vascular collapse is begun by introducing a plastic catheter into a peripheral or central vein, preferably through unburned skin. Cut-downs are rarely necessary. Blood is drawn for cross-match, blood count, electrolytes, glucose, creatinine and urea nitrogen. Arterial blood gases and pH are obtained if there is any suspicion of inhalation injury or respiratory dysfunction; monitoring of the blood acid–base balance will also aid the fluid resuscitation. An infusion of electrolyte solution is begun at a rate dependent on the size of the burns, as discussed in the next section. Initial monitoring of the resuscitation is performed by inserting an indwelling urinary catheter attached to a closed draining system.

Following airway stabilization and the initiation of resuscitation, the adequacy of respiration is evaluated. If respiratory distress is present, an early cause could be a deep burn with an unyielding eschar about the anterior and lateral chest walls. When present, it is relieved by a chest escharotomy to release the restriction of rib motion and increase thoracic excursion, thus improving ventilatory function. Inhalation of steam or noxious gases can cause epiglottal or pharyngeal oedema, resulting in upper airway obstruction requiring intubation; either the oral or nasal tracheal route may be utilized. Tracheostomy is best avoided in the emergency treatment unless mandated by associated injuries such as severe facial fractures.

An encircling eschar can cause vascular embarrassment to the extremities owing to the development of subcutaneous oedema in the presence of a stiff, inelastic burn eschar. Elevation of the extremities can help to limit tissue oedema, but a surgical escharotomy may be necessary. The need for release to prevent avascular necrosis and the adequacy of escharotomy can be monitored by repeated checking of distal capillary refill or by the use of a Doppler flow meter. Tissue compartment pressures can be monitored simply by hooking up an 18-gauge needle to a pressure tubing and a pressure transducer, and inserting the needle into the tissues. Tissue pressures of 30 mmHg or greater indicate the need for immediate escharotomy to preserve the limb.

Relieving pain and anxiety should be considered once the state of shock and the respiratory status have been evaluated. Analgesics are given intravenously since intramuscular absorption is unpredictable during the period of decreased cardiac output and massive fluid shifts. Small, frequently repeated dosages of narcotics and tranquillizers are quite effective; continuous infusion of short-acting agents such as fentanyl (a narcotic) and midazolam or lorazepam (sedatives) can be titrated to effect. For dressing changes, bolus doses may be added. These medications may contribute to decreased gastrointestinal motility, worsening the effect of splanchnic vasoconstriction in producing ileus. A nasogastric tube is used both for feeding and for monitoring gastric residual volumes.

Tetanus prophylaxis and antistreptococcal measures are instituted for moderate and major burns, as outlined for minor burns. However, further infection prophylaxis is necessary for the larger and deeper burn wound. Reverse isolation measures are used aseptically to begin the burn wound management. Cold saline or water for 15–20 min is helpful in decreasing oedema and pain in the wound. Blisters are best debrided since they are hard to maintain intact in the larger burn wounds. If the blister is broken, serum and desquamated cells form a crust that is susceptible to bacterial invasion. Following debridement, the wound is dressed with a topical antibacterial agent. In choosing the initial burn wound management, it is helpful to know the preferences of the physicians who will provide definitive treatment, since the various wound dressings have different advantages and disadvantages.

Once these initial steps are complete, consideration of transfer to a definitive care facility is undertaken. The sample categorization listed in Table 4.5 can help to determine where the patient will receive definitive care. Transfer procedures and treatments *en route* are best agreed on prior to the individual event, so that this aspect of the victim's care can proceed smoothly.

Definitive treatment

Resuscitative fluid management

Initial guidelines regarding the amount and rate of fluid replacement are provided by the weight of the patient and percentage of the TBSA injured. However, these are only guidelines and it is more important to understand the pathophysiology of decreased cardiac output and extracellular fluid volume loss. Rigid application of the various formulae that have been proposed is not useful and ignores the individual variability of patients.

To determine the resuscitative fluid replacement, it is important to realize that the greatest loss of fluid occurs during the first 8–12 h postburn and then continues more slowly over the next 12–16 h. Simultaneous measurements of the cardiac output, plasma volume and extracellular fluid have demonstrated that plasma volume replacement and the return of a normal cardiac output depend on the rate of fluid replacement. Because of the increased capillary permeability, colloid replacement seems to be of no benefit in the immediate postburn period. Osmotic pressure cannot be built up over a freely permeable membrane. Therefore, since sodium seems to be the ion that is lost to the circulation in disproportionate amounts, sodium ions (and not colloid) appear to be the key to resuscitation.

Many formulae have been advanced to predict how and when the sodium ion-containing solution is best administered. Critical analysis of the formulae reveals that the total volume replacement varies by only 2% over 48 h and the total millimoles (milliequivalents) of sodium vary by only 6% during the same period. All formulae give approximately 0.52 mmol of sodium/kg body weight/% body burn. In order to compensate for the obligatory loss from the vascular compartment, this must be given at a rate exceeding 4.4 ml/kg/h. When the sodium ion is replaced in this amount and at this rate, cardiac output returns to normal by 24 h postburn. This occurs whether the sodium ion is in a hypotonic, an isotonic or a hypertonic solution.

Following return of the cardiac output at 24 h, there remains a plasma gap. This amounts to approximately 0.35–0.5 ml/kg/% body burn. By 24 h capillary integrity returns and Starling's hypothesis appears to be restored. Therefore, colloid can be used to replete the plasma volume.

By 30 h, both cardiac output and plasma volume should be returned to normal and effective resuscitation completed. Further administration of sodium appears only to aggravate the oedema. Therefore, from 30 h until gastrointestinal peristalsis returns, free water can be given to maintain a normal serum sodium level and cover the obligatory insensible losses.

Acute resuscitation is begun with a buffered balanced salt solution given at a rate calculated at 2–4 ml/kg body weight times the per cent TBSA burn. Approximately half of this volume will be required in the first 8 h following injury, and the remaining volume in the succeeding 16 h. The administered volume is titrated hourly depending primarily on the urinary output but, in addition, the pulse and blood pressure, haematocrit and base deficit determined on blood gas analysis. Resuscitation is continued for 24 h and at that time dextrose and water replace the salt solution. Colloid is added to replace the remaining plasma volume deficiency. This approach covers all fluid, protein and electrolyte losses in the adult and generally leads to an adequately resuscitated patient. There is great variability in the response of patients to thermal injury, however, and continuous monitoring is essential.

Adequacy of fluid and electrolyte resuscitation is determined by clinical observation and not by the ability to fulfil an arbitrary formula. A urine output of 30–50 ml/h in the adult or 1 ml/kg/h in the child is the best monitoring parameter. If the urine output does not reach these levels, the fluid input must be increased. Urine flow in excess of these parameters prior to mobilization of the oedema reflects fluid overload. In addition to the urine output, the burns victim who is being adequately resuscitated should have a clear, lucid sensorium, a pulse rate less than 120 beats/min and a haematocrit less than 60%. Blood acid–base balance may be followed; a mild metabolic acidosis is tolerated but a progressive increase in the base deficit indicates the need for increased fluids.

The use of a central venous pressure-monitoring catheter and, in particular, Swan-Ganz monitoring of the pulmonary wedge pressure has not proved routinely useful in the acute resuscitation period. Because of the total body capillary leak and the tendency for the left ventricle to go in and out of failure for brief periods, these pressure indices do not necessarily reflect true intravascular volume.

In the child of 10 kg body weight or less, the maintenance fluid requirements are often greater than those required for burn loss replacement. Therefore, in these children the maintenance fluid requirements are calculated using 100 ml/kg body weight of a fluid containing 3 mmol sodium ion/100 ml and 2 mmol potassium ion/100 ml. In addition, 2 ml/kg/% body surface burn are required to replace the loss due to thermal injury. Plasma may be useful in infants to provide passive immunization, so one-quarter of their burn fluid loss may be replaced with plasma.

Respiratory management

Major burns victims should receive supplemental oxygen during the burn shock period. They should receive an inspiratory oxygen fraction (F_{I,O_2}) of 100% if there is evidence of carbon monoxide intoxication; high oxygen should be continued until the carboxyhaemoglobin (COHb) level falls to less than 5%. All patients with major burns should be monitored with periodic arterial blood gas determinations during the first 18–24 h postburn.

Upper airway oedema of the pharynx, epiglottis and vocal cords is evaluated. This is easily done by indirect laryngoscopy or, when available, by fibreoptic bronchoscopy. If mild oedema is noted, intermittent positive pressure breathing with a bronchodilator may be a useful adjunct to the humidified oxygen. Meticulous pulmonary toilet must also be carried out. If significant laryngeal oedema is seen, intubation is recommended via the nasotracheal or orotracheal route with a low-pressure cuffed endotracheal tube.

Emergency escharotomy of the chest may be required if ventilatory pressures rise because of the stiff chest wall eschar and the underlying oedema. Electrocautery should be used if available to avoid excessive haemorrhage. An effective escharotomy may require multiple incisions in both the vertical and transverse directions and the incisions may need to extend into the neighbouring unburned tissues.

These measures should suffice for the uncomplicated burns victim. Patients with inhalation injury or who develop progressive pulmonary insufficiency or other respiratory problems will be discussed under 'Pulmonary complications'.

Metabolic and nutritional needs

To overcome the negative nitrogen balance attendant with the major burn, at least 20 g of nitrogen/m^2 body surface area burn/day during the first month postinjury and approximately 15 g N$_2$/m^2/day during the second month must be given to the patient. Since maintenance of the burns victim in a cool, dry environment adds to the metabolic needs and nitrogen catabolism, it is best to avoid this. Environmental temperatures between 32 and 34°C have been demonstrated to decrease the urinary excretion of nitrogen.

In addition to the protein needs, non-protein calories must be provided. A popular formula to estimate nutritional needs has been to give 25 kcal/kg body weight plus 40 kcal/% body surface area burn to the adult. In many cases this will lead to excessive caloric delivery, and caloric needs are decreased if adequate protein is delivered. The child needs more calories/kg body weight and the infant needs as much as 90–100 kcal/kg. Feeding regimens that utilize high calories and inadequate protein may not improve nitrogen balance and may promote hyperglycaemia and excessive carbon dioxide production. A high protein diet containing a calorie:nitrogen ratio of 100:1 appears to help to counter the hypermetabolic response and achieve nitrogen balance. In the victim with a major burn, the nutritional requirements are best met by administering continuous enteral feeding via a nasogastric tube or feeding tube. Solutions containing up to 1.5 kcal/ml with an osmolar concentration of not more than 600 are well tolerated. This regimen decreases the need for parenteral hyperalimentation. In fact, parenteral nutrition increases the mortality in burns patients and should be utilized only as a last resort.

Vitamin supplementation and fat must be provided. One gram of ascorbic acid, 50 mg of thiamine, 50 mg of riboflavin and 500 mg of nicotinamide plus twice the daily requirements of vitamins A and D appear to be sufficient. The standard tube feedings contain adequate amounts of fat but elemental diets and parenteral regimens may be deficient. Trace metals must also be provided if less than full tube feedings are used for alimentation.

As noted in the 'Response' section, continuous metabolic monitoring of patients who are on ventilators appears to be most effective in predicting caloric needs on a daily basis (Figure 4.8).

Protecting the gastrointestinal tract

Even though the complications of the gastrointestinal tract are not due strictly to true hyperacidity following burns, controlled studies have shown that neutralization of the gastric contents and maintenance of the gastric pH above 7.0 protects against clinically significant complications of stress ulceration (antacids or H_2 blockers). However, the greatest protection is offered by starting enteral alimentation at the earliest opportunity.

Immune considerations

The concept of using immunotherapy to prevent or correct the defects in host response has been popular, although evidence of beneficial effects is limited. The early use of whole blood or plasma may passively affect the immune response but this has not been of documented value except possibly in infants. γ-Globulin

injections have also been tried in children at a dose of 1 ml/kg body weight on alternate days during the first week postburn.

The use of hyperimmune or convalescent serum to provide passive immunization has been documented experimentally. However, this carries the risk of allergic reaction or anaphylaxis, as does the use of any antiserum. Active immunization by vaccination has had several recent trials. If this is used for specific bacterial species such as *Pseudomonas aeruginosa*, it must be a polyvalent vaccine because of the tendency for new strains emerging for which the vaccine is not effective. Even large clinical series reporting the use of polyvalent vaccines have concluded that active immunization is not a very effective means of preventing the infectious complications in the burns victim.

One of the most useful and practical means of boosting the immune system is by providing adequate nutritional support. Failure of the body's response to common skin antigens and prolonged acceptance of skin allografts have been used as proof of impaired cellular immunity in the burns victim. Anergy can be best treated by preventing or correcting the negative nitrogen balance, which is best done by enteral feeding. Similarly, the well-nourished patient appears to reject skin allografts at a normal rate. Therefore, close attention to metabolic and nutritional needs will serve a double purpose.

The burn wound

Attention to the burn wound must not take precedence over the life-saving support of other systems in the burn wound victim. Therefore, discussion of the treatment of the burn wound has been reserved to this point. However, the *sine qua non* of treatment of the burns victim is treatment of the wound itself, and the eventual success or failure of how the other systems respond will depend on how well one treats the burn wound. Proper treatment of the wound begins with causing no harm to the injured cells so that any tissue still viable after the initial thermal event can survive. As these protected, surviving, injured cells are recovering, the necrotic cells not capable of recovery must be removed and replaced. **Closure of the wound with viable tissue or cells to provide a functional and aesthetically satisfactory coverage as rapidly as possible is the goal of burn wound treatment**.

Initial cooling, cleaning and debridement of the burn wound were discussed above under 'Emergency department treatment'. The definitive care team must determine which part of the wound is non-viable and when the wound should be closed. Determination of wound viability and predicting healing is one of the most difficult problems facing the burn surgeon. No method to determine the depth of burn is absolute. Therefore, since it is important to cause no harm to the remaining viable cells, an absolute approach to burn wound management is difficult. This is not a serious problem in the small circumscribed burn wound or even in one up to 15–20% of TBSA. For these wounds, if one feels that they include dead cells deep into the reticular dermis even though they may not be full thickness, one is justified in early excision of the necrotic tissue and closure of the wound.

Excision of burn wounds and grafting are now performed reasonably early after injury. Although massive wound excisions can be performed, many centres limit the wound area excised and grafted during one procedure to 20% of body surface area. Excisions are associated with significant and in some cases extensive blood losses. When excisions are performed relatively early, bleeding is generally less than when excision is delayed for a week or longer. The early burn is still in the ischaemic phase and haemorrhage is limited. Early burn excision and wound closure have essentially eliminated burn wound sepsis as a clinical problem.

Based on the concentric zones of injury elucidated by Jackson, an intradermal or a tangential excision has evolved, first reported by Janzekovic in a clinical series of 4370 patients treated by tangential excision and grafting 3–5 days postburn. She lists as advantages for this method:

- removal of only necrotic tissue
- salvage of injured tissue that would otherwise have progressed to necrosis
- preservation of the biological properties of the dermis
- prevention of contractures by immediate skin grafting.

In addition, when the amount of donor site tissue is limited, this technique can remove necrotic tissue to the level of viable cells and temporary coverage can be provided while the surviving deep dermal elements recover to provide skin continuity. This approach is presently the standard practice in many burn centres in the USA. However, the timing of excision still varies greatly.

The theoretical advantage of full-thickness excision of truly necrotic skin and partial-thickness excision of deep dermal burns is ideal for the treatment of the burn wound. Tangential excision increases blood losses, and direct excision to fascia in large, full-thickness burns minimizes blood losses but requires more operative time. It is also deforming, since all subcutaneous tissues is removed. For the large, partial-thickness injury, tangential debridement should be beneficial. In most centres it has appeared to reduce the morbidity and mortality. However, all the theoretical advantages are difficult to attain in the practical clinical situation. Removal of **only** dead tissue is not easy. In fact, several pathological studies have been reported showing that up to 50% of the tangential shavings contain viable skin. Bleeding can be of staggering amounts and portals of infection are opened if the tangential debridement is performed after the wound has been colonized. Graft take in controlled studies has been documented to be suboptimal on the tangentially excised wound. However, the decreased mortality, decreased hospital stay and increased cost-effectiveness suggested by propo-

nents of this treatment have shown its effectiveness in centres that have the necessary expertise and support.

When the burn wound exceeds 35–40% of the body surface area, full-thickness excision and autografting become an arithmetic problem. Available donor sites for coverage decrease as the size of excision increases, and subsequently skin substitutes are often required.

Since determination of definitely non-viable tissue is difficult and the various types of excision and closure have not proved to be a panacea in all centres, an alternative approach is available. This approach allows the patient to be supported while the burn wound evolves and reversibly injured cells heal. It demands protection of the wound from bacterial invasion, the major deterrent to healing. The skin is never sterile and cannot be readily sterilized. It is colonized by both resident and transient flora. These bacteria are in the depths of the skin, in tubules of sebaceous glands and around hair follicles. Therefore, cultures of the skin surface rarely reflect the skin's bacterial population. For major burns, topical antimicrobials are used to prevent an increase in colonization from exogenous transient flora or proliferation of resident flora to levels sufficient to cause burn wound sepsis.

The choices for burn treatment include excision with skin dressing as previously discussed, occlusive dressings, exposure and semi-open techniques with topical chemotherapy. True occlusive dressing methods are infrequently used today. To be effective, the dressing must be carefully constructed and applied using meticulous aseptic technique. Following careful cleaning and debridement of the wound, an inner layer of fine mesh or impregnated gauze is placed next to the burn to allow drainage. Next, a bulky absorptive material is applied and carefully immobilized by a non-distensible inelastic wrap. The dressing remains intact to protect the wound and is only changed if wound exudate soaks through it, or odour, pain or fever demands wound inspection. This method is based on the concept of protecting the wound from exogenous bacteria. However, since all skin contains a bacterial level of 10^3 organisms/g of tissue, the occlusive dressing does not prevent multiplication of these organisms in a warm, moist environment or wound sepsis from endogenous sources.

To reverse the problem seen with occlusive dressings, exposure therapy was introduced in the UK by Wallace in 1949. With this method, a dry eschar forms over the burn wound and acts as a physiological dressing. This prevents access of bacteria to the underlying wound and the dryness of the eschar will not support bacterial growth on its surface. To use this method, a reverse isolation technique is necessary to attempt to decrease the exposure to exogenous contamination, especially during the time required for eschar formation. In Sweden, circulating warm air beds hasten the eschar formation.

Several major disadvantages prevent universal acceptance of this method. As with the occlusive dressing method, the only bacteria from which the victim is protected are those from exogenous sources and these are not the major offenders. The eschar does not remain an intact barrier but often develops cracks that break the theoretical barrier. In addition to not being a totally effective means of infection prophylaxis, there is evidence that desiccation of the injured cells in the zone of stasis is deleterious to their survival and that burn wounds treated by exposure become deeper over the first 24–48 h. Chiefly because neither the occlusive dressing nor the exposure methods were effective in preventing the complications of burn wound sepsis, the semi-open technique with topical chemotherapy has evolved. Once it was realized that the prevention of infection in the burn wound involved the maintenance of an equilibrium between endogenous as well as exogenous bacteria and factors of host resistance, it became obvious that the goal was to prevent the numerical proliferation of bacteria. As the balance of bacteria is upset by the burn injury, organisms proliferate to levels greater than 10^5 organisms/g of tissue and migrate through the tissue. These proliferating organisms surround and occlude blood vessels, leading to thrombosis and an avascular burn wound sepsis. Topical chemotherapy seems to be the only rational approach to prevent the numerical proliferation of bacteria and, therefore, is the mainstay of infection prophylaxis in most centres today.

Any topical chemotherapeutic agent suitable for treatment of the burn wound should prevent desiccation, not produce pain, be non-allergenic and non-toxic and, most importantly, be bactericidal but not injure viable cells in the burn wound. Unfortunately, none of the topical agents currently available fulfils all of these criteria. All have advantages and disadvantages. **None has totally prevented bacterial proliferation. The three most commonly used topical chemotherapeutic agents world-wide are silver sulfadiazine, silver nitrate solution and mafenide acetate.**

Regardless of the topical agent chosen to be used in the semi-open method for infection prophylaxis, its efficacy should be monitored by constant surveillance of the bacterial flora of the burn wound. This is most effectively achieved by quantitative and qualitative analysis performed on burn wound biopsies. The bacteria isolated from the biopsies can be tested against the various topical agents available. The test bacteria are spread over an agar plate and the topical chemotherapeutic agents are placed into wells in the agar. Zones of inhibition predict an agent's effectiveness. Using objective results of bacterial control, one can decide which agent is best for a given victim at a given time. The problem with this approach is that testing of the topical agents is not as easy as for standard antibiotics, since agents such as silver sulfadiazine are relatively water insoluble and do not diffuse through the agar.

There is no chemotherapeutic agent of choice and there can never be one. The bacterial flora of a given wound in a given burns unit are continuously changing and must be monitored for effective infection prophy-laxis. Microbial resistance to silver sulfadiazine, in particular, has become common.

If early excision of the necrotic tissue is not elected and topical chemotherapy is the method of burn wound treatment, the non-viable tissue still must be removed. Historically, eschar separation occurred spontaneously between 10 and 14 days postburn. This spontaneous separation was due to bacterial autolysis in the subeschar spaces. Successful control of wound sepsis by topical chemotherapy has resulted in prolonged adherence of the eschar. Therefore, it is necessary to make a definitive plan to remove the necrotic tissue as soon as non-viability has been established. Physical removal of the non-viable tissue may take the form of full-thickness excision, intradermal debridement, daily surgical cleaning of the loosening eschar or enzymic dissolution of the eschar.

Daily debridement following removal of the topical agent can be carried out in hydrotherapy, in a dedicated treatment room or at the bedside. The eschar will gradually soften and the non-viable tissue can be gently debrided. Pain medication must be administered as necessary. Enzymic agents periodically gain popularity as a means to debride necrotic tissue. These enzymes are used to digest denatured collagen and other dermal material while sparing viable collagen. A major deterrent to their use is the potential accelerated bacterial proliferation when enzymes are used to dissolve the eschar. This tendency towards sepsis can be controlled if the enzymic agent is used concomitantly with topical antibacterial agents, or when wound areas are limited to approximately 10% of the body surface area.

Once the necrotic tissue has been removed from the burn wound, either in the first few days or up to 10–14 days later, closure can proceed. If the injury is superficial partial thickness in depth, closure will occur spontaneously by regeneration from epidermal elements in the dermis. The deep partial-thickness and full-thickness defects will require closure by autografts. When donor sites are not sufficient for autograft coverage, temporary closure of the burn wound is achieved with biological dressings. These temporary biological dressings applied to the burn wound render it less painful, reduce fluid and protein loss from the wound surface and preserve bacteriological control while donor sites re-epithelialize prior to reuse.

Allograft skin, xenograft skin and amniotic membranes have been demonstrated to be effective as temporary biological dressings. The material most widely accepted for extensive wounds is cadaver allograft, available in fresh, frozen or preserved forms from local or distant tissue banks. These materials are applied to the burn wound following removal of the eschar and remain in place from 48 to 96 h. Unfortunately, the use of human tissues presents the problem of potential transmission of viral diseases such as hepatitis and acquired immunodeficiency syndrome (AIDS). Consequently, synthetic and biosynthetic dressings are becoming more important and more available in serving as temporary skin substitutes. Among these is a bilaminate composite dressing comprised of nylon mesh and silicone bonded to a collagen peptide coating. A variant of this is the use of the same material incorporating laboratory-grown human fibroblasts to form a 'tissue' analogue. It must be remembered that these biological and biosynthetic dressings are only temporary, and permanent closure with autograft skin is the ultimate goal of burn wound treatment.

Sheets of autograft skin should be used for permanent wound closure whenever possible. Priority areas for grafting should be the face, especially the eyelids, the neck, the hands and the various flexion creases of the body, e.g. the popliteal and antecubital fossae. When donor sites are limited, the sheet graft can be meshed so that it can be expanded from 1.5 to nine times its original size. Meshed grafts are a compromise to the best wound closure and should not be used on the face. Successful skin grafting requires that the grafts be applied to a satisfactory bed; that is, a bed that contains 10^5 or fewer bacteria of tissue and no streptococci. This can be determined preoperatively by quantitative and qualitative bacterial cultures of tissue biopsies from the wound bed. It also can be predicted by the successful application of a skin allograft applied as a test or a prognosticator of autograft acceptability. Following application of the autograft to a properly receptive bed, several days of immobilization are necessary. This combination of therapeutic manoeuvres should result in greater than 95% success in permanent closure of the burn wound.

Preservation of function

Successful treatment of the burns victim means not only survival but also the return to society as a functional human being. Contraction is a normal component of wound healing. Fibroblasts with contractile properties are found in the granulating wound following thermal injury. If the contracture is severe enough, a pathological contracture results. Prevention of contracture, therefore, becomes an important part of the definitive care of the burns victim. Prevention is more desirable and effective than later correction of deformity. The principles of prevention of contracture and preservation of function are practised immediately upon admission. These include splinting in the optimal position at all times to avoid contracture. Larson has shown that the position of comfort is the position of contracture and that the burn wound will shrink until it meets an opposing force. Positioning, splinting and range-of-motion exercises are begun immediately and continued until wound closure.

At the time of wound closure, adequate amounts of skin are applied while maintaining the proper positioning and splinting. Following adherence of the grafts, prolonged pressure is applied by specially constructed elastic garments. The pressure appears to reduce hypertrophic scarring, increase pliability and preserve contouring. Splints are maintained, especially at night, and range-of-motion exercises continued until the newly healed collagen has matured. By maintaining a closely regulated schedule for 9 months to 1 year following

wound closure, a much more functional result is obtained and the need for reconstructive procedures markedly reduced.

Common complications due to burn injuries

The previous section discussed treatment of the major burns victim when only the normal physiological responses to thermal trauma were present. Complications can occur in every physiological system secondary to burn injury. Many of these complications are unique; thus, their management must be understood to care successfully for the burns victim.

Renal failure

Acute renal failure can occur only after prolonged and profound shock from unrecognized or untreated hypovolaemia following the thermal burn. It should rarely occur if the principles of resuscitation are understood. Following an acute burn, oliguria or anuria should not be diagnosed as renal failure but only as insufficient volume replacement. Increasing the resuscitation solution to an adequate amount to achieve 30–50 ml/h urine flow will maintain renal function. If fear of overloading is present, central venous pressure or pulmonary wedge pressure can be monitored. Only if filling pressures are high should the increased rate of resuscitation be slowed. This may occur particularly in the elderly, who may have poor cardiac function. Diuretics are of little help in this situation and should be reserved until hypovolaemia is fully corrected.

Inhalation injury

Inhalation of heat, noxious gases and incomplete products of combustion may be the most lethal component of thermal injury. Several syndromes are associated with inhalation and cause complications to the pulmonary response. The first group of victims develops pulmonary complications within moments of injury and often dies at the site of the fire. This is due to asphyxia because the combustion consumes the oxygen available to the victim. Davies reported that the UK Fire Research Station has shown that the concentration of oxygen close to the seat of a fire can be as low as 2%. At this concentration, death ensues in 45 s. The problem is worsened because the oxygen-deficient inspired air contains carbon monoxide, which combines with the haemoglobin molecule, thus further decreasing the availability of oxygen to the tissue. COHb levels can reach 30 000 ppm, which causes death within minutes. Adding to the hypoxia is the inhalation of hydrocyanide contained in smoke. This causes rapid tissue hypoxia and profound metabolic acidosis.

Another immediate complication arising from inhalation is the oedematous response discussed in the previous section. This can become worsened if, in addition to the heat, noxious gases such as sulfur dioxide and hydrochloric acid are present to cause bronchial spasm. This combination of oedema, laryngeal spasm and bronchospasm often causes immediate death.

The next group of patients with pulmonary complications develops respiratory symptoms several hours after admission. These are the patients suspected on initial evaluation to have suffered significant inhalation injury. This group develops progressive hypoxia and hypercarbia, and may have high levels of COHb. Initial high-flow humidified oxygen may not suffice as treatment. Further hypoxaemia, restlessness, tachypnoea and wheezing occur. This degree of significant inhalation injury may be diagnosed by fibreoptic bronchoscopy or by a radioactive xenon lung scan. However, these are not necessary and a clinical diagnosis is suggested by an oxygen tension (Po_2) of less than 10 kPa (75 mmHg) within 72 h postburn in a well-resuscitated patient or a rapidly falling Po_2 in the presence of a slowly increasing carbon dioxide tension (Pco_2). In these patients, vital capacity, minute ventilation, maximum expiratory flow volume curves and effective compliance must be maintained. When high flow oxygen, continuous positive airway pressure (CPAP) mask and bronchodilators fail to cause improvement, intubation may be required. An increasing pulmonary resistance and right-to-left pulmonary shunt along with increased work of breathing may require mechanical ventilation. The goal of ventilation is to use the lowest $Fi_{,O_2}$ level possible to maintain a $Pa_{,O_2}$ greater than 7.3 kPa (55 mmHg). The $Fi_{,O_2}$ should be maintained at less than 40–50%. If this cannot be done, one must add positive end-expiratory pressure. Steroids have not been shown to be helpful in treating smoke inhalation and in several studies have been shown to be harmful. Secondary bacterial invasion of the injured lungs must be watched for and treated when it occurs, based on deep sputum cultures.

Other pulmonary complications may occur that are not necessarily related to inhalation. These are atelectasis, pneumonia, pulmonary emboli, emphysema, bronchiectasis, pneumothorax and pulmonary oedema. Therefore, meticulous toilet must be maintained throughout the course of treatment of the burns victim and bronchoscopy should be utilized when appropriate. Finally, respiratory failure can occur with systemic sepsis as part of the multiple organ failure syndrome. These patients require intubation and mechanical ventilation. However, despite high oxygen concentrations, high ventilatory pressures and increased positive end-expiratory pressures, the patient sometimes cannot be adequately ventilated and succumbs.

Complications of hypermetabolism and nutrition

A catecholamine-mediated hypermetabolism is manifested by tachycardia and hyperdynamic cardiac activity with resultant increase in the myocardial oxygen requirements. Although a degree of hypermetabolism is a normal response to injury, severe uncontrolled supermetabolism can be associated with death. A syndrome of hyperglycaemia, glycosuria, acute dehydration, shock, coma and renal failure may be seen. Hyper-glycaemia is common following trauma because of the increased catecholamine response and a decreased sensitivity to insulin. Combined with the hyperglycaemia resulting from the necessary high calorie replacement of a major burn, a syndrome of pseudodiabetes can occur. Careful monitoring of the blood sugar and liberal use of insulin usually can control the hyperglycaemia. A constant insulin infusion may be most efficacious.

Gastrointestinal complications

Despite the initial intubation and subsequent treatment with antacids, gastroduodenal ulceration occurs in upwards of 80% of patients with major burns. However, clinically significant bleeding is becoming less common as burn wound sepsis is controlled and enteral nutrition is established. Once bleeding occurs, it is usually brisk and difficult to control. Neutralization of gastric contents to above pH 7.0 may help. However, if bleeding cannot be rapidly controlled, operative intervention is necessary. Gastric resection is reported to be the most effective management of significant bleeding, except in children, in whom vagotomy and drainage have been successful.

Lower intestinal bleeding can also complicate the burn injury. Ulcers of the mucosa and muscularis mucosa of the colon have been reported. Colonoscopy can identify the source of bleeding. Intra-arterial pitressin may control colonic bleeding. The question of *Candida* in the aetiology of these ulcerations has been raised since it has not been seen in a centre where antifungal oral medication is a routine part of the management of all burns victims.

Enteral feeding appears to maintain the integrity of the gastrointestinal tract by an as yet undefined mechanism. An oral diet preserves gut mucosal mass and maintains digestive enzyme content. Other studies have verified that oral feeding stimulates the gut to elaborate trophic hormones. Enteral calories initiate greater insulin release than parenteral nutrition, and insulin appears to promote anabolism. Consequently, enteral feedings serve to protect the gastrointestinal tract, providing further indication for prompt institution.

In addition, bacterial translocation through the gastrointestinal tract has attracted attention as a source of infection and inflammation in trauma patients. This phenomenon has been studied in numerous animal studies. An exaggerated systemic inflammatory response, driven by endotoxin and cytokines, may contribute to hypermetabolism, catabolism, tissue injury and multiple organ failure. In a retrospective review of necropsies in burns patients by Desai *et al.*, (1991) 85 out of 161 adults and 30 out of 49 children were noted to have ischaemic intestinal pathological findings, ranging from superficial necrosis to full-thickness mucosal necrosis. More than 80% of these patients were septic at the time of death, with endogenous intestinal flora species most frequently identified as the causative agent.

Compression of the distal portion of the duodenum by the superior mesentery artery may result in partial or complete duodenal obstruction in the debilitated catabolic patient. This results in postfeeding fullness, bile-stained vomitus and failure to gain weight. The syndrome is entirely preventable by the initiation of prompt enteral feeding. Once the symptoms begin, the diagnosis is confirmed by cinefluoroscopy of the duodenum following ingestion of a barium meal. Treatment often can be effective by passing an intestinal tube by fluoroscopy beyond the obstruction and instituting enteral hyperalimentation. Failure to pass the tube requires parenteral hyperalimentation. If operation becomes necessary, a duodenojejunostomy relieves the problem.

Biliary stasis leading to acalculous cholecystitis may occur in the immobile burns victim who is being hyperalimented. It is rare in the burns patient who receives constant enteral nourishment. This syndrome should be suspected in patients with right upper quadrant pain, unexplained vomiting or fever of an unknown origin. It appears more commonly in patients with sepsis who may develop metastatic emboli to their gallbladder. Perforation can occur without warning and emergency cholecystectomy or cholecystostomy becomes necessary.

Hepatitis may occur in the burns victim who survives the initial hospitalization. Multiple blood transfusions add to the risk of infection with hepatitis B and C. In addition, multiple anaesthesias may be required during the course of management, exposing the patient to the dangers of drug-induced hepatitis. This complication must be considered during the convalescent period and 1 year postburn.

Infectious complications

The most frequent complications of the major burn are due to bacterial, viral or fungal infection. As infection in the burn wound is beginning to be understood and controlled, pulmonary infections have become the leading cause of morbidity and death. The pulmonary infection supervenes on the lung, which may already be compromised by the inhalation of noxious gases and smoke. These will not be reiterated here. World-wide, the leading infectious complication remains burn wound sepsis. However, in burn centres that practise early wound excision, generalized burn wound sepsis has become rare.

Burn wound sepsis is an imbalance in the normal equilibrium between microbes and host resistance, resulting in a vast numerical increase in microbes. As microbes increase from the normal level of up to 10^3 organisms/g of tissue to levels of greater than 10^5/g, they break out of the hair follicles and sebaceous glands and migrate through the tissue, colonizing the dermal–subcutaneous interface. Levels of growth in excess of 10^5 microbes/g of tissue constitute 'burn wound sepsis', and levels of 10^8–10^9 microbes/g may be associated with lethal burns. Surface swabs are deceptive since the process of proliferation occurs in the subeschar plane. Blood cultures may also be deceptive since lethal burn wound sepsis can occur without

spread of viable organisms into the blood stream and without secondary visceral lodgement. This is especially likely to be the case for Gram-negative organism burn wound sepsis. If the burn wound sepsis is due to Gram-positive organisms, bloodstream invasion is more likely, although negative blood cultures do not provide security.

Burn wound sepsis can occur from microbes arising in the wound from both exogenous and endogenous sources. Regardless of the source of microbes, quantitative bacterial cultures of wound biopsies have been a useful guide to management. These biopsies must contain the eschar-viable tissue interface. In addition, histological biopsies processed to determine the depth of invasion may be helpful, although these are less frequently utilized. The presence of microbes in adjacent unburned tissue determines invasive burn wound sepsis. There are clinical aids to the diagnosis; these include sudden discoloration or mottling of the burn wound, surrounding oedema and erythema, increased odour from the wound, and increased or greenish drainage. When gastric retention occurs after tube feeding has been well tolerated for some time or when residual amounts are increasing, the cause may be a developing ileus, which could herald burn wound sepsis, particularly caused by Gram-negative bacteria.

Several clinical signs suggestive of the systemic response to burn wound sepsis are valuable. Hyperthermia or hypothermia must be considered a possible sign of sepsis, especially if the temperature is greater than 39°C or less than 36.5°C. Pulmonary oedema or other evidence of acute respiratory distress in the patient who is not considered to be fluid overloaded may be secondary to wound sepsis. The onset of unexplained ileus after 48 h postburn is suggestive of sepsis. An onset of mental confusion or a mental status change requires that sepsis be considered. Finally, a deepening or worsening of the burn wound is probably due to microbial proliferation and invasion.

Laboratory aids that are helpful in diagnosing systemic sepsis include the presence of greater than 10^5 bacteria or fungi/g of tissue on biopsy of the wound or histological evidence of invasion of bacteria/fungi into normal tissue. Blood cultures are helpful when positive. Blood glucose levels have been helpful, since levels of over 7.28 mmol/l (130 mg%) are statistically associated with septicaemia from Gram-positive organisms, whereas the presence of a blood glucose of less than 6.16 mmol/l (110 mg%) suggests Gram-negative septicaemia. A reduced white blood cell count of less than 4000/mm^3 or a markedly elevated count of greater than 30 000/mm^3 suggests sepsis. Azotaemia without dehydration or history of nephrotoxic drugs is often associated with burn wound sepsis. In the immediate postburn period, thrombocytopenia and transient disseminated intravascular coagulopathy are common, but usually correct themselves by 24 h. The presence of thrombocytopenia, hyperfibrinogenaemia or fibrin split products in the blood after 24 h is an indication of sepsis.

The infections discussed up to this point have been bacterial in origin. Fungi and viruses may also cause infection in the burns patient. Prominent among these is *Candida*. *Candida* pneumonia and wound invasion has accompanied the increased use of prolonged courses of multiple antibiotics that disturb the patient's microbial ecology. The presence of *Candida* in the burn wound may not have clinical significance but the finding of it in the blood stream or in the urine of a non-catheterized patient should be considered an indication for antifungal therapy. Although exceedingly rare, the presence of a fluffy yellow exudate seen on the patient's retina is diagnostic of candidaemia. Viral burn wound sepsis also occurs. The reported cases carry an extremely high mortality. The presence of vesicular lesions at the periphery of the wound should raise the suspicion of viral invasion, which is most commonly herpes.

The treatment of burn wound sepsis begins with prevention. The standard treatment of debridement, tetanus prophylaxis, topical chemotherapy, timely removal of necrotic tissue and adequate enteral nutrition to maintain the immune response are all means of preventing burn wound sepsis. Since these measures have become routine in most burn centres, the incidence of burn wound sepsis has markedly deceased. The trend towards earlier excision and wound closure, especially when this can be effected with autograft skin, has helped to eliminate the severity of burn wound sepsis seen when eschar was allowed to remain in place for a period of weeks. However, if the bacteria proliferate to larger numbers in the burn wound, invasive sepsis into the systemic circulation must be treated. The early sign of invasion is at the subeschar uninjured tissue interface. Once systemic sepsis is present, the entire burns victim must be supported. Haemodynamic support is necessary to prevent vascular collapse. The cardiac decompensation, pulmonary oedema and respiratory distress may require intubation and ventilatory support. Nutrition must be maintained and this becomes difficult since ileus accompanies the sepsis. Parenteral alimentation may be necessary, but should only be instituted if all efforts at supplying enteral nutrition fail.

Systemic antibiotics are of little value in trying to control the bacterial or fungal levels in the burn wound following the oedematous phase. The vascular changes of the full-thickness burn with local occlusion of small vessels prevent the adequate delivery of potent systemic antibiotics to the foci of microbial growth. Even though they are not helpful in controlling infection confined to the burn wound, systemic antibiotics are necessary when systemic sepsis develops. Close monitoring of antibiotic blood levels is necessary because proper blood levels are difficult to maintain in the hypermetabolic burns victim.

The burn wound may require excision to control the septic focus. Other foci must be sought. Most common of these is suppurative thrombophlebitis. Where systemic sepsis occurs in the burns patient and the burn wound is not the source, all veins that have been previously cannulated should be examined and, if suspicious, should be opened or excised. Other foci of infection often overlooked in the burns victim are the heart valves and the meninges. Reports of acute bacterial endocarditis and meningitis are becoming more frequent as understanding of the burn wound infection control is improving. In addition, as mentioned above, the development of ileus demonstrated by difficulty in delivering enteral feedings or radiographic changes with bowel dilation merits consideration of ischaemic enteritis, with the possibilities of translocation of bacteria and perforation. Infection of indwelling catheters should be considered, and catheters should be changed frequently since their infection rate is exceedingly high in burns patients.

Catheter infections are frequent in burns patients, probably because of intermittent bacteraemia from the wounds and perhaps the gastrointestinal tract. Central catheters should be rotated frequently, at least every 72 h, between the subclavian, jugular and femoral regions. If catheters are rewired instead of fresh insertion sites chosen, it is good practice to monitor microbial counts on the catheter tips using quantitative bacteriology. A catheter tip which cultures 15 organisms is considered infected, and if that catheter was wired for placement of a new catheter, a new anatomic site should be chosen.

Differences seen in chemical burns and electrical injury

Chemical burns

Tissue damage secondary to a chemical depends on:

- the concentration of the agent
- the quantity of the agent
- the length of time for which the agent is in contact with the tissue
- the degree of tissue penetration
- the specific mechanism of action.

The principal difference between thermal burns and chemical burns is that with chemical burns, tissue destruction continues as long as contact is maintained unless the agent is inactivated by its reaction with the tissue. This means that chemical burns are usually deeper than they initially appear and progress with time.

The initial treatment of a chemical burn is dilution of the chemical with water. This is best delivered by continuous running water or by prolonged hydrotherapy in large volume tanks for as long as several hours. Care should be taken to avoid hypothermia. Neutralizing agents should not be used since they may cause exothermic reactions and thereby increase tissue damage. Following the initial dilution, local care of the wound with debridement, topical chemotherapeutic agents and eventual wound closure is the same as for the thermal burn. The exception is the chemical burn involving the eyes. These injuries require initial copious irrigation with saline and consultation with the ophthalmologist.

Electrical injury

Electrical injury is the result of the flow of electrons through a conductor. Electrons seek the path of least resistance through the conductor. Collisions of electrons with conductor particles change electrical energy into thermal energy or heat. If the conductor is tissue in the human body, this produces an electrical injury.

The effects of passage of an electric current through the body depend on the type of current, the voltage of the current, the resistance offered by the tissue, the amperage of current flowing through the tissue, the pathway of the current through the body and the duration of contact. The relationship between the current flow in amperage, voltage and resistance measured in ohms is expressed by Ohm's law (current = voltage/resistance). More importantly, the actual heat generated by passage of current through a conductor is determined by Joule's law (heat = voltage × current). Combining the two laws, one can predict the damage occurring with electrical injury. Tissue resistance to electrical current increases from nerve to vessel to muscle to skin to tendon to fat to bone.

Several types of injury are seen after contact with an electrical source. The arc injury is a localized injury caused by intense heat or flash at the termination of current flow. This often occurs on flexor surfaces of joints where current exits and re-enters skin, attempting to find the shortest pathway. The major type of injury is that due to heat generated as current flows through tissue. This type of injury is worse in tissue with high resistance. The vessels thrombose as current passes rapidly along them. The full extent of this type of current injury is insidious and not immediately appreciated. The third type of injury is the flame burn, which occurs if the heat generated from the electricity is high enough to cause ignition of the victim's clothing.

There are some special effects of electrical injury that differentiate it from other thermal trauma. Anoxia and ventricular fibrillation can cause immediate death. Although both early and delayed cardiac rhythm abnormalities may occur, there is increasing evidence that the presence of a normal electrocardiogram on admission is assurance that cardiac damage has not occurred and further cardiac monitoring is unnecessary. There is a risk of renal failure if severe muscle injury results in myoglobinuria, which can damage the renal tubules. This requires a higher urine flow (75–100 ml/h in adults) to 'wash out' the myoglobin from the tubules. The urine should be alkalinized to keep the myoglobin in a more soluble state. A problem arises since most clinical laboratories cannot differentiate haemoglobin from myoglobin in the urine sample; haemoglobin is far less toxic to the kidneys than is myoglobin. Tetanic muscle contractions accompany the passage of electricity and may be strong enough to fracture bones, especially the spine. Spinal cord damage can occur secondary to such a fracture, and spinal cord and peripheral nerve damage can also occur late owing to a delayed demyelinating effect of the current. Intraperitoneal damage can occur to the gastrointestinal tract secondary to the current,

and may lead to bowel perforation and peritonitis. Because of the progressive vessel thrombosis, electrical burns tend to deepen over days and delayed rupture of major vessels has been reported. Finally, late effects can accompany these injuries. Chief among these is cataract formation, which is delayed for days to months following injury.

Treatment for the victim of an electrical injury may begin with cardiopulmonary resuscitation if cardiac standstill or ventricular fibrillation occurs. Fluid replacement is begun with a buffered salt solution at a volume and rate to achieve a urine output of 75–100 ml/h. No type of replacement formula can serve even as a rough guideline because the injury is more extensive than can be predicted by the skin damage. Monitoring is generally easier in the electrical injury since total capillary permeability does not occur. Therefore, the use of central venous pressure monitoring is more helpful than in a major thermal injury in which capillary leaking is predominant. An osmotic diuretic such as mannitol may be prescribed if haemoglobinuria or myoglobinuria is present, although it is better to maintain high urinary flow with fluids alone, since diuretics may produce a rebound hypovolaemia. Associated injuries, such as bony fractures, must be treated. For wound management, the non-viable tissue is debrided early. This may have to be repeated as the progressive destruction continues. Intravenous fluoroscein and illumination of the wound with ultraviolet light have proven helpful in delineating viable and non-viable tissue at the time of debridement. The best topical chemotherapeutic agent for the electrical injury is one with the best penetrating ability and the one most effective against *Clostridia*. These characteristics describe mafenide acetate cream (Sulfamylon) better than other agents. Fasciotomies should be performed liberally if the underlying muscle compartments are oedematous. However, despite release of compression, vascular thrombosis frequently leads to major amputations since major vessels may be damaged.

Future trends for improving treatment of the burns victim

The greatest chance to improve statistics for burns victims in the future is prevention. Advances in the USA such as the routine use of non-flammable materials for children's nightclothes have reduced the severity of injury. Laws to make all clothes non-flammable seem to be an attainable goal. Similarly, legislation to govern the amount of heat delivered from household hot water systems would decrease the number of scald burns occurring in the home. Finally, fabrication standards to prevent public meeting areas from being constructed with materials known to produce toxic substances upon incineration will prevent severe smoke inhalation. More widespread use of sprinkler systems and smoke alarms in buildings will also decrease injuries. Burn-prevention educational efforts in the workplace can be increased.

Severe major blocks in solving the plight of the burns victims are obvious. All treatment and prognoses are based on the amount of injured tissue present. Although charts are available to determine the extent of the burn wound, these are prone to inaccuracies. New techniques of planimetry and computer analysis can lead to more accurate and reproducible mapping of the surface extent of the burn. However, there are still no effective means available to determine the depth of the wounds. Dyes such as fluoroscein have not been reliable at differentiating depth. Work with a fibreoptic perfusion fluorometer may improve this usage in the future. Reflected light imaging, laser Doppler fluorimetry, high-frequency ultrasonic imaging and portable xenon-133 washout scans are being evaluated as means to predict adequately which cells are non-viable postburn. Magnetic resonance imaging may prove valuable in evaluating the presence of viable versus non-viable tissue.

Once the amount of truly non-viable tissue can be determined, the zones of injury in the burn wound can be accurately delineated. It may be possible to manipulate pharmacologically the cells in Jackson's zone of stasis to increase their survival. Pilot studies in this field have shown that the progressive sludging and thrombosis in the zone of stasis are not affected by antisludging or anticoagulant drugs such as heparin or low molecular weight dextran. However, inhibitors of certain arachidonic acid metabolites seem to prevent sludging and decrease the progressive dermal ischaemia. Agents that inhibit prostaglandin and thromboxane synthesis can experimentally increase dermal perfusion and salvage the zone of stasis. Other mediators of the inflammatory response such as histamines, leukotrienes, vasoactive amines and free oxygen radicals have been demonstrated to be present in the burn wound early after injury. Understanding the role of these mediators and modulating their effects pharmacologically may significantly lessen the volume of tissue destroyed by thermal trauma.

Manipulation of the immune defence mechanisms may alter the course of the burns victim. Many of the immune defects seen following a major burn and thought to be inherent in the burn injury have been reversed by providing adequate nutrition to the patient. The study of several factors found in the serum of burns victims that result in immune suppression and cardiac dysfunction may lead to treatments that may improve survival. Immunomodulators that can specifically reverse various lymphocyte and phagocyte abnormalities seen following burns are being evaluated in clinical trials. Examples of immunomodulators being examined are various colony stimulating factors to treat the bone marrow, and inhibitors of cytokines such as TNF and various interleukins. However, it may be difficult to treat isolated immune defects in the burns victim, while other mediators continue to be active, and expect to improve patient outcome.

Finally, if a burn wound of any size could be covered without further stressing the burns victim, then the morbidity and mortality would rapidly diminish. The present need to use autograft skin is often the difference between survival and death. Several exciting experimental developments are underway. Epidermal and dermal cells are being grown in tissue culture, and sheets of cultured skin can be applied to the wound. Thus far, the process is very expensive and successful 'take' of the cultured grafts is frequently less than desirable. Further improvements in cultured skin are underway in many laboratories. The use of allograft skin (from cadaveric donors) has been shown to be useful as a temporary skin replacement, but it is eventually rejected. Artificial skins are being investigated in many laboratories and burn centres world-wide. Living dermal tissue composed of matrix supports of various types and containing cultured fibroblasts appears to improve the anchoring of keratinocytes to the wound surface. Another attempt for a skin substitute is the use of cadaver skin to cover the excised wound, followed several weeks later by scraping or dermabrasion to remove the antigenic epidermal layer. The dermal base can then accept a cultured graft or a thin-meshed autograft. These new substitutes for the victim's own skin may ease the plight of the burn surgeon.

Guide to futher reading

Desai, M. H., Herndon, D. N., Rutan, R. L. *et al.* (1991). Ischemic intestinal complications in patients with burns. *Surg Gynaecol Obstet* **172**, 247.

Jackson, D. McG. (1953). The diagnosis of the depth of burning. *Br J Surg* **40**, 588.

Infected patients

'In acute disease it is not quite safe to prognosticate either death or recovery' – Hippocrates, Aphorisms II, c. 460–377 BC

The biological factors involved in infection (infestation in the case of parasites) are:

▢ the virulence of the invading microbe
▢ the size of the infecting inoculum
▢ the state of the host's defence system.

At its most basic level, infection represents an adverse shift of balance in favour of microbial invasion that overwhelms the host defence system. In immunologically competent individuals the invasion is determined by the product of the virulence and the size of the inoculum of the pathogenic organisms. In immunocompromised patients low-virulence organisms and even commensals that are not normally considered pathogenic can obtain a foothold and cause serious infections [see Module 1, Vol. I].

Section 5.1 • Classification and consequences of infections

Classification

From a practical standpoint infections in surgical patients are best categorized as:

▢ community-acquired infections
▢ nosocomial (hospital) acquired infections that cover (i) common postoperative infections; and (ii) infections in critically ill patients, usually in intensive care units (ICU).

This distinction is important for various reasons, e.g. varying spectrum of infectious disease within the two settings, frequent presence of immune deficiency in hospital patients and significantly higher prevalence of infections by antibiotic resistant organisms in hospital-acquired infections.

Nosocomical (hospital-acquired) infections afflict 3–5% of patients and are the most important contributors to prolonged hospital stay, increased costs and death after surgical treatment. On average, a postoperative wound infection increases the costs of an operation by 300–400%. Infections that arise following discharge from hospital are not reported consistently and probably account for half of the infections after surgical treatment. These postdischarge infections have assumed greater importance to the overall assessment of surgical morbidity and costs with the significant increase in ambulatory and short-stay surgical care. A minimum of 45 days of follow-up is necessary to obtain a valid assessment of wound infection rates.

Community-acquired infections cover a wide range, with some being primarily medical in the first instance, e.g. respiratory infections, meningitis, acquired immunodeficiency syndrome (AIDS) and viral hepatitis, and others surgical, e.g. abscesses, appendicitis and peritonitis. Thus, surgical community-acquired infections require emergency surgical treatment [see Module 17, Vol. I].

Consequences of nosocomial infections

The importance of nosocomial infections is highlighted by the statistic that in 1990 they were the sixth leading cause of death in the USA, and hospital surveys indicate a rising incidence, with many being caused by antibiotic-resistant bacteria. In addition, nosocomial infections incur added costs and increase the discomfort and disability experienced by patients following elective operations. For patients who sustain serious injury and those who require critical care, infection is frequently lethal. The onset of bacterial or fungal infection contributes, as an independent causative factor, to the development of multiple organ systems failure.

Section 5.2 • Postoperative surgical infections

Evaluation of postoperative pyrexia

Pyrexia is a common feature of postoperative infections, although it may be absent in immunologically compromised patients. Its important features are:

- time of onset
- degree of pyrexia and type (persistent, intermittent)
- accompaniments, particularly rigors (shivering) and haemodynamic change.

Most early postoperative fevers are due to non-infectious causes, particularly pulmonary collapse. Early wound infections (occurring within 18–24 h) tend to be of a serious nature (see below). Rigors indicate bacteraemia or viraemia and always necessitate blood culture in addition to physical examination. A flushed appearance with a hyperdynamic circulation is also indicative of bacteraemia and usually signifies the early stages of septic shock. Intermittent pyrexia is indicative of an abscess.

If a patient develops a high temperature in the postoperative period, the following are necessary in all patients: physical examination of the lungs, wound, calves and urine. In addition, most would advise a chest X-ray. Leucocytosis is a feature of the early postoperative period when cultures are usually negative. Thus, these laboratory tests [white blood cell count (WBC), total and differential] and culture screen (sputum, urine, blood and wound) are undertaken on a selective basis and in response to specific clinical findings:

- fever that persists beyond the first 24 h
- fever that recurs after a period without fever (intermittent)
- fever that arises after the first 24 h
- fever accompanied by rigors, haemodynamic change or chest/abdominal signs.

Procurement of material for culture

This is an important practical aspect of management as it ensures valid culture results and aids recovery of organisms that are difficult to culture.

- The first principle is to retrieve an uncontaminated specimen in a sterile container that does not contain air if anaerobes are thought to be involved in the infection. Thus, material from intra-abdominal abscesses that often contains anaerobic organisms should be aspirated into a sterile syringe and all the air expelled. The specimen should then be transferred to an anaerobic transfer container or left in the syringe for direct inoculation into culture media in the bacteriology department.

- Gram staining of the infected material provides an important immediate evaluation while the results of culture are awaited.

- The request form accompanying the specimen should give sufficient details and, in particular, indicate the pathogens suspected whenever possible.

- Blood cultures should be obtained in duplicate, 20–30 ml per set obtained from different sites in adults. The skin overlying the venepuncture site should be scrubbed with antiseptic (povidone iodine) for 2 min beforehand and sterile gloves worn to prevent contamination.

- The wound surface should be cleaned with sterile water (not bacteriostatic saline) before obtaining the specimen, which is best obtained by scraping. Sometimes a small biopsy is needed for culture. Swabs of wounds or fluids are undependable, as they may not represent the fluid content of the wound accurately. Bullous lesions are aspirated after gentle surface cleaning.

- Body fluids (ascites, pleural effusions) are aspirated into a syringe after disinfection of the wound surface with povidone iodine.

- In some situations, quantitative cultures are needed, e.g. clean catch specimens of urine and burn sepsis.

Common spectrum of infection

The common postoperative infections include:

- wound infections [Module 18, Vol. I]
- pneumonia [Module 18, Vol. I]
- urinary tract infections
- central venous line infections
- intra-abdominal abscess
- infection of implanted material.

Urinary tract infections

These are most commonly associated with catheterization of the bladder (indwelling and 'in and out'). Symptoms include dysuria and frequency and, sometimes, the onset of incontinence. Loin pain and tenderness are only found in patients with severe upper urinary tract infections. The specific diagnosis of urinary infection is made with the recovery of more than 10^5 organisms per ml of urine. The most common organisms cultured in nosocomial urinary infections are *Escherichia coli*, *Pseudomonas aeruginosa* and coagulase-negative *Staphylococcus* spp.

Central venous line infection

This is encountered in 3–5% of patients who have monitoring lines in place and those receiving parenteral nutrition. Fever in such patients is an indication for inspection of the puncture site for signs of inflammation and for changing the line. For temporary lines removal and replacement to another site are indicated. Replacement over a guide wire may permit preservation of a valuable access site. Permanent lines may occasionally be salvaged, temporarily, by a course of systemic antibiotics. However, if signs of infection have not resolved completely within 48 h, the catheter should be removed. The tip of all removed catheters should be cultured. **The presence of more than 15 colonies is indicative of line infection.** Episodes of line sepsis can be prevented by meticulous attention to cleanliness of nutrition support lines [see Module 8, Vol. I].

Intra–abdominal abscess

Intra-abdominal abscess can arise in:

- patients undergoing a major operation involving the alimentary tract. The abscess results either from contamination at the time of surgery or from suture line leakage
- critically ill patients from failure of intraperitoneal host defences and the gut barrier function with translocation of intraluminal bacteria into the peritoneal cavity (sometimes referred to as **tertiary peritonitis**)
- patients with acute abdominal conditions requiring emergency operations, e.g. trauma, perforated viscus or severe gangrenous perforated appendicitis. These patients have a 6–10% risk of developing intra-abdominal abscesses.

Signs and symptoms of postoperative abdominal abscess usually arise between the fifth and tenth postoperative day and include intermittent fever, localized tenderness and absent bowel sounds. In some instances the abscess is palpable abdominally or rectally (pelvic collection). Persistent drainage from an abdominal wound infection that has been opened indicates that this is being fed from an intra-abdominal site. Patients with intra-abdominal abscess may develop signs of sepsis such as hypotension, hyperdynamic circulation, respiratory distress and other features of the multiple organ failure/SIRS syndrome.

Plain radiology may show an elevated immobile hemidiaphragm in patients with subphrenic abscess and visible gas may be seen, especially in patients who have sustained anastomotic dehiscence or have developed a pancreatic abscess, but diagnosis is nowadays based on ultrasound scanning and especially computed tomography (CT). Both are usually performed, one after the other. CT provides more detailed information on the precise location and anatomy of the abscess cavity.

CT-guided drainage is now used as the first line of treatment in these patients, with surgery being reserved for large multiloculated abscesses containing a large amount of slough. Systemic antibiotics are indicated to forestall the systemic effects of bacteraemia that may occur before, during or after the abscess drainage.

The key issue relates to the role of laparotomy in septic patients with SIRS and multiorgan failure. In the past, this was recommended in all these patients on the premise that the detection and evacuation of abscesses was followed by improvement or reversal in 50% of patients. This view is now not generally accepted, as the majority of patients with SIRS do not have an intra-abdominal focus of infection. The current consensus is that laparotomy is used selectively in patients who are in the early stages of the disease, especially those in whom the organ failure was precipitated by intra-abdominal infection in the first instance, i.e. detection of residual collections. Laparotomy is not indicated in patients in the late hypodynamic decompensated stage of the disease unless there are specific signs of intra-abdominal infection.

Infection of implanted prosthetic material

Infection is an ever-present risk when prosthetic material or implants are used, whether this is simple mesh for hernia repair or a more complex implant, e.g. joint prosthesis, vascular grafts, cardiac valves or pacemaker devices. The clinical evidence of infection of implanted materials ranges from subtle to catastrophic. Thus, implanted intravenous lines may exhibit only fever and local erythema at the puncture sites, whereas infected aortic grafts may present with life-threatening haemorrhage due to anastomotic disruption or acute aorto-enteric fistula.

In nearly all instances, removal of the implant is necessary to control infection. Removal and replacement of implanted devices such as pacemakers to another site with systemic antibiotic cover is needed. For infected vascular grafts removal with a new prosthesis tunnelled through uncontaminated tissue (extra-anatomical bypass) is usually performed, e.g. axillobifemoral grafts for infected abdominal aortic grafts. In some patients, the threat to life or anticipated disability may prohibit removal of the implant, e.g. infected thoracic aortic graft. Irrigation of the infected area with antibiotic solutions in addition to systemic antibiotics may buy time but does not provide permanent control of the infection.

A growing percentage of nosocomial infections is associated with medical devices. One solution to this problem is to coat the device with anti-infective coating. Antibiotic coating has been used especially for vascular grafts. In this instance the polymer is impregnated with gelatin, which then binds antibiotics such as rifampicin. This approach has a number of limitations. In the first instance, each antibiotic is effective only against certain bacteria. Secondly, there is the problem of bacterial resistance and, thirdly, antibiotic coating tends to be effective only for short periods (days to weeks). A more recent technology involves **oligo-dynamic iontophoresis** (OI). This is an electrochemical process whereby minute amounts of silver ions are released from the device into the surrounding tissue fluid, thereby preventing bacterial colonization and infection of the implant. OI-enhanced materials (OIE) are polymers impregnated with silver, platinum and carbon particles. These components, following implantation of the device, set up an electrochemical reaction once in contact with the crystalloid tissue fluid, with the silver and platinum particles acting as the electrodes of a battery. The result of this reaction is the release of bactericidal silver ions that lasts for several months. Currently, OIE central line catheters are being evaluated in randomized trials.

Section 5.3 • Principles of antibiotic therapy

Antibiotics are rarely used as the sole agents to eradicate surgical infections; in most instances they constitute adjuvant treatment to surgical and radiological interventional procedures, e.g. excision of the infecting focus, drainage of abscesses, debridement or lavage of infected serous cavities. They are certainly no substitute for effective surgical management of these disorders. The use of antibiotics as prophylactic agents to cover certain operations is well established and of proven value [see Module 18, Vol. I]. **The adverse effects of antibiotics, particularly the emergence of resistant strains of organisms, limit their overall usefulness, especially in critically ill patients.**

Antibiotic policy

Certain principles governing antibiotic therapy in hospital practice are agreed and in general usage.

- Each hospital has its own drug formulary that includes an antibiotic policy (first-line antibiotics to be used for specific conditions) based on cost efficacy, the pharmacokinetic properties and the hospital's known resistant species. This policy covers both the treatment of established infections and the use of specific antibiotics for prophylaxis of infection in patients undergoing surgery. By agreement, certain antibiotics are kept in reserve for serious infections.
- For established infections, the sensitivity of the organisms cultured to antibiotics is performed routinely and the first-line antibiotic regimen used may need to be changed accordingly.
- For certain antibiotics, therapeutic drug monitoring is necessary to (i) establish adequate serum concentrations, and (ii) identify potentially lethal concentrations. Nowadays, this applies particularly to aminoglycosides (gentamicin, netilmicin, tobramycin and vancomycin) and flucytosine. The desirable levels of aminoglycosides vary according to the nature and severity of the infection. Dose adjustment is essential in patients with renal impairment, when advice should be sought from the clinical pharmacist. The volume of distribution of aminoglycosides is increased in critically ill patients and, for this reason, suboptimal dosing is common.
- In some infections synergistic combinations of antibiotics are indicated. Antimicrobial synergy occurs, for example, when an aminoglycoside is combined with penicillin for treatment of certain staphylococcal or enterococcal infection, and with

ticarcillin for enhanced activity against *Pseudomonas* spp. For surgical patients, the traditional treatment of potentially life-threatening infections, e.g. pneumonia, suppurative cholangitis, peritonitis and burn sepsis, has been with combinations of aminoglycosides and other drugs such as cephalosporins, clindamycin and metronidazole.

- Infected collections negate antibiotic activity owing to changes in tissue pH, oxygen tension, levels of magnesium and calcium, and the production by various organisms of substances that inactivate antibiotics, such as β-lactamase which inactivates penicillin. Thus, drainage and debridement will improve antibiotic effectiveness as well as reduce the bacterial inoculum.
- In serious infections in critically ill patients, discussion with and advice from the hospital clinical bacteriologist is essential.
- Special nursing measures and isolation of patients with methicillin-resistant *Staphylococcus aureus* infections (MRSA) are necessary.

Additional measures for enhancing antibiotic action include:

- altering body fluid pH, e.g. urine
- delaying excretion of the drug, e.g. use of probenecid with penicillin
- changing the route of administration, e.g. intravenous from oral
- increasing the dose of antibiotic (effective in cephalosporins). This can be achieved by increasing the absolute dose or the total dose (increase duration of therapy), or by reducing the dosing interval
- using substances that block bacterial-inactivating enzymes, e.g. clavulinic acid.

Types of antibiotic

Penicillins

The use of penicillins has been eclipsed by other antibiotics because of the emergence of resistant organisms that produce penicillinase, as well as the emergence of MRSA. Penicillins as a group are effective against Gram-positive organisms and *Neisseria gonorrhoea*. The aminopenicillin group (ampicillin, amoxycillin) also has limited Gram-negative activity. Penicillinase-resistant penicillins are useful against resistant staphylococci.

More recent penicillin classes include the carboxypenicillins (carbenicillin, ticarcillin) and ureidopenicillins (mezlocillin, azlocillin and piperacillin). The main advantage of carboxypenicillins is their effectiveness in *Pseudomonas* spp. and *Proteus* spp. infections. Ureidopenicillins are effective against *Pseudomonas* and *Klebsiella* spp. Resistance of β-lactamase-producing *Staphylococcus* spp. and *Haemophilus influenzae* is common. Reports of decreasing activity of ureidopenicillins with increasing inoculum size are important.

As a group, penicillins may produce allergic reactions that range from rashes (relatively common) to anaphylaxis (rare). Ampicillin is associated with diarrhoea.

Haemolytic anaemia, drug fever, granulocytopenia and hepatitis are unusual but important side-effects.

Cephalosporins

These were first introduced in the 1950s and are usually classified into three generations:

- **first-generation cephalosporins**: cefadroxil, cephalexin, cephadrine, cefazolin, cephalothin, cephapirin
- **second-generation cephalosporins**: cefaclor, cefamandole, cefonicid, ceforanide, cefotetan, cefoxitin, cefuroxime
- **third-generation cephalosporins**: cefoperazone, cefotaxime, ceftazidine, cefizoxime, ceftriaxone.

First-generation drugs are available in both oral and parenteral forms. Cefazolin has been used widely as a prophylactic drug in high-risk elective operations. Only one second-generation cephalosporin is available for oral use (cefaclor); this is active against *H. influenzae*.

The major advantage of second-generation cephalosporins is improved activity against Gram-negative organisms such as *E. coli* and *Proteus* spp. Activity against *Streptococcus pneumoniae* and *Streptococcus pyogenes* is equal to the first-generation drugs. Cefoxitin is a useful drug for surgical patients because of its activity against *Bacteroides fragilis* and persistent high tissue levels lasting for 3–4 h. The level of activity against anaerobes is shared by cefotetan. Cefoxitin is useful as a primary drug directed against suspected mixed infections within the peritoneal cavity and is commonly used in trauma patients.

Third-generation cephalosporins have improved activity against Gram-negative organisms. Thus, some of the drugs in this category have been suggested as primary single-drug therapy for difficult infections such as nosocomial pneumonia and peritonitis. The major advantage of these drugs over combinations of aminoglycosides with earlier generations of cephalosporins for nosocomial infections is the lack of toxicity and lack of need to monitor drug levels. However, clinical studies have not documented a superior outcome in pneumonia or peritonitis when third-generation cephalosporins are compared with combination therapy with aminoglycosides. Toxic side-effects of third-generation cephalosporins are unusual. Moxalactam is associated with prolongation of the prothrombin time.

Aminoglycosides

This group has a wide spectrum of activity against a large number of organisms and has consistently been shown to be useful in many difficult clinical infections, particularly pneumonia and peritonitis. Toxicity is the major drawback, involving renal damage and ototoxicity, the latter producing deafness and vestibular dysfunction. Gentamicin, tobramycin and amikacin are most often used. The drugs are given parenterally because of poor intestinal absorption.

Serum drug level monitoring is essential to determine effective tissue levels of the drug. Timing of the blood-level assay is important. One level should be drawn within 30 min of beginning an infusion of drug, with the second (peak) level being drawn 30 min after the end of the infusion. Peak levels above 5 μg/ml are associated with improved survival from serious infections. With pneumonia, higher levels in the range of 10 μg/ml may be required.

Clindamycin

This antibiotic is useful in infections caused by *B. fragilis*. The drug suppresses protein synthesis by bacterial ribosomes and binds to the same subcellular site as chloramphenicol. Thus, simultaneous use of these two drugs is highly inadvisable. Clindamycin-associated diarrhoea, rarely progressing to pseudomembranous colitis, is an adverse side-effect.

Vancomycin

This has assumed major importance in the treatment of surgical infections due to resistant microorganisms, particularly methicillin-resistant *S. aureus* and *S. epidermidis* and *Corynebacterium diphtheriae*. In MRSA infections, the addition of aminoglycosides or rifampicin may be necessary (sometimes all three). Vancomycin should be administered over a 1-h period to avoid hypotension and a red rash over the upper body (red man syndrome). Vancomycin is also used in the treatment of pseudomembranous colitis caused by *Clostridium difficile*. Resistance to vancomycin is now well documented amongst nosocomial infections.

Carbapenems

This group, which is related to the penicillins, is active against a variety of Gram-negative organisms and anaerobes. The most commonly used antibiotic of this group is imipenem-cilastin. Cilastin is a toxicity-free additive that inhibits the dehydropeptidase enzyme that catalyses the reaction leading to rapid excretion of imipenem by the kidney. Another member of the group is meropenem. These antibiotics are valuable in the treatment of serious abdominal and pulmonary infections caused by Gram-negative bacteria.

Monobactams

The only member of this group that is used clinically is aztreonam, which exhibits marked activity against aerobic Gram-negative organisms. Studies have confirmed outcomes equivalent to combination therapy with aminoglycosides in infections due to *E. coli*, *Klebsiella pneumoniae*, *Streptococcus marcescens*, *P. aeruginosa*, *Enterobacter* spp., *Proteus* spp. and *Providencia* spp. Combined with clindamycin, this drug has been effective in the treatment of aspiration pneumonia.

Beta–lactamase inhibitors

The binding of the β-lactamase inhibitor clavulinic acid to certain antibiotics, e.g. ticarcillin, enhances their activity. Co-amoxiclav (amoxycillin + clavulinic acid) is effective against aspiration and postoperative pneumonia and peritonitis.

Quinolones

This group includes ciprofloxacin and norfloxacin. These drugs have a wide spectrum of activity against Enterbacteriaceae and may be administered orally and parenterally. Occasional nausea, vomiting and diarrhoea represent the most common side-effects.

Metronidazole

Originally introduced for the treatment of protozoal infections (*Trichomonas vaginalis*, *Giardia lamblia*, *Entamoeba histolytica*), this is the most effective agent against anaerobic Gram-negative infections, *Bacteroides* and *B. fragilis*, and is often used in combination with cephalosporins and aminoglycosides for mixed infections. Metronidazole is also effective in pseudomembranous colitis cause by *C. difficile*.

Section 5.4 • Infections in critically Ill intensive care unit patients

Patients in ICUs are two to five times more likely to develop nosocomial infections than the general hospital population (where 5% prevalence is regarded as the norm). The acknowledged risk factors include:

- **age > 70 years**
- **shock**
- **steroids**
- **chemotherapy**
- **ICU stay > 3 days**
- **previous antibiotics**
- **mechanical ventilation**
- **invasive monitoring**
- **indwelling urinary catheter > 10 days**
- **acute renal failure**
- **surgical vs medical patient.**

Invasive monitoring poses a real dilemma and the value of the widespread used of the pulmonary floatation catheters has been questioned recently. Selective use only in patients who require this invasive cardiac monitoring is a sensible option [**see Module 19, Vol. I**]. The consequences of infection in ICU patients are always serious, with an established association with multiple organ systems failure and a fatal outcome.

Detection of infection in intensive care unit patients

Evaluation of the critically ill patient for infection is often difficult. The two problems are (i) differentiation between colonization and invasive infection, and (ii) localization of the site of infection. In the search for infection, a systematic head-to-toe approach is needed. The prior condition of the patient is also taken into consideration, i.e. pre-existing medical diseases and the surgical procedures that have been performed. Frequently, the occurrence of infection in ICU patients is closely associated with complications of surgical interventions. In this context, the nature of the operation is important, e.g. anastomotic dehiscence and intra-abdominal abscesses after gastrointestinal surgery, mediastinitis after cardiac surgery. Other hospital-acquired infections must also be excluded:

- **head and neck**: sinusitis, meningitis, ventriculitis, etc.
- **chest**: aspiration, pneumonia, lung abscess, empyema
- **abdomen**: *C. difficile* pseudomembranous colitis, urinary tract infection
- **catheter-related infections**: arterial catheters, central venous catheters, Swan–Ganz catheters.

Sinusitis is most commonly associated with nasotracheal intubation but may also complicate indwelling nasogastric tubes. The overall reported incidence in ICU patients is 2%. Facial trauma is a predisposing factor. The maxillary sinuses are involved in 50–75% of cases. The mechanism by which the sinusitis occurs is usually obstruction of the sinus ostia by the tube, hence the sinus involved is almost always on the same side as the nasal tube. The diagnosis, once suspected, is established by a CT scan (Figure 5.1). The bacteria involved are usually Gram-negative bacilli, *S. aureus* or anaerobes. Treatment includes removal of the nasal tube, decongestant sprays, antibiotics and drainage of the sinus.

Meningitis and ventriculitis are most commonly related to intracranial surgery, head trauma or the placement of intracranial pressure monitors. The most common organisms causing these infections are Gram-negative bacilli, *Staphylococcus* spp. and *Streptococcus* spp. The use of prophylactic antibiotics in patients with intracranial monitoring devices remains controversial.

Chest infections in intensive care unit patients

These are very common and include pneumonia, lung abscess, empyema and mediastinitis (after cardiac surgery). Pneumonia is by far the most common. Lung abscess usually arises against a background of pneumonia, and empyema is most commonly encountered

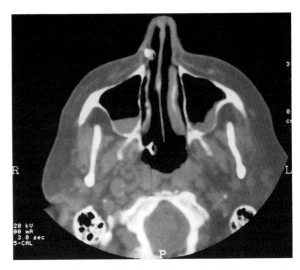

Figure 5.1 CT scan of the head in a patient who was septic from sinusitis. Note the air–fluid levels in the maxillary sinuses.

in trauma patients with chest tube drainage and oesophageal perforation or leaks. The majority of ICU-acquired pneumonias reflects the ICU's bacterial flora. Within a short time of arriving in the ICU, the patient's own bacterial flora is replaced by the ICU flora, which often contains antibiotic-resistant strains. The risk factors for pneumonia are:

- age
- aspiration
- head injury
- smoking
- intubation and mechanical ventilation
- lung injury: adult respiratory distress syndrome (ARDS) and pulmonary contusion
- prior use of antibiotics
- prolonged preoperative hospital stay
- pulmonary oedema
- use of H_2 blockers and proton-pump inhibitors
- upper abdominal and chest incision.

Patients on mechanical ventilation are particularly at risk as normal protective mechanisms such as mucociliary clearance mechanism and coughing are breached. The mechanism by which pneumonia occurs in ICU patients is thought to be by aspiration of upper airway and oropharyngeal secretions in most instances, as evidenced by the bacteriology. Thus, approximately 70–75% are caused by aerobic Gram-negative bacilli, 15–20% by *S. aureus* and 5–15% by *Candida*. Only 2–15% of normal humans have Gram-negative bacilli colonizing their upper airways, but in critically ill patients, the colonization of the upper airway occurs within the first few days of ICU stay in 55–75% of patients.

The diagnosis of pneumonia in critically ill patients may be difficult. Chest X-ray may not be helpful as many of these patients already have pulmonary infiltrates from other causes, e.g. ARDS or pulmonary contusion (trauma patients). Thus, diagnosis is based on: (i) quantity and quality of sputum, (ii) Gram staining, and (iii) sputum culture. The presence of copious purulent sputum containing, leucocytes and intracellular bacteria on Gram staining is enough to make a diagnosis pending the results of culture. Initial therapy is based on sputum Gram staining as follows:

- **Gram–negative bacilli**: third-generation cephalosporin, extended spectrum penicillin, monobactam, aminoglycoside
- **Gram–negative bacilli with suspicion of *Pseudomonas***: imipenem or cilastatin, penicillin + aminoglycoside, third-generation cephalosporin + aminoglycoside
- **Gram-positive cocci in clumps**: nafcillin, vancomycin for methicillin-resistant *S. aureus*
- **Gram-positive cocci in chains**: penicillin G
- **yeast**: amphotericin B, fluconazol.

The results of sputum culture may not be representative of the infection because of contamination by oral flora. To overcome this, samples may be obtained by transtracheal aspiration through the cricothyroid membrane via an angiocath (in non-intubated patients) or via a flexible bronchoscope with a protected brush technique for sputum sampling.

Catheter-related infections

Patients in the ICU are more likely to develop catheter-related sepsis than those in hospital wards. However, it is unclear whether this is due to the patient's underlying illness or to the fact that these patients tend to have catheters that are often inserted under emergency conditions, are *in situ* for long periods and are frequently manipulated. Catheter-related bacteraemia is encountered when the number of colony-forming units (CFU) cultured from the tip is 15 or more. The changing of catheters to prevent this bacteraemia and sepsis remains controversial, with several regimens being recommended:

- change catheter to a different site every 3–7 days
- change the catheter over a guide wire every 3–7 days
- do not change unless there is a problem.

In practice, no advantage has been documented to favour any one of these policies and the most important factor in the protection against catheter-related sepsis is the adoption of a strict aseptic technique when placing and caring for catheters. Several adjunctive techniques have been used to minimize the incidence of catheter-related sepsis: bonding antibiotics and silver compounds to the catheters, sterile protective plastic sleeves, silver ion-impregnated collagen cuffs, etc. Especially in ICU patients, catheter-related sepsis may have potentially lethal consequences, such as subacute bacterial endocarditis and suppurative thrombophlebitis.

The algorithm for management of catheters in critically ill patients is shown in Figure 5.2.

Fungal infections

These are important in ICU patients for two reasons.

- **Disseminated fungal infections constitute a grave prognostic marker of critical illness.**
- **Despite newer fungal agents, the mortality (usually from multisystem organ failure) remains high, ranging from 33 to 75%.** By far the most common organism responsible in ICU patients is *Candida albicans*. Much less commonly, other fungi, e.g. *Aspergillus* spp., *Torulopsis glabrata*, *Mucor* spp., are responsible.

The risk factors for colonization and invasive infections are:

- multiple antibiotic usage over a prolonged period
- immune depression
- steroid therapy
- parenteral nutrition
- concomitant bacteraemia.

MANAGEMENT PROTOCOL FOR CENTRAL AND ARTERIAL CATHETERS

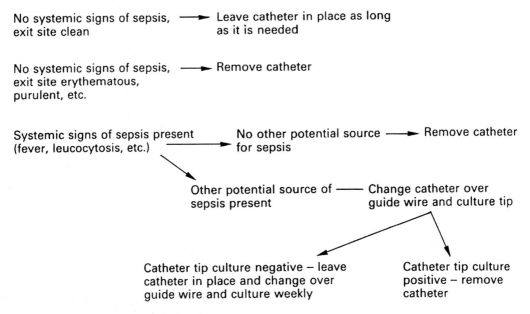

Figure 5.2 Algorithm for the routine care of intravascular catheters.

Section 5.5 • Specific bacterial infections of surgical importance

Gas gangrene and related anaerobic infections

Gas gangrene

Gas gangrene is extremely rare in civilian practice (0.1/100 000 per annum). The essential factor required for spore germination and production of illness is reduced oxygen tension. This may result from severe contusion and laceration with necrotic tissue, devitalization of a wound by compression, impaired blood supply, foreign bodies implanted in the depths of a punctured wound, e.g. shrapnel or pieces of clothing and soil, which induces tissue necrosis as a result of its high ionized calcium salts and silicic acid. The oxygen tension of a wound may be further lowered by coexisting infection with pyogenic organisms. Gas gangrene has been reported following injection of adrenaline into the buttocks where the skin is often contaminated by clostridial spores from the patient's faeces.

Bacteriology and pathology
Gas gangrene is a mixed clostridial infection by saccharolytic (pathogenic) and proteolytic (saprophytic) organisms. The true pathogens are *Clostridium perfringens* (*C. welchii*), *C. novyi* (*C. oedematiens*) and *C. septicum*. Type A *C. perfringens* is the most important human pathogen. It produces α-toxin, which is a lecithinase and breaks down the phospholipid constituents of red cells with the production of haemolysis. Other exotoxins produced by some strains of *C. perfringens* include haemolysin, collagenase, hyaluronidase and deoxyribonuclease.

These exotoxins produce a cellulitis and a progressive myonecrosis. They ferment the muscle carbohydrate, with the production of lactic acid and gas (H_2, CO_2). The discharge from the wound is initially odourless. Spread of the necrosis occurs as a result of exotoxin release and ischaemia from pressure by gas and exudate within tight muscle compartments. The affected area becomes tense, oedematous and crepitant. At first, the dead muscle is odourless and brick red in colour. Progressive putrefaction by saprophytic clostridia (*C. sporogenes*, *C. histolyticum*) of the dead muscle completes the pathological process with the production of the characteristic fishy odour and the greenish-black appearance of the established disease.

The profound toxaemia is due to the circulating exotoxins and results in shock, haemolytic anaemia, renal failure and jaundice. The organisms themselves do not invade the blood stream except as an agonal event, and this accounts for the foamy liver and gas bubbles found in other organs at necropsy.

Clinical features
The majority of gas gangrene infections are exogenous and result from contamination of large wounds as occurs in agriculture tractor injuries, severe comminuted compound fractures sustained in road traffic accidents and battle casualties. An appreciable number

of cases in civilian practice is, however, endogenous in origin from contamination by bowel organisms. In the West, endogenous gas gangrene is most commonly encountered following amputation for peripheral vascular disease. Risk factors in this group include diabetes and incontinence. Other instances of gas gangrene may result from criminal abortion and infections following intestinal, and less commonly, biliary operations.

The incubation period between the initiating incident and the onset of the clostridial infection varies from 1 day to 4 weeks. Its duration carries an inverse relationship with the severity of the illness and the mortality. The demonstration of gas (Figure 5.3) is not essential for the diagnosis as non-gas forming clostridial infections of wounds are well documented. Indeed, the most useful clinical classification is into gas-forming and non-gas-forming clostridial infections. **The most important factor that determines whether the infection remains localized and non-crepitant, or becomes invasive with severe toxaemia and gas formation, is the presence of dead muscle.**

- **Non-gas-forming infections**: the disease is mild and apart from pyrexia, there is minimal toxicity. The wound is oedematous and erythematous, and may develop a brownish discoloration. Crepitus is absent; pain and tenderness are not severe and the mortality due to the clostridial infection is negligible.
- **Gas-forming infections**: the incubation period is usually less than 3 days and the onset acute. The condition declares itself by severe pain in the region of the wound and rapid development of toxaemia, drowsiness, fever and tachycardia. The affected area becomes swollen, tense, oedematous and extremely tender. The discharge may be serous or blood stained. It is variable in amount and initially odourless but subsequently becomes sweet to foul smelling. Gas is detected by crepitus and radiological examination. The overlying skin goes through a series of changes from intense white to inflammatory erythema with ecchymosis, bullae formation and frank greenish-black gangrene (Figure 5.4). In severe cases, jaundice, haemolysis and renal failure develop and contribute to the death of the patient. The overall mortality is 40% but the mortality due to overwhelming clostridial infection is 10–15%.

(a)

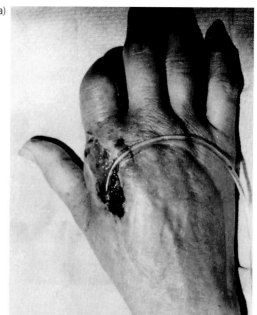

(b)

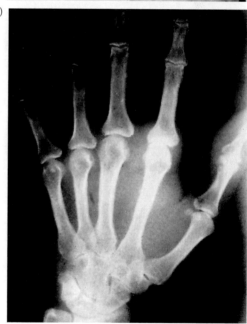

Figure 5.3 (a) Gas gangrene of the hand; (b) radiograph of the same hand showing gas in the soft tissues.

Treatment

The treatment consists of general resuscitative measures for shock and specific therapy, i.e. antibiotics, antitoxin, surgical treatment and, when available, hyperbaric oxygen.

- **Antibiotic therapy** is used both in the prophylaxis and in the treatment of established disease. For prophylaxis, the antibiotic therapy must be started immediately before the operation, e.g.

amputation for peripheral vascular disease or soon after the injury, and should be continued until the healing is complete if the risk is high. The benefit of antibiotic therapy in established disease remains doubtful, largely because of poor antibiotic penetration into ischaemic tissue. None the less, it constitutes part of the orthodox therapy. Initially, parenteral benzyl penicillin is administered in large doses (1–2 mega units 4–6 hourly) to all patients except for those with a known history of penicillin sensitivity, when metronidazole, clindamycin, vancomycin or chloramphenicol is used instead.

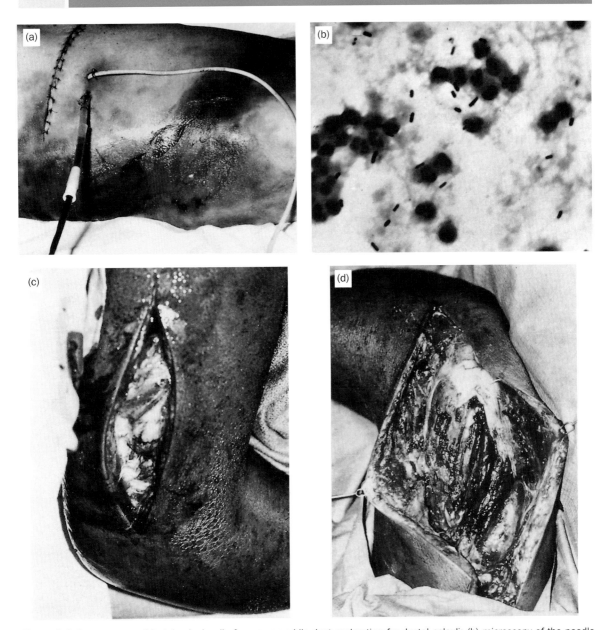

Figure 5.4 Gas gangrene: (a) abdominal wall after common bile-duct exploration for ductal calculi; (b) microscopy of the needle aspirate from the same patient showing clostridial organisms; (c) gas gangrene of the upper arm: note bulging of oedematous tissues after incision of the skin; (d) same patient: extensive necrosis of upper arm muscles.

Tetracycline and erythromycin exhibit moderate activity against most clostridial species but rapid development of drug resistance is a problem. The treatment is continued for a minimum of 7 days and the antibiotic regimen may need to be changed, depending on the bacteriology and sensitivity tests.

Surgical treatment

Surgical treatment must be carried out immediately after resuscitation and commencement of antibiotic therapy and is delayed only if facilities for hyperbaric oxygen therapy are available (see below), when operative intervention is postponed until completion of the first hyperbaric treatment. The aim of surgical treatment is the excision of all necrotic tissue regardless of anatomical defects thus produced. Pus is evacuated and the completely debrided wound is irrigated with hydrogen peroxide solution. **The complete excision of all dead and infected tissue at the first operation is crucial to the survival of the patient**. In limb infections, this may necessitate amputation. No attempt is made to provide skin cover and the wound is packed with gauze soaked in isotonic saline solution. The patient is returned to the operating theatre 24–48 h later for a dressing change under general anaesthesia. Any residual necrotic areas are excised down to bleeding tissues, after which the wound is dressed as before. Reconstructive surgery and skin grafting are delayed until the infection has been totally eradicated.

■ **Hyperbaric oxygen therapy** benefits patients with pure clostridial infections, and may result in rapid improvement in the clinical condition and in limb salvage. Hyperbaric oxygen therapy is started soon after the initial resuscitation and before surgical intervention. It consists of repeated treatments of 1.5–2 h at a pressure of 250 kPa (2.5 atm).

Clostridial enterocolitis

This results from the ingestion of improperly cooked food contaminated by *C. perfringens*. The disease is usually self-limiting and causes severe colicky abdominal pain and diarrhoea. The organism is present in the stool in high counts. Occasionally, the condition is more severe and leads to widespread necrosis of the bowel (primarily of the small intestine) and is then referred to as enteritis necrotica. In addition to severe abdominal pain, vomiting and diarrhoea, the patient exhibits signs of peritonitis with profound toxaemia and shock. The condition carries a very high mortality.

Infective non-clostridial gangrene

Various clinical syndromes have been described as infective non-clostridial gangrene. The most common causative organisms are anaerobic streptococci, but necrotizing infections with *E. coli* and bacteroides are well documented. The most common member of the bacteroides species responsible for infective gangrene is *Fusiformis fusiformis*, which is often accompanied by *Borrelia vincenti*, although it is doubtful whether the latter plays any part in the disease process.

These gangrenous conditions usually arise against a background of debility, atherosclerosis and diabetes mellitus. The causative anaerobes often act in association with *S. pyogenes*, staphylococci and coliform bacilli. However, in some well-documented cases, a causative organism cannot be identified. In some cases a precipitating factor, e.g. trauma, operation or viral infection, initiates the condition; in others, particularly in diabetic patients, the morbid process arises spontaneously.

A commonly favoured pathological classification is into:

■ cutaneous gangrene (progressive bacterial gangrene)
■ subcutaneous gangrene (necrotizing fasciitis)
■ subfascial infective gangrene.

In cutaneous gangrene, the necrosis is limited to the skin only and systemic signs are usually minimal, although the disease may extend to the deeper tissues. In subcutaneous gangrene, the necrotic process primarily involves the subcutaneous fat and/or the deep fascia, usually sparing the underlying muscle layer. Necrosis of the skin is secondary to the development of thrombosis of the perforating vessels as they course through the necrotic infected deeper layers. Subcutaneous gangrene is a serious, rapidly spreading disease, which is accompanied by toxaemia and may prove fatal. Subfascial infections consist of myositis and myonecrosis.

The above classification, although useful in outlining the pathology and prognosis in the majority of these infections, does not cover the entire spectrum of these infections, some of which cannot be readily placed in either of these two categories. In addition, a cutaneous infection may spread to involve the subcutaneous and subfascial compartments. Thus, a more comprehensive clinical classification of infective non-clostridial gangrene is:

■ cutaneous gangrene (Meleney's progressive bacterial gangrene)
■ subcutaneous gangrene: necrotizing fasciitis and Meleney's undermining ulcer
■ infected vascular gangrene
■ cancrum oris and noma vulva: protein calorie malnutrition
■ streptococcal myositis
■ human bite infections.

Cutaneous gangrene (Meleney's progressive bacterial gangrene)

This is usually a synergistic infection with two microbial species that differ in their requirements for oxygen. In classic cases, the microorganisms involved are microaerophilic streptococci and aerobic staphylococci, although bacteroides and a variety of Gram-negative aerobic bacteria can be involved. Bacterial inoculation most frequently follows minor trauma, or a postoperative consequence of a surgical drain or mass closure with deep tension sutures. It often follows drainage of abscesses, particularly in patients with diabetes mellitus and severe atherosclerosis. In most instances, 1 or 2 weeks elapse before the onset of clinical manifestations. At that time, the skin surrounding the wound becomes red, oedematous and very tender. As the cutaneous infection extends outwards, the central area becomes necrotic, turning to eschar that ulcerates (Figure 5.5). A thin, foul-smelling discharge simulating dishwater emanates from the ulcer. At this stage, the patient becomes systemically toxic. Broad-spectrum antibiotics and surgical excision are necessary for survival. The most favoured first-line antibiotic combination is benzyl penicillin, metronidazole and gentamicin. At operation, the infected necrosis is found to be limited to the skin and subcutaneous fat, but the fascia and underlying muscle are spared except for in advanced cases. Following complete excision, the wound is left open and packed with gauze soaked in a bactericidal agent. Debridement may have to be repeated. Secondary wound closure or skin cover by grafting is only attempted after the infection has been completely eradicated and healthy granulation tissue has formed.

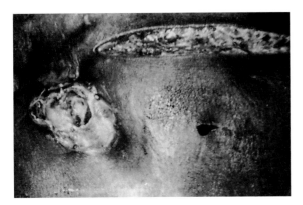

Figure 5.5 Meleney's progressive bacterial gangrene. Culture revealed *S. aureus* and a microaerophilic streptococcus.

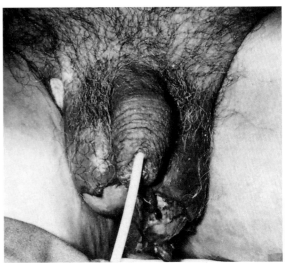

Figure 5.7 Fournier's gangrene with necrosis of scrotal skin.

Subcutaneous gangrene

The most important example of this is necrotizing fasciitis, also known as haemolytic streptococcal gangrene, hospital gangrene and gangrenous erysipelas. It includes conditions such as perineal phlegmon (Figure 5.6) and Fournier's scrotal gangrene (Figure 5.7). It is caused by haemolytic streptococci, and less commonly, haemolytic staphylococci. Various other organisms have been identified in some of these infections including coliforms, bacteroides, diphtheroids and *Pseudomonas*. Most commonly, the condition arises following surgery or trauma. Spontaneous cases have been described, although in some of these patients, the preceding trauma may have been so slight as to be ignored by the

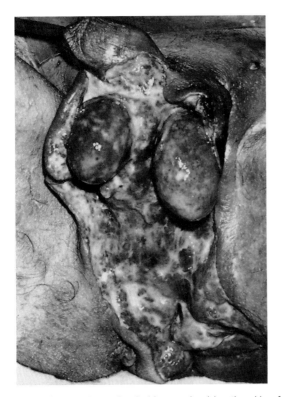

Figure 5.6 Extensive perineal phlegmon involving the skin of the scrotum and penile shaft.

patient. The most commonly affected sites are the extremities, followed by the lower trunk, including the external genitalia and the perineum. The exact mechanism for the subcutaneous necrosis is unknown but appears to be related to the binding of the mucopeptide fraction of the bacterial cell wall with dermal collagen. The necrosis does not involve the muscle layer and skin involvement is secondary to thrombosis of the perforating vessels coursing through the infected necrotic area.

The disease is always serious and carries a definite mortality. The affected part is initially very painful but then becomes numb owing to the involvement of sensory nerve fibres. The process spreads rapidly through the subcutaneous fatty/fascial plane with reddish discoloration, inflammatory oedema (sometimes bullous), necrosis and eventual sloughing of the overlying skin (Figure 5.8). Systemic manifestations are always present and the toxaemia may be severe with pyrexia, tachycardia and shock. Blood cultures should always be taken in these patients. Treatment includes resuscitation with crystalloids and blood, antibiotics using a triple regimen (benzyl penicillin, metronidazole and aminoglycoside), and early wide surgical excision and drainage with delayed skin cover.

Meleney's chronic undermining ulcer results from infection by a microaerophilic streptococcus and usually develops after surgery on the intestinal and genital tracts. The infection and necrosis start in the subcutaneous tissues (Figure 5.9) but the disease progressively affects the deeper tissues to involve the pelvis. Treatment is with a combination of benzyl penicillin and metronidazole, together with surgical excision and delayed skin cover.

Infected vascular gangrene

A significant proportion of these necrotic infections occur in diabetic patients. Infected vascular gangrene has a gradual onset. The affected part (usually the foot)

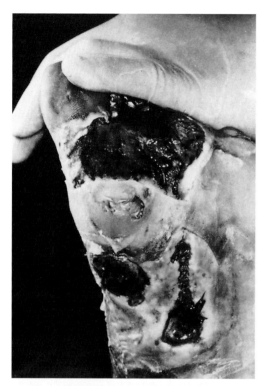

Figure 5.8 Necrotizing fasciitis of the sole of the foot.

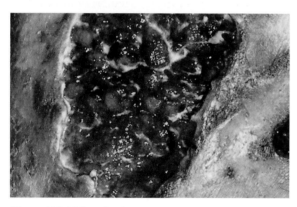

Figure 5.9 Meleney's chronic undermining ulcer in the right iliac fossa in a renal transplant patient.

becomes painful, swollen, black and foul smelling. Radiographs show extensive gas formation in the tissues of the involved foot. The infection is a mixed one with faecal organisms, most commonly *B. fragilis* and *Peptostreptococcus*. The severity of the toxaemia is variable.

Streptococcal myositis

This represents a unique infection that can usually be distinguished from clostridial infections by the presence of pronounced skin reaction: cyanotic discoloration, blebs containing foul-smelling fluid teeming with Gram-positive cocci, and islands of frankly gangrenous skin. After instituting supportive care and antibiotics, treatment is with a generous incision, exploration and

drainage of all the infected muscle groups, aptly termed the 'fillet' procedure. Only occasionally is myonecrosis present and this requires excision. The wound is kept open and packed with saline gauze. Prognosis is surprisingly good if the infection is managed before the onset of myonecrosis.

Cancrum oris and noma vulvae

These are instances of mucocutaneous gangrene affecting the mouth (cancrum oris) or the vulva (noma vulvae). Both arise against a background of malnutrition in children and are usually preceded by an infectious illness, such as measles. The infection is often a mixed one, but the protagonists are either anaerobic streptococci or members of the bacteroides species. The disease results in slow but relentless necrosis of the perioral or vulval tissues, and in cancrum oris death may result from inhalation pneumonia. Correction of the underlying malnutrition is essential, in addition to antibiotic therapy. Skin cover and plastic reconstruction are delayed until the infection has been cleared and the patient's nutritional status has improved.

Human bite infections

The anaerobic infections caused by human bites can be particularly virulent and cause marked tissue destruction. The infection is usually a mixed one, the causative organisms being a combination of two or more of the following: *Bacteroides melaninogenicus*, *Fusobacterium* spp., anaerobic cocci and spirochetes. The first line antibiotic is penicillin, which is administered in high doses. The importance of tetanus prophylaxis in these patients must not be forgotten.

Tetanus

In the vast majority of cases, tetanus is an exogenous infection, although rare instances of endogenous infections are documented after septic abortions and operations on the gastrointestinal tract. The conditions governing the germination of spores of *Clostridium tetani* are identical to those of gas gangrene and necessitate local hypoxia. The most common portal of entry world-wide is the umbilical stump following the application of dung to this region in newborn babies that is practised in some developing countries. Elsewhere, the lower limbs constitute the most common portal of entry. Usually, the wound is a minor one but it is always penetrating in nature. **In some 25% of cases in the West, the portal of entry is not evident at the time of diagnosis.** Other sources of infection include piercing of the ear lobes, tattooing, burns, parenteral injections including vaccination, skin lesions, especially leg ulcers, nasal foreign bodies and ear infections. The disease is well recognized in drug addicts.

Clostridium tetani (Figure 5.10) produces two exotoxins. The most important is a neurotoxin called tetanospasmin that is responsible for the disease. A haemolytic toxin called tetanolysin acts on the peripheral neuromuscular junctions but does not play a

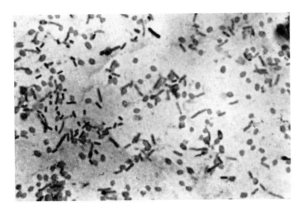

Figure 5.10 *Clostridium tetani* organisms.

significant role in the disease. Tetanospasmin reaches the central nervous system (CNS) along the axons of motor trunks, probably in the tissue spaces between the nerve fibres, and acts by blocking the inhibitory impulses at the motor synapses. This results in two forms of contractions of striated muscles: tonic (spasm), characteristic of the early disease, and clonic (convulsions), indicating severe established disease.

The overall mortality of tetanus is 10–15%. Adverse factors include extremes of age, short incubation period, type of injury and severity of the illness. Thus, whereas mild to moderate tetanus carries a small mortality, death from the disease occurs in 30–40% of patients with severe tetanus. Death usually results from asphyxia from involvement of the muscles of respiration and from cardiovascular complications resulting from sympathetic overactivity.

Clinical features
Neonatal tetanus is by far the most common type in developing countries, where it accounts for 70% of cases. It is best considered separately from the disease in children and adults.

Neonatal tetanus
The clinical picture is characteristic and the disease usually becomes manifest on the eighth day, hence the popular name 'eighth-day disease'. It starts with failure to suckle on the third day. This is followed quickly by spasm of the facial muscles (risus sardonicus) and masseter (lockjaw), and progression to generalized clonic spasms with flexion of the arms, clenched fists, extension of the lower limbs and plantar flexion of the toes.

Children and adults
The majority of patients (95%) who develop tetanus have not been previously immunized. The incubation period ranges from 4 to 10 days, and the shorter the interval the more severe the disease. The progress of the disease (the time from the first symptom to the onset of tetanus) varies according to the severity of the disease but the full-blown picture is reached by the third day in 70% of cases.

The condition declares itself by stiffness, twitching and cramps limited to the same spinal segment as the area of infection (local tetanus). Other early symptoms and signs include muscle pains, headaches, irritability, restlessness, constipation, sweating and tachycardia. This is followed by the development of spasm of the masseter muscles, facial musculature and muscles of deglutition (dysphagia). In the full-blown picture, there are generalized clonic convulsions that may be triggered by mild external stimuli (sound, movement of personnel, etc.). As the extensor muscles are more powerful than the flexor muscles, the patient classically assumes a position of opisthotonos. It is characteristic of tetanus that the muscles do not relax between convulsive attacks, and this distinguishes tetanic convulsions from those caused by strychnine poisoning.

Tetanus is classified into:

- mild: no dysphagia or respiratory distress
- moderate: presence of dysphagia and respiratory distress
- severe: gross spasticity and major spasms.

Treatment
Prophylaxis
The best method of prevention is by active immunization with tetanus toxoid (a formolized preparation of the exotoxin adsorbed on aluminium hydroxide or phosphate). Three injections are administered, with the second injection 6 weeks after the first, and the third injection 6–12 months later. A booster injection is given at 10-year intervals and at times of wounding. Booster toxoid injections are not necessary if a patient sustains a wound within 5 years of completion of an active immunization course or booster dose. However, if the period since the last toxoid injection exceeds 5 years, but is less than 10 years, a booster dose should be administered. In the absence of a history of active immunization, or if the period since the last toxoid injection exceeds 10 years, passive immunization with human tetanus immunoglobulin (tetanus immune globulin, TIG) in a dose of 250 units intramuscularly is indicated. This single dose provides immunity for about 4 weeks. If the wound has not healed by this time, a second dose is administered. Active immunization with toxoid should be started at the same time (using a different limb) in those not previously immunized, or a single booster dose is administered to those patients who had allowed their active immunization to lapse for more than 10 years. The use of equine antitetanic serum (ATS) is no longer practised because of the risk of anaphylactic reactions. Active immunization with tetanus toxoid of the pregnant female will protect the infant from neonatal tetanus.

Treatment of established disease
Specific measures include surgical attention to the wound if present with excision and open packing with antibiotic or hydrogen peroxide-soaked gauze. Benzyl penicillin is administered in a dose of 2 mega units

every 4 h for 7 days, and TIG is given in a dose of 2000–4000 units intramuscularly. Metronidazole (500 mg orally every 6 h or 1.0 g rectally 8-hourly) may be used instead of penicillin and is reported to be more effective. In neonatal tetanus, good results have been obtained with intrathecal TIG and predisolone.

For mild tetanus, the patient only requires sedation with diazepam. Tracheostomy and sedation are necessary for patients with moderate tetanus. In severe disease, the patient has to be treated with neuromuscular blockade and positive pressure ventilation. The very severe cases with sympathetic overactivity and cardiovascular complications (tachycardia, labile hypertension, vasoconstriction, myocardial instability) require general anaesthesia, mechanical ventilation and adrenergic blockade.

Chronic bacterial infections

These are produced by the species of the order Actinomycetales, so named because the bacterial cells may branch to form hyphae. With some species, e.g. *Actinomyces israelii*, this branching tendency is marked and simulates the appearance of a fungal growth (*actino* = radial, *myces* = fungus). The composition of the order Actinomycetales is shown in Table 5.1. Streptomycetaceae are not pathogenic to humans. The genus *Streptomyces* is, however, of medical importance as it contains many species valuable for the production of antibiotics (streptomycin, tetramycin, etc.). Most species of *Nocardia* are harmless and live on decaying organic matter in the soil. A few species, e.g. *N. asteroides*, can cause infection of the lung that is often fatal and may be mistaken for tuberculosis. Other species (*N. madurae*, *N. brasiliensis*) are known to produce a chronic disease of the hands or feet similar to actinomycosis.

Tuberculosis

In conjunction with all of the mycobacteria, the tubercle bacilli are non-sporing, immobile, aerobic and Gram-positive. **Differential staining methods are used to identify the mycobacteria since, after heat staining with carbol fuchsin, these bacteria, with the exception of *Nocardia* spp., are unique in resisting decoloration after treatment with strong acids and alcohol, i.e. are acid fast.**

There are several strains of non-pathogenic saprophytes in the soil and on plants (e.g. *Mycobacterium phlei*)

and on the human skin (*M. smegmatis*). The pathogenic status of several other species is variable but some are often found in tuberculosis-like disorders or in association with established tuberculosis, especially in immune-suppressed individuals. They are referred to variously as atypical, environmental, anonymous or MOTT (mycobacteria other than typical tubercle) to differentiate them from the established pathogens, i.e. *M. tuberculosis* and *M. bovis*.

The precise differentiation of the various mycobacteria is important. Culture is usually performed on Löwenstein–Jensen medium and requires 6 weeks, although faster growth can be obtained in Dubois medium. No single test is said to be reliable in the identification of *M. tuberculosis* and *M. bovis*, although tests for virulence in guinea-pigs (*M. tuberculosis*) and rabbits (*M. bovis*) are amongst the most reliable of the diagnostic tests. *Mycobacterium tuberculosis* is the only species known to produce niacin on culture.

Following the eradication of tuberculous herds and the introduction of pasteurized milk, bovine tuberculosis is rarely encountered in the West, and most of the reported cases are pulmonary infections. The vast majority of cases in these countries are caused by *M. tuberculosis*, usually as a result of inhalation of organisms present in fresh droplets or dust contaminated with dried sputum by a patient with open pulmonary tuberculosis. Both bovine and human infections are still common in economically deprived areas, such as parts of the African continent, Latin America and India. The global increase in tuberculosis that occurred during the 1980s and 1990s was associated with a re-emergence of resistance to antituberculous drugs (isoniazid and multidrug).

Pathology
It has been estimated that 90% of all tuberculous infections involve the lungs, but the infection may affect practically any organ or tissue. The most commonly recognized extrapulmonary infections include tuberculosis of the skin, lymph nodes, bones and joints, genitourinary tract, abdomen and intestines, and CNS.

Tuberculous lesions assume one of two forms:

- proliferative: the tubercle follicle
- exudative.

The most common proliferative lesion that is usually encountered in the lungs and solid organs is the

Table 5.1 The actinomycetales

Order	Family	Genus	Pathogenic species
Acinomycetales	Mycobacteriaceae	Mycobacterium	M. tuberculosis
			M. leprae
	Actinomycetaceae	Actinomyces	A. israelii
		Nocardia	N. asteroides
			N. madurae
	Streptomycetaceae	Streptomyces	–

tubercle follicle. This consists of an area of coagulative necrosis (caseation) due primarily to hypersensitivity to the tuberculoprotein, surrounded by epithelioid and Langerhans giant cells (both derived from macrophages), and an outer zone of small, round cells consisting mainly of lymphocytes and fibroblasts.

The exudative form of tuberculosis is typically encountered in infections of the serous cavities, e.g. tuberculous pleurisy/peritonitis, and epithelial surfaces (sterile pyuria in renal tuberculosis). It results in the formation of a cellular exudate rich in fibrin, together with a dense infiltration of the tissues with lymphocytes.

Childhood tuberculosis is characterized by marked involvement of the regional lymph nodes, as exemplified by the primary complex (Ghon focus at the periphery of the lung midzone and hilar lymphadenopathy) and tabes mesenterica, where a small focus in the intestine is associated with marked enlargement of the mesenteric lymph nodes, which at times rupture causing tuberculous peritonitis. By contrast, in the adult, lymph node enlargement is not marked and the disease either heals by fibrosis or extends locally by caseation, liquefaction and cavitation, with little tendency to blood stream dissemination. This altered tissue response in the adult appears to be the result of tissue maturation.

Softening and liquefaction of the caseous material underlies the development of tuberculous 'cold' abscesses. The liquefied debris may track along fascial planes, as in the psoas abscess originating from spinal

tuberculosis (Figure 5.11), or point to the surface with the eventual formation of tuberculous sinuses, e.g. collar-stud abscess in the neck from tuberculous lymphadenitis and scrotal sinuses from tuberculous epididymitis.

Involvement of a pulmonary vein by a tuberculous focus in the lung may lead to blood stream dissemination and miliary tuberculosis, especially if the resistance is lowered by poor nutrition, debility, old age or immune deficiency from any cause. If the blood stream inoculum is small, the bacilli may be destroyed by the cells of the monocyte–macrophage system. Failing this, they may either produce metastatic disease immediately or remain quiescent with reactivation some years later. These lesions are referred to as local metastatic tuberculosis or secondary tuberculosis and account for the majority of tuberculous infections encountered in surgical practice.

Clinical features
The general symptoms of active tuberculous infections include malaise, asthenia, weight loss, mild fever and night sweats. The symptomatology is, however, extremely varied and the disease may simulate many other disorders. The specific symptoms relate to the organ involved in the disease.

Tuberculosis is a disease of malnutrition and overcrowding. Other predisposing factors include poor general health, chronic disease, silicosis and diabetes. Certain ethnic groups, such as the Australian Aborigines, Black Africans and native Americans, are particularly susceptible.

Allergy (hypersensitivity) and acquired immunity
Tuberculous infection, subclinical or otherwise, results in the development of a cell-mediated allergy (delayed hypersensitivity) to tuberculoprotein that causes caseation and an accelerated macrophage response. This hypersensitivity, which indicates present or past infection, can be determined by the tuberculin skin reaction,

(a)

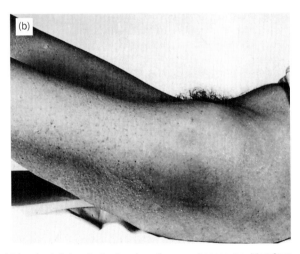

(b)

Figure 5.11 Tuberculous abscess: (a) left iliac fossa; (b) femoral triangle: infrainguinal extension of psoas abscess resulting from spinal disease.

which consists of the intracutaneous injection of purified protein derivative (PPD) that is derived from and has replaced Koch's old tuberculin (OT). The delayed hypersensitivity, although closely related, is not the mechanism of the acquired immunity to tuberculosis. This immunity, which is only partial, is cell mediated by sensitized lymphocytes. Active immunization with bacille Calmette–Guérin (BCG) is generally recommended for tuberculin-negative individuals. Complications of BCG vaccination are rare and include local abscess formation, regional lymphadenitis and, rarely, systemic infection with progressive pulmonary disease. The latter has been reported following immunotherapy with BCG in patients with malignant disease.

Treatment

Effective modern chemotherapy is followed by an almost universal cure rate without the necessity for long-term follow-up. It has eliminated the need for sanatorium management. The drugs available include streptomycin, para-aminosalicylic acid (PAS), isoniazid, rifampicin, pyrazinamide and ethambutol. *Mycobacterium bovis* is intrinsically resistant to pyrazinamide. The resistance to isoniazid in the UK now averages 5.5% and multidrug resistance 1.35%. Both isoniazid and multidrug resistance rates are higher in patients known to be infected with human immunodeficiency virus (HIV) (13.5% isoniazid and 6.1% multidrug) [see Disorders of the Respiratory System, Vol. II].

Leprosy

It is estimated that 15 million people in the world have leprosy, which is common throughout most of Africa, southern Asia, the Far East, and South and Central America. There are about 400 active cases registered in the UK. However, no case of indigenously contracted leprosy has been reported in Britain.

Mycobacterium leprae, the causative organism, is a slender and acid-fast rod, occurring singly or in clusters (globi) in the reticuloendothelial (macrophage) cells. This slowly multiplying organism has been grown in the footpads of mice and the armadillo but not in an artificial culture medium. The infectivity of leprosy is a function of the concentration of leprosy bacilli in the body of the patient, and the chances of bacteria emerging and remaining viable and pathogenic to susceptible contacts. Leprosy is not a very contagious disease. It is frequently contracted in childhood or adolescence, revealing itself in symptoms and signs some years later. This silent period is commonly 2–5 years and often longer. Bacilli-laden nasal discharge is probably the main source of infection, but bacilliferous ulcerations, sweaty hairy skin and maternal milk may contain viable bacilli. Infection may be acquired by inhalation or through abrasions in the skin.

Pathology

The pathological lesions depend on the type and extent of the immune response. If cell mediated immunity is strong, **tuberculoid** lesions form. The reaction consists of non-specific accumulation of giant cells, epitheloid cells, histiocytes and lymphocytes. Lymphocytic infiltrations are observed around and within nerve bundles. Bacilli are scanty (**paucibacillary disease**) and the lepromin test is positive.

When cell-mediated immunity is depressed, **lepromatous** leprosy (multibacillary disease) results. The whole dermis is replaced by highly bacilliferous tissue that invades the adnexa and eventually destroys superficial nerves, pigment-forming cells, sweat and sebaceous glands and hair follicles. The target tissues are the Schwann cells, endothelial cells and muscle cells. Bacilli may also be found in the liver, bone marrow, spleen, kidneys and lungs. Acute vasculitis caused by immune complexes may give rise to erythema nodosum leprosum, or other manifestations such as iritis, neuritis, orchitis, lymphadenitis and myositis. Long-standing lepromatous leprosy can result in chronic nephritis and amyloidosis.

Clinical features

Leprosy encompasses a whole spectrum of disease between the two main types, lepromatous and tuberculoid. The earlier manifestation, which is qualified as indeterminate, consists of a small hypopigmented macule, 2–5 cm, appearing anywhere in the body and often healing spontaneously. Determinate lesions that progress to clinical disease may arise out of indeterminate ones or *de novo*. Their subsequent features will depend on whether the disease is predominantly tuberculoid or lepromatous in nature.

Tuberculoid leprosy: in this type (Figure 5.12), there are a few or solitary skin lesions measuring 2–5 cm in diameter, often with a raised edge. The lesions are dry, hairless and anaesthetic. They are hypopigmented in dark-skinned and coppery in white-skinned individuals. Local or distant cutaneous nerve thickening occurs. The most common nerves involved are the ulnar nerve at the elbow, the median nerve at the wrist, the common peroneal in the popliteal fossa, the posterior tibial around the medial malleolus and the greater auricular nerve over the sternomastoid muscle. Sensory, motor and autonomic nerve trunks are affected. Nerve damage occurs early in tuberculoid leprosy.

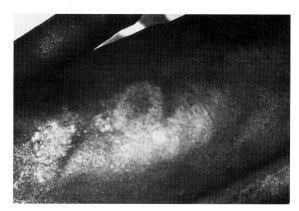

Figure 5.12 Tuberculoid leprosy.

Lepromatous leprosy: this presents as a widespread symmetrical macular rash, slightly hypopigmented or erythematous, affecting the face, extensor surface of the limbs and the upper trunk. The midline of the back, the axillae, groin and scalp are usually spared. There is congestion and discharge from the nose, the mucosa of which is thickened and yellow. Iritis may occur.

As the disease progresses, the skin, especially of the face, becomes thickened and nodular with thinning or loss of the eyebrows (Figure 5.13). Symmetrical enlargement of the peripheral nerves occurs, with widespread peripheral anaesthesia and muscular weakness. Painless neuropathic ulceration, absorption of the extremities of the digits, wrist drop, foot drop and claw hand occur (Figure 5.14). Nerve damage is observed late in lepromatous leprosy. Although acute exacerbations are found in all kinds of leprosy, they are most serious in the lepromatous type. An acute relapse is often heralded by an attack of erythema nodosum leprosum, and manifests widespread sensitivity phenomena in the skin, uveal tract, nerves, lymph nodes and joints.

Borderline leprosy: the presenting features are not typical of either tuberculoid or lepromatous leprosy.

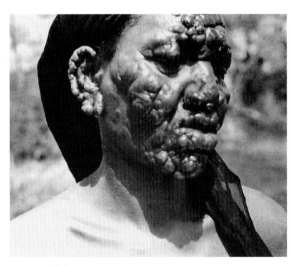

Figure 5.13 Lepromatous leprosy.

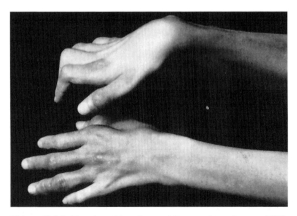

Figure 5.14 Claw hand in advanced lepromatous leprosy. With early treatment this lesion should never be seen.

The disease may be arrested at this stage or progress in either direction. In borderline tuberculoid leprosy, the lesions are more numerous and varied than in the pure tuberculoid disease. The peripheral nerves are thickened and sensation is impaired. It is a common presentation in Africans. Asians and Europeans usually present with borderline lepromatous leprosy. Symmetry of the skin lesions is less constant, while the nodules are often discrete, red and fleshy. Nerve damage occurs early.

Diagnosis

Examination of dermal material obtained by the slit-scrape method reveals numerous bacilli in lepromatous and borderline lepromatous leprosy, while in pauci-bacillary disease (tuberculoid and borderline tuberculoid) bacteria are scanty and difficult to demonstrate. The dermal fluid is placed on a slide, dried and stained with a modified Ziehl–Neelsen's method. Bacilli are also found in the nasal discharge. Histological examination of biopsies confirms the diagnosis.

Treatment

Multibacillary disease: the treatment of lepromatous and borderline lepromatous leprosy is by a combination of (i) rifampicin 600 mg once monthly, (ii) dapsone 100 mg daily, and (iii) clofazimine 50 mg daily with an additional monthly dose of 300 mg. Where clofazimine is unacceptable because of its effects on skin colour, it is replaced with ethionamide 250 mg. This triple drug therapy is given for a minimum of 2 years, preferably until such time as the patient has achieved skin smear negativity. Acute exacerbations of multibacillary disease require hospitalization with complete physical and mental rest. If the symptoms are not relieved by aspirin 0.6 g three times a day, chlorpromazine is administered for 5 days. Patients with severe symptoms or those who develop erythema nodosum leprosum lesions require treatment with prednisolone or clofazimine or thalidomide.

Paucibacillary disease: tuberculoid and borderline tuberculoid leprosy are treated with (i) rifampicin 600 mg once monthly, and (ii) dapsone 100 mg daily for 6 months.

Actinomycosis

This is a rare chronic infection caused by *A. israelii*, most commonly in the region of the lower jaw (cervicofacial). The disease is characterized by the formation of loculated abscesses with marked induration and sinus formation (Figure 5.15).

Pathology

Actinomyces israelii occurs as a normal commensal in the human mouth. The organism is anaerobic and Gram-positive but not acid fast. Although the precise conditions that result in the development of this endogenous infection are not known, the disease often follows trauma such as extraction of a carious tooth. The traumatic implantation of the organism in suffi-

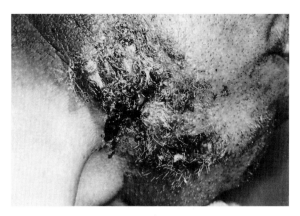

Figure 5.15 Cervicofacial actinomycosis.

cient numbers appears necessary for the establishment of the disease, and cases following human bites or penetrating hand injuries resulting from violent contact with human teeth (punch actinomycosis) are well documented. The disease starts as an area of acute suppurative inflammation that persists as a chronic process with the formation of multiple loculated abscess cavities surrounded with dense fibrosis. Colonies of the organism occur in the pus as small greyish-yellow granules (sulfur granules), and consist of a densely felted mass of filaments surrounded by radially disposed club-shaped excrescences (Figure 5.16).

The disease spreads mainly by direct contact, with considerable destruction of tissue and multiple sinus formation. Blood-borne spread is important, as exemplified by the spread of ileocaecal actinomycosis via the portal vein to the liver, with the development of multiple intercommunicating liver abscesses (honeycomb liver). Pulmonary infection may also disseminate via the blood stream to other organs such as bones, kidneys and CNS. In most instances, actinomycosis starts in the cervicofacial region (70%). In other instances, the primary infection occurs in the ileocaecal region (20%) or lungs (10%).

Treatment
The organism has a wide spectrum of sensitivity to commonly used antibiotics such as penicillin and lincomycin. Prognosis is good following prolonged antibiotic treatment [**see Gastrointestinal Disorders, Vol. II**].

Syphilis
This venereal disease is caused by *Treponema pallidum* and is transmitted by sexual intercourse. The most common portal of entry is the genital region, followed by the mouth or lips. Transmission by fomites is rare since the organisms are destroyed by rapid drying, but can occur. Placental transmission of *T. pallidum* is well documented with prenatal infection. In addition, infants may acquire extragenital infection during delivery from a mother with acute syphilis. Infants with congenital syphilis have lesions at birth or acquire them soon afterwards.

Pathology and clinical course
Following penetration of the skin or mucous membrane, the spirochetes spread along the lymphatics and lymph nodes to reach the blood stream within hours of exposure. The primary lesion, which appears some 2–4 weeks later, is known as the chancre, and is found most often in the genitalia, lips and mouth. It consists of a painless, indurated papule that breaks down to form a typically flat hard ulcer (Figure 5.17) and heals completely even without treatment. The associated regional lymphadenopathy is also painless.

The disease becomes generalized (**secondary syphilis**) within 2–3 months of infection. A widespread skin eruption (papular, vesicular or bullous) develops predominantly on the face, palms and soles. In addition, other lesions such as condylomata lata, mucous patches and serpiginous ulcers occur, usually at mucocutaneous junctions. Constitutional symptoms include low-grade fever, sore throat, headaches, joint and muscle pain, generalized lymphadenopathy, iridocyclitis and anaemia. The disease remains highly infective during this stage. All secondary lesions heal spontaneously.

Tertiary syphilis is characterized by destructive lesions of a localized or diffuse nature that probably result from hypersensitivity to the spirochetal antigens. The classical localized lesion is the gumma, which consists of an area of coagulative necrosis surrounded by a zone of lymphocytes, plasma cells and macro-

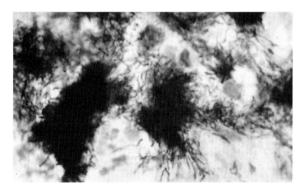

Figure 5.16 Microscopy of the sulfur granules from a patient with cervicofacial actinomycosis.

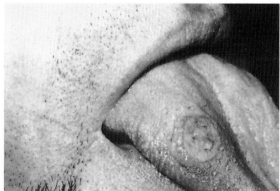

Figure 5.17 Syphilitic ulcer of the tongue: primary lesion.

phages. Adjacent arteries exhibit marked endarteritis obliterans. The most common sites of gumma include the testes, liver and bones (nose, palate, skull, clavicle, ulna and tibia). The bony lesions account for the deformities of tertiary syphilis, e.g. saddle nose (Figure 5.18). The diffuse tertiary lesions of syphilis include syphilitic aortitis and vasculitis, cerebral syphilis (meningovascular and parenchymatous) and diffuse syphilitic osteitis. The vascular lesions lead to weakening of the media with aneurysm formation and, in the case of the ascending aorta, with aortic regurgitation.

Meningovascular syphilis is characterized by focal meningitis, vascular episodes due to endarteritis and isolated cranial nerve palsies. Parenchymatous neurosyphilis comprises tabes dorsalis and general paralysis of the insane. In the former, there is degenerative demyelination and gliosis affecting the posterior columns of the spinal cord and posterior spinal nerve roots, resulting in the characteristic high stepping gait. General paralysis of the insane is a chronic syphilitic meningoencephalitis. The disease affects the frontal lobes most severely.

Diffuse syphilitic inflammation of bones in tertiary syphilis is exemplified by the sabre tibia (Figure 5.19), where the apparent bowing is due to the deposition of new periosteal bone, and the worm-eaten appearance of the skull that results from the combined effects of destruction and new bone formation.

Diagnostic tests

Treponema pallidum cannot be cultured. The organism can be identified from the exudate of primary and

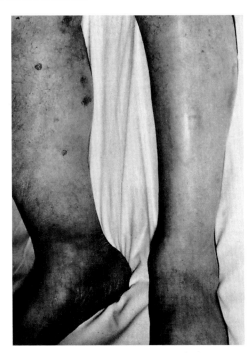

Figure 5.19 Diffuse syphilitic osteitis resulting in a sabre tibia.

secondary lesions by dark-ground illumination after fluorescent antibody staining. Serological tests are based on either the Wasserman or the treponemal antibodies. The former include the Kahn and Venereal Disease Research Laboratories (VDRL) flocculation tests, and the latter the Reiter protein complement-fixation test, the *Treponema pallidum* immobilization test (TPI) and the fluorescent treponemal antibody test (FTA). The serological tests using the treponemal antibody are more specific (fewer false-positive reactions).

Treatment

Both primary and secondary syphilis responds readily to adequate treatment, which is usually by intramuscular penicillin.

Gonorrhoea

This is caused by *N. gonorrhoea* and, in the vast majority of cases, transmission is by sexual intercourse.

Clinical features

In the female, the disease causes an acute purulent inflammation of the vulva, cervix, uterus and adnexa. Presentation with acute pelvic peritonitis and tubo-ovarian abscess is common. Secondary involvement of the rectum (proctitis) is found in 50% of females. Rarely, the rectum is the primary site of infection. In adult life the vagina is relatively resistant to gonococcal infection. This is not so in prepubertal girls, probably because of the immature and non-keratinized vaginal epithelium. Thus, gonococcal vaginitis and vulvo-vaginitis may occur in this age group. However, most cases of vulvovaginitis in prepubertal girls are not venereal in origin but result from endogenous infection

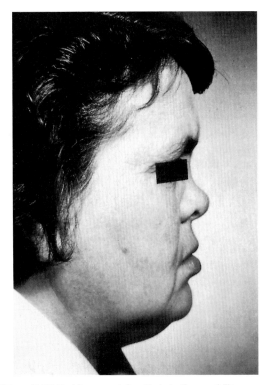

Figure 5.18 Saddle nose deformity in tertiary syphilis.

with *Neisseria* spp. (*N. sicca*, *N. flava*, etc.) from the upper respiratory tract, the organisms being introduced into the vagina by dirty hands, towels, clothing, etc. Vulvovaginitis in both children and adults can be caused by *C. albicans* and *T. vaginalis*.

In the male, infection with *N. gonorrhoea* results in inflammation of the urethra but often also involves the epididymis, seminal vesicles, bladder and prostate. The untreated urethral inflammation may lead to stricture formation of the bulbar or spongy urethra.

In both genders the disease may result in infertility due to stricture of the fallopian tubes in the female and vas deferencs in the male. One of the disastrous consequences of gonococcal infection in the female used to be infection of the eyeballs of the neonate during delivery (gonococcal ophthalmia neonatorum), which led to blindness in infancy. This is rarely encountered nowadays, with the advent of effective chemotherapy and routine instillation of silver nitrate or other antiseptic into the eyes of the newborn.

Treatment
Gonococcal infections are usually sensitive to penicillin. Tetracyclines are used for resistant infections, which account for 25% of cases.

Lymphogranuloma venereum

Lymphogranuloma venereum (LGV), also known as tropical bubo, is caused by *Chlamydia trachomatis*. Chlamydiae are obligate intracellular parasites and for this reason used to be considered as viruses. However, they have all the characteristics of bacteria, including a complex cell wall, but lack the metabolic enzymes necessary for an independent existence. *Chlamydia trachomatis* has three serotypes that cause LGV and others that are responsible for oculogenital infections.

LGV is common in tropical countries and is contracted by sexual intercourse, the reservoir of infection being the cervix in the asymptomatic female and the rectal mucosa in the asymptomatic homosexual male. It produces a papular, ulcerative or bullous lesion in the genital region that is not often painful and which heals spontaneously. This is followed within 1–6 weeks by gross lymphadenopathy (buboes). The enlarged lymph nodes in the ilio-inguinal region suppurate and subsequently ulcerate, discharging seropurulent material. The disease may involve the pelvic organs and rectum in the female. It often becomes chronic with extensive scarring leading to elephantiasis and fibrous strictures of the rectum, vagina and urethra. Sulfonamide therapy (5 g daily for 7 days) gives good results in early cases. Tetracyclines are indicated for resistant cases. Surgical treatment should only be undertaken after an adequate course of chemotherapy. Abscesses should be aspirated and incision avoided.

Granuloma inguinale

This is found in certain tropical countries and the southern USA. It is an infection with Donovan bodies (Donovania granulomatosis). Although infection is generally acquired by sexual intercourse, extragenital inoculation may occur. The primary lesion is a papule that ulcerates subsequently. In the male, it is usually found on the penis but other sites are well documented in both genders. However, the majority of primary lesions occurs in the genital, perineal, perianal or pubic regions. A 5-day course of streptomycin (4 g daily) is curative in most instances. Aureomycin, tetracycline and chloramphenicol are also effective.

Chancroid (soft chancre)

This is caused by *Haemophilus ducreyi* and is transmitted by sexual contact. The infection is more common and more severe in males. The disease starts as a soft macule, usually in the foreskin, 3–10 days after exposure. The lesion subsequently becomes necrotic and produces a ragged ulcer that may result in substantial penile destruction. These ulcers may be multiple and vary considerably in size. In the female, ulcerative lesions are found in the vulva and vagina. The inguinal lymph nodes become enlarged and painful and may suppurate. Treatment is by sulfonamides and tetracycline in the first instance. Resistant cases respond to cephalothin.

Condylomata acuminata

The term 'condylomata acuminata' (genital warts) is used to differentiate these pointed warts from the flat condylomata lata of syphilis. Genital warts result from infection with the human papilloma virus (HPV) and occur in the genital, perineal and perianal regions (Figure 5.20), and may be followed by the appearance of warts elsewhere in the body. Treatment is by the application of 10% podophyllin or excision.

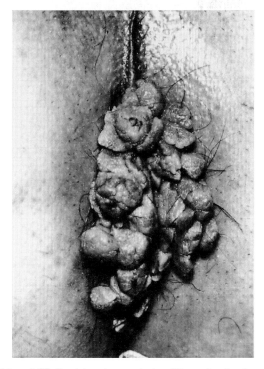

Figure 5.20 Condylomata acuminata of the perianal region.

The important infections in surgical practice are the Herpetoviridae, human papilloma virus, viral hepatitis and AIDS.

Herpetoviridae infections

This family comprises a large number of viruses but only four are pathogenic to humans. These are the herpes simplex virus (HSV), varicella zoster virus (VZV), cytomegalovirus (CMV) and Epstein–Barr virus (EBV). They are important because of their common and ubiquitous occurrence, and because of their association in some instances with the development of certain neoplastic conditions. Moreover, they can cause serious and at times fatal infections in debilitated and immunocompromised patients.

These viral infections cause an initial, often mild and inconsequential, primary infection, following which the virus remains dormant in a non-infectious state (latent) at certain sites, e.g. sensory ganglia in HSV and probably in VZV. From time to time, reactivation of the virus with occurrence of clinical manifestations, such as cold sores or shingles, may follow a febrile illness, operation, menstruation, radiotherapy, etc. The latency site for the EBV genome is thought to be the B-lymphocytes, whereas the CMV genome appears to persist in the renal tubules, leucocytes (particularly polymorphs), parotid gland and cervix.

Herpes simplex infections
There are two recognized strains: HSV-1, which is responsible for the majority of non-genital infections, and HSV-2, which accounts for most of the ocular and genital infections. HSV infections are widespread and prevalence rates range from 50 to 100% depending on socioeconomic status. The infection is acquired in the first instance by close personal contact, and genital herpes is now one of the well-recognized venereal diseases in the West, with a rising incidence such that in the UK genital herpes is twice as common as syphilis.

Labial herpes: this is the most common type of infection caused by HSV-1. The portal of entry is the mouth, and vesicular lesions occur most commonly on the lips, as cold sores, but may be severe, especially in the neonate, debilitated and immunocompromised, where they may cause extensive gingivostomatitis with intraoral/pharyngeal ulceration, fever and cervical lymphadenopathy. Rarely, the infection may disseminate to the brain, liver and adrenals, and is then usually fatal. Labial herpes is the most common recurrent type. Precipitating factors include fever, exposure to sunlight and menstruation. Each crop of labial vesicles is preceded by a burning sensation in the skin of the affected site.

Cutaneous herpes: although HSV does not penetrate intact healthy skin, infections may occur in patients with skin disorders and in the presence of burns and lacerations leading to an extensive vesicular eruption (eczema herpeticum). In burn patients, the infection may become widely disseminated and lead to severe and often fatal pneumonia.

Ocular herpes: most of these infections are due to HSV-1 except for those acquired in the neonatal period from an infected mother. The eye lesions include follicular conjunctivitis that may progress to corneal involvement with the formation of dendritic ulcers and corneal opacities. Corticosteroids enhance the eye damage caused by the virus and should be avoided in these infections.

CNS infections: HSV infections may cause encephalitis, radiculitis, myelitis and meningitis. The encephalitis is usually the result of reactivation of latent infection.

Genital herpes: although the majority of genital herpes infections is due to HSV-2, some are caused by HSV-1. The disease, which is usually sexually transmitted, has an incubation period of 2–20 days with an average of 6 days. The primary infection is followed by recurrent attacks that are usually less severe with intervening periods of latency during which the patient feels well and has no clinical manifestations. The risk of transmission of the disease is highest during an acute attack but asymptomatic individuals may pass on the disease to their sexual partners. There is strong evidence linking herpes simplex infection of the cervix with the development of cervical cancer and a four-fold increased risk is encountered in females with genital herpes. An association between cancer of the vulva and genital herpes has also been suggested, although the evidence linking the two conditions is inconclusive at present.

A primary attack is heralded by systemic symptoms due to the viraemia: malaise, fever and myalgia. The lesions are found on the penis and perianal region in the male, and labia, clitoris, vagina, cervix, perineum and perianal region in the female. They consist of painful vesicles that ulcerate, then crust and heal spontaneously. Neuralgia is often present. The severe pain during an attack may precipitate acute retention of urine.

Treatment of herpes simplex virus infections
As the virus is metabolically inactive during a latency period, treatment is futile at this stage. Effective therapy with the antiviral agent Acyclovir is possible provided it is started early during a first or recurrent attack. There is a preferential uptake of the drug by the infected (virally colonized) cells, where it is activated by a virus-specific thymidine kinase forming acyclovir triphosphate, which inhibits the viral DNA polymerase.

Varicella zoster virus infections
The painful clinical condition known as zoster (formerly herpes zoster) is always the result of a reactivation of the same virus that causes chickenpox. Although in some instances no apparent cause for this activation

is clinically obvious, in others a state of depressed cell-mediated immunity is present due to trauma, malignancy and immunosuppressive drugs, particularly in transplant patients. In severely immunocompromised patients, the infection may be systemic, with the development of pneumonia and involvement of other organs such as the liver, CNS, adrenals and pancreas. The systemic disease carries a very high mortality.

In the more usual condition, an exanthematous rash develops over a dermatome supplied by a specific dorsal nerve root or extramedullary nerve ganglion. The dermatomes supplied by the third dorsal to the second lumbar segment of the spinal cord are the ones most commonly affected, followed by that supplied by the fifth cranial nerve. Pain and paraesthesiae often pre-date the development of the vesicular rash. The most distressing feature of the disease is the development of neuralgia (St Anthony's fire), which may persist for several weeks and require specialist treatment.

Cytomegalovirus infections

The pattern of infection with CMV varies with the socioeconomic state of the country. In poor, developing countries with overcrowding and poor sanitation, the disease is acquired early in life and by the age of 5 years, the vast majority of children becomes sero-positive for the virus. In the West neonatal infection is rare and most primary infections are acquired in adolescence, mainly from kissing and sexual intercourse, such that the prevalence of seropositive individuals rises to 60–70% by the age of 60 years. The disease can be transmitted by the transfusion of blood products, particularly fresh blood and pooled platelet donations, and organ and bone marrow transplantation. It is thus a real hazard in transplant patients and in patients with leukaemia, since the transmission of the virus may be followed by serious infection due to the immunocompromised state, leading to hepatitis, haemolytic anaemia, leucopenia and thrombocytopenia. The average reported mortality of this generalized CMV disease is 2% but can be as high as 15–20%, especially in bone marrow transplant recipients.

The infection may be transmitted to the fetus across the placenta. This may result in intrauterine death and spontaneous abortion. The vast majority of congenitally infected babies appears normal at birth, but 10–30% of them will suffer brain damage (microcephaly) and mental retardation. A few babies show the classical cytomegalic inclusion disease, the features of which are similar to those of the generalized disease encountered in immunosuppressed adults.

Infection in a normal adolescent may be asymptomatic or the individual may develop fever, sore throat, lymphadenopathy and hepatosplenomegaly. The clinical picture is very similar to that of glandular fever but the Paul Bunnell test is negative. The blood may contain the characteristic intranuclear inclusions (owl eye) within atypical mononuclear cells. Anti-CMV antibodies can be demonstrated following the primary infection.

In susceptible immunocompromised patients, the risk of CMV infection may be reduced by using blood and organs from CMV-negative donors, transfusion of leucocyte-free blood and administration of high titre anti-CMV immunoglobulins to the recipients.

Epstein–Barr virus infections

This gammaherpes virus was the first virus to be identified in human neoplastic cells. In excess of 90% of the world population becomes infected with EBV before adolescence. Aside from causing glandular fever (infectious mononucleosis), infection with EBV leads to the development of a number of tumours, e.g. lymphoproliferative disorders (endemic Burkitt's lymphoma, opportunistic lymphoma, nasal natural killer cell lymphoma), gastric carcinoma (10–15% of case world-wide), nasopharyngeal carcinoma and spindle cell tumours (in immunocompromised hosts) [see Gastrointestinal Disorders, Vol. II].

Individuals that become infected with EBV become life-long carriers. The virus homes on two target cell types, B-lymphocytes (latent virus) and the epithelial cells of the oropharynx (replicating virus), which are thus the main site of intermittent production of infectious virus, the B-lymphocytes becoming infected by circulating within the oropharyngeal mucosa. The infected B-lymphocytes then carry the virus elsewhere, with infection of other epithelial sites.

Infectious mononucleosis is a disease of the West with a peak incidence in adolescence and young adult life. It is transmitted in the saliva by kissing and is often referred to as the 'kissing disease'. The incubation period varies from 4 to 7 weeks and is followed by the development of malaise, fever, asthenia, sore throat, lymphadenopathy and splenomegaly. The blood picture shows a lymphocytosis with more than 10% atypical monocytes. The Paul Bunnell test, which detects the presence of heterophile antibodies to sheep red cells, is positive. The liver function tests are often deranged during the first week of the illness, which usually lasts for 3–4 weeks. However, prolonged asthenia and debility for several months after the acute illness are quite common.

Human papilloma virus

The human papilloma virus (HPV) is a DNA virus and there are more than 60 different types that can cause various types of lesions in squamous epithelium. Common warts found on the feet and hands are caused by HPV types 1 and 2, whereas genital warts are commonly caused by types 6 and 11, although several other types may be responsible. Anogenital papilloma virus is transmitted by sexual activity but the epidemiology is poorly understood owing to difficulties in obtaining accurate information.

Epidemiological data and molecular biology studies have shown a clear association between both female genital cancer and anal squamous cell cancer and a sexually transmitted agent. Nucleic acid hybridization techniques have demonstrated that various types of

HPV are integrated into the genome of these tumours. In addition to being responsible for anogenital warts, they are known to be the causative agent in premalignant intraepithelial neoplasia of the cervix (CIN), vulva (VIN), vagina (VAIN) and anus (AIN).

Viral hepatitis

There are many viruses that can infect the human liver and cause hepatitis of varying severity (Table 5.2). Some are essentially hepatotropic, i.e. the liver is the primary site of infection. At least six distinct viruses fall into this category: A, B, C, D, E and G. In addition, others are still undefined and are referred to as non-A and non-B (NANB).

Viral hepatitis is the most common liver disease today and constitutes a world-wide problem. Following the acute illness that may progress to fulminant liver failure, persistence of the virus leads to chronic liver disease, the severity of which varies from healthy asymptomatic carrier to ongoing chronic active disease with progression to cirrhosis and, in the case of

Table 5.2 Viruses causing acute hepatitis

Hepatitis A (HAV)	Enteral transmission, rarely causes liver cell necrosis
Hepatitis B (HBV)	Transmitted by blood products, needles, tattooing, sexual activity, mothers to babies, aerosol (dental treatment); can progress to liver cell necrosis and chronic liver disease
Hepatitis C (HCV)	Transmitted sexually and by blood products, can progress to liver cell necrosis; high incidence of progression to chronic liver disease
Hepatitis Delta (HDV)	Incomplete hepatotropic virus; capable of infection only when activated by HBV. Acquired either as a coinfection with HBV or as superinfection in HbsAg carriers
Hepatitis E (HEV)	Enteral transmission. Mild self-limiting disease. Does not progress to chronic liver disease
Hepatitis G (HGV)	Transmitted by blood products. Uncertain clinical significance
Epstein–Barr virus (EBV)	Agent of infectious mononucleosis. Hepatitis rare and usually mild
Cytomegalovirus (CMV)	Immunosuppressed patients and infants
Yellow fever virus	Can cause liver cell necrosis when mortality is high
Ebola and Marburg virus	Causes African haemorrhagic fever, consisting of papular rash, DIC, pancreatitis and hepatitis. Spread by needles and person to person. High mortality. No specific therapy available
Others	

hepatitis B and C disease, the development of hepatocellular carcinoma.

Hepatitis A

Hepatitis A virus (HAV) is also known as enterovirus type 72 and the disease was formerly known as infectious hepatitis. The virus is shed in large numbers in the faeces for a few weeks before the overt clinical illness, which varies in severity. The IgM antibody to the virus (anti-HAV) is present in high titres in the serum early on during the acute disease and is detected for 6 months after an acute infection. The IgG antibody indicates past infection and is present in 40–50% of the urban population in Britain. Hepatitis A rarely gives rise to chronic liver disease and carries a low mortality.

Hepatitis B

Hepatitis B virus (HBV) infection is caused by a double-stranded DNA virus that replicates by reverse transcription. Hepatitis B is endemic in the entire human population and hyperendemic in many parts of the world. The extent of the infection is indicated by the estimated 300 million people who have persistent infection with the virus. The transmission of the acute disease is by the parenteral route and was formerly common as a complication of blood transfusion; hence the old terminology of 'serum or post-transfusion hepatitis'. With the testing of donors for the HBV, and the heat-inactivation methods for the preparation of the protein fractions, hepatitis B after transfusion of blood and blood products has been virtually eliminated. The HBV has great infectivity and is transmitted by needle sharing in drug misusers, in whom it is prevalent. It has caused disease in surgeons and nurses as a result of accidental injuries by 'sharps'.

The HBV has been fully characterized. The whole virus (virion) is known as the Dane particle and consists of a core covered by surface antigen (HbsAg). The latter is formed in excess as separate tubules and spheres. The centre of the virus contains a core antigen (HbcAg) that is never found in the circulating blood, the 'e' antigen (HbeAg), double-stranded DNA and a DNA polymerase. Antibodies are formed to the various antigens and can be detected in the peripheral blood at some time in all patients during the acute infection and in some carriers. The HbeAg is encountered early on during the course of the acute hepatitis, and is usually associated with high titres of HbsAg and the presence of Dane particles (complete HBV). It is the best marker of probable infectivity, and is usually replaced by the anti-HbeAg antibody soon after the jaundice develops. Anti-HbsAg denotes recovery from acute infection and immunity. Anti-HBcAg is detected in the peripheral blood early on during the acute infection. It is not protective and is found in all carriers. Anti-HbeAg is present in convalescent patients and in the majority of carriers. This antibody is associated with a low probability of infectivity. The interpretation of the various serum markers of hepatitis B is shown in Table 5.3.

Hepatitis B may be followed by chronic liver disease,

Table 5.3 Guide to the interpretation of serum markers of hepatitis B

HbsAg	HBeAg	Anti-HBe	Anti-HBc	Anti-HBs	Interpretation
+	+	−	−	−	Incubation period or early acute hepatitis B
+	+	−	+	−	Acute hepatitis B or persistent carrier
+	−	+	+	−	Late acute hepatitis B or persistent carrier
+	−	−	+	−	Late acute hepatitis B or persistent carrier
−	−	+	+	+	Convalescent acute hepatitis B
−	−	−	+	+	Past infection

which in some types progresses to cirrhosis and end-stage liver disease requiring liver transplantation. It is also responsible for the development of hepatocellular carcinoma. The viral genome (DNA) of HBV becomes incorporated in the host DNA and this integration has been shown to be a necessary step in the development of primary hepatocellular carcinoma (HCC). The important role of HBV infection in the development of HCC is now well established in hyperendemic areas.

Chronic hepatitis B
Chronic infection with HBV occurs in 5–10% of adult patients who are unable to eliminate the HbsAg within 3 months from the acute infection. The previous classification of chronic hepatitis B into the healthy HbsAg carrier state and patients with chronic B hepatitis (chronic persistent and chronic active) has been superseded by a more valid classification that has therapeutic and prognostic implications. The new classification is based on (i) the presence or absence of HBV replication (assessed by measuring HBV-DNA or HbeAg in the serum, or HbcAg in the liver), and (ii) the presence or absence of liver cell inflammation by assay of the serum aminotransferase activities, ASAT or SGOT. Replication of HBV is usually associated with raised ASAT or SGOT. Three categories are thus recognized:

- chronic HbeAg-positive hepatitis (CHBe$^+$)
- chronic HbeAg-negative hepatitis with normal aminotransferase activity (CHBe$^-$/ASAT$^-$)
- chronic HbeAg-negative hepatitis with raised aminotransferase activity (CHBe$^-$/ASAT$^+$).

Chronic HbeAg-positive hepatitis
Antigen-positive disease with evidence of viral replication comprises 15% of patients. The disease is usually associated with continued liver cell inflammation (raised transaminases) and is symptomatic. On follow-up seroconversion from HBe$^+$ to HBe$^-$ occurs in about 50% of patients during the ensuing 5 years, with improvement in symptoms and normalization of the liver function tests. However, subsequent reactivation (with seroconversion to HBe$^+$) occurs in 5% of patients. The overall 5-year mortality is 10%.

Chronic HBeAg-negative hepatitis with normal aminotransferase activity
The 'normal carrier' state accounts for the majority of cases (60%). These patients have no viral replication or symptoms and their liver function tests are normal. The outcome of this group of patients is good and the mortality is low but they are subject to superinfection with HDV (see below). The reactivation with seroconversion to HBe$^+$ is low in these patients.

Chronic HbeAg-negative hepatitis with raised aminotransferase activity
This is encountered in 25% of patients and forms a heterogeneous group with either ongoing HBV replication (liver HbcAg$^+$ despite being seronegative for HbeAg) or other hepatic disease, e.g. concomitant HDV infection, autoimmune reactivity, alcohol misuse, drug-related hepatitis, hepatocellular carcinoma or schistosomiasis. The outcome in the individual patient depends on the exact aetiology. Symptomatic decompensated cirrhosis is highest in this category and develops in 20–30% of patients.

Vaccination against hepatitis B
There is now an official recommendation that health-service workers, particularly all doctors and nurses, should undergo active immunization against hepatitis B. Within the UK all students seeking admission to medical schools must also undergo this vaccination. The licensed vaccines that are available are prepared either by means of genetic engineering (recombinant hepatitis B vaccine) or from fully purified formalin-inactivated B surface antigen (HbsAg) obtained from the plasma of known carriers. Both types of vaccine are safe and effective. The vaccination programme consists of three doses administered at zero time, 2 months and a booster at 6 months. This regimen is effective in preventing the development of hepatitis B if immunization is started within a few weeks of exposure, that is after an interval which is less than the incubation period of the disease. It is the recommended treatment in non-immunized medical and nursing staff who sustain accidental injury by 'sharps' contaminated with blood from an infected patient. Some also advise the administration of hepatitis B specific immunoglobulin for additional (passive) immunization. The previous concern that some of these commercial IgG preparations were unsafe because of contamination by HIV has been abolished by HIV testing of donors and the introduction of rigorous techniques that ensure viral inactivation during the processing of the donated plasma.

Hepatitis C

Hepatitis C virus (HCV) is a lipid-enveloped, circular, single-stranded RNA virus. Hepatitis C is transmitted by blood products. Thus, approximately 80% of patients with NANB hepatitis and haemophiliacs are HCV positive by antibody testing. Hepatitis C is also frequently encountered in dialysis patients (20%) and is common in drug addicts. It causes acute hepatitis that progresses to chronic hepatitis and cirrhosis. HCV is a major cause of chronic liver disease and hepatocellular carcinoma world-wide. Following the acute infection, 85% of patients develop chronic infection with persistent viraemia. The chronic hepatitis may run a mild course with fluctuating levels of transaminase levels over several years, but progression to cirrhosis is encountered in 30% of cases. The variable course is thought to be the result of host factors, e.g. route and size of the infecting inoculum, patient's gender, age at time of infection and alcohol consumption. Thus, severe chronic disease is rare in females, whereas chronic alcohol consumption and increasing age at the time of infection are strong risk factors for disease progression. Cirrhosis due to HCV is now the most common indication for liver transplantation in the West. Recurrence of HCV in the grafted organ is very common and 50% of transplanted patients develop chronic hepatitis. Early intervention with interferon and ribavirin may prevent or delay the progression of HCV-related graft disease. As with HBV, there is a strong link between persistent HCV infection and the development of hepatocellular carcinoma. Thus, anti-HCV antibodies are found in over 70% of non-hepatitis B patients who develop this tumour.

Hepatitis delta virus disease

Hepatitis delta virus (HDV) is an incomplete hepatotropic virus that is unable to replicate on its own. It is thus capable of infection only when activated by the presence of HBV, when it forms a virion particle consisting of an outer coat (from the HBs antigen of HBV) and an inner core of HDAg and RNA genome. The disease may be acquired either as a coinfection together with HBV in previously normal individuals or as superinfection in carriers of HBsAg. Special subsets of HbsAg carriers are at high risk of superinfection. These include those individuals who are exposed to multiple blood and interpersonal contacts such as intravenous drug addicts, haemophiliacs, institutionalized patients, prisoners and homosexuals. Parenteral inoculation appears to be the most efficient mode of transmission. It is now known that blood that is negative for the HBsAg may transmit HDV at a frequency of 1 in 3000 transfusions.

Coinfection in previously normal individuals usually leads to a self-limiting hepatitis with a variable clinical presentation. Both IgM (during acute illness) and IgG (in the convalescent period and for 1–2 years after clearance of the HBsAg) anti-HDAg antibodies appear in the plasma in moderate to severe disease, which may progress to fulminant hepatic failure. The more usual mild form of coinfection causes little or no serological response.

In superinfection, the HDV aggravates pre-existing type B hepatitis (chronic aggressive hepatitis) or induces new HDV disease in healthy HBsAg carriers. In the latter group, the hepatitis is often severe and may progress to fulminant hepatic failure. There is good evidence that therapy with interferon can eradicate HDV infection.

Hepatitis E

Hepatitis E virus (HEV) consists of a non-enveloped single-stranded RNA, which causes enterally transmitted hepatitis. The epidemiological features are similar to those of hepatitis A but the E virus is serologically different and it can infect individuals who have recovered from hepatitis A. The disease is spread by contamination of drinking water with sewage and by person-to-person contact. Hepatitis E is extremely common in developing countries, where it accounts for over 50% of cases of acute viral hepatitis. Although the disease is usually mild to moderate, HEV infection tends to be particularly severe and is associated with a high mortality in pregnant women.

Non-A and non-B hepatitis

This term is reserved for hepatitis by as yet unidentified viruses and the diagnosis is made by exclusion of the known hepatotropic viruses and CMV. Hepatitis C was grouped within this category before its isolation and cloning. NANB hepatitis (with unidentified viruses) remains the problem facing the transfusion of blood and blood products (as there are no tests to screen donors who may harbour these viruses). It accounts for the vast majority of all-transfusion related hepatitis and approximately 7–10% of transfused patients develop the infection. NANB is also transmitted by clotting factor concentrates (factors VIII and IX) and for this reason is very common in haemophiliac patients. Outbreaks following intravenous administration of immunoglobulin have been reported. The incubation period of NANB hepatitis varies widely but averages 8 weeks. The disease is clinically indistinguishable from hepatitis A and B and may indeed cause fulminant liver failure. However, in most instances the hepatitis is mild and may only be represented by an elevation of the serum aminotransferase enzymes. None the less, significant cohorts of patient who contract NANB infection go on to develop chronic liver disease. The clinical significance of the recently isolated hepatitis G virus (HGV) reported in patients after blood transfusion remains uncertain.

Acquired immunodeficiency syndrome and related conditions

There is no doubt regarding the world-wide devastation caused by AIDS and its allied conditions: persistent generalized lymphadenopathy (PGL) and AIDS-related complex (ARC). Since the first few cases were recognized in the USA in 1981, estimates from the World Health Organization from 180 countries show that over 10 million people are infected with the virus (HIV positive) but are currently well. The majority of these will, in time, develop the disease and eventually die from it. AIDS has particular relevance to surgeons and other health-care workers who, by virtue of their occupation, are at risk, although with suitable precautions the risk of acquiring the infection from patients is small.

Virology and immune deficiency

The first virus was isolated in France from a patient with lymphadenopathy and was therefore called lymphadenopathy-associated virus (LAV). In the USA the virus was first isolated from AIDS patients and was thus named human T-cell lymphotropic virus type III (HTLV III) to distinguish it from other known lymphotropic viruses (home in on lymphocytes) such as HTLV-I and HTLV-II. The former is associated with a special form of leukaemia/lymphoma. There is now international agreement that the term HIV should be used to describe the agent responsible for AIDS and allied conditions (PGL, ARC). More recently, a variant, HIV-2, has been isolated from African patients, but there does not appear to be any material difference in the disease potential between these two viruses and the collective term HIV is recommended for either agent.

The structure of HIV is shown in Figure 5.21. It is a retrovirus, i.e. its genome contains only RNA, and to replicate once it invades the host cell, the viral RNA is transcribed into DNA by a special viral enzyme called reverse transcriptase, i.e. new viral RNA is made using the host DNA as the template (reverse of the normal process: DNA makes RNA makes protein). Once introduced into the blood stream, HIV homes in on the T-helper lymphocytes, monocytes and macrophages that carry the surface receptor, CD4, on to which the virus latches. The T-helper lymphocytes (CD4) thus colonized are progressively destroyed. By contrast, the colonized macrophages, although providing a reservoir for continued viral replication, seem to be resistant to its destructive effects. HIV also colonizes the neural tissue and this accounts for the dementia that develops in some patients. The T-suppressor/cytotoxic lympho-

Table 5.4 Parameters of immunodeficiency disorder in AIDS, PGL and ARC

- Decreased CD4-positive lymphocytes and lymphopenia
- Decreased ratio CD4:CD8 lymphocytes
- Reduced cytotoxic response
- Reduced monocyte function
- Increased immunoglobulins
- Decreased blastogenic response of lymphocytes to mitogens
- Cutaneous anergy to multiple skin-test antigens
- Increased levels of circulating immune complexes

cytes are not colonized because they contain a different receptor (CD8). The replication and expression of the virus in the T-helper lymphocyte terminates when the cell dies prematurely. The longitudinal consequence of this HIV–T-helper lymphocyte interaction for the infected patient are impaired function and progressive gradual depletion of the T-helper lymphocytes, reversal of the helper/inducer (CD4) to suppressor/cytotoxic (CD8) cell ratio and progressive decrease in the level of detectable virus in the blood. The immunological depression is characterized by several abnormal parameters (Table 5.4).

Laboratory evidence of human immunodeficiency virus infection

The current routine tests are based on the detection of antibodies to circulating HIV. Following infection, antibodies to the various antigens appear in the circulation. These do not appear to confer any benefit but are used in the diagnosis (HIV antibody testing). Regrettably, there is a long period (usually 6 weeks but sometimes several months) between infection and the appearance of antibodies. There is, therefore, a long 'window' when an individual may have negative antibody testing to HIV and still be infected.

Other tests include viral cultivation from the patient's lymphocytes, detection of circulating viral P-24 antigen (useful in helping to establish infection in an infant whose HIV antibodies may be maternal) and the use of the polymerase chain reaction (PCR), by which the very small amount of viral DNA in infected cells can be greatly amplified. The PCR method is the gold standard test for the confirmation of HIV infection.

Transmission of human immunodeficiency virus infection

The proven vehicles of infection are blood, semen and vaginal secretions. The disease is transmitted by penetrative unprotected sexual intercourse (homosexual and heterosexual), needle sharing by drug misusers and blood products. Prior to the introduction of HIV testing of donors, a large proportion of haemophiliacs were infected by contaminated clotting factor concentrates, as were a few patients who received blood transfusion

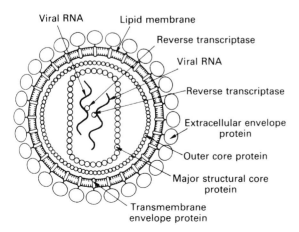

Viral RNA
Lipid membrane
Reverse transcriptase
Viral RNA
Reverse transcriptase
Extracellular envelope protein
Outer core protein
Major structural core protein
Transmembrane envelope protein

Figure 5.21 The structure of HIV.

to cover surgical procedures, especially cardiac operations. With the introduction of testing of blood donations, this route of transmission has now been eliminated but regrettably many of the infected haemophiliacs have died of AIDS and some have transmitted the disease to their legitimate sexual partners. The largest two groups contracting HIV infection are still active homosexuals (especially those with multiple partners) and drug addicts and users, in whom HIV is spread by sharing contaminated needles.

Babies of HIV-positive mothers have a 25% risk of contracting the infection *in utero* or perinatally and by breast feeding. By contrast, parents of infected children have not been shown to be at risk. Oral zidovudine during late pregnancy and labour reduces the rate of mother to child transmission of HIV by 51%. The longer course reduces it by 67%. Breast feeding in the short course remains a problem, as this is responsible for one-third of the maternal transmission. Thus, in short-course prevention, breast feeding has to be replaced by formula feeding of the babies.

There is no evidence that HIV is transmitted by non-sexual social contact (including sharing meals), accidental contamination with blood during participation in contact sport or by blood-sucking insects. Transmission by human bites is possible and occurs if blood is transmitted.

The risk of transmission to health-care workers is due to certain mishaps:

- **direct percutaneous inoculations of infected blood, e.g. accident by sharps (needle pricks, scalpel stab injuries, etc.)**
- **spillage of infected blood on to skin may introduce infection through minute scratches or abrasions**
- **contamination of mucosal surfaces by infected blood, e.g. accidental splashing of eyes**
- **transfer of infected material via environmental surfaces, e.g. blood-contaminated equipment and instruments.**

The question concerning the risk involved in mouth to mouth resuscitation in an emergency remains unsettled, although there have been no such reported incidents to date.

Clinical features of human immunodeficiency virus infection

The majority of patients does not develop any symptoms after the infection and is discovered to be HIV positive with testing. A small proportion of individuals acquires a self-limiting illness which resembles infectious mononucleosis a few weeks to months after the infection and others exhibit a transient encephalitis. Several months later, some infected subjects develop a more lasting generalized enlargement of the lymph nodes, PGL. Significant symptoms start to appear with disease progression and these include weight loss, chronic diarrhoea, minor opportunistic infections and candidiasis. The deterioration in health and physique is clear cut with progression to full-blown AIDS, the clinical features of which vary in accordance with the type of indicator illness that develops. The average incubation period from the time of infection to full-blown AIDS is 8 years, although faster progression is well documented. At present, the available evidence suggests that eventually most HIV-positive subjects will develop AIDS, although the time frame is variable and there are prospects that aggressive antiretroviral therapy may delay or stop the development of the disease. The clinical markers associated with an increased risk of progression to AIDS are: constitutional symptoms, oral candidiasis and oral hairy leucoplakia. The laboratory indices which are also predictive of progression to AIDS include anaemia, lymphopenia, neutropenia, raised erythrocyte sedimentation rate (ESR), reduced T-helper (CD4) lymphocytes, raised CD8 lymphocytes, elevated viral antigenaemia (P24) and reduced anti-P24 antibodies.

The following clinical definitions are now accepted.

- **AIDS: acquired immunodeficiency syndrome is defined as a syndrome in which a person has a reliably diagnosed disease that is at least moderately indicative of an underlying cellular immune deficiency (e.g. an opportunistic infection or Kaposi's sarcoma in a person aged less than 60 years) but who, at the same time, has no known underlying cause of cellular immune deficiency or any other cause of reduced resistance reported to be associated with that disease.** The reliably diagnosed disease is referred to as the indicator disease. The nature of this varies according to the absence (Table 5.5) or presence of laboratory evidence of HIV infection (Table 5.6). Absence of laboratory evidence may arise because the tests for HIV were not performed (for any reason) or gave inconclusive results. In the UK, the most commonly diagnosed indicator illness for AIDS is pneumonia due to *Pneumocystis carinii*.
- **PGL: persistent generalized lymphadenopathy is defined as lymphadenopathy at two or more non-contiguous, non-inguinal sites for 3 months or longer in the absence of any current illness or medication known to cause enlarged lymph nodes.**
- **ARC: AIDS-related complex is defined as weight loss of more than 10%, intermittent fever of more than 38°C, intermittent or continuous diarrhoea, fatigue and malaise, night sweats and PGL.**

In addition, both PGL and ARC must be accompanied by at least two abnormalities indicative of an immune deficiency/disorder. With the above definitions and criteria, an alternative useful clinical classification of HIV infection, which embraces all stages, is shown in Table 5.7.

Table 5.5 Indicator diseases for case definition of AIDS for surveillance purposes without laboratory evidence regarding HIV infection (Centers for Disease Control, Atlanta, Georgia)

1. Candidiasis of the oesophagus, trachea, bronchi or lungs
2. Extrapulmonary cryptococcosis
3. Cryptosporidiosis with diarrhoea > 1 month
4. Cytomegalovirus disease of an organ other than liver, spleen or lymph node in a patient > 1 month of age
5. Herpes simplex virus infection causing a mucocutaneous ulcer that persists longer than one month; or bronchitis, pneumonitis or oesophagitis for any duration affecting a patient > 1 month of age
6. Kaposi's sarcoma affecting a patient < 60 years of age
7. Primary lymphoma of the brain affecting a patient < 60 years of age
8. Lymphoid interstitial pneumonia and or pulmonary lymphoid hyperplasia affecting a child < 13 years of age
9. *Mycobacterium avium* complex or *M. kansasii* disease, disseminated (at a site other than or in addition to lungs, skin, cervical or hilar lymph nodes)
10. *Pneumocystis carinii* pneumonia
11. Progressive multifocal leucoencephalopathy
12. Toxoplasmosis of the brain affecting a patient > 1 month of age

Table 5.6 Indicator diseases for case definition of AIDS for surveillance purposes with laboratory evidence regarding HIV infection (Centers for Disease Control, Atlanta, Georgia)

1. Bacterial infections, multiple or recurrent (any combination of at least two within a 2-year period), of the following types affecting a child < 13 years of age: septicaemia, pneumonia, meningitis, bone or joint infection, or abscess of an internal organ or body cavity (excluding otitis media or superficial skin or mucosal abscesses), caused by *Haemophilus*, *Streptococcus* or other pyogenic bacteria
2. Coccidioidomycosis, disseminated (at a site other than or in addition to lungs or cervical or hilar lymph nodes)
3. HIV encephalopathy (HIV/AIDS dementia)
4. Histoplasmosis, disseminated (at a site other than or in addition to lungs or cervical or hilar lymph nodes)
5. Isosporiasis with diarrhoea persisting > 1 month
6. Kaposi's sarcoma at any age
7. Primary lymphoma of the brain at any age
8. Other non-Hodgkin's lymphoma of B-cell or unknown immunological phenotype
9. Any mycobacterial disease caused by mycobacteria other than *M. tuberculosis*, disseminated (at a site other than or in addition to lungs, skin, or cervical or hilar lymph nodes)
10. Disease caused by *M. tuberculosis*, extrapulmonary (involving at least one site outside the lung, regardless of whether there is a concurrent pulmonary involvement)
11. *Salmonella* (non-typhoid) septicaemia, recurrent
12. HIV wasting syndrome (emaciation, slim disease)

Tumours in acquired immunodeficiency syndrome

The tumours that develop in AIDS patients are Kaposi's sarcoma, primary cerebral lymphoma and non-Hodgkin's lymphomas. Kaposi's sarcoma is one of the most common manifestations of AIDS and carries a high mortality (usually from severe opportunistic infections) with a median survival of 18–24 months. The tumour is a multifocal metastasizing malignant reticulosis, with features resembling those of angiosarcoma. It involves principally the skin (multiple red violaceous nodules), mucous membranes and lymph nodes, although visceral lesions are sometimes encountered. The disease in AIDS sufferers differs in several respects from Kaposi's sarcoma developing in immunocompetent individuals. There is now an established association of AIDS Kaposi's sarcoma with CMV infection. Significant palliation can be obtained by local radiotherapy.

The non-Hodgkin's lymphomas which develop in AIDS patients are of either B-cell or indeterminate origin and of certain histological types: small non-cleaved lymphoma (either Burkitt or non-Burkitt), immunoblastic lymphoma, large-cell lymphoma, diffuse histiocytic lymphoma, diffuse undifferentiated lymphoma and high-grade lymphoma.

Antiviral therapy for acquired immunodeficiency syndrome

The antiviral drug in established clinical use is 3'-azido-3'deoxythymide (zidovudine, azidothymidine, AZT). It acts as a chain-terminator in DNA synthesis. The 3'-azido group prevents the formation of further 5'-3' phosphodiester linkages and, for this reason, DNA synthesis is halted. AZT therapy in patients with AIDS results in both clinical and immunological improvement. The latter is indicated by increased CD4 helper lymphocytes, reduction in the circulating antigenaemia and restoration of cutaneous delayed-type hypersensitivity in previously anergic patients. AZT is particularly effective in promoting recovery in patients who develop *P. carinii* pneumonia. The accumulated clinical experience with AZT indicates that therapy, which has to be continued indefinitely, extends the life expectancy of AIDS patients but does not cure the disease. Unfortunately, AZT is very toxic and causes bone-marrow depression (anaemia and neutropenia), nausea and vomiting, and CNS complications (headaches, confusion, fits and Wernicke's encephalopathy). Combination therapy with other antiviral agents such as acyclovir seems to result in potentiation but is also attended by increased toxicity. AZT has also been used in combination with interferon. Several other chemotherapeutic agents with similar actions to AZT (inhibit reverse transcriptase) are being evaluated, e.g. 2',3'-dideoxycytidine and ansamycin. Active immunization may protect against disease progression. At present, two types of vaccine are being developed: inactivated whole virus vaccines and anti-idiotype vaccines (block CD4 receptors).

Acquired immunodeficiency syndrome and hospital surgical practice

Experience in Britain and other countries suggests that the risk to health-care workers is low provided certain universal and specific precautions are adopted routinely. As many infected individuals are unaware that they are HIV positive, all patients should be assumed to be infectious for HIV and other blood-borne pathogens. It is unsafe to apply universal precautions only in high-risk groups and in patients known to be HIV positive. The universal precautions (Table 5.8) apply to all health workers exposed to the following body fluids: blood, amniotic fluid, pericardial fluid, peritoneal fluid, pleural fluid, synovial fluid, cerebrospinal fluid, and semen and vaginal secretions. Universal precautions do not apply to exposure to faeces, nasal secretions, sputum, sweat, tears, urine and vomit. Although saliva is not regarded as a risk vehicle, precautions are needed in dental and oral work, as the saliva is then likely to be contaminated with the patient's blood.

When blood samples are obtained the doctor should wear disposable gloves. Plastic aprons and eye protection are needed when splashing or spurting is likely. Blood should be collected preferably with Vacutainers and on no account must the needle be resheathed. In high-risk cases, all specimens sent to the laboratory must be sealed in a plastic bag and marked with a red hazard sticker, as for hepatitis B. Accidental spillage of blood should be treated with 1% sodium hypochlorite solution.

The specific guidelines for operating-theatre staff are outlined in Table 5.9. All staff involved in the operating theatre should wear plastic aprons, disposable gowns, goggles, gloves and impermeable leg and footwear.

Table 5.7 Alternative useful clinical classification of HIV infection

Group I	Acute infection: infectious mononucleosis-type illness
Group II	Asymptomatic infection: asymptomatic HIV-positive subjects
Group III	Persistent generalized lymphadenopathy (PGL)
Group IV	A: Constitutional disease: fever, diarrhoea and weight loss lasting > 1 month B: Neurological disease: dementia, myelopathy and peripheral neuropathy C: Secondary infectious disease: opportunistic C_1: Specified in CDC surveillance definition of AIDS C_2: Other infections: oral hairy leucoplakia, nocardiosis, oral candidiasis, etc. D: Secondary cancers: Kaposi's sarcoma, non-Hodgkin's lymphomas, primary cerebral lymphoma E: Other conditions: other disorders attributable to HIV infection

Table 5.8 Universal precautions against the spread of AIDS

1. These apply to all patients irrespective of risk category or HIV status (known or unknown)
2. Care in the handling of sharps: needles, scalpels, sharp instruments, etc.
3. All cuts and abrasions on patients and staff should be covered with a waterproof dressing. Personnel should wear plastic aprons and disposable gloves when dealing with blood or secretions
4. Parenteral procedures should be kept to a minimum
5. External surfaces of equipment and bench surfaces which may have been contaminated by blood and other secretions should be wiped with a fresh preparation of sodium hypochlorite solution 1% (10 000 ppm available chlorine) or 2% activated gluteraldehyde. Contaminated gloves, paper tissues and cotton wool should be incinerated.
6. In the event of a death of a person with AIDS, the body should be wrapped in impermeable plastic sheeting or a polythene cadaver bag before coffining
7. Equipment being sent for maintenance and servicing should be disinfected with gluteraldehyde before leaving the ward or theatre
8. Disposable equipment should be used wherever possible, and reusable equipment immersed in 2% gluteraldehyde for 1 h before being returned for processing
9. Walls and floor should be cleaned with soap and water

Action in the event of an accident involving possible transmission to medical and nursing staff

The rate of transmission resulting from accidental inoculation of health-care workers with blood from individuals known to be infected has been reported to be of the order of 0.13–0.55, i.e. 1:770 to 1:200 chance of infection as a result of any single event. When such an accident occurs, the following procedure is necessary.

■ **Contaminated areas (spillage and splashes) or injury site (from sharps) should be immediately and thoroughly washed with soap and water.**
■ **The incident is reported to the Occupation Health Officer.**
■ **If the HIV status of the source patient is not known, the patient consent's for HIV testing is obtained. This is usually forthcoming but if the patient declines consent, the statement by the General Medical Council becomes relevant: 'Only in the most exceptional circumstances, where a test is imperative in order to secure the safety of persons other than the patient, and where it is not possible for the prior consent of the patient to be obtained, can testing without explicit consent be justified.' In such a difficult situation, this statement implies that HIV testing of a blood specimen that had previously been**

Table 5.9 Guidelines for operating-theatre staff

- It is justifiable to set aside a theatre and staff solely for HIV-positive patients.
- Shaving should be avoided
- The anaesthetic room staff should wear disposable masks, plastic aprons, gloves and overshoes
- The anaesthetic machine and work surfaces should be stripped of all but essential equipment
- All theatre staff should wear impermeable overshoes, which must not be taken out of the theatre
- All staff, scrubbed and unscrubbed, should wear disposable gowns, plastic aprons, goggles and gloves (double for the surgeons and scrub nurse)
- Disposable drapes should be used. Swabs should be counted on a polythene sheet on the floor, not on the swab rack
- Only disposable scalpels are used. All instruments should be handed to and from the surgeon on a tray such that the surgeon or nurse picks the instrument without any direct transfer from nurse to surgeon and vice versa
- Suction bottles should be half filled with freshly prepared 2% gluteraldehyde solution
- Spilt blood or body fluids must be diluted with fresh 2% gluteraldehyde and mopped up with white paper towels. All consumables should be placed in a watertight bag for plastic incineration
- Splashes of blood or body fluids or accidental puncture wounds should be immediately and thoroughly washed with soap and water and the consultant should then inform the Occupational Health Service of such an incident
- The operating nurse must ensure that the patient's skin is completely free of blood after the operation
- The patient should wear a clean operating gown before transfer back to the ward

obtained from the patient for other purposes is permissible.

■ The exposed health worker should be counselled and expert advice sought. Consent for HIV testing from the individual concerned should be obtained, in which event, an immediate specimen (baseline) followed by others at intervals are necessary. Seroconversion usually occurs within 3 months.

Section 5.7 • Fungal infections of surgical importance

From the clinical standpoint, fungal infections are best divided into cutaneous, subcutaneous and deep. Risk factors include prolonged antibiotic therapy that encourages growth of commensal fungal organisms, and leucopenia and T-helper lymphocyte (CD4) depression that are associated with invasive and potentially fatal fungal disease.

The **cutaneous** (superficial) mycoses have a worldwide distribution and include dermatophytosis (ringworm), superficial candidosis (thrush) and pityriasis versicolor. The **subcutaneous** fungal infections are lar-

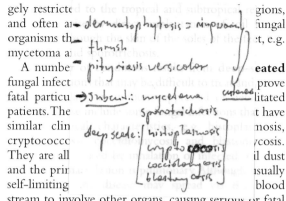

gely restricted to the tropical and subtropical regions, and often are caused by soil fungal organisms that live in the soil or on the soles of the feet, e.g. mycetoma and sporotrichosis.

A number of these deep-seated fungal infections may be difficult to treat and prove fatal particularly in myceloma cutaneous debilitated patients. The sporotrichosis conditions that have similar clinical histoplasmosis mosis, cryptococco crypto cocci ycosis. They are all coccidiomycosis il dust and the prim blastomycosis isually self-limiting... but may spread via the blood stream to involve other organs, causing serious or fatal illness. Many of the histological features of these deep-seated fungal infections are similar to those found in tuberculosis.

Finally, **systemic mycoses** may arise from superficial and deep-seated fungal infections when the patient's immune response is depressed or the patient is critically ill. These are commonly encountered in ICU patients.

Candidosis (candidiasis)

The *Candida* species of fungi occur as commensals in the mouth, alimentary tract and vagina. Infection with *C. albicans* is common in clinical practice, and usually arises as an opportunistic superinfection in debilitated or critically ill and immunosuppressed patients.

The infection is encountered in several clinical forms. Oral candidosis (thrush) and the vaginal and perianal infections are common and usually occur as a consequence of antibiotic therapy (Figure 5.22). Vaginal candidosis is also found in conditions that result in a low pH of the vaginal secretions from excess glycogen in the vaginal cells, e.g. pregnancy, diabetes and females on the contraceptive pill. Cutaneous circumoral infection (perlèche) and chronic paronychia may also occur in these patients.

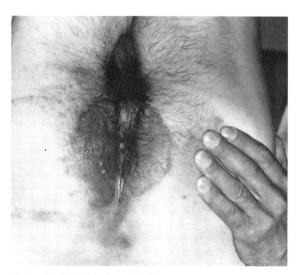

Figure 5.22 Perianal candidosis.

Alimentary and pulmonary candidosis

The oral infection may extend to involve the gastro-intestinal tract, particularly the oesophagus, following prolonged therapy with broad-spectrum antibiotics. Both alimentary and pulmonary candidosis may arise as opportunistic infections in the presence of impaired cell-mediated immunity, e.g. immunosuppression from illness, malignancy or drugs.

Generalized (systemic) candidosis

This is the most serious form and is characterized by blood-stream spread to any organ, but most commonly to the lungs, kidneys and the endocardium. This serious systemic infection is encountered in patients on parenteral nutrition, patients with prosthetic devices, transplant patients and critically ill patients.

The general clinical features of systemic candidosis include high fever, hypotension, rigors and renal impairment. The reported overall survival following appropriate systemic antifungal therapy is 65–70%.

Pulmonary candidosis

There are two types of pulmonary candidosis: monilial bronchitis and monilial pneumonia.

Monilial bronchitis occurs in infancy, fibrocystic lung disease and debilitated elderly patients. The bronchial walls are studded with greyish-yellow plaques containing fibrin, hyphae and spores. Clinically, there is an irritating cough productive of scanty, 'milky' sputum. The chest X-ray may be normal or show basal striations.

Monilial pneumonia is a necrotic pneumonia that occurs in critically ill and debilitated patients, giving patchy, ill-defined shadows on the chest X-ray. The patient has a high fever with tachycardia, dyspnoea and cough productive of blood-stained sputum.

The treatment is with 5-flucytosine, which is the drug of choice if the organism is sensitive; otherwise, intravenous or inhaled amphotericin B may be tried (see below).

Chronic mucocutaneous candidosis

Several types of primary immunological disease affecting the T-lymphocyte function are associated with widespread development of chronic mucocutaneous candidosis. The immunological deficit varies from patient to patient.

Treatment of systemic fungal infections

General considerations are important since antifungal therapy alone may be insufficient. Thus, infected prosthetic implants need to be removed or replaced. Whenever possible, the immune depression is reversed at least partially by dose reduction of any immunosuppressive drug. Variable and conflicting results have been obtained by the administration of transfer factor and transfusion of leucocytes.

Intravenous amphotericin B remains the mainstay of therapy for systemic fungal infections. It is administered in 5% dextrose, initially in a dose of 0.25 mg/kg/24 h and increasingly gradually over a period of 4–6 days to 1.0 mg/kg/day. The daily dose is administered over a period of 3–4 h. Since it deteriorates rapidly in solution on exposure to sunlight, the intravenous solution must be shielded. Treatment is monitored by blood levels, which should be kept in the 1–3 µg/ml range. The main disadvantage of amphotericin B is its toxicity: rigors, hypotension, phlebitis, hepatic damage, renal damage, anaemia, leucopenia and hypokalaemia. The prior intravenous administration of either hydrocortisone (50–100 mg) or chlorpheniramine (10 mg) is said to reduce some of the early side-effects. In order to minimize toxicity, amphotericin B is often administered in a reduced dose in combination with other drugs. Various combinations are used, including amphotericin B + 5-flucytosine for cryptococcosis, rifampicin + amphotericin B for candidosis and blastomycosis. Altering the rate of infusion and alternate-day treatment may help to reduce the incidence and severity of side-effects. Other measures that are used to reduce toxicity include heparin infusion against phlebitis, and mannitol and bicarbonate to minimize renal damage.

5-Flucytosine is a synthetic antifungal agent that can be administered orally or intravenously. It is active mainly against *Candida* and *Cryptococcus*. Apart from its side-effects (diarrhoea, rashes, leucopenia and hepatitis), its main disadvantage is the rapid emergence of resistance.

A number of imidazoles has significant antifungal activity. The two most often used are ketoconazole, which is administered orally (200–600 mg), and miconazole, which is given intravenously since it is poorly absorbed after oral administration. Ketoconazole has fewer side-effects than miconazole, which may cause rashes, phlebitis, ventricular tachycardia and anaphylaxis. Drug resistance to the imidazoles is rare and they have a broad spectrum of activity against many fungi (except for aspergilli) and some Gram-positive bacteria. All other imidazoles (clotrimazole, econazole, tioconazole) are mainly used as topical antifungal agents. Oral ketoconazole is advocated as prophylaxis in transplant patients.

Treatment of cutaneous fungal infections

Topical polyenes (natamycin, nystatin, candicidin) are used as 1–2% creams or ointments, as suspensions or tablets (oral or vaginal). The topical imidazole preparations are also effective. In chronic mucocutaneous candidosis associated with T-lymphocyte immune defects, treatment with transfer factor gives varying results.

Mycetoma

This is a localized infection of the skin and subcutaneous tissues of the extremities, usually of the feet and less frequently of the hands. It is found in developing countries. The infection is caused by organisms normally resident in the soil, which are implanted by thorn and similar injuries in individuals who walk barefooted. **Bacterial mycetoma** is caused by infection with species of nocardia or acintomyces (actinomycetoma). **Fungal mycetoma** (eumycetoma, maduromycosis) is endemic in certain countries, e.g. India, and is caused by various fungi including *Madurella mycetomi*, *Allescheria boydii* and *Aspergillus nidulans*. The disease results in chronic suppuration with severe tissue destruction and multiple discharging sinuses (Figure 5.23). In both bacterial and fungal mycetoma, osteomyelitis of the bones of the foot may develop.

In bacterial mycetoma, treatment with the appropriate antibiotics together with surgical drainage and debridement may prove efficacious. The fungal mycetomas, by contrast, seldom respond to antifungal chemotherapy as the organisms acquire a protective cement sheath or develop thickened cell walls. None the less, a trial of treatment with an antifungal agent, e.g. griseofulvine, 5-flucytosine or ketoconazole, may be effective in patients with early and limited disease,

and without bone involvement. In most instances, however, amputation is necessary to eradicate the disease.

Section 5.8 • Parasitic infestations of surgical importance

Hydatid disease

The disease can be caused by one of three species of the genus *Echinococcus*: *E. granulosus*, *E. multilocularis* and *E. oligettas*. Since the epidemiological and pathological features of these three tapeworms are very similar, a detailed description of *E. granulosus* only is given here. Hydatid disease, which is caused by the larval form of *E. granulosus*, has a cosmopolitan distribution, being particularly prevalent in sheep- and cattle-raising areas.

Parasitology

The adult echinococcus is a small tapeworm that inhabits the upper part of the small intestine of canines, especially dogs and wolves. When the ova, which are passed in the faeces, are swallowed by humans or other intermediate hosts, e.g. sheep and cattle, the enclosed embryo is liberated in the duodenum. It penetrates the intestinal mucosa to reach the portal circulation, and is usually held up in the liver to develop into a hydatid cyst. If the embryo passes through the liver filter, it enters the general circulation and thus reaches the lungs and other parts of the body. Two main varieties of cyst occur: unilocular and multilocular. The unilocular hydatid cyst (Figure 5.24) develops a wall with two layers: an outer, thick, laminated layer and an inner (germinal) layer, which is composed of a protoplasmic matrix containing many nuclei. Around the cyst there is a connective-tissue capsule formed by the tissues of the host. Bulb-like processes known as brood capsules arise from the germinal layer. The brood capsules undergo localized proliferation and invagination of their walls to form scolices (tapeworm heads). Each scolex has suckers and hooklets. Some of the brood capsules separate from the walls and settle to the bottom of the cyst as fine granular sediment 'hydatid sand'. As the hydatid cyst enlarges, invaginations of the wall may give rise to daughter cysts. In some cases in which no effective encapsulation occurs, the daughter cysts develop as a result of evaginations of the cyst wall,

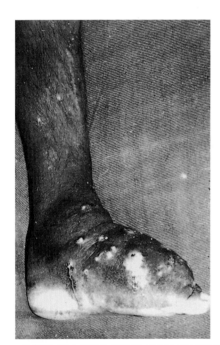

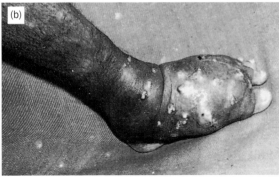

Figure 5.23 (a, b) Fungal mycetoma of the foot showing swelling, chronic induration with multiple sinuses and fungal granules. (Courtesy of Dr D. M. Muthukumarasamy, Kilpauk Medical College, India.)

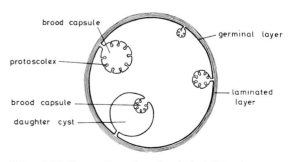

Figure 5.24 Composition of a unilocular hydatid cyst.

producing the multilocular or alveolar hydatid cysts. This variety of cyst is caused by *E. multilocularis*.

When the hydatid is eaten by definitive hosts, e.g. dogs, foxes or wolves, the numerous larvae develop into sexually mature worms in a few weeks. Dogs are usually affected when they eat the infected viscera of sheep or cattle (Figure 5.25). Humans acquire hydatid disease when they swallow infected ova as a result of their close association with dogs. Although infection is usually acquired in childhood, clinical symptoms do not appear until adult life. The dog faeces contaminating the fleeces of sheep can also be an indirect source of human infection.

Pathology

When the ingested ovum reaches the duodenum, the hexacanth embryo is released and penetrates the intestinal mucosa to reach the portal circulation and thence the liver, most commonly the right lobe. Hydatid cysts are usually single but may be multiple and involve the left lobe. Larvae may pass through the liver to infect other organs, e.g. lungs (71%), muscle (5%), brain (5%), spleen (2.5%), kidneys (2%), other abdominal organs (5%), bone (0.5%) and rarely the heart. During the stage of migration, there may be a mild reaction with fever and urticarial skin rash. There is an eosinophilic reaction to the larva itself, which

subsides as the host's fibrous tissue capsule thickens. In humans the hydatid cyst may be the classical unilocular, the osseous or the alveolar.

The alveolar multiloculated hydatid cyst is usually found in the liver and has a sponge-like appearance (Figure 5.26). In the brain it resembles a bunch of grapes (Figure 5.27). The alveolar multiloculated cyst may metastasize.

The classical unilocular hydatid cyst may be sterile but is usually fertile and surrounded by a fibrous capsule. Rupture of fertile cysts, depending on their site, causes dissemination of daughter cysts with the formation of secondary metastatic hydatids. The escape of the cyst fluid and 'hydatid sand' may cause a severe allergic reaction with urticarial lesions, pruritus, fever, abdominal pain, dyspnoea, cyanosis, delirium and syncope. In addition, there is marked eosinophilia.

In bone the usual fibrous capsule of the host is not formed and, instead of being round, the cyst assumes an irregular branching shape as it penetrates the bony canals. Erosion of bone occurs and the medullary cavity is eventually invaded, when the cyst assumes its normal spherical form. The more highly vascularized areas, the epiphyses of long bones and the centres of the vertebral bodies, ilium and ribs, are the most frequently affected sites. Radiologically, they appear as rounded areas of rarefaction. Spontaneous fractures may occur.

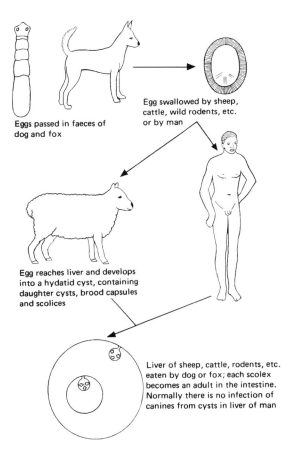

Figure 5.25 Life cycle of *Echinococcus granulosus*.

Eggs passed in faeces of dog and fox

Egg swallowed by sheep, cattle, wild rodents, etc. or by man

Egg reaches liver and develops into a hydatid cyst, containing daughter cysts, brood capsules and scolices

Liver of sheep, cattle, rodents, etc. eaten by dog or fox; each scolex becomes an adult in the intestine. Normally there is no infection of canines from cysts in liver of man

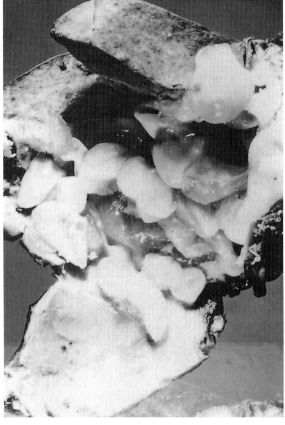

Figure 5.26 Hydatid disease of the liver.

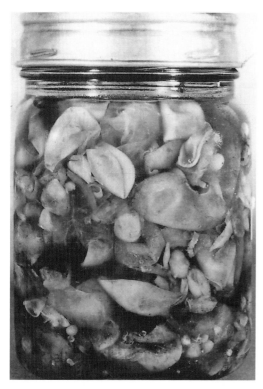

Figure 5.27 Hydatid cysts removed from the brain at necropsy.

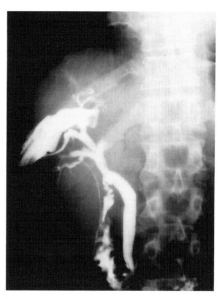

Figure 5.28 Hydatid cyst of the liver communicating with the right biliary tract.

Clinical features

The liver and lungs are the organs involved in the disease in over 90% of cases and hepatic hydatid disease accounts for 75% of these. Although the infection is usually acquired in childhood, a hepatic hydatid cyst may not produce symptoms until adult life and the interval between infection and manifestation of symptoms may exceed 30 years. At presentation the majority of cysts occurs in the right lobe. Exogenous cysts may communicate with the biliary tract and these contain bile-stained fluid (Figure 5.28). Secondary infection may occur with *Salmonella* and pyogenic organisms.

Rupture of the cyst may result from secondary infection or trauma and may be accompanied by severe allergic manifestations that can be life threatening. Rupture may involve the peritoneal cavity, the gallbladder, biliary tract, pleural cavity or hepatic veins, when secondary metastatic cysts develop in the lungs.

The alveolar cyst may occur in the liver but is most frequently found in the lungs in children. Infection of the cyst results in a chronic pulmonary abscess. The cyst may rupture as a result of coughing or secondary infection. The cyst may rupture into the bronchus, when scolices may be detected in the sputum, into the mediastinum or pleural cavity, with secondary dissemination and the development of pneumothorax and haemothorax.

In the brain, the cysts are usually single and present with symptoms of a space-occupying lesion. Rupture may disseminate the lesions in the subarachnoid space of the spinal cord, which may also be involved by extension of a hydatid cyst involving the vertebrae or

paravertebral tissues. Cerebral emboli secondaries have been reported from primary hydatid cysts in the lung, liver and heart.

Hydatid disease of the heart may be first discovered at autopsy. During life, the cysts may rupture into the pericardium or into the chambers of the heart, with consequent pulmonary metastases or systemic embolization causing thrombosis, infarction or aneurysm formation. Constrictive pericarditis may complicate rupture into the pericardium.

Occasional involvement of the spleen and kidneys by solitary cysts is well documented. In the kidney rupture into the renal pelvis results in renal colic and dysuria, with passage of hydatid material in the urine. Rarely, there is involvement of other sites, e.g. orbit, ovaries, broad ligament and uterus.

Investigations

Moderate eosinophilia ($300–2000/\text{mm}^3$) is usually present and the immunoglobulin level is elevated. Hydatid contents (hooklets, scolices) may be detected in the faeces, sputum or urine if the cyst ruptures. A plain radiograph of the chest and abdomen may be suggestive (Figure 5.29), although more information is obtained by ultrasound examination and especially by CT, which gives valuable information on the contents, size and precise location of the cyst (Figure 5.30). CT is the best method of establishing the diagnosis of liver, pulmonary and cerebral hydatid disease.

The Casoni test using crude sterile hydatid fluid is unreliable. An intradermal test antigen made from an extract of lyophilized material of *E. multilocularis* from experimental infections in gerbils is preferable. The detection of circulating scolex antigen by countercurrent immunoelectrophoresis (CIE) or the enzyme-linked immunosorbent assay (ELISA) gives the most

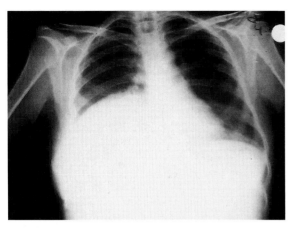

Figure 5.29 PA chest radiograph outlining a large liver with marked elevation of the diaphragm caused by hydatid cyst of the right lobe.

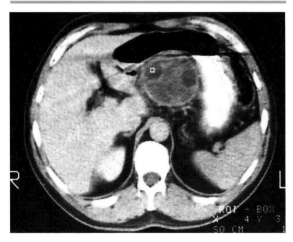

Figure 5.30 CT scan showing a large hydatid cyst of the pancreas containing daughter cysts. The pancreas is a rare site of involvement by hydatid disease. (Courtesy of Dr Moh'd Saad, Adan Hospital, Kuwait.)

reliable results. The dot-ELISA test is a field test for hydatid disease that can be carried out rapidly without specialized equipment. It detects antibody to purified parasite antigen (bound to strips of nitrocelluose paper) in a small finger-prick sample.

Treatment

The methods used to control the disease are aimed at prevention of access to infected carcasses by dogs, and registration and regular treatment of dogs with effective antihelmintics.

The use of mebendazole often results in death and shrinkage of the hydatid disease, thereby avoiding the need for surgical intervention. Serum levels greater than 1100 ng/ml 1–3 h after an oral dose may be required to kill the parasite. To achieve this, a dose of 200 mg/kg/day of mebendazole in three divided doses is required for about 16 weeks. Albendazole, a more absorbable derivative, is even more effective. It is administered in a dose of 12–15 mg/kg/day for 28 days **[see Hepatobiliary and Pancreatic Disorders, Vol. II]**.

Amoebiasis

The disease is caused by *E. histolytica*. The parasite lives in the large intestine, causing ulceration of the mucosa with consequent diarrhoea. Secondary lesions may occur, most commonly in the liver, but other tissues may be affected, e.g. lung, brain, genital organs and skin. Amoebiasis has a world-wide distribution but clinical disease occurs most frequently in tropical and subtropical latitudes. It is found in countries where standards of personal and environmental sanitation are low.

Parasitology

The amoeba, which multiplies by binary fission, lives in the lumen of the large intestine where, under suitable conditions, it invades the mucosa/submucosa and ingests red blood cells. When diarrhoea occurs, amoebae are expelled and can be detected in freshly passed fluid stools. In the absence of diarrhoea and when other conditions are favourable for encystation, the amoebae cease feeding, become spherical and secrete a cyst wall, and the nucleus divides twice to form the characteristic mature four-nucleate cyst. This is the infective form and, when ingested, the cyst hatches in the lower part of the small intestine/proximal colon and a four-nucleate amoeba emerges. After a series of nuclear and cytoplasmic divisions, each multinucleate amoeba gives rise to eight uninucleate parasites that establish themselves and multiply in the large intestine.

In endemic areas, the prevalence is stable and the morbidity rate from the disease is low. The disease is spread by cyst passers, who fall into two groups: (a) convalescents who have recovered from an acute attack, and (b) individuals who can recall no clinical symptoms or signs of infection. Poor sanitation is more important than climate in the predominance of overt infection in the tropics. Carrier rates of *E. histolytica* among symptomless subjects vary from 20 to 80% in different communities. The parasite can be transmitted by direct contact through contaminated hands of cyst carriers. It is also transmitted indirectly through contaminated food, e.g. raw vegetables.

Pathology

The primary sites of infection in order of frequency are the caecum, colonic flexures, descending colon and rectum. The appendix is sometimes involved and rarely the ileum. Macroscopically, the large intestine becomes studded with discrete ulcers with overhanging edges, the intervening mucosa being relatively normal. The ulcers spread laterally in the submucosa and become confluent. Large areas of mucosa thus become devitalized and form greenish shaggy sloughs. The necrotic process may involve the muscularis propria and even extend to the serosa in severe cases. In patients in whom the host–parasite balance has been altered by drugs, concurrent disease or pregnancy, the entire mucosa may be sloughed. The wall of the bowel is thickened and friable (Figure 5.31).

The amoebae spread laterally beneath the intestinal epithelium and form large 'flask-shaped' or 'water-bottle' ulcers that have overhanging edges and consist of a zone of necrosis surrounded by chronic inflammatory infiltrate of lymphocytes and macrophages with a variable fibroblastic reaction. Amoebae are found at the periphery of the lesion in the submucosa and muscle layers and in the necrotic tissue itself (Figure 5.32).

Liver abscess (Figure 5.33) is the most common extraintestinal complication. The abscess is usually solitary but multiple abscesses are not uncommon. The right lobe of the liver is most frequently affected. Bile appears to destroy the amoebae and for this reason the gallbladder is never affected. In over 50% of patients with amoebic liver abscess, there is no evidence of amoebic infection on stool examination. The amoebae cause lysis of the liver parenchyma, primarily in the periportal region. An expanding area of necrosis ensues and the abscess cavity may reach large proportions. The cavity contains sterile, chocolate-coloured fluid, granular debris and a few inflammatory cells. Amoebae may or may not be present in the pus. Histologically, the wall of the abscess consists of necrotic tissue and compressed liver parenchyma containing a variable infiltrate of monocytes, plasma cells, lymphocytes and fibroblasts.

Clinical features

The classical disease is amoebic dysentery, the symptoms of which appear within 1–2 weeks of infection

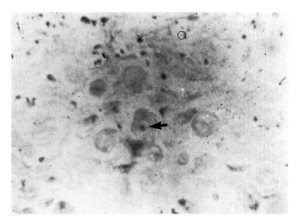

Figure 5.32 Amoebic colitis section of colon. Note *E. histolytica* trophozoites.

but may be delayed for months to years. The onset is usually gradual, with some looseness for a few days followed by evacuation of six to 12 mucoid, blood-stained motions per day. Colic and tenesmus are unusual unless there is a lesion immediately inside the anus. Physical examination may be negative. Occasionally during an acute attack, there is palpable thickening of the caecum or left colon with tenderness on palpation. Pyrexia is absent and there is little prostration. The duration of an attack of average severity may be a few days but it may linger on for some weeks. The attack usually subsides spontaneously. There follows a period of remission varying from a few days to several months, even years. During remission, the patient is often constipated. Another attack of dysentery then follows. This sequence of relapses and remissions may continue for several years and is typical of the

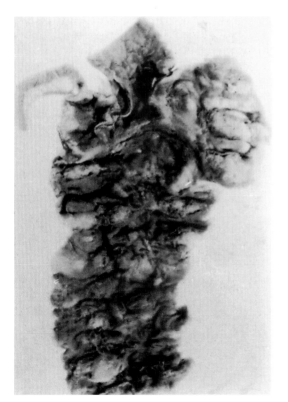

Figure 5.31 Fulminating amoebic colitis resulting from the use of steroids given for a mistaken diagnosis of ulcerative colitis.

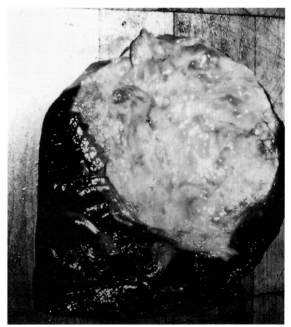

Figure 5.33 Large single amoebic abscess of the liver.

disease. Complications, e.g. liver abscess, may develop at any time. Complications are encountered in 20% of neglected cases.

In malnourished individuals or in patients with comorbid disorders, the attacks may be prolonged, severe and even fatal. Fulminating amoebiasis is also encountered in immunosuppressed patients. The fulminating disease has a sudden onset with swinging pyrexia, chills, sweating and very severe dysentery with rapid dehydration and prostration. In such cases the stools are watery with flecks of faecal matter and variable amounts of blood and mucus. There may be severe intestinal haemorrhage or perforation with amoebic peritonitis. The mortality of these cases is high.

The direct complications of an intestinal infection are haemorrhage from erosion of a large intestinal blood vessel, transmural extension of the infection with the formation of amoebic granulomas (amoebomas) and frank intestinal perforation. In addition, a form of slow intestinal leakage through extensively diseased bowel may result in localized peritonitis. This should be suspected in patients whose condition deteriorates and in whom there is increased abdominal distension with signs of ileus. Plain radiology reveals free gas under the diaphragm. Other local complications include amoebic strictures that may occur in any part of the colon and intussusception, which is rare. All of these complications are unusual in the common attacks of average severity.

The clinical features of amoeboma include a palpable mass, usually in the right iliac fossa, low-grade fever, tenderness, and symptoms and signs of intestinal obstruction. Clinically, such a lesion may be indistinguishable from a neoplasm, ileocaecal tuberculosis, appendix mass or actinomycosis.

In the early stages of an amoebic liver abscess, the patient complains of discomfort and fullness in the liver region. The liver enlarges and becomes tender. Moderate fever develops, at first intermittent and subsequently remittent. Sweating is severe, especially at night. The patient becomes anorexic and loses weight. The liver tenderness is maximal over the site of the abscess, usually in the right intercostal region laterally. The enlarged liver may cause obvious bulging of the chest wall and upper abdomen. Chest-wall movement is restricted on the affected side. Breathing is painful and the patient develops shallow tachypnoea. The liver dullness is increased upwards and radiology reveals a raised, immobile hemidiaphragm. The liver edge is usually palpable well below the costal margin, and is firm and tender. Jaundice is uncommon. Most patients have a moderate polymorphonuclear leucocytosis. The ESR is raised. Signs of pulmonary involvement (collapse and pleural effusion) are usually limited to the base of the right lung. When the abscess ruptures through the diaphragm into the lung, the abscess contents discharge into the bronchial tree and the patient develops a cough with expectoration of the classical 'anchovy sauce' sputum. Untreated, the abscess

may involve other regions, e.g. pericardial sac, peritoneal cavity and parieties. Embolic spread may result in abscess formation in other organs, including the brain. Although usually secondary to liver disease, primary amoebic abscesses of the lung and brain are well documented.

The diagnosis of amoebiasis is established by the identification of *E. histolytica*. Microscopic examination of stool specimens during an acute attack will reveal motile amoebae. In asymptomatic infections and during remissions, the stools contain *E. histolytica* cysts. Repeated stool examinations (minimum of six) should be made before absence of infection can be assumed. Culture methods may assist diagnosis in scanty infections. Sigmoidoscopy often yields useful information. The appearances consist of small yellow ulcers with surrounding hyperaemia, and a normal mucosa in between the ulcers. In chronic cases, amoebic lesions may appear as 'pin-point craters' that are irregularly disposed.

The diagnosis of extraintestinal amoebiasis can be difficult as concomitant dysentery is only present in 5–10% of patients. PA chest radiography shows abnormalities in 75% of cases: elevated diaphragm, basal collapse, patchy opacities and pleural effusion. Ultrasound or CT examination of the liver is necessary for establishing the diagnosis and for percutaneous aspiration of the abscess (Figure 5.34).

Serological tests are useful in suspected cases of amoeboma and in those patients diagnosed as ulcerative colitis who have been to the tropics. The serodiagnostic tests include direct immunofluorescence, ELISA and an isoenzyme electrophoretic technique that differentiates the invasive from the non-invasive form of *E. histolytica*.

Treatment
Medical

Metronidazole is the standard treatment for acute amoebic dysentery and for amoebic liver abscess. Tinidazole is also effective. Asymptomatic intestinal amoebiasis can be treated with either diloxanide furoate (furamide) or di-iodohydroxyquinoline (diodoquin).

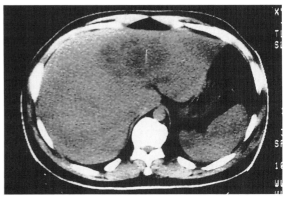

Figure 5.34 CT scan of amoebic abscess of the liver.

Surgical

Surgical intervention may be necessary in:

- fulminating amoebic colitis
- amoebic perforation of the colon
- amoebic liver abscess.

Fulminating amoebic colitis: surgical treatment is indicated when the patient deteriorates despite medical therapy, in the presence of radiological evidence of toxic dilatation, and the onset of an acute episode, e.g. perforation, severe bleeding. The operative treatment consists of resection of the diseased segment with exteriorization of the bowel ends.

Amoebic bowel perforation: this occurs in 1–2% of patients hospitalized for the disease. Although any segment of the small and large intestine may be involved, the most common sites are the caecum, ascending and sigmoid colon. Multiple localized or diffuse perforations are encountered in 25% of cases presenting for surgery. Three types of perforation are recognized: extraperitoneal, perforation of a granuloma or ulcer without acute dysentery, and perforation associated with fulminant disease. Antiamoebic therapy is the primary treatment for all localized extraperitoneal perforations. Surgery is indicated only if the patient's condition deteriorates and rupture appears imminent. Diversion of the faecal stream by an ileocolic anastomosis beyond any colonic involvement and local drainage is the recommended treatment, except in perforations associated with gangrene and fulminant colitis.

Amoebic liver abscess: the majority of amoebic liver abscesses respond to therapy with metronidazole with or without percutaneous CT or ultrasound-guided aspiration. Surgical treatment is reserved for when medical therapy and percutaneous aspiration have failed and for certain specific indications that include:

- frank or impending rupture
- onset of complications, e.g. secondary infection or haemorrhage
- abscess in the left lobe because of difficulties in aspiration in this area and the risk of rupture into the pericardial sac.

In general, patients requiring surgical drainage have advanced disease and the overall mortality of this group is high (30%). A period of therapy with metronidazole lasting for a minimum of 4 days before surgical intervention has been shown to reduce mortality significantly. Transbronchial rupture is usually well tolerated and is often curative, although rarely it may cause fatal pneumonia or lung abscess. Rupture into the pleural cavity is accompanied by shock, respiratory distress and empyema. This situation requires urgent intervention to drain the abscess and the empyema, and to ensure early re-expansion of the collapsed lung. Intraperitoneal rupture requires adequate peritoneal toilet in addition to drainage of the abscess cavity.

Complications following surgical drainage: apart from respiratory complications and shock, these include liver failure, biliary peritonitis and fistulas. Massive haemorrhage is rare and amoebiasis of the skin is unusual if adequate antiamoebic therapy is started before surgery.

Shistosomiasis

The three species infecting humans are *Shistosoma haematobium*, *S. mansoni* and *S. japonicum*. About 200 million people are affected in various parts of the world. *S. haematobium* occurs in many parts of Africa, parts of the Middle East and a few foci in southern Europe (Portugal). *Shistosoma mansoni* is found in the Nile delta, Africa, South America and the Caribbean. *Shistosoma japonicum* occurs in China, Japan, the Philippines and other foci in the Far East. Other schistosomes that infect humans include *S. bovis*, *S. matthei* and *S. intercalatum*.

Parasitology

These worms are trematodes with the peculiar morphology whereby the male is folded to form a gynaecophoric canal in which the female is carried. The adult worms are found in the veins: *S. haematobium* predominantly in the vesical plexus, *S. mansoni* in the inferior mesenteric vein and *S. japonicum* most commonly in the superior mesenteric vein.

The female lays eggs, which pass through the bladder or bowel into urine or faeces. A proportion of the eggs remains in the tissues and some are carried to the liver, lungs and other organs. If an excreted egg lands on water, it hatches and produces a free-living form, the miracidium, which swims about by ciliary activity. It next invades an intermediate host, a snail of the appropriate species. Within the snail, it undergoes asexual multiplication, passing through intermediate stages of redia and sporocyst to become the mature cercaria. This is the infective larval stage for humans. It emerges from the snail and swims, being propelled by its forked tail. On contact with humans, the cercaria penetrates the skin, sheds its tail and becomes a schistosomule that migrates to the usual site for mature adults of the species. The respective life cycles are shown in Figures 5.35–5.37.

Humans are the reservoir of *S. haematobium* but naturally acquired infection with *S. mansoni* has been found in various animals, including primates. *Shistosoma japonicum* is widely distributed in various animals (cats, dogs, cattle, pigs, rats, etc.) and these constitute a significant part of the reservoir. Humans acquire the infection by wading, swimming, bathing or washing clothes and utensils in polluted waters. The age and gender distribution of schistosomiasis varies from area to area. One common pattern is of high prevalence rates of active infection in children who excrete large quantities of eggs, and a lower prevalence of active infection among adults, with the latter exhibiting late chronic manifestations of the disease. The load of infection is an important factor in determining the severity of the pathological lesions and the disease.

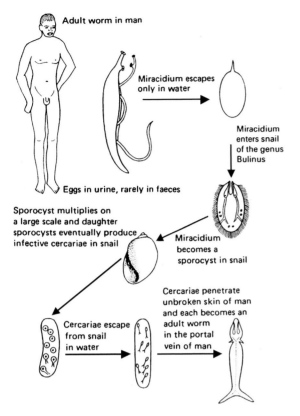

Adult worm in man

Miracidium escapes only in water

Miracidium enters snail of the genus Bulinus

Eggs in urine, rarely in faeces

Sporocyst multiplies on a large scale and daughter sporocysts eventually produce infective cercariae in snail

Miracidium becomes a sporocyst in snail

Cercariae penetrate unbroken skin of man and each becomes an adult worm in the portal vein of man

Cercariae escape from snail in water

Figure 5.35 Life cycle of *S. haematobium*.

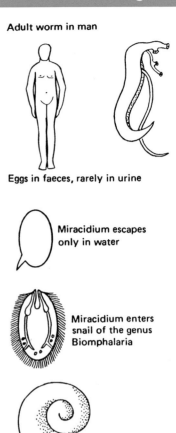
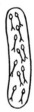

Adult worm in man

Eggs in faeces, rarely in urine

Miracidium escapes only in water

Miracidium enters snail of the genus Biomphalaria

Miracidium becomes a sporocyst in snail

Sporocyst multiplies on a large scale and daughter sporocysts eventually produce infective cercariae in snail

Cercariae escape from snail in water

Cercariae penetrate unbroken skin of man and each becomes an adult worm in the portal vein of man

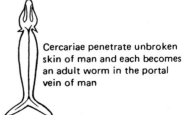

Figure 5.36 Life cycle of *S. mansoni*.

Pathology

Shistosoma haematobium

This affects mainly the urinary tract. The bladder lesions include acute and polypoid lesions, fibrous plaques, 'ground-glass' lesions, sandy patches, ulceration, stricture, leucoplakia and cystitis glandularis, fibrosis, calcification of the bladder wall and bladder neck obstruction. However, the bladder may appear normal macroscopically even in fairly severe infections, and mucosal biopsies and press preparations are necessary if *S. haematobium* is suspected.

In the acute stage the bladder may only be hyperaemic, with or without petechial haemorrhages. Ova retained in the vesical tissues, most commonly in the subepithelial layer, result in the formation of pseudotubercles, when the bladder becomes studded with small, yellow, seed-like bodies surrounded by a zone of hyperaemia. They are most frequently situated in the trigone, with the base and lateral walls next most commonly affected. Adult schistosomes are often present in the neighbouring vesical veins. Nodules or polyps may be formed by coalescence of these tubercles, hyperplasia of the mucosa, and early fibrosis and hypertrophy of the muscle. These papillomatous or granulomatous lesions are responsible for the filling defects seen on cystography in the early stages (Figure 5.38). They subsequently shrink to form white fibrous plaques as the ova become calcified. The bladder

Adult worm in man, horses, cattle, etc.

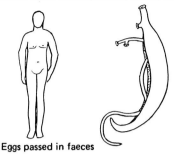

Eggs passed in faeces

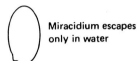
Miracidium escapes only in water

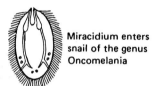
Miracidium enters snail of the genus Oncomelania

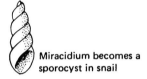
Miracidium becomes a sporocyst in snail

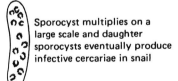
Sporocyst multiplies on a large scale and daughter sporocysts eventually produce infective cercariae in snail

Cercariae escape from snail in water

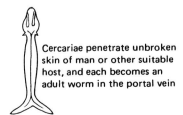
Cercariae penetrate unbroken skin of man or other suitable host, and each becomes an adult worm in the portal vein

Figure 5.37 Life cycle of *S. japonicum*.

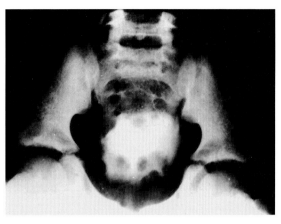

Figure 5.38 Granulomatous lesions in *S. haematobium* infection seen radiologically as bladder-filling defects.

mucosa may eventually present a ground-glass appearance as a result of the mucosal atrophy and submucosal fibrosis. A fibrocalcific type of polyp is also encountered. It forms a small, usually solitary lesion consisting of dense fibrous tissue surrounding dilated capillaries and calcified ova and without a covering epithelium. Villous polyps may also form but are less common. They have club-shaped fronds covered by hyperplastic epithelium.

The most common lesion encountered in vesical schistosomiasis is the 'sandy patch'. This late lesion is seen in the trigone, where the mucosa appears roughened, raised and greyish-brown in colour (Figure 5.39). The overlying epithelium may be irregularly thickened or atrophic with areas of metaplasia. In the submucosa and muscularis, pseudotubercles and foreign body granulomas surround ova in various stages of disintegration or calcification, but the predominant feature is dense fibrosis.

The bladder epithelium may undergo atrophy or become hyperplastic. Foci of leucoplakia may be present. Epithelial downgrowths into the submucosa

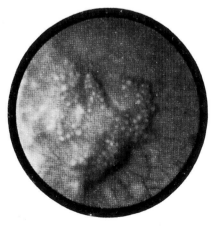

Figure 5.39 Sandy patches of the bladder in *S. haematobium* infection. (Courtesy of Thieme Verlag.)

(Brunn's nests) are a common feature and they may become vesicular (cystitis glandularis). Squamous metaplasia may supervene. Intractable ulceration leads to bacterial infection that may spread to involve the entire urinary tract with abscess formation and septicaemia. The urethra is often involved with stricture formation.

Varying degrees of ureteric involvement, usually the lower two-thirds, are encountered in 70% of cases and are more common in males. Linear calcification in the lower end of the ureter is pathognomonic. In addition, there may be secondary changes in the ureters induced by the bladder lesions, e.g. vesicoureteric reflux and hydronephrosis. Obstructive renal failure may result from ureteric involvement. Renal lesions directly due to the parasite are rare.

Shistosoma mansoni and Shistosoma japonicum
Ova are discharged in the faeces but some are retained in the tissues and excite an eosinophilic reaction with the formation of multiple abscesses. In the large intestine, the mucosa is reddened and granular, with pinpoint yellowish elevations surrounded by a hyperaemic zone. Shallow ulcers may form. The inflammatory reaction in the submucosa leads to the formation of sessile or pedunculated polyps. These are found in 17–20% of Egyptian patients. The muscular and serosal layers are also involved with pseudo-tubercles and these may be associated with a focal peritonitis and intestinal adhesions. Inflammatory masses may be produced in the intestinal wall (bilharzioma). With progressive fibrosis, the intestinal wall becomes rigid and the lumen stenosed. The mesentery is thickened and thrombosis of its veins may occur. Granulomatous lesions may form in the mesenteric and retroperitoneal nodes. These form masses that may simulate a neoplasm (pseudotumour); caecocolic intussusception, intestinal obstruction and rectal prolapse may supervene. With secondary infection, ischiorectal and anorectal abscesses and fistulas may form.

Pyloric obstruction has been described in *S. japonicum* infections, and lesions may be found in the stomach, peritoneum and pancreas. Infection of the appendix is common and rarely the small intestine may be more affected than the colon.

As the ova are released into the portal system, the liver is invariably involved. Hepatic involvement is more severe in *S. japonicum* owing to the larger number of ova produced by this schistosome. The liver may be enlarged or contracted and its surface shows a fine to coarse nodularity. Its consistency is firm and the cut surface exhibits white 'clay-pipe stem' fibrosis. This fibrosis is produced by ova in and around the portal venous radicals (Figure 5.40). The ova are usually trapped in the portal venous radicals and only occasionally reach the hepatic sinusoids. The affected portal venules become obstructed from thrombophlebitis. Thin-walled vascular channels form

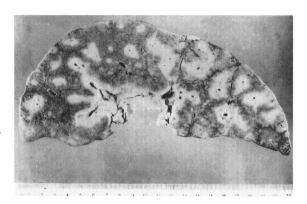

Figure 5.40 Gross appearance of the cut liver surface in *S. japonicum* infection.

in the fibrosed portal tracts (angiomatoids) and result either from recanalization of thrombosed veins or as adaptive communications between the portal and arterial circulations. An increase in the number and size of the intrahepatic branches of the hepatic artery accounts for the maintenance of a normal liver blood flow in the majority of patients. The parenchymal cells of the liver are usually unaffected and the overall liver function remains good despite established portal hypertension.

The pulmonary changes are usually encountered in the late stages of *S. japonicum* and *S. mansoni* infections. They include widespread fibrosis with the development of cor pulmonale and chronic respiratory failure.

Cerebral involvement is more common in *S. japonicum* and spinal disease in *S. mansoni*. Small tubercles are found in the meninges and in the white and grey matter of the brain and spinal cord.

Clinical features
During the stage of invasion and maturation of the worm, which lasts for 12 weeks, the patient may develop a generalized illness with fever, malaise, exhaustion and sometimes diarrhoea and abdominal discomfort. Urticaria may supervene and eosinophilia is invariably present. This initial illness is known as Katayama syndrome and is thought to result from a temporary state of antigen excess that exists until the host's antibody production is mobilized. It may occasionally be very severe and fatal. This stage occurs in all three infections.

Shistosoma haematobium
The stage of established infection occurs 10–12 weeks after cercarial penetration and is manifested by frank haematuria with egg extrusion. The haematuria is intermittent and often transitory. Episodes of haematuria continue to be experienced by untreated patients, although the attacks become less severe with time. Microscopic examination of urine reveals red blood cells between attacks.

Bladder: initially, the patient complains of dysuria, frequency and urgency of micturition. Bladder ulceration is accompanied by suprapubic and perineal pain. Two clinicopathological entities have been described: (i) sloughing of polypoid patches in early active disease, and (ii) chronic ulceration at sites of heavy egg deposition. Increasing frequency accompanies vesical fibrosis and contraction of the bladder. Occasionally, the bladder is large and atonic. This may result from reduced blood supply or bladder neck obstruction.

Kidneys and ureters: ureteric involvement is common and is usually bilateral. Loin pain results from hydroureter and hydronephrosis. Proximal bacterial infection and stone formation are frequent complications. Pyelonephritis is thus frequent. Two varieties of nephrotic syndrome have been described in Egypt and Brazil. In Egypt, the nephrotic syndrome is related to *Salmonella* septicaemia and the glomerular lesions are proliferative and reversible. *Shistosoma haematobium* infection in Egypt predisposes the patient to the development of a carrier state for *Salmonella typhi* and *S. paratyphi*. In Brazil, the lesions are predominantly membranoproliferative and irreversible with no association with *Salmonella* infection. Bacteriuria is often present in hospital patients and the urine contains eosinophils.

Calculi: these are common in Egypt, where they occur in 25% of infected patients, but are rare in other parts of Africa. They occur in the bladder, ureters, kidneys and urethra and consist of a central core of oxalate surrounded by an outer coat of urate incorporating ova. These stones may disappear following successful medical therapy and this is most likely to happen in young patients in whom fibrosis and irreversible stenosis are absent.

Association with vesical cancer: this is now established. Schistosomal bladder cancer is frequently of the squamous cell type (40–75%) and arises commonly from the trigone and superior apical regions. It is diffuse (multicentric) in one-third of cases. Various theories have been proposed to explain the association but the most favoured is the β-glucuronidase hypothesis. The enzyme β-glucuronidase is excreted in the urine of patients with active *S. haematobium* infection (from the adult worm). The increased urinary β-glucuronidase may hydrolyse inactive carcinogenic glucuronides, releasing active carcinogens. Thus, in Egypt raised levels of urinary metabolites of tryptophan, serotonin and the carcinogen 3-hydroxyanthranilic acid have been demonstrated in the urine of infected patients, and very high levels in patients with established bladder cancer.

Hepatic involvement: the clinical picture is dominated by bleeding oesophageal varices. The spleen is invariably massively enlarged in these patients who have good liver function despite the portal hypertension (Child A or Child B).

Shistosoma mansoni and Shistosoma japonicum

The onset of egg laying in a first infection is accompanied by bloody diarrhoea. The lesions in the colon are variable. There may be segmental roughening of the mucosa with congestion, small ulcers and, in the late stages, sandy patches. Polyps may develop, especially in *S. mansoni* infections. Polyp formation is due to high localized egg burden damaging the muscularis mucosa. These polyps are therefore inflammatory in nature and are thus reversible with medical treatment.

In some cases, severe dysentery with frank ulceration and massive haemorrhage occurs and is often fatal.

Perforation and stricture of the colon are uncommon complications. Rectal prolapse is usually associated with polyps. Pseudotumour results from an excessive connective tissue reaction to schistosomal granulomas. It may be located within or outside the intestinal lumen and may be palpable. Pseudotumour often causes stenosis.

Hepatosplenic schistosomiasis occurs in patients with a heavy worm load about 5–15 years after infection. Ova are deposited in the terminal radicles of the portal vein with granuloma formation and fibrosis of the portal tracts leading to portal hypertension, massive splenomegaly and ascites. These patients often have associated HBV infection. *Shistosoma mansoni* infections may be associated with chronic *Salmonella* infection and the nephrotic syndrome.

Diagnosis

Diagnosis is established by the demonstration of living schistosome eggs in the urine (*S. haematobium*) or stools (*S. mansoni, S. japonicum*) or biopsy material. Dead eggs only signify past infection.

Medical treatment

The only broad-spectrum antischistosomal agent that is effective against all *Shistosoma* species is praziquantel. Oxamniquine is only effective against *S. mansoni*, while metriphonate is only effective against *S. haematobium*.

Praziquantel is the drug of choice and is given in the following dosage:

- *S. haematobium*: 30 mg/kg (single dose)
- *S. mansoni* with acute intestinal infection: 20 mg/kg daily for 3 days
- *S. mansoni* with colonic polyposis: 20 mg/kg twice daily for 3 days
- *S. mansoni* with hepatosplenic disease: 30 mg/kg daily for 6 days
- *S. japonicum*: 20 mg/kg three times for 1 day.

Surgical aspects

The need for surgical intervention in schistosomiasis may arise from the development of complications of the disease.

Portal hypertension

Schistosomiasis causes a parenchymal block, usually without significant hepatocellular dysfunction or reduction of the hepatic blood flow. Minor degrees of portal hypertension and hypersplenism may be reversed with antihelmintic therapy. Treatment for oesophageal varices is only required if bleeding has occurred. Many of these patients may be managed with sclerotherapy or banding of the varices. Surgical intervention is indicated if bleeding cannot be controlled in this way, or recurs after repeated sclerotherapy. Portacaval shunts are contraindicated in these patients because of the high risk of severe encephalopathy. Selective decompression by a Warren shunt gives good results. The favoured procedures are, however, either splenectomy with porta-azygos disconnection or the more extensive devascularization operation of Sugiura [see Hepatobiliary and Pancreatic Disorders, Vol. II].

Bilharzial granuloma of the gastrointestinal tract

This complication predominantly affects the large bowel, with small intestinal and appendiceal lesions being uncommon. Small bowel granuloma usually presents with acute intestinal obstruction, or more rarely with mesenteric infarction.

The clinical features of large bowel bilharzial granuloma are varied. The patient may have chronic symptoms, e.g. vague abdominal pain, palpable mass in the lower abdomen, passage of blood and mucus, anaemia and rectal prolapse. In these cases, the diagnosis is usually made by sigmoidoscopy and biopsy. Less commonly, the patients present with large bowel obstruction and at operation a lesion in sigmoid or descending colon or rectum is found (pseudotumour) that is macroscopically indistinguishable from carcinoma. Resection without primary anastomosis is performed in these patients. In the elective situation after adequate bowel preparation resection with primary anastomosis is safe.

Obstructive uropathy

Cystoscopy should be avoided when possible because of the risk of introducing secondary infection. It is reserved for diagnostic problem cases, e.g. exclusion of neoplasm. The surgical treatment of obstructed ureters remains controversial. An accurate assessment of the extent of the disease and the state of the bladder by intravenous pyelography and ultrasound is essential. Adequate excision of the diseased segment with direct reimplantation or by means of ileal conduits with vesicoileal anastomosis gives the best results. More severe ureteric and bladder disease requires major surgical treatment (ileocaeco-urethroplasty, etc.) in specialized urological units.

Malaria

Malaria is still the most widely spread communicable disease in the topics. About one billion of the

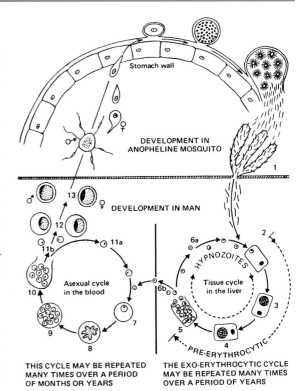

Figure 5.41 Life cycle of *P. vivax* and *P. malariae*. The life cycle of *P. falciparum* is similar but hypnozoites do not occur. (1) Sporozoites entering salivary glands of mosquito; (2–5) pre-erythrocytic cycle in the liver; (6a) hypnozoites in liver responsible for initial invasion of erythrocytes and for subsequent relapses; (6b–11a) erythrocytic schizony; (11b) immature gametocytes awaiting ingestion by anopheline mosquito.

world's population are still at risk. The two most common parasites are *Plasmodium vivax* and *P. falciparum*.

Parasitology

The complete life cycle of the human malaria parasite embraces a period of development within the mosquito and a period of infection in humans (Figure 5.41). After ingestion of infected human blood, a period of development (10–14 days) occurs in the mosquito, resulting in the production of sporozoites. A mosquito bite infects the human host with these forms, which remain in the circulating blood for 30 min, then enter tissue cells, notably the liver. During the next 7–9 days, the sporozoites develop in the hepatocytes. This stage of development is known as the pre-erythrocytic cycle. The cryptozoic schizonts that form rupture and release numerous merozoites, most of which enter the circulation to invade the erythrocytes, thus starting the erythrocytic cycle. No symptoms of malaria are experienced during the pre-erythrocytic cycle. The plasmodium first appears in red cells as a small speck of chromatin surrounded by scanty cytoplasm and soon becomes a ring-shaped trophozoite. As the parasite develops, pigment particles appear in the cytoplasm and the chromatin becomes more prominent. Chromatin division then proceeds and, when complete, the mature schizont containing daughter merozoites has formed. The parasitized red blood cells now rupture, releasing merozoites, the majority of which re-enter erythrocytes to reinitiate erythrocytic schizogony. In *P. falciparum* infection, the erythrocytic cycle takes 36–48 h (subtertian); in *P. vivax* and *P. ovale* infection 48 h (tertian) and *P. malariae* 74 h (quartan). The extent of the red cell infection differs from parasite to parasite, being highest (15%) with *P. falciparum*.

In response to an unknown stimulus, a number of the merozoites released when the red cells rupture develop into male and female gametocytes that are inert in the human but provide the reservoir of infection, enabling mosquitoes to perpetuate the malaria cycle. A certain proportion of the merozoites liberated in the pre-erythrocyte phase do not enter the blood stream. Instead, they re-enter the liver cells to produce metacryptozoic schizonts that are responsible for the persistence of the exo-erythrocytic cycle (EE) that occurs in *P. vivax*, *P. ovale* and *P. malariae* but not *P. falciparum*. The EE cycle is responsible for the reappearance of malaria some years after clinical cure. The exception to this is *P. falciparum*, where relapses are not encountered after adequate medical treatment.

Clinical features

Plasmodium falciparum: this is the only type of malaria that may be directly fatal. The clinical picture is extremely variable. A common misconception concerns the periodicity of the fever which, especially in first attacks, is irregular and occurs daily. Headaches, malaise, nausea, vomiting and generalized joint pains are frequent, presenting symptoms of an uncomplicated attack. On physical examination, there is hepatosplenomegaly and a variable degree of anaemia. This rather non-dramatic clinical picture can deteriorate suddenly into one with severe manifestations and a fatal outcome. Abdominal presentation resembling acute appendicitis can occur. The severe manifestations include cerebral malaria, algid malaria, severe malarial anaemia, hyperpyrexia, jaundice, pulmonary oedema and malarial haemoglobinuria. Patients are usually dehydrated and may have herpes labialis.

Plasmodium malariae: this produces the nephrotic syndrome in children with long-standing infection.

Plasmodium vivax: fever is the most constant sign. Initially remittent, the pattern changes to intermittent, regularly recurring fever every second day. In children convulsions occur when the fever is high. The classical features of the attack, i.e. cold stage, hot stage and sweating, are unusual in infants and children. General symptoms are similar to those of *P. falciparum* but milder. The spleen enlarges early in the disease, some degree of anaemia may be present and there is often mild leucopenia. The disease is rarely fatal unless the spleen ruptures.

A conclusive diagnosis of malaria is made by detection of the parasite in the blood.

Table 5.10 Chemoprophylaxis of malaria

- Chloroquine-sensitive areas   Chloroquine 300 mg once weekly, or
  Proguanil 200 mg daily

- Chloroquine-resistant areas   Chloroquine 300 mg once weekly and Proguanil 200 mg daily, or
  Mefloquine 250 mg once weekly

Treatment

Treatment consists of antiparasite chemotherapy and supportive management of the various manifestations. Only *P. falciparum* has become resistant to chloroquine. The drugs used in chloroquine resistant areas include quinine, Fansidar, Metakelfin, mefloquine (Lariam) and halofantrine (Halfan). In areas with resistance to both chloroquine and Fansidar, treatment is with quinine + tetracycline or mefloquine or halofantrine. Chemoprophylaxis is important for visitors to endemic regions and is outlined in Table 5.10. The prophylactic treatment should be started 1 week before departure and continued for 4 weeks after returning from the endemic area.

Filariasis

The more common of the several species of filarial parasites transmitted by various arthropod vectors include *Wuchereria bancrofti*, *Onchocerca volvulus*, *Brugia malayi* and *Loa loa*. Some of these essentially tropical and subtropical diseases produce filarial elephantiasis of the lower limbs and genitalia as a result of the occlusion by sclerosis of the lymphatics by adult worms resulting in gross lymphoedema. Many manifestations remain subclinical.

The life history of the various parasites that infect humans follows a common pattern, although details vary from species to species. The adult male and female worms of the infected person reproduce in the skin or lymphatics. The long, thin larvae are known as microfilariae. These enter the peripheral blood stream at specific hours depending on the filarial species and the feeding habits of the associated arthropod vector. In the insect (mosquitoes, blackflies, midges, etc.), the microfilariae mature and migrate to the biting structures of the arthropod and thus enter the blood stream or skin of the next victim of the insect bite. Further maturation occurs in the human, where the adult worms congregate into masses causing granulomatous painful swellings. *Wuchereria bancrofti* is the main cause of elephantiasis and hydrocele.

Elephantiasis of the lower limbs occurs in certain areas of East Africa and Ethiopia where there is no filariasis. These cases of non-filarial elephantiasis of the lower limbs are the result of an obstructive lymphopathy of the peripheral lymphatics caused by aluminosilicate and silica absorbed from the soil through the skin of the feet.

Guide to further reading

Ahrenholtz, D. H. (1988). Necrotizing soft tissue infections. *Surg Clin N Am* **68**: 199–214.

Bizollon, T., Ducerf, C. and Trepo, C. (1999) Hepatitis C virus recurrence after liver transplantation. *Gut* **44**: 575–578.

Connor, E. M., Sperling, R. S., Gelber, R., *et al.* (1994). Reduction of maternal–infant transmission of human immunodeficiency virus type I with zidovudine treatment. AIDS Clinical Trials Group Protocol 076 Study Group. *N Engl J Med* **331**: 1173–80.

Eyer, S., Brummitte, C., Crossley, K. *et al.* (1990). Catheter-related sepsis: prospective study of three methods of long-term catheter maintenance. *Crit Care Med* **18**: 1073–1076.

Fry, D. E. (1988). Antibiotics in surgery – an overview. *Am J Surg* **155**: 11–15.

Fukayama, M., Chong, J.-M. and Kaizaki, Y. (1998). Epstein–Barr virus and gastric carcinoma. *Gastric Cancer* **1**: 104–114.

Irish, C., Herbert, J., Bennett, D. *et al.* (1999). Database study of antibiotic resistant tuberculosis in the United Kingdom, 1994–96. *BMJ* **318**: 497–498.

Peters, W. and Gillis, H. M. (1989). *A Color Atlas of Tropical Medicine and Parasitology*, 3rd edn, Wolfe Medical Publications, London.

Pories, S. E., Gamelli, R. L., Mead, P. B. *et al.* (1991). The epidemiologic features of nosocomial infections in patients with trauma. *Arch Surg* **126**: 97–102.

Anaemia, hypovolaemia and oedema

'There is more wisdom in your body than in your deepest philosophy – Freidrich Nietzsche, 1844–1900'

This module covers the pathophysiology and management of patients who have a reduced haemoglobin load (anaemia), sustain a sudden reduction in the circulatory blood volume (hypovolaemia) or accumulate abnormal amounts of fluid in the interstitial space or serous cavities (oedema). Transfusion of blood and blood products is also covered in this module.

The spectrum of disorders covered in this module is wide and of variable surgical urgency, e.g. the patient with iron-deficiency anaemia requiring elective surgery for a right-sided colon cancer, the emergency management of a patient with profound hypotension from major ongoing blood loss, and patients with generalized oedema due to cardiac, hepatic or renal disease.

Section 6.1 • Anaemic patients: types, pathophysiology and management

Definition and types of anaemias of surgical importance

Anaemia is defined as a reduced level of circulating haemoglobin (Hb). Minor degrees are asymptomatic as the oxygen-carrying capacity of the blood, although reduced, is sufficient to meet the needs for daily activities. Below a certain level of Hb (8.0 g/dl), the oxygen-carrying capacity is sufficiently compromised as to be unable to meet the oxygen needs except at rest and the patient becomes symptomatic (symptomatic anaemia). The primary symptoms are those of oxygen lack (asthenia, lethargy, tiredness, diminished exercise, tolerance, etc.); others follow from the compensatory mechanism which consists essentially of a fast hyperkinetic circulation giving rise to palpitations, buzzing in the ears and angina. Severe anaemia may indeed cause heart failure. The types of anaemia are summarized in Table 6.1. In surgical practice, by far the most common is iron-deficiency (hypochromic microcytic) anaemia due to chronic occult blood loss (low serum ferritin and iron, high serum transferrin with low percentage saturation) exemplified by carcinoma of the right colon or stomach. In right colon cancer, hypochromic microcytic anaemia with positive faecal occult blood is the only early manifestation of the disease.

Megaloblastic anaemia arises from deficiency of vitamin B_{12}, folate or both. In a surgical context, megaloblastic anaemia is important from the preventive aspect, i.e. the need for vitamin B_{12} replacement therapy after gastrectomy and distal ileal resection/disease; its occurrence (due to folate deficiency) in patients on chemotherapy for cancer and in those on chronic dialysis prior to renal transplantation. Pernicious anaemia (megaloblastic anaemia + atrophic gastritis

Table 6.1 Types of anaemia

- Iron deficiency (hypochromic microcytic)
- Sideroblastic (hypochromic microcytic + ringed sideroblasts in the marrow)
- Anaemia of chronic disease (normocytic normochromic)
- Macrocytic normoblastic
  Liver disease
  Alcoholism
  Reticulocytosis secondary to haemolysis
- Macrocytic megaloblastic
- Congenital haemolytic (various morphological types, splenomegaly)
  Red cell membrane defects: hereditary spherocytosis, hereditary elliptocytosis
  Red cell enzyme defects: glucose-6-phosphate deficiency, pyruvate kinase deficiency
  Haemoglobinopathies (abnormal Hbs): sickle cell disease, thalassaemia
- Acquired haemolytic
  Idiopathic warm autoimmune haemolysis (active at 37°C, IgG antibodies)
  Idiopathic cold autoimmune haemolysis (active at lower temperatures, IgM antibodies)
  Drug-induced immune haemolysis
  Haemolytic disease of the newborn (RhD incompatibility)
- Aplastic/hypoplastic (bone marrow stem cell failure/depression)

with achlorhydria + parietal cell antibodies and impaired absorption of vitamin B_{12} corrected by oral intrinsic factor) assumes surgical importance because of the high risk for gastric cancer in these patients.

Anaemia associated with chronic disorders (normocytic normochromic) is commonly encountered in surgical practice in patients with malignant disease. It often does not respond to haematinics and then requires blood transfusion. Iron-deficiency anaemia and the anaemia of chronic disease may coexist. Patients with marrow failure (leukaemia, high-dose chemotherapy and malignant infiltration) require haematological support with blood transfusion, other component transfusion (platelets, granulocytes, clotting factors) and marrow rescue agents (recombinant colony-stimulating factors).

Anaemia and blood volume

The blood transfusion requirements of the anaemic patient are very different from those of the patient with acute blood loss. The crucial difference between anaemia and hypovolaemia (from acute haemorrhage) concerns the circulating blood volume (CBV), which is maintained or increased in anaemic individuals irrespective of the morphological type and aetiology of the anaemia (even when due to chronic blood loss). The deficit in anaemia thus relates to the haemoglobin load and hence to the oxygen-carrying capacity of the blood. This reduced haemoglobin level in symptomatic anaemia, even when fully saturated (oxygen saturation = 100%), is insufficient to provide normal tissue oxygenation. The compensatory mechanism consists of a hyperkinetic circulation with tachycardia and fast circulation time. In itself, this persistent tachycardia may contribute to anaemic cardiac failure due to deficient oxygenation of the myocardium (reduced diastolic interval).

During transfusion of anaemic patients, therefore, the prime consideration from the therapeutic safety standpoint is the prevention of circulatory overload and congestive cardiac failure. The objective of the transfusion is thus to raise the Hb load in a volume and during a time scale (slow transfusion over a 4-h period) that can be tolerated by the patient. A transfusion of red cells of 4 ml/kg will raise the circulating haemoglobin concentration by approximately 1.0 g/dl. Thus, each unit of red cells (300 ml) should raise the circulating Hb in a 70 kg adult by this amount. As the reason for transfusion of anaemic patients is to increase the oxygen-carrying capacity of blood, the red cell concentrates should be less than 14 days old as these have near normal levels of 2,3-diphosphoglycerate (2,3-DPG).

Section 6.2 • Nature, causes and consequences of hypovolaemia

Nature, causes and response

Nature and causes
Hypovolaemia is defined as a reduced CBV (= 70 ml/kg in adults; 80 ml/kg in infants) and can be either true or apparent. True hypovolaemia results from contraction of the CBV as a result of losses (blood from haemorrhage, plasma in the burnt patient and dehydration from deficits of water and saline). Apparent hypovolaemia ensues from an increased vascular capacity, usually due to loss of the peripheral resistance in the muscular arterioles (sepsis, adrenal insufficiency, anaphylaxis, neurogenic factors), although in some of these conditions, e.g. sepsis, the situation is more complex as the increased capillary permeability induces intravascular fluid losses into the interstitial space.

Response to hypovolaemia
Ultimately, the adverse effects of hypovolaemia are due to an inadequate (not necessarily reduced) cardiac output and hence inadequate cellular perfusion. To appreciate the pathophysiological consequences of hypovolaemia, one has to appreciate the normal control of cardiac output. Overall cardiac output (CO) is determined by the stroke volume (SV) and heart rate (HR) as follows: $CO = SV \times HR$. In a young, fit adult at rest, each ventricle fills during diastole to reach an end-diastolic volume of 120 ml of blood. With each ventricular contraction (systole), 70 ml is ejected from each ventricle. This amount is known as the ejection fraction, which is normally 60% of the volume of blood present in each ventricle at the end of diastole. In accordance with Starling's law (force of cardiac contraction increases with the diastolic stretch of the cardiac muscle fibres), the more the heart fills during diastole, the greater the amount of blood expelled with each beat (stroke volume), but the ejection fraction remains fairly constant. Cardiac output is then determined by:

- **Preload**, i.e. venous filling, venous return: determined by the CBV and venous tone. The peripheral veins, especially the venules of the liver and spleen (capacitance vessels) act as a large reservoir and contain 45% of the intravascular volume, while the large central veins hold about 18%. Hence, preload is reduced significantly in hypovolaemia. To some extent, the compensatory venous vasoconstriction due to the release of noradrenaline from the sympathetic nerve endings in the vein walls may help to maintain an adequate preload up to a certain deficit in the CBV.

Two other mechanisms facilitate the venous return: respiratory excursions and skeletal muscle activity. During inspiration, the diaphragm descends, increasing the intra-abdominal pressure that is transmitted to the intra-abdominal veins. At the same time, the intrathoracic pressure falls, lowering the right atrial pressure, the net effect being to accentuate venous return. This mechanism remains operative in hypovolaemia, unless complicated by chest injuries, which preclude normal ventilation (flail chest, haemopneumothorax and ruptured diaphragm). The contraction of the skeletal muscles within their fascial compartments is the main contributor of venous return in the lower limbs (the muscle pump). The contracting muscle bulk restrained by the overlying fascial sheath directly compresses the deep veins and encourages flow from the superficial to the deep venous systems. The efficiency of the muscle pump is dependent on the integrity of the venous valves. The muscle pump is lost in the prostrated hypovolaemic patient, but because of the supine or head-down position in which these patients are nursed, the loss of the muscle pump is not an important factor in the reduced preload.

- **Cardiac contractility** is diminished in hypovolaemia as a consequence of the reduced end diastolic filling/volume of the ventricles (and thus stretch of the cardiac muscle fibres).
- **Afterload**, i.e. peripheral arterial resistance: this acts as an impediment to cardiac ejection and thus a reduced afterload (e.g. by vasodilator therapy) tends to favour an increase in the cardiac output, but only in the presence of an adequate CBV. In the hypovolaemic patient, peripheral resistance is initially increased (sympathetic and adrenal response) so that the percentage fall in the blood pressure is always an underestimate of the drop in the cardiac output. Thus, for example, in previously healthy young adults, the acute loss of 20% of the blood volume reduces, on average, the arterial pressure by 15% and the cardiac output by 41%.
- **Heart rate**: within limits, tachycardia increases the CO but extreme heart rates reduce output by diminishing ventricular filling and coronary artery nutrient blood flow to the myocardium.

The response of an individual to blood loss varies considerably. Indeed, some young, healthy individuals, by virtue of the intense vasoconstriction they can mount in response to volume deficits, can lose as much as 25% of the CVB without any significant change in the arterial blood pressure. The response is influenced by age, duration and severity, pre-existing myocardial disease, anaemia and associated trauma. In the accident victim, the additional trauma alters the neuroendocrine and metabolic response. Thus, trauma victims with mild to moderate hypovolaemia may have a normal or even an elevated CO, and they may be normotensive or even hypertensive after the accident. Even the heart-rate response is variable in these patients, with either a tachycardia or bradycardia at the time of resuscitation.

Consequences of hypovolaemia

Diminished tissue perfusion, tissue hypoxia, anaerobic glycolysis and lactic acidosis

The immediate consequence is hypovolaemic shock, defined as a state of inadequate cellular perfusion [**see Module 18, Vol. I**]. The delivery of oxygen (D_{O_2}) to the tissues is reflected by the product of cardiac output × arterial oxygen content (C_{aO_2}) adjusted to the patient's build (indexed):

$$D_{O_2} \ (\text{ml/min/m}^2) = CO \times C_{aO_2} \times 10$$

The arterial oxygen content depends on the Hb level and the percentage oxygen saturation. Under normal physiological conditions, D_{O_2} ranges from 500 to 720 ml/min/m^2 and the oxygen consumption (V_{O_2}) between 100 and 160 ml/min/m^2, representing an oxygen extraction ratio of 22–30%. This level of tissue oxygenation ensures aerobic metabolism of glucose with the production of ATP, CO_2 and H_2O via pyruvate so that the blood lactate is very low (> 2.0 mmol/l) unless there is sustained muscular exertion when a certain amount of anaerobic metabolism is incurred with the production of lactate. This tendency to acidosis shifts the oxyhaemoglobin to the right, favouring dissociation, i.e. increased release of oxygen. Thus, any fall in the D_{O_2} is compensated for by increased extraction of oxygen. Tissue oxygenation is disturbed in all forms of shock.

D_{O_2} is reduced in hypovolaemic shock and is accompanied by an increased extraction, so that V_{O_2} is not markedly depressed unless the hypovolaemia is extreme. The severity of the lactic acidosis and the extent of reduction of the mixed venous haemoglobin saturation in the pulmonary artery, S_{vO_2} (obtained by pulse oximetry of a blood sample from the distal lumen of a Swan–Ganz catheter) depend on the severity of the hypovolaemia and on adequate early restoration of the blood volume.

Acute renal failure

Every organ incurs hypoxic damage from sustained hypovolaemia. The intense peripheral and splanchnic vasoconstriction that occurs in response to blood volume losses to redistribute the available blood to the brain puts the kidneys at particular risk of ischaemic damage: acute renal failure (ARF). Initially (prerenal or potential ARF), the renal function is simply responding to the prerenal deficits and intense vascular shut down, with low perfusion pressure and reduced oxygen delivery. There is 'physiological' oliguria with the production of small volumes of concentrated urine and low fractional sodium excretion. Renal tubular function is relatively well maintained. Urine osmolality is still greater than serum osmolality (urine/plasma osmolality ratio > 1.05). There are no structural changes and recognition of the problem at this stage with adequate correction of the prerenal deficits can prevent the development of established acute tubular necrosis (ATN), sometimes also referred to as acute reversible intrinsic renal failure (ARIRF).

With established renal ischaemia, metabolites and autocoids are released within the kidneys. Some, such as PGF_2 and prostacyclin, have direct cytoprotective properties for tubule cells and vasodilator effects improving blood flow to zones at risk. Others, such as endothelin released from endothelial cells, reduce further the glomerular blood flow and potentiate the renal failure. There is an early reversible phase of structural tubular cell injury characterized by cell swelling, exfoliation of tubular cells, brush border effacement and loss of transporting polarity. The exfoliation of tubular cells is thought to be due to redistribution of the integrin adhesion molecule receptors from the basolateral to the apical membranes. The exfoliated cells adhere downstream to other tubular cells to form casts. Irreversible cell damage is indicated by the appearance of nuclear pyknosis, mitochondrial calcifications and cytoplasmic membrane disruption. The ARF tubular damage is found predominantly in the outer medulla where oxygen delivery is always borderline. Changes in the cortical tubules are less marked, partly because cortical blood flow, and hence transporting workload, fall quickly after the ischaemic insult. The renal impairment results from (i) fall in the whole kidney glomerular filtration rate, (ii) obstruction of tubules by casts, and (iii) back-leakage of filtrate across the damaged tubules into the interstitium.

Recovery of acute reversible intrinsic renal failure

Clinically, recovery of sufficient renal function for independent survival after oliguric ARIRF takes 2–4 weeks. Old age, sepsis, jaundice and cardiorespiratory failure are adverse factors that usually prevent recovery of renal function.

Management of ARIRF
[See Module 11, Vol. I.]

Section 6.3 • Management of hypovolaemia

The management of the hypovolaemic patient entails:

- detection of the hypovolaemia, its cause and severity
- arrest of haemorrhage [Module 2, Vol. I]
- establishing good intravenous access with large-bore peripheral cannulae (two if hypovolaemia is severe)
- replacing the deficit
- repeating clinical observations and monitoring the patient.

Detection of hypovolaemia, its cause and severity

Although in the majority of patients the diagnosis of hypovolaemia is obvious, in some patients it is less clear-cut because of previous partial resuscitation and variable degrees of vasoconstriction. Diagnosis and assessment are thus based on clinical assessment, including careful history, clinical examination, estimation of observed losses, haemodynamic measurements (heart rate, pulse volume, arterial and venous pressures and haematocrit) and indices of tissue perfusion (nail bed capillary refill, peripheral skin temperature, urine output and level of consciousness). It must be stressed that the haemodynamic measurements are complementary to the clinical assessment, as a normotensive patient with a normal heart rate may still be hypovolaemic.

The severity of hypovolaemia correlates with the volume lost and is reflected in the clinical signs. In general, contraction of the CBV by more than 25% (1.5 litres) is regarded as severe hypovolaemia. The severity of the hypovolaemia is much more difficult to assess clinically when the hypovolaemia is secondary to deficits of water and saline. In these instances, careful reappraisal of the fluid balance charts gives the best estimate of the losses incurred.

Intravenous access and replacement of deficits

The principle of volume replacement, 'replace like with like', needs to be qualified in respect of the cause of the hypovolaemia. It applies fully to hypovolaemia associated with fluid and electrolyte losses [see Module 7, Vol. I]. Burn patients may require blood in addition to crystalloids and protein solutions [see Module 4, Vol. I]. A previously healthy adult is able to tolerate a blood loss of 25% of the CBV (1.5 litres) with volume replacement by crystalloids or plasma expanders only. Beyond this loss, blood transfusion becomes necessary as the oxygen-carrying capacity of the blood is then compromised by the significant reduction in the Hb content of the blood.

Although good intravenous access for volume replacement is an obvious necessity, it is often compromised by inability to insert an appropriately sized cannula (or two in severe hypovolaemia) because of the collapsed veins. Valuable time is often lost in persisting with efforts to cannulate percutaneously a peripheral upper limb vein. In these cases, a cut-down is made over a suitable vein.

Hypovolaemia due to acute blood loss

The management entails:

- replacing the volume at the same time as controlling the bleeding. Blood samples are taken for blood group/antibody screening, urea and electrolytes and haematology, i.e. Hb, packed cell volume (PCV) and platelet count. Rapid intravenous infusion is commenced with crystalloid solutions, e.g. isotonic saline or colloids (protein solutions or non-plasma colloid volume expanders). Several clinical trials have confirmed that colloid solutions are not superior to crystalloids for resuscitation but much larger volumes of crystalloids are needed. Resuscitation with isotonic saline should be avoided in patients with severe liver disease in view of risk of sodium overload. For the same reason, only salt-poor albumin solutions should be administered to these patients. Dextran and hetastarch (Hespan, HES) should be limited to 1.5 litres/24 h
- blood transfusion if losses exceed 1.5 litres
- administering oxygen by face mask or nasal catheter
- requesting early coagulation screen
- repeating clinical observation and monitoring of the patient.

Massive blood transfusion

Massive blood transfusion is defined as that which is equivalent to or exceeds the patient's own blood volume within 12 h. It carries high morbidity and mortality rates, primarily because of the underlying condition that necessitates the massive blood transfusion and, to a lesser extent, because of the adverse acute changes that are caused by the rapid infusion of large amounts of cold stored blood. Patients requiring massive blood transfusion form a heterogeneous group: young, previously healthy trauma victims, patients with major bleeding disorders, obstetric complications, etc. The nature of the underlying condition and the age of the patient largely determine the survival. Pre-existing renal and liver disease and old age militate against recovery.

Aside from being cold, stored blood has an acid pH, contains citrate anticoagulant, and has an elevated plasma K^+ and ammonia and a reduced 2,3-diphosphoglycerate (2,3-DPG). The metabolic consequences therefore include hypothermia, acidosis, hyperkalaemia and an increased affinity of the transfused Hb for oxygen (reduced 2,3-DPG), thereby contributing to the tissue hypoxia. The reduced oxygen-carrying capacity is not a real problem nowadays with the use of modern anticoagulant preservative solutions that ensure adequate concentration of 2,3-DPG in stored blood for up to 14 days. For this reason, blood that is less than 14 days old is recommended for massive blood transfusions. The reduced oxygen-carrying capacity is likely to be important only in anaemic patients and in those with pre-existing cardiac disease. The hypothermia may lead to cardiac arrhythmias including ventricular fibrillation and asystole. For this reason, patient warming (heating blankets, etc.) and blood warming are necessary if the transfusion rate exceeds 50 ml/min. Unfortunately, the heating coils increase the resistance of the oxygen-giving circuit, but their use is essential in these patients. Citrate intoxication is due to the chelation of ionized calcium, which may result in the prolongation of the QT interval, but this does not materially affect cardiac function and the ionized calcium level rapidly returns to normal after the transfusion as the excess citrate is metabolized and excreted. Thus, the use of supplemental calcium is not justified, particularly as it may itself give rise to arrhythmias. Hyperkalaemia is seldom a problem as the excess plasma K^+ enters the red blood cells (RBCs) with warming to body temperatures. It is, however, a consideration in patients with acidosis and renal failure when calcium is administered as the physiological antidote.

Clotting factors and other blood component deficiencies (Table 6.2) that arise as a result of massive blood transfusion are more important than the metabolic complications. Stored blood is deficient in factors V and VIII and beyond 48 h contains practically no functioning platelets. The situation is further compounded by the dilution that occurs in these patients because of infusion of crystalloids and plasma

Table 6.2 Haematological consequences of massive blood transfusion

- Clotting factor deficiency, especially factors V and VIII
- Thrombocytopenia
- Disseminated intravascular coagulation
- Reduced plasma colloid osmotic pressure

expanders before or in between units of blood. The breakdown of some of the transfused cellular components (RBCs, platelets, leucocytes) releases thromboplastin-like material and thus can trigger disseminated intravascular coagulation (DIC).

Adult respiratory distress syndrome (ARDS) may complicate massive blood transfusion and is often multifactorial. Its incidence is influenced by the underlying condition (sepsis and major trauma), but microemboli from white cell and platelet aggregates and reduced plasma oncotic pressure (dilution) can contribute to the development of the syndrome. ARDS can also develop as a result of transfusion-related acute lung injury (TRALI; see below).

The modern practice of 'safe' massive blood transfusion is outlined in Figure 6.1. Previous standardized regimens have been replaced by component treatment based on repeated coagulation screens and haematological tests. Platelets are, however, inevitably required when 1.5 litres or more of the patient's blood volume has been replaced. The amount of platelets needed by these patients averages 1 unit of platelet concentrate/10 kg body weight. Fresh-frozen plasma (FFP) is used to treat defined defects outlined by the coagulation screen. DIC is presumed if the thrombin time is more than double the control value. In these cases, 10 units of cryoprecipitate are administered in addition to FFP to correct the deficiency of clotting factors (V, VIII).

Monitoring of the hypovolaemic patient

The primary objectives of monitoring are to ensure that the CBV has been replaced and that tissue perfusion has been restored to normal. In addition, in the unstable patient monitoring provides early signs of either renewed bleeding or cardiac decompensation and thus the need for inotropic support. The extent of monitoring needed depends on the severity of the hypovolaemia, associated comorbid cardiorespiratory disease or trauma and cardiovascular stability of the patient.

Basic monitoring of the otherwise stable patient who recovers quickly with volume replacement includes:

- **arterial blood pressure, core temperature and pulse rate**
- **central venous pressure (CVP)**: if values are equivocal, the effect of a fluid challenge on the CVP (100–200 ml over 2–3 min) will determine

---

Management of Patients Undergoing Massive Blood Transfusion

- Replace and maintain blood volume – *use stored blood less than 14 days old*

- Maintain haemostasis – *based on coagulation screen (platelet count, thrombin time and prothrombin time)*

- Maintain oxygen carrying capacity – *ensure packed cell volume > 20 or Hb > 80g/L (repeat haematological testing)*

- Keep the patient warm – *heating coils on the blood circuit, heated blanket, etc.*

- Correct or avoid metabolic complications – *see text*

- Maintain a normal plasma protein concentration – *avoid excessive crystalloid infusions and monitor plasma albumin level*

Figure 6.1 Management of patients undergoing massive blood transfusion.

---

whether the patient is still hypovolaemic (CVP remains unchanged or may even drop as the vasoconstriction subsides) or is likely to be overloaded (sharp elevation in CVP)
- **hourly urine output**: an output > 30 ml urine/h indicates adequate renal perfusion
- **pulse oximetry**: preferably one that also displays the pulse plethysmogram in addition to percentage saturation of the Hb.

More intensive monitoring is required in cardiovascularly unstable patients, including those who sustain major trauma. This includes (in addition to the above):

- **insertion of a radial artery cannula** for continuous monitoring of the arterial pressure and to obtain samples for blood gas analysis
- **core–peripheral temperature gradient**: a useful, non-invasive indicator of peripheral perfusion
- **insertion of a pulmonary artery flotation catheter** (PAFC, Swan–Ganz catheter): this allows monitoring of the right atrial pressure, pulmonary artery pressure and pulmonary capillary wedge pressure, measurement of the cardiac output (by thermodilution) and sampling of the mixed venous blood for oxygen saturation (Sv,O_2). A number of important derived variables can be obtained

from these measurements in conjunction with the results of blood gas analysis. These are pulmonary vascular resistance, systemic vascular resistance, oxygen extraction ratio and systemic oxygen consumption [see Module 19, Vol. I].

Section 6.4 • Gastrointestinal haemorrhage

It is customary to consider gastrointestinal (GI) bleeding as occurring from either the upper or the lower GI tract. This classification, although in established usage, is not entirely satisfactory as it omits a group of disorders, albeit less common, that present with bleeding from lesions in the midgut (from the duodenojejunal junction to the proximal transverse colon). In the upper/lower GI classification, right colonic bleeding lesions are grouped with lower GI bleeding. The causes of GI bleeding by topographical site in the gut are outlined in Table 6.3.

Irrespective of site, GI bleeding is best addressed from a clinical standpoint in accordance with presentation of the patient:

- **chronic occult blood loss**: the patient is unaware of the bleeding, presents with iron-deficiency anaemia and has a positive faecal occult blood

- **overt minor episodes of blood loss** which prompt the patient to seek medical advice from the general practitioner: common presentation of patients with haemorrhoids, rectal tumours and inflammatory bowel disease
- **acute episode of GI bleeding** that cause varying degrees of hypovolaemia, in some cases life-threatening
- **recurrent obscure GI bleeding**.

Chronic occult gastrointestinal bleeding

Presentation with anaemia is common in patients with gastric and especially right colon cancer. The management of patients with these tumours is covered in Volume II. Occult bleeding forms the only proven basis of screening for colorectal cancer. Using the standard haemoccult test, which has a sensitivity for cancer of around 50%, it has been shown that screen-detected tumours have a much better prognosis than tumours that present with symptoms. More importantly, randomized population-based studies have shown categorically that groups offered faecal occult blood screening have a significantly reduced mortality for colorectal cancer. Screening theory is covered in **Module 15, Vol. I; 'Diseases of the Colon and Rectum', Vol. II**.

Some patients present with dyspeptic symptoms and are found to be anaemic on examination, e.g. reflux oesophagitis, peptic ulceration. Other causes of occult bleeding are much less common and usually present diagnostic problems requiring special investigations (recurrent obscure GI bleeding).

Elective presentation with episodes of gastrointestinal bleeding

Nowadays, this presentation relates most commonly to patients with colorectal disease, e.g. polyps, cancers, inflammatory bowel disease and haemorrhoids. Both cancers and inflammatory bowel disease (ulcerative colitis, Crohn's colitis, indeterminate colitis, dysentery) are usually associated with alteration in bowel habit. The various disorders are covered in Volume II.

Acute upper gastrointestinal bleeding

Epidemiology

The overall incidence varies widely in Western countries (40–150/100 000), with regional differences within each country. Thus, within the UK, Aberdeen has an incidence of 116/100 000 whereas Oxford, at 47/100 000, pales by comparison. Irrespective of regional differences, the epidemiology of acute upper GI bleeding has changed during the past 40 years. The highest prevalence is nowadays encountered in the elderly. This is the main reason why mortality from

Table 6.3 Causes of gastrointestinal bleeding by topographical site

Foregut	Midgut	Hindgut
Oesophagitis	Ulcers: usually drug induced	Colorectal tumours/polyps
Oesophageal varices	Small bowel tumours	Inflammatory bowel disease
Gastritis	Vascular anomalies: right colon and small bowel	Diverticular disease
Peptic ulcer: DU, GU	Hereditary telangiectasia	Angiodysplasia
Tumours: adenoca, smooth muscle, lymphoma	Peutz–Jeger polyps	Ischaemic colitis
Vascular anomalies	Jejunal diverticula	Trauma
Hereditary telangiectasia	Meckel's diverticulum: infants and children	Endometriosis
Anastomotic suture line: postoperative	Aortoenteric fistula: patients with aortic grafts	Anastomotic suture line: postoperative
Mallory–Weiss syndrome	Crohn's disease	Portal hypertension
Trauma: including iatrogenic	Anastomotic suture line: postoperative	Haemorrhoids
Anal fissure		
Haemobilia	Portal hypertension: includes bleeding from stomal varices	Bleeding disorder[a]
Chronic pancreatitis: aneurysms, sectorial portal hypertension	Parasitic infestations	
Bleeding disorders	Endometriosis	
	Right colon cancer/polyps	
	Bleeding disorder[a]	

[a]In at least 25% of patients bleeding occurs from a pre-existing lesion, e.g. ulcer.

acute upper GI bleeding has not declined significantly despite better and earlier diagnosis by endoscopy and advances in endoscopic control of bleeding and in blood transfusion practice. The fact is that elderly people do not tolerate severe hypovolaemia and are less likely to recover if they require operative intervention than young, fit patients. Age-specific data from the Office for Population Census Statistics (OPCS) for deaths from bleeding duodenal and gastric ulcer in England and Wales demonstrate the very significant effect of increasing age, with death rates rising 400-fold between the age ranges 0–49 years and 80+ years (Figure 6.2).

Causes of acute upper gastrointestinal bleeding

The causes of upper GI bleeding in descending order of frequency are outlined in Table 6.4. Duodenal and gastric ulcer account for the majority. The mortality is higher in patients with bleeding gastric ulcer, again attributable to the older age group. In some 20% of patients, the diagnosis is not clear at presentation despite urgent upper GI endoscopy. This arises because (i) there is too much blood in the stomach to permit adequate inspection, (ii) the lesion is missed (e.g. Mallory–Weiss tear or Dieulafoy submucosal aneurysm), (iii) the lesion has healed, or (iv) the source of bleeding is outside the stomach and proximal duodenum (upper jejunal, haemobilia, etc.).

Bleeding due to aspirin and non-aspirin non-steroidal anti-inflammatory drugs

Much of the misinformation concerning aspirin and non-aspirin non-steroidal anti-inflammatory drugs (NSAIDs) has arisen because of the poor quality of the early reports, which relied on contrast radiology for diagnosis and lacked proper controls. **All of these drugs cause drug-induced peptic ulcers in the stomach and duodenum** more commonly than acute gastric erosions, which account for only a small percentage of diagnosed cases. Aspirin increases the risks for both gastric and duodenal ulcers by two to four times, and according to the results of a study by Faulkner *et al.* (1988), one in every 10 ulcer bleeds in patients aged 60 years or over is induced by aspirin.

The non-aspirin NSAIDs (e.g. fenbufen, benoxaprofen, indomethacin, piroxicam, ibuprofen) pose a particular problem because they carry a higher risk of peptic ulceration than aspirin, and are taken largely by elderly patients who may be at increased risk of ulcer complications and death. Calculations based on published series indicate that 20% of all bleeding ulcers in patients over 60 years are caused by non-aspirin NSAIDs. A more recent case–control study reported in 1997 demonstrated that the situation had not changed a decade later. Emergency admissions were more likely to be NSAID users than controls (31% vs 16%) and had significantly higher blood transfusion requirement, although NSAID usage did not influence mortality. On the basis of these data, it has been estimated that there are 65 000 emergency upper GI hospital admissions (perforation, bleeding, acute pain) per annum in the UK and of these 12 000 are caused by NSAID use, with 2230 deaths. A further 300 attributable deaths occur in the community (patients not admitted to hospital).

Overall, 30% of ulcer bleeds in patients aged above 60 years are due to aspirin or non-aspirin NSAIDs.

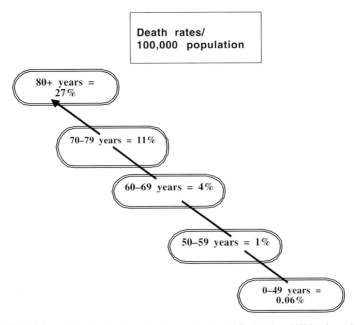

Figure 6.2 Deaths per 100 000 from bleeding duodenal and gastric ulcer in England and Wales in various age groups. Note the 400-fold increase between the age ranges 0–49 years and 80+ years.

Table 6.4 Causes of acute upper gastrointestinal bleeding: percentage distribution by disease category (average figures for the UK)

Disease category	Percentage Distribution
Duodenal ulcer	29
Gastric ulcer	22
Oesophagitis and ulcer	12.0
Acute gastric lesions	7.0
Mallory–Weiss	7.0
Oesophageal varices	5.0

Prevention of non-steroidal anti-inflammatory drug gastrointestinal toxicity and the cyclooxyenase system

Many agents, e.g. sucralfate, high-dose H_2 blockers and, more recently, proton-pump inhibitors, have been shown to be effective in reducing duodenal lesions caused by NSAIDs, but all have been less successful in preventing gastric mucosal damage. This approach, although in established practice, is not the answer to the epidemiological problem. During the past decade there has been considerable pharmacological research aimed at the development of NSAIDs that are free of significant GI toxicity (bleeding and perforation). This has led to significant new information on the cyclooxygenase (COX) system responsible for the production of prostaglandins, and has also resolved the previous apparent paradox that prostaglandin production protects as well as injures tissues. It has been known since the initial proposal by Vane that aspirin acts by inhibiting the COX enzyme and thus the synthesis of prostaglandins. COX was thought to be a single enzyme, but research has now confirmed that there are two isoforms of COX: COX1 and COX2. COX1 (also known as constitutive cyclooxygenase) is always present and is responsible for most of the physiological prostaglandin production involved in cytoprotection, especially of the gastric mucosa. In contrast, COX2 (inducible cyclooxygenase) is involved in the synthesis of prostaglandins that mediate the inflammatory response (including joint inflammation). Thus, specific inhibitors of COX2 suppress the inflammatory response, while preserving the cytoprotective function of COX1. The first COX2 inhibitor to be launched in Europe is meloxicam. The early reports indicate a significant reduction in GI toxicity in regular users but confirmation of this breakthrough awaits confirmation with large endoscopy-based studies.

Clinical presentation of acute upper gastrointestinal bleeding

Most patients are admitted as emergencies with haematemesis, melaena or both. Severity is dictated by the presence and extent of hypovolaemia into:

- **mild**: no significant hypovolaemia, includes patients who are anaemic
- **moderate**: hypovolaemia that responds to volume replacement (crystalloids and blood) and, thereafter, the patient is stable
- **severe**: active continued major bleeding rendering resuscitation with transfused blood difficult or recurrent major bleeding after successful resuscitation from the initial bleed. These are the patients at risk and include patients with bleeding oesophageal varices. In elderly patients with atherosclerosis, the hypotension may precipitate myocardial infarction or cerebrovascular accident.

Although this classification is useful as it dictates management, the category can change after initial assessment from mild to severe. Thus, complacency must be avoided and repeat clinical observation monitoring is essential even in patients with mild upper GI haemorrhage. This situation is best exemplified by the patient who develops an aortoenteric fistula after aortic replacement by a prosthetic graft. The initial (secondary) bleeds may appear trivial, yet they are warning manifestations of an impending catastrophic haemorrhage that is often fatal.

Some insist on differentiating between recurrent and persistent bleeding. The former is defined as a second episode of haematemesis or melaena associated with evidence of hypovolaemia after the initial successful resuscitation and a period of haemodynamic stability. In patients with ulcers, the endoscopic stigmata associated with increased risk of recurrence are an active spurting vessel, a visible vessel (Figure 6.3) and adherent clot. Persistent bleeding is diagnosed when the patient requires 8 units (> 60 years) or 12 units (< 60 years) or more over a 48-h period to maintain the Hb at 10 g/dl. In practice, both require measures to control the bleeding and the important decision is whether these patients should be treated endoscopically or surgically.

In addition to the severity of the bleed, the patient must be examined for stigmata of chronic liver disease that may indicate variceal haemorrhage, although these patients could equally bleed from ulcers or portal hypertensive gastropathy [see The Liver in Hepatobiliary and Pancreatic Surgery, Vol. II]. Also necessary is clinical examination of the cardiovascular and respiratory systems with appropriate investigations (chest X-ray and electrocardiogram). Significant cardiac and respiratory disease are important determinants of morbidity and mortality and influence the approach used to control bleeding.

Management of acute upper gastrointestinal bleeding

The action plan is outlined in Figure 6.4. Diagnosis is based on upper GI endoscopy carried out within 24 h of admission in haemodynamically stable patients and following resuscitation. The policy that all patients with

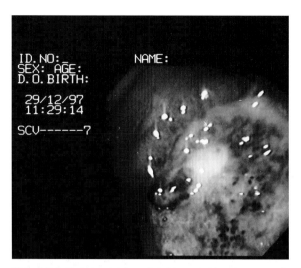

Figure 6.3 Endoscopic view of visible vessel in a large gastric ulcer.

acute upper GI haemorrhage should have a joint consultation by a surgeon and gastroenterologist soon after admission has much to commend it. Patients with severe continued bleeding require surgery concomitantly with volume replacement through two large-infusion cannulae.

All patients are kept on nil by mouth at least until endoscopy has been performed. The practice of insertion of a nasogastric tube is popular with surgeons but not gastroenterologists. If a tube is used, it should be of the Salem sump suction variety. Lavage through the tube with ice-cold saline to induce gastric mucosal vasoconstriction is practised in some North American centres but has never caught on in the UK. Without doubt, a nasogastric tube cannot be relied on to diagnose recurrent bleeding and certainly is no substitute for clinical observation and regular monitoring of pulse, blood pressure, CVP, pulse oximetry and urine output. Aside from this, nasogastric tubes may cause mucosal trauma. Thus, the case for nasogastric suction 'to keep the stomach empty', although established by surgical tradition, is by no means proven.

Pharmacological control of bleeding

The agents used are H_2 blockers, sucralfate, proton-pump inhibitors, vasopressin (or analogues), somatostatin and tranexamic acid.

There has never been any material evidence that acid suppression with H_2 blockers imparts any benefit in patients with acute upper GI bleeding, although proton-pump inhibitors may help. Likewise, there is no evidence that vasopressin and somatostatin are useful in ulcer bleeds. By contrast, tranexamic acid (oral or intravenous) has been confirmed by controlled, randomized studies to reduce the transfusion requirements, rebleeding rates (by 30%), need for surgical intervention (by 30–40%) and mortality (40%). The current recommended regimen consists of intravenous tranexamic acid for the first 3 days followed by oral administration for a further 3 days. To date, tranexamic acid is not widely used outside Scandinavia except as perioperative treatment for elective surgery in Jehovah's Witness patients.

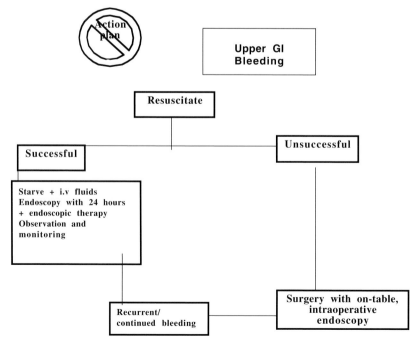

Figure 6.4 Action plan for patients with acute upper GI bleeding.

Both vasopressin (and analogues) and somatostatin have been shown to be effective in the initial control of variceal bleeding [see Module 10, Vol. I; Hepatobiliary Surgery, Vol. II].

Endoscopic treatment

Control of bleeding in the majority of patients (unless severe or catastrophic) is achieved with interventional flexible endoscopic techniques carried out by experts in a dedicated endoscopy suite with the necessary cardiovascular monitoring. Large-diameter instrument channels (3.4 mm or greater) or twin-channel endoscopes (Figure 6.5) are used, as the standard endoscopes (instrument channel 2.8 mm) are very easily blocked by blood clots. The twin-channel endoscope has one channel for therapy and the other for suction. Its disadvantage lies in the large overall diameter of the instrument and consequent reduced flexibility. For this reason, some prefer the single large-diameter instrument-channel endoscope and, if aspiration of luminal contents proves difficult when the therapeutic device is inserted, a nasogastric tube is passed alongside the endoscope for suction and irrigation.

The endoscopic techniques used for visible vessels and active bleeding can be classified as thermal, electrocoagulation, photocoagulation and injection therapy (Table 6.5). Sometimes, a combination of techniques, e.g. adrenaline injection therapy with electrocoagulation or photocoagulation, is used and is reported to be beneficial by allowing a clearer target for the endoscopist and by reducing the heat-sink effect when thermal energy is applied [see Module 20, Vol. I].

Vascular embolization

Vascular embolization is used for endoscopically or surgically inaccessible bleeding sites, e.g. liver in haemobilia, bleeding from pancreas (usually postpancreatic necrosis) and some lesions in the small intestine [see Module 20, Vol. I].

Indications for surgical treatment

With the expansion and increased efficacy of endoscopic techniques for the control of acute GI bleeding, fewer patients are treated surgically. None the less, there are clear-cut clinical situations where surgical treatment remains the patient's only hope of survival. The important determinant of survival in these seriously ill patients is a timely decision that surgical treatment is needed. Persistence with conservative management or endoscopic control until the patient's condition is seriously compromised by prolonged hypovolaemia inevitably results in demise of the patient, usually from multisystem organ failure.

The patients with acute upper GI bleeding who require surgical treatment are:

■ **patients admitted with exsanguinating haemorrhage** such that resuscitation by volume

replacement cannot keep up with the losses. An on-table endoscopy after tracheal intubation and induction of anaesthesia is usually carried out and can be useful (e.g. detection of oesophageal varices), but often the endoscopy is unrewarding because of too much blood and clots in the stomach. Some would also include patients with an active arterial spurter in the surgical category requiring immediate surgery. Intraoperative enteroscopy (small bowel endoscopy by a long colonoscope introduced orally and guided by the surgeon

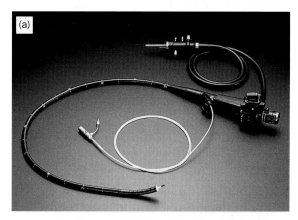

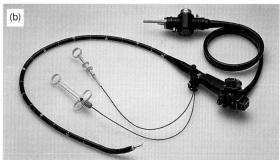

Figure 6.5 Large biopsy channel endoscopes: (a) single and (b) twin instrument channel. (Courtesy of Olympus, Japan.)

Table 6.5 Techniques for endoscopic control of upper gastrointestinal bleeding

- Injection therapy: vasopressors, sclerosants, thrombin, mixtures
- Banding: alternative to injection sclerotherapy for oesophageal varices
- H-F electrocoagulation: unipolar, bipolar, argon ion plasma coagulation
- Heater probe
- Photocoagulation: gas vapour lasers, diode array lasers
  - non-contact (laser beam)
  - contact (with sapphire tip)

through the duodenum and dudodenojejunal flexure) may need to be done during the course of the operation, if the exact site of bleeding cannot be determined at laparotomy. This has replaced previous surgical manoeuvres, e.g. application of bowel clamps to different sections of the GI tract, to locate the bleeding source

■ **elderly patients (> 60 years)**: the survival of these patients is compromised by surgical delay. Most surgeons would advise surgery if (i) more than 4 units of blood are necessary during the initial resuscitation of the hypovolaemia on admission, (ii) the patient has one recurrence of bleeding after initial successful endoscopic control of bleeding, and (iii) there is persistent bleeding requiring 8 units of blood transfusion within 48 h

■ **younger patients (< 60 years)**: these usually tolerate bleeding better and therefore the threshold for surgical treatment is set higher: (i) patients requiring 8 or more units of blood during the initial resuscitation, and (ii) persistent bleeding requiring 12 units of blood over a 48-h period.

For details of surgical treatment of these patients see **Module 16, Vol. I; Gastrointestinal Surgery, Vol. II**.

Lower gastrointestinal bleeding

Epidemiology
Because rectal bleeding is common and as it rarely occasions admission to hospital, true rates are not easily ascertained. However, recent questionnaire studies indicate that about 80% of the population experience at least one episode of rectal bleeding at some stage during their lives, and at any one point, about 7% of the population will have noticed rectal bleeding within the last 6 months. Clearly, this has very significant implications for the investigation and management of this condition.

Causes of rectal bleeding
It is useful to think of causes of rectal bleeding in terms of anatomical sites, i.e. anus, rectum, colon and upper GI tract. It is very important to remember that any lesion in the stomach, duodenum or small bowel that bleeds may present with overt rectal bleeding, if the rate of blood loss is fast enough. The causes of rectal bleed-

ing are shown in Table 6.6. These conditions are covered in detail in Volume II **[see Gastrointestinal Surgery, Vol. II]**.

Of the common causes, haemorrhoids bleed because of trauma to the engorged vascular cushions; proctitis and colitis bleed from mucosal ulcerations; tumours bleed from dilated, fragile neoplastic vessels; and diverticular disease from erosion of a vessel at the mouth of a diverticulum. Most overt rectal bleeding is minor in terms of amount, but occasionally, it can be massive. When this occurs, it is usually caused by diverticular disease, angiodysplasia or upper GI source, such as a small bowel vascular malformation or a duodenal ulcer.

Clinical presentation of lower gastrointestinal bleeding
Unlike upper GI bleeding, the vast majority of patients presenting to surgeons with rectal bleeding are seen at clinic, and only a minority is admitted as emergencies. In general, rectal bleeding can be categorized as:

■ trivial
■ troublesome
■ suspicious
■ massive.

Trivial: this type of bleeding is common and consists of occasional smears of blood seen on the toilet paper with no other symptoms. Often, there are no clinical findings, although the patient may have first- or second-degree haemorrhoids.

Troublesome: this is usually bright red, and when caused by haemorrhoids, it typically occurs after defecation and may drip into the toilet pan. This can be quite alarming, and when profuse and frequent, it may lead to anaemia. Anal fissure also causes bright-red bleeding associated with defecation, but unlike haemorrhoids, it is usually accompanied by severe anal pain.

Suspicious: this type of bleeding should raise the clinical suspicion of colorectal cancer. Typically, rectal cancer causes quite fresh bleeding often associated with tenesmus. Left-sided colon cancer is more likely to present with dark blood mixed with or on the surface of the stool, and is frequently associated with change of bowel habit and/or lower abdominal pain. It should be noted that right-sided cancers tend not to cause overt bleeding or change of bowel habit, but rather present

Table 6.6 Causes of rectal bleeding by anatomical site

Anal causes	Rectal causes	Colonic causes	Upper GI causes
Haemorrhoids	Polyp	Polyp	Peptic ulceration
Fissure	Carcinoma	Carcinoma	Meckel's diverticulum (ectopic ulceration)
Perianal abscess/fistula	Proctitis	Diverticular disease	Small bowel vascular lesion
Anal carcinoma	Rectal prolapse	Colitis (idiopathic, infective or ischaemic)	
		Angiodysplasia	

with iron-deficiency anaemia. This is because the faeces in the right side is still liquid, and the caecum and ascending colon are capacious and distensible. Thus, blood is well mixed with stool and obstructive symptoms are late to develop, except when the ileocaecal valve is involved.

Massive: in this case, the patient presents with profuse rectal bleeding and symptoms and signs of hypovolaemia. In many cases such bleeding stops spontaneously, but if it does not, it constitutes a life-threatening surgical emergency. The most common cause of massive rectal bleeding is diverticular disease, but it may originate from vascular lesions of the colon or small bowel and from more proximal lesions, especially posterior duodenal ulcers. Blood acts as a cathartic, and rapid upper GI haemorrhage can pass rapidly through the small and large bowel and appear as fresh rectal bleeding. Traces of food, tablets, etc., in the blood suggest a source in the stomach or duodenum.

Management of lower gastrointestinal bleeding

Investigation
The investigation of lower GI bleeding depends on the clinical presentation (Figure 6.6). For the young patient with trivial rectal bleeding, a digital rectal examination is normally sufficient, whereas in older patients a rigid sigmoidoscopy should be carried out. With typical haemorrhoidal bleeding, a proctoscopy and rigid sigmoidoscopy should be carried out in all cases, and if no cause is found or there is no response to treatment of haemorrhoids, a barium enema is ordered. If this is also negative, consideration should be given to flexible sigmoidoscopy and, finally, colonoscopy.

In the patient with bleeding that is suspicious of neoplasia, a thorough examination of the whole colon with barium enema and flexible sigmoidoscopy is mandatory, and if no cause is found, with colonoscopy. Barium enema alone is not satisfactory, as the rectum is not well seen and a tortuous sigmoid colon is difficult to interpret radiologically. If polyps are seen on barium enema or sigmoidoscopy, then total colonoscopy should be arranged to visualize the whole colonic mucosa and perform polypectomy. It may be argued that colonoscopy should be carried out as a primary investigation instead of barium enema and sigmoidoscopy, but (i) it is more painful, (ii) there is a higher risk of perforation, and (iii) in most countries the facilities and expertise for this policy are not widely available.

In massive rectal bleeding, the priority is resuscitation, but investigation must proceed promptly, usually during the resuscitation. The first step must be to exclude bleeding haemorrhoids by means of proctoscopy, and this should be followed by upper GI endoscopy. If these do not give the diagnosis and the patient remains unstable, most authorities recommend urgent mesenteric angiography, since if the bleeding is

brisk enough (> 0.5 ml/min), this will locate the bleeding point precisely. There is a school that favours acute colonoscopy with or without colonic lavage through a nasogastric tube, but this has been found to be impractical, and it cannot provide any degree of localization of small bowel lesions. For bleeding which is intermittent and does not show up on angiography, radionuclide-labelled red cell scanning may be used. Here, the patient's own red cells are labelled with ^{51}Cr and reinjected so that a gamma camera can be used to localize pooling of blood in the intestine. This, however, is of very limited practical value as it is necessary to carry out very frequent scans over a prolonged period (see Figure 6.6d).

Treatment
Medical: the only situation where colonic bleeding can be treated effectively with drugs is an acute exacerbation of inflammatory bowel disease. The mainstay is high-dose steroid therapy [see Gastrointestinal Surgery, Vol. II].

Endoscopic: endoscopic treatment is used in the management of bleeding haemorrhoids in the form of sclerosant injection or banding, but it has little place in the treatment of acute colonic bleeding. There have been occasional case reports of injection therapy for bleeding diverticular disease using a colonoscope, and angiodysplasia can be treated by electrocoagulation and photocoagulation, but not usually in the acute bleeding phase.

Radiological: as with upper GI lesions, colonic bleeding can be treated by means of radiological embolization. However, more than with the small bowel, this is associated with a risk of necrosis and perforation of the bowel wall.

Surgical: the elective surgical treatment of haemorrhoids, anal fissure and colorectal causes of bleeding, such as large bowel cancer, is covered in Volume II [see Gastrointestinal Surgery]. In the patient with massive bleeding from the colon or small bowel, appropriate surgical resection after attempts at preoperative localization is required. If the source is in the small bowel, it is helpful if the radiologist can leave a superselective catheter close to the bleeding site so that the surgeon can inject methylene blue down the catheter at the time of laparotomy to highlight the segment of bowel to be removed.

Occasionally, it is necessary to proceed to laparotomy without preoperative angiography, and in this case it is wise to perform intraoperative colonoscopy with on-table antegrade colonic lavage to try to localize the bleeding lesion. If this is impossible or unsuccessful, and blood appears to be confined to the colon, then colectomy and ileostomy, preserving the rectal stump for later re-anastomosis, is the safest option.

Recurrent obscure gastrointestinal bleeding

This applies to patients who experience recurrent episodes of GI bleeding (both acute and chronic) in

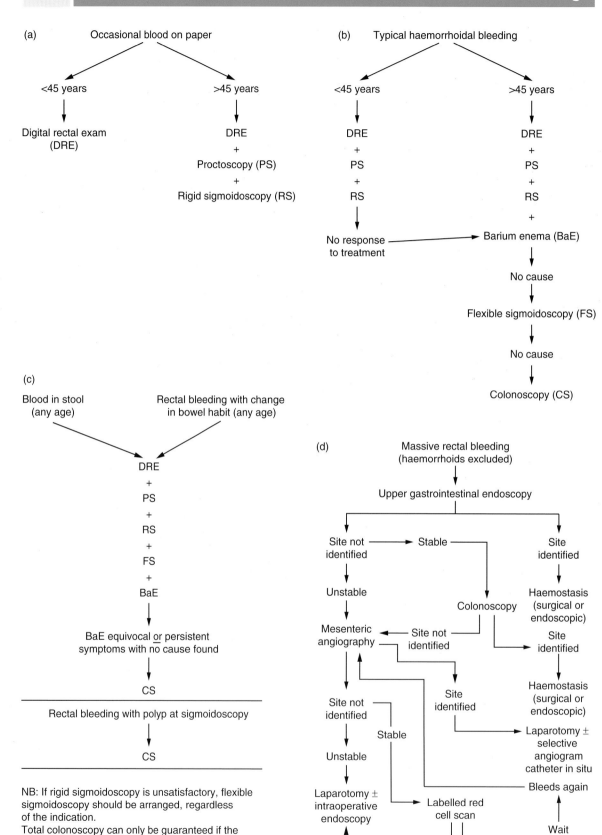

Figure 6.6 Investigation of lower GI bleeding.

whom no identifiable cause can be established despite full routine, often repeat investigations. Although fortunately rare, these patients often present a management problem. The presentation may be with:

- recurrent melaena
- fresh rectal bleeding
- anaemia
- haematemesis (rare).

In the majority of these patients, the source of the recurrent blood loss is in the midgut, i.e. small bowel below the duodenojejunal junction and the proximal colon. However, some are caused by missed lesions in the foregut. This is exemplified by the Dieulafoy lesion, which is a submucosal gastric microaneurysm or unusually large artery that runs in close contact with the mucosa. In more than 80% of patients, the lesion is situated within 6.0 cm of the gastro-oesophageal junction where it is easily missed. Haemobilia is another (albeit rare) cause of obscure recurrent GI bleeding.

Within the small bowel, the most common cause is small bowel ulceration (drug induced or associated with systemic disease, e.g. systemic lupus erythematosus, polyarthritis nodosa, rheumatoid arthritis, Henoch–Schonlein purpura). Small bowel tumours account for only 2–3% of cases and the lesion is then most commonly an adenocarcinoma. Peutz–Jeghers jejunal polyps and other syndromes associated with GI polyposis [see Gastrointestinal Surgery, Vol. II] often present with recurrent occult bleeding. Vascular anomalies of the small bowel can be a cause of recurrent obscure GI bleeding and are being increasingly recognized with the advent of small bowel enteroscopy. Telangiectasia, either as part of the hereditary condition (Rendu–Weber–Osler syndrome) or as isolated flat intramucosal telangiectasia or haemangioma, can likewise cause GI bleeding from the small bowel. One of the most common causes of acute bleeding in children is Meckel's diverticulum from ulceration of ectopic gastric mucosa. Jejunal diverticulosis can bleed and usually presents with recurrent episodes of melaena. Other causes include radiation enteritis, aortoenteric fistula (grafted patients) and endometriosis in females.

However, the most common source of recurrent obscure GI bleeding is the proximal colon and the most frequent lesion responsible is angiodysplasia. Tiny areas of angiodysplasia (about 2 mm) are easy to miss, particularly in the caecum [see Lower GI Bleeding and Gastrointestinal Surgery, Vol. II].

Management

The primary objective is to establish the cause of the bleeding. A vast array of specialized investigations is used to elucidate the cause in the elective situation. It is important that a sensible sequence is adopted to minimize patient inconvenience and to reduce costs. In the acute bleeding situation, the investigative options of practical benefit are fewer and essentially consist of emergency angiography and on-table enteroscopy and colonoscopy (see Figure 6.7 for action plan).

Angiography (aortic, selective visceral arteries) plays a crucial role in these patients and is the most effective investigation. Its exact role depends on the clinical situation. In patients with active bleeding, contrast angiography seeks to demonstrate the bleeding site by documenting extravasation of contrast, whereas in the elective situation (chronic bleeding), the aim is to detect abnormal vascular patterns (Figure 6.8). The success rates of angiography in acute haemorrhage depend on bleeding rate. Thus, if aortic injection is used, the lesion has to be bleeding at the rate of at least 5.0 ml/min. With selective visceral artery cannulation, however, localization can be obtained with lower bleeding rates (0.5–2.0 ml/min).

Barium meal and follow-through is virtually useless in these patients. Much higher yields are obtained, especially for the detection of small bowel tumours, ulcers and strictures, by enterocylsis (small bowel enema) with compression fluororadiology. Radio nuclide scanning is used for three purposes: (i) to quantify blood loss in the chronic situation (5-day test using ^{51}Cr-labelled autologous RBCs); (ii) for localizing blood loss by technetium-99m (^{99m}Tc)-sulfocolloid in the first instance, followed by labelled autologous RBCs; and (iii) for the diagnosis of bleeding Meckel's diverticulum (when ^{99m}Tc-pertechnetate is used to display the ectopic gastric mucosa (not the ulcer or the bleeding point itself). Endoscopic retrograde cholangiopancreatography (ERCP) is useful in cases suspected of haemobilia or if the bleeding is likely to be of pancreatic origin.

Ultimately, the treatment depends on the nature of the lesion, its surgical accessibility, the severity of the clinical situation and the condition of the patient. In general, all patients with life-threatening bleeding from the gut itself require laparotomy. Those where bleeding is from liver and pancreas are best managed with radiological embolization in the first instance.

Section 6.5 • Retroperitoneal haemorrhage

Retroperitoneal haemorrhage is always caused by a serious condition and, aside from hypovolaemia, which may be extreme and life threatening, it is also often accompanied by adynamic ileus. Common clinical settings include patients with leaking abdominal aneurysms [see Module 10, Vol. I; Vascular Surgery, Vol. II] and victims of retroperitoneal trauma involving pancreas, duodenum and kidney [see Module 4, Trauma, Vol. II]. Retroperitoneal bleeding, which is particularly difficult to control is encountered in some patients as a complication of

Management of patients with obscure recurrent gastrointestinal bleeding

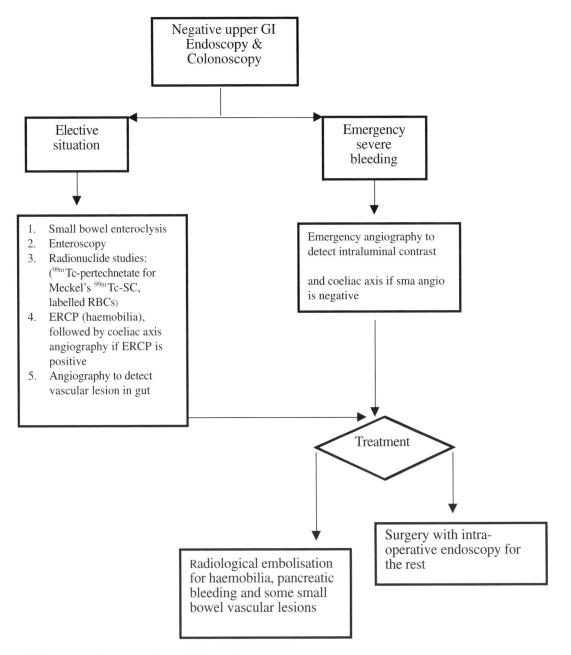

Figure 6.7 Action plan for recurrent obscure GI bleeding.

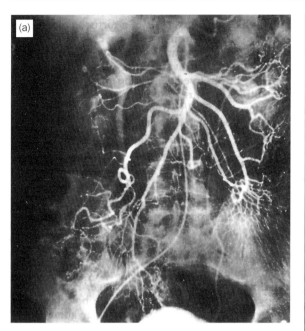

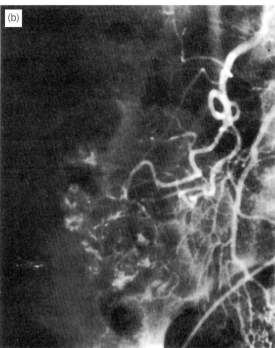

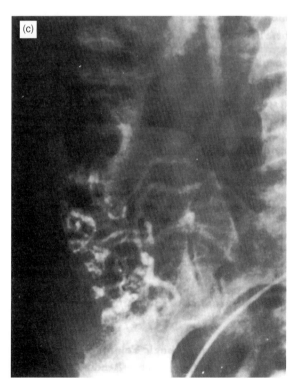

Figure 6.8 Selective superior mesenteric angiogram in chronic bleeding demonstrating vascular abnormality in the caecum. The angiographic features are: (a) prominent and early filling of clusters of irregularly dilated small vessels with the caecal wall supplied by the ileocolic artery; (b) persistence of contrast within the clusters of small blood vessels; and (c) early and profuse filling of enlarged draining veins from the affected area.

severe necrotizing pancreatitis [see Hepatobiliary and Pancreatic Surgery, Vol. II]. This combination is often fatal. An iatrogenic cause of retroperitoneal bleeding that has been responsible for some fatalities is aortoiliac trauma inflicted most commonly by the Veress needle during the induction of a closed pneumoperitoneum, although some of these injuries have been caused by the first (optical) trocar/cannula. These mishaps are entirely preventable by adoption of the proper technique, use of open laparosocopy or visually guided insertion systems [see Module 21, Vol. I].

Section 6.6 • Transfusion of blood and plasma products

Rather than the administration of whole blood, modern blood transfusion is based on the selective intravenous infusion of the required component of the blood that is necessary in a particular patient. This practice ensures safe, economic use and increases the therapeutic scope. Thus, a single donation may be used for treating a variety of disorders.

Essentials of safe blood transfusion practice

Modern safe blood transfusion practice is based on:

- careful selection of donors
- quality assurance testing of blood and blood products prepared and issued by the transfusion centres
- blood grouping, antibody screening and cross-matching
- standardized blood-ordering policies
- strict guidelines for administration and monitoring of patients receiving blood products by the clinicians
- local and central reporting of adverse effects when encountered.

Two blood samples (clotted and anticoagulated in EDTA) are sent with the completed request form to the blood transfusion department once the decision is taken that the patient needs a transfusion. The patient's red cells are grouped for ABO and Rh (D). The antibody screen is carried out on all serum samples to detect the presence in the recipient of any clinically important antibody that would haemolyse the transfused cells. Cross-matching entails testing the red cells from the donor units against the patient's serum. This constitutes the final safeguard against incompatibility. In some countries cross-matching is considered unnecessary if detailed blood group and screening have been performed, but within the UK it remains, by general consensus, standard practice.

The final step in the safe administration of blood is the check by two people that the information on the transfusion request form, the labels on the unit of blood and the patient identification (from case notes and wrist band) all agree. Regrettably, this remains the weakest link in the safety chain and most deaths from blood transfusion in the UK are tragic consequences of errors in identification.

General and medicolegal aspects

Different regulations concerning the transfusion of blood and plasma products apply within various countries. In the UK, plasma products fall within the scope of the UK Medicines Act (1968) and the associated European Community Legislation. All such plasma products have thus to be licensed and thereafter are considered as prescription only medicines (POM, i.e. can only be prescribed by a fully qualified medical practitioner); each must be accompanied by an approved summary of product characteristics (SmPC).

In contrast, whole blood and blood components are exempt from the UK Medicines Act (1968) and are therefore supplied by the regional blood transfusion centres as unlicensed products. However, blood components are considered in clinical practice as POM. It is a medicolegal requirement within the UK that details of any blood component infusion are fully documented in the patient's case notes: **indication, date/time of issue, donation number, ordering physician, duration of infusion, who gave the infusion, who checked it prior to administration and time the infusion was commenced. The written procedures for infusing blood and blood components are issued by the hospital blood transfusion department. The hospital management is responsible for ensuring that the written procedures are updated and made available to all staff (medical and nursing) who may have to administer transfusions.**

In the UK, all blood and plasma products are derived from voluntary, non-remunerated donors aged 18–65 years. In accordance with the policy of the Department of Health, donors are carefully selected and all donations are tested for known markers of disease. Currently, these are syphilis, human immunodeficiency virus-1 (HIV-1), HIV-2, hepatitis B and hepatitis C. Sterilization of other transmitting agents not detected by donor screening is not guaranteed. Thus, the risk of disease transmission, although very low, cannot be ignored. Pertinent examples of this include the transmission of acquired immunodeficiency syndrome (AIDS) to haemophilic patients and their partners in the recent past. The current concern is with the recently identified hepatitis G virus, although it is not yet known whether this virus causes significant disease.

Plasma products

Plasma products are produced at protein fractionation centres from pools derived in the UK from voluntary, non-remunerated donors. These products (Table 6.7) do not require ABO compatibility with the patients and are used in clinical practice for the following purposes:

- **as coagulation factors** for specific deficiency states, either to stop spontaneous bleeding or to cover an operation/intervention in a patient with such a deficiency, e.g. haemophilia A (congenital factor VIII deficiency) **[see Module 19, Vol. I]**
- **to provide passive immunity** to non-immunized individuals exposed to a serious infective agent (viral or bacterial), e.g. human tetanus immunoglobulin **[see Module 5, Vol. I]**
- in the prophylaxis of haemolytic disease of the newborn due to Rhesus incompatibility and sensitization of Rh (D)-negative women. Human anti-D immunoglobulin is also used in the management of Rh (D)-incompatible blood transfusion following the accidental transfusion of Rh (D)-negative individuals with Rh (D)-positive blood
- **in the management of autoimmune thrombocytopenic purpura (AITP).** High-dose intravenous human immunoglobulin can produce remissions of varying duration. IgG is also used to treat acute haemorrhage from this condition when conventional therapies have failed and to cover patients with ITP requiring surgery including elective splenectomy **[see Surgery of Spleen and Lymph Nodes, Vol. II]**
- **as volume replacement fluid (ALBA 4.5%), as a plasma volume expander and in short-term management of hypoproteinaemic patients (human albumin solution 20%).**

Intravascular (serum) albumin accounts for 40–45% of the total body albumin. Under normal conditions, albumin has a half-life of 15–20 days. The normal level is achieved by a balance between synthesis (in the liver) and breakdown (predominantly intracellularly by lysosomal proteases) through a feedback regulation controlled by the oncotic pressure of the hepatic extravascular space. Serum albumin is a key protein in circulatory and transport physiology. In the first instance, it accounts for more than 50% of the total plasma proteins and for this reason, it is the principal agent responsible for the plasma oncotic pressure essential for the exchange of fluid (and thus oxygen, nutrients and waste products) between the microcirculation and the interstitial fluid space. Albumin, through its oncotic action, ensures the re-entry of fluid from the interstitial space to the capillary bed and, in this fashion, it stabilizes the CBV. Hypoalbuminaemia from any cause thus results in fluid sequestration in the interstitial space and serous cavities (oedema/ascites) with contraction of the effective circulatory blood volume. Serum albumin also provides an important transport service as a carrier for hormones, enzymes, drugs, metabolites (e.g. bilirubin) and toxins. The combination with albumin renders all of these substances water soluble and inactive.

ALBA 4.5% is iso-osmolar and is supplied in bottles of 400 ml containing approximately 45 g/l plasma protein of which ≥ 95% is albumin. It is indicated in acute blood volume loss (instead of or with crystalloids), and in the treatment of burns after the first 24 h (when crystalloids are preferred) to maintain a plasma albumin close to 25 g/l. This is necessary to ensure a colloid osmotic pressure above 20 mmHg (2.7 kPa) and thus the return of fluid to the circulation at the venous end of the capillaries. ALBA 4.5% is also useful in surgical practice in conditions characterized by severe acute albumin losses, e.g. acute pancreatitis and small bowel infarction. Rapid infusion of ALBA 4.5% can cause vascular overload with pulmonary oedema in patients with diminished cardiorespiratory reserve or hypertension. Thus, administration in these patients should be cautious and always monitored by a CVP line. Less than 10% of the infused albumin leaves the intravascular compartment during the first 2 h after infusion. Thus, the CBV will increase from 1 to 3 h after administration and CVP monitoring in these patients should continue for at least 4 h after the albumin infusion has been stopped.

Human albumin solution 20% is an aqueous solution containing 20% w/v protein in 100 ml with albumin forming 95% or more of the protein. The solution is hyperosmolar, i.e. it acts as oncotic agent, drawing fluid from the extravascular compartment to the intravascular compartment. Hence, there is a real danger of overload in susceptible patients, e.g. patients with diminished cardiorespiratory reserve and hypertensive patients. For this reason, human albumin solution 20% is usually contraindicated in patients with severe anaemia or cardiac failure. Human albumin solution 20% is indicated in the short-term management of severely hypoproteinaemic patients with diffuse oedema that is resistant to diuretic therapy (e.g. nephrotic syndrome) and in the initial management of patients with leakage due to damage of major lymph trunks in the chest or peritoneal cavities (chylous ascites, chylothorax) following surgical interventions (usually radical resections for oesophageal and gastric cancer). In this instance, human albumin solution 20% is administered to maintain the serum albumin above 25 g/l until surgical treatment designed to secure the intrathoracic or intra-abdominal lymph leak is carried out as a matter of some urgency because of the daily profound losses. Surgical control is much preferable to peritoneovenous shunting for chylous ascites, as it constitutes definitive therapy and prevents the risks of peritoneovenous shunting, which include episodes of DIC and infection. Human albumin solution 20% is also used in patients with hypoproteinaemia associated with refractory ascites and peripheral oedema due to chronic liver disease, and in the clinical management of patients with severe burns where plasma volume expansion is required.

Table 6.7 Plasma products used in clinical practice

Plasma product	Indication	Route of administration	Shelf-life	Storage
Coagulation factors				
Factor VIII concentrate	Haemophilia A	i.v.	24 months	Light-protected storage at +2 ± 8°C
Factor IX concentrate	Single/multiple congenital deficiency of factor IX, II or X Single/multiple acquired prothrombin complex factor deficiency (including reversal of Coumarin anticoagulant therapy)	i.v.	36 months	Light-protected storage at +2 ± 8°C
Immunoglobulin products				
Human immunoglobulin	X-linked primary hypogammaglobulinaemia Late-onset hypogammaglobulinaemia Hypogammaglobulinaemia secondary to haematological malignancies Children with symptomatic HIV infection who have recurrent bacterial infections Idiopathic thrombocytopenic purpura Kawasaki's disease In allogeneic bone marrow transplant to prevent infections and graft-vs host disease	i.v.	Lyophilized product = 24 months. Used immediately after reconstitution	Light-protected temperature not exceeding 25°C
Human normal immunoglobulin (250 mg protein per vial, 90%+ = IgG)	Hepatitis A prophylaxis Prevention of measles in immunocompromised patients Replacement therapy in primary immunodeficiency syndromes	Deep i.m.	36 months	Light-protected storage at +2 ± 8°C
Human hepatitis B immunoglobulin (1000 IU per via)	Prophylaxis of hepatitis B after parenteral exposure or contamination of a wound/conjunctive by blood/secretions containing HbsAg, recent sexual contacts of diagnosed hepatitis B cases, Newborn babies whose mother has had acute hepatitis B in the last trimester or is a known HbsAg-positive carrier	Deep i.m.	36 months	Light-protected storage at +2 ± 8°C
Human tetanus immunoglobulin (250 IU per vial)	Used in conjunction with tetanus toxoid in patients with 'at-risk wounds' of tetanus and who have not been adequately immunized against tetanus or whose immune status is in doubt	Deep i.m.	36 months	Light-protected storage at +2 ± 8°C
Human anti-D immunoglobulin (various strengths)	Rh (D) sensitization in Rh (D)-negative mothers and Rh (D) incompatible blood transfusion	Deep i.m.	24 months	Light-protected storage at +2 ± 8°C
Human varicella zoster immunoglobulin (250 mg MVZ immunoglobulin per vial)	Prophylaxis of immune compromised individuals/patients exposed to varicella or zoster	Deep i.m.	36 months	Light-protected storage at +2 ± 8°C
Human rabies immunoglobulin (800 IU per vial)	Used in conjunction with rabies vaccine in individuals exposed to rabies and who are not considered adequately immunized	Deep i.m.		Light-protected storage at +2 ± 8°C
Albumin products				
Human albumin solution 4.5%	Acute blood volume loss. Severe burns after first 24 h. Therapeutic plasmapheresis Severe acute albumin losses	i.v.	36 months	Light-protected storage below 25°C
Human albumin solution (20%)	Short-term management of hypoproteinaemic patients Chronic liver disease with refractory ascites and peripheral oedema Severe burns requiring plasma volume expansion	i.v.	18 months	Light-protected storage below 25°C

Table 6.8 Other plasma products

- High-purity factor IX concentrate
- Human immunoglobulin (for intravenous use) 10 g dose size
- Fibrin glues
- Human fibrinogen concentrate
- Human thrombin
- Intravenous tetanus immunoglobulin
- Intravenous cytomegalovirus immunoglobulin
- Intravenous hepatitis B immunoglobulin

Other plasma products

Other plasma products are listed in Table 6.8. The important ones, from a surgical standpoint, are fibrin glue, intravenous human immunoglobulin, tetanus immunoglobulin [see Module 5, Vol. I] and intravenous hepatitis B immunoglobulin [see Module 5, Vol. I].

Human fibrin glue

There is a number of proprietary preparations of this glue based on a similar formulation (Tisseal-Immuno; Fibrin Sealant Kit-SNBT). The authors' clinical experience is with the Scottish National Blood Transfusion (SNBT) product. The two solutions (thrombin and fibrinogen) are derived from pooled non-remunerated donations and heat inactivated against all known human viruses. The two solutions have to be reconstituted immediately prior to use and special delivery sets for both open and laparoscopic surgery are needed for application to the bleeding surface or suture line. Essentially, the delivery sets consist of twin syringes (one for each of the two solutions) with a Y-connection to a twin barrel segment, with the two barrels joining at the end to allow mixing of the two solutions and thus the polymerization of fibrinogen to fibrin [see Module 2, Vol. I].

Human immunoglobulin for intravenous use

Human immunoglobulin for intravenous use (IVIgG) can be used in the following:

- **patients with AITP** to cover surgery and childbirth
- **antibody-deficient states**, e.g. primary and secondary hypogammaglobulinaemia (due to myeloma and chronic lymphatic leukaemia and children with AIDS) to prevent recurrent bacterial infections.

IVIgG is not a substitute for orthodox management of AITP including steroids and splenectomy (when steroid therapy fails). It is used in the management of thrombocytopenic bleeding where high-dose therapy (1–2 g/kg over 1–5 days) can produce a significant rise in the platelet count but this is of a variable duration.

When a patient with AITP requires surgery (including splenectomy), IVIgG is administered preoperatively if the platelet count is very low. High-dose IVIgG can cause renal failure, especially in the elderly. Thus, it is administered cautiously and only when strictly necessary in the elderly and in patients with pre-existing renal disease.

Blood components

Whole blood and blood components are prepared in regional transfusion centres from individual donations or pools of a small number of donations. The ABO and Rh (D) of each unit of whole blood and cell preparations are stated on the pack label of each unit and these products can only be administered after cross-matching to ensure compatibility with the patient's serum, except in dire life-threatening emergencies, when non-cross-matched group O Rh (D)-negative blood may be given. The ABO group of platelet concentrates is usually compatible with that of the patient but, although highly desirable, this is not essential. Platelets from Rh (D)-positive donors may produce anti-Rh (D) antibodies when transfused to Rh (D)-negative patients (important in a female of childbearing age). The ABO group of FFP should be compatible with that of the patient. The ABO compatibility of cryoprecipitate with that of the patient is desirable, although not essential.

Ordering of blood

Emergency situation

See management of hypovolaemia.

Elective situation

Unnecessary ordering of cross-matched blood constitutes bad practice and is wasteful of a limited resource. Many operations do not usually require a perioperative blood transfusion, others may do and some incur a need for red cells as a matter of routine. Nowadays, blood for elective surgery is ordered in accordance with the 'blood tariff' policy. This is based on the average requirement of a particular operation (Table 6.9).

Type and screen (group and hold, group and save) is all that is required for all operations that do not usually require blood. The patient's ABO and RhD type are determined and the serum is screened for IgG antibodies against red cells. The patient's serum is kept in the blood transfusion laboratory for 7 days. Should blood be required, cross-matched red cell units can be available in 15 min.

Predeposit

The benefit of this approach (autologous as distinct from allogeneic transfusion) is the elimination of disease transmission, allergic and incompatible reactions (other than procedural errors). There are established UK guidelines for autologous blood transfusion.

Table 6.9 Blood tariff for elective surgery

		Blood requirements		
	Operation	Routine tariff group and screening procedure (G + S), no units cross-matched	Increased tariff Increased tariff considerations	Indication leading to increased tariff
General surgery				
	Abdominoperineal resection	4		
	Bowel resection	3		
	Breast biopsy/lumpectomy	G + S		
	Cholecystectomy	G + S		
	Partial gastrectomy	G + S		
	Total gastrectomy	3	4	Thoracotomy
	Haemorrhoidectomy	G + S		
	Hernia repair	G + S		
	Ileostomy	G + S		
	Laparotomy	G + S	2	Malignancy
	Liver biopsy	G + S		
	Radical mastectomy	2		
	Simple mastectomy	G + S		
	Splenectomy (elective)	2		
	Thyroidectomy	G + S		
	Vagotomy (truncal, RSV)	G + S		
	Varicose vein operations	G + S		
Urology				
	Partial cystectomy	2		
	Total cystectomy	4		
	Transurethral resection of bladder lesions	G + S	2	Larger tumours
	Nephrectomy	2		
	Nephrolithotomy	2		
	Prostatectomy	2		
Thoracic surgery				
	Oesophagogastrectomy	4		
	Hiatus hernia	G + S		
	Pneumothorax	G + S		
	Thoracotomy for pulmonary resection	3	4	Reoperation
	Mediastinoscopy	2		
Arterial surgery				
	Aortic aneurysm	6	10–12	Ruptured
	Femoropopliteal bypass	3		

After Napier *et al.* (1985) *BMJ* **291**: 799–801, courtesy of the editor.

Patient selection includes establishing the fitness of the patient for the procedure. Predeposit is arranged through the blood transfusion department and between 2 and 4 units can be harvested preoperatively. The blood is collected, labelled and stored as in allogeneic (donor) voluntary donations, and the autologous units ABO and Rh D are grouped and cross-matched with the patient's serum. Despite the initial enthusiasm, the experience with predeposit has been disappointing. It is more expensive that allogeneic blood transfusion. The blood is wasted if the patient does not need perioperative transfusion as it cannot be administered to other patients, and if the patient requires blood in excess of the predeposited units, all possible advantage is lost. Currently, autologous blood transfusion seems a sensible option in fit patients (aged 18–65 years, free from cardiovascular, cerebrovascular and respiratory disease, no sepsis, malignancy or haematological abnormality) requiring an operation that is very likely to require modest amounts of perioperative blood transfusion and who live near the hospital.

Controlled haemodilution

In this procedure, the patient is bled immediately before surgery (after induction of anaesthesia) down to haematocrit of 25–30% with CVP monitoring while the blood volume is maintained by infusion of crystalloids. The collected autologous blood is transfused after the operation. Aside from reducing the need for donor blood, controlled haemodilution by preoperative isovolaemic bleeding has a number of advantages, which emanate from the reduction in the blood viscosity: increased capillary perfusion, and lower incidence of deep vein thrombosis and postoperative renal failure. Controlled haemodilution is used extensively in cardiothoracic surgery and for patients undergoing major orthopaedic operations. It is practised less frequently in general surgery.

Intraoperative blood salvage

This includes automated blood salvage by the cell-saver equipment (Haemonetics) and more simple manual systems for storage and reinfusion of red cells, as exemplified by the Solcotrans autologous collection system. Both techniques are only applicable to clean operative sites without bacterial, bowel or tumour cell contamination. The Haemonetics cell-saver system is a completely automated device that aspirates, anticoagulates and filters the extravasated blood from the operative field. The red cells are then washed before being transfused in a PCV of 0.50. It is used extensively during liver transplantation and in Jehovah's Witness patients undergoing major surgery.

The manual techniques have limited capacity (a few units), such that their usefulness is suspect, and it has been argued that in many instances they are employed under circumstances in which blood transfusion was probably unnecessary.

Transfusion of fresh blood

The transfusion of fresh blood for bleeding disorders has been largely replaced by FFP and therapy with other blood components, depending on the nature of the deficiency as determined by the coagulation screen.

Whole blood

Whole blood has a haematocrit of 0.35–0.45. The cells are suspended in 300 ml of a 4:1 mixture of donor plasma and a nutrient citrate anticoagulant solution. With storage (maximum 35 days at 2–6°C), changes occur in both the composition of the supernatant solution and the haematocrit. Thus, at expiry the K^+ level averages 9.0 mmol (1.0 mmol for fresh blood), the lactate 10.0 mmol (1.0 mmol for fresh blood) and the hydrogen ion activity 55.0 nmol (20 nmol for fresh blood). Thus, with storage, whole blood becomes increasingly acidotic. The deterioration is much more rapid when whole blood is kept out of the refrigerator or blood transport box. If the unit of whole blood has been left out at room temperature for more than 30 min prior to commencement of infusion, the unit should be discarded. The transfusion of each unit of blood should be complete within 4 h of spiking the pack. A blood warmer is used when large volumes of whole blood are transfused over a short time and when the patient's plasma contains cold acting antibodies. Whole blood is not suitable for the correction of symptomatic or critical anaemia.

Red cell preparations

As with whole blood, each unit of red cells is obtained from a single donor and consists of RBCs suspended in a total volume of 300 ml. There are minor differences in the red cell preparations from various regional transfusion centres. The Scottish National Blood Transfusion Service (SNBTS) supplies two preparations: Red Cells and Red Cells in Additive Solution. A unit of Red Cells has a haematocrit of 0.65–0.75 with 80 ml of a 4:1 mixture of donor plasma and a nutrient citrate anticoagulation solution. A unit of Red Cells in Additive

---

Investigation of an acute haemolytic transfusion episode

1. Report incident to the Blood Transfusion Department

2. Establish that the unit has been issued to the patient receiving it

3. Obtain fresh samples of patient's blood (clotted and in EDTA) for re-cross-matching and serological testing

4. Sent sample of the blood unit for culture

5. Return unit to the Blood Transfusion Department

6. Obtain further blood samples from patient for clinical chemistry (electrolytes, urea, free Hb) and coagulation screen

7. Discuss any further transfusion requirements with the Blood Transfusion Officer

Figure 6.9 Action plan after incompatible blood transfusion reaction.

solution has a haematocrit of 0.55–0.65 with 100 ml of storage medium and only a small residue of anticoagulated plasma. Both preparations have a much lower Na^+ (15–20 mmol) and hydrogen ion activity (2–5 nmol) than whole blood. They are used primarily to increase tissue oxygenation after haemorrhage and in patients with anaemia. They are both stored at 2–6°C and their maximum shelf-life at this temperature is 35 days. The same precautions on safe usage apply as with transfusion of whole blood.

Platelets

Platelet preparations are available as concentrates from single or multiple donors, with each unit containing 55×10^9 platelets suspended in 50–69 ml of a 4:1 mixture of donor plasma and nutrient anticoagulant solution. They can also be prepared from a single donor by an apheresis procedure (platelet apheresis). Each unit of the latter contains at least 240×10^9 platelets suspended in 120–250 ml of a 4:1 mixture of donor plasma and a nutrient anticoagulant solution. Patients with platelet alloimmunization (usually because of previous sensitization) can only receive platelet apheresis units and these have to be human leucocyte antigen (HLA) compatible or be cross-matched and shown to be compatible with the patient's serum. Patients with profound cellular immunodeficiency or those receiving transfusions from related donors should be transfused with irradiated platelets.

Infusion of platelets is indicated (usually prophylactically) in thrombocytopenia or in the presence of a functional abnormality of the platelets (e.g. Glanzman's disease) when these are associated with bleeding problems. In surgical practice, platelet cover is needed when the count falls below 50 000. In AITP, human IgG is administered to raise the platelet count before platelet transfusion is considered. The indications for platelet transfusion are summarized in Table 6.10.

The development of antibodies to HLA class I antigens occurs in approximately 50% of patients who receive intensive blood product support. These antibodies cause febrile reactions, reduce successful take of a bone marrow transplant in patients with aplastic anaemia, and can also lead to platelet refractoriness. This is diagnosed if the patient's platelet count fails to rise by at least 10×10^9 on the day after a platelet transfusion. Platelet refractoriness due to alloimmunization can be prevented to some extent by leucocyte-depleted platelet transfusion (by either platelet-pheresis or the use of filters to remove the leucocytes).

Fresh-frozen plasma

Each unit is obtained from a single donation and consists of 200–300 ml of plasma with 40–60 ml of citrate anticoagulant nutrient mixture. The plasma proteins in FFP are in similar concentrations as in normal plasma. FFP is stored at −30°C and with this frozen storage has a shelf-life of 12 months. It is thawed rapidly at 37°C

Table 6.10 Indications for platelet transfusion

- Surgical
  Bleeding and thrombocytopenia
  Cover for operative interventions: platelet count
  < 50 000, platelet dysfunction[a]
  Acute disseminated intravascular coagulation (with FFP)
  Massive blood transfusion
  Postcardiac bypass thrombocytopenia

- Medical
  Marrow suppressed patients (intensive cy)
  Aplastic/hypoplastic anaemia

[a]Disorders of platelet function: Glanzmann's disease, Bernard–Soulier syndrome, platelet storage pool deficiency.

immediately before use and infused intravenously through a standard blood component transfusion set containing an on-line filter. The ABO group of the FFP must be compatible with that of the recipient. The infusion of 1 unit of FFP should be completed within 4 h of thawing.

FFP is used in the following clinical situations:

- to correct isolated plasma protein deficiencies, e.g. isolated deficiencies of factors II, V, VII, X, XI, XIII, pseudocholinesterase, antithrombin III and C1 esterase inhibitor

- to reverse oral anticoagulation with warfarin/coumarin compounds if prothrombin complex concentrate is not available. Normally, reversal of anticoagulant is indicated in the presence of bleeding

- in patients with liver disease, major hepatic resections and severe liver injuries to provide haemostatic support and to cover operations and interventions

- in the treatment of patients with DIC to replace factors consumed by the pathological process

- in patients who develop a bleeding diathesis after large-volume blood transfusion. In this situation, however, platelet transfusion is more commonly needed first

- in the treatment of thrombotic thrombocytopenic purpura (TTP), where FFP is usually combined with plasma exchange.

Cryoprecipitate

Cryoprecipitate is a concentrate of factor VIII, von Willebrand's factor and fibrinogen, and is obtained by freezing and thawing plasma. One unit of cryoprecipitate consists of 20 ml containing 150–300 mg of fibrinogen and 80–120 IU of factor VIII. It is stored at −30°C and at this temperature has a shelf-life of 12 months. It is thawed rapidly at 37°C immediately before use and infusion should be complete within 4 h of thawing.

Cryoprecipitate is used for the following conditions:

- fibrinogen deficiency and dysfibrinogenaemia
- uraemic bleeding
- von Willebrand's disease **[see Module 19, Vol. I]**.

Special blood components

These include irradiated components, frozen, thawed and washed red cells, components for neonatal use, leucocyte-depleted cellular components, CMV-negative cellular components, apheresis plasma and cryosupernatant. Washed red cells are used in patients who develop non-haemolytic transfusion reactions. Frozen, thawed and washed red cells are indicated in patients who have rare antibodies.

As infection with cytomegalovirus (CMV) can be lethal in patients following bone marrow transplantation, leucocyte-depleted components or CMV-negative cellular components are administered in these patients if they are CMV negative. CMV-negative cellular components are also administered in all patients with haematological malignancy until their CMV status is known. CMV-negative cellular components are also indicated in patients undergoing solid organ transplantation where both donor and recipient are CMV negative.

Adverse effects of transfusion of blood and blood products

It is the recommended clinical practice that every patient is monitored closely during the first 15–30 min of the infusion of each unit of blood. This enables the early detection of the clinical manifestations of severe acute reaction due to incompatibility or bacterial infection, when the infusion is stopped and the necessary action taken (see below).

Within the UK, the Serious Hazards of Transfusion (SHOT) group set up a voluntary confidential reporting system for serious adverse effects excluding infectious complications in 1966. The objectives of this confidential reporting system are (i) to increase awareness of the serious adverse events; (ii) to determine the factors which contribute to their occurrence (risk analysis); and (iii) to issue reports based on the centralized database that recommend the necessary changes in practice designed to improve the safety of blood transfusion. The practice of SHOT is equivalent to that adopted by high-risk industries (e.g. aerospace) over many years to prevent accidents due to both malfunction and human error, thus achieving the ALARP (risk is As Low As is Reasonably Possible) endpoint. The medical co-ordinator of SHOT is Dr Elizabeth Love at the Manchester Blood Centre (Tel. 0161 273 7181, confidential fax 0161 236 6904). The reporting service set up by SHOT is not designed to replace the advice and investigation of any adverse event by the local blood transfusion centre. Infectious complications must be reported to the local blood transfusion centre as soon as the diagnosis is suspected. Complications that develop in patients receiving fractionated plasma products should be reported to the Committee for Safety of Medicines using the existing yellow card system.

As the mechanisms involved in transfusion-related complications are varied, these are usually classified under separate aetiological categories. In addition, some of the adverse effects are immediate (acute), whereas others are late (Table 6.11).

Non-haemolytic febrile transfusion reactions

The routine establishment of quality control in the manufacture of both intravenous fluids and disposable giving sets has virtually eliminated pyrogenic reactions. Pyrexia following blood transfusion is nowadays the result of alloimmunization to leucocyte and platelet antigens in patients who have been immunized by previous blood transfusion or pregnancy (antibodies to class I HLA antibodies). The symptoms are rigors followed by fever, usually within 30–60 min after the start of the transfusion. The management includes cessation or slowing of the transfusion and the administration of an antipyretic such as paracetamol.

Patients who require repeated transfusions and who have experienced non-haemolytic febrile transfusion reactions (NHFTR) are pretreated with paracetamol 1.0 g orally before the start of the transfusion, with a second dose 4 h later. The patient is kept warm and the transfusion is administered slowly (4 h for red cells and 2 h for platelets). Leucocyte-depleted cell components (buffy coat depleted red cells or filtered red cells; apheresis platelets) are given if the above measures fail.

Table 6.11 Complications of transfusion of blood and blood products

- Acute
  Allergic
  Anaphylaxis
  Haemolytic
  Metabolic
  Transfusion-related acute lung injury
  Circulatory overload
  Non-haemolytic febrile transfusion reactions
  Haemostatic: dilution of clotting factors and thrombocytopenia
  Septic shock (bacterially infected units)

- Late
  Delayed haemolytic transfusion reactions
  Sensitization/alloimmunization
  Haemolytic disease of the newborn
  Immune suppression
  Graft-vs-host disease
  Transfusion iron overload (haemosiderosis)

- Infective
  Bacterial (brucellosis, syphilis, Chagas disease)
  Helminthic (filariasis)
  Protozoal (babesiosis, kala azar, malaria, trypanosomiasis, toxoplasmosis)
  Rickettsial (relapsing fever, Rocky Mountain spotted fever)
  Viral (human parvovirus B19, cytomegalovirus, Epstein–Barr virus, HIV- and -2, HTLV-I and -II, hepatitis A, B, G and yellow fever)

Allergic reactions and anaphylaxis

The other non-haemolytic reactions include **allergic reactions** and **severe anaphylaxis**. The symptoms of allergic reactions are urticarial rash and itch within minutes of the start of the transfusion. Treatment is with antihistamines (chlorpheniramime 10 mg by slow intravenous or intramuscular injection) and reduction of the transfusion rate with observation of the patient. If symptoms do not progress over the next 30 min the transfusion is continued. Patients who had previously experienced allergic reactions to transfusion are pre-treated with chlorpheniramine 8.0 mg orally 30 min before the transfusion.

Severe anaphylaxis is a rare (1:20 000 transfusions) but potentially fatal reaction. Occasionally, it is caused by antibodies to IgA in patients who have extremely low levels of this immunoglobulin in their plasma. Whatever the cause, anaphylaxis results in the release of vasoactive peptides and activation of complement with the development of profound hypotension, laryngeal oedema and or bronchospasm and cutaneous flushing. Anaphylaxis is treated with immediate termination of the transfusion, intravenous crystalloids, maintenance of airway, oxygen, adrenaline, intravenous antihistamines and salbutamol. The adrenaline (0.5–1.0 mg) is given immediately by the intramuscular route and the dose repeated, if necessary, every 10 min, depending on the improvement in the blood pressure and pulse. Chlorpheniramine 10–20 mg is administered by slow intravenous injection after the adrenaline treatment and is continued for 24–48 h. Salbutamol is administered by nebulizer. Because of its delayed action, hydrocortisone is of secondary value in this severe complication but its (controversial) use may prevent further deterioration. Severe anaphylaxis can only be predicted in patients with low serum IgA. Transfusion should be avoided, if at all possible, in these patients. If deemed essential they can only receive special products.

Acute haemolytic reactions

These are usually the result of ABO incompatibility resulting from human error at the bedside (blood given to the wrong patient) or in the laboratory (faulty cross-matching). The transfused cells react with the patient's own anti-A or anti-B antibodies or other alloantibodies to red cell antigens.

Incompatible blood transfusion is a serious complication and carries an average mortality of 3%, or higher if more than 200 ml of incompatible blood are administered. The reaction is usually most severe if group A red cells are administered to a group O patient. The syndrome is caused by the release of the polypeptide products of complement (C3a, C4a, C5a) in the plasma. These cause contraction of smooth muscle and degranulation of mast cells with release of vasoactive peptides (bradykinin and serotonin). Procoagulant substances are released from the stroma of the lysed red cells. These, together with antigen–antibody complexes, initiate DIC. The clinical features in the conscious patient include pain at the infusion site and along the vein, facial burning, chest and back pain, fever, rigors and vomiting. The patient becomes restless, breathless, flushed and hypotensive, and develops oozing from vascular access sites and wounds (DIC). The only manifestations of incompatible blood transfusion in unconscious or anaesthetized patients are sudden hypotension and bleeding due to DIC. The extensive intravascular haemolysis results in haemoglobinaemia and haemoglobinuria. Oliguria rapidly supervenes and progresses to ARF. The differential diagnosis is between incompatibility and the infusion of bacterially contaminated blood.

The management entails immediate recognition **with cessation of the transfusion and replacement of the giving set**. Adequate hydration is maintained by intravenous infusion of crystalloids (isotonic saline or Hartmann's solution). An attempt is made to force diuresis with intravenous large-dose frusemide (150 mg). If this fails, a 20% solution of mannitol (100 ml) is administered. If diuresis is obtained, a high urine output is maintained (100 ml/h) by large-volume crystalloid infusions. Often, however, these patients progress to ARF, necessitating haemodialysis. The other problems that require immediate support are bleeding from DIC (blood component therapy guided by clinical state and coagulation screen) and hyperkalaemia. Intravenous glucose–insulin (50 ml 50% glucose + 10 units of insulin) is administered if the serum K^+ rises above 6.0 mmol/l. This is followed by an intravenous infusion of 10% glucose containing 10 units of insulin over a period of 4 h. **After the initial resuscitation is completed, the investigation of such an incident is essential and is outlined in Figure 6.9.**

Acute haemolytic reactions giving a similar picture may arise from acute haemolysis caused by preformed antibodies in the patient's blood (anti-Rh D, Rh E, Rh C and Kell, etc.) as a result of alloimmunization to minor blood group antigens in the donated unit. These may be encountered in patients requiring repeated blood transfusions. Those caused by anti Rh D (rare nowadays since patients receive Rh D compatible cells) are not usually severe as they do not activate complement.

Delayed haemolytic transfusion reactions (DHTR) are rare but can occur in patients whose level of antibodies to the blood group antigen is so low that it escapes detection by the pretransfusion screen. Following transfusion, the secondary immune response raises the antibody titre to a level that results in the delayed destruction of the transfused cells. Thus, the manifestations, which include fever, falling Hb, jaundice and haemoglobinuria, appear some 5–10 days after the transfusion. DHTRs are seldom fatal.

Transfusion-related acute lung injury

TRALI is one cause of ARDS and was previously thought to result from pulmonary microvascular occlusion by microaggregates of platelets, leucocytes and fibrin (50–200 μm), which are known to be present in stored blood. For this reason, microaggregate filters were recommended for transfusions in excess of 5 units of blood. A more definite cause is donor blood containing antibodies to the patient's leucocytes (nearly always donations from multiparous women). Following transfusion, the patient develops fever, increasing breathlessness, non-productive cough and hypoxaemia. The chest X-ray shows the typical features of ARDS with perihilar infiltrates leading to a whiteout in severe cases. The management is that of ARDS [see Modules 13 and 19, Vol. I].

Metabolic and haemostatic complications

These complications are confined to patients who, because of severe haemorrhage, receive a massive blood transfusion of stored blood. **Massive blood transfusion is defined as that which is equivalent to or exceeds the patient's own blood volume within 12 h.** Aside from being cold (4°C), stored blood has an acid pH and a reduced 2,3-DPG, and contains citrate anticoagulant, elevated plasma potassium and ammonia. The metabolic consequences therefore include hypothermia, acidosis and an increased affinity of oxy-haemoglobin for oxygen that is not readily released to the tissue, thereby contributing to defective tissue oxygenation. The hypothermia may lead to cardiac arrhythmias including ventricular fibrillation and asystole. For this reason, blood warming is necessary if the transfusion rate exceeds 50 ml/min. Unfortunately, the heating coils increase the resistance of the giving circuit, but none the less their use is essential in these patients. Citrate intoxication is due to the chelation of ionized calcium, which may result in prolongation of the QT interval, but this does not usually materially affect cardiac function and the ionized calcium levels rapidly return to normal after the transfusion as the excess citrate is metabolized and excreted. Thus, the use of supplemental calcium is not justified, particularly as it may itself give rise to arrhythmias. Hyperkalaemia is seldom a problem as the excess plasma K^+ enters the RBCs with warming to body temperature. It is, however, a consideration in patients with acidosis and renal failure when calcium is administered as the physiological antidote.

Stored blood is deficient in platelets and labile clotting factors (V and VIII). For this reason, massive transfusion of stored blood induces a dilution of the labile clotting factors in addition to a moderate thrombocytopenia. The deficiency of the labile clotting factors can be circumvented by the administration of 2 units of FFP for every 8 units of blood.

Platelet-specific alloantibodies may cause **post-transfusion purpura** (PTP), which is most commonly encountered in females and may prove fatal. The syndrome becomes manifest some 5–9 days after the transfusion with severe bleeding associated with extreme thrombocytopenia. Initially treatment is with high-dose corticosteroids and high-dose intravenous immunoglobulin. If platelets are needed they have to be compatible with the patient's alloantibodies.

Circulatory overload

This is encountered when blood is administered too rapidly or in large volumes. It is most commonly encountered during the transfusion of anaemic patients, particularly those with severe and chronic anaemia. These patients must be transfused very slowly and only with packed cells (with or without concomitant diuretic therapy). In addition, transfusion is restricted to 1 unit in any 12-h period. In some patients, an exchange transfusion has to be carried out to avoid severe congestive failure.

Pulmonary oedema consequent on left ventricular failure is common after massive blood transfusion and must be differentiated from ARDS.

Immune suppression

There is no doubt concerning the immunosuppressive effect of blood transfusion which, indeed, was employed specifically for this purpose in patients before renal transplantation to improve graft survival prior to the introduction of cylcosporin, the effective immunosuppression of which has made prerenal transplant transfusion unnecessary. In the context of general surgery, perioperative blood transfusion, by virtue of this immunosuppressive effect, which is additive to that inherent to the operative trauma, has undoubted undesirable consequences. Aside from the risk of circulatory overload, perioperative blood transfusion enhances the risk of infective complications (proven), and may increase recurrence rate and reduce disease-free survival in patients after extirpative surgery for cancer. Although the latter is unproven, there is circumstantial evidence for this adverse effect, especially in patients undergoing resections for colorectal cancer.

Transfusion haemosiderosis

Every unit of blood contains 250 mg of iron that is retained by the body. Iron overload of the mono-cyte–macrophage system is caused by repeated red cell transfusions over many years and becomes significant after 100 units have been administered, when the liver, pancreas, myocardium and the endocrine glands become damaged. It is especially a problem in childhood anaemias (e.g. thalassaemia) and in patients with chronic refractory anaemia. The iron overload is reduced in these patients by iron chelation therapy with desferrioxamine.

Graft-versus-host disease

This is a rare but usually fatal complication that occurs mainly in immunodeficient patients, e.g. recipients of allogeneic marrow transplants and fetuses receiving intrauterine transfusions. However, graft-versus-host disease (GvHD) has also been documented in immunocompetent patients after transfusion of blood from a relative. The disease is caused by the T-lymphocytes and starts some 4–30 days after the transfusion. The patient develops a high fever and a diffuse erythematous skin rash progressing to erythroderma and desquamation, GI symptoms, severe hepatic dysfunction and panocytopenia. GvHD is prevented by administering gamma-irradiated cellular components to immune-deficient patients. Similarly, blood donated from relatives should be gamma irradiated.

Transmission of infectious disease

A wide spectrum of infectious disease can be transmitted by the transfusion of blood and blood products, although with the modern practice of screening of blood donors and heat treatment of blood protein products, the risk is extremely small. The most commonly transmitted viral disease is hepatitis C (< 1 per 30 000 components transfused). Post-transfusion hepatitis B is now extremely rare in the UK. Hepatitis A can very occasionally be transmitted by blood products. Hepatitis G has only been recently identified. Currently, it can only be identified by gene amplification technology and there is no screening test. It is not known whether hepatitis G can cause serious disease and whether the existing plasma fractionation and heat treatment inactivate it, although this is thought likely.

Human parvovirus (HPB) B19 may not be activated by current plasma fractionation and heat treatment. It causes depressed erythropoiesis in some patients. Human T-cell leukaemia virus (HTLV)-related disease following transfusion is extremely rare in the UK and for this reason, donors are not screened for HTLV-I/II infection. However, the prevalence of HTLV-I is high in some countries, notably Japan and the Caribbean. HTLV-I causes neurological disease and a rare form of adult T-cell leukaemia, usually for many years after the transfusion.

CMV is a problem as 50% of UK donors have antibodies to CMV, but fortunately only a fraction of antibody-positive donations transmits the virus. Post-transfusion CMV is important in premature infants born to CMV antibody-negative mothers and in CMV-negative recipients of bone marrow allografts from CMV seronegative donors. These patients should receive CMV-negative products or leucocyte-depleted blood components. The HIV problem has largely been resolved by donor selection and testing.

Transfusion of bacteriologically contaminated or infected blood

This disastrous complication is fortunately rare in the UK (2 per million units transfused). The pathogens are usually cold-growing strains of *Pseudomonas fluorescens* or *Yersinia enterocolitica*. Skin organisms such as *Staphylococci* can proliferate in platelet concentrates stored at 20–22°C. The clinical picture is similar to that of ABO-incompatible blood transfusion reaction. Despite aggressive supportive therapy, the majority of patients does not survive this complication.

Section 6.7 • Solutions for intravenous infusion

These include colloid solutions (ALBA 4.5% and synthetic colloids), isotonic crystalloid solutions, hypertonic saline solutions and red cell substitutes. There has been debate regarding the comparative efficacy of crystalloids versus colloids for volume replacement in the resuscitation of critically ill patients. A recent meta-analysis of published randomized trials indicated that resuscitation with colloids is associated with an increased absolute risk of mortality of 4%, i.e. four extra deaths for each 100 patients resuscitated. **This systemic review does not support the continued use of colloids.**

Synthetic colloid solutions: plasma expanders

Synthetic colloids are preferred to ALBA during resuscitation of hypovolaemic patients (except in burn patients), largely on the grounds of costs. Thus, for example, 1 unit of ALBA 4.5% costs £35, whereas the equivalent 500 ml solution of gelatin retails at £3–4. Synthetic colloidal solutions are used, as an alternative to isotonic crystalloids, in the resuscitation of hypovolaemic patients before blood is available or when it is unnecessary. Three types of preparation are available: dextrans, gelatins and hetastarch (hydroxyethyl starch, HES) (see Table 6.12).

The clinical effects of a synthetic colloid depend on its colloid osmotic pressure, its plasma half-life and its capillary permeability. The colloid osmotic pressure is expressed by the molecular weight and concentration of the colloid, but as these are non-uniform solutions (particles are not of uniform weight), their molecular weight is better expressed by the 'number average' (M_n) rather than 'weight average' (M_w). M_n represents the mean osmotically active particle weight and is compared to the molecular weight of albumin (70 000).

Dextrans

These are solutions of inert glucose polymers produced from hydrolysed starch, which are available in various molecular sizes (dextran 40, dextran 70, etc.). As the

Table 6.12 Synthetic colloid solutions: plasma expanders

Product	Nature	M_n	COP (mmH$_2$O)	Half-life
Dextran 70	Hydrolysed starch	70 000	268	12 h
Hetastarch, Hespan, HES	Hydroxyethyl maize starch	70 000	350	17 days
Gelofusine	Succinylated Gelatin	22 600	465	4 h
Haemaccel	Polygeline	24 500	350–390	5 h

COP, colloid osmotic pressure.

renal threshold for these inert polysaccharides is in the order of 50 000, dextran 40 molecules are filtered through the glomeruli, whence they may block the renal tubules and cause ATN, especially in patients with reduced renal blood flow. For this reason, dextran 40 is rarely used nowadays. Dextran 70 is free from this side-effect and can be used for volume replacement (up to 1.5 l/24 h in an adult). It is available either in saline (0.9%) or in 5% dextrose (when added Na^+ is undesirable). The colloid osmotic pressure of dextran 70 is 268 mmH_2O (lower than those of other plasma substitutes), but because of its half-life (12 h), its effect is relatively prolonged.

Dextran 70 infusion affects the coagulation system by inhibiting platelet aggregation and rendering fibrin more susceptible to fibrinolysis. For these reasons, dextran 70 is used in some centres in the prophylaxis of postoperative deep vein thrombosis. Large infusions (more than 20 ml/kg/day) can reduce factor VIII levels and induce capillary oozing. This limit of 1.5 litres of dextran 70 must not be exceeded during volume replacement. As dextran 70 interferes with blood cross-matching by inducing rouleux formation *in vitro*, a blood sample should be obtained before the infusion is commenced.

Adverse effects of dextran infusion are well documented. These are usually mild anaphylactoid reactions (1:2000 infusions) but serious reactions can occur, although they are rare (1:6000 infusions).

Hetastarch (Hespan)

This is not frequently used in the UK but is widely employed in the USA, where gelatin preparations are not available. It consists of a 6% solution of hydroxyethyl starch (chemically modified maize starch) in 0.9% saline. Its average particle size (M_n = 70 000) and colloid osmotic pressure are equivalent to those of 5% albumin. Although the smaller molecules are removed by glomerular filtration (40% within 24 h), the larger polymers undergo slow hydrolysis by plasma α-amylase, and some are then filtered once the size is reduced below the renal threshold. Approximately 30% of the infused dose ultimately leaves the vascular compartment and is taken up by the monocyte–macrophage system, predominantly in the liver and spleen. There are some concerns over the potential for impaired function (blockade) of this system following large infusions of Hetastarch. In any event, the final elimination from the body is a slow process, and at 4 months, the plasma concentration averages 1% of the original value. The half-life of Hetastarch in the plasma is considerably longer than any of the other plasma substitutes and averages 17 days. In animals, infusions of hydroxyethyl starch exceeding 20 mg/l (equivalent to 1500 ml in a 70 kg patient) impair platelet function and coagulation. Hetastarch administration may be followed by a rise in the serum amylase but there is no evidence of any pancreatic damage. In a recent report, one serious and 13 mild reactions were encountered in 16 000 infusions.

Gelatin solutions

The modern preparations consist of solutions of heat-degraded cattle bone gelatin: succinylated gelatin (Gelofusine) and polygeline (Haemaccel). Although both are made up in balance crystalloid solution, the calcium concentration is different. Haemaccel contains over 10 times more calcium (6.25 mmol/l) and potassium (5.1 mmol/l) than Gelofusine. The high calcium content of Haemaccel can lead to clotting in the warming coils when this colloid is mixed with citrated blood or FFP. Whereas the colloid osmotic pressure of Haemaccel (350–390 mmH_2O) is similar to that of plasma, that of Gelofusine is greater (465 mmH_2O), i.e. it tends to draw fluid into the intravascular compartment from the interstitial space. As their particle weight is small (Haemaccel M_n = 24 500; Gelofusine M_n = 22 600), they are rapidly filtered by the renal glomeruli and cause an osmotic diuresis which is beneficial. This too accounts for their short half-life: 5 h for Haemaccel and 4 h for Gelofusine. As neither preparation affects either the bleeding time or coagulation time (except by dilution), they are perfectly safe for large-volume colloid replacement. There is some evidence that some of the gelatin complexes may leave the vascular compartment and become sequestered in the interstitial space, particularly the lung. These extravasated complexes may contribute to the increased lung water, which may retard the return of pulmonary gas exchange to normal.

The original version of Haemaccel led to a number of histamine-induced adverse reactions when the solution was infused rapidly, but since 1981, the manufacturing process has been altered to reduce the amount of cross-linking agent responsible for the plasma histamine released. The incidence of minor reactions with the modified Haemaccel is 9 per 1334 infusions. The reported serious anaphylactoid reactions with Gelofusine infusion vary from 1:6000 to 1:12 000. Within the UK, the concern with gelatin solutions is their bovine origin, possible contamination with the prion protein responsible for bovine spongiform encephalopathy (BSE) and the possible development of new-variant Creutzfeldt–Jakob disease (CJD) but, to date, no health warnings have been issued. Presumably, the heat-degradation process destroys the prion protein. It seems likely that the original gelatin will be obtained from BSE-free herds in the future.

Crystalloid solutions

These are isotonic balance salt or dextrose solutions (Table 6.13). The two most commonly used for volume replacement are isotonic saline (0.9%) and Ringer's lactate (Hartmann's solution), which approximates most closely to the electrolyte composition of plasma. This and the less acidic pH of Hartmann's solution (6.5 vs 6.1) account for its preferment over isotonic saline by some surgeons, while others consider the lactate content of Hartmann's solution to be a disadvantage since shock is accompanied by elevated blood lactate, and for this reason, prefer isotonic saline. Amidst this minor controversy, all are agreed that 5% dextrose has no place in resuscitation. It is equivalent to the safe intravenous administration of water and the little dextrose it contains is not metabolized. As distinct from colloid following intravenous infusion, crystalloid solutions are rapidly distributed between the intravascular and interstitial spaces roughly in the proportion of 3:1. This is not a disadvantage, as in shock both compartments are contracted. However, the amount required to restore the CBV is significantly larger (at least by a factor of 3) then when colloid solutions are used. Thus, the replacement of 1.0 litre of circulating blood requires the infusion of 3.0 litres of Hartmann's or isotonic saline, as opposed to 1.0 litre of colloid. The extent of expansion of the body fluid compartments limits the magnitude of losses that can be replaced solely by crystalloid solutions.

Combined crystalloid–colloid blood replacement

The current widely practised compromise for blood volume replacement entails the infusion of a mixture of crystalloids and synthetic colloids in a ratio of 2:1. Stored blood or red cell concentrates are added when the blood loss exceeds 1.5 litres or if the haematocrit falls below 25%.

Hypertonic saline

Intravenous infusions of hypertonic crystalloid solutions (500 mmol/l) have been reported to have beneficial effects in patients with refractory shock, in whom they may increase the survival rate. Several formulations have been proposed. The Sackford solution contains the following in mmol/l: Na^+ 250, Cl^- 100, lactate 63, K^+ 4 and Ca^{++} 9. These hypertonic solutions increase cardiac output and possibly improve cerebral oxygen delivery in severely shocked patients. The exact mechanism of action is unknown but is possibly vagally mediated by the arrival of the hypertonic bolus in the pulmonary vasculature. Some reports indicate that hypertonic solutions reduce the peripheral resistance and are accompanied by a lesser weight gain than ordinary isotonic crystalloid solutions. The duration of the effect on the circulation of hypertonic solutions is short

lived and probably does not exceed 1 h. These solutions, although promising, are still undergoing evaluation and cannot be considered as routine resuscitative therapy.

Red cell substitutes

These solutions, still largely experimental, are intended for oxygen carriage from the lungs and its delivery to the tissues, as substitutes for blood. They include haemoglobin solutions and the perfluorocarbons.

Hb solutions prepared from bovine blood are not favoured because of the risk of contamination with prion protein causing BSE. Two preparations are now available for experimental evaluation: modified haemoglobin solutions and microencapsulated haemoglobin.

The modified haemoglobin solutions consist of polymerized Hb complexed with pyridoxine-5-phosphate and dialysed to remove vasoconstrictor substances present in the red cells. When haemoglobin is extracted from the RBCs, it rapidly loses its 2,3-diphosphoglycerate (2,3-DPG), which is necessary for its low affinity for oxygen (essential for the release of oxygen to the tissues). This problem is overcome by complexing the Hb with pyridoxine-5-phosphate, which restores the normal oxygen affinity. Polymerization is necessary to increase the molecular size as non-polymerized Hb rapidly leaves the vascular compartment and is filtered through the glomeruli into the urine. However, the previously held view that Hb is nephrotoxic has been shown to be incorrect. Renal damage is caused by the red cell stroma and not the released Hb. The polymerization process is also viricidal and results in a four-fold increase in the half-life of the Hb (20 h). Modified haemoglobin solutions contain up to 150 g Hb/l. An alternative approach is to encapsulate the Hb-pyridoxine-5-phosphate in lipid membrane microspheres of equivalent size to the RBCs. The half-life of solutions made of Hb containing microspheres is similar to that of polymerized Hb solutions. Experimental studies in animals have demonstrated survival after replacement of 90% of the red cell mass by either Hb solution.

In contrast to the chemical reaction involved in oxygen transport by Hb, emulsions of perfluorocarbons carry oxygen in physical solution at high partial oxygen pressures, although they readily release the oxygen when the Po_2 is low, i.e. at tissue level. The need for high partial oxygen pressure required for adequate oxygen uptake from the lung limits their clinical usefulness, although some of the newer formulations have overcome this problem to some extent. Perfluorocarbons have a short intravascular half-life and, following extravasation, are taken up by the cells of the monocyte–macrophage system. One advantage of these solutions is their low viscosity, which offers advantages in some clinical situations, e.g. limb salvage and patients with myocardial infarction. Recent solutions consist of combinations of

Table 6.13 Crystalloid solutions for intravenous use (mmol/l)

Solution	Na^+	K^+	Cl^-	HCO_3^-	Ca^{++}
Isotonic (N) saline	154	–	154	–	–
Dextrose 5% N saline	154	–	154	–	–
Dextrose 5% N/2 saline	77	–	77	–	–
Hartmann's solution (Ringer lactate)	131	4	110	(28)[a]	3
Ringer's solution	147	4	155	–	4
Dextrose 5%	–	–	–	–	–

[a]As lactate.

a mixture of three perfluorocarbons with hydroxyethyl starch. The 20% solution requires inspired oxygen of 100%, but the 35% solution can be used with 60% inspired oxygen, rendering it more acceptable for general clinical use. To date, the clinical experience with these solutions has been limited and little is known about their long-term toxicity.

Section 6.8 • Oedema

Oedema is defined as the excessive accumulation of tissue fluid, mainly in the interstitial but also in the intracellular space. Under physiological conditions, the Starling forces (capillary pressure and plasma oncotic pressure) ensure the orderly bidirectional movement of fluid between the intravascular compartment (more specifically the effective circulatory volume, ECV) and the interstitial space. Thus, during the course of one day, some 20 litres of fluid leave the capillaries at the arteriolar end and 18 litres are absorbed back across the capillary membrane at the venous zone of the capillary network, leaving an excess of 2 litres, which is returned to the circulation by the lymphatics. Oedema represents a breakdown of this balanced fluid transport with a net accumulation of tissue fluid.

Oedema may be **localized** (e.g. inflammatory, neurogenic, local hypersensitivity reaction), when only an imbalance of the Starling forces and other locoregional factors (e.g. increased vascular permeability) are operative, or **generalized**, when the role of the kidney is of paramount importance, irrespective of the aetiology (cardiac, hepatic or renal disease).

Mechanisms of generalized oedema formation

Chronic disease
The basic mechanisms that are common to all disorders accompanied by excessive water and salt retention causing oedema with or without ascites or hydrothorax are outlined schematically in Figure 6.10. In addition, other factors that are disease specific may be involved, e.g. hypoalbuminaemia in chronic liver and renal disease and relative excess of aldosterone (secondary hyperaldosteronism) in cirrhosis, but these are less important in the aetiology of interstitial tissue fluid overload.

In heart failure, chronic hepatic and renal disease the raised capillary pressure is due to an elevated venous pressure that is transmitted to the capillary bed. This reduces the amount of fluid reabsorbed from the interstitial space back into the intravascular compartment. The net result is a contraction of the plasma volume which, in itself, would tend to limit the pathological process. However, the low-pressure volume receptors in the atrium and pulmonary vessels detect a reduction in the ECV and trigger the excess reabsorption of water and NaCl by the kidneys, so that the plasma volume is restored. The net outflow of fluid to the interstitial space is continued until a steady state is reached.

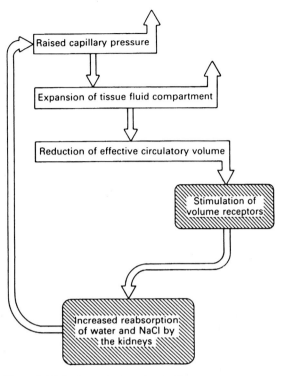

Figure 6.10 Basic mechanisms involved in generalized oedema.

This occurs when the pressure in the interstitial space is raised sufficiently to counter the elevated capillary pressure. In essence, this means that tissue perfusion is impaired.

In some disorders, the oncotic pressure is reduced. This may be due to the reduction in the serum albumin from increased permeability of the glomerular capillaries in certain forms of renal disease (e.g. nephrotic syndrome) or to defective synthesis (e.g. chronic liver disease) or protein malnutrition (e.g. kwashiorkor). The reduced oncotic pressure augments the effect of the raised capillary pressure in the net accumulation of tissue fluid in liver and kidney disease.

Clinically, oedema is often dependent, and for this reason, is commonly found around the ankles in ambulant patients or over the sacral area when the patient is bed-bound. The cause of this distribution can be directly ascribed to the greater venous (and hence capillary) pressures in these regions and to the effects of gravity. Oedema is also prominent in patients with renal disease in the periorbital regions, where the tissues are lax. Certain individuals, usually female, suffer from a deficiency of renal handling of sodium and this leads to cyclical oedema manifesting in puffiness of the hands, feet and face.

Critically ill patients
Generalized oedema is often encountered in critically ill patients on ventilatory and inotropic support (major trauma and advanced sepsis). This is usually multifactorial, e.g. excess crystalloid infusion with patho-

logical expansion of the interstitial space, third space losses, low cardiac output, increased capillary permeability and low plasma oncotic pressure (dilution). The concept of the 'third space' arose from the observation that surgical trauma and inflammatory disease resulted in increased capillary permeability and sequestration of extracellular fluid in the traumatized or inflamed tissue (e.g. oedematous bowel in intestinal obstruction or peritonitis). The generalized oedema of critically ill patients responds to intravenous fluid restriction (haemodynamic monitoring permitting) if the patient's condition improves. Diuretics are seldom indicated as most of these patients are in renal failure. Haemodialysis with hyperosmolar dialysate may be necessary.

Mechanisms of localized oedema formation

Here, the important pathological variables are vasodilatation and increased permeability of the capillary endothelium. The vasodilatation of the precapillary sphincters results in elevation of the capillary pressure with excess transudation over reabsorption across the capillary membrane.

Inflammatory oedema

The increased permeability of the capillary endothelium, which is caused by the cytokine cascade, components of complement following activation by the classic or alternative pathway, kinins, prostaglandins, proteases (e.g. granulocyte elastase), etc., results in the escape of both fluid and albumin in the interstitial space. The extravasated albumin, by raising the oncotic pressure of the tissue fluid, further accentuates the net accumulation of fluid in this compartment. These mechanisms operate irrespective of the aetiology of the condition: bacterial inflammation, inflammatory oedema of healing wounds, oedema due to anaphylaxis, neurogenic oedema, etc.

Apart from its local and systemic effects, inflammatory oedema is important from a technical aspect in relation to tissue approximation (closure of wounds and intestinal anastomosis). Oedematous tissue sustains a marked reduction in its tensile strength and, for this reason, when the edges are approximated by sutures, there is a tendency for the sutures to cut through with breakdown of the wound or dehiscence of the anastomosis. Thus, special techniques are needed to deal with this situation [see Module 2, Vol. I].

Limb oedema

In patients with oedema affecting one limb, the usual cause can be found in some problem within the deep venous system. Often, this is the result of previous deep venous thrombosis, which leads to the post-phlebitic syndrome (marked lower limb oedema, eczema, pigmentation and ulceration). In a small proportion of patients, compression of the left common iliac vein by the right common iliac artery may be responsible for left-sided leg oedema [see Module 10, Vol. I].

Less commonly, limb swelling may arise from lymphoedema owing to blockage or insufficiency of the lymphatic trunks draining the limb. The most common variety is secondary lymphoedema from blockage or disruption due to trauma, surgical excision of lymph nodes (postmastectomy), radiotherapy for cancer, infiltration by malignant disease, parasitic infestations, e.g. filariasis, etc. In primary lymphoedema, the mechanism is insufficiency rather than obstruction (hypoplastic or incompetent lymphatics) [see Module 10, Vol. I].

Whatever the cause of lymphoedema, the accumulated fluid has a high protein content, which induces a fibrotic reaction in the subcutaneous region and is particularly prone to infection, especially by streptococcal organisms. These inflammatory episodes aggravate the subdermal fibrosis so that the skin becomes thick, dry, scaly and rough (elephantiasis). Long-standing lymphoedema does not pit on pressure, although early lymphoedema does.

Other unusual causes of limb swelling include: **disuse oedema** when the patient holds the limb completely immobile for long periods, **post–traumatic osteodystrophy** (very painful swelling such as to make the limb useless, accompanied by osteoporosis, also known as Sudeck's atrophy), and **local gigantism**, which may be due to arteriovenous malformations or Klippel–Trenaunay syndrome (combination of congenital varicose veins, abnormal deep veins and capillary naevi).

Angioneurotic oedema

This is caused by the congenital absence of C1 esterase inhibitor. As a result of this deficiency, afflicted individuals are prone to episodes of unchecked activation of complement with marked oedema formation that often affects the upper airway, leading to life-threatening asphyxia. Acute episodes are treated by infusion of C1 esterase inhibitor derived from plasma and antihistamines. Patients may require endotracheal intubation or tracheostomy.

Guide to further reading

Blower, A. L., Brooks, A., Fenn, G. C. *et al.* (1997). Emergency admissions for upper gastrointestinal disease and their relation to NSAID use. *Aliment Pharmacol Ther* **11**: 283–291.

Contreras, M., ed. (1990). *ABC of Transfusion*. BMJ Publication.

Donnelly, M. T. and Hawkey, C. J. (1997). Review article: COX-II inhibitors – a new generation of safer NSAIDs? *Aliment Pharmacol* **11**: 227–236.

Faulkner, G., Pritchard, P., Somerville, K. and Langman, M. J. S. (1988). Aspirin and bleeding peptic ulcer in the elderly. *BMJ* **297**: 1311–1313.

Henry, D. A. and O'Connell, D. L. (1989). Effects of fibrinolytic inhibitors on mortality from upper gastrointestinal haemorrhage. *BMJ* **298**: 1142–1146.

HMSO (1996). *Handbook of Transfusion*, 2nd edn, HMSO, London.

Schierhout, G. and Roberts, I. (1998). Fluid resuscitation with colloid or crystalloid solutions in critically ill patients: a systemic review of randomised trials. *BMJ* **316**: 961–964.

Stael von Holstein, C. C. S., Eriksson, S. B. S. and Kallen, R. (1987). Tranexamic acid as an aid to reducing blood transfusion requirements in gastric and duodenal bleeding. *BMJ* **294**: 7–10.

Patients with metabolic disorders

1 • Fluid and electrolyte balance

2 • Acid–base balance

'Experience is a good teacher, but she sends in terrific bills' – Minna Antrim

The detection and correction of metabolic and acid–base disturbances is an integral part of surgical practice, and assumes special importance in emergency and postoperative situations. A knowledge of the underlying physiological principles is necessary and comorbid pulmonary and/or renal disease complicates management. Inadequate fluid and electrolyte/acid–base balance may have serious, at times fatal consequences.

Section 7.1 • Fluid and electrolyte balance

Distribution of body water and electrolytes

In males, water makes up around 60% of the body mass, and in females the figure is nearer 50% owing to the greater fatty tissue component. Thus, in a 60 kg woman, the total body water would be 30 litres. This can be divided into intracellular fluid (ICF) and extracellular fluid (ECF) compartments, which consist of two-thirds (20 litres) and one-third (10 litres) of the total body water, respectively. The extracellular compartment has two components: interstitial and intravascular (plasma) (Figure 7.1). The plasma accounts for around one-quarter of the ECF, thus amounting to 2.5 litres in the 60 kg woman. A variable amount of

water is also present is body spaces (gut, renal tract, peritoneal and pleural cavities, etc.) which, under normal circumstances, amounts to around 500 ml. This is termed transcellular water.

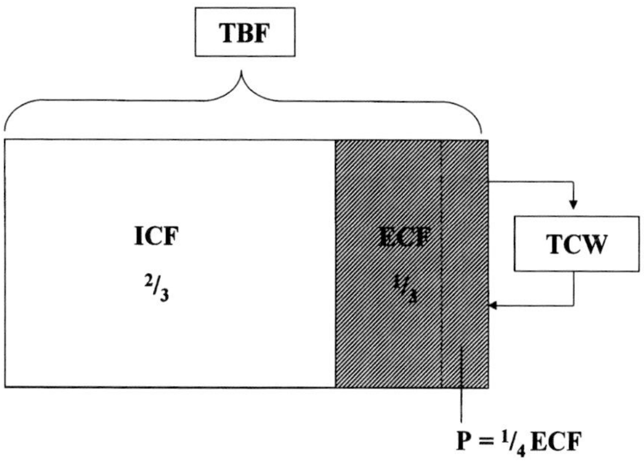

Water can pass freely among the ICF, ECF and plasma, and its distribution depends on pressure gradients across the cell membranes that separate the ICF from the ECF, and the capillary walls which separates the interstitial fluid (ISF) from plasma. These pressure gradients are in turn dependent on the net effect of hydrostatic and osmotic pressures. However, because osmotic pressure differences are determined by species which cannot diffuse from one compartment to another, and because the cell membrane and the capillary wall have very different permeabilities, the regulation of ICF and ECF is determined by charged ions, whereas the regulation of ISF and plasma is dependent on proteins.

Charged ions do not easily cross the lipid cell membrane, and so the concentration or osmolarity of the extracellular electrolytes is the main determinant of the distribution of the ICF and the ECF. The main extracellular cation is Na^+; its normal concentration in ECF is 140 mmol/l, whereas its concentration in the ICF is usually about 10 mmol/l. This ratio is reversed with K^+ (Table 7.1). These concentrations are maintained by

Figure 7.1 Fluid compartments of the body. TBF, total body fluid; ICF, intracellular fluid; ECF, extracellular fluid; P, plasma; TCW, transcellular water.

Table 7.1 Concentrations (mmol/l) of ions in extracellular and intracellular fluid

Ion	ICF	ECF (and plasma)
Na^+	10	140
K^+	150	4.5
Cl^-	Trace	105

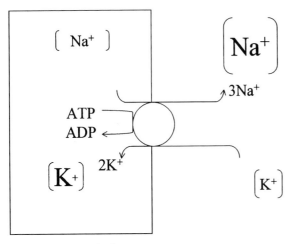

Figure 7.2 The Na^+/K^+ pump.

active transport in the healthy cell membrane, the energy for which comes from the hydrolysis of ATP (the Na^+/K^+ pump; Figure 7.2).

Unlike ions, proteins do not diffuse rapidly across the capillary wall, so the distribution of fluid between the plasma and the interstitial compartments of the ECF is determined by the transcapillary protein concentration gradient as well as the hydrostatic pressure (see section on 'Oedema'). It must be appreciated, however, that protein only accounts for around 1% of the total plasma osmolarity.

Glomerular filtration

Urine is formed by the nephrons within the kidney. Each nephron consists of a glomerulus, which is made up of a tuft of capillaries surrounded by Bowman's capsule. This is where plasma is initially filtered and the resulting fluid is modified by both secretion and reabsorption as it passes in turn through the proximal convoluted tubule, loop of Henle, the distal convoluted tubule and the collecting duct. The resultant urine is collected in the renal pelvis and discharged through the ureter (Figure 7.3).

The driving forces involved in the initial filtration are the hydrostatic and osmotic pressure gradients between the capillaries in the glomerulus and Bowman's capsule. Because of the large glomerular surface area and the low resistance to fluid movement across the glomerulus there is a high glomerular filtration rate, which normally equals about 120 ml/min. Although this is remarkably constant, it is subject to modification by factors that increase the glomerular capillary hydrostatic pressure, the glomerular capillary flow rate or the glomerular capillary surface area. Regulation of renal blood flow is important for maintaining normal filtration as this is the main determinant of capillary pressure and capillary flow. The blood supply to the kidneys is in the region of 1.2 l/min and is maintained at this level over a wide range of arterial pressures because of autoregulation of the blood flow. Thus, if systemic arterial pressure falls, dilatation of the afferent arterioles reduces the renal vascular resistance, tending to maintain the blood flow. However, at very low pressures (systemic arterial pressure less than 80 mmHg) autoregulation fails and the renal blood flow declines rapidly. Further reduction in the glomerular blood flow is caused by reflex stimulation of the sympathetic supply to the kidney. This accounts for the reduction in urine output during systemic hypotension.

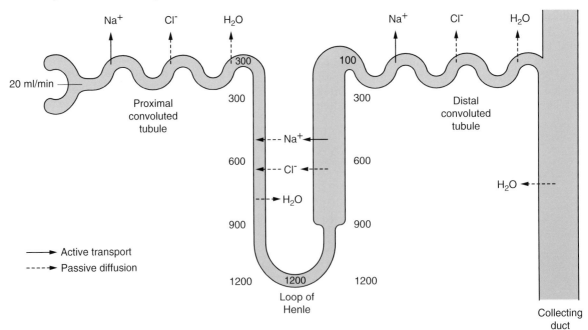

Figure 7.3 Diagram of a nephron indicating sodium and water reabsorption and changes in osmolality. This is controlled by hormonal influences (see Figure 7.4). Numbers refer to osmolarity (mosmol/l) in the tubular fluid and the renal parenchyma. Solid arrow, active transport; dotted arrow, passive diffusion or osmosis.

Modification of glomerular filtrate

This is outlined in Figure 7.3. After the production of the filtrate, which is protein free but otherwise plasma like, it is modified by reabsorption and secretion as it passes through the rest of the nephron. In the **proximal convoluted tubule** active transport drives sodium across the tubular epithelium into the peritubular fluid. Chloride ions follow passively and the resulting osmotic gradient draws water out of the tubule, leading to a net reabsorption of a sodium, chloride solution, which is essentially iso-osmotic with plasma. Thus, the volume of the filtrate is decreased but there is no change in its osmolality.

In the **loop of Henle** the thick portion of the ascending limb is impermeable to water but actively transports sodium out of the filtrate, thus raising the concentration of sodium chloride and thus the osmolality in the medullary fluid around the whole of the loop of Henle. The thin descending limb is permeable to both ions and water so that the fluid from the proximal convoluted tubule descending through the medulla is both concentrated and reduced in volume by the passive influx of sodium and chloride and the osmotic removal of water. This solution becomes more dilute as it ascends the opposite limb of the loop of Henle due to the active removal of the solute, so that the solution entering the distal convoluted tubule has a lower osmolality than that leaving the proximal tubule.

The most important effect of the loop of Henle is to increase the osmolality of the interstitial fluid in the medulla of the kidney, and this can reach 1200 mosmol/l at the bottom of the loop. This leads to the subsequent reabsorption of water from the collecting ducts. In the distal convoluted tubule, most of the remaining sodium is actively reabsorbed from the filtrate so that less than 1% of the initially filtered sodium reaches the collecting duct and is excreted in the urine. As the fluid entering the collecting ducts is of low osmolality, further water reabsorption occurs from the collecting ducts as they descend through the medulla towards the renal pelvis. As this reabsorption occurs without any active ion transport, the volume of the urine is decreased and its osmolality is increased. For the same reason, the reabsorption is entirely dependent on the permeability of the collecting ducts to water.

Control of fluid and electrolyte excretion

Excretion of water and electrolytes by the kidney, and hence the regulation of ECF volume and osmolality is precisely controlled by three hormones: aldosterone, antidiuretic hormone (ADH) and atrial natriuretic hormone (Figure 7.4).

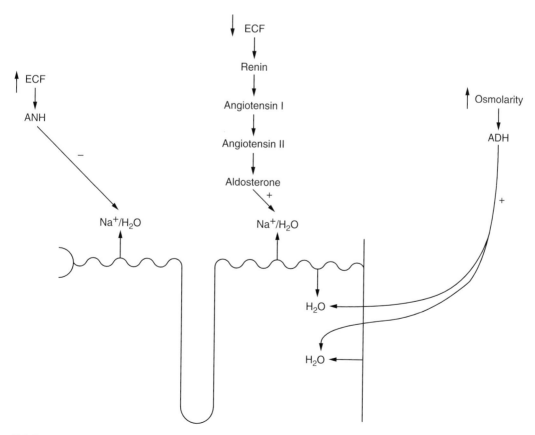

Figure 7.4 Endocrine control of sodium and water reabsorption by the nephron. ECF, extracellular fluid; ADH, antidiuretic hormone; ANH, atrial natriuretic hormone.

Aldosterone

Aldosterone is a steroid, which is produced in the adrenal cortex and stimulates reabsorption of sodium and water from the distal convoluted tubule. Its control (Figure 7.4) depends on the release of renin from the juxtaglomerular apparatus. This is activated by:

- a fall in the afferent arterial pressure
- reductions in the amount of filtered sodium caused by reduced plasma concentrations of sodium or reduced glomerular filtration
- stimulation of the sympathetic nerve supply to the kidney.

When the renin has been released into the circulation, it catalyses the conversion of the plasma protein angiotensinogen into angiotensin I. This is further converted to angiotensin II by angiotensin-converting enzyme in the vascular endothelium. Angiotensin II in turn stimulates the release of aldosterone. The effect of aldosterone is to increase the ECF volume and this is supplemented by the independent effects of angiotensin II, which include:

- enhanced systemic arteriolar vasoconstriction
- release of ADH
- central stimulation of thirst.

It should also be noted that aldosterone stimulates the rate of secretion of potassium in the distal convoluted tubule. This is the most important regulator of plasma potassium as adrenal cortical secretion of aldosterone is stimulated by potassium.

Antidiuretic hormone

ADH is a peptide hormone synthesized by the paraventricular nucleus of the hypothalamus and released from the posterior pituitary.

Its secretion is stimulated by:

- decreased circulating blood volume detected by cardiovascular volume receptors
- decreased arterial pressure detected by cardiovascular baroreceptors
- increased osmolality of the ECF detected by osmoreceptors in the hypothalamus.

ADH increases the permeability of the collecting ducts to water and this promotes reabsorption of water under the influence of the osmolality in the renal medulla. The final result is therefore to increase the ECF volume. ADH also causes direct vasoconstriction, which increases the systemic arterial blood pressure, hence its alternative name of vasopressin.

Atrial natriuretic hormone

Atrial natriuretic hormone is another peptide hormone that is released from the atria of the heart in response to an increase in the ECF volume. It leads to increased glomerular filtration and inhibits the tubular reabsorption of sodium. This results in increased excretion of sodium (natriuresis) and water, which in turn results in reduction of the ECF volume.

Fluid and electrolyte balance and its clinical implications

Maintenance of fluid and electrolyte balance is important for optimal function of the organism. The effects of disorders of fluid and electrolyte balance are described in the next section. The term fluid balance indicates the relationship between fluid output and fluid intake; excess intake is described as a positive fluid balance while excess loss constitutes a negative fluid balance. Maintaining fluid balance is an important part of patient care, particularly in the postoperative period.

Fluid output varies widely from a maximum of around 7 litres in 24 h down to a minimum of 1 litre in 24 h. Fluid loss occurs in the following ways.

- **Urinary excretion.** This usually varies between 1 and 2 l/day but may rise when there has been a high fluid intake. The minimum urine output necessary for adequate excretion of toxic waste materials is in the region of 500 ml/day.
- **Insensible fluid loss.** This is due to the continuous evaporation of fluid from the surface of the skin and the airways. Normal daily losses are in the region of 500 ml but this can be increased during assisted ventilation. The other situation where insensible fluid loss increases dramatically is during laparotomy.
- **Sweating.** Sweating is related to insensible skin losses but responds to strenuous exercise, environmental temperature or fever. Under extreme circumstances it can be the main reason for fluid loss, with daily volumes exceeding 5 litres.
- **Intestinal excretion.** The amount of fluid lost in faeces under normal circumstances is about 100 ml/day but abnormalities such as vomiting, diarrhoea or intestinal obstruction can lead to much greater losses.

As described in the previous section, the fluid output is regulated by the kidney and this in turn depends on aldosterone, ADH and atrial natriuretic hormone.

To maintain homeostasis fluid output must be balanced by fluid intake and water is incorporated into the body by two main mechanisms. Drinking (or eating water-containing foods) leads to fluid being absorbed by the intestinal tract and this is controlled by the thirst centre in the hypothalamus, which is stimulated by increased osmolarity of the ECF. Another source of water comes from the metabolic production of water from oxidation in body cells (e.g. hydrocarbon metabolism). This source accounts for about 300 ml of metabolic water each day.

Under normal circumstances the fluid balance is maintained quite precisely but in the surgical patient it has to be monitored carefully. As a baseline a normal 60 kg adult would require in the region of 2 litres of water per day. The normal intake of sodium would be in the region of 100 mmol/day, although this can be considerably less owing to the sodium-conserving powers of the kidney. As potassium is exchanged for sodium, obligatory renal losses of potassium are greater than for sodium and average about 50 mmol/day. Thus, by maintaining a patient on intravenous fluid consisting of 500 ml of normal saline (154 mmol sodium per litre), 1.5 litres of isotonic water as 5% dextrose and 60 mmol potassium should be adequate under uncomplicated circumstances.

It must be appreciated, however, that the surgical patient is likely to have lost fluid by insensible loss and may also be losing fluid via nasogastric aspiration, sequestration of fluid in the small bowel, losses from fistulae, etc. It is therefore of great importance to monitor the adequacy of fluid replacement, and this is best done by measuring urine output. As the kidney is exquisitely sensitive to ECF control mechanisms, the volume of urine is a good measure of the adequacy of fluid replacement and a minimum urine output of 30 ml/h should be achieved. Haemodynamic stability must also be maintained, and for this reason, it is also important to monitor pulse, blood pressure and, where appropriate, central venous pressure.

When urine output drops it is important to distinguish between a response to reduction in the ECF volume (prerenal failure) and renal disease. Prerenal failure may go on to acute tubular necrosis secondary to prolonged hypotension, and if there is any doubt regarding the distinction between prerenal and renal failure, it is useful to measure the urine osmolality and the urine sodium levels. In prerenal failure the urine osmolality will be greater than that of plasma and in the region of 500 mmol/l. The urine sodium will be less than 10 mmol/l. When acute tubular necrosis has become established the urine osmolality will approximate to that of plasma and will be less than 500 mmol/l. The urine sodium concentration will be greater than 50 mmol/l.

Fluid and electrolyte disorders and their correction

The major abnormalities of fluid and electrolyte balance can be categorized as follows:

- water lack
- water excess
- ECF lack
- ECF excess
- potassium lack: hypokalaemia
- potassium excess: hyperkalaemia.

Because the regulation of sodium is so integral with that of water, isolated problems of sodium balance are not commonly relevant. Severe disturbances of plasma sodium levels indicate a general problem of cellular homeostasis and cannot be corrected by simple fluid or electrolyte therapy.

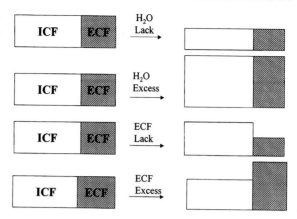

Figure 7.5 Relative shifts in intracellular fluid (ICF) and extracellular fluid (ECF) compartments in fluid and electrolyte disorders.

Water lack

Lack of water is caused either by poor intake of water or by diabetes insipidus, where posterior pituitary damage compromises the secretion of ADH. This results in a decrease in the whole body fluid volume (Figure 7.5). The clinical features are those of thirst, confusion and hypothermia but the patient is not clinically dehydrated, as the drop in ECF volume is balanced by a drop in ICF volume. The diagnosis can be confirmed by a raised plasma sodium and urea. Treatment is by the administration of oral water or intravenous isotonic water in the form of 5% dextrose.

Water excess

Under these circumstances the total body fluid volume increases (Figure 7.5). This is caused by excess intake of water either from abnormal drinking patterns or from infusion of too much 5% dextrose. It can also be caused by inappropriate or ectopic ADH secretion (e.g. by hormone-producing tumours). The clinical features are those of confusion and hypothermia but there are no obvious clinical signs, again because the increase in ECF is balanced by an increase in ICF. Here the diagnosis may be confirmed by a low plasma potassium and a low plasma urea. Treatment is by a combination of water restriction and infusion of hypotonic sodium chloride. Diuretics should not be used as these will merely decrease the ECF volume.

ECF lack

In this situation, only the ECF volume drops, leaving the ICF volume intact (Figure 7.5). The causes here are essentially related to diversion of transcellular water (vomiting, diarrhoea, intestinal obstruction, etc.) or to excessive insensible loss or sweating. The clinical features are those of dehydration and hypovolaemia and although the plasma urea is high, the sodium concentration is normal. The diagnosis is made by the observation of a negative fluid balance or, in extreme cases, the development of clinical features of hypovolaemia. The condition is treated by the replacement of ECF (essentially normal sodium chloride).

ECF excess

Here there is an increase in the ECF compartment without any changes in the ICF compartment (Figure 7.5). ECF excess is usually caused by excessive infusion of saline in the face of impaired excretion. **This will lead to the clinical features of raised central venous pressure, cardiac failure and/or peripheral oedema and the diagnosis is usually made clinically.** It may be confirmed by the chest X-ray appearances of cardiac failure and the observation of a positive fluid balance. Treatment is best effected by a combination of fluid restriction and administration of loop diuretics such as frusemide.

Potassium lack

Hypokalaemia is caused most commonly by gastrointestinal losses (vomiting, diarrhoea, mucus secretion) where replacement has been inadequate. Diuretics may also be responsible. The clinical features are those of confusion and weakness, and arrhythmias may result. The diagnosis is made by the finding of a low plasma potassium and the ECG will show a shallow T-wave (Figure 7.6). **If the potassium level drops to < 2.5 mmol/l, treatment is urgent owing to the risk of fatal cardiac arrhythmias.** This consists of intravenous potassium replacement, given at no more than 20 mmol/h in a solution of no more than 40 mmol/l. More rapid replacement may give rise to hyperkalaemic complications (see below). Replacement should be even more cautious if there is oliguria.

Potassium excess

In the surgical patient, this is most commonly caused by acute renal failure or excess intravenous replacement. Another common cause is diabetic ketoacidosis. The patient will tend to be confused and weak and again cardiac arrhythmias can be a problem. The diagnosis is made from a high plasma potassium level and a peaked T-wave can be seen on the ECG (Figure 7.6). In this situation, potassium must be restricted and high levels of potassium must be brought down rapidly using glucose and insulin infusion combined with ion-exchange resins. In the patient with acute renal failure, haemodialysis may be necessary.

In the patient with a plasma potassium of >6.6 mmol/l the following regime should be observed:

- 10 ml 10% calcium chloride i.v. for cardioprotection
- 15 units soluble insulin with 50 ml 50% glucose
- polystyrene sulfonate resin 30 g/h as an enema.

Oedema

Oedema is swelling caused by accumulation of interstitial fluid. To understand its pathogenesis it is important to appreciate the mechanisms that are responsible for filtration and absorption of fluid across the capillary wall.

The hydrostatic pressure gradient between the capillary pressure and the interstitial fluid pressure acts to filter fluid out of the capillary. In contrast, the osmotic pressure gradient, which is generated by virtue of the fact that the capillary wall acts as a semipermeable membrane such that water can cross the capillary but plasma proteins cannot, acts to draw water into the capillary. This osmotic pressure is often called the colloid osmotic pressure or the oncotic pressure of the plasma. It must be remembered that protein accounts for only a very small fraction of the total osmolality of plasma, which is largely caused by dissolved electrolytes. However, as the capillary wall is permeable to the smaller molecules and ion proteins are the only relevant osmotic influence, the direction of fluid transfer at any point along the capillary is determined by the net filtration pressure gradient. Capillary hydrostatic pressure falls from about 35 mmHg at the arteriolar to about 15 mmHg at the venular end. Interstitial fluid pressure is close to atmospheric pressure or slightly below (−2 mmHg). Thus, the hydrostatic gradient acting out of the capillary has a mean value of around 25 mmHg. The colloid osmotic gradient does not vary along the length of the capillary and under normal circumstances is about 27 mmHg. Thus, the total filtration along the length of the capillary usually exceeds absorption and the additional filtered fluid is returned to the circulation by means of the lymphatic system, so maintaining the interstitial fluid volume (Figure 7.7).

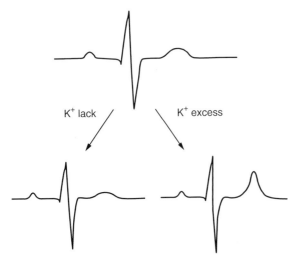

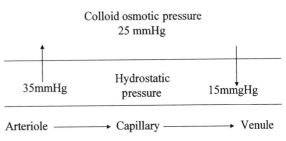

Figure 7.6 ECG changes in potassium disorders.

Figure 7.7 Effect of hydrostatic pressure and colloid osmotic pressure on fluid shifts across the capillary wall.

Thus, it can be seen that oedema may be due to one of three factors.

- **Increases in the hydrostatic gradient** may be due to anything that causes increased venous pressure, such as prolonged standing, cardiac failure or venous obstruction. Decreases in interstitial fluid pressure may also cause oedema and this accounts for oedema during prolonged air flights.
- **Reductions in the osmotic gradient** will reduce absorption and thus increase net filtration. This is usually due to a low plasma protein concentration because of malnutrition, renal disease or liver failure. It may also be due to increased capillary permeability to protein as seen in the inflammatory responses to infection or trauma.
- **Lymphatic obstruction** leads to a reduction in the clearance of both fluid and protein from the interstitial tissues. The swelling that results from this abnormality is usually referred to as lymphoedema [see Module 6, Vol. I].

Section 7.2 • Acid–base balance

The normal pH ($-\log_{10}[H^+]$) of ECF is 7.4 and the maintenance of this normal level is very important as enzyme function is sensitive to changes in the concentration of hydrogen ions. The main factors that control the pH are the acid–base buffers systems, renal control of pH and respiratory control of pH.

Buffers

There are three important acid–base systems that act as pH buffers in the blood: bicarbonate, proteins and phosphates.

Bicarbonate

Carbon dioxide (CO_2) and water (H_2O) can react reversibly to form carbonic acid (H_2CO_3), which then dissociates releasing hydrogen ions (H^+) and bicarbonate (HCO_3^-). The chemical equation that describes this process can be written as follows:

$$CO_2 + H_2O \leftrightarrow H_2CO_3 \leftrightarrow H^+ + HCO_3^-$$

This reaction is catalysed by carbonic anhydrase in the red blood cells. When H^+ is added to blood it reacts with HCO_3^- to form carbonic acid, thus keeping the pH constant. Under normal situations, the buffering power of the HCO_3^- is greatly increased because the additional CO_2 formed is cleared by the respiratory control mechanisms that regulate arterial P_{CO_2}. This permits the chemical reaction to continue moving to the left, thus continuing to remove H^+ ions from the solution. Respiratory and renal control mechanisms (see below) adjust the CO_2 and HCO_3^- concentrations to assist maintenance of the acid–base balance.

Proteins

Acidic and basic amino acid residues in both red cell proteins and plasma proteins can act as buffers. The haemoglobin in the red cells provides more buffering capacity than any other single buffer but, unlike the bicarbonate buffer system, it cannot be regulated to compensate for excessively abnormal acid–base conditions.

Phosphates

Phosphates both in the cells and in the ECF can act as buffers, but under normal conditions these make a relatively small contribution to the total buffering capacity of blood.

Combined buffer mechanisms

The combined effect of these buffers is dramatic. The addition of 1 mmol of H^+ to 1 l of solution at a pH of 7.4 would cause the pH to reduce to 3.0 in the absence of buffers. However, in normal blood the addition of 1 mmol of H^+ would only reduce the pH to 7.38 as long as a normal P_{CO_2} was being maintained by ventilation.

The means whereby buffers regulate pH can be described by the Henderson–Hasselbalch equation:

$$pH = pK_a + \log_{10}[\text{Base}]/[\text{Acid}]$$

where K_a is the dissociation constant for the acid and $pK_a = -\log_{10}K_a$. If this is applied to the bicarbonate buffer system, we have:

$$pH = pK_a + \log_{10}[HCO_3^-]/[H_2CO_3]$$

where K_a is the dissociation constant for carbonic acid. In practice, the concentration of carbonic acid is not easy to measure, but as it represents the product of the reaction between CO_2 and H_2O it can be expressed in terms of [CO_2]. This in turn can be expressed as P_{CO_2} as the concentration of gas in aqueous solution is proportional to the partial pressure of the gas as stated in Henry's law. Thus, the Henderson–Hasselbalch equation for the bicarbonate buffer system can be expressed as:

$$pH = pK' + \log_{10}[HCO_3^-]/[P_{CO_2}]$$

where K' is a new constant. By examining this equation, it can be seen that plasma pH can be controlled by regulation of both [HCO_3^-] and [P_{CO_2}], and this forms the basis of the renal and respiratory control of acid–base balance, as described below.

Renal control of pH

The kidney regulates extracellular pH through the tubular secretion of H^+, a process that is directly linked to the absorption of HCO_3^-. This maintains a normal pH in the face of metabolic acidosis, as H^+ ions are excreted in exchange for HCO_3^- ions and these make up the most important pH buffer in the blood.

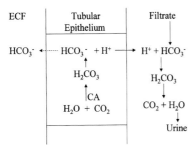

Figure 7.8 Regulation of extracellular pH through renal secretion of H^+ and absorption of HCO_3^-. Tubular secretion of H^+ leads to reabsorption of filtered HCO_3^-. CA, carbonic anhydrase.

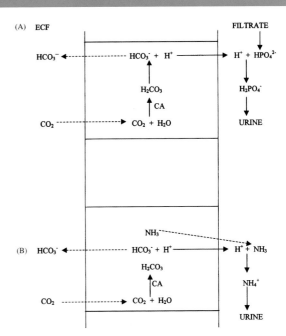

Figure 7.9 Secreted H^+ can combine with filtered phosphates (A) or secreted ammonia (B) and be excreted in the urine. The remaining HCO_3^- from the dissociation of carbonic acid in the tubular epithelium is absorbed into the extracellular fluid (ECF), thus increasing its HCO_3^- concentration.

H^+ ions and HCO_3^- ions are formed within the renal tubular epithelial cells via dissociation of carbonic acid formed by the combination of CO_2 and water. This latter reaction is catalysed by carbonic anhydrase. The H^+ ion is then transported actively into the tubular fluid and the HCO_3^- diffuses out into the renal capillaries, maintaining electrical neutrality inside the cell. In the tubular fluid, the H^+ ion combines with filtered HCO_3^- to form CO_2 and H_2O and the CO_2 can diffuse across the cell membrane, thus completing the cycle (Figure 7.8). The end result of this process is reabsorption of filtered HCO_3^- that is conserved rather than being excreted. In a metabolic alkalosis, however, where the plasma concentration of HCO_3^- rises, urinary excretion of HCO_3^- also increases as there is more HCO_3^- filtered than can be exchanged for the secreted H^+.

H^+ ion secretion not only serves to conserve filtered HCO_3^-, but can lead to an increase in the total body HCO_3^- in response to acidosis. This takes place when H^+ ion reacts with urinary buffers other than HCO_3^- in the tubular fluid (e.g. HPO_4^{2-} and NH_3). The $H_2PO_4^-$ and the NH_4^+ ions cannot cross the lipid membrane of the tubular epithelia and are thus excreted in the urine. The HCO_3^- produced by dissociation of the carbonic acid within the tubular cells then diffuses into the ECF and serves to increase the total HCO_3^- (Figure 7.9).

Under normal circumstances, therefore, the urine is acid and the kidney excretes between 50 and 80 mmol of H^+ every 24 h. However, any change in plasma H^+ concentration leads to compensatory changes in the rate of both tubular acid secretion and HCO_3^- absorption. When the H^+ concentration increases, H^+ is effectively exchanged for HCO_3^-, but this does not all come from the tubular fluid. HCO_3^- exchange can continue by means of generation of additional HCO_3^- within the tubular epithelial cells after all the filtered HCO_3^- has been reabsorbed. The mechanisms whereby this takes place are described above. Thus, the kidney can increase the HCO_3^- concentration during a prolonged respiratory acidosis and this tends to return the pH to normal levels. Similarly, the opposite effect takes place

during a sustained respiratory alkalosis, where H^+ secretion decreases and there is a parallel fall in HCO_3^- absorption leading to a decreased plasma concentration of HCO_3^-. Thus, these mechanisms provide metabolic compensation for respiratory acidosis and alkalosis (see below). This form of compensation may take several days.

Respiratory control of pH

As a result of the bicarbonate buffer system, CO_2 in the blood influences pH by forming carbonic acid, which then dissociates to form H^+. Thus, any rise in P_{CO_2} will lead to a fall in pH while a fall in P_{CO_2} will lead to a rise. As the arterial levels of CO_2 are dependent on inspired P_{CO_2}, respiratory function has an important role in the regulation of pH. The respiratory system maintains a constant arterial P_{CO_2} as an appropriate rate of ventilation is controlled by respiratory chemoreceptors sensitive to CO_2. Failure of these mechanisms can lead to an abnormal arterial P_{CO_2}, leading to a respiratory acid–base disorder.

Arterial pH can affect ventilation through chemoreceptors sensitive to hydrogen ions, which alter the P_{CO_2} in order to compensate for pH changes of metabolic origin. Thus, ventilation is stimulated by a metabolic acidosis, which leads to a reduction in P_{CO_2} and inhibited by a metabolic alkalosis, leading to an elevated P_{CO_2}. This respiratory compensation for metabolic acid–base disorders may take several hours to take effect fully.

Biochemical assessment of acid–base balance

Acid–base balance is normally investigated using arterial pH, P_{CO_2}, HCO_3^- and the base excess. These are described below.

pH

The normal pH in an arterial blood sample is 7.4. Variations from this indicate either acidosis (low pH) or alkalosis (high pH). The underlying cause of the abnormality can be established by measurements of the other parameters listed below.

P_{CO_2}

The normal value of arterial P_{CO_2} is 5.3 kPa (40 mmHg) and variations in this indicate a respiratory contribution to the acid–base disturbance, either as a positive factor or as a compensatory mechanism.

HCO_3^-

The normal concentration of HCO_3^- in the arterial blood is 25 mmol/l. In metabolic acidosis this will fall as the increase in concentration of the hydrogen ions will drive the bicarbonate buffering reaction towards the carbonic acid, thus reducing the HCO_3^- concentration. Likewise, a metabolic alkalosis drives the reaction to release HCO_3, with a consequent rise in its concentration. However, changes in P_{CO_2} can also affect the concentration of HCO_3. An increase in P_{CO_2} would lead to increased formation of carbonic acid and HCO_3^-; conversely, a low P_{CO_2} would lead to lowered HCO_3^-. This effect is small when compared with metabolic changes in HCO_3^- concentration and it can be avoided by using the standard HCO_3^- concentration. This is the expected concentration if the arterial blood sample has been equilibrated to a normal P_{CO_2}.

Base excess

This is derived by titration of arterial blood sample with a strong base or acid until a normal pH level is achieved. In order to remove any respiratory contribution to an acid–base abnormality, the blood is equilibrated at the normal P_{CO_2} level. As the base excess causes reflex alterations in the total buffer base (only about half of which is accounted for by HCO_3^-), the value provides a more accurate measurement of the metabolic contribution to any abnormality. Base excess is normally 0 and a positive base excess indicates alkalosis, while a negative base excess (base deficit) indicates a metabolic acidosis.

Disturbances of acid–base balance

Abnormalities of acid–base balance can be divided into four main groups: respiratory acidosis, metabolic acidosis, respiratory alkalosis and metabolic alkalosis. These are summarized in Table 7.2.

Table 7.2 Abnormalities of arterial biochemistry in acid–base disorders

(i) Acidoses (pH low)

Type	Resp	Resp	Mixed	Metab	Metab
Compensation	None	Metab		None	Resp
P_{CO_2}	↑	↑	↑	↔	↓
$[HCO_3^-]$	↔	↑	↓	↓	↓

(ii) Alkaloses (pH high)

Type	Resp	Resp	Mixed	Metab	Metab
Compensation	None	Metab		None	Resp
P_{CO_2}	↓	↓	↓	↔	↑
$[HCO_3^-]$	↔	↓	↑	↑	↑

Resp, respiratory; Metab, metabolic.

Respiratory acidosis

This is a feature of respiratory failure and is characterized by a high arterial P_{CO_2} leading to a fall in pH. If the respiratory acidosis is prolonged, metabolic compensation results from increased renal absorption of HCO_3^- in exchange for secreted hydrogen ions. This gives rise to a secondary increase in the concentration of HCO_3^-. This metabolic compensation takes several days to develop, however, and is a feature of chronic respiratory failure rather than acute respiratory failure.

Metabolic acidosis

This may be caused by increased amounts of acid such as lactic acidosis produced by anoxic metabolism or ketoacidosis in severe diabetes mellitus. The other cause may be due to loss of alkali from the body, as will occur in diarrhoea. Renal failure can produce metabolic acidosis as there is inadequate secretion of acid and reabsorption of HCO_3^-. Prolonged metabolic acidosis stimulates ventilation, leading to a reduction in P_{CO_2}. The effect of this respiratory compensation tends to increase the pH.

Respiratory alkalosis

This occurs with increased ventilation due to hysterical overbreathing or some lung diseases such as pneumonia. It leads to a reduction in P_{CO_2} and metabolic compensation may occur by means of decreased reabsorption of HCO_3^- by the kidney, leading to a reduction in the plasma concentration of HCO_3^-.

Metabolic alkalosis

This may be caused by a loss of acid as in persistent vomiting or excess alkali as in the therapeutic administration of antacids. It gives rise to an increase in the concentration of HCO_3^- and the base excess. A metabolic alkalosis will decrease ventilation so that respiratory compensation occurs by a rise in the arterial P_{CO_2}.

MODULE 8
Malnourished patients

**'Tell me what you eat and I will tell you what you are'
– Anthelme Brillat-Savarin, 1755–1826**

This module describes the causes, recognition and clinical consequences of malnutrition. The principles of artificial nutrition support are discussed. The indications and clinical management of the techniques of enteral and parenteral nutrition are outlined, with particular reference to the surgical patient.

Section 8.1 • Pathology of protein energy malnutrition

The development of disease may be accompanied by a loss of appetite, intestinal malfunction associated with the impaired absorption of nutrients and in some cases metabolic changes leading to tissue wasting. Thus, in many patients there is an inadequate supply of nutrients which, in combination with the influence of inflammatory mediators, leads to weight loss and defective organ function. This process is described by the term **disease-associated malnutrition**.

The normal feeding–fasting cycle is characterized by the postprandial deposition of glycogen and fat and protein synthesis, modulated by the secretion of insulin. Subsequently, a reduction in the secretion of insulin and increase in the secretion of glucagon facilitates the mobilization of glucose from glycogen, and proteolysis and lipolysis to provide energy substrates.

During prolonged starvation the supply of glycogen is rapidly exhausted and glucose, an essential fuel for the brain, is formed in the liver from amino acids derived from muscle protein (gluconeogenesis). As the insulin concentrations fall, lipolysis liberates free fatty acids; these compete with glucose for cellular uptake and are used for the generation of energy by organs including muscle and the liver, thereby minimizing the requirement for glucose. Within the liver, fatty acids are converted to ketone bodies; unlike fatty acids, ketones gain access to the central nervous system and supply some energy to the brain, further reducing the requirement for gluconeogenesis. Thus, the wasting of muscle tissue is minimized. The amount of muscle tissue metabolized for the production of glucose is reduced from 75 g on day 3 to 20 g on day 40 of starvation. Nevertheless, tissue wasting, which progresses during the course of starvation, involves the respiratory muscles, the heart and the intestine, in addition to the adipose stores.

In the previously fit subject death from complete starvation occurs after the loss of 30–40% of the initial body weight, usually by 60–70 days, when organ impairment may be irreversible. In the hospital the rate of nutritional depletion is influenced by several factors. Many patients experience partial starvation when nutritional decline is slower, similar to the Minnesota experiment in which previously fit males were given a 1600 kcal diet for 12 weeks. Patients may receive a diet that is inadequate not only in the energy content but also in the range of nutrients. The historic view that the provision of carbohydrate without protein leads to Kwashiorkor, through increased insulin concentrations and the suppressed breakdown of muscle protein, thereby depriving the liver of amino acids for albumin synthesis, is no longer tenable. The deficiency of antioxidant micronutrients, in addition to the generation of cytokines, is the more likely cause of this nutritional disorder. Cytokines, small peptides, notably tumour necrosis factor and insulin-like growth factor-1 (IGF-1), which originate from lymphoid and haemopoietic cells in response to tissue damage, promote lipolysis and proteolysis.

Infections, burns and trauma, including surgical operations, lead to accelerated nutritional decline. Although this has been explained by a presumed increase in energy requirements in the stressed patient, and the humoral response to stress, most of the observed changes are attributable to the release of cytokines. Energy requirements in critical illness have previously been overestimated; any increased energy needs are often matched by a reduction in mobility. Cytokines such as interleukin, tumour necrosis factor

Table 8.1 Some examples of the metabolic effects of cytokines

- Anorexia
- Pyrexia
- Release of amino acids from muscle tissue
- Increased glucose transport
- Stimulation of hepatic lipid synthesis
- Promotion of acute-phase protein synthesis
- Reduced albumin synthesis
- Increased vascular permeability
- Immune cell availability

and interferons, which are principally responsible for the metabolic changes, share multiple activities, some of which are listed in Table 8.1. Furthermore, in severely ill patients, especially those in intensive care, the effect of the initial pathology may be compounded by the secondary effect of the breakdown in the gut mucosal barrier, with increased permeability to microbial toxins, and enhanced translocation of bacteria, continuing cytokine generation and leading to greater tissue and organ damage. Data to support the concept that such a breach of intestinal barrier function promotes the systemic inflammatory response in this manner have largely been derived from the animal model.

The diseases that are commonly associated with protein energy malnutrition include:

- any disorder that impairs the ingestion, digestion or absorption of food
- diseases associated with a prolonged inflammatory response
- diseases which cause an increased energy expenditure.

Some common examples are listed in Table 8.2. There are usually several factors leading to weight loss in each

patient. For example, the patient with chronic obstructive pulmonary disease may have difficulty eating because of dyspnoea and the effect of medication such as theophylline, chronic infection due to bronchiectasis, and increase in respiratory workload associated with airways obstruction.

Section 8.2 • Consequences of malnutrition

The syndrome of malnutrition is associated with a poor outcome in hospital patients. Prolonged hospital stay and increased morbidity and mortality have been documented in affected surgical patients who are at increased risk of infection and poor wound healing.

The adverse consequences of malnutrition stem from: (i) protein energy deficit; (ii) vitamin deficiencies; and (iii) deficiencies of trace elements.

Protein energy malnutrition

Malnutrition impairs organ function (Table 8.3). Mental function can be affected, and patients become withdrawn and apathetic. Malnourished patients are often reluctant to co-operate with their treatment. Muscles become weaker and fatigue more rapidly. These effects can be demonstrated in normal people during dietary restriction of only 2 weeks' duration. Not only may such changes affect the mobilization of patients after operative procedures and illness, they may also contribute to respiratory and cardiac failure.

There is a failure of antibody production and phagocyte function. Other aspects of the immune response may be impaired; thus, malnourished patients are at increased risk of infection. Thermoregulation is also defective and this may lead to hypothermia, especially in the elderly.

Children are particularly vulnerable to the effects of starvation, which results in growth failure. Protein energy malnutrition in children is associated with thymic atrophy and similar changes affect other lymphoid tissues.

Table 8.2 Some causes of disease-associated malnutrition

Anorexia	Depression
	Chronic disease
Inability to eat	Neurological disorders
	Oropharyngeal disease
	Oesophageal disease
	Gastric surgery/resection
Intestinal disease	Inflammatory bowel disease
	Radiation enteritis
	Gluten enteropathy
	Hollow visceral myopathy
Inflammatory response to infection/trauma	Intra-abdominal sepsis
	AIDS

Table 8.3 Some of the effects of protein energy malnutrition

Impaired mental function	Apathy
	Fatigue
	Inability to co-operate with treatment
Impaired muscle function	Respiratory failure
	Delayed mobilization
Impaired immune function	Increased incidence of infection

Table 8.4 Some examples of the roles of vitamins and the clinical effect of vitamin deficiencies

Vitamin	Biochemical function	Clinical features of deficiency
Vitamin A	Tissue growth and differentiation	Xerophthalmia, impaired dark adaptation
Vitamin D	Calcium absorption	Rickets in children, osteomalacia in adults
Vitamin E	Membrane antioxidant	Haemolytic anaemia, neuropathy, myopathy
Vitamin K	Synthesis of coagulation factors and osteocalcin	Coagulation defects, possible bone disease
Vitamin B_1, Thiamin	Decarboxylation in carbohydrate, fat and alcohol metabolism	Beri-beri: cardiac and neurological effects, Wernicke–Korsakov syndrome
Vitamin B_2, riboflavin	Oxidative metabolism	Lesions of the mouth and skin
Vitamin B_6, pyridoxine	Transamination of amino acids	Anaemia, lesions of the lips and skin
Vitamin B_{12}, cyanocobalamine	Recycling of folate coenzymes	Megaloblastic anaemia, demyelination
Vitamin C	Antioxidant, iron absorption, collagen synthesis	Impaired wound healing, scurvy
Biotin	Carboxylase reactions in lipogenesis and gluconeogenesis	Scaly dermatitis, hair loss
Folate	Purine and pyrimidine metabolism	Megaloblastic anaemia, growth retardation
Niacin	NAD/NADH in oxidative metabolism	Pellagra: rash, weakness and diarrhoea

Vitamin deficiencies

Some patients demonstrate features of specific nutrient deficiencies, in particular vitamin and trace element deficiencies. Examples of vitamin deficiencies include thiamin and Wernicke's encephalopathy, folate and megaloblastic anaemia, and ascorbic acid and scurvy. Thiamin has an important role in the metabolism of carbohydrates and alcohol. Patients who misuse alcohol and eat a poor diet are at particular risk of deficiency, which might be exposed by the use of a glucose infusion in the fasted hospital patient. Vitamin replacement should precede carbohydrate loading in such patients. Examples of the role of vitamins and the effects of vitamin deficiencies are summarized in Table 8.4.

Deficiencies of trace elements

Deficiencies of trace elements may also lead to specific features, e.g. zinc depletion is associated with skin rashes, impaired sense of taste and immune dysfunction, copper deficiency can cause a microcytic anaemia and selenium depletion leads to a myopathy, which also affects cardiac muscle (Table 8.5). Cardiomyopathy due to selenium depletion was identified as the cause of premature deaths in the Keshan province in China, where the soil content of selenium is very low. Other deficiencies became apparent when patients first received prolonged parenteral nutrition without adequate micronutrient supplementation.

Section 8.3 • Assessment of nutritional status

There is evidence that malnutrition is common in hospital patients and that nutritional status deteriorates during hospital stay. The nutritional status of the patient

Table 8.5 Some examples of the functions of trace elements and the clinical effects of deficiencies

Trace element	Biochemical function	Effect of deficiency
Chromium	Insulin activity, lipoprotein metabolism	Glucose intolerance, weight loss, peripheral neuropathy
Copper	Cytochrome oxidase, superoxide dismutase, encephalins	Hypochromic anaemia, neutropenia, cardiac dysrhythmia
Fluoride	Bone mineralization	Dental caries
Iodine	Thyroxine	Cretinism in children, hypothyroidism in adults
Iron	Haemoglobin myoglobin cytochrome system	Anaemia
Manganese	Mitochondrial superoxide dismutase	Lipid abnormalities, anaemia
Selenium	Glutathione peroxidase	Myopathy, pseudoalbinism
Zinc	Enzymes of intermediary metabolism and protein synthesis	Diarrhoea, skin rashes, immune deficiency, growth retardation

is not assessed in routine clinical practice and malnutrition is not recognized in the majority of affected patients. Thus, many patients do not receive appropriate nutritional management. Recognition of nutritional depletion is made difficult by the lack of suitable clinical indices of malnutrition and consequent functional impairment.

Malnutrition is identified after clinical assessment supported by anthropometric measurements and some laboratory investigations. An adequate history includes enquiry about the appetite and changes in the diet and the normal body weight. Examination may reveal evidence of muscle wasting as well as features of micronutrient deficiency, such as bruising, rash and glossitis.

Measurement of body composition

The traditional method of measuring body composition from body density determined by underwater weighing and the use of sophisticated techniques such as dual-energy X-ray absorptiometry (DEXA) are inappropriate or unavailable for routine clinical practice.

Anthropometric measurements

The measurements of weight and height are important. Fluctuation in body weight in the long term may reflect nutritional changes, and in the critically ill patient acute weight change is caused by changes in fluid balance. The measurement of height will determine growth velocity in the child, a sensitive marker of nutrition and disease. In the adult, knowledge of height and weight allows the calculation of the body mass index (BMI) from the weight (kg)/height (m)^2. The normal range for BMI is between 19 and 25. BMI values below 19 represent malnutrition, patients with a BMI in excess of 25 are overweight and those with values of 30 are described as obese.

Fasting in the patient who is not metabolically stressed leads to preferential mobilization of fat stores that are measured by skin-fold callipers. In the stressed patient proteolysis leads to muscle wasting measured by calculating the mid-arm muscle circumference (MAMC). The MAMC (cm) is derived from the mid-arm circumference – triceps skin-fold thickness × 0.314.

These measurements are useful for the identification of malnourished patients, monitoring patients who are at nutritional risk as well as those who are receiving long-term nutritional support. Variation in technique between observers and changes in the patient's hydration status can also influence the measurements. Furthermore, in relation to the effect of nutritional depletion and possible need for nutritional intervention, it is the change in nutritional status over time, rather than one single measurement, that is important. For example, a preoperative patient may have suffered from an involuntary weight loss of more than 10%, with an attendant increased risk of operative morbidity, yet still have a BMI within the normal range.

Bioelectrical impedance analysis (BIA)

BIA is a non-invasive method of assessment, which depends on the difference in electrical conductivity of fat and fat-free mass. The impedance of the body to an electrical current is measured, and is assumed to be proportional to the square of the height of the subject divided by the volume. The resistance between the right wrist and right ankle is measured and used to calculate the conductivity. From the impedance, total body fat and body water are calculated. However, the technique assumes a normal hydration state. This may not be the case in many patients, although there have been attempts to produce prediction equations for different disease states, including general surgical patients. Further validation is needed before this technique can be accepted into routine clinical practice.

Measurement of organ function

Malnutrition leads to impaired muscle strength and increased fatigability. The laboratory methods employed for these measurements using graded electrical stimuli are not suitable for clinical practice. Studies have shown that impaired muscle function can be reversed with nutritional support before improvement in clinical nutritional indices is observed. This observation led to the reappraisal of handgrip dynamometry (Figure 8.1). Handgrip dynamometry, determined by the highest value of three readings recorded with a dynamometer gripped in the non-dominant hand, will give a value that reflects nutritional state when compared with values standardized for age and gender. However other influences, notably the willingness of the patient to co-operate, reduce the specificity and thus the clinical usefulness of the technique. Tests of respiratory function have also been used for the determination of nutritional status. Unfortunately, the results are influenced by three variables: nutritional state, co-operation and pulmonary disease.

Malnutrition leads to anergy, with the loss of cutaneous responses to antigens traditionally determined by the Mantoux response. Many diseases have the same effect. The total lymphocyte count is depressed in malnutrition and has been used to monitor nutritional support. These measurements are little used in this context.

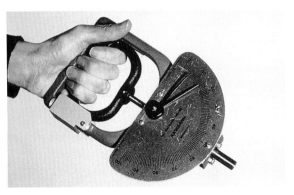

Figure 8.1 Handgrip dynamometer.

Laboratory investigations

Protein calorie malnutrition causes a decrease in the rate of albumin synthesis. Traditionally, the serum albumin concentration has been advocated as a nutritional marker. Whereas there is evidence to support the use of albumin as a prognostic indicator, in that patients with low serum albumin values have prolonged hospital stay and increased morbidity and mortality, albumin correlates poorly with nutritional status. In the Minnesota experiment the total circulating albumin was reduced by only 2% after 24 weeks of reduced protein and energy intake. This was associated with a 10% reduction in serum albumin concentrations, which may have reflected other influences.

Children with marasmus and adults with anorexia nervosa maintain serum albumin concentrations until the terminal stages of their illness. Conversely, in well-nourished patients who become septic the albumin concentrations fall rapidly, reflecting changes in vascular permeability and fluid retention, as well as a reduction in albumin synthesis caused by the influence of the cytokine responses to infection or tissue damage.

Albumin has a very long half-life of 21 days. Consequently, other proteins have been advocated for diagnosis and nutritional monitoring. They include transferrin, thyroxin-binding prealbumin and retinol-binding protein, with respective half-lives of 8 days, 2 days and 12 h. These are also influenced by other factors, such as the iron and vitamin A status, and the acute-phase response. The insulin-like growth factors are a family of low-molecular-weight peptides produced by the liver. Studies have suggested that IGF-1, which has a half-life of a few hours, may be a useful marker of nutritional status. Reduced serum concentration may reflect a general decrease in protein synthesis with malnutrition and, unlike the other factors, it is thought not to be influenced by the acute-phase response. Currently, this is an expensive assay that requires further validation to define any role in clinical practice.

Clearly, there is no single laboratory marker of nutritional status. However, the laboratory has an important role in the identification of single nutrient deficiencies. The serum values of iron, calcium, magnesium and potassium are commonly measured, along with vitamins such as folic acid, vitamin B_{12} and 25-hydroxy-vitamin D, as a guide to replacement during nutritional support, in depleted patients, and in specific disorders of absorption. The measurement of other micronutrients, such as selenium, copper, chromium and manganese, is usually only available in supraregional laboratories. This information is required in severely depleted patients who are receiving prolonged nutritional support, including patients treated by home parenteral nutrition. There is often difficulty in interpretation, blood values do not necessarily correlate with body content and serum values may fall in the context of an acute illness.

Section 8.4 • Principles of artificial nutrition support

Artificial nutrition support (ANS) may be employed to prevent starvation or to treat malnutrition in patients who are unable to eat or to digest and absorb sufficient nutrients. The potential role of ANS in modifying the inflammatory and immune responses to disease through the provision of specific nutrient substrates – 'immunonutrition' – is currently under evaluation.

The need for ANS should be recognized early because impaired organ function can be demonstrated within 2 weeks of starvation, the restoration of nutritional status in the depleted patient is a prolonged process and nutritional repletion may not be achieved in the context of significant illness.

ANS may be delivered by the enteral route by oral supplements or enteral tube feeding, or intravenously by parenteral nutrition. Enteral nutrition should be employed wherever possible; it is cheaper, safer and more physiological than parenteral feeding. The intestine has an important immune and barrier function. Luminal nutrition appears to be important for the stimulation of gastrointestinal motility, secretory IgA and the integrity of the mucosal barrier. Glutamine and short-chain fatty acids are important substrates for the enterocyte and colonocyte, respectively; they are not given in standard parenteral nutrition.

Nutritional requirements depend on the nutritional status of the patient, the nature of the underlying disease and the adequacy of organ function. Any nutrition derived from the oral diet must also be taken into consideration and during enteral feeding the effect of intestinal impairment on energy needs should be considered. In patients who are malnourished some allowance is needed for nutritional repletion, unless the patient is metabolically stressed as a result of sepsis or trauma. The aim in these patients is to maintain nutritional status or minimize tissue loss; repletion is achieved during the recovery phase of the illness. Initial hypocaloric feeding should be considered in patients who are severely wasted to minimize the risk of the refeeding syndrome (see below).

There is no satisfactory bedside method for the measurement of energy requirements. Approximate values can be estimated from the Schofield equation and adjusted for stress, activity and desired energy balance to reflect nutritional status. For the majority of patients 25–35 kcal and 0.2 g nitrogen/kg is sufficient; as a rule, provision should not exceed 40 kcal and 0.3 g nitrogen/kg in the adult. Some patients in the intensive care unit receive lipid energy through medication with Propofol, which must be considered when calculating energy needs. The previous views about large energy needs were based on inaccurate methodology; furthermore, it would seem that any increased energy needs associated with illness are balanced by a reduction in energy expenditure through reduced mobility. Excess nutrient delivery leads to futile cycling with lipogenesis, increased production of carbon dioxide, and the consequences of hyperglycaemia and hyperlipidaemia. Cyclical feeding, in which there is an interval free of infusion, has physiological advantages. In comparison with continuous feeding it reduces sodium and water retention, and it may also lead to less fat accretion by avoiding the continuous stimulation of insulin.

Some patients with intestinal disease are able to maintain energy and nitrogen balance, but not electrolyte balance. Patients with Crohn's disease frequently develop hypomagnesaemia, and patients with a high jejunostomy become salt and water depleted. This reflects the leaky junctions in the jejunal epithelium, which allow sodium to pass into the intestinal lumen down a concentration gradient. Such patients need additional fluids and electrolytes. Some can be managed satisfactorily with isotonic solutions of sodium and carbohydrate, in which the sodium concentration is approximately 100 mmol/l, provided they avoid drinking hypotonic solutions without sodium, which increase the stomal losses. However, parenteral administration may be required.

Most of the enteral feeds contain the average daily recommended requirement of micronutrients, vitamins and trace elements in a volume of 2 litres. Some commercial trace element and vitamin preparations are compounded with the other nutrients, amino acids, glucose, lipids and electrolytes, for parenteral nutrition. The need for additional supplements in depleted patients should be considered. For example, malnourished alcoholic patients will need additional thiamin, while very malnourished patients who receive nutritional support may require additional phosphate, potassium and magnesium. Electrolyte requirements are also influenced by the administration of drugs such as amphoteracin, which can increase the renal excretion of potassium and magnesium, and the presence of impaired organ function, including liver cardiac and renal disease. Under these circumstances the parenteral prescription will need adjustment or special enteral products may be used (see below).

Section 8.5 • Enteral nutrition

Oral supplements

When used correctly and taken between meals, oral supplements can substantially increase nutrient intake without reducing the consumption of the oral diet.

Supplements are useful in anorectic patients and patients with dysphagia pending treatment of oesophageal disease. They have also been shown to reduce morbidity in elderly patients with fracture of the neck or femur, and following abdominal surgery.

Most supplements are milk based, while some are based on soya protein and are fruit flavoured. Not all are nutritionally complete in relation to micronutrients. A complete supplement should be prescribed if it comprises a substantial proportion of the nutritional intake. The dietician selects the product according to the taste preferences of the patient. Nevertheless, compliance remains a problem, especially in patients with malignant disease.

Enteral tube feeding

Indications
Enteral tube feeding is needed in:

- patients with profound anorexia
- patients who are unable to eat or swallow
- some patients with impaired intestinal function.

Anorexia may be a feature of many diseases. Such patients are unable or unwilling to ingest sufficient food or supplements. However, after the initiation of enteral feeding the appetite frequently improves. Oropharyngeal disease, cerebrovascular disease and motor neuron disease are common indications for tube feeding. Tube feeding may also be useful in the postoperative or critically ill patient with gastric paresis, when jejunal feeding may need to be combined with gastric aspiration. Supplemental nocturnal tube feeding is a useful method of exploiting the residual intestinal function in patients with Crohn's disease and to increase nutrient intake in patients with cystic fibrosis.

Intestinal access
Access to the intestine will depend on the duration of feeding and gastric function. In the short term and in critically ill patients, fine-bore nasal tubes are convenient. In the long term and for the mobile patient, percutaneous tubes are more suitable. Patients with disease of the oesophagus, impaired gastric function and recent surgery to the upper alimentary tract will need access to the jejunum. The routes of access are summarized in Table 8.6.

There is increasing use of percutaneous endoscopic gastrostomies (PEG) in patients with chronic neuro-

Table 8.6 Intestinal access for enteral tube feeding

Route of entry	Tip position	Method of placement
Nasal	Nasogastric	Patient or nurse
	Nasojejunal	Endoscopist or surgeon
Percutaneous	Percutaneous gastrostomy	Endoscopist, radiologist or surgeon
	Percutaneous gastrojejunostomy	Endoscopist
	Percutaneous jejunostomy	Surgeon or endoscopist

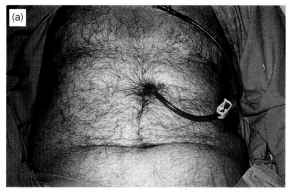

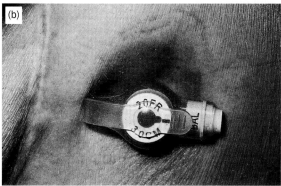

Figure 8.2 (a) Percutaneous endoscopic gastrostomy (PEG); (b) button gastrostomy.

logical disease; once the track has formed the PEG tube can be replaced with a button gastrostomy (Figure 8.2), which is more convenient for the mobile patient. The use of jejunostomy tubes following oesophagogastric surgery can avoid the need for the more expensive and hazardous option of parenteral nutrition.

Nutrient solutions

A wide range of nutrient solutions is available for enteral tube feeding and the types of feed are summarized in Table 8.7.

The cheaper whole-protein polymeric diets are preferred for the majority of patients. They comprise whole protein, hydrolysates of starch and long-chain triglycerides (LCT). LCT contains linoleic acid, which is metabolized to arachidonic acid, the precursor of series 2 prostanoids and series 4 leukotrienes that induce inflammation and increase immunosuppression. In contrast, the omega-3 fatty acids lead to the production of series 3 prostanoids and series 5 leukotrienes

Table 8.7 Types of enteral feed solution

- Oral dietary supplements
- Polymeric feeds
- Predigested chemically defined
- Specialized diets
- Disease-specific feeds

that have anti-inflammatory and immune-enhancing effects. Some special diets are now available that contain omega-3 fats and additional glutamine. Clinical benefit has been demonstrated in the context of burn injury. Other special diets have a reduced sodium content and are useful in some patients with sodium retention associated with cardiac and liver disease.

Chemically defined diets contain peptides instead of whole protein, and some also contain medium-chain triglycerides. They are used to promote absorption in patients with severe intestinal disease. Disease-specific diets include formulae enriched in branched-chain amino acids for patients with portal systemic encephalopathy due to liver disease, and diets in which a large proportion of the non-protein energy is supplied as lipid for patients with respiratory failure. The clinical evidence to support the use of these disease-specific products is not very convincing.

Nutrient delivery

The need to deliver the nutrient solution at the appropriate rate and to avoid bacterial contamination by the use of clean procedures merits emphasis. Infusion is commenced at 50 ml/h and increased, according to tolerance, to 100 ml/h in the majority of patients who are receiving gastric tube feeding. An initial rate of 25 ml/h may be preferred for critically ill patients, and when initiating feeding in the postoperative patient via a nasojejunal tube. Conversely, flow rates of up to 180 ml/h may be employed in some patients who are receiving enteral tube feeding at home.

Enteral feeding is given by enteral pump infusion, rather than bolus feeding, which is associated with increased gastrointestinal intolerance. When gastric feeding is considered and gastric motility is in question gastric residual volumes are measured. Volumes of up to 400 ml in the critically ill patient do not necessarily preclude gastric feeding, but the volumes should be checked 2 h after initiating the infusion. This is not necessary with postpyloric feeding. The feeding is given overnight or for longer periods. One further theoretical advantage is that it allows the gastric pH to fall when the buffering effect of the infusion is withdrawn, thus minimizing the tendency to gastric colonization, which might be a factor in the development of infection.

Contamination of the enteral feed should be avoided by the use of a commercial feed, selection of an appropriate reservoir and giving set, and the observance of a protocol when administering the feed. Episodes of infection in the critically ill have been directly related to enteral feeds, and there is the risk of infection with specific intestinal pathogens such as *Salmonella* sp., bacterial translocation in the presence of impaired intestinal and immune function, and bacterial overgrowth, which reduces the efficiency of the feed.

Complications

The complications of enteral feeding can be considered in three groups:

- nutritional and metabolic
- complications of nutrient delivery
- gastrointestinal complications.

Patients require monitoring with respect to fluid and electrolyte status, biochemical parameters and nutritional progress. In particular, fluid retention and electrolyte balance may require attention; hyperglycaemia and hyperkalaemia may be encountered in diabetic subjects and patients with renal impairment. Hypophosphataemia may occur during the refeeding syndrome in the severely malnourished patient. If it is not recognized, the patient may present with thrombocytopenia, cardiac dysrhythmia and mental confusion. Hyomagnesaemia and hypokalaemia are other features of this syndrome, which may reflect rapid cellular uptake with the switch of energy source from endogenous lipid in the starving patient to exogenous carbohydrate. Thiamin deficiency precipitated by glucose infusion represents another example of this problem and is especially relevant in the alcoholic subject.

Complications of delivery are common, especially with nasogastric tubes. More than half of these tubes become displaced and there is a risk of incorrect positioning with the tube in the bronchial tree. Pulmonary aspiration occurs with too rapid infusion or impaired gastric emptying. Complications of the percutaneous tubes include the complications of placement, peritonitis if there is a leak of feed or intestinal contents through the incorrect appositioning of the alimentary tract and the abdominal wall at the site of the tube, and stomal infection.

Diarrhoea is a common problem. Possible causes include bacterial infection of the feed, concomitant antibiotic administration and hypoalbuminaemia. Continuous intragastric infusion of feed has been shown to cause a secretary response in the ascending colon, which is thought to reflect the absence of a normal cephalic phase in tube feeding with an absence of the normal stimulated postprandial peptide YY response. This colonic secretion can be overcome by the instillation of short-chain fats in the caecum; these are normally produced by the action of anaerobic bacteria on dietary fibre. This provides a rationale for the use of fibre-containing feeds and one explanation for the association of antibiotics with diarrhoea. The use of intermittent feeding may allow the gastric pH to fall when the buffering effect of the feed is withdrawn for a period. This may be helpful in reducing gastric and consequently intestinal bacterial colonization, although adequate data to support this suggestion are lacking. Nevertheless, intermittent feeding will minimize fluid and fat accretion in comparison with continuous feeding owing to the effect on insulin secretion.

Section 8.6 • Parenteral nutrition

The term total parenteral nutrition is frequently used. This implies that the complete range of nutrients is being administered by the parenteral route, which is normally the case, and that nutrition is being delivered exclusively by vein, which is often not the case. Consequently, the term parenteral nutrition is preferred. Parenteral nutrition is often employed to supplement enteral nutrition when there is limited intestinal tolerance or function.

Indications

Examples of common indications for short-term and long-term parenteral nutrition are given in Tables 8.8 and 8.9.

In the majority of these patients parenteral nutrition will be supplemental. Whereas many patients with wasting due to acquired immunodeficiency syndrome (AIDS) have been treated with long-term parenteral nutrition, there is minimal evidence of benefit. Patients with untreatable cancer should only be considered for parenteral nutrition if they are not terminally ill and when the problem is due to untreatable intestinal obstruction and not simply cachexia.

Venous access

The realization that nutrient needs are less than they were previously considered to be, the recognition that most patients receive parenteral nutrition in hospital for less than 2 weeks and the availability of lipid-containing nutrient mixes have led to the use of peripheral veins for the administration of parenteral nutrition. Access may

Table 8.8 Some indications for short-term parenteral nutrition

- Severe inflammatory bowel disease
- Mucositis following chemotherapy
- Severe acute pancreatitis
- Some patients with multiorgan failure
- Following major excisional surgery
- Prior to major surgery in malnourished subjects

Table 8.9 Some causes of intestinal failure in adults, for which prolonged parenteral nutrition may be needed

Inflammatory disease	Crohn's disease
	Gluten enteropathy
	Radiation enteritis
Motility disorders	Hollow visceral myopathy
	Scleroderma
Short bowel syndrome	Mesenteric infarction
	Crohn's disease
Miscellaneous disorders	Inoperable intestinal obstruction
	AIDS

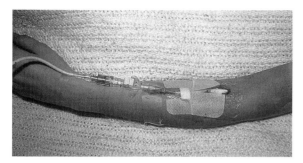

Figure 8.3 Peripheral feeding catheter with Interlink connection device.

be by conventional venflon, which should be resited every 1–2 days before thrombophlebitis occurs, or 15-cm ultrafine catheters, which are inserted in one of the antecubital veins (Figure 8.3). The peripheral line should be reserved exclusively for the administration of nutrition and it requires the same standard of care as a central line. Under these circumstances peripheral access will last for 2 weeks or longer.

Central parenteral nutrition is needed when prolonged treatment is envisaged, there are unusual nutritional requirements with volume restriction and a hyperosmolar solution, or in the absence of adequate peripheral veins. Central access is normally via tunnelled central catheters. For mobile patients and long-term treatment of more than 2 months, cuffed catheters are preferred (Figure 8.4). Some of the latter patients who need home parenteral nutrition may favour an implanted subcutaneous port. More recently, the peripherally inserted central catheter has gained popularity. Central catheters should be placed with the tip in the distal superior vena cava, but not in the right atrium.

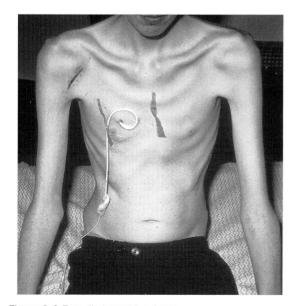

Figure 8.4 Tunnelled central catheter.

All access devices must be managed by staff trained in aseptic procedures following written protocols. This is the only way to ensure the prevention of dangerous and avoidable complications such as catheter-related sepsis.

Nutrients

The nutrients are compounded in a multilayer plastic bag under sterile conditions in the pharmacy. The needs of the majority of patients can be met from a range of standard nutrition solutions. Commonly used parenteral solutions provide 9 or 14 g of nitrogen as amino acids, and 1600 or 2200 non-protein calories as glucose and lipid in 2.5–3.0 litres of water, with 80 mmol of sodium and 60 mmol of potassium. Calcium, magnesium and phosphate are also included, as are commercial preparations of vitamins and trace elements. These provide the currently recommended daily requirements of micronutrients. The need for additional supplements should be considered in patients who are severely depleted when parenteral nutrition is initiated, and in those patients who do not receive a nutrient bag every day. Some patients, especially those with Crohn's disease, have suffered from selenium depletion. Conversely, it used to be thought that more manganese is absorbed from the diet than is the case. This led to the formulation of preparations that supplied too much manganese for intravenous administration. Such problems are more common in patients who receive parenteral nutrition at home.

The most common adjustments to the nutrient prescription include fluid and electrolytes in patients with increased losses, or reduced tolerance with renal impairment. Considerations of lipid stability limit the addition of electrolytes, especially divalent ions. A separate electrolyte infusion is sometimes needed.

Nutrient delivery

The nutrients are delivered via an infusion pump. As with enteral nutrition, cyclical feeding is preferred in the stable patient, but continuous infusion may be required in the stressed patient. Cyclical infusions facilitate mobilization, and are associated with less fluid retention and fat deposition. Catheter patency is maintained with a heparin lock when the patient is disconnected from the infusion.

All catheter procedures must be undertaken according to strict aseptic protocols to minimize the risk of complications.

Complications

Complications of parenteral nutrition may be considered in three groups:

- nutritional and metabolic
- catheter-related
- effect on other organ systems.

Nutritional and metabolic complications

Fluid overload, hyperglycaemia and electrolyte imbalance are common potential problems, especially in unstable patients. Patients who are severely malnourished may suffer from the refeeding syndrome (see above). Additional electrolytes may need to be given to some patients; this applies particularly to phosphate, potassium and magnesium. Stressed patients are prone to hyperglycaemia so some of the energy should be provided as lipid and insulin may be needed. Rebound hypoglycaemia can occur after discontinuing the infusion of concentrated glucose solutions until endogenous insulin levels fall. Tapering the rate of infusion before disconnection minimizes this problem.

Long-term patients who receive little nutrition from other sources are at risk of micronutrient deficiencies. Whereas the profile of commercially available trace element solutions has been changed to cover previous deficiencies such as selenium, it is worth remembering that amounts delivered in each nutrition bag are designed to meet estimated daily needs. Thus, patients with initial depletion or who do not require a nutrition bag every day (this applies to many of the patients who receive parenteral nutrition at home) are at risk of deficiency and monitoring is important. The excessive accumulation of aluminium from protein hydrolysates and manganese from incorrectly formulated trace element solutions, leading to bone and neurological disease, respectively, should no longer occur.

The overprovision of macronutrients such as glucose and amino acids is harmful. Excess glucose will lead to hepatic steatosis and is accompanied by increased respiratory demands and the stimulation of the sympathetic nervous system. The excessive administration of amino acids has been associated with cholestasis in paediatric practice and possible alterations in bone metabolism.

Catheter-related complications

Complications associated with catheter insertion are common. They include pneumothorax, damage to adjacent vascular structures and incorrect positioning of the catheter tip. Placement with the aid of screening is important and the use of ultrasound is helpful in minimizing these risks. After correct placement there are four important catheter-related complications:

- infection
- thrombosis
- occlusion
- fracture.

Catheter-related infection

Three types of infection can be recognized: exit-site infection, tunnel infection and catheter-related septicaemia (CRS).

Exit-site infections usually respond to local dressing complemented by systemic antibiotic therapy. However, clearance will not be successful if there is a Dacron cuff, which lies adjacent to the exit site (rather than half way along the tunnel) when it becomes contaminated. **Infection of the tunnel**, which can complicate exit-site infection, is characterized by pain and redness; it does not respond to treatment and is an indication for catheter removal. Rarely, tunnel infections may arise from retrograde spread of infection from an infected central vein. This is a very serious problem, which reflects previous inadequately treated catheter-related sepsis.

Catheter-related septicaemia is the most serious infection and can be fatal. In the short term, microbes may gain access from the exit site, but after 2 weeks the hub is the most common site of contamination. The problem is usually heralded by pyrexia and rigors during infusion. Diagnosis can be difficult, especially in patients with other sources of sepsis; there may also be other reasons for pyrexia, and these include venous thrombosis. When this complication is suspected, catheter removal is the safest course of action. However, if venous access is difficult and the need for continuing central parenteral nutrition is anticipated, drawback and peripheral blood cultures should be obtained. Semiquantitative cultures have been used to implicate the line as the primary source of infection; however, the use of the endoluminal brush promises more precise and reliable information. While awaiting the results of culture, the central catheter should be locked and the patient is given systemic antimicrobial cover against the most likely infecting organisms; vancomycin and gentamicin is a suitable regime in the short term. Catheter salvage is possible using antibiotic and urokinase locks. There are insufficient data to recommend specific guidelines in relation to the dose of urokinase and type of antibiotic. One approach involves the insertion of a 2000 U/ml urokinase lock for 1 h before the infusion of antibiotics; pending the results of blood cultures, vancomycin and gentamicin administered twice a day cover likely pathogens, although blood antibiotic concentrations should be monitored. The antibiotic prescription may need to change according to microbiological results. Salvage should not be attempted when *Candida* and *Staphylococcus aureus* infections are identified: it is unlikely to succeed with subcutaneous ports, and the potential risk of recrudescence and metastatic infection, including endocarditis and osteomyelitis, should be considered.

The emphasis must be on prevention. The development of catheter care protocols and management by nutrition support teams has almost eliminated the problem. The use of antimicrobial agents as additives in the nutrient solution cannot be recommended for routine practice and requires further study, but may help in the management of the difficult patient who is prone to recurrent infection.

Central vein thrombosis

Central vein thrombosis tends to develop after treatment for a few weeks (Figure 8.5). It may be heralded by pyrexia, pulmonary embolism, subclavian vein thrombosis or occlusion of the superior vena cava with facial swelling. This is a serious problem, which impairs venous access and can prove fatal.

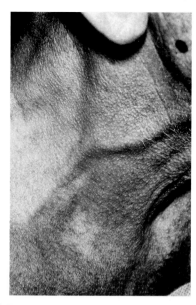

Figure 8.5 Venous thrombosis associated with central parenteral nutrition.

The diagnosis should be confirmed by bilateral upper limb venography. Rarely in adult practice does the thrombus involve the heart; however, if any new cardiac murmur is heard transoesophageal echocardiography is recommended.

Thrombosis accompanies the use of concentrated glucose regimens and a proximal location of the catheter tip in the superior vena cava; thrombotic tendency is reduced by the administration of lipid emulsions. Patients with coagulation disorders such as antithrombin III deficiency and patients with Crohn's disease are more likely to develop this problem.

Treatment with thrombolytic drugs such as streptokinase is effective in restoring venous patency. Streptokinase is infused for 48 h, when repeat venography will usually demonstrate recanalization. The patient is then given heparin and ultimately warfarin. There is a theoretical risk of inducing pulmonary embolism from fragmented thrombi. The use of heparin alone does not lead to significant recanalization in the short term.

Many authorities use heparin in the nutrient solution as a prophylactic measure. Evidence suggests that there is a need for at least 3 units of heparin per millilitre of feed solution, although the possible effect on the stability of the emulsion must be considered. There is insufficient evidence to support the routine use of heparin in all patients. Low-dose warfarin may be an effective alternative, notwithstanding interactions between warfarin and the vitamin K derivatives, which occur in the lipid emulsions. The need for prophylaxis will depend on individual circumstances. For example, prophylaxis will be required in patients with a thrombotic disorder and in patients who have already developed venous thrombosis. Conversely, anticoagulation is unwise in some patients with active inflammatory disease in whom there is a significant risk of bleeding.

Catheter occlusion

Catheter occlusion may be due to kinking or luminal deposition of fibrin, lipid sludge or amorphous debris. This is a particular problem with lipid mixes, the tendency to which may be reduced by the use of an ethanol flush before the application of the heparin lock.

When occlusion occurs a chest X-ray should be obtained. Providing the position of the catheter is satisfactory, attempts at line salvage can be considered. When there is evidence for fibrin occlusion, after blood flashback or with a fibrin sleeve, urokinase can be used to clear the catheter. Streptokinase is reserved for the management of serious central vein thrombosis to avoid sensitizing the patient. When occlusion develops with the use of lipid mixes, an ethanol lock may restore the patency of an incompletely occluded catheter.

Catheter damage

The use of connection devices or extension sets reduces the need to clamp the catheter and prolongs catheter life. Repair kits are available if fracture occurs. Subcutaneous ports eventually leak. This becomes apparent when the patient complains of pain around the infusion site. New ports can be attached to the existing catheter.

Effect of parenteral nutrition on other organ systems

Parenteral nutrition may affect the hepatobiliary system, the immune system and the skeleton. Any theoretical detrimental effect must be weighed against the known impairment of organ function associated with the malnutrition that this treatment seeks to prevent or reverse.

Changes in organ function may be a reflection of the underlying disease, malnutrition, drug treatment and lack of oral or enteral nutrition, as well as the effect of parenteral nutrition. The development of hepatobiliary disease in patients who are treated with prolonged parenteral nutrition illustrates this point. Some forms of hepatobiliary disease occur more commonly in patients with inflammatory bowel disease; the lack of oral nutrition leads to biliary sludge and possible changes in intestinal permeability with toxin absorption. The administration of excessive amounts of glucose may cause hepatic steatosis and in neonatal patients the excessive prescription of amino acids has been incriminated in the development of cholestasis. Metabolic bone disease in some patients is attributable to previous malnutrition and exposure to corticosteroid therapy. The influence of parenteral nutrition on bone metabolism is controversial.

Catheter complications can cause serious disease in other systems. Endocarditis and osteomyelitis have been described following catheter-related sepsis, and pulmonary embolism can complicate central vein thrombosis. With due care and the observance of good written protocols parenteral nutrition is relatively safe, and is life saving for a significant group of patients with short- or long-term intestinal failure.

Guide to further reading

Heatley, R.V., Green, J. H. and Losowsky, M. S., eds (1994). *Consensus in Clinical Nutrition*. Cambridge University Press, Cambridge.

Payne, J. J., Grimble, G. and Silk, D., eds (1995). *Artificial Nutrition Support in Clinical Practice*. Edward Arnold, London.

Pennington, C. R. (1997). Disease and malnutrition in British hospitals. *Proc Nutr Soc* **56**: 393–407.

Rombeau, J. L. and Rolandelli, R. H., eds (1997). *Clinical Nutrition: Enteral and Tube Feeding*. W.B. Saunders, Philadelphia, PA.

Rombeau, J. L. and Caldwell, M. D. (1993) *Clinical Nutrition: Parenteral Nutrition*, 2nd edn. W.B. Saunders, Philadelphia, PA.

MODULE 9

Obese patients

1 • Body mass index

2 • Diseases associated with obesity

3 • Medical management of obesity

4 • Surgical management of morbid obesity

'Imprisoned in every fat man, a thin one is wildly signalling to be let out' – Cyril Connolly (1903–1974), *The Unquiet Grave.*

Section 9.1 • Body mass index

'Overweight' and 'obesity' are terms often used to describe individuals with an increased body fat. Measuring fat accurately in humans requires specialist equipment and so usually excess weight is defined by measuring the body mass index (BMI).

BMI is calculated by measuring a person's weight in kg and then dividing by that person's height in metres squared (kg/m^2).

For example, an adult weighing 90 kg with a height of 1.80 m has a BMI of $90/1.80^2 = 27.8$ kg/m^2.

The advantage of BMI as an index rather than the use of weight alone is that BMI takes into account height, such that small and tall people of similar proportions but differing height have similar BMI. There are individual cases where this index can fail, such as a muscular body builder whose raised BMI is due not to fat excess but to muscular tissue. However, overall there is a good correlation between BMI and body fat.

The internationally accepted range of BMI in **adults** is as follows:

	BMI	WHO classification
Acceptable range	18.5–24.9	
Overweight	25.0–29.9	Grade 1 overweight
Obese	30.0–39.9	Grade 2 overweight
Morbid obese	≥40	Grade 3 overweight

Occasionally, one might read the term ideal body weight (IBW), which is defined as 100%, with overweight then defined as 101–119% and obese as 120% or greater above ideal.

For **children,** weight excess may also be classified according to the BMI. The BMI of each child is compared to standardized reference curves of BMI against age. A child whose BMI is above the 99.6 percentile for age is usually considered overweight and requires remedial action. Nevertheless, the child with a BMI 98–99.6% might also have a weight problem, but in certain individuals, such as boys who are stocky and muscular, the BMI may appear in the 'high' range and yet not be indicative of excess fat. This makes the BMI in children far less reliable as an indicator of excess fat that in adults.

Body fat measurement

Body fat may be measured using a number of techniques.

- The simplest method is to use BMI and age fitted into the **Deurenberg formula**:

Body fat % = 1.2 (BMI) + 0.23 (age in years) − 10.8 (1 = male; 0 = female) − 5.4

Example for a 40-year-old man of BMI 36:

Body fat = 1.2 (36) + 0.23 (40) − 10.8 (1) − 5.4 = 36.2%

The Deurenberg formula accounts for 80% of the variation in body fat between individuals and indicates that one becomes fatter with age and that women have 10% more fat than men.

- Another simple method involves measuring **skinfold thickness** at four sites (biceps, triceps, subscapular and suprailiac) using a spring-loaded calliper. The values are then applied to published equations to calculate body fat.
- More accurate methods employ **underwater weighing** or the isotopic measurement of **whole body potassium** content, which is an index of lean (non-fat) mass, but both methods require complex equipment not found except in specialized units.
- A more readily available method is that of **impedance analysis**. This depends on the difference in electrical resistance between lean tissue and fat, which are good and poor conductors, respectively. A weak current is applied across the body and the resistance measured between two electrodes from which the lean and fat mass can be calculated using published equations. The range of body fat content of a normal adult is 10–20% in men and 20–30% in women.

Abdominal fat can be measured using:

- **computed tomographic (CT) or magnetic resonance imaging (MRI)** scans of the abdomen
- the easier and inexpensive method of measuring the **sagittal diameter** (i.e. front to back) across the abdomen at the level of lumbar vertebrae 4/5 using special callipers and then to apply appropriate equations. This technique equals the accuracy of a single-slice CT scan at the same level.

Body fat distribution

Two types of fat distribution are recognized in adult obesity:

- some adults store their fat mainly around the hips and thighs, giving them a 'pear' shape known as **gynoid** distribution, as this is characteristic of women
- the second type is the storage of fat primarily in the abdomen, producing an 'apple' shape known as **android** distribution. This latter abdominal distribution of fat may also be seen in overweight but non-obese people and is important to document as it is more closely related to disease risk than the BMI alone.

To check for abdominal obesity the **waist:hip ratio** is measured. This ratio is derived from the waist circumference divided by the hip circumference, both in centimetres. The waist circumference is usually measured halfway between the superior iliac crest and the rib cage in the mid-axillary line, whereas the hip circumference is measured one-third of the distance between the superior iliac spine and the patella. The disease risks associated with abdominal obesity, described in detail in the next section, include hypertension, hyperlipidaemia, hyperuricaemia, diabetes mellitus and cardiovascular diseases, which as a group some have named as the Reaven's syndrome. Abdominal obesity is a risk to health if the waist:hip ratio is > 0.95 in males or > 0.8 in females.

Recently, research has indicated that measurement of **waist circumference** alone might suffice to define disease risk of intra-abdominal fat as follows:

	Increased risk	**Substantial risk**
Men	≥94 cm	≥102 cm
	(= 37 inches)	(= 40 inches)
Women	≥80 cm	≥88 cm
	(= 32 inches)	(= 35 inches)

Aetiology of obesity

Excess weight in the population appears to depend on certain factors:

- **familial and genetic predisposition** play a role in weight gain. There is a number of known genetic conditions, which produce a syndrome complex associated with obesity. The best known is Prader–Willi syndrome, which is associated with deletions on chromosome 15, resulting in excessive appetite. Such are rarities and have little relevance to the causation of obesity in the general population. Studies on families with obesity have implicated over 20 genes on at least 12 chromosomes, emphasizing the polygenic influence on the development of obesity. The contribution to weight gain of transmission in susceptible families ranges from 25 to 40%, with the heritable determination of selective intra-abdominal fat deposition being greater at 30–50%. This transmission is derived from both the maternal and paternal lines, with an accumulative influence down the generations such that the progeny are more obese than their parents if they are also obese
- **certain drugs** may contribute to weight gain, such as corticosteroids, tricyclic antidepressants, sulfonylureas for diabetes, some steroidal contraceptives and valproate used in epileptic therapy
- **defined endocrine causes** are rare, probably accounting for less than 1% of all weight gain in the population. Cushing's syndrome due to excess corticosteroid production causes substantial weight gain, especially in the abdominal region. Some hypothalamic tumours such as craniopharyngiomas are associated with development of obesity, whereas hypothyroidism causes weight gain, possibly by reducing the metabolic rate
- **age**: weight increases with age at least up to 60 years and may be related to declining physical activity (see below)
- **gender**: women have a higher prevalence of excess weight than men, especially when older than 50 years
- **ethnicity**: some groups have a high prevalence, such as Pima Indians and Naurians
- **education and income**: in industrialized countries there is a higher prevalence in those with less education and/or low income
- **parity**: on average, weight increases by 1 kg per pregnancy
- **fat intake**: prevalence is higher in those on high-fat intake, especially in those snacking on energy-dense foods, which are often high in fat and sugar but low in bulk
- **alcohol**: moderate consumption may be associated with excess weight as it provides substantial caloric energy
- **smoking**: cessation increases weight. The average weight gain is 2.8 kg in males and 3.8 kg in females; nevertheless, the risk for health of continued smoking is so substantial that a rise in weight of 11 kg would be required to negate the benefit of giving up smoking 20 cigarettes/day
- **physical activity**: declining physical activity predisposes to weight gain, such as sedentary jobs and certain pastimes (e.g. watching television and computer games). Decreasing activity with age can be as much as 700 kcal (2.9 MJ)/day for the sports-keen young man compared with the inactive retired person of 65 years.

Prevalence of obesity

The proportion of the population in the UK with obesity has doubled since 1980. In 1980 some 6% of men and 8% of women had a BMI of 30 or greater, whereas by 1993 these figures were 13% in males and 16% in females.

The **prevalence** of excess weight in the **UK adult** population is as follows:

	Overweight	Obese	Total with excess weight
Men	44%	14%	58%
Women	32%	17%	49%

Other **European countries** have a greater problem, especially in women, with a prevalence of obesity in females of 30% in southern Italy (18% in males), 32% in Poland (13%), 19.3% in the former West Germany (17.2%), 26.8% in East Germany (20.5%) and 44% in Russia (13%). The **USA** has a prevalence of obesity in females of 24.7% (1994) and 19.7% in males. Prevalence is lower in The Netherlands (8.3% in females and males) and in Finland (11% females, 14% males).

Section 9.2 • Diseases associated with obesity

Mortality and morbidity

Mortality

There is now extensive evidence that links excessive body weight with overall mortality. This is well illustrated by the prospective Nurses Health Study in a cohort of 115 195 women from the USA. These women were 30–55 years of age and healthy when enrolled in 1976. During 16 years of follow-up there were 4726 deaths, some 881 from cardiovascular causes, 2586 from cancer and 1259 from other aetiologies.

In the analysis of those women who had never smoked the relative risk of death is not only seen in those with frank obesity, but the risk rises with modest gains in weight. For instance, the relative risk of death was 1.3 in those with a BMI 25.0–26.9, 1.6 in those with a BMI 27.0–28.9 and was doubled (2.1) for those with a BMI of 29.0–31.9. Among women with a BMI above 32 and who had never smoked, the risk of death from cardiovascular disease was 4.1 and from cancer was 2.1. In terms of attributable risk some 53% of all deaths in this study among women with a BMI of 29 or greater could be attributed directly to their obesity.

Although coronary heart disease is a major cause of weight-related death, the obese often develop other conditions that further predispose to their mortality. This relative mortality is highest for diabetes mellitus and next for digestive diseases, including cancer. Table 9.1 shows this relative mortality risk of obesity reported in a study of 750 000 men and women in the USA. In this study, the mortality for cancer was highest for colorectal cancer in males (1.73 in males, 1.22 in females), whereas in females this was in endometrial cancer, followed by cancer of the gallbladder and biliary passages. In addition, in those with substantial obesity there was an increased risk from cervical, breast and ovarian cancers. Smoking appreciably elevates overall mortality such that those who smoke 20 or more cigarettes per day have double the risk of non-smokers throughout the weight range, and this is especially apparent in males.

Recent evidence indicates that a weight loss of > 9 kg in women is associated with a 25% reduction in all causes, diabetic, cardiovascular and cancer mortality. If the obese person has already developed a weight-related disease then intentional weight loss of any amount has been shown to reduce mortality by 20%. This is most marked for cancer, with a 40–50% reduction, and for diabetes, with a 30–40% fall in mortality. It is important to emphasize 'intentional' weight loss, as

Table 9.1 Mortality risk in obesity

		Males	Females
Diabetes mellitus		5.19	7.90
Digestive diseases		3.99	2.29
Coronary heart disease		1.85	2.07
Cerebral vascular disease		2.27	1.52
Cancer	All sites	1.33	1.55
	Colorectal	1.73	1.22
	Prostate	1.29	
	Gallbladder/biliary	3.58	
	Endometrium	5.42	
	Cervix	2.39	
	Ovary	1.63	

The table compares the risk of those weighing 140% or more above an ideal weight (100%) with those weighing 90–109% of ideal.

much confusion has arisen in the past from the inclusion of non-intentional, i.e. disease-driven weight loss, which pre-empts death from many conditions.

Morbidity

Excess weight is associated with a multiplicity of problems, as outlined in Table 9.2, hence the categorization of obesity as a distinct disease in many countries. The beneficial effects of 10% weight loss are outlined in Table 9.3.

Table 9.2 Morbidity complications of obesity

Cardiovascular	*Hypertension*
	Coronary heart disease
	Cerebrovascular disease
	Oedema and varicose veins
	Deep venous thrombosis
	Hypertension
Respiratory	Breathlessness
	Sleep apnoea
	Hypoventilation syndrome
Gastrointestinal	Hiatus hernia
	Gallstones and cholelithiasis
	Fatty liver and cirrhosis
	Haemorrhoids, herniae
	Cancer colorectal
Metabolic	Hyperlipidaemia
	Insulin resistance
	Diabetes mellitus
	Polycystic ovarian syndrome
	Hyperandrogenization
	Menstrual irregularities
Neurology	Nerve entrapment
	Headaches due to raised intracranial pressure
Renal	Proteinuria
Breast	Breast cancer
	Male gynaecomastia
Uterus	Endometrial cancer
	Cervical cancer
Urological	Prostate cancer
	Benign prostatic hyperplasia
	Stress incontinence
Skin	Sweat rashes, Fungal infections
	Lymphoedema
	Cellulitis
	Stasis ulcers
	Acanthosis nigracans
Orthopaedic	Osteoarthritis of hip, knee and feet
	Gout
Endocrine	Growth hormone and IGF-1 reduced
	Reduced prolactin response
	Hyperdynamic ACTH response to CRH
	Increased urinary free cortisol
	Altered sex hormones
Pregnancy	Pre-eclampsia
	Gestational diabetes
	Preterm labour
	Caesarean section, forceps delivery, breech presentation
	Episiotomy infection
	Deep venous thrombosis
	Perinatal mortality
	Large babies
	Neural tube defects
Social	Disability on low income
	Reduced employment prospects

Table 9.3 Benefits to the obese of a 10% weight loss

Mortality	20–25% fall in total mortality
	30–40% fall in diabetes-related deaths
	40–50% fall in obesity-related cancer deaths
Blood pressure	Fall of 10 mmHg systolic pressure
	Fall of 20 mmHg diastolic pressure
Angina	Reduces symptoms by 90%
	33% increase in exercise tolerance
Lipids	Fall by 10% in total cholesterol
	Fall by 155% in LDL-cholesterol
	Fall by 30% in triglycerides
	Increase by 8% in HDL-cholesterol
Diabetes	Reduces risk of developing diabetes by > 50%
	Fall of 30–50% in fasting glucose
	Fall of 15% in HbA$_{1c}$
Rheology	Decreases blood viscosity by 20–27%
	Decreases red cell aggregation by 20%

Diabetes mellitus

About 75% of type II diabetic patients are overweight in most studies. In the Nurses Health Study the BMI, after adjustment for age, was the dominant predictor of the risk for diabetes. In females the risk rises above a BMI of 22, with a five-fold increased risk at a BMI of 25, a 28-fold risk at BMI of 30, and a 93-fold higher risk above a BMI of 35. Compared with those of stable weight, a gain of 8–10.9 kg increases the risk of diabetes by 2.7-fold. In contrast, those women who lose more than 5 kg reduce their risk of developing diabetes by 50% or more. These results were also independent of any family history of diabetes. In a study of 51 529 men then aged 40–75 years in 1986 and subsequently followed up for 5 years, the risk for diabetes increased for all BMI levels of 24 or above. Even men with a slight excess weight were more likely to develop diabetes than those with a BMI of less than 23 kg/m^2. The risk adjusted for age was increased 2.2-fold in those with BMI 25–26.9, 6.7 in those with BMI 29–30.9 and 42 in those with BMI of 35 or more. The BMI at age 21 years and the absolute weight gain during adulthood were independent risk factors for diabetes development. A BMI of 27 at age 21 years increased the risk 6.4-fold, whereas a gain in weight of 9 kg from the age of 21 years further raised the risk 3.5-fold. Fat distribution measured by the waist circumference was also independently associated with diabetes development. A waist circumference above 100 cm (40 inches) alone increased the risk by 3.5-fold, even after control for BMI.

These results are in keeping with a major Finnish study in Oslo on the 10-year follow-up of 3751 men aged 40–49 years at the outset. The percentage developing diabetes was 0.6% in normal-weight men but 23.4% in those 25% or more overweight. Weight loss improves this risk in males and females. In the Nurses study, a 5 kg weight loss reduced the risk of developing diabetes by 50% or more. Weight loss also improves mortality in those with established diabetes. A 9 kg weight loss reduces diabetes-related mortality by 30–40%, whereas a 5% weight loss reduces HbA_{Ic} by 7% and decreases fasting blood glucose by 15%. A loss of 10–20% in weight in type II diabetic patients can normalize metabolic control and possible life expectancy.

Cardiovascular disease, blood pressure, lipids and rheology

A number of cardiovascular risk factors is influenced by overweight, namely hypertension, impaired glycaemic control, hyperlipidaemia, and haemostatic and rheological factors. Until recently, it was thought that only severe degrees of excess weight increased the risk of **coronary heart disease**, but recent evidence shows a clear association with modest weight gain. In the Nurses study the risk of coronary heart disease was increased two-fold in those women of BMI 25–28.9 and 3.6 for a BMI of 29 or more. Weight gain from age 18 years increased the risk 1.6-fold for an 8–10.9 kg gain and 1.9-fold for an 11–19 kg gain. In males a 10% increase in weight will increase the risk of coronary heart disease by 38%, whereas a 20% weight rise corresponds to an 86% increased risk.

Blood pressure is increased by 6 mm systolic and 4 mm diastolic for a 10% gain in body fat, with those genetically more susceptible showing the greater effect. A weight loss of 11 kg has been reported to decrease both systolic and diastolic pressure by 20% in hypertensive patients, even when the sodium intake was kept constant. As a general rule, blood pressure is reduced by 1 mm systolic and 2 mm diastolic for each 1% reduction in body weight.

The characteristic **lipid** disorder in obesity is elevated total cholesterol and triglycerides, high low-density lipoprotein (LDL)-cholesterol and low high-density lipoprotein (HDL)-cholesterol. A meta-analysis has indicated that for every 1 kg of weight lost, there is a corresponding reduction by about 1% in total cholesterol and LDL, a rise by 1% in HDL and a reduction by 3% in triglycerides.

A number of **haemostatic factors** is associated with weight gain, particularly factors VII and X, which may relate to thrombosis and the risk of fatal myocardial infarction. A 15% weight loss is associated with a decrease in blood viscosity by 27%, in red cell aggregation by 20% and in haematocrit by 5.5%, whereas plasma fibrinogen remains unaffected. Such data on blood pressure, lipids and haemostatic factors probably account for the reduction in morbidity and mortality from cardiovascular diseases with modest weight loss. A 10 kg weight loss over 1 year may reduce symptoms of **angina** by 91% with a 33% increase in exercise tolerance. **Cerebrovascular disease** is also common in the obese. In the Whitehall study involving 17 753 men aged 40–64 years, the risk of stroke associated with obesity for male non-smokers was increased 2.6-fold.

Digestive diseases

Gallbladder disease is the most common form of digestive disease in obese individuals. A study of 73 532 obese women in the USA and Canada reported a 2.7-fold increase in the prevalence of gallbladder disease. There is a progressive linear increased risk of gallstones from a BMI of 20 upwards, which is twice as high in women as in men, increases with age and rises with the number of pregnancies. Weight and age appear additive, with obesity being six-fold more important than age. Weight loss may actually exacerbate gallbladder disease. In the Boston Nurses study, women who lost 4–10 kg had a 44% increased risk for detectable gallstone disease, whereas weight loss above 10 kg increased this risk to 94%. This may be associated with the rise in the body pool of circulating cholesterol as adipose tissue stores are mobilized and the increase in rate at which cholesterol is excreted in the bile in the obese individual. The development of gallstones depends on the precipitation of cholesterol from a supersaturated bile. Dieting with a low intake of dietary fibre further decreases the solubilization of excreted cholesterol, increasing gallstone formation.

Liver abnormalities have been described in the obese, mainly as a result of fatty infiltration. However, in the morbidly obese with BMI greater than 40, only 2% have normal livers, 56% show fatty infiltration alone, whereas 42% have fatty infiltration associated with fibrosis or cirrhosis. In the American Cancer Society study of 750 000 men and women in the USA, **colorectal** cancer was the principal site of excess cancer mortality in obese males (see Table 9.1), whereas cancer of the gallbladder and biliary passages was more prevalent in obese females. The relative mortality rates of **cancer of the stomach and pancreas** were higher in obese males (1.88 and 1.62, respectively) than in females, where the mortality rate for stomach cancer (1.03) was reported similar to the non-obese and that for pancreatic cancer (0.61) significantly lower. The relative risk of **endometrial cancer** is more than doubled in women aged 60–69 years with a BMI of 25–29 kg/m^2 and is increased 5.4-fold in those with significant obesity.

Chronic abdominal compartmentation syndrome

Abdominal obesity, especially in the morbid obese individual, can result in the **chronic abdominal compartmentation syndrome**. It is thought that the mass of omental fat increases intra-abdominal pressure, resulting in high intravesical pressure (> 20 mmH_2O), resulting in stress incontinence, as well as increased gastric acid reflux. The tenting of the diaphragm can increase intrathoracic pressure, raising right atrial pressure, with associated pulmonary hypertension and subsequent breathlessness, dependent oedema with stasis ulcers and headaches due to increased intracranial pressure. The acute form of this syndrome has been described after bariatric surgery, where an acute rise in intra-abdominal pressure may result in reduced urine output, rise in jugular venous pulse, increased pulmonary wedge pressure and falling cardiac output.

Breast cancer

The relationship between breast cancer and obesity is not clear. In the American Cancer Society study the mortality ratio for breast cancer was not significantly raised for those 120–139% above ideal body weight (IBW = 100%), but was 1.63 for those > 140% IBW. However, age has a significant impact on the risk of developing breast cancer. Premenopausal obese women have the same risk as lean women but in the post-menopause, obese women exhibit a higher risk. Abdominal obesity and a positive family history increase this risk. It has been conjectured that this association with obesity and especially central adiposity is associated with enhanced conversion of androgens to oestrogen in the fat mass and a reduced sex-hormone-binding globulin (SHBG), which adds to an increase in free oestradiol levels.

Arthritis and bone mass

It is not easy to find objective evidence for the improvement of the arthritic condition with weight loss, especially in the elderly. Whereas there is evidence that obesity is associated with osteoarthritis of the hip and knee, extensive literature does not indicate that weight loss in modest obesity had any measurable clinical benefit on this condition other than some modest relief of pain in the lower back, ankles and feet. Bone mass is increased in the obese but bone mass can decrease by 3–15% with weight loss. Some suggest that this loss recovers with weight regain but this may not occur in postmenopausal women. Uric acid levels also increase with weight, precipitating gout, but also acutely rise with dieting. Musculoskeletal problems result in increased disability and the need for time off work, seen even in those with modest overweight.

Endocrine abnormalities and psychological factors

The production of sex steroids is altered in the obese. Obese women, especially those with central adiposity, have increased levels of free testosterone and are hyperandrogenic with marked insulin resistance, the latter implicated in the development of polycystic ovarian syndrome. In obese men visceral adiposity is associated with a reduced testosterone level. Growth hormone is also reduced in obesity and insulin-like growth factor-1 (IGF-1) is negatively associated with increasing visceral adiposity. It has been conjectured that these hormonal abnormalities may be secondary to an increased activity of the hypothalamic–pituitary–adrenal axis. Those who have visceral obesity exhibit a hyperdynamic adrenocorticotropic hormone (ACTH) secretion to corticotrophin-releasing hormone (CRH) as well as increased cortisol release from the adrenals, whereas those with gynoid obesity show a lesser response, identical to that observed in naturally thin individuals. Urinary free cortisol levels have also been reported to be positively associated with increasing visceral adiposity. As cortisol and insulin both increase fat accumulation, whereas growth hormone and testosterone promote lipid metabolism, the abnormalities noted in the obese would have the effect of promoting fat deposition, especially of visceral fat.

This overactivity of the hypothalamic–pituitary axis has been conjectured as being due to higher influences possibly related to certain socioeconomic factors and psychological problems, which appear to be more prevalent in the visceral obese. In population studies, men and women with a higher waist:hip ratio (more visceral obesity) report ill more often, have more frequent peptic ulcers and stomach bleeding, and have more general health complaints. These individuals use more tranquillizers and antidepressant tablets, have more time off work for sickness, and suffer stress-related symptoms, sleepiness and nightmares. They tend to be from the lower socioeconomic groups, have poorer education, impaired personality, extraversion, low achievement, aggression, low dominance and a need for sociability. Such inability to cope with life events in those with a genetic propensity for a certain fat distribution may produce a permanent hyperarousal response, which stimulates certain brain peptides, especially CRH, which then drive the pituitary–adrenal axis to produce a raised cortisol output. Such would also be implicated in neuropeptide Y release, one of the brain's most potent peptides for the stimulation of appetite, especially for carbohydrates. This peptide could potentiate CRH release, producing a vicious cycle, driving the individual onwards to store visceral fat. This obesity cascade is outlined in Figure 9.1.

Respiratory problems

There are several ways in which obesity affects lung function. An increased amount of fat in the chest wall and abdomen limits respiratory excursion, reducing lung volume. This is accentuated in the supine position, increasing the mechanical work of breathing by 30% in modest obesity and by three-fold in **obesity-hypoventilation syndrome**, sometimes called the Pickwickian syndrome. A ventilation perfusion disturbance resulting in abnormal gas exchange is often observed in extremes of obesity with underventilated but overperfused lower portions of the lungs. This results in hypoxia with normal arterial carbon dioxide levels, the degree of hypoxia worsening in the supine position. This hypoxia expands the pulmonary blood volume, which adds strain to ventricular function. These changes in respiratory function are exacerbated during sleep, where there is a reduction in arterial oxygen saturation and a rise in carbon dioxide tension in all individuals, but especially marked in the obese. Irregular respiration and occasional apnoeic episodes often occur in lean people during sleep but obesity, with its influence on respiratory mechanics, increases

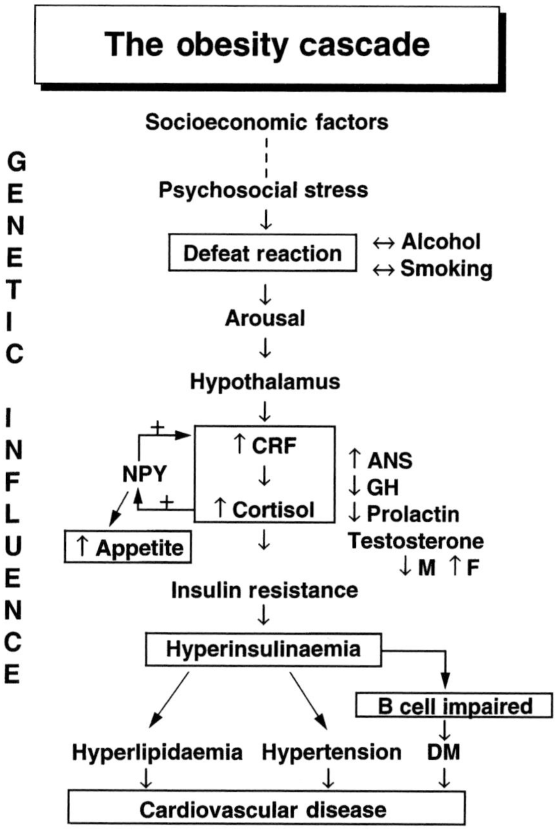

The obesity cascade

Figure 9.1 The obesity cascade. NPY, neuropeptide Y; CRF, corticotrophin-releasing factor/hormone; ANS, autonomic nervous system; GH, growth hormone; M, male; F, female; DM, diabetes mellitus.

their frequency and may result in severe hypoxia with resultant arrhythmias and cardiac dysfunction.

In many with uncomplicated obesity these ventilation perfusion defects are countered by increased ventilation, which restores blood gases to normal but, in some cases, depression in both hypercapnic and hypoxic respiratory drives with an accompanying irregular pattern of breathing and apnoeic episodes result in obesity-hypoventilation syndrome. Frequent awakening and the resultant sleep deprivation produce **daytime somnolence**. Persistent hypoxia further blunts the hypoxic drive, resulting in the development of **pulmonary hypertension** and eventual **right ventricular failure,** which further worsens the hypoxia. Continuous recorded monitoring of arterial oxygen saturation using an ear-lobe oximeter will diagnose those at risk.

Pregnancy

Obese women have a higher risk of obstetric complications. Women who are significantly obese (i.e. > 135% IBW) have a 6.6-fold increased risk for the development of gestational diabetes, 1.9-fold risk for pregnancy-induced hypertension and 1.4-fold risk for urinary tract infections. Other complications include pre-eclampsia (1.5-fold risk), thrombophlebitis, postpartum haemorrhage and wound or episiotomy infections. Obese women have an increased risk of Caesarean delivery owing to a variety of factors such as fetal size, especially macrosomia (birth weights > 4000 g), an increase in maternal pelvic soft tissue narrowing the birth canal, late deceleration of the fetal heart rate, intrapartum meconium staining, prolonged labour, malpresentations and cord incidents. This increased prevalence of Caesarean section occurs in pregnancies with or without antenatal complications. In the latter, the rate has been reported as high as 19.6% in the morbidly obese compared with 10.1% in normal weight and 12.4% in moderate obesity. Fetal weight appears to be directly proportional to maternal size, with more than 50% of obese women having babies who weigh greater than 3600 g. Maternal weigh when not associated with antenatal complications is not associated with an increased perinatal mortality, but the latter is increased by as much as three-fold if there has been an antenatal complication. Recently, an increased risk of neural tube defects, especially spina bifida, has been reported in women with BMI greater than 29 (odds ratio 1.9).

Section 9.3 • Medical management of obesity

Clinical assessment is important at the outset of the management of excess weight. This assessment (Table 9.4) includes the comorbid risk factors, BMI, waist circumference, certain relevant biochemical parameters and psychological evaluation (by questionnaire). Psychological disorders such as an eating disorder or depression should be professionally managed before dieting proceeds. In those needing to lose weight,

Table 9.4 Assessment of the obese patient

History
- Smoking habit
- Current drug therapies; drugs that affect weight, e.g. valproate, steroids
- Alcohol intake
- Risk factors such as angina, myocardial infarction, stroke, intermittent claudication

Examination
- BMI; weight in indoor clothing without shoes; height without shoes
- Waist circumference
- Blood pressure

Tests
- Urinalysis
- GGT; for alcoholic liver disease
- Lipid profile
- Thyroid-stimulating hormone
- Blood glucose; random or fasting
- Psychological
- Depression and eating disorders
- GGT, γ-glutamyl transferase.

the first goal at the outset is to achieve a modest weight loss of 10%, as research indicates that this is sufficient to achieve a significant improvement in health (illustrated in Table 9.3). As it is highly unlikely that an ideal weight will be achieved in many, to strive for this is likely to demoralize both the patient and their advisor! Once 10% weight has been lost another goal can be set (e.g. a further 10% loss) by mutual agreement. Although substantial weight loss might be required clinically for some, this is still best achieved by the 10% rule, the speed at which this loss is required being the guiding influence to the method chosen.

The medical management of weight can be considered in four approaches based on the most recent advice given by the Royal Colleges of Physicians in Scotland and England.

Weight reduction

This aims to provide a 3-month structured management plan designed specifically to the needs of each individual patient. This comprises:

- support from a trained health-care professional in a **group setting.** There is a greater weight loss using groups than with individual consultations, possibly due to the interplay and mutual support of the individuals in the group, e.g. 15 kg weight loss at 3 months in groups compared with 8 kg with individual sessions
- diet consisting of a **moderate reduction in energy intake** of about 600 kcal (2.5 MJ) less than expenditure assessed on weight, gender and age using published formulae. This produces a greater weight loss than more strict diets due to improved compliance. For example, the weight loss in one trial where the diet was restricted by 600 kcal (2.6 MJ) was 5 kg, compared with just 3 kg on a standard 1000 kcal (4.2 MJ) diet, which contrasts with the predicted weight loss of 6 and 13 kg, respectively, if complete adherence had occurred. Most diets aim to reduce fat intake. The dietary change should involve the entire patient's household where appropriate, for often the dietary education of the household needs rectification if long-term progress is to be made. Starvation diets are now dismissed as potentially dangerous, owing to sudden death from heart disease exacerbated by profound loss in muscle mass and the development of arrhythmias secondary to elevated free fatty acids and deranged electrolytes
- **behavioural modification therapy**, which is designed to support a process of change in the individual's attitude, perception and behaviour as regards food intake, life-style and physical activity. Each session, usually conducted in a group, emphasizes specific topics
- promotion of **increased physical activity**, which can be maintained long term. Such exercise

need not be overexertional, as health gain is achieved at modest exercise levels as long as these are maintained throughout life. Walking briskly for 30 min each day can contribute 100–200 kcal (0.4–0.8 MJ) of energy expenditure daily, resulting in an additional weight loss of 1 kg/month.

Weight maintenance plan

The weight reduction is then followed by a 3-month structured programme emphasizing weight maintenance, although continued weight loss is often an option for many. This again emphasizes therapy in groups with continued behavioural therapy, promotion of exercise and diet modification.

Exercise is designed to prevent weight regain once lost by dietary restriction. For example, moderate exercise of 30 min of brisk walking each day can maintain a weight of 70 kg, whereas without such extra activity the weight would plateau out on 77 kg on the same dietary intake.

Drug therapy

Appetite suppressants

Appetite-suppressant drugs belong to two groups. The first act on the hypothalamus, influencing the catecholaminergic pathway, and include **amphetamine, diethylpropion, phentermine and mazindol**. However, because of their cerebral stimulant properties and potential misuse all are restricted in use by the Misuse of Drugs Regulation 1985. The second group of anorectic agents acts on the hypothalamic serotonergic system, namely DL-**fenfluramine** and its dextro isomer **dexfenfluramine**, neither of which has cerebral stimulant or addictive activity. These two drugs were used world-wide for many years until their withdrawal in 1997 owing to a previously unforeseen complication. Echocardiography demonstrated that some patients given a combination of fenfluramine with phentermine developed an unusual heart condition involving both left- and right-sided heart valves producing regurgitation. Some also developed pulmonary hypertension. Those valves removed surgically had a glistening white appearance with plaque-like encasement of the leaflets and chordae, histopathological features identical to those seen in carcinoid syndrome, a condition also associated with raised 5-hydroxytryptamine (5-HT, serotonin).

Sibutramine, which reduces food intake through β_1- and 5-HT$_{2A/2C}$ receptor agonist activity is likely to be available shortly in the UK. This drug also enhances metabolic rate via stimulation of β_3 peripheral receptors. Weight loss is improved 3–5 kg more than placebo after 6 months of therapy and is associated with an improvement in the lipid profile. Side-effects include dry mouth, constipation and insomnia, whereas the noradrenergic effects of the drug can increase heart rate and blood pressure in some.

Fat absorption inhibitor: orlistat

Orlistat, which has recently been marketed, inhibits pancreatic and gastric lipases, decreasing ingested triglyceride hydrolysis. This produces a 30% reduction in dietary fat absorption, which can contribute to a caloric deficit of about 200 kcal (0.8 MJ)/24 h. A trial of orlistat over 1 year while on a hypocaloric diet restricting fat to 30% of energy intake resulted in a 10.2% (10.3 kg) weight loss, compared with 6.1% (6.1 kg) on placebo. During the second year the patients were given a eucaloric diet. Those continued on the drug regained some weight but this was on average some 2.4 kg less than those continued on placebo. After 2 years of continuous orlistat treatment, 57% maintained a greater than 5% weight loss, compared with 37% in those on placebo. Pooled data indicate that after 1 year on orlistat some 20% lost 10% or more of their body weight, compared with 8% on placebo (mean difference 3.2 kg). In type II diabetic patients 1 year of therapy resulted in a weight loss of 6.2 kg, compared with 4.3 kg on placebo. Twice as many patients receiving orlistat lost 5% (49% vs 23%) and also 10% (17.9% vs 8.8%) of their weight. In both non-diabetic and diabetic patients there were improvements in lipid profile but these were only slight (0.36% reduction in total cholesterol and 8.6% decrease in the LDL:HDL ratio in non-diabetics).

Adverse side-effects are mainly related to the effect of the fat malabsorption on the gut: loose, oily stools (20%), faecal urgency (22%), flatus with discharge (24%), increased defecation (11%) and faecal incontinence (8%). The incidence of gastrointestinal adverse events decreases with prolonged use and in trials resulted in only 3.5% premature withdrawals. Treatment with orlistat may impair the absorption of fat-soluble vitamins A, D, E, K and β-carotene. Although levels of these vitamins remained within the normal range in most patients after 2 years of therapy, a diet rich in fruit and vegetables is advised, with consideration given to the prescription of a multivitamin taken at bedtime (not with orlistat, which is taken with meals).

Contraindications to the usage of orlistat include chronic malabsorption states, cholestasis and hepatic failure, pregnancy, breast feeding and children. The product licence for orlistat advises that the drug should only be prescribed if diet alone has achieved a weight loss of 2.5 kg over a period of 4 consecutive weeks. This is to ensure dietary compliance and hence reduce subsequent adverse events due to a high fat intake. The licence also states that the drug should cease if the patient fails to lose at least 5% of their weight after 12 weeks of drug therapy.

A recent report from the Royal College of Physicians in the UK regarding the use of any weight-reduction drug suggests that such therapy should only be considered in those with a BMI > 30 who have failed to lose 10% weight after at least 3 months of a structured weight reduction programme consisting of dietary advice, behavioural modification and exercise, as described above in the 'Weight reduction' section.

The College Report advises that an obesity-reduction drug might then be prescribed for 3 months in the first instance as long as there are no contraindications to its usage. If after 3 months of therapy the patient fails to lose 5% weight while on the drug, then the drug should be withdrawn. If, however, weight loss exceeds 5% loss then the drug may be continued for as long as its licence indicates, with careful monitoring for adverse events.

Antidepressive drugs

Treatment of depressed obese patients with **tricyclic antidepressants** often produces weight gain, resulting in drug non-compliance. The new class of antidepressants, which inhibit serotonergic uptake (**SSRI**), such as fluoxetine, also reduce weight in a dose-dependent and time-limited manner. Weight is lost for about 6 months on this class of drug but then is regained for reasons unknown and, therefore, is not recommended for the treatment of obesity without depression.

Bulk-forming drugs and **diuretics** should not be used to enhance fat loss. **Thyroid replacement** therapy should only be used in the obese person when there is evidence of biochemical hypothyroidism and not otherwise.

Very-low-calorie diets

Very-low-calorie diets (VLCD) produce weight losses of 1.5–2.5 kg/week, compared with 0.5 kg on conventional diets. VLCD are mainly used for short-term, rapid weight loss, and are often used for 12 weeks in the first instance, although compliance is often incomplete, with the patient reverting to ordinary food using the VLCD intermittently. In the UK the recommendation is that VLCD should only be considered by those with BMI > 30 and under supervision by an experienced physician/nutritionist.

Contraindications to use include:

- cardiac disease, unstable angina, recent myocardial infarction, significant cardiac arrhythmias, decompensated congestive cardiac failure
- cerebrovascular disease: recent stroke
- unstable epilepsy
- major organ system failure
- protein wasting conditions
- active substance misuse
- untreated endocrine condition, e.g. hypothyroidism
- pregnant women, during breast feeding and in children.

The composition of the diet should ensure a minimum of 50 g of protein each day for men and 40 g of protein for women to minimize muscle degradation. Energy content should be minimum 400 kcal (1.65 MJ) for women of height < 1.73 m (68 inches) and 500 kcal (2.1 MJ) for all men and women taller than 1.73 m. Most use a liquid feed, although VLCD made of solid food are used but are less successful.

Side-effects may be a problem in the early stages of the diet, especially orthostatic hypotension, headache, diarrhoea and nausea, but short-duration therapy is generally well tolerated.

Section 9.4 • Surgical management of morbid obesity

The surgeon involved in the management of morbid obesity is part of a **multidisciplinary team** that consists of a physician with special interest in the obesity syndrome, a psychologist and a dietician. No patient should undergo bariatric (antiobesity) surgery before:

- medical investigation and treatment
- psychological assessment has excluded significant disorders and confirmed that the patient can cope with the severe dietary restriction imposed by the surgery.

Weight reduction on medical therapy indicates compliance with the enforced dietary restriction after surgery. In addition, it makes surgical intervention easier, whether this is conducted by the open or laparoscopic approach. The patient must realize that surgery is part of an altered lifestyle that involves not only a drastic revision of eating habits but also a commitment to daily exercise.

Indications

In most, if not all cases, the decision for surgery is a joint one between the physician and surgeon. The ideal patient is one who has no major perioperative risk factors, a stable personality and no eating disorders, and who has come down to a BMI of 35 or less with medical management.

Contraindications

Bariatric procedures have to be considered as major surgical interventions with a risk (albeit small) of perioperative death and a significant early and late morbidity. In the authors' practice bariatric surgical treatment is contraindicated in the following:

- patients in the major risk category for perioperative cardiac complications [Modules 3 and 20, Vol. I]
- patients in the moderate risk category for perioperative cardiac complications with poor myocardial reserve on testing [Modules 3 and 20, Vol. I]
- significant chronic obstructive or restrictive lung disease [Modules 13 and 16, Vol. I]
- non-compliance with medical therapy
- psychological instability/disorders
- eating disorders
- hiatus hernia/established gastro-oesophageal reflux disease.

Preparation for surgery

A full and detailed explanation of the procedure and how this fits into the overall treatment and exercise programme is essential. The provision of a booklet that contains all of the information has been found to be very helpful and motivational. Aside from routine preoperative assessment [Module 16, Vol. I], spirometry is essential in these patients. Preoperative breathing exercises are beneficial in reducing the incidence and severity of postoperative pulmonary insufficiency. Single-dose antibiotic prophylaxis (co-amoxiclav or cefuroxime) is administered after induction of anaesthesia. These patients fall in the high-risk category for perioperative thromboembolic disease and must receive the appropriate prophylactic measures [Module 16, Vol. I]. As most run into respiratory problems immediately postoperatively and require ventilatory support with intermittent positive pressure ventilation (IPPV), nursing in an intensive care unit in the first instance is mandatory. The use of bilevel positive airway pressure (BiPAP system) during the first 24 h postoperatively has been shown to reduce significantly pulmonary dysfunction after gastroplasty and accelerates re-establishment of preoperative pulmonary function.

Operative procedures

Some operations such as jejunoileal bypass are of historical interest, as they are no longer practised because of their significant long-term morbidity and mortality (liver failure and cirrhosis). It is obvious from the number of procedures practised (Table 9.5) that the ideal operation for morbid obesity has not been developed. The procedures that are used either restrict intake, e.g. Mason procedure, laparoscopic adjustable banding, or induce malabsorption, e.g. biliopancreatic diversion, or both, e.g. resectional gastric bypass, biliopancreatic diversion with duodenal switch. All procedures are accompanied by a significant morbidity (see below) and a mortality that varies between 1 and 5%. Bariatric surgery has to be considered as a subspecialty of surgical gastroenterology. The Cancun statement of the International Federation for Surgery of Obesity (IFSO) details the requirements for clinical competence and standards, and these include dedicated specialist exper-

Table 9.5 Bariatric (antiobesity) procedures

- Insertion of intragastric silicon balloons
- Vertical banded gastroplasty (Mason procedure): open or laparoscopic
- Roux-en-Y gastric bypass: open or laparoscopically assisted
- Resectional gastric bypass (subtotal gastrectomy with Roux-en-Y)
- Biliopancreatic diversion (Scopinaro's procedure)
- Leeds procedure
- Adjustable gastric banding (laparoscopic)

tise within a multidisciplinary team. **Thus, bariatric operations should not be undertaken outside this set-up**. Despite the morbidity, the Swedish Obese Subjects (SOS) trial comparing bariatric surgery versus conventional weight reduction has demonstrated clear and significant improvement in the health-related quality of life (HRQL) at 2 years only in the surgical arm. This is the first time that the superiority of bariatric surgery over conventional therapy has been confirmed.

Intragastric balloon

The principle behind this intervention is the reduction of the gastric volume by a silicon balloon that has a valve to which is docked a detachable filling tube. The deflated balloon is inserted into the stomach under intravenous sedation and local pharyngeal anaesthesia (midazolam). The position of the balloon is checked by flexible endoscopy. The balloon is then filled with 800 ml of saline and the filling tube detached from the valve. The position of the filled balloon is checked radiologically (Figure 9.2) and following a period of 12 h observation, oral intake is commenced. Initial reports suggest that these balloons are well tolerated and result in significant weight loss prior to bariatric surgery. Intragastric balloons were never intended as a permanent solution but as a temporary expedient over a period of 3–4 months to enable weight loss and give the patient the opportunity to adjust to a reduced dietary intake.

The initial promise of intragastric balloons has not been fulfilled and the authors have abandoned their use. In the first instance, the weight loss is variable and on average less than that obtained by VLCDs. Secondly, there are problems and complications with their use:

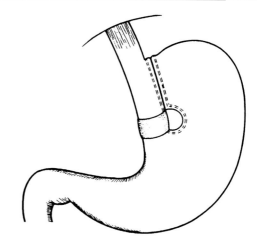

Figure 9.3 Vertical banded gastroplasty.

- deflation and removal may be difficult and often require more than one endoscopic session
- complications can occur, e.g. intestinal obstruction requiring laparotomy.

Vertical banded gastroplasty

Vertical banded gastroplasty (VBG) is the most commonly performed operation (Figure 9.3) and can now be undertaken by the laparoscopically assisted approach. Its positive features include simplicity and ease of performance, which are reflected in a low postoperative mortality rate (1%). However, the revision rate requiring further surgical interventions is high and averages 30%. Specific complications include bolus obstruction, disruption of the staples partitioning off the pouch (reduced by double stapling), pouch dilatation and band erosion into the channel between the pouch and distal stomach. The procedure does not increase significantly the incidence of gastro-oesophageal reflux in patients with a competent O-G junction. The operation can be reversed.

Roux-en-Y gastric bypass

This procedure (Figure 9.4) is more certain in achieving significant weight loss than VBG but it is a more major, although still reversible procedure. In expert hands the perioperative mortality, although higher than VBG, is acceptable at 2%. There is still an appreciable revision rate, albeit lower than VBG, in patients undergoing Roux-en-Y gastric bypass.

Resectional gastric bypass

This operation has been advocated recently and consists of subtotal gastrectomy with Roux-en-Y reconstruction (Figure 9.5). It virtually guarantees weight loss by a combination of reduced intake and malabsorption. It, is, however, a major specialist operation and is irreversible. Its other benefit is the virtual abolition of gastro-oesophageal reflux. The only reported series on 85 patients showed excellent results with no postoperative mortality. The series included 38 patients with

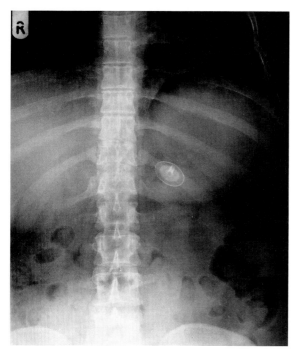

Figure 9.2 X-ray showing saline-inflated intragastric balloon.

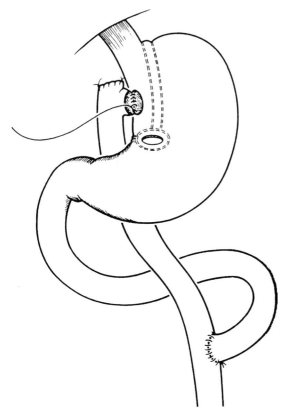

Figure 9.4 Roux-en-Y gastric bypass.

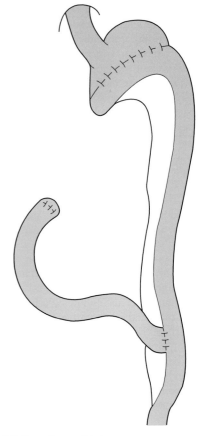

Figure 9.5 Resection gastric bypass.

previous failed or problematic bariatric operations. Currently, this operation has to be regarded as a remedial procedure to be undertaken for failures after less major bariatric operations. Patients who have undergone resectional gastric bypass (RGB) require long-term vitamin B_{12} replacement and oral iron therapy. These patients are also prone to postgastrectomy bone disease.

Biliopancreatic diversion
This intervention, first reported by Scopinaro in 1978 (Figure 9.6), is popular on the European continent and results in substantial weight loss (average 70% at 2 years). The operation consist of a distal two-thirds gastrectomy with closure of the duodenal stump followed by a reconstruction that essentially results in a duodenal switch. The ileum is then transected 250–350 cm from the ileocaecal valve (depending on the length of the small bowel). The distal end (alimentary limb = 250–350 cm) is closed and brought up for end-to-side anastomosis with the gastric remnant. The proximal end (biliopancreatic limb) is anastomosed end-to-side to the alimentary limb some 50 cm from the ileocaecal valve. The procedure is technically demanding with an operative mortality of 2% and a major perioperative morbidity of 10%. Specific long-term complications of biliopancreatic bypass include anastomotic ulceration (10%) and protein malnutrition in (4%).

Leeds operation
Also referred to as the 'magenstrasse and mill' procedure, this intervention separates the lesser curvature from the O–G junction to the antrum by suturing or linear cutting staplers (Figure 9.7). The procedure is physiologically attractive but no large published series has used this procedure.

Laparoscopic adjustable gastric banding
Laparoscopic adjustable gastric banding (LAGB) (Figure 9.8) is the latest addition to the surgical armamentarium. Definitive conclusions on the efficacy of LAGB are not possible because experience with the technique is limited in most centres. The obvious merits of the procedure are that:

- it avoids open surgery and thus expedites recovery
- the anatomy of the upper gastrointestinal tract is undisturbed, except for the silicon band below the O–G junction
- the procedure is completely reversible.

The disadvantages are that:

- the technique is still evolving and good results are dependent on experience with the procedure
- it aggravates existing gastro-oesophageal reflux.

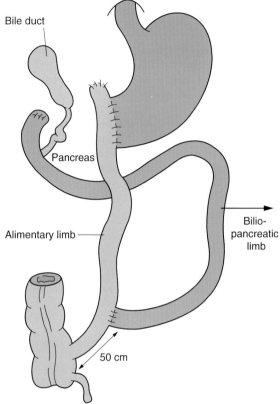

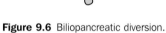

Figure 9.6 Biliopancreatic diversion.

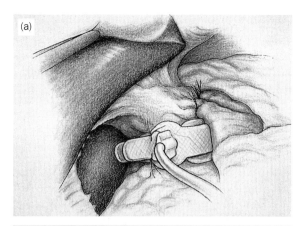

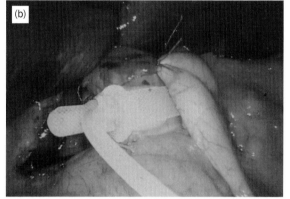

Figure 9.8 Laparoscopic adjustable banding.

In general, all of the reports, including the present authors' experience, have been favourable and most favour the Swedish band (Figure 9.9). The only unfavourable report (insufficient weight reduction) has been with another type of adjustable band. A clinical trial comparing LAGB with VBG has shown equal efficacy in terms of weight loss at 6 months.

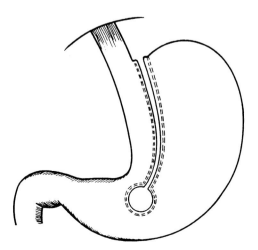

Figure 9.7 Magenstrasse and Mill (M&M) procedure.

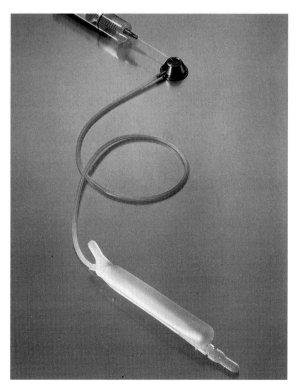

Figure 9.9 Swedish band for laparoscopic treatment of morbid obesity.

Outcome after bariatric surgery

Benefit

The results of the SOS trial have documented that despite the morbidity and failures, bariatric operations impart a significant benefit, with weight loss and improved HRQL that are substantially better than conventional weight-reduction measures. Peak improvements were documented in the surgical arm at 6 and 12 months after the intervention, with a slight to moderate decrease in the HRQL at 2 years. The degree of improvement in the HRQL correlated with the magnitude of weight loss in the individual patient. In the Dutch controlled cross-sectional study, the quality of life (QoL) was significantly improved by bariatric surgery and this improvement was not related to the type of surgical procedure. This study also documented some deterioration in the QoL with time. Good QoL is maintained if the patient continues to exercise daily and permanently alters his or her eating habits. Another study involving psychometric testing of patients before and after bariatric surgery demonstrated that the psychopathology (depression, denial of emotional stress, social incompetence, indifferent attitude) was reversed by surgery, with the exception of somatization. This indicates that the preoperative psychological disturbances are the result rather than the cause of morbid obesity.

Specific improvements include reduction in oral hypertensive medication and antidiabetic therapy by 6 months. Significant lowering of the serum cholesterol and triglyceride levels also occurs, particularly after biliopancreatic diversion. Hepatic steatosis is often improved, but at the expense of an increase in the incidence of inflammatory lobular hepatitis. The improvement in respiratory function (lung volumes on spirometry and respiratory muscle power) contributes to the increased exercise tolerance. Morbidly obese patients with sleep apnoea benefit from bariatric surgery.

Morbidity

The greatest problem remains the frequent need (20–30%) for reinterventions because of failures or complications, e.g. pouch dilatation, disruption of staple lines, erosion of band around the conduit from the pouch in the Mason procedure and anastomotic ulcers after biliopancreatic diversion.

Gastro-oesophageal reflux and oesophagitis are aggravated in patients with pre-existing incompetence after VBG and LAGB. Arthralgia and arthritis are common after intestinal bypass operations. They are much less frequent, but still occur, in approximately 4% of patients undergoing the current bariatric interventions. Although joint pain and disorder is an integral part of the obese syndrome, it does appear that the 'arthritis vasculitis syndrome' can develop after surgery, particularly following biliopancreatic diversion.

Incisional hernia is a common complication after all open bariatric operations. Protein malnutrition and thiamine deficiency leading to Wernicke's encephalopathy have been documented and stress the need for long-term dietary supervision.

Guide to further reading

Cowan, G. S., Jr (1998). The Cancun IFSO statement on bariatric surgeon qualifications. International Federation for Surgery of Obesity. *Obes Surg* **8**: 87.

Curry, T. K., Carter, P. L., Porter, C. A. and Watts, D. M. (1998). Resectional gastric bypass is a new alternative in morbid obesity. *Am J Surg* **175**: 367–370.

Finer, N., ed. (1997). Obesity – a series of expert reviews. *Br Med Bull* **53**: No. 2.

Jung, R. T. (1990). *A Colour Atlas of Obesity*, Wolfe-Mosby-Times Publications, London.

Karlsson, J., Sjostrom, L. and Sullivan, M. (1998). Swedish obese subjects (SOS) – an intervention study of obesity. Two-year follow-up of health-related quality of life (HRQL) and eating behaviour after gastric surgery for severe obesity. *Int J Obes Relat Metab Disord* **22**: 113–126.

Lew, E. A. and Garfinkel, L. (1979). Variations in mortality by weight among 750,000 men and women. *J Chronic Dis* **32**: 563–576.

Lundell, L., Ruth, M. and Olbe, L. (1997). Vertical banded gastroplasty or gastric banding for morbid obesity: effects on gastroesophageal reflux. *Eur J Surg* **163**: 525–531.

Manson, J. E., Willett, W. C., Stampfer, M. J. *et al.* (1995). Body weight and mortality among women. *N Engl J Med* **333**: 677–685.

Noya, G., Cossu, M. L., Coppola, M. *et al.* (1998). Biliopancreatic diversion for treatment of morbid obesity: experience in 50 cases. *Obes Surg* **8**: 61–66.

Obesity in Scotland – integrating prevention with weight management. Scottish Intercollegiate Guidelines Network Number 8 (1996), Royal College of Physicians, Edinburgh.

Van Gemert, W. G., Severeijins, R. M., Greve, J. W. *et al.* (1998). Psychological functioning of morbidly obese patients after surgical treatment. *Int J Obes Relat Metab Disord* **22**: 393–398.

Patients with peripheral vascular disease

1 • Assessment of patients with peripheral arterial disease

2 • Occlusive peripheral arterial disease

3 • Dilating peripheral arterial disease

4 • Chronic venous disease

5 • Lymphoedema

'But when I don't smoke I scarcely feel as if I'm living. I don't feel as if I'm living unless I'm killing myself' – Russell Hoban, *Turtle Diary*, Ch. 7

Section 10.1 • Assessment of patients with peripheral arterial disease

The term 'peripheral arterial disease' refers to conditions affecting the whole arterial tree with the exception of the heart and coronary arteries. Atherosclerosis, however, affects the whole arterial tree, peripheral and coronary, and so patient assessment must reflect this. Patients with arterial disease should be expected to have significant occlusive disease referable to several areas of the arterial system and these may affect treatment options. They are generally elderly and may also have other significant comorbidity affecting other organs and systems (e.g. chronic pulmonary disease, diabetes and chronic renal failure). A full clinical assessment in every case is therefore mandatory in order to determine the most appropriate treatment plan.

The great majority of patients presenting with symptoms of peripheral arterial disease suffer from atherosclerosis. Other pathological conditions should not be forgotten, however. These include Buerger's disease (thromboangiitis obliterans), other forms of arteritis (such as Takayasu's disease), cystic medial necrosis and intimal hyperplasia. The pattern of the disease may be stenotic, dilating or a combination of the two.

History

When taking a patient's history, clearly the first item on which to concentrate is the primary complaint. As will be indicated, it is important to determine factors such as the severity, duration and speed of onset of symptoms, any progression and their effect on the patient's lifestyle. It is necessary to ask about the other common areas affected by arterial disease; depending on the primary complaint these will include cerebrovascular disease, upper limb ischaemia, ischaemic heart disease,

cardiac failure, symptomatic aortic aneurysm, mesenteric ischaemia and lower limb ischaemia. Enquiries are made about the risk factors for arterial disease, i.e. diabetes mellitus (age of onset, insulin dependency, complications), hypertension (quality of control, drugs used), hyperlipidaemia (diet, medication), family history and smoking (age on starting, still smoking, age when stopped, number of cigarettes a day). Other conditions common in this group, such as chronic respiratory disease, peptic ulceration and renal impairment, are specifically asked about, along with any other medical history. A detailed chronological history of previous vascular reconstruction is required, as well as any other operations that the patient may have undergone. A list of current medication is made, specifically asking about cardiovascular drugs, aspirin and anticoagulants. Finally, an assessment of the patient's level of function is required: their type of accommodation, who lives with them, do they need help at home, can they attend to their own cooking and cleaning, can they walk far enough to do their own shopping, and are they dyspnoeic on walking, climbing a flight of stairs, getting dressed or talking.

With practice, a careful history can be taken quickly. It will provide a diagnosis and a good indication of the patient's general fitness, and will largely determine how appropriate any proposed intervention would be. Vascular surgery is a highly systematic specialty and, starting with the history, it is best not to cut corners, no matter how obvious the presenting complaint may be.

Clinical examination

Examination of a patient with peripheral vascular disease should include the whole vascular tree and should be performed in the same systematic fashion as taking the history. Starting with the upper limb, the hands are inspected generally, looking for such signs such as ischaemia (uncommon), muscle wasting (thoracic outlet syndrome) or scleroderma (Raynaud's). The pulses (radial, ulnar, brachial and axillary) are all palpated bilaterally and the blood pressure is measured in both arms, the higher reading being the correct measurement. The carotid pulses are then palpated and bruits sought over them and over the subclavian artery (in the supraclavicular and infraclavicular fossae). The heart and chest are examined as usual and the abdomen is palpated. The aorta is often palpable, and with practice it is generally possible to determine whether or not it is aneurysmal. If there is any doubt, an ultrasound should be requested. Auscultation in the flanks and in the iliac fossae may reveal bruits, although such a finding does not necessarily imply a stenosis of any specific vessel. The lower limb pulses (femoral, popliteal, dorsalis pedis and posterior tibial) are palpated and the legs examined for signs of acute or chronic ischaemia. The difficult popliteal pulse may be examined in a number of ways, one of which involves placing the thumbs of both hands over the tibial tuberosity. The fingers of both hands then meet in the popliteal fossa between the heads of gastrocnemius. The examiner then passively flexes the knee to about 30°, the initial amount of pressure applied to the palpating fingers being that required to lift the leg. Keeping the fingertips together, they are then moved from side to side searching for the popliteal pulse which is felt by applying varying degrees of compression against the tibia. It is important not to tense the skin in this manoeuvre, but to keep it lax, otherwise the artery may not be felt. When feeling all pulses, an assessment is made of the nature of the arterial wall, particularly with respect to calcification. The calcified, pulseless femoral artery may be felt in the groin as a hard, rod-like structure. An absent femoral pulse is highly significant as it has important implications for investigation and treatment. Bruits are sought over the femoral artery in the groin and over the adductor hiatus in the lower thigh. Assuming that too much pressure is not being applied to the stethoscope, the presence of a bruit suggests a stenosis. The absence of a bruit, however, means little as the underlying vessel may be normal or tightly stenosed.

Non-invasive vascular assessment

Basic principles
The basis of non-invasive vascular assessment is Doppler ultrasound. The probe emits a high-frequency signal (5 MHz for deeper structures such as the femoral vessels, 8 MHz for those which are more superficial) which is reflected off tissues. A receiver within the probe picks up the reflected signal and any shift in the frequency between the emitted signal and the received signal is detected. The probe is held over the vessel being studied at 60° towards the angle of blood flow. Sufficient gel is used so that pressure need not be exerted on the probe. The 60° angle is important to maximize the frequency shift: stationary tissues reflect the signal and do not change its frequency, whereas moving

red cells within the vessel also reflect the signal but their movement shifts the signal frequency (increasing it if blood is flowing towards the probe and decreasing it if blood is flowing away).

The simplest devices convert the frequency shift into an audible signal; hand-held devices are available which, in addition to the audible signal, indicate with an arrow in a small display whether blood is flowing towards or away from the probe; more sophisticated devices incorporate a monitor that displays the frequency shift pattern as a continuous waveform plotted against time.

The normal arterial Doppler waveform is triphasic. During systole there is a rapid increase in the velocity of blood flow towards the probe. This produces the first rapid rise in the waveform and corresponds to the first 'whoosh'. At the end of systole the velocity of blood flow reduces to zero (the waveform returns to the baseline) and the first whoosh dies down. The elastic arteries then recoil after having been stretched in systole and as the aortic valve closes there is a short period of reverse flow. This is shown as a short and small-amplitude wave below the baseline on the monitor and is heard as a short whoosh. There is then an even shorter period of forward flow, which is visible on the monitor and heard as the third, rapid whoosh.

With progressive atherosclerosis, arterial wall elasticity is lost. This is detected with Doppler by a loss of the third component of the waveform: the triphasic wave becomes biphasic. With more loss of elasticity the biphasic wave becomes monophasic. As stenoses progress proximally the monophasic wave changes from being peaked with a rapid rise and fall to one which is flatter with a gradual rise and fall, until eventually it is no longer detectable. Using a hand-held Doppler is an extension of the clinical examination and gives valuable information on the location of disease.

Ankle:brachial index
Physiological quantification of the severity of arterial disease can be obtained by measuring the blood pressure at the ankle and comparing it to brachial pressure, i.e. the ankle:brachial index. Brachial pressure is measured in the usual fashion with a sphygmomanometer, using a Doppler probe to detect systolic blood pressure. If there is a discrepancy between the two arms, the higher pressure should be used. The sphygmomanometer cuff is then placed around the lower calf just above the ankle and the pressure in the dorsalis pedis and posterior tibial arteries measured. The ankle:brachial index is then calculated using the higher of the two ankle pressures. Pressure at the ankle should be the same as, or slightly greater than, that in the arm, and the normal ankle:brachial index is between 0.9 and 1.1; as proximal stenoses progress the ratio falls, reaching perhaps 0.7 in a claudicant and 0.4 in a patient with severe claudication or rest pain. A word of caution – the ankle:brachial index is unreliable in those with exces-

sive vascular calcification, particularly diabetic patients. An excessively high cuff pressure is required to occlude flow in these patients, resulting in a falsely high ankle:brachial index. The use of toe cuffs and a laser Doppler probe detecting capillary flow can resolve this problem.

Pre-exercise and post-exercise pressures

There are some patients in whom the history of leg pain is not typical of claudication and others in whom the pain sounds like claudication but the resting ankle:brachial index is normal. Non-invasive vascular assessment can be a great help here. The ankle:brachial indices are measured with the patient at rest. The patient then undertakes a standardized exercise regimen on a treadmill (e.g. 1 min at 3 km/h up a 10% gradient) and the ankle:brachial index is measured again. In the normal vascular tree there will be no fall compared with pre-exercise levels. The extra blood flowing into the vasodilated muscle bed (reduced peripheral vascular resistance) is easily accommodated by the normal vessels, which continue to provide a normal pressure at the ankle. Consider a mild proximal stenosis, however. At rest the relatively high muscle vascular resistance helps to maintain pressure in the main vessel below the stenosis and the ankle:brachial index is normal. After exercise the muscle vascular resistance is lowered, the downstream 'squeeze' that maintained pressure in the main artery is lost and the ankle:brachial index falls. In this way, pre-exercise and post-exercise pressures can help to resolve diagnostic difficulties.

Segmental pressures

Another way in which non-invasive assessment can help to determine the physiological effect of stenoses is by providing segmental pressures. These give an assessment of the blood pressure at different levels in the limb (upper thigh, above knee, below knee, ankle, or the equivalent in the upper limb). There may be a stenosis visible on angiography, the significance of which is uncertain. The segmental pressure immediately below the level of the stenosis will indicate how much of a pressure drop, if any, has occurred across it. To measure segmental pressures, appropriately sized cuffs are placed around the limb at the sites mentioned. A Doppler probe detects blood flow at the ankle and the first cuff (high thigh) is inflated over systolic pressure. As the cuff is deflated below the systolic pressure at the high thigh, blood will flow down to the ankle and will be detected by the Doppler probe. Any stenoses or occlusions distal to the cuff do not matter as it is simple blood flow at the ankle that is being detected. This process is then repeated with the other cuffs in sequence, resulting in figures that give a good indication of the anatomical level of significant stenoses or occlusions. Another word of caution – the high thigh pressure may be falsely low if there is a proximal superficial femoral occlusion and either a common femoral or profunda femoris stenosis.

Colour flow duplex assessment

The duplex scanner combines B-mode ultrasound (real-time anatomical scanning) with Doppler information in one imaging system. Arteries, bypasses and veins can be scanned and any stenoses can be visualized anatomically, while their effect on blood flow can be shown using the Doppler information. Blood flow information is superimposed on the anatomical image with blood flowing towards the probe shown as red and away from the probe as blue (or vice versa). If blood flow is turbulent, as at a stenosis, the colour changes through orange to white when turbulence is maximum. The actual velocity of blood flow can be measured at different sites, as can the frequency of the reflected signal. This information is used to calculate the percentage stenosis and this technique is widely used to determine the degree of carotid artery stenosis and to detect stenoses in vein bypass grafts. It is also applied in some centres to reduce the need for angiography in lower limb disease, although scanning a whole leg can be time consuming and is operator dependent.

Invasive vascular assessment

The keystone of diagnosis in occlusive arterial disease is the patient's history, augmented on occasion by pre-exercise and post-exercise ankle:brachial indices. The other non-invasive tests and all of the invasive tests are used to help to delineate the anatomical pattern of disease as a prelude to treatment: an angiogram cannot diagnose claudication. If treatment is not being planned, angiography should not be requested. This is particularly the case since all angiography carries a finite, if low, risk to limb and even to life. The overall complication rate of radiological peripheral vascular intervention is around 0.7% and the mortality rate about 0.09%.

Intra-arterial digital subtraction angiography

Intra-arterial digital subtraction angiography (IADSA) is the standard method of performing angiography in most units. Intra-arterial access is obtained most commonly in the groin (occasionally in the arm) using the Seldinger technique. A hollow needle is inserted into the artery and free back-flow of arterial blood confirmed. A soft-tipped guide wire is passed through the needle to the site where the contrast injection is required. The needle is removed and a pigtail catheter inserted over the guide wire to the appropriate site. The guide wire is then removed and a pump filled with contrast medium connected to the catheter. The image intensifier then takes a control image of the area being studied, following which the contrast is automatically injected under pressure. The machine continues taking images until the contrast has passed through the area of interest. The initial control image is then digitally subtracted from the subsequent images to leave a detailed angiographic image (Figure 10.1). Using this technique it is possible to obtain excellent quality images of all the

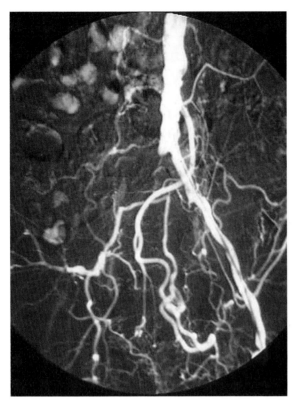

Figure 10.1 Intra-arterial digital subtraction angiogram showing occlusion of the right iliac system.

arteries down to and including those in the foot. It is important that the patient stays still during each image run, otherwise the digital subtraction works less well. In some patients this may be difficult as the contrast injection causes quite an intense burning sensation down the limbs being studied.

The usual study for the lower limbs is known as a peripheral angiogram in which contrast is injected into the aorta just above or just below the renal arteries (moving the catheter distally gives a greater concentration of contrast in the lower limbs). An antegrade puncture of the femoral artery (a single femoral angiogram) places the catheter tip in the superficial femoral artery and is used either for more detailed views of a single leg or as a prelude to angioplasty. With the catheter placed in the aortic arch (an arch angiogram), views of the arch and great vessels are obtained. The subclavians are seen to beyond the vertebral artery origin and the carotids to beyond their bifurcation. Selective angiograms of either carotid or subclavians can be taken as required, although the risk of distal embolization increases. Selective views may also be taken of the mesenteric and renal arteries (with lateral projections for the former).

The risks of angiography include direct arterial trauma either at the entry site or anywhere along the path of the catheter. The trauma may result in acute vessel occlusion, distal embolization or perforation. Other entry site complications are bleeding or false aneurysm

formation. The dose of contrast used has to be monitored, although volume is not usually an issue with intra-arterial studies. Some patients are allergic to the contrast and the medium is nephrotoxic. Patients with pre-existing renal impairment should be well hydrated prior to angiography and their renal function carefully monitored afterwards. Contrast medium interacts with metformin and there is a risk of metabolic acidosis. Because of this, metformin should be stopped around the time of angiography and the diabetes controlled by other means.

Intravenous digital subtraction angiography

Intravenous digital subtraction angiography (IVDSA) is performed either by placing a large-bore, short-length cannula in a good arm vein or by placing a peripherally inserted central venous catheter. An infusion pump rapidly injects a large volume (200 ml) of contrast in a single bolus. The digital subtraction technique is again used, but the image acquisition is timed to coincide with the bolus passing through the arteries in the area of interest. Further runs and bolus injections are used to obtain a full sequence of pictures.

The advantages of this technique over intra-arterial studies are that no arterial puncture is required, so reducing many of the risks of angiography. It is important, however, that the patient has a good cardiac output, otherwise the contrast bolus becomes too dilute on its passage through the lungs to give useful pictures. In addition to this reason, cardiac failure is a relative contraindication because of the injection volumes used (up to 1000 ml). Renal failure is another relative contraindication because of the volume load and the increased risk of contrast-induced nephrotoxicity. The images obtained are not as good as with an intra-arterial injection and detail of the calf vessels is difficult to obtain. There is a role for the technique, however, and some units use it in preference to intra-arterial injections because of the lower risk of arterial complications.

The future of angiography

Special reconstructions of contrast-enhanced computed tomographic (CT) studies can give useful information about the state of arteries, but most promise in the area of non-invasive angiography lies with gadolinium-enhanced magnetic resonance imaging. Advances in image acquisition technology may allow magnetic resonance angiography to take over from intra-arterial digital subtraction angiography in the not too far distant future.

Section 10.2 • Occlusive peripheral arterial disease

Cerebrovascular ischaemia

Stroke is the third leading cause of death in the UK, as well as being a major cause of morbidity. The advent of CT scanning enabled the differentiation to be made between haemorrhage and infarction as the cause of stroke: in the Western world, the majority of strokes is due to cerebral infarction. Cerebral infarction is caused by one of two events:

- occlusion of a cerebral artery (in an area of poor collateralization) by embolus or by thrombosis *in situ* on underlying atherosclerosis
- global reduction in blood flow to an area of the brain (less common).

Embolic disease arising from atherosclerosis at the carotid bifurcation is a common cause of stroke and is amenable to preventive treatment.

History
Embolic disease from the carotid bifurcation can result in a series of symptoms of increasing severity.

Amaurosis fugax is at the milder end of the scale and results when a platelet embolus originating on the carotid bifurcation travels along the ophthalmic artery (the first branch of the internal carotid artery) and then into the central retinal artery. It may lodge here or in a more distal branch. Occlusion of the central retinal artery results in transient blindness affecting the whole visual field of the eye ipsilateral to the source of the embolus. The patient often describes the event as a curtain coming down over the eye. If a more distal branch in the retina is occluded then only part of the visual field will be lost. Either way, the other eye is not affected: this important point can help to distinguish amaurosis fugax from a recovered homonomous hemianopia. When the embolus breaks up, the visual field is recovered, providing the duration and depth of ischaemia were not too great. If the embolus does not break up, or if the ischaemia is too severe, then recovery does not occur and the patient may lose part or all the visual field in that eye. In these cases an ophthalmological opinion is useful to visualize the embolus on fundoscopy and so diagnose the cause of the visual field loss.

A transient ischaemic attack is defined as a focal neurological deficit lasting for less than 24 h with full recovery. In these cases the embolus passes into the cerebral circulation to cause sensory or motor symptoms on the side contralateral to the side of origin of the embolus. Commonly, the patient reports a hemiplegia or monoplegia, expressive dysphasia (Broca's area is in the dominant left hemisphere in right-handed people), a hemianopia if the optic radiation is involved or unilateral sensory disturbance. The symptoms all relate to the internal carotid territory on the side of origin of the embolus. The vertebral territory is not affected. With recovery, either the embolus breaks up or the collateral circulation is recruited and no permanent neurological damage results. A history of a motor transient ischaemic attack can generally be taken as evidence of embolic disease, usually from the carotid bifurcation. A purely sensory transient ischaemic attack may result from embolic disease, but there is a higher chance that another pathology may be the cause, such

as epilepsy or even a cerebral tumour. In such cases, it is recommended that a CT brain scan or a neurological opinion is sought before advising surgery.

A patient suffers crescendo transient ischaemic attacks when three or more occur in rapid succession. The same territory is often involved in all of the attacks, giving rise to similar symptoms each time. The significance of crescendo transient ischaemic attacks is that a full-blown stroke becomes much more likely.

The concept of resolving ischaemic neurological deficit (RIND) has been introduced to describe those focal neurological deficits that take longer than 24 h but less than 1 week to recover fully, while that of stroke in evolution describes an event in which the neurological deficit has not yet stabilized.

In a full stroke there is persistent neurological deficit beyond 1 week. This may be permanent or even fatal; alternatively, slow recovery may occur for up to 1 year following the event.

Examination
Clinical examination follows the plan outlined above. In addition, it is important to make a neurological assessment to document any pre-existing deficit. As mentioned, fundoscopy can be useful on occasion to identify a retinal embolus.

Investigation
The primary investigation in many units is now a colour-flow duplex scan (Figure 10.2). As described above, this gives a good indication of the degree of stenosis at the carotid bifurcation and also gives information on the plaque type: it is becoming apparent that the type of plaque (friable, ulcerated, fibrous) may give an important indication as to the risk of future stroke.

The 'gold standard' investigation, however, is still selective carotid angiography, if only because the studies that demonstrated the value of carotid

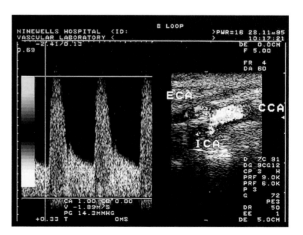

Figure 10.2 Duplex scan of the carotid bifurcation showing a moderate stenosis. The Doppler flow pattern is also shown. CCA, common carotid artery; ICA, internal carotid artery; ECA, external carotid artery.

endarterectomy used this imaging modality. The draw-back with this investigation is a 1–3% stroke rate, related to catheter manipulation within the carotid arteries. Contrast injection into the aortic arch over-comes this and has a significantly lower stroke risk, although the images obtained are less clear. Duplex tends to overestimate the degree of stenosis compared with angiography and there can be wide variations between the two modalities. Because duplex scanning is operator dependent it is important that the results are regularly scrutinized. Unless confidence in the duplex results is high, those patients who are shown to have a high-grade stenosis on duplex scanning should probably undergo confirmatory angiography.

Management

The current treatment choices lie between optimal medical management (control of all risk factors and antiplatelet therapy with aspirin, or the new adenosine diphosphate receptor inhibitor, clopidogrel) and carotid endarterectomy. Surgery has always been more popular in the USA than in Europe, but there was little hard evidence to support its role until 1990, when the results of two large randomized trials (one in Europe, the other in North America) became available. These trials demonstrated convincingly that patients with recent (within 6 months) amaurosis fugax, transient ischaemic attack or stroke with good recovery and an internal carotid stenosis of 70–99% had a lower risk of further stroke after carotid endarterectomy than on medical treatment. This finding held true as long as the com-bined operative stroke and mortality risk was less than 6%. Both studies also showed that if the internal carotid artery stenosis was less than 30% then medical therapy was the safest option. The European study went on to show that medical therapy was also the best option for those with a 30–69% stenosis.

Carotid endarterectomy is usually performed under general anaesthesia, although regional blockade is used in some units. The endarterectomy extends from the distal common carotid to the end of the plaque in the internal carotid and also includes the origin of the external carotid. Much work has been performed on the value of placing an intra-arterial shunt during the procedure and on selecting those patients who would benefit from a shunt. Various methods are used to make this selection (e.g. stump pressure, transcranial Doppler, cerebral oximetry, electroencephalography), but no one method has achieved universal acceptance. The arteri-otomy may be closed either directly or with a patch (Dacron or vein), depending on the size of the internal carotid artery.

Apart from perioperative stroke, the local complica-tions of the procedure include numbness around the angle of the mandible, hypoglossal nerve palsy, recur-rent laryngeal nerve palsy and neck haematoma with possible associated stridor due to laryngeal oedema. Myocardial infarction is also a significant complication and reflects the correlation that exists between carotid and coronary atherosclerosis.

Chronic lower limb ischaemia

Consider the scenario of a patient with slowly progres-sive atherosclerosis affecting one or more lower limb arterial segments. The first complaint that such a patient will have will be intermittent claudication at a certain distance. The pain is generally felt at the level below that of the arterial disease and extends distally: aortic disease causes buttock, thigh and calf claudica-tion, iliac disease results in thigh and calf claudication and superficial femoral disease causes calf claudication. Intermittent claudication is described as a cramp-like or toothache-like pain associated with weakness of the affected muscle group (weakness is a particular feature in diabetic patients with neuropathy). It occurs after a certain distance, which will be shorter if the patient walks quickly or uphill, and is relieved by standing still. The pain rarely takes longer than 5 min to resolve, fol-lowing which the patient can walk the same distance again. A patient's claudication distance is generally sta-ble in the medium term; therefore, a patient with leg pain after walking 20 m on one day, after walking 200 m on another and occasionally at rest is unlikely to be suffering from intermittent claudication.

It is important to distinguish intermittent claudication from the pain of spinal stenosis. In the latter, disc pro-trusion or osteophyte formation results in a narrowing of the spinal canal. The ensuing pressure on the cauda equina produces referred pain in the lower limb. The pain is precipitated by prolonged standing and is often felt in the calf. It is being upright that results in the pain, and as it is more common to walk when upright than to stand still for a length of time the patient complains of the pain on walking. This pain can therefore be very similar to that of intermittent claudication, but there are distinct differences. The pain of spinal stenosis is only relieved by sitting or lying down; simply standing still provides no respite. Spinal stenosis pain takes longer to resolve than intermittent claudication, often 20 min or more. Intermittent claudication is only brought on by walking, whereas the pain of spinal stenosis occurs when standing, for example in a queue. Confusingly, the pain of spinal stenosis is sometimes called spinal claudication; however, there is no ischaemic aetiology to it.

About 60% of patients with intermittent claudica-tion reach a certain level of activity at which their symptoms stabilize. The claudication can improve in about 20% of cases if the patients are encouraged to exercise regularly within the limits of their pain and if their risk factors are all addressed. Any improvement is brought about by collateral vessels enlarging and carry-ing more blood flow around stenoses and occlusions. In the other 20% there will be a deterioration in the symptoms over time. These patients report a decreasing claudication distance over a period of weeks to months. Eventually, they are unable to walk around the house without discomfort. The next stage is nocturnal ischaemic pain. This often occurs before daytime rest pain, for three reasons: cardiac output and blood pres-sure are lower at night, so further reducing the perfusion of tissue distal to a tight stenosis or occlusion; lying down elevates the legs compared with the upright posture, further increasing the perfusion pressure required to cross a stenosis; and the feet are warmer in bed at night than during the day and so the basal metabolic rate of the soft tissue is increased: in the absence of adequate perfusion lactate builds up and results in pain. Patients woken with nocturnal pain will hang their foot over the side of the bed to increase perfusion pressure and to cool the tissues down. They may find more relief from placing their foot on a cold surface (such as a tiled floor) or, paradoxically, from walking around. Walking increases the perfusion pressure more because of the upright posture and the rise in blood pressure. Some patients may have to sleep in a chair and the resulting dependency leads to ankle oedema. The oedema reduces tissue perfusion further by acting as a diffusion barrier between the capillaries and the tissues. As arterial disease progresses further rest pain is felt during the day and it is not relieved by any of the above factors. Both nocturnal and rest pain are felt in the foot, generally in the forefoot. This is because the foot is the most distal part of the limb and the furthest away from any collateral circulation that has developed.

As ischaemia progresses further, tissue loss results, in the form of either ulceration or gangrene (Figure 10.3). Gangrene tends to start in the toes, while ulceration is often the result of minor trauma, as intact skin

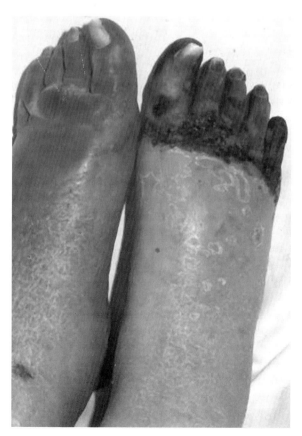

Figure 10.3 Chronic ischaemia with gangrene of the right forefoot and super-added acute changes in the left foot.

requires a lower blood supply to remain intact than a wound does to heal. Secondary infection originating at a site of tissue loss can worsen the ischaemia: tissue oedema increases interstitial pressure, which may rise higher than the low capillary perfusion pressure of a severely ischaemic limb. Blood then thromboses in the microcirculation and the effect can spread proximally to the small arteries.

Management

The treatment of chronic lower limb ischaemia is conservative unless claudication is incapacitating or limb loss is threatened (nocturnal pain, rest pain, tissue loss). Conservative management consists most importantly of controlling the risk factors associated with vascular disease, particularly stopping smoking and control of hypertension, hyperlipidaemia and diabetes. In this way, the 'early warning' symptom of claudication may enable treatment to delay or prevent more significant vascular disease in the coronary or cerebral circulation. All patients should be placed on 75 mg of aspirin as antiplatelet therapy (the role of clopidogrel, the new adenosine monophosphate receptor blocker, has yet to be delineated) unless there are contraindications and the patient should be encouraged to take up as much walking exercise as possible within the limits of their pain. The majority of claudicants can be managed in this way and a proportion of them (up to 80%) will suffer no further deterioration in their symptoms.

The decision to investigate patients with claudication is taken hand in hand with the decision to offer treatment if an appropriate lesion is found. This has to balance the degree of disability with the risk of any radiological or surgical intervention. Equivalent walking distances will clearly have different effects on an elderly person with coexisting cardiac failure and osteoarthritis than on a young, otherwise fit and active person. A good guiding principle here is that if the patient is able to manage at their symptom level, then they are best treated in a conservative fashion. If the patient is unable to manage and a trial of conservative treatment has failed then investigation is appropriate.

The anticipated site of the lesion responsible for the symptoms also has a bearing: the more proximal the lesion the more likely it is that treatment will be successful, and the less likely it is that a limb-threatening complication will ensue. This is where segmental pressures and waveform analysis can be of great help. Major abdominal surgery carries more systemic risk than infrainguinal reconstruction. If the patient is generally fit, then investigation is therefore appropriate if the lesion is thought to be in the aortoiliac segment. Patients with femoropopliteal disease can be investigated and treated for claudication, but long-term clinical success is not as likely as with aortoiliac disease. Patients with tibial vessel disease are rarely, if ever, offered treatment for claudication as the risks of bypass on to, or angioplasty of, these small arteries outweigh the benefit of being merely being able to walk further.

The decision as to whether to investigate a claudicant is therefore based on the patient's symptoms, the anticipated site of the lesion and on the surgeon's own philosophy regarding the risks of treatment. When a patient has critical ischaemia, however, the norm is to offer investigation and treatment. The only exceptions would be those patients with significant coexisting morbidity whose life expectancy (with or without treatment of their critical limb ischaemia) is expected to be very short, or those in whom the general risks of surgery are judged to be too great. This latter group particularly includes patients requiring aortoiliac reconstruction. In cases of critical ischaemia the risk of limb loss with conservative treatment justifies the risks of bypass or angioplasty of tibial vessels.

Once the decision to investigate has been made, an angiogram is obtained. The principles determining reconstruction (either angioplasty or surgery) are a good inflow, a good outflow and the availability of a suitable means to deal with the lesion itself. Combinations of treatment modalities may be used, e.g. iliac angioplasty to improve the inflow prior to femoropopliteal bypass.

Lesions most suitable for angioplasty are short, concentric, not heavily calcified and are situated in an otherwise healthy arterial segment. Angioplasty of lesions over 10 cm in length is unlikely to result in long-term patency.

Some lesions are best stented after angioplasty. These include those lesions at the aortic bifurcation and those in which angioplasty alone has produced a less than optimal result, particularly if there is a dissection flap.

Bypass surgery is undertaken if angioplasty is not appropriate and if the risk–benefit analysis for that patient suggests that it is appropriate. Possible inflow sites for the bypass are the aorta, the iliacs, the common, superficial or profunda femorals, the popliteal and rarely (for critical ischaemia) the calf vessels. Potential outflow sites are the iliacs, the common, superficial or profunda femorals and the above- or below-knee popliteal. The anterior or posterior tibial and peroneal are also outflow sites suitable for use in critical ischaemia.

The ideal conduit for infrainguinal reconstruction is the ipsilateral long saphenous vein. The contralateral long saphenous vein, the short saphenous veins or arm veins may also be used if necessary. Vein bypasses (either reversed or non-reversed) have superior long-term patency rates to prostheses, with the possible exception of the above-knee femoropopliteal bypass. If the patient is able to tolerate aspirin, the long-term patency of a prosthesis at this level is similar to that of a vein bypass. If a prosthesis has to be used in a below-knee femoropopliteal bypass, its chances of long-term patency can be improved using a vein cuff at the distal anastomosis.

Acute lower limb ischaemia

Acute occlusion of the lower limb vessels may result either from an embolus or from thrombosis developing *in situ* on underlying arterial disease. An embolus may lodge in an otherwise normal arterial tree or in vessels already affected by atherosclerosis. The clinical picture will differ in the two cases.

The patient with severe acute ischaemia

These are the patients with the well-known classical presentation of acute lower limb ischaemia: the patient develops a sudden onset of pain, paralysis, paraesthesiae (or anaesthesia), 'perishing' cold, pallor and pulselessness (the '6 ps'). In such a case, the patient is in agony; the leg is white, cold and paralysed, and the patient is unable to move it and unable to feel anything touching it (Figure 10.4). Such a severe degree of ischaemia results when there is sudden occlusion of the inflow to the entire leg: the embolus usually lodges in the common femoral artery. The symptoms may be bilateral if a larger embolus lodges at the aortic bifurcation (a 'saddle' embolus). In order for the degree of ischaemia to be so severe, there have to be few, if any, collateral vessels capable of carrying blood around the acute occlusion. The patient has an otherwise healthy arterial tree and there is no history of previous intermittent claudication. Classically, these are patients who have had previous rheumatic fever with resulting mitral stenosis and atrial fibrillation. As such patients are becoming increasingly rare, the classical presentation of severe acute ischaemia is also becoming more uncommon.

The treatment of severe acute ischaemia due to an embolus is emergency exploration of the femoral artery. There is no time to be wasted, as the degree of muscle ischaemia is so severe that changes become irreversible after about 6 h. An arteriotomy is made in the common femoral artery and the inflow assessed. A Fogarty balloon catheter is passed proximally into the aorta, the balloon inflated and the catheter withdrawn. This removes any proximal thrombus/embolus and should restore normal inflow. The Fogarty catheter is then passed distally down the superficial femoral and deep femoral arteries, again withdrawing any thrombus or embolus from these vessels. The arteriotomy is closed, with a vein patch if necessary, and flow restored to the leg. The 'pinking-up' of the foot should be immediately apparent. An on-table angiogram should then be performed, injecting contrast through a needle puncture of the common femoral artery. This should confirm free flow of contrast and the absence of

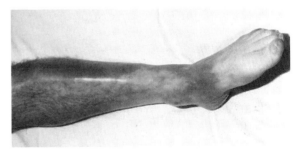

Figure 10.4 Severe acute ischaemia.

thrombus/embolus in the superficial femoral, popliteal and calf arteries. If there is a residual filling defect, the Fogarty catheter should be repassed. The patient should then be anticoagulated for life, if there are no contraindications.

The patient with less severe acute ischaemia

Most patients presenting with acute ischaemia are elderly with a degree of underlying arterial disease. The causes of acute ischaemia in this group are either embolus or thrombosis *in situ* on underlying atherosclerotic plaques. The presence of pre-existing arterial disease and the associated development of a collateral circulation result in a paradox, in that an acute event in these patients does not result in such severe ischaemia as it does in a patient with an otherwise normal arterial tree. The collateral circulation allows some perfusion around the acute occlusion. The extent of this collateral circulation modulates the classical presentation of severe acute ischaemia to a greater or lesser degree.

Patients with this disease pattern will often have a history of claudication in the affected or contralateral limb and also evidence of vascular disease elsewhere. The patient will complain of an acute onset of pain in the affected limb. While the initial pain is severe, it may improve with time as the collateral circulation opens up. This may result in a delay in the patient seeking medical attention. The other changes of severe acute ischaemia are present to a greater or lesser degree. Sensory disturbance is usually present, with paraesthesiae being more common than the anaesthesia of severe acute ischaemia. Muscle paralysis is a bad sign and an inability to move the toes is an indication that the ischaemia is severe. Tenderness affecting the calf muscles often indicates muscle necrosis and serious consideration should be given in such cases as to whether revascularization or amputation is the better option.

The total pallor of the limb in severe acute ischaemia gives way to a mottled appearance when the ischaemia is less severe. There are areas of pallor (where there is no blood in the microcirculation), of cyanosis (where flow is so sluggish that maximal deoxygenation of haemoglobin occurs) and of rubor (where the microcirculation has opened up and there is reactive hyperaemia), resulting in the 'marbled' appearance. Buerger's test in these patients is very useful. The limb should be elevated and inspected. If the ischaemia has not yet destroyed capillary integrity then the limb will blanch. Any stubborn areas of cyanosis can be further tested while the limb is elevated by examining for the presence of capillary refill. Skin that blanches under these circumstances is viable. If, however, there are bluish areas that will not blanch then this implies that capillary integrity has been destroyed and that the patch of skin is no longer viable. The patient then sits up and hangs the limb in a dependent position. Viable skin becomes bright red owing to reactive hyperaemia. The longer this takes the more critical is the ischaemia.

The combination of sensory loss, degree of paralysis, calf muscle tenderness and skin colour changes (particularly fixed skin mottling) is used to gauge the degree of severity of the ischaemia. This is then used to help to determine the type and urgency of treatment.

Angiography should be performed first. This will give information on the proximal circulation, the level of the occlusion and the extent of the collateral circulation. The distal circulation may not be well opacified because of poor flow, and patent vessels may be present even if they do not show on the angiogram. On occasion, the angiogram may show an embolus occluding a more distal vessel (e.g. the popliteal). In such cases the cut-off is sharp and if there is little atherosclerosis, embolectomy should be performed. More commonly, there is generalized atherosclerosis and the acute occlusion is caused by thrombosis *in situ*. Vascular calcification may be seen and the cut-off is more gradual than with an embolus. Even if an embolus is suspected, embolectomy should only be performed after careful consideration if there is significant atherosclerosis, as withdrawal of the balloon will traumatize the vessel, making it thrombogenic.

Embolectomy is not appropriate in the majority of cases. The treatment choice then lies between thrombolysis and bypass. If there are contraindications to thrombolysis (bleeding diathesis or long-term anticoagulation treatment, recent bleeding ulcer or active peptic ulceration, stroke within 3 years, any cerebral haemorrhage, recent surgery) or if the degree of ischaemia is so severe that tissue loss is considered imminent then surgical bypass will be required. The choice of inflow vessel is determined by the angiogram. The outflow vessel may be demonstrated on the angiogram; if it is not, then surgical exploration of the vessels considered most likely to be suitable should be performed. If a suitable vessel is identified (possibly with the assistance of on-table angiography or even on-table bolus thrombolysis into a thrombosed run-off vessel) then a bypass can be constructed.

If the degree of ischaemia is not so severe then thrombolysis may be considered. This is delivered through an intra-arterial catheter placed with its tip in the thrombus. Streptokinase, tissue plasminogen activator or urokinase may be used as either a low-dose continuous infusion or a high-dose bolus regime (pulse spray), which may act more quickly. Check angiography is performed every 8–12 h and the catheter tip repositioned if necessary. After dissolution of the thrombus the underlying cause for the thrombosis is usually apparent and this has to be dealt with by angioplasty or surgery.

Intra-arterial thrombolysis is a major intervention with significant complications and it should not be undertaken lightly. Its advantage, however, is that it can unmask the underlying cause of the acute ischaemia and thereby reduce the magnitude of the revascularization procedure (angioplasty or bypass) that is required.

Mesenteric vascular ischaemia

This phenomenon is difficult to diagnose in either the chronic or the acute situation. Chronic mesenteric vascular ischaemia results in postprandial abdominal pain (mesenteric angina) and weight loss. It is a difficult diagnosis to make on clinical grounds alone and is often made by exclusion after a series of investigations. Of the three mesenteric arteries (coeliac axis, superior and inferior mesenteric arteries), two generally have to be occluded to support this diagnosis. Although duplex scanning can give an indication of the pattern of disease, angiography is required with lateral views of the aorta to show the anterior origins of these vessels. Treatment is by balloon angioplasty if the lesion is considered suitable or by bypass, usually on to the superior mesenteric artery with inflow from the aorta.

Acute mesenteric ischaemia presents as a sudden onset of abdominal pain with or without rectal bleeding. The pain is often worse than the physical findings may suggest, but it is related to the extent and degree of ischaemia. At the milder end of the scale, the pain and rectal bleeding are self-limiting, as the mucosa of the descending colon has infarcted and sloughed but the remainder of the colonic wall has remained viable. Such patients may end up with either ischaemic colitis or a postischaemic fibrotic stricture. At the other end of the scale the patient has generalized peritonitis and emergency laparotomy shows extensive gangrene of the small and large bowel. The only surgical option in these cases is resection, if this is considered appropriate. On rare occasions, emergency laparotomy will show severe but recoverable small bowel ischaemia due to either an embolus lodging in the superior mesenteric artery or thrombosis occurring *in situ*. The former is amenable to treatment by mesenteric embolectomy, closing the arteriotomy with a vein patch; the latter may be amenable to bypass.

Upper limb ischaemia

Upper limb ischaemia is much less common than ischaemia in the lower limb. The upper limb vessels are much less likely to be affected by atherosclerosis, so the pattern of aetiology is different. Probably the most common cause is embolic, followed by iatrogenic trauma during cardiac catheterization via the brachial route. A more rare cause is the thoracic outlet syndrome. Finally, Raynaud's affects the fingers to a greater extent than the toes.

Upper limb embolus

Upper limb emboli tend to lodge at the bifurcation of the brachial artery and cause symptoms similar to acute ischaemia in the lower limb. The arm, however, has a great capacity to recover by the recruitment of collaterals or the break up of the embolus. If, on presentation, the arm is clearly viable (no or little sensory loss, no paralysis or muscle tenderness, capillary refill present) then treatment may be conservative with heparinization to reduce the propagation of thrombus.

If there is any doubt as to the viability of the arm then exploration of the brachial artery through a 'lazy-S' incision in the antecubital fossa should be performed. The Fogarty catheter is inserted through a transverse brachial arteriotomy. The brachial artery is cleared of embolus/thrombus, as are both the radial and ulnar arteries. On-table angiography should confirm clearance of the vessels.

An alternative approach aimed at minimizing the long-term risk of claudication is to compare the radial artery pressure (measured with a sphygmomanometer cuff placed on the forearm and a portable Doppler probe) in the symptomatic arm with that in the normal arm. If the ratio is 0.6 or less then claudication is likely in the long term and embolectomy should be performed.

Catheterization trauma

Repair of catheterization trauma usually requires a vein patch or occasionally a bypass. The decision to perform a repair follows the same principles as deciding whether to perform an embolectomy.

Thoracic outlet syndrome

A narrow space between scalenus anterior and the first rib or an abnormal cervical rib can cause compression of the T1 nerve root and subclavian artery. The arterial symptoms include claudication, especially with the shoulder abducted, and a Raynaud's pattern of finger discoloration due to microembolization from a post-stenotic dilatation of the subclavian artery. Physical examination may demonstrate a reduction or abolition of the radial pulse with the shoulder abducted and externally rotated (Allen's test) and a reproduction of the symptoms when the patient repeatedly makes and relaxes a fist with the shoulder abducted (Roos test).

Treatment involves scalenotomy, excision of the first rib and of the cervical rib, if present. If there is a subclavian dilatation causing embolization then this has to be resected with either end-to-end anastomosis or bypass.

Raynaud's

The term Raynaud's refers to the typical skin colour changes of white, blue and red. These are caused by digital artery spasm or occlusion resulting in a white digit. As sluggish flow returns the digit becomes cyanosed owing to the high concentration of deoxygenated haemoglobin. When normal flow is re-established there is redness due to reactive hyperaemia.

Raynaud's may be primary or secondary. Primary Raynaud's is not associated with any systemic condition, is generally bilateral and affects young women most commonly. It is benign and tissue loss is not a feature. Secondary Raynaud's may be associated with systemic conditions such as scleroderma, in which case it is also bilateral, or with local conditions such as a subclavian aneurysm, in which case the symptoms are unilateral. The outlook in secondary Raynaud's is not as good, however, and tissue loss is a feature.

Section 10.3 • Dilating peripheral arterial disease

Abdominal aortic aneurysms

Pathogenesis

An aneurysm may be defined as an abnormal dilatation of an artery to greater than 1.5 times its normal diameter. An aneurysmal artery usually has a thin wall and is typically lined with laminated thrombus. The expansion of an aneurysm appears to be governed by the law of Laplace: tension = pressure × radius. As an aneurysm expands the wall tension increases. Clinical experience confirms that larger aneurysms are more likely to rupture. Aneurysms are generally associated with atherosclerosis, although whether this is a causative effect is debatable. There is a possibility that they are caused by an imbalance of collagen and elastin metabolism in the media.

Epidemiology

The prevalence of aneurysms in the normal population is 2.4%. High-risk groups include those with peripheral vascular disease (prevalence 10–14%) or hypertension (10.7%) or a sibling with known aneurysm (20%).

Age has a strong effect, increasing the prevalence of aortic aneurysms in both genders. There is a 100-fold increase in the mortality from aortic aneurysm between men below 55 and those above 85 years of age, with a 10-fold increase between the 55–64 age group and those above 85 years of age. Aneurysms in younger people (< 40 years) are usually associated with connective tissue disorders such as Marfan's syndrome and type IV Ehlers–Danlos syndrome. Smoking is associated with abdominal aortic aneurysm and with death due to abdominal aortic aneurysm.

Natural history

The annual growth rate of aortic aneurysms has been shown to be approximately 0.3–0.5 cm, although individual aneurysms have different growth rates and the speed of expansion also varies at different times. Although it is not possible to predict the growth rate of an individual aneurysm, in general, large aneurysms expand more quickly than small ones.

Rupture is associated with diastolic hypertension and chronic obstructive airways disease. The presence of a small aneurysm raises the annual death rate by 230%. Larger aneurysms carry a greater 5-year rupture risk, with 6 cm aneurysms carrying a risk of 60%, 7 cm of 70% and 8 cm of 80%. The actual site of rupture is thought to be a localized weakness or bleb on a more diffusely weakened aneurysm wall. Most aneurysms rupture posterolaterally into the retroperitoneal space and on extremely rare occasions a patient may survive for weeks or months with a contained rupture.

Four per cent of patients with abdominal aortic aneurysms will have aneurysms at other sites such as popliteal and femoral. Conversely, a patient presenting with a popliteal aneurysm has a 6% probability of having an abdominal aortic aneurysm.

Diagnosis

Most abdominal aortic aneurysms are asymptomatic. They are often only identified as part of a routine physical, ultrasound or radiographic examination. The expansile pulsation is usually found above and to the left of the umbilicus.

Aneurysms may become symptomatic, either with the development of abdominal or back pain with or without rupture or, more rarely, due to distal embolization. Rupture is usually characterized by abdominal pain associated with collapse. Any elderly patient who develops a new acute onset of abdominal pain and collapse should be assumed to have ruptured an aortic aneurysm until proven otherwise. The pain may also be felt in the back, the loins (mimicking ureteric colic) and even into the groins. Very rarely, an aneurysm may rupture into an adjacent structure to produce an aortoenteric fistula or aortocaval fistula. The former is characterized by a small herald bleed which, unless the clues are picked up, is generally followed 24–48 h later by exsanguinating haemorrhage. Rarely, an aortoenteric fistula may present as chronic low-grade gastrointestinal blood loss. An aortocaval fistula is characterized by congestive cardiac failure and a loud abdominal bruit.

Small aneurysms are difficult to detect by palpation and even large ones may be missed in the obese patient. Plain anteroposterior or lateral radiographs will provide the diagnosis in 80–90% of patients showing calcification in the aneurysmal arterial wall. B-mode ultrasound is the routine method of investigation and is reliable in determining the size and site of an aneurysm (Figure 10.5). Ultrasound is less reliable for determining the exact relationship of the aneurysm to the origin of the renal arteries and for visualizing the iliac vessels. B-mode ultrasound is the investigation of choice for serial long-term follow-up. CT is more sensitive. It allows the visualization of renal artery origins and can be used with contrast enhancement to diagnose contained ruptures and dissections. It will also make possible the diagnosis of inflammatory aneurysm

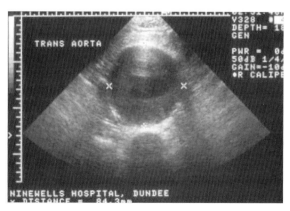

Figure 10.5 Ultrasound scan of an aortic aneurysm.

by showing the thickened wall of the sac. The use of angiography is generally restricted to the assessment of coincidental arterial disease affecting the visceral or peripheral arteries as part of the preparation for surgery.

Selection for and timing of surgery

Patients presenting with aortic aneurysms are elderly and, when the surgeon is weighing the operative risk, may be assumed to have multisystem disease. Age should be regarded as a risk factor but must be considered as part of the patient's general condition. Other factors leading to exclusion from surgery include renal and cardiac failure, malignancy and cerebrovascular disease. There is a fine balance between surgical intervention, the estimated probability of rupture, age, the presence of risk factors, anticipated quality of life and expected survival unrelated to the aneurysm.

Up to one-third of aneurysms present with rupture without previous symptoms. There is strong justification for carrying out repair of aortic aneurysms greater than 5.5 cm in diameter in otherwise fit individuals.

Operations for aortic aneurysm

It is fortunate that approximately 90% of abdominal aortic aneurysms arise below the level of the renal arteries and can therefore be treated surgically without directly disturbing the blood supply to the kidneys or other viscera. Downward extension of the ectatic process to involve the iliac arteries is very common, occurring in approximately two-thirds of cases.

Preoperative assessment

The repair of an aortic aneurysm is a prophylactic procedure (i.e. not all patients will inevitably die from the disorder). The procedure must therefore be significantly of less risk to the patient than the disease. Patients in whom a repair of an aortic aneurysm is anticipated require careful preoperative evaluation. The three main areas of concern are the cardiac, pulmonary and renal status. An initial clinical assessment is made based on the patient's symptoms. Unstable angina, angina at rest, recent (< 6 months) myocardial infarction and congestive cardiac failure are all symptoms of real concern and militate against repair. Even if these are absent, some form of formal cardiac assessment is required owing to the age of the patient. This usually takes the form of radionuclide ventriculography or echocardiography at rest, or preferably some form of stress testing. If a reversible defect is found then coronary angiography should be considered.

Poor pulmonary function is also an area of concern. In patients with a poor respiratory reserve, preoperative pulmonary function tests (forced expiratory volume in 1 s and vital capacity) are required, as is a blood gas estimate. A raised creatinine (> 260 mol/l) is also a risk factor for perioperative death. Careful discussion between the surgeon and anaesthetist is required.

Complications of aneurysm repair

In addition to the predictable range of complications to be expected in a population of elderly and atherosclerotic patients, there is a number of hazards to which aneurysm patients are particularly susceptible.

Early complications include haemorrhage, distal embolization, renal failure, mesenteric and spinal cord ischaemia.

Haemorrhage from suture lines in friable aorta can usually be controlled. Venous bleeding in the region of the neck of the aneurysm may be more difficult to manage, especially in emergency operations, when difficulties due to the haematoma will be compounded by coagulation disorders resulting from massive bleeding and large-scale volume replacement.

Large aneurysms invariably accumulate large amounts of thrombus within the sac and surgical manipulations can result in embolism. Thrombus may also form distal to the arterial clamps. More troublesome is microembolization into the distal arterial tree giving rise to 'trash foot', which in severe cases may result in tissue loss or even major amputation.

There are several mechanisms whereby the kidneys may be damaged during aneurysm surgery. Anatomical variations in the renal arteries are frequent. These vessels may be unavoidably damaged by the aneurysm process or by surgery. It may be necessary to clamp the aorta above normally sited renal arteries in difficult cases and renal damage is liable to occur if the warm ischaemia time exceeds 30 min. Renal artery stenosis is a common finding on preoperative aortograms in patients with aortic aneurysms and the kidneys are thereby more vulnerable to damage. The ectatic aorta contains atheromatous debris and thrombus, which may embolize into the kidneys during dissection or when the aorta is cross-clamped. Perioperative hypovolaemic or cardiogenic shock may result in acute tubular necrosis.

The inferior mesenteric artery is often obliterated by the expanding aneurysm, but if still patent at the time of operation will need to be either ligated or, occasionally, reimplanted into the graft. Usually, without implantation, the collateral circulation is sufficient to sustain colon viability. Mild ischaemic damage to the large bowel follows aneurysm surgery not uncommonly, but it is severe in around 2% of cases. Diarrhoea in the early postoperative period is the most consistent sign and if bloody, this implies a serious degree of necrosis of the gut wall.

In the case of infrarenal aneurysm, although it is often necessary to oversew a number of lumbar arteries, clinically apparent spinal cord ischaemia seldom results. The paraplegia rate is less than 1%.

The **late complications** of aortoiliac reconstructions by synthetic graft, whether for aneurysm or for occlusive disease, are rare but important because they are life threatening. They include infection, aortoenteric fistula and sexual dysfunction.

Infection in a synthetic graft may occur at any stage in the postoperative course from the early postoperative period to many years later. Bacteria have been cultured from sac thrombus in 8% of asymptomatic and 20% of ruptured aneurysms, but no relationship has been demonstrated between thrombus bacteriology and early or late graft infection. The patient with graft infection may present with the symptoms of bacteraemia or septicaemia with malaise, pyrexia and rigors. Alternatively, the patient may be relatively well and the manifestations entirely local. Abscess formation with eventual secondary haemorrhage may occur at one of the suture lines or there may be distal embolization of the infected thrombus. Complete removal of the infected graft is mandatory. Flow is re-established with construction of a fresh extra-anatomic bypass, or the use of an *in situ* replacement using an antibiotic-impregnated graft is becoming more accepted. This complication carries both a high mortality and a high amputation rate.

A patient known to have had abdominal arterial reconstruction who presents with gastrointestinal blood loss should be assumed to have an aortoenteric fistula until proven otherwise. As with graft infection, it can occur at any stage after operation. The bleeding into the gastrointestinal tract associated with aortoenteric fistula is often surprisingly slight and insidious, at least to start with, becoming partially sealed with thrombus, but sooner or later it becomes massive. In a patient with a graft *in situ* and upper gastrointestinal bleeding emergency upper gastrointestinal endoscopy should be performed. Oesophageal varices and peptic ulcer having been excluded, laparotomy should be undertaken by an experienced vascular surgeon.

Sexual dysfunction is not uncommon following aortic surgery. It is due to damage to the autonomic nerves or the blood supply to the pelvis.

Surgical results

A low mortality can be achieved for operations performed as planned procedures, of 1–5%. Following rupture, even with surgical repair, the number of patients dying in the community (and hospital) with and without a correct diagnosis means that the true overall mortality may approach 95%. Further, there is wide variation in the reported perioperative mortality of emergency repair (usually defined as 30-day mortality) in the last 15 years, with figures ranging from 40 to 60%.

Long-term survival following aneurysm repair approaches that of the normal population. There is no statistical difference in the long-term postoperative survival between the ruptured and non-ruptured groups.

Inflammatory aortic aneurysm

Between 5 and 10% of abdominal aortic aneurysms are termed inflammatory. These aneurysms are a variant of the condition of periaortitis, a spectrum that includes idiopathic retroperitoneal or mediastinal fibrosis and perianeurysmal retroperitoneal fibrosis.

The macroscopic appearance is of a thick (2–3 cm), white-walled aneurysm with dense perianeurysmal fibrosis involving adjacent structures (duodenum, left renal vein and ureters). Patients with inflammatory aneurysms are predominately male, with a mean age similar or younger to that of 'atherosclerotic' aneurysms. Pain is a common feature (occasionally leading to the erroneous diagnosis of rupture), along with weight loss. Symptoms may also arise from the compression of adjacent structures such as the inferior vena cava, duodenum and ureter. The erythrocyte sedimentation rate is often raised. CT is the investigation of choice, allowing assessment not only of the aortic wall but also of adjacent structures.

The treatment of inflammatory aneurysm is dependent on the symptoms and size of the aneurysm. There is a reduced tendency for inflammatory aneurysms to rupture, although precise rates in relation to size are not available. The preferred method is by graft replacement using the inlay method, with careful and limited dissection of surrounding structures. Surgical treatment of ureteric involvement is not performed at the time of aneurysm surgery owing to the risk of creating a urinary fistula. Subsequent ureteric surgery may not be necessary as spontaneous regression of the fibrosis may follow graft replacement. Severe ureteric compression may be alleviated by preoperative ureteric stents or by percutaneous drainage. The use of steroids is a matter of debate.

Thoracic aortic aneurysm

Thoracic aneurysm is less common than infrarenal aneurysm. Historically, the most common type was aneurysm of the ascending aorta, associated with tertiary syphilis. Syphilitic aneurysms are the result of periarteritis and mesoarteritis, which weaken the media and give rise to dilatation of the vessel, usually in the thorax. Another rare cause of thoracic aneurysm is cystic medial necrosis, usually in Marfan's syndrome. Two very rare inflammatory causes are giant cell arteritis and Takayasu's disease. Giant cell arteritis occurs in older patients and, as the name suggests, is characterized by giant cell infiltration and medial degeneration. Takayasu's disease occurs in a younger age group and is characterized by a generalized inflammatory reaction in the aortic wall.

Aneurysms associated with atherosclerosis are the most common. The prognosis has been shown to be a 20–50% 5-year survival if left untreated. The diagnosis is most often an incidental finding on a plain chest radiograph, 25% being asymptomatic, although thoracic aneurysms may cause cough, respiratory obstruction and pneumonia due to local pressure. Stretching of the recurrent laryngeal or phrenic nerve may cause symptoms and occasionally vertebral body erosion may produce back pain or spinal nerve compression. Finally, there is cardiac insufficiency, secondary to aortic valve stretching or compression of the pulmonary artery or right ventricle. The diagnosis is confirmed and the extent of the aneurysm delineated by aortography and CT scanning. Up to 12% of patients with abdominal aortic aneurysm have a thoracic extension or involvement of the origins of visceral arteries. Surgical treatment is the only effective option. although there is a significant risk of paraplegia and death.

Popliteal aneurysms

Popliteal aneurysms are the most common peripheral arterial aneurysm. As mentioned previously, there is an association with other aneurysms. A popliteal aneurysm should be suspected when a popliteal pulse is unusually easy to feel. The diagnosis is made using B-mode ultrasound, with its size and the presence of mural thrombus being noted. If a popliteal aneurysm is identified then the aorta should also be scanned. A diagnosis is usually made when the popliteal artery is over 2 cm in diameter. An angiogram is indicated if surgical repair is being considered.

The concern is primarily over distal embolization or thrombosis with a high (30%) incidence of leg loss. Rarely, popliteal aneurysms may rupture. As with aortic aneurysms the larger a popliteal aneurysm the more likely it is to cause morbidity. The size at which an aneurysm should be repaired is a matter of debate, but given modern peripheral vascular techniques repair should be considered at > 2.5 cm in diameter.

Following repair the long-term outlook for the affected limb is good, with very high graft patency and limb salvage rates.

False aneurysms

These arise following trauma to an artery. If bleeding from the site of trauma is restricted by the surrounding tissues a cavity will form that is in communication with the arterial lumen. Blood eddies to and fro within this cavity, leaving and re-entering the arterial lumen. The pressure within the cavity compresses the surrounding tissue to form a capsule or sac. This is the essential difference between a false aneurysm and a true aneurysm: the wall of the latter is comprised of arterial wall, whereas the wall of a false aneurysm is made of the surrounding tissues compressed into a capsule.

The trauma resulting in a false aneurysm is most commonly iatrogenic, following radiological intervention or surgical reconstruction, although any form of penetrating trauma can be responsible. The diagnosis is made clinically and confirmed with duplex scanning or angiography. False aneurysms can be painful and they are generally best repaired if the patient is medically fit. In the past, surgical repair (suture, patch or a fresh bypass) was used exclusively. Currently, if the defect is small, duplex-guided compression of the false aneurysm can close the defect and if the pressure is maintained for 15–20 min, the blood within the cavity can thrombose. Resorption then takes place over time.

Section 10.4 • Chronic venous disease

Between 20 and 40% of individuals have varicose veins. Unfortunately, up to 10% of varicose vein operations are for recurrent varicose veins. In the majority of these cases there is a significant element of surgical technical inadequacy at the primary procedure. Similarly, a lack of understanding of the potential factors operating in patients with chronic leg ulceration may also lead to inadequate, inappropriate or even dangerous treatment.

Varicose veins

Venous anatomy

The superficial venous system can usefully be divided into three parts; the long saphenous vein, the short saphenous vein and the perforating or communicating veins. Superficial venous anatomy shows marked diversity, including vein duplication.

The long saphenous vein is the longest vein, commencing on the medial side of the foot and passing anterior to the medial malleolus. It then passes up the medial side of the leg and terminates in the femoral vein in the groin. There are normally four to six tributaries joining the vein at the groin, but unfortunately there are numerous variations. There is duplication of the long saphenous vein in 5–10% of individuals. The saphenous branch of the femoral nerve joins the long saphenous vein at the level of the knee. It lies posterior and in close relationship to the vein.

The short saphenous vein arises at the outer border of the foot behind the lateral malleolus. It ascends the calf in the midline posteriorly to empty into the popliteal vein in about 60% of cases, into the long saphenous vein in about 20% and elsewhere in the remainder. In the lower third of the leg the sural nerve is in close proximity.

The perforator veins join the deep and superficial systems. Their function is to carry blood from the superficial to the deep system. In the thigh the perforators tend to communicate directly with the deep veins, while below the knee this communication tends to be indirect via venous plexuses.

Physiology of venous drainage

Venous valves are usually semilunar in shape and bicuspid. A normal valve can resist a retrograde flow pressure of up to 300 mmHg. The system is designed to allow blood flow from superficial to deep and from distal to proximal.

The foot muscle pump works by weight compression of the venous plexus in the sole of the foot that occurs with walking. The calf muscle pump functions by compression of the sinusoids and deep veins. The resting pressure within the deep veins is about 125 cmH$_2$O but this falls to less than 30% of that value on walking.

Aetiology

Varicose veins can be usefully defined as abnormally dilated and tortuous superficial veins of the leg. This is in response to a pathological increase in their intraluminal pressure. This increase in intraluminal pressure is due to the higher intraluminal pressures of the deep veins (necessary to allow movement of blood out of the leg) being abnormally transmitted from the deep to the superficial venous system.

The structures that fail and allow the transmission of this pressure load are the valves within the veins, classically the saphenofemoral valve in the groin, although the same can occur at the saphenopopliteal junction or via one of the perforating veins.

Most varicose veins are primary (no preceding pathology). Varicose veins are more common following multiple pregnancies. An occupation that involves a lot of standing is probably only significant in that once the patient has varicose veins they are more likely to be symptomatic. The evidence that varicose veins run in families is poor.

Deep venous thrombosis can lead to deep venous occlusion, deep venous incompetence or both. Deep venous occlusion forces blood into the superficial system from the deep. This in turn leads to superficial venous hypertension and hence to varicose veins. Deep venous incompetence results in an increased deep venous pressure. This is transmitted to the superficial veins when the valves fail in the perforators.

Klippel–Trenaunay syndrome is a congenital malformation of veins with varicose veins, limb hypertrophy and port-wine staining.

Presentation

'Beauty is in the eye of the beholder' and likewise, it can be said, so is imperfection. This may extend to normal veins, particularly those over the dorsum of the foot. Cosmetic worries may be due to the lumpiness of dilated veins or spider veins/flares, which are dilated capillaries or venules.

The pain or discomfort associated with varicose veins may be localized to dilated veins or be more generalized, involving the whole leg. The patient may also complain of heaviness. All of these symptoms may be worsened by prolonged standing, premenstrually and in the summer. Relief may be gained by the use of support stockings, walking or elevation of the affected leg.

Unilateral lower leg swelling is associated with varicose veins and is usually accompanied by aching. If there is no ache then primary lymphoedema is a possible differential diagnosis.

Thrombophlebitis is not a significant problem except in the unusual situation when the thrombosis passes proximally along the long saphenous vein. Possible extension into the deep veins should be prevented by urgent saphenofemoral ligation. Severe discomfort can be treated by incision and avulsion of both the affected vein and the causative clot, but most cases can be managed conservatively.

Substantial subcutaneous bruising or even gross bleeding may occur with direct trauma to a varicosed vein. This should be treated by external compression and leg elevation.

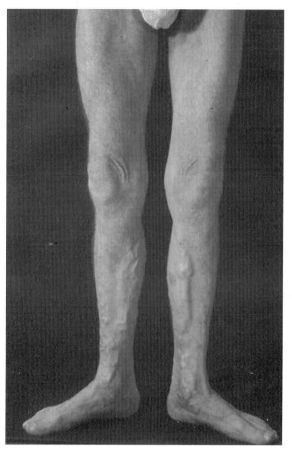

Figure 10.6 Varicose veins affecting the long saphenous systems of both calves.

Clinical evaluation

A full history is important, specifically with respect to previous deep venous thrombosis. Symptoms of pain, fatigue, aching and heaviness may be present.

The patient should be examined standing as even fairly gross varicose veins may not be seen at all with the patient lying down. The distribution of the veins is noted, along with their relationship to the long and short saphenous veins (Figure 10.6).

Signs of chronic venous insufficiency, such as swelling, pigmentation and oedema localized in the gaiter area, may also be evident.

The Brodie–Trendelenburg test is a good method of demonstrating valvular incompetence. The patient should lie down with the leg elevated to empty the varicose veins. A tourniquet is placed around the upper thigh. The patient then stands. If the veins are totally controlled by the tourniquet with a full rapid return on release then the problem is above the site of the tourniquet (saphenofemoral incompetence). If they fill despite the tourniquet and on release of the tourniquet no difference is apparent, then the incompetence is situated below the tourniquet (saphenopopliteal or perforator incompetence). A combination of initial partial filling and further filling on release implies problems both above and below the tourniquet.

Continuous wave Doppler

A hand-held Doppler probe is used to augment manual examination. Compression and release of the calf will enable any reverse flow due to valvular incompetence to be detected. There is a signal on compression and if there is significant incompetence a second signal on release of the calf as the blood 'falls' back down the vein. The probe can interrogate the saphenofemoral and saphenopopliteal junction.

Radiological evaluation

Radiology is usually used in two circumstances. The first is to decide whether or not the varicose veins are secondary: is there a pre-existing deep venous occlusion that is producing varicose veins as a compensatory mechanism? Any clinical history suggestive of a possible deep venous thrombosis should have some form of assessment of deep veins. This can be performed using either ascending venography or duplex evaluation. The second area is to evaluate the role of the short saphenous vein in the presence of primary varicose veins. This latter question is best answered by duplex scanning.

Management

A significant number of patients with varicose veins do not require surgery. However, the patient may perceive this approach as unacceptable.

Injection sclerotherapy is of some use for isolated, small, below-knee varicosities and to tidy up following definitive surgery. The treatment depends on promoting an inflammatory reaction within the varicosity and compressing the site to encourage postinflammatory organization and obliteration. Large varicosities, varicosities above the knee and when there is saphenofemoral incompetence are not suitable. The sclerosant (sodium tetradecyl sulfate) is injected to produce the required superficial thrombophlebitis and small foam pads under compression dressings are used to close the vein. The compression is maintained for 3–6 weeks. Complications include anaphylaxis, skin staining and ulceration.

The aim of surgery is two-fold: firstly to disconnect the deep and superficial systems where there is incompetence (saphenofemoral junction, saphenopopliteal junction or above-knee perforators) and secondly to remove superficial varicosities.

It is therefore vital to delineate the site of deep to superficial incompetence. Prior to surgery the patient is stood up and the varicose veins to be removed are marked with an indelible pen. The marks should outline the vein on either side of the varicosities, as marking and then stabbing through the mark can produce unsightly tattooing.

In order to disconnect the deep and superficial systems at the groin effectively, the common femoral vein must be dissected free on its anterior and medial surfaces and all tributaries ligated and divided. The tributaries should be taken back to their first divisions and these divided. The saphenofemoral junction, once iso-

lated, is clamped and divided, and the proximal end flush transfixed.

The long saphenous vein should be stripped to the level of the knee, as this will reduce the recurrence rate from 35 to 19% when compared with a saphenofemoral disconnection alone. The reason for this is that the mid-thigh perforators are destroyed by stripping and these are common sites for recurrent incompetence.

Previously marked superficial varicosities are removed through small (2–3 mm) stab incisions.

Ten per cent of cases have an element of short saphenous vein incompetence. When operating on the short saphenous vein the site of the saphenopopliteal junction should be marked preoperatively, having been identified by duplex scan on the morning of the procedure. Care must be taken to identify and protect the sural nerve. The fascia must be repaired, otherwise the fat of the popliteal fossa may herniate through the deficit and produce an unsightly bulge.

The large wounds are closed in layers with an absorbable fascial and subcuticular suture. The stab wounds can be closed with sticky paper strips. The leg is bandaged to minimize bruising and to compress any residual varicosities, for the same reason as with sclerotherapy.

The bandage is replaced by a full-length support stocking on the next day and the patient should wear this for 3–6 weeks. The patient is also encouraged to take daily exercise.

Recurrent varicose veins

Technically, good groin surgery, performed understanding the principles by which varicose veins occur (abnormal pressure transmission between deep and superficial veins), should virtually eliminate the possibility of recurrent varicose veins based on a persistent abnormal connection at the groin. Unfortunately, recurrence rates following varicose vein surgery have been cited as 20–40%. Of these, two-thirds have been shown to be due to poor primary groin surgery. In these circumstances a potentially technically awkward re-exploration of the groin is required.

Classification of recurrent varicose veins

The most recent classification revolves around the need to explore the groin and the source of recurrent incompetence. Type 1 refers to groin incompetence (there is a need to re-explore the groin) and type 2 to non-groin recurrence (mid-thigh perforators or cross-groin recurrence). There is a subdivision within each type to describe more precisely the nature of the recurrence:

- type 1A: via the saphenofemoral junction
- type 1B: via tributaries of the saphenofemoral junction
- type 2A: cross-groin recurrence (via the pudendal vein)
- type 2B: via mid-thigh perforators.

From the above it can be seen that a patient can have a combination of different types of recurrence (e.g. type 1A, 2B: an intact saphenofemoral junction with a mid-thigh perforator).

Chronic venous insufficiency

Chronic venous insufficiency is a common cause of considerable morbidity. It is a state where the mechanism of venous drainage for the lower limb is failing and there is a relative venous hypertension. This can be due to deep venous occlusion, deep or superficial venous valvular incompetence or any combination of these conditions. Chronic venous insufficiency can therefore result from primary varicose veins, following a deep venous thrombosis or owing to primary deep venous valvular incompetence.

As mentioned previously, the venous pressure at the ankle when standing is approximately 125 cmH$_2$O; the distance from the diaphragm to the ankle. On walking, this falls to 30% of this value. This is due to the three elements required for adequate venous drainage of the lower limb: an unobstructed conduit, the foot and calf pumps and the presence of competent valves. If the deep or superficial valves are incompetent or the deep veins occluded (or, worse still, occluded deep veins and the collateral pathways of secondary varicose veins surgically removed) the venous ankle pressure will rise, producing venous hypertension.

The classical changes are varicose eczema, lipodermatosclerosis (thickened, pigmented skin) and ulceration. The manner by which venous hypertension produces the changes of chronic venous insufficiency is unclear. Theories to account for the changes include a fibrin cuff produced by protein leakage from capillaries acting as a nutrient diffusion barrier. A more recent theory is the trapping and activation of white blood cells, resulting in local tissue damage through the release of cytokines.

Clinical presentation

The patient may complain of any combination of swelling, itching, restless legs or the skin changes outlined above. Up to 40% of patients will have isolated superficial varicose veins.

A full history is vital in all patients. It is important to establish any possible history of deep vein thrombosis or any other medical problems such as diabetes, hypertension or peripheral arterial disease.

Clinical examination

The distribution and pattern of incompetence of any varicose veins should be noted and skin changes should be recognized. The most common site for a chronic venous ulcer is just above the medial malleolus.

The presence or absence of peripheral pulses must also be recorded, as should a full neurological examination of the leg, paying particular attention to any sensory deficit. Where pulses are diminished or absent the patient's ankle:brachial index should be evaluated and recorded.

Investigation

The key issue in investigation is to delineate the state of the deep and superficial venous drainage of the leg.

Non-invasive plethysmographic tests

These techniques (photoplethysmography, strain gauge plethysmography, foot volumetry) are a measure of venous function. They assess venous function by measuring the volume of the leg or foot or by interrogating the capillary refill time. The patient exercises the foot, promoting venous return and thereby reducing the volume of the foot. On stopping, a rapid return to the resting state means that blood is filling the leg from both arterial and venous sides of the circulation (there is significant venous valvular incompetence). If the refill time is slowed by a high tourniquet then it can be inferred that the superficial system is responsible.

Duplex scanning

Duplex scanning can be used to visualize and assess the direction of flow within the deep and superficial veins. It is not, however, a quantitative technique. The deep veins are examined for occlusion and incompetence and the superficial veins for incompetence and sites of deep to superficial incompetence, particularly following previous varicose vein surgery.

Phlebography

Phlebography has two main modalities. The first is ascending venography to assess for deep venous obstruction when the results of duplex are in doubt or when that modality is unavailable. The second is varicography, where a distal significant varix is cannulated and contrast injected. The contrast can then be followed to the site of deep to superficial incompetence. This investigation is normally reserved for recurrent varicose veins. The disadvantage of phlebography is that it is invasive and carries a very small risk of deep venous thrombosis. The patient is also exposed to ionizing radiation.

Management of chronic venous ulceration

The management of chronic venous insufficiency depends on the constellation of findings. Patients with a contribution from superficial venous incompetence (as determined by plethysmography) should have standard varicose vein surgery as described above. Patients with sloughy ulcers will benefit from bed rest with leg elevation to reduce the associated exudation and cleansing with a combination of dressings.

Patients with isolated deep venous insufficiency due to either incompetence or obstruction require compression bandaging but have a high rate of ulcer recurrence.

Compression bandaging and hosiery have multiple beneficial effects including improving venous return. These effects only operate while the compression is applied. The current recommendation is for four-layer compression bandaging for active ulcer healing. This applies a more consistent pressure gradient with higher pressure at the ankle (40 mmHg) and lower pressure higher up the calf (15 mmHg). There is no evidence that compression hosiery or bandaging has any extra effect if it is extended into the thigh.

Patients with mixed arteriovenous ulceration may benefit from improvement with some form of revascularization. It must, however, be borne in mind that the long saphenous vein is likely to be useless as a conduit and a prosthetic graft may be required. In the presence of an open leg ulcer there is a significantly increased chance of graft infection and consequent amputation. The presence of arterial disease with an ankle:brachial index of less than 0.8 militates against the use of compression hosiery as there is then a real risk of inducing significant ischaemia.

There is no place for routine systemic antibiotics unless spreading cellulitis or systemic effects such as pyrexia are present.

Section 10.5 • Lymphoedema

This is a failure of the transport mechanism of protein-rich fluid (lymph), which results in its abnormal collection in the tissues, i.e. lymphoedema. There are two broad groups, primary and secondary.

Primary lymphoedema may be due to either obstruction of flow or reflux. Obstruction of flow can result from congenital aplasia (15%) or from hypoplasia (70%). The remaining 15% of cases of primary lymphoedema are caused by incompetent and dilated channels. There are three types related to the age of presentation. Congenital lymphoedema presents at birth; Milroy's disease is a distinct subgroup of this, which has a familial sex-linked incidence. Lymphoedema praecox and tarda manifest in adolescence and middle age, respectively. Lymphoedema praecox accounts for 80% of cases.

Secondary lymphoedema is due to the obliteration of channels. This may follow repeated episodes of lymphangitis, resulting in fibrosis, surgical removal lymphadenectomy, radiotherapy, tumour infiltration or, most commonly on a world-wide basis, infestation by filarial worms (*Wucheria bancrofti*).

Clinical features

Lymphoedema is characterized by the insidious onset of painless ankle oedema, which gradually ascends the leg. Initially, it may pit to pressure but as subcutaneous fibrosis occurs there is less pitting and the leg may become brawny and hyperkeratotic. Early onset is suggestive of a severe form of the disease.

The main complaints are the cosmetic appearance, heaviness of the limb, and skin problems such as cracks and ulceration.

Management

There is no cure for this disorder. The aim should be supportive, with compression hosiery and leg elevation. Pneumatic compression may also be used in severe cases. Skin infections should be treated to reduce lymphangitis and fibrosis. Lymph node clearance in combination with radiotherapy can be anticipated to cause lymphoedema and should only be used if the benefits are worth the consequences.

Surgical debulking with excision of subcutaneous tissue and redundant skin is very rarely employed. Other interventions have not stood the test of time.

Guide to further reading

Beard, J. D. and Gains, P. A., eds (1998). *Vascular and Endovascular Surgery*, W.B. Saunders, Philadelphia, PA.

Rutherford, R. B., ed. (1998) *Vascular Surgery*, 3rd edn, W.B. Saunders, Philadelphia, PA.

Tibbs, D. J., Sabiston, D. C., Davies, M. G. *et al.* (1997). *Varicose Veins, Venous Disorders and Lymphatic Problems in the Lower Limbs*, Oxford University Press, Oxford.

Jaundiced patients

'Jaundice from the French jaune, meaning yellow' – Lord Cohen of Birkenhead, Professor of Medicine, University of Liverpool

Jaundice is a syndrome, the hallmark of which is yellowish discoloration of the tissues owing to the accumulation of bilirubin (conjugated or unconjugated). It has varied aetiology and mechanisms, and the different disorders contribute to the individual symptoms and signs. Jaundice can be detected clinically when the serum bilirubin exceeds 40.0 mmol/l. A useful practical approach is to determine at the outset whether the yellow discoloration arises against a background of established liver disease (most commonly cirrhosis). Patients with a previously normal liver fall into two subgroups: medical (diffuse intrahepatic disease) and surgical caused by 'extrahepatic' or 'large bile duct' obstruction.

Section 11.1 • Hepatobiliary physiology

The liver is the largest and most metabolically active organ in the body, and in ancient times it was considered to be 'the seat of life', hence its name. It is functionally interposed between the gut, from which it receives macronutrients and micronutrients, and the other organs to which it supplies energy sources in exchange for metabolites that are either incorporated into complex molecules or degraded. Toxic endogenous and exogenous substances (xenobiotics) are detoxified and excreted into the bile or blood stream for disposal through the kidneys. In addition, the liver is responsible for the synthesis of specific proteins, e.g. albumin, clotting factors, immunoglobulins and lipoproteins, and plays a crucial role in bilirubin metabolism.

Hepatic circulation

The normal hepatic blood flow, 100–120 ml/min/100 g, accounts for 25% of the cardiac output. The liver receives this large blood supply via the portal vein (75% at a pressure of 6–10 mmHg) and hepatic artery (25% at systemic arterial pressure). Both systems feed into the low-pressure (2–4 mmHg) sinusoidal bed. There is evidence that reduction in the portal blood flow is compensated by a consequent increase in the arterial inflow. The portal vein has an average oxygen saturation of 85%, and for this reason, supplies 50% of the oxygen to the liver in the fasting state. The portal pressure is largely determined by the state of the splanchnic arteriolar circulation and the intrahepatic resistance.

The hepatic microcirculatory (functional) unit is the hepatic acinus, which is distinct from the histological lobule. The hepatic acinus is a three-dimensional mass of liver cells perfused by a terminal portal venule and a terminal hepatic arteriole. The unit has three functional zones (1, 2, 3) and its blood flow is centripetal, i.e. from the acinar axis to the periphery, where the sinusoidal blood drains into one or two terminal hepatic venules (Figure 11.1). Regulation and distribution of flow through the hepatic acini is effected by precapillary (presinusoidal) sphincters, predominantly on the terminal hepatic arterioles. Under physiological conditions, the hepatic parenchyma extracts less than 40% of oxygen supplied by the portal vein and hepatic artery (in equal amounts). Increased oxygen requirement is met by increased oxygen extraction rather than vasodilatation and increased blood flow.

Drugs and hormones may influence the hepatic circulation directly or indirectly by alterations in the cardiac output or splanchnic circulation. Portal pressure and liver blood flow are increased by adrenaline and decreased by β-adrenergic blockade. Somatostatin lowers the portal pressure in patients with portal hypertension, mainly by increasing the flow through the portasystemic collaterals. Vasopressin lowers both portal pressure and liver blood flow by reducing cardiac output and inducing splanchnic vasoconstriction.

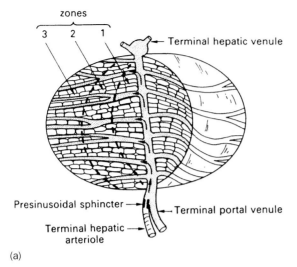

(a)

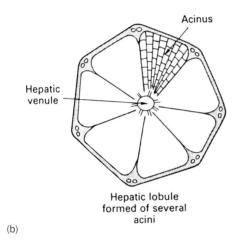

(b)

Figure 11.1 (a) Functional microcirculatory unit of the liver. The hepatic acinus is a three-dimensional mass of liver cells perfused by a terminal portal venule and a terminal hepatic arteriole. The unit has three functional zones (1, 2, 3) and its blood flow is centripetal. (b) Several of these acini form a hepatic lobule in which the draining hepatic venule appears at the centre of the rosette.

Hepatic metabolism

Energy sources and supply

Metabolites reach the liver from the gut. The liver stores, metabolizes and distributes these to the peripheral tissues to meet the daily requirements. In addition, during fasting and exercise, the hepatic parenchyma receives metabolites transported from the peripheral tissues. These include fatty acids and glycerol from adipose tissue, lactate and pyruvate from the erythrocytes and skeletal muscles, the latter also releasing branched-chain α-keto acids. The liver exports energy to the tissues in the form of two substrates: glucose and acetoacetate. Glucose is derived from hepatic glycogenolysis from stored glycogen and by synthesis (gluconeogenesis) from lactate, pyruvate, glycerol, etc. Acetoacetate is derived from acetyl-coenzyme A (CoA) formed from the oxidation of fatty acids. This crucial

role of energy storage and supply is controlled and modulated by complex neuroendocrine biofeedback systems involving several key hormones (insulin, glucagon, adrenaline) and adrenergic neural influences. It is disturbed to a varying extent by hepatocyte malfunction or failure which, when extreme, results in hypoglycaemia, accumulation of certain α-ketoacids and other metabolic derangements.

Synthesis and metabolism of nitrogenous compounds

Ammonia is derived from two sources: catabolism of proteins and nucleic acids, and from urea by the action of bacterial urease in the gut. The liver is the major site of metabolism of ammonia. The hepatocytes convert ammonia to urea by means of the urea cycle and its enzymes. In addition, ammonia is used by the hepatocytes in the synthesis of glutamine, which is then transported to the peripheral circulation (where it accounts for 20% of the amino acid pool) for delivery to other organs that are able to release ammonia by the action of glutaminases. Ammonia is also used for the synthesis of non-essential amino acids. The liver also synthesizes key substances, e.g. creatinine and carnitine, that are needed by other organs such as skeletal muscles, heart and brain.

Protein synthesis
The liver synthesizes a vast array of proteins. These fall into two broad categories: integral membrane proteins for cell membranes and subcellular organelles, and secretory proteins. The latter are exported by the liver and include albumin, immunoglobulins, clotting factors and other proteases. All of these secretory proteins are synthesized as precursor molecules containing 15–30 extra amino acids in the N-terminal segment. Cleavage of this polypeptide chain imparts full biological activity. Liver protein synthesis is depressed by fasting and protein calorie malnutrition. The action of hormones is complicated and is influenced by the nutritional state, but in general, hepatic protein synthesis is diminished by glucagon and stimulated by insulin, growth hormone, thyroxine and glucocorticoids. The latter act by enhanced processing and nucleocytoplasmic transport of specific mRNAs for certain proteins.

Lipoprotein synthesis and lipid metabolism
Lipoproteins are complex lipids that are bound to specific proteins known as apoproteins. They are characterized by size and density into: chylomicrons, very low-density lipoproteins (VLDL), low-density lipoproteins (LDL) and high-density lipoproteins (HDL). The chylomicrons, which are rich in dietary cholesterol, are formed in the gut and then transported in the blood, where peripheral lipolysis by plasma lipoprotein lipase produces chylomicron fragments. LDL and VLDL are formed exclusively in the liver and essentially provide endogenous triglyceride transport. Peripheral lipolysis of VLDL in the plasma produces LDL, the main function of which is the transport of cholesterol esters

Table 11.1 Hepatic metabolism of lipids and lipoproteins

Synthesis
  Lipids
    Triglycerides, cholesterol, phospholipids and bile acids
  Enzymes involved in lipid metabolism
    Hepatic triglyceride lipase
    Cholesterol acyltransferase
  Apoproteins
  Lipoproteins VLDL and HDL (nascent)

Metabolism
  Chylomicron remnants, LDL and HDL

Excretion
  Phospholipids and cholesterol

to the peripheral cells. The peripheral lipolysis of chylomicrons and VLDL in the plasma results in the transfer of surface lipids and proteins to nascent HDL (newly produced by the intestine and liver). These high-density lipoproteins are important as, through the action of the enzyme acyltransferase, they provide the mechanism by which excess cholesterol from the peripheral tissues is transported to the liver where it is used in the synthesis of compounds, e.g. bile acids, or degraded or excreted in the bile. The important role of the liver in lipid and lipoprotein metabolism is summarized in Table 11.1.

Hepatic synthesis and secretion of bile acids
The main primary bile acids manufactured in the liver are cholic acid (CA) and chenodeoxycholic acid (CDCA). They are synthesized from cholesterol and this process involves the addition of hydroxyl groups, removal of the double bond and the addition of a side-chain. The important rate-limiting step in the synthesis of bile acids from cholesterol is the addition of the hydroxyl group in the 7-α position by the enzyme 7-α hydroxylase. The activity of this enzyme is altered by changes in the bile salt pool via a poorly understood biofeedback mechanism. Thus, increased 7-α hydroxylase activity occurs with reduction of the pool. By this mechanism, the liver can enhance the synthesis of bile acids 10–20-fold whenever losses are incurred. Following synthesis, CA and CDCA are conjugated with glycine and taurine before being excreted in the bile. A small fraction of the secreted bile is stored in the gallbladder; the remainder enters the intestine where recycling through the entero-hepatic circulation occurs both during the fasting interdigestive state and after meals.

Hepatic control of blood coagulation and fibrinolysis

The key and central role of the liver in haemostasis, physiological anticoagulation and fibrinolysis is expressed by five major functions:

- synthesis of clotting factors
- synthesis of inhibitors of coagulation: antithrombin III, protein C, protein S, C1 inhibitor, α_1-antitrypsin
- synthesis of fibrinolytic proteins: plasminogen

- synthesis of inhibitors of fibrinolysis: antiplasmin
- clearance and catabolism of activated clotting factors and plasminogen activators by the reticuloendothelial Kupffer cells.

Synthesis of clotting factors
The liver synthesizes and secretes into the blood several clotting factors, including a low molecular weight procoagulant portion of factor VIII (antihaemophilic globulin). The clotting factors are secreted as inactive precursors and, when activated in the plasma, function as serine proteases in the complex coagulation cascade. The hepatic synthesis of certain clotting factors is vitamin K dependent: factor II, factor VII, factor IX and factor X. In addition, the hepatic synthesis of some anticoagulants, protein C and protein S, is also vitamin K dependent. It is this group of clotting factors and proteins that is particularly depressed in liver disease. These vitamin K-dependent glycoproteins all contain γ-carboxyl glutamic acid, which confers calcium-binding properties essential for the coagulation process. The key step in their synthesis by the hepatic parenchyma is the γ-carboxylation of the glutamic acid residues near the N-terminus. This requires molecular oxygen, CO_2 and reduced vitamin K (hydroquinone form) that acts as the cofactor for the vitamin K-dependent carboxylase. In this process, the hydroquinone is converted to 2,3-vitamin K epoxide but the reduced vitamin is then regenerated by the activity of the enzyme, vitamin K epoxide reductase (Figure 11.2). In the absence of vitamin K (obstructive jaundice) and in chronic liver disease, acarboxyl derivatives are formed and secreted by the hepatocytes. These abnormal proteins do not bind calcium and thus lack coagulant activity. Indeed, high levels of abnormal proteins accumulate in the blood of a patient with chronic liver disease and the prothrombin time is unchanged by the administration of vitamin K. By contrast, the prolonged prothrombin and partial thromboplastin times in patients with obstructive jaundice are reversed to normal within 24 h of parenteral administration of vitamin K analogue. The oral anticoagulants (coumarin and warfarin) inhibit the γ-carboxylation of the glutamic acid residues in addition to blocking the action of vitamin K epoxide reductase, thereby preventing the regeneration of the reduced enzyme.

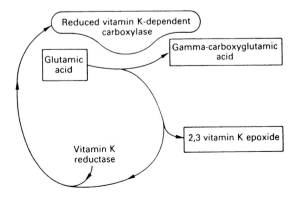

Figure 11.2 Hepatic vitamin K cycle.

Synthesis of inhibitors

The liver synthesizes antithrombin III (ATIII), protein C, protein S, α_2-plasmin inhibitor and C1 inhibitor. ATIII is the major inhibitor of thrombin, activated factor IX (IXa) and activated factor X (Xa). The activity of ATIII is depressed in patients with diffuse hepatic disease such as cirrhosis. α_2-plasmin inhibitor is the main inhibitor of plasmin and thus prevents lysis of fibrin clot. Its concentration is decreased in cirrhosis, thereby contributing to the enhanced fibrinolysis. C1 inhibitor inhibits kallikrein, XIIa and the first component of complement. The level of this inhibitor is not altered in chronic liver disease. Congenital deficiency of C1 inhibitor is the underlying cause of hereditary angioneurotic oedema.

Clearance of activated factors and degradation products

Hepatic decompensation, acute and chronic, is attended by diminished clearance of activated clotting factors, especially Xa, plasminogen activators and plasmin. The latter is responsible for the increased fibrinolysis. A more common abnormality in severe and acute liver disease is the accumulation of high levels of fibrinogen and fibrin degradation products (FDPs). The exact mechanism for this is uncertain but it is likely to be multifactorial: disseminated intravascular coagulation (DIC), increased catabolism and fibrinolysis. The high FDP levels antagonize thrombin, interfere with fibrinogen polymerization and impair platelet function, resulting in prolonged coagulation and bleeding times.

Detoxification

Detoxification of metabolically useless or harmful metabolites and drugs is an important function of the hepatic parenchyma. It is achieved by three mechanisms: oxidation–reduction, conjugation and hydrolysis. In general, oxidation–reduction by oxidoreductases is used for the disposal of lipophilic compounds as by this process they are converted to polar derivatives (water-soluble) and are thus capable of excretion in the bile or urine. Some oxidoreductases are located in the cytosol, e.g. alcohol and aldehyde dehydrogenases, and others in the mitochondria, e.g. monoamine oxidases, or microsomes, such as cytochrome P-450. Others have several subcellular locations (reductases). The cytochrome P-450 system plays a crucial role in the detoxification of a large spectrum of lipophilic exogenous compounds, e.g. alkanes, aromatic hydrocarbons, aliphatic amines, heterocyclic amines, amides, ethers (indomethacin and phenacetin) and sulfides (chlorpromazine).

Although oxidation–reduction reactions produce water-soluble derivatives that are often less toxic, metabolites are also formed by this mechanism that have greater reactivity and, in some instances, enhanced toxicity. The conjugating systems and, to a lesser extent, hydrolysis complete the process of detoxification of many xenobiotics. Conjugation is a process by which a suitable chemical group is donated to the toxic metabolite to render it less toxic and more water soluble. Various enzymes mediate these conjugation reactions (Table 11.2).

Table 11.2 Hepatic conjugating systems involved in the detoxification of xenobiotics

Chemical group	Enzyme systems	Xenobiotic (e.g.)
Glucoronidation	UDP-glucoronyl transferase	Morphine, bilirubin
Sulfation	Sulfotransferases	Propranolol, retinol
Thioether[a]	Glutathione S-transferases	Isothiocyanates
Methylation	Methyltransferases	Dopamine, adrenaline
N-Acetylation	N-Acetyltransferases	Sulfonamides, isoniazid
Amino acids[b]	Acyl ligases	Benzoate derivatives

[a]Forming mercaptopuric acid derivatives.
[b]Glutamine, glycine, taurine and ornithine conjugates.

Metabolism of haem and bile pigments

Haem, which is a complex of iron with protoporphyrin IX, is derived largely from haemoglobin released by effete red blood cells and, to a lesser extent, from the breakdown of other haemoproteins (myoglobin, tissue cytochromes, etc.). The breakdown of haem involves cleavage of the porphyrin ring by the enzyme haem oxygenase in the spleen and the Kupffer cells of the liver with the formation of biliverdin. This is then reduced to bilirubin by a specific enzyme, bilirubin reductase. Bilirubin, which is toxic and relatively insoluble at normal pH, is carried bound to albumin in the plasma. Aside from providing an effective plasma transport system, albumin binding reduces the toxicity of bilirubin. This protective mechanism prevents brain damage (bilirubin encephalopathy, kern icterus) in the newborn unless bilirubin production is excessive and exhausts the albumin-binding capacity. Certain drugs, e.g. sulfonamides, displace bilirubin from the albumin-binding sites and can therefore induce bilirubin encephalopathy in the newborn.

On reaching the liver, the bilirubin dissociates from the albumin and attaches to a plasma membrane receptor on the hepatocytes, entering these cells by a process of facilitated diffusion. Although some of the intracellular bilirubin may diffuse back into the plasma, most becomes bound to cytosolic ligands known as binding proteins Y and Z. These trap bilirubin and other organic anions before conjugation to monoglucuronides and diglucuronides by the enzyme uridine diphosphoglucuronoside (UDP-glucuronosyl transferase) (see Figure 11.3). Bilirubin diglucuronide is the major pigment present in human bile.

Enterohepatic circulation of bile salts

In health, 95% of the bile acids entering the gut are reabsorbed. Passive reabsorption occurs to a limited extent throughout the small intestine, but the major fraction is reabsorbed by active (energy-dependent) mechanisms involving high-affinity receptors that are located in the terminal ileum. Limited bacterial dehy-

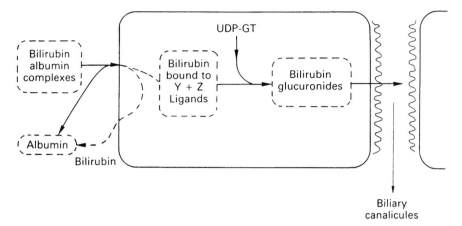

Figure 11.3 Bilirubin metabolism by the hepatocyte. On reaching the liver, the bilirubin dissociates from the albumin and enters the hepatocyte by a process of facilitated diffusion. Although some of the intracellular bilirubin may diffuse back into the plasma, most becomes bound to cytosolic ligands (proteins Y and Z). These trap bilirubin before its conjugation to monoglucuronides and diglucuronides by UDP-glucuronosyl transferase.

droxylation of the primary bile acids in the 7 position occurs in the lower ileum and proximal colon with the formation of deoxycholic acid (DCA) from CA and lithocholic acid (LCA) from CDCA. These are known as secondary bile acids. The bile acid composition of bile in health is therefore: CA = 45%, CDCA = 35%, DCA = 15% and LCA = 5%. Following intestinal absorption into the portal blood stream, LCA (which is toxic) is sulfated in the liver, but the rest (CA, DCA and CDCA) are resecreted unchanged into the bile, thereby re-entering the small intestine. Sulfated LCA is poorly absorbed and is thus excreted in the faeces. The enterohepatic circulation has two reservoirs: the gallbladder and the lumen of the small intestine. The relative functional size of these alters between fasting and the postprandial state, when the gallbladder reservoir is emptied and the intestinal luminal reservoir expanded (Figure 11.4). An average-size meal is attended by two cycles; the bile acids after completion of their role in the absorption of fats are reabsorbed in the terminal ileum on each occasion. The recycling process continues in the interdigestive state, with bile being propelled by the migratory motor complexes. An effective normal enterohepatic circulation reduces the level of hepatic synthesis of bile acids to the amount needed to replace the 5% daily losses. However, when abnormal losses are experienced with reduction in the bile salt pool (malabsorption), the hepatic synthesis is increased by stimulation of 7-α hydroxylase activity. Three consequences result from impaired absorption when this overwhelms the capacity of the liver to compensate such that the bile salt pool is contracted. The first is malabsorption of fats and fat-soluble vitamins. The second is diarrhoea (which adds to the steatorrhoea) due to the dehydroxylation and deconjugation of the bile salts by colonic bacteria. The third consequence is increased cholesterol secretion in the bile that becomes supersaturated as the bile acid content is reduced at the same rate as the increased cholesterol content.

Bile secretion

The liver secretes 600 ml of bile daily. The mechanisms concerned are complex and only partially understood. However, bile secretion is made up of two components: the bile acid-dependent and bile acid-independent fractions. The former represents the passive flow of water and electrolytes across the canalicular epithelium in response to osmolar forces generated by the secretion of bile acids by the hepatocytes. The bile acid-independent fraction is thought to be due to the movement of inorganic ions across the bile canaliculi and the epithelium of the bile ductules with concomitant passive water flux via the transcellular and paracellular routes. The bile acid-independent fraction is enhanced by secretin. The bile secreted by the liver is mostly stored in the gallbladder, where it is concentrated and periodically discharged into the small intestine both during fasting

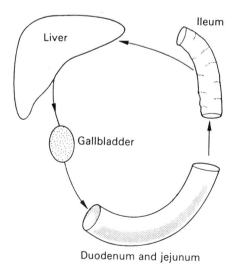

Figure 11.4 Enterohepatic circulation of bile acids. The system has two reservoirs: the gallbladder and the lumen of the small bowel. Reabsorption of the bile acids in the terminal ileum is crucial to the integrity of the circulation and maintenance of the bile acid pool.

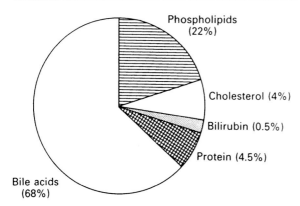

Figure 11.5 Schematic representation of the percentage composition of organic solutes in human bile.

and, in large quantities, after meals. The composition of human bile is shown in Figure 11.5. Biliary cholesterol is held in solution as a result of molecular aggregation with bile salts and phospholipids (micellar suspension). The relative proportion of these constituents is essential for the maintenance of cholesterol solubility. If excessive cholesterol or insufficient bile acids are secreted, the bile becomes supersaturated with cholesterol, which then precipitates out as cholesterol crystals and hence gallstone formation **[see Hepatobiliary and Pancreatic Disorders, Vol. II]**.

Sinusoidal cell system
There are four types of hepatic sinusoidal cell: endothelial, fat-storing, pit and Kupffer cells. Only the endothelial and Kupffer cells are in direct contact with the sinusoidal blood stream. The pit cells are the least numerous and possess both neuroendocrine and natural killer cell activity, although little is known about their physiological activity. Collectively, the various cell types form a highly organized system that interacts with the hepatic parenchyma and is involved in the defence against microbial invasion, immune surveillance, lipid metabolism and storage of vitamin A (retinoids). Some of the components of the system (endothelial and fat-storing cells) have been implicated in the pathogenesis of hepatic fibrosis and cirrhosis.

Endothelial cells
The endothelial cells, which line the sinusoids, function as a selective filter. They have fenestrations that permit entry of a wide range of solutes to the space of Disse and liver parenchyma (up to 250 000 molecular weight) but exclude large particles such as chylomicrons. Reduction in size by lipolysis in the blood stream is required before chylomicrons resulting from fat absorption by the small intestine can pass through the endothelial fenestrations for uptake by the liver parenchyma. Other important functions of the endothelial sinusoidal cells include endocytosis, synthesis of effector substances, energy metabolism, degradation by lysosomal enzymes and metabolism of lipoproteins. Endocytosis is a process by which the cell binds particles and large, complex molecules to specific high-affinity cell-surface receptors

before they are internalized and subsequently degraded by intracytoplasmic lysosomal enzymes. Physiologically, endocytosis by the hepatic endothelial sinusoidal cells is important in the turnover and catabolism of circulating glycoproteins, mucopolysaccharides (heparin) and modified low-density lipoproteins. The important role of the endothelial sinusoidal cells in the metabolism of lipoproteins is further illustrated by a specific surface receptor for hepatic lipase. This enzyme is elaborated and secreted by the parenchymal hepatocytes and then attaches to the surface of the endothelial cells, where it is involved in the breakdown of circulating lipoproteins with the release of cholesterol. The important effector substances synthesized by the endothelial sinusoidal cells include eicosanoids derived from arachidonic acid (prostaglandin E_2 and prostacyclin), angiotensin converting enzyme and various signal molecules.

Fat-storage cells
These are also known as Ito cells or lipocytes. Their main function is storage of vitamin A and its other retinoid derivatives and, for this reason, the cells contain high levels of binding proteins for both retinol and retinoic acid. Other fat-soluble vitamins (E and K) have been detected in the storage lipid droplets of the sinusoidal fat-storage cells. In addition, fat-storage cells, which morphologically resemble fibroblasts, synthesize collagen fibres.

Kupffer cells
These are fixed macrophages and constitute the largest component (80%) of the monocyte–macrophage system. They are predominantly located within the lumen of the sinusoids, being anchored to the endothelial lining by long cytoplasmic processes. They are avid phagocytes and play a vital role in the defence against invading microorganisms, clearance of particulate matter and endotoxins, immune surveillance, hepatic microcirculation, and catabolism of lipids and glycoproteins (Table 11.3).

Kupffer cells modulate and protect hepatocytes by the release of various mediator substances and cytokines. Thus, they stimulate the hepatocytes to synthesize fibrinogen and α_2-macroglobulin, and they secrete erythropoietin and colony stimulating factor that regulates the proliferation of granulocytes. Kupffer cell function is suppressed whenever there is inadequate perfusion of the sinusoids by portal blood (hypovolaemia), hypoxaemia, portal hypertension with intrahepatic portasystemic shunting and cirrhosis.

Endotoxin derived from the gut microflora is normally present in the portal venous blood. Under physiological conditions, it is cleared by the Kupffer cells by receptor-mediated pinocytosis such that there is no spillover of endotoxin into the blood stream. This important protective function is lost or depressed in severe obstructive jaundice and chronic liver disease, in both of which endotoxinaemia is often encountered in the absence of bacteraemia. In addition, the Kupffer cells are involved in some of the pathogenetic mechanisms involved in chronic liver disease:

Table 11.3 Function of Kupffer cells

Phagocytosis of particulate matter, senescent red blood corpuscles, bacteria and viruses
Detoxification of endotoxin
Secretion of mediators, including cytokines
Prolongation of life of hepatocytes
Regulation of hepatic microcirculation
Antigen processing and mediation of immune reactions
Catabolism of lipids and glycoproteins including certain enzymes

- development of virally induced chronic liver disease, when viral replication proceeds unchecked because of impaired macrophage function. Furthermore, continuous release of viral antigen into the circulation takes place
- diminished antigen sequestration by a depressed Kupffer cell system resulting in an augmented antibody response to dietary and enteric bacterial antigens. This accounts for the polyclonal hypergammaglobulinaemia of hepatic cirrhosis
- the loss of immune surveillance resulting from depletion of the Kupffer cell population in cirrhosis, which has been implicated in the development of hepatocellular carcinoma.

Section 11.2 · Pathophysiology of jaundice

Mechanisms of jaundice

The hyperbilirubinaemia may be either conjugated or unconjugated. Itching is a distressing symptom most commonly encountered in patients with conjugated hyperbilirubinaemia, and is thought to be caused by the retention and accumulation of bile salts. The various mechanisms, alone or in combination, that lead to the hyperbilirubinaemia are:

(i)   Excess bilirubin production: haemolysis, ineffective erythropoiesis, etc.
(ii)   Impaired uptake and transport by the hepatocytes
(iii) Failure of conjugation
(iv)   Impaired secretion of conjugated bile into the bile canaliculi
(v)   Impairment of bile flow subsequent to secretion by the hepatocyte.

Thus, in essence there are three categories of jaundice:

- haemolytic: mechanism (i)
- hepatocellular: mechanisms (ii–iv)
- cholestatic or obstructive: mechanism (v).

Cholestatic jaundice may be intrahepatic (hepatic disease impairing transport of conjugated bilirubin from the hepatocyte to bile canaliculi and intrahepatic ducts) or extrahepatic (from large bile duct obstruction). The latter is also referred to as surgical jaundice. Malignant jaundice is sometimes considered as a separate category,

and may be purely obstructive (mechanism v), e.g. periampullary cancer, or the result of extensive hepatic infiltration, most commonly secondary tumour deposits (mechanisms ii–iv).

Congenital disorders of bilirubin transport

Unconjugated hyperbilirubinaemia is encountered in various situations. These include neonatal hyperbilirubinaemia (increased production and delayed maturation of the liver), increased bilirubin production due to haemolytic disorders (e.g. sickle cell disease, spherocytosis), ineffective erythropoiesis (e.g. thalassaemia, megaloblastic anaemia) and hereditary disorders such as Gilbert's and Crigler Najjar syndromes (types I and II). In Gilbert's and Crigler Najjar type II, hepatic bilirubin UDP-glucuonosyl transferase activity is reduced, whereas in the more serious type I Crigler Najjar disease, this enzyme is totally absent.

Other congenital disorders of bilirubin metabolism are characterized by conjugated hyperbilirubinaemia, as exemplified by the Dublin–Johnson and the Rotor syndromes. The former is characterized by defective hepatocyte transport of conjugated bilirubin that diffuses back into the plasma, abnormal black discoloration of the liver owing to the deposition of a melanin-like pigment and, in some patients, factor VII deficiency. The Rotor syndrome is a more benign disorder. It consists of defective hepatic storage and increased reflux of conjugated bilirubin into the plasma.

Section 11.3 · Medical jaundice

Within the context of hepatocellular disease, clinical jaundice indicates substantive encroachment of liver function and hepatic reserve. In the acute situation, it reflects the severity of the underlying situation. In chronic liver disease jaundice carries a poor prognosis.

The important medical disorders that cause jaundice are:

- hepatitis: acute and chronic
- drug-induced liver disease (DILD)
- liver failure
- cirrhosis.

Acute hepatitis

Acute hepatitis is a disorder of varied aetiology. In the majority of cases the disease is mild and self-limiting and is characterized by hepatocellular jaundice (hyperbilirubinaemia and marked elevation of the transaminases indicative of acute inflammation or injury of the hepatocytes) with full recovery and no long-term sequelae. In some cases, however, the injury proceeds to massive liver cell necrosis when the patient develops acute fulminant liver failure. This carries a high mortality despite modern supportive therapy and may require liver transplantation for survival. Certain forms of viral hepatitis lead on to a chronic carrier state where the individual has persistence of the viral agent and can transmit the infection to others. This carrier state may be associated with normal liver function or with the development of chronic liver disease (chronic hepatitis). The most common causes of acute hepatitis are viruses and drugs (including alcohol).

The viruses known to cause acute hepatitis are:

- **hepatitis A (HAV)**: enteral transmission, rarely causes liver cell necrosis
- **hepatitis B (HBV)**: transmitted by blood products, needles, tattooing, sexual activity, mothers to babies, aerosol (dental treatment); can progress to liver cell necrosis and chronic liver disease
- **hepatitis C (HCV)**: transmitted sexually and by blood products; can progress to liver cell necrosis; high incidence of progression to chronic liver disease
- **hepatitis delta (HDV)**: incomplete hepatotropic virus; capable of infection only when activated by HBV. Acquired either as a coinfection with HBV or as a superinfection in HbsAg carriers
- **hepatitis E (HEV)**: enteral transmission; mild self-limiting disease; does not progress to chronic liver disease
- **hepatitis G (HGV)**: transmitted by blood products; uncertain clinical significance
- **Epstein–Barr virus**: agent of infectious mononucleosis. Hepatitis rare and usually mild
- **cytomegalovirus**: infection occurs in immunosuppressed patients and infants
- **yellow fever virus**: can cause liver cell necrosis when mortality is high
- **Ebola and Marburg virus**: causes African haemorrhagic fever consisting of papular rash, DIC, pancreatitis and hepatitis. Spread by needles and person to person. High mortality; no specific therapy available
- **others**.

[see Module 5, Vol. I]

Chronic hepatitis

The term chronic hepatitis includes three syndromes, all of which are characterized by hepatomegaly and persistent abnormalities of the liver function tests.

Chronic persistent hepatitis (CPH): in this condition, there is continued inflammation of the portal tracts without necrosis and normal architecture after an attack of acute hepatitis. The transaminases remain mildly elevated but other liver biochemistry is normal. The majority of patients has a good prognosis but some progress to chronic active hepatitis and cirrhosis.

Chronic active hepatitis (CAH): this is characterized by chronic hepatic inflammation of the hepatic lobules that is progressive for up to 6 months. The inflammation extends beyond the confines of the portal tracts and there is accompanying piecemeal necrosis. The liver function tests are abnormal, with raised bilirubin, AST, ALT and alkaline phosphatase and γ-glutamyl transpeptidase. CAH usually follows hepatitis B, C or D, but may also be drug induced. It

often progresses to cirrhosis and end-stage liver disease and is associated with a high risk of hepatocellular carcinoma.

Autoimmune chronic active hepatitis (ACAH): in this instance, the chronic hepatitis is associated with hyperglobulinaemia, non-organ specific autoantibodies and existence of other autoimmune disorders, e.g. rheumatoid arthritis, ulcerative colitis and Hashimoto's thyroiditis.

Drug-induced liver disease

There is a wide spectrum of DILD: acute hepatitis, CAH, hepatic fibrosis, fulminant liver failure and hepatic neoplasia. DILD accounts for 40% of hospitalized patients with acute hepatitis and 20% of patients with fulminant liver failure. Some of the common types of DILD are shown in Table 11.4.

Liver failure

Liver failure is also referred to as hepatic encephalopathy, as the hallmark symptom is a diminished level of consciousness and coma. It covers a spectrum of neurological disorders that afflict patients suffering from liver disease and/or portasystemic shunting. Hepatic coma always indicates severe decompensation and carries a significant but variable mortality, depending on type.

Hepatic coma is encountered in:

- **acute liver failure**: acute fulminant encephalopathy
- **subclinical chronic liver failure**: intellectual impairment, reduced level of consciousness, abnormal psychometric tests in chronic liver disease
- **overt chronic liver failure**: recurrent episodes of coma (often precipitated by bleeding) accompanied by cortical atrophy
- **shunt encephalopathy**: after portasystemic shunting.

Acute (fulminant) liver failure is defined as severe encephalopathy occurring within 6–8 weeks of the onset of illness. Essentially, it consists of acute massive hepatocellular necrosis in a previously normal liver caused by drugs (e.g. acetaminophen, halothane), viral infection (A, B, C) or poisoning (e.g. *Amanita phalloides*). It is more common in females, irrespective of aetiology. This female prevalence is thought to be associated with the level of the sex hormone binding globulin (SHBG), high levels of which are associated with severe fulminant disease and the development of a chronic carrier state. Acute liver failure carries a high mortality despite newer methods of hepatic support and liver transplantation. Acute fulminant liver failure is accompanied by multisystem involvement: cerebral oedema (contributes to the coma), bleeding from clotting failure, loss of peripheral vascular resistance, renal impairment and severe depression of the immune defence system with extreme susceptibility to serious respiratory infections. Acute pancreatitis may also develop in these patients.

Table 11.4 Drug-induced liver damage

Category	Example	Hepatic lesion
Antibiotics	Tetracyclines, especially after i.v. use, dose related	Fatty infiltration
	Penicillins: hypersensitivity	Hepatitis
	Chloramphenicol	Hepatitis
	Sulfonamides: hypersensitivity	Granulomas, focal hepatocellular necrosis
Analgesics and anti-inflammatory drugs	Paracetamol: dose dependent	Centrilobular necrosis: massive liver necrosis
	Phenylbutazone: hypersensitivity	Hepatitis with granuloma, may progress to cirrhosis
	Carbamazepine	Cholestasis
	Salicylates: dose related	Focal hepatic necrosis
Psychotropic drugs	Monoamine oxidase inhibitors	Hepatitis, may progress to massive hepatic necrosis
	Phenothiazines: hypersensitivity	Hepatitis and cholestasis
	Tricyclic antidepressants	Cholestatic hepatitis, more usually mild elevation of transaminases only
Steroids	Testosterone and anabolic steroids	Cholestasis, peliosis hepatis, hepatic tumours
	Oestrogens	Cholestasis, gallstones, hepatic tumours
Anaesthetic agents	Halothane	Hepatitis which may progress to massive liver cirrhosis
Antituberculous drugs	PAS: hypersensitivity	Hepatitis
	INAH: occurrence related to acetylator status	Focal to severe hepatic necrosis
	Rifampicin: dose related	Defective bilirubin transport, mild hepatitis
Cytotoxic and immunosuppressive drugs	Azathioprine	Cholestasis and peliosis hepatis
	6-Mercaptopurine: dose related	Hepatitis
	Methotrexate: long-term therapy	Fatty change, fibrosis of the portal tracts and cirrhosis
Others	Benzothiazine diuretics	Cholestatic hepatitis
	Phenindione	Cholestatic hepatitis
	Chlorpropamide	Cholestatic hepatitis
	Phenytoin	Hepatocellular necrosis

Chronic liver failure arises against a background of cirrhosis and is often referred to as end-stage chronic liver disease. It is characterized by overt chronic encephalopathy with severe mental impairment, muscle wasting, fluid and salt retention, bleeding tendency, splenomegaly with thrombocytopenia and episodes of variceal haemorrhage from portal hypertension.

Cirrhosis

Liver cirrhosis is the end result of hepatocyte death and needs to be distinguished from hepatic fibrosis, which can occur in the portal regions from chronic bile duct obstruction, as a congenital condition, in schistosomiasis, or around the central veins in chronic heart failure. In cirrhosis, there is a confluent necrosis of zones 1 and 3 of the hepatic lobules leading to the formation of fibrotic bridges. The regeneration of the surviving hepatocytes (regenerative nodules) results in further distortion of the hepatic architecture. Three morphological types of cirrhosis are recognized:

- **micronodular**: small regenerating nodules separated by thick fibrous septa: alcoholic cirrhosis, malnutritional cirrhosis, cryptogenic cirrhosis (aetiology unknown). Mallory hyaline change is often present in alcoholic cirrhosis
- **macronodular**: nodules of variable size with normal histological appearances within the larger nodules (diagnosis may be missed on liver needle biopsy): posthepatitic cirrhosis
- **mixed**: results from regeneration in a micronodular cirrhosis.

In terms of its aetiology, the cirrhosis is termed as:

- **cryptogenic**: cause unknown or cannot be established
- **posthepatitic**: most commonly after hepatitis B or C
- **alcoholic**
- **primary biliary cirrhosis.**

Primary biliary cirrhosis is a disease of unknown aetiology in which the intrahepatic bile ducts are progressively destroyed by an immunological process. It affects females predominantly, with age of onset about 40 years. Circulating antibodies against mitochondrial constituents are found in all patients. The symptoms include weight loss, malaise, itching and icterus. The disease runs a variable course but ultimately ends up in end-stage liver disease. Liver transplantation is indicated for progressive disease before stage C is reached.

Irrespective of morphological type, disease severity in cirrhotic patients (and hence prognosis) is based on assessment of clinical condition and biochemical profile. Two severity scores are commonly used: (i) Child–Pugh score/grading (modified from the initial

Table 11.5 Child–Pugh classification of disease severity in cirrhotic patients

Parameter	A	B	C
Albumin (g/dl)	> 3.5	3.0–3.5	< 3.0
Bilirubin (mol/l)	< 25	25–40	> 40
Prothrombin time (s > normal)	< 4.0	4–6	> 6[a]
Prothrombin level (%)	> 64	40–65	< 40[a]
Ascites	None	Controlled	Refractory
Encephalopathy	None	Minimal	Advanced

[a]In the original Child–Turcotte classification, nutrition was used, but this has been substituted with prothrombin activity.

The bilirubin has to be adjusted for patients with primary biliary cirrhosis (A = 5–7, B = 8–10, C = 11+).

Table 11.6 Paul Brousse Hospital classification system

Parameter	Number of criteria
Albuminaemia < 3.0 g/100 ml	1
Hyperbilirubinaemia > 30 mol/l	1
Encephalopathy	1
Clinical ascites	1
Coagulation factor II and V 40–60%	1
Coagulation factors II and V < 40%	2

A, none of the criteria; B, one or two criteria; C, three or more criteria.

Child–Turcotte) and (ii) the Paul Brousse Hospital classification system (Tables 11.5 and 11.6).

Portal hypertension

This results from obstruction to the portal venous flow and in the vast majority of cases (80%) arises against a background of cirrhosis. Much less commonly, the increased resistance to portal blood flow is caused by some form of hepatic fibrosis or from occlusion of inflow (portal and splenic veins) or outflow vessels (hepatic) veins. Thus, the characterization of portal hypertension is as follows:

- **prehepatic or preparenchymatous:** due to primary portal vein thrombosis
- **hepatic or parenchymatous:** postsinusoidal occlusion of blood flow in the liver most commonly by regenerating nodules of cirrhosis, less commonly by hepatic fibrosis. In cirrhosis, the increased splanchnic blood flow also contributes to the hypertension
- **posthepatic:** occlusion of the small (veno-occlusive disease) or large hepatic veins, i.e. Budd–Chiari syndrome.

Irrespective of type, obstruction to the portal blood flow is followed by enlargement of natural portasystemic communications (Figure 11.6) and by *de novo* collateral channels at surgically constructed mucocutaneous junctions (colostomy, ileostomy). The major risk

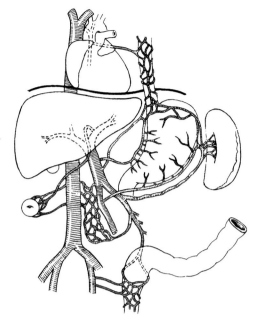

Figure 11.6 This shows the portal venous drainage from the gastrointestinal tract and demonstrates the major anastomotic sites between the portal and systemic systems: the cardio-oesophageal junction leading up to the azygos system, the retroperitoneum, the umbilicus and in the inferior rectal plexus.

of haemorrhage is from oesophageal varices (left gastric to azygous enlarged venous communications).

It should be stressed that not all patients with chronic liver disease develop portal hypertension. Estimates vary from 15 to 40%. In addition, only 30% of patients with varices suffer variceal haemorrhage within 2 years of diagnosis and thereafter only a smaller fraction bleeds each year.

Aside from gastrointestinal (variceal) haemorrhage, portal hypertension is associated with fluid and salt retention/ascites and hypersplenism (thrombocytopenia and haemolysis).

Variceal bleeding is always a serious situation since the resultant hypovolaemia results in further deterioration of the hepatic and renal function. In addition, the blood within the lumen of the gastrointestinal tract provides a massive protein load from which ammonia and other toxic products produced by bacterial action are absorbed, causing encephalopathy. Recovery is dependent on control of the bleeding and the Child–Pugh status, with a high mortality in C patients.

Section 11.4 • Surgical jaundice

The causes of surgical jaundice are

- ductal calculi
- gallstones
- pancreatic and biliary malignancy
- non-malignant strictures
- external compression of bile duct by lymph nodes and tumour masses
- parasitic infestations of the biliary tract.

Gallstones and ductal calculi

Gallstones are very common world-wide. The prevalence in the western hemisphere is 18.5%, with a female preponderance (2:1). The currently accepted classification recognizes three main types of gallstone [see Hepatobiliary and Pancreatic Disorders, Vol. II]:

- **cholesterol stones**: essentially metabolic stones that form in the gallbladder and are preceded by biliary sludge. Account for 75% of stones in the West
- **black pigment stones**: form in the gallbladder and are more common in Far Eastern countries; account for 25% of stones in the West. Can be associated with haemolytic states. Consist of bilirubin polymers with varying amounts of cholesterol (3–25%) in a matrix of organic material. Associated with infection in less than 20%
- **Brown pigment stones**: form in the bile ducts (primary ductal stones) and are associated with obstructive lesions and infections and infestations of the biliary tract. Bacteria are present in the crevices and pits of the amorphous soft stones that consist of calcium bilirubinate and palmitate bound in a matrix of organic material.

Spectrum of symptomatic gallstone disease

The symptomatology and pathogenic potential of gallstones vary widely. Most surveys on necropsy findings have shown that silent (symptomless) gallstones heavily outnumber the symptomatic ones. When symptomatic, gallstones can cause:

- chronic symptoms due to stones associated with chronic cholecystitis: jaundice is rare
- acute biliary colic/acute obstructive cholecystitis: jaundice occurs in 20–40%
- jaundice due to large bile duct obstruction: jaundice in 100%
- cholangitis and septicaemia: jaundice in 100%
- acute gallstone-associated pancreatitis: conjugated hyperbilirubinaemia in 50%
- biliary fistulous disease
- gallstone ileus
- carcinoma of the gallbladder (strong association).

Ductal calculi

The pathogenic potential of ductal calculi consists of the triad: jaundice, cholangitis and acute gallstone-associated pancreatitis.

Ductal calculi can result from migration of gallstones through a patent cystic duct. These are referred to as **secondary** ductal calculi (cholesterol or black pigment), as distinct from **primary** ductal stones, which arise *de novo* within the bile ducts and are brown pigment stones. These are associated with biliary tract colonization by glucuronidase-secreting bacteria, e.g. *Escherichia coli*, usually in the presence of subclinical obstruction at the distal end of the common bile duct. Calculi may also form around foreign bodies within the lumen of the common bile duct. These become encrusted with calcium bilirubinate. A common example of this nowadays is caused by the internalization of titanium metal clips used to secure the medial end of the cystic duct stump during laparoscopic cholecystectomy (LC). The exact pathology for this eventuality is not known but pressure necrosis by the clip that included the adjacent wall of the common bile duct is thought to be involved. The patients present several months after an uneventful LC with jaundice and/or cholangitis.

Several other clinical terms are used in relation to ductal calculi: unsuspected, missed or retained, and recurrent. **Unsuspected stones** are those discovered accidentally during cholecystectomy for symptomatic gallstone disease when routine intraoperative cholangiography (IOC) is performed. The stones are usually small and floating, and the common bile duct is of normal calibre. The liver function tests are normal, although some patients may have a mild elevation of the alkaline phosphatase that is either missed or attributed to other causes. The estimated incidence of unsuspected stones is 5–10% of patients undergoing cholecystectomy.

The terms **missed** and **retained** are synonymous and indicate that the intervention (surgical or endoscopic) failed to achieve complete ductal clearance. By custom, ductal calculi that present or are diagnose within 2 years of the intervention are designated as missed or retained. Most are, in fact, detected much earlier. The insertion of T-tube or cystic duct drainage cannulae after surgical ductal clearance (open or laparoscopic) permits the performance of a postoperative tube choledochogram as a check for complete ductal clearance.

Recurrent ductal stones present at least 2 years after the first intervention. These tend to be primary ductal stone (brown pigment) and are almost always associated with significant dilatation of the common bile duct, indicating a fibrotic or dysfunctional terminal segment of the common bile duct. **There is a mistaken belief that endoscopic sphincterotomy is sufficient to overcome this obstruction.** This is not the case as the Vaterian segment (containing the entire choledochal sphincter complex) cannot be completely divided by an endoscopic sphincterotomy (essentially a papillotomy), however generous. If fit, these patients are best managed by ductal clearance and an internal surgical drainage procedure, most commonly a choledochoduodenostomy, which can be open or laparoscopic [see Hepatobiliary and Pancreatic Disorders, Vol. II].

Pancreatic and biliary malignancy

The clinical picture of both pancreatic and biliary cancer is dominated by jaundice (large bile duct obstruction) and itching. In pancreatic ductal adenocarcinoma weight loss is also an important clinical feature, as is recent onset of diabetes.

Pancreatic cancer

It is important to distinguish between pancreatic adenocarcinoma (head, body, tail) and periampullary tumours because of their vastly different prognosis.

Mortality rates from pancreatic cancer have been increasing, and in Europe deaths from pancreatic cancer range from 8 to 12:100 000 males and 4–6:100 100 females annually. Risk factors include smoking (strongest), chronic pancreatitis, familial predisposition and cystic fibrosis. K-ras mutations are involved in the development of pancreatic adenocarcinoma. The prognosis of non-endocrine pancreatic carcinoma is poor, with a 5-year overall survival of < 5%, in part due to the advanced stage at the time of diagnosis. Survival is significantly better in patients undergoing potentially curative resection for small node-negative tumours [**see Hepatobiliary and Pancreatic Disorders, Vol. II**].

Periampullary cancers
These include cancers of the ampulla of Vater, distal common bile duct and peri-Vaterian duodenum. By far the most common presentation is painless progressive jaundice and itching. Rarely, presentation is with hyperamylasaemia, pancreatitis or grey stools (gastrointestinal blood loss). Prognosis after resection is good, with 30–50% 5-year survival, and is stage dependent, being very good in T1 and T2, node-negative tumours [**see Hepatobiliary and Pancreatic Disorders, Vol. II**].

Biliary tract cancers

Carcinoma of the gallbladder
This is the most common malignancy of the biliary tract and accounts for 3–4% of all gastrointestinal malignancies. It is a disease of old age and carries a uniformly poor prognosis. Gallstones are present in 75–90% of cases. The clinical presentation is with jaundice and/or acute cholecystitis [**see Hepatobiliary and Pancreatic Disorders, Vol. II**].

Bile duct cancers: cholangiocarcinomas
These tumours of the biliary tract, all of which present with jaundice, usually occur in the elderly but some occur as early as the fifth decade. They are classified by the anatomical site of origin:

■ **intrahepatic**: from minor hepatic ducts, often multicentric and usually classified with primary liver tumours
■ **proximal**: from right and left hepatic ducts, hilar confluence and proximal common hepatic ducts
■ **middle**: from the distal common hepatic duct, cystic duct and its confluence with common bile duct
■ **distal**: included with periampullary tumours.

Most of these tumours are of the scirrhous variety and some can be very acellular, such that histological confirmation may be difficult. Radiologically, they give rise to a 'stricture' with proximal dilatation (Figure 11.7).

Benign bile duct strictures

Most benign bile duct strictures are the result of iatrogenic injury during cholecystectomy. The constriction and compression of the intrapancreatic segment of the common bile duct by the pseudotumour of chronic

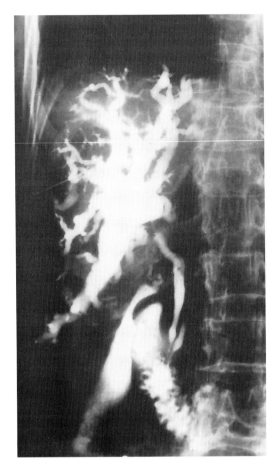

Figure 11.7 Percutaneous transhepatic cholangiogram in a 75-year-old female showing a hilar cholangiocarcinoma. The patient presented with jaundice and itching.

pancreatitis can result in jaundice that complicates the course of this disease in some patients. This situation usually poses a diagnostic problem, as it may be very difficult to exclude an associated pancreatic malignancy, even on histology. Strictures can also be caused by parasitic infestations of the biliary tract and may complicate acquired immunodeficiency syndrome (AIDS). Multiple strictures are the hallmark of sclerosing cholangitis, an obscure disorder of uncertain aetiology, which results in progressive fibrous obliteration of the biliary tract and has a well-established association with ulcerative colitis.

The exact incidence of iatrogenic stricture following cholecystectomy is not known. The estimated incidence based on published retrospective series averages 1:500 open cholecystectomies. There appeared to be an increased incidence following the introduction of laparoscopic cholecystectomy, but this has levelled off, and reports from large national audits indicate that the bile duct damage rate is now of the same order as that following open cholecystectomy. The pathological anatomy of postoperative iatrogenic bile duct strictures is based on the level of the stricture and thus the presence and length of an extrahepatic residual bile duct (Figure 11.8). Iatrogenic bile duct injuries require expert remedial surgery in tertiary referral centres because of serious

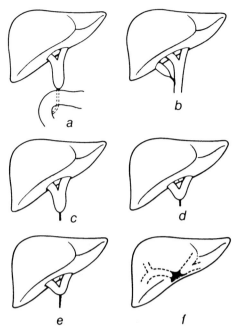

Figure 11.8 Pathological anatomy of postoperative bile duct strictures. (a) Distal bile duct stricture; (b) stricture of an anomalous branch of the right hepatic duct; (c) low stricture of the common hepatic duct (> 2.0 cm); (d) mid common hepatic duct stricture (< 2.0 cm); (e) high stricture with intact confluence of the right and left hepatic ducts; (f) obliteration of the entire common hepatic duct and confluence.

consequences: recurrent cholangitis, hepatic fibrosis, secondary biliary cirrhosis and portal hypertension.

Section 11.5 • Malignant jaundice

This term is used to describe jaundice due to malignant large bile duct obstruction, e.g. biliary and pancreatic cancer, or jaundice occurring in association with hepatic malignancy, which can be primary (hepatocellular carcinoma) or secondary from a primary in another site. **The presence of jaundice in association with liver tumours indicates extensive involvement of the liver parenchyma, with the patient being incurable and unlikely to benefit from any form of treatment.** Undoubtedly, surgical treatment and chemotherapy are both contraindicated in jaundiced patients who harbour hepatic malignancy.

Hepatocellular carcinoma

Primary liver cancer (liver cell carcinoma, hepatocellular carcinoma) may arise in a morphologically normal liver or complicate established cirrhosis (cirrhomimetic hepato cellular carcinoma). It is extremely common in some parts of the world (Middle and Far Eastern countries) but is less common in the West. The aetiology is varied but the vast majority is the result of viral hepatitis, particularly HBV and HCV, and integration of the virus into the genome of the tumour has been documented. Association of some cases with oral contraceptives and androgenic steroids is well documented. Ingestion of

food contaminated with aflatoxins produced by the fungus *Aspergillus flavus* has been incriminated in some cases. There is also a high incidence of the disease in patients with certain familial/congenital disorders such as α_1-antitrypsin deficiency and tyrosinaemia. The fibrolamellar variant of the disease is encountered predominantly in young patients without cirrhosis and carries a good prognosis after complete resection.

The symptoms include pain in the right hypochondrium, hepatic enlargement and ascites. The latter indicates advanced disease. In some cases the tumour gives rise to systemic manifestations. These include polycythaemia, carcinoid syndrome, hypoglycaemia and hypercalcaemia. Raised α-fetoprotein is present in 60–70% of cases [**see Hepatobiliary and Pancreatic Disorders, Vol. II**].

Hepatic metastases

Metastatic liver disease is a major unresolved problem and in Western countries 90% of hepatic tumours are metastatic, notably from primaries in the gastrointestinal tract, pancreas, lung and breast. The most common, by far, are secondary hepatic deposits from primary colorectal cancer and these account for the majority of deaths from this disease.

Morphologically, on laparoscopic inspection, secondary hepatic deposits may be:

- **discretely nodular**: single, multiple, unilateral or bilateral
- **miliary**: widespread small seedling deposits
- **diffusely confluent**: disease involving multiple segments or lobes.

Only discretely nodular disease is potentially curable by surgical resection. Overall, about 5% of patients with hepatic metastases are suitable for this treatment. Palliation and some prolongation of survival can be obtained by systemic chemotherapy and by *in situ* ablation techniques provided the extent of hepatic involvement is < 25–30%.

From the clinical standpoint, hepatic metastases can be:

- **occult**: present but undetectable by current imaging tests at the time of resection of the primary. Detected at subsequent follow-up
- **asymptomatic**: known to be present but with no symptoms or jaundice, although the alkaline phosphatase or γ-glutamyl transpeptidase may be elevated. Some of these may be potentially curable by resection.
- **symptomatic**: the patient has a large liver, pain in the right hypochondrium and overt clinical jaundice/malignant ascites. These cases are untreatable.

Section 11.6 • Investigation of the jaundiced patient

General algorithm

There is a set protocol that must be followed in all jaundiced patients. This will always lead to a definite diagnosis of the underlying cause or disease in the individual case. The surgeon must always remember that jaundice may signify the presence of (i) liver disease, (ii) biliary tract disorder, e.g. stones, tumours, strictures, parasites, (iii) pancreatic disease, or (iv) acquired or congenital haemolytic disease.

The work-up is geared to answer the following four questions.

- Is the jaundice cholestatic or hepatocellular?
- Has the patient any evidence of parenchymatous liver disease?
- Is there any evidence of malignancy on clinical examination?
- Is the biliary tract dilated on ultrasound examination?

These questions are answered by the algorithm shown in Figure 11.9. All patients with medical jaundice are managed by gastroenterologists and hepatologists and will not be discussed further.

History

In all patients with jaundice a careful history and physical examination will result in the correct diagnosis in 80% of patients. The important aspects of history that must be obtained in every patient include:

- abdominal pain, weight change and fever
- drug intake
- injections
- alcohol misuse
- transfusion of blood and blood products
- contact with jaundiced individuals
- travel to hepatitis-endemic areas
- sexual activity: when appropriate
- ingestion of raw shellfish and wild mushrooms.

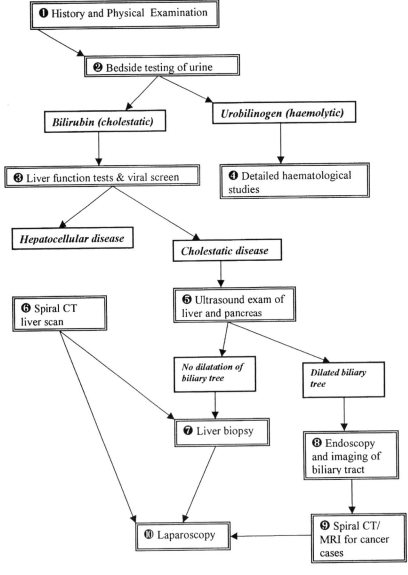

Figure 11.9 Algorithm for jaundiced patients.

Physical examination

The physical examination of the jaundiced patient should commence with the detection or exclusion of evidence of weight loss and stigmata of chronic liver disease:

- hepatosplenomegaly: enlargement of spleen signifies portal hypertension
- spider naevi: cutaneous endarterioles in the drainage area of the superior vena cava. Fill from centre outwards when compressed. More than one is clinically significant
- evidence of clotting disturbance: bruising
- water and salt retention: oedema/ascites
- muscle wasting: triceps, interosseous muscles, quadriceps
- palmar erythema: can be difficult to interpret in the individual case
- parotid enlargement: not always present
- gynaecomastia and testicular atrophy in males: unreliable owing to great individual variation
- liver tremor: indicates advanced disease and encephalopathy.

The neck should always be palpated for enlarged lymph nodes. The abdomen is examined for enlarged liver and spleen, palpable gallbladder, abdominal masses and ascites. A digital rectal examination should be carried out in all patients.

Investigations

The initial investigations are examination of urine for bilirubin (obstructive/cholestatic jaundice) or excess urobilin (haemolysis), liver function tests, serology (for viral antibodies) and an ultrasound examination of the liver, biliary tract and pancreas. Patients with surgical jaundice will exhibit a cholestatic biochemical profile (conjugated hyperbilirubinaemia with marked elevation of bile duct enzymes such as alkaline phosphatase and γ-glutamyl transpeptidase, only mild elevation of the transaminases) and a dilated biliary tract on ultrasound examination. If the ultrasound examination does not demonstrate dilatation of the biliary tract, the jaundice is medical, i.e. hepatocellular disease. It should be noted that as gallstones are so common, their presence, although indicative of calculous obstruction, does not exclude biliary or pancreatic malignancy.

All jaundiced patients with large bile duct obstruction (dilated biliary tree on ultrasound) must undergo:

- spiral computed tomographic (CT) scan
- endoscopic retrograde cholangiopancreatography (ERCP) or magnetic resonance cholangiopancreatography (MRCP)
- laparoscopy if biliary or pancreatic cancer is suspected.

Spiral CT with intravenous contrast enhancement (Figure 11.10) is essential in all patients with suspected tumours. The alternative is magnetic resonance imaging (MRI) of the liver and pancreas with intravenous superparamagnetic ferric oxide

(Endorem), which yields even greater definition (Figure 11.11). This shows liver tumours as white areas (no Kupffer cells) against a black background (contrast in Kupffer cells).

ERCP and MRCP: ERCP has an established diagnostic role in patients with cholestatic jaundice. Periampullary tumours can be visualized and biopsied (Figure 11.12). The cholangiogram confirms the diagnosis in carcinoma of the pancreas (Figure 11.12). However, in recent years the development of MRCP, which is completely non-invasive and does not require injection of contrast, has challenged the established role of diagnostic (as opposed to interventional) ERCP because a number of comparative trials have confirmed equal diagnostic yield (Figure 11.13). The other controversial issue is whether laparoscopy should follow or precede ERCP. This controversy is likely to be resolved when MRCP replaces ERCP for diagnostic purposes.

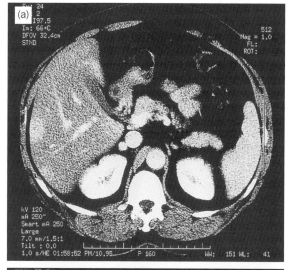

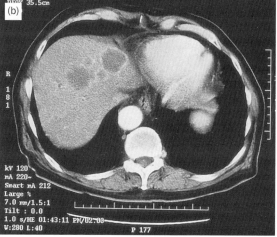

Figure 11.10 Spiral contrast enhanced CT scanning of liver: (a) multiple carcinoid tumour deposits that enhance with the contrast because of their vascularity; (b) non-enhancing secondary deposits with rim enhancement at the periphery of the tumour (blood supply mainly from the hepatic artery).

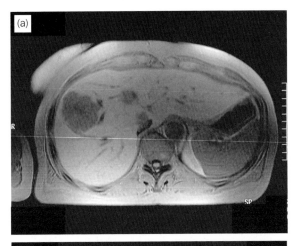

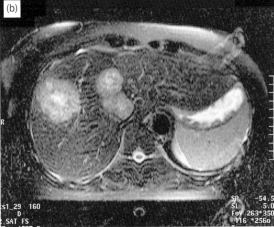

Figure 11.11 MRI imaging of the liver: (a) scan prior to Endorem (superparamagnetic ferric oxide) infusion; (b) after Endorem infusion – the tumour deposits appear as white lesions (no Kupffer cells) and the hepatic parenchyma as black (Kupffer cells take up the Endorem).

Laparoscopy with laparoscopic contact ultrasonography: undoubtedly this provides the most sensitive and reliable assessment, staging and operability of hepatic (primary or secondary), biliary and pancreatic cancers, and should precede laparotomy in all such cases. Patients confirmed to be inoperable can, if expertise is present, be palliated by the laparoscopic approach. Laparoscopic palliation, as opposed to endoscopic stenting, is indicated in patients with non-resectable pancreatic cancer in whom the disease burden is not extensive and whose general condition is good, and for these reasons they are expected to survive for several months. Another indication for surgical palliation (laparoscopic or open) is the presence of duodenal obstruction requiring a gastrojejunostomy.

Percutaneous transhepatic cholangiography (PTC): even with use of a skinny needle, this technique carries a certain morbidity. It is therefore used when ERCP is not technically feasible or fails to demonstrate the intrahepatic biliary tract because of an obstructing lesion at the hilum (Figure 11.14). The approach can be used therapeutically to insert stents

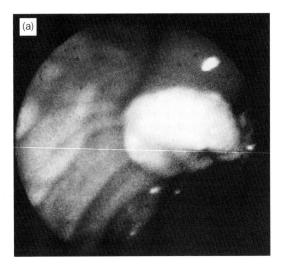

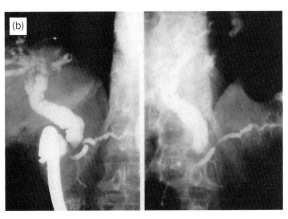

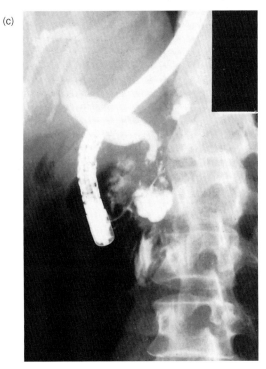

Figure 11.12 (a) Endoscopic view of a periampullary carcinoma; (b) cholangiopancreatogram of the same patient; (c) ERCP showing a carcinoma of the head of the pancreas.

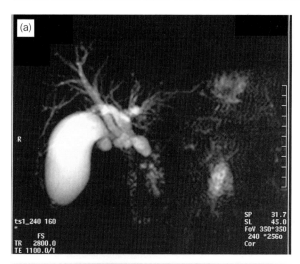

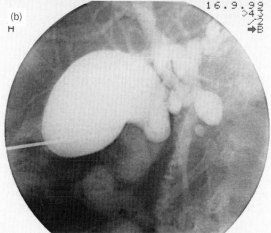

Figure 11.13 (a) MRCP in a patient with pancreatic cancer; (b) cholecystocholangiogram of the same patient taken during laparoscopic staging and palliation.

(endoprosthesis) through proximal inoperable cholangiocarcinomas.

Biopsy of tumours of liver, bile ducts and pancreas: this can be performed under image guidance, during laparoscopy or laparotomy. **Biopsy for tumours (by any approach) that are considered resectable is ill advised as it may cause dissemination and local implantation.** As surgeons we must do nothing that may jeopardize outcome, even if this results in a suspected but unconfirmed diagnosis. **Biopsy is, however, mandatory when the tumour is considered inoperable, as absolute proof is essential before confirming a death sentence.**

Endoscopic ultrasonography (EUS): with the considerable advances in transducer technology and related image-processing software, endoscopic ultrasonography has been shown in a number of studies to be extremely useful for the diagnosis and staging of bile duct and proximal pancreatic pathology. A more recent development is intraductal ultrasonography (IDUS), where a fine transducer probe is introduced in the bile or pancreatic duct at ERCP.

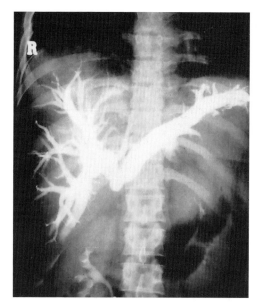

Figure 11.14 PTC showing high bile duct stricture with an intact confluence (Corlette-Bismuth type d).

Section 11.7 • Management of patients with surgical jaundice

General considerations

In the first instance, these patients fall into the category of urgent to emergency cases. Certainly, the patient with cholangitis needs urgent drainage, which is most commonly done nowadays with endoscopic sphincterotomy, stenting or nasobiliary drainage. Secondly, prolonged jaundice from unrelieved large bile duct obstruction (from any cause) adds to the perioperative morbidity and recovery, especially if hepatic conjugation ceases completely, such that at operation the patient is found to have unpigmented (white) bile that essentially reflects canalicular secretion.

Even without delays patients with obstructive jaundice undergoing surgery are subject to specific risks that require prophylactic measures:

- infections: cholangitis, septicaemia, wound infections
- bleeding: non-coagulant acarboxyl derivatives of vitamin K-dependent factors
- renal and liver failure
- fluid and electrolyte abnormalities.

Thirdly, certain disorders that cause large bile duct obstruction are best treated in tertiary hepatobiliary pancreatic units as this ensures the best outcome following surgical treatment. The special expertise necessary relates to case selection for the appropriate treatment, the surgical expertise in conducting complex and major operations and the necessary supportive care, which includes the services of a hepatologist and an interventional radiologist.

The disorders that are best managed in established hepatobiliary pancreatic units are:

- pancreatic and biliary cancers
- chronic pancreatitis
- bile duct strictures
- hepatic tumours.

Specific treatment

Gallstones and ductal calculi

Cholecystectomy (usually laparoscopic) is only indicated for symptomatic gallstones and their complications (acute cholecystitis, acute pancreatitis, jaundice due to ductal calculi). There is now firm evidence from several prospective, randomized trials that 'early' cholecystectomy' for acute cholecystitis, i.e. operation within the same hospital admission, is superior to 'interval or delayed' cholecystectomy at a subsequent admission some 2–3 months after resolution of the attack, provided the patient is fit for surgery and anaesthesia **[see Modules 3 and 16, Vol. I]**. The benefits of early cholecystectomy include reduced overall morbidity, reduced hospital stay and prevention of further attacks that may occur in patients managed by the delayed/interval cholecystectomy policy. The laparoscopic approach in patients with acute cholecystitis starts as an assessment of the severity of the inflammation and hence the feasibility and safety of an operation conducted laparoscopically. The vast majority will be eminently suitable (tense, inflamed gallbladder with minimal to moderate oedema of the cystic pedicle). Others, such as inflammatory phlegmon, empyema and gallbladder with gangrenous patch, are better and more safely conducted by conversion to the open approach.

Unfit patients (ASA III) should be treated conservatively in the first instance with the expectation that the acute cholecystitis will resolve in 80% of cases. In those that do not, including patients with empyema, an ultrasound, a laparoscopically guided cholecystostomy or the Burhenne minicholecystostomy (under ultrasound guidance) will tide the patients over the critical illness. Once recovered, these patients can be assessed to quantify the risk imposed by their underlying comorbid disease, on which is based the decision for or against an interval cholecystectomy.

The current orthodox treatment for patients with concomitant ductal calculi is preoperative endoscopic stone extraction followed by cholecystectomy, preferably during the same hospital admission. Single-stage laparoscopic cholecystectomy and ductal stone clearance, either by the transcystic route (distal stones < 6 mm) or by laparoscopic supraduodenal direct common bile duct explorations (large or occluding stones), is performed in some centres instead of the two-stage approach. The recently reported final results of a randomized clinical trial demonstrated equal efficacy in stone clearance, similar morbidity and mortality but reduced hospital stay in the single-stage laparoscopic arm.

Pancreatic disease

Surgical resection (pancreatoduodenectomy) is undertaken if the tumour is resectable and the patient is fit for major surgery. Most periampullary cancers are resectable and this is attended with a good prognosis, the extent of which is stage dependent. By contrast, most proximal pancreatic adenocarcinomas are not resectable and are managed palliatively with stenting (by interventional endoscopy or interventional radiology) or by surgery (open or laparoscopic). Expandable metallic wall stents made of nickel–titanium shape-memory alloy give better palliation than plastic stents. There is some debate as to whether surgical palliation should always include a gastroenterostomy in addition to biliary bypass, with some surgeons opting for both and others including a gastroenterostomy when there are clinical symptoms of gastric outlet obstruction or obvious duodenal involvement at surgery. Current chemotherapy regimens impart little benefit or survival advantage in patients with inoperable pancreatic cancer. There is some evidence from phase II studies that lithium–linolenic acid may delay disease progression and thus the time to death. Radiotherapy (interstitial or external supervoltage) may benefit some tumours. By and large, however, 90% of patients with pancreatic adenocarcinoma are dead within 12 months of the diagnosis.

In patients with jaundice thought to be due to chronic pancreatitis, when the disease is particularly pronounced in the head of the pancreas (pseudotumour), the options are between a formal pancreatoduodenectomy or subtotal resection of the head leaving a rim of pancreas in the duodenal curve and releasing the transpancreatic duct (Beger's procedure). A modification of Beger's procedure involves transection of the bile duct just above the pancreas with reimplantation into the duodenum. Both operations preserve the duodenum. If there is doubt concerning the diagnosis, the appropriate procedure is a formal pancreatoduodenectomy.

Biliary malignancy

Carcinoma of the gallbladder is a miserable disease that is virtually always incurable when diagnosed clinically. Palliation of the jaundice and itching due to involvement of the common hepatic duct is achieved by endoscopic or radiological stenting with plastic or nickel–titanium expandable stents. In the rare instance when the disease is resectable and the patient is fit, resection is indicated, although cure is rarely obtained. If the tumour invades the hepatic parenchyma (T$_3$ lesion), a right hepatectomy with resection of the common bile duct and nodal clearance is performed in selected cases. If the lesion is confined to the gallbladder (T$_1$, T$_2$) with no obvious hepatic involvement, the liver resection is limited to the gallbladder bed.

A not uncommon situation is the discovery by pathological examination of an unsuspected carcinoma of the gallbladder after laparoscopic cholecystectomy. Opinions vary on the management of these patients. If the gallbladder was extracted through an unprotected port wound (which is usually the case), then all patients, irrespective of tumour stage, should have formal block excision of the abdominal wall around and including the port wound as there have been many reported instances of port site deposits. One instructive report on a case of prophylactic abdominal wall excision demonstrated tumour cells in the excised block of tissue. A more aggressive approach is favoured by some. In addition to the excision of the abdominal wall, a laparotomy is performed with nodal clearance and excision of the gallbladder bed. This seems sensible if the tumour involves the muscularis propria of the gallbladder (T_2 lesion).

Middle and distal bile duct tumours are resected with removal of the pancreas and duodenum. The proximal resection margin must be well clear of the tumour because of submucosal spread, and for middle-third tumours; this corresponds to the hilar bifurcation. Proximal (hilar) tumours may be resected if the patient's condition is good despite age. The resection extends beyond the bifurcation and must always include the caudate lobe. This requires a combined anterior and posterior dissection of the hilar plate with control of the hepatic vein draining the caudate lobe. Non-resectable or inoperable bile duct tumours can be either stented or bypassed surgically: segment III bypass for left lobe, segment V bypass for right lobe [**see Hepatobiliary and Pancreatic Disorders, Vol. II**].

Hepatic tumours

Only patients who are not jaundiced, have no evidence of disease elsewhere (including hepatic nodes) and are otherwise fit with good liver function are suitable for hepatic resection.

For primary resectable hepatocellular carcinoma, the appropriate operation is a hepatectomy on the affected side. The best outcome is obtained after resection of well-differentiated fibrolamellar carcinomas. Hepatectomy is not usually possible in patients who develop the disease on a background of cirrhosis (cirrhomimetic hepatocellular cancer), although if small and the hepatic reserve is judged to be reasonable (A or B), resection of the involved segments may be possible in selected patients. Otherwise, treatment is by *in situ* ablation or embolization.

Secondary tumours, usually from colorectal cancer, are a much more common problem. There is a definite place for surgical resection if the disease is confined to one side and there are no more than three deposits. Many reports now indicate a 5-year survival of 25–30%. The resection may involve right or left hepatectomy or anatomical segmentectomies depending on size, number and location. The most important factor influencing outcome after surgical resection is a tumour-free margin of at least 1.5 cm. Resection combined with *in situ* ablation by cryosurgery or radio-frequency thermal ablation is a recent development that is applicable to bilateral disease.

Systemic chemotherapy, most commonly based on high-dose infusion of 5-fluorouracil (5-FU) with folinic acid (de Gramont regimen), induces disease regression in some 30%, although the benefit is measured in months in those patients that respond. Newer agents active against colon cancer include Ririnotecan, which may achieve a response in patients who do not obtain regression or exhibit renewed growth after 5-FU/folinic therapy. There is no evidence that regional hepatic intra-arterial therapy with external infusion pumps or implantable devices (Infusaid) is any more effective than systemic chemotherapy.

Laparoscopic or image-guided percutaneous *in situ* ablation can be achieved by (i) alcoholinization (small lesions, <2.0 cm), (ii) cryosurgery with high-efficiency liquid nitrogen needle probes, (iii) radiofrequency thermal ablation, and (iv) interstitial laser hyperthermia. Only patients with less than 30% of liver involvement, with good general condition and liver function and absence of disease elsewhere in the body are currently considered candidates for *in situ* ablation. The advantage of percutaneous or laparoscopic *in situ* ablation is that it can be repeated if new lesions or recurrence at the treated sites are detected on follow-up. The early results of a combination of *in situ* ablation with systemic chemotherapy in phase II studies look very promising.

Bile duct strictures

Management is best conducted in tertiary referral units without delay and in particular without an attempt at surgical correction by surgeons with little experience in the surgery and management of these problems. Treatment depends on the pathological anatomy of the stricture, the presence of bile or abscess collections and the condition of the patient [**see Hepatobiliary and Pancreatic Disorders, Vol. II**]. A combined interventional radiological–surgical approach or a purely surgical or purely interventional radiological management is indicated in the individual case.

Combined interventional–surgical approach: interventional radiology before definitive surgical treatment is often necessary to drain bile and infected fluid collections or abscesses. In patients with major injuries and poor general condition, percutaneous drainage may be needed. In some instances, the radiologist is able to negotiate the stricture and insert plastic endoprostheses, which are preferable to external drainage. The radiological information provides an excellent road map for the surgeon.

Surgical treatment: the aim of remedial surgery is to establish an anastomosis between the biliary tree and a jejunal Roux-en-Y limb through healthy unscarred bile ducts. If there is a serviceable extrahepatic duct stump (after bringing down the hilar plate), a single anastomosis between the upper common hepatic duct and the jejunal loop (**single hepatojejunostomy**) suffices to restore normal liver function. In high strictures, however, the bifurcation is involved and the anastomosis involves joining the two ducts (sometimes three, in the case of trifurcation) separately to the jejunal loop (**multiple hepatojejunostomy**). In all instances, a precise single-layer mucosa-to-mucosa anastomosis is the best guarantee against restenosis.

Temporary stenting of the anastomosis is indicated if the surgeon is not completely sure of complete mucosa-to-mucosa anastomosis and for multiple hepatojejunostomy. A sensible measure in these cases consists of fashioning an access jejunostomy attached to the anterior abdominal wall, the site of which is marked by metal clips. This enables percutaneous access to the anastomosis for percutaneous dilatation in the event of restenosis.

Interventional radiological treatment: as these patients have benign disease and usually have a long life expectancy, stenting is not a viable option other than as a temporary measure (see above). However, good reports comparable to open surgery have been reported with radiologically guided percutaneous balloon dilatation in patients with high uncomplicated partial strictures. These may require more than one dilatation.

Portal hypertension

Treatment is indicated only if varices bleed. Control of variceal haemorrhage is by endoscopic sclerotherapy or endoscopic banding in the first instance. Some centres also advocate the use of intravenous infusion of somatostatin. Balloon tamponade is only indicated if endoscopic control fails. Measures to reduce encephalopathy are instituted at the time of bleeding. These include enemas, lactulose or neomycin (not both) to reduce ammonia absorption from the gut, correction of fluid and electrolyte balance, withdrawal of any sedative or opiate drugs and 10% dextrose infusions. Hypokalaemia must be prevented at all costs as this converts ammonium ion (NH_4^+) to ammonia (NH_3), which passes easily through the blood–brain barrier. Most of these patients have renal failure and may require haemofiltration or dialysis.

Further management depends on the Child–Pugh stage. Child A and good B patients are best managed with distal shunt (Warren shunt) as an elective operation. Child C patients requiring hepatic transplantation are decompressed while they are waiting for the transplant by trans internal jugular portasystemic shunt (TIPSS, introduced radiologically through the neck (Figure 11.15). Experience with TIPSS has now shown a high occlusion rate beyond 6 months and they are therefore unsuitable for decompression of portal hypertension in patients with good liver function not requiring hepatic transplantation.

Guide to further reading

Bismuth, H., Houssin, D., Ornowski, J. and Meriggi, F. (1986). Liver resections in cirrhotic patients: a western experience. *World J Surg* **10**: 311–317.

Bret, P. M. and Reinhold, C. (1997). Magnetic resonance cholangiopancreaticography. *Endoscopy* **29**: 472–486.

Cuschieri, A. (1988). Laparoscopy in the management of pancreatic disease, in *Surgical Diseases of the Pancreas*, 3rd edn (J. Howard, Y. Idezuki, I. Ishe and R. Prinz, eds), Williams & Wilkins, Baltimore, MD, pp. 111–119.

Cuschieri, A., Croce, E., Faggioni, J., *et al.* (1999). EAES ductal stone study. Results of the multicentre prospective randomized trial comparing two-stage vs single-stage treatment. *Surg Endosc* (in press).

Furukawa, T., Oohashi, K., Yamao, K., *et al.* (1997). Intraductal ultrasonography of the pancreas: development and clinical potential. *Endoscopy* **29**: 561–569.

Kuoiwa, M., Tsukamato, Y., Naitho, Y., *et al.* (1994). New technique using intraductal ultrasonography for the diagnosis of bile duct cancer. *J Ultrasound Med* **13**: 189–195.

Mahfouz, A., Hamm, E. and Taupitz, B. (1997). Hepatic magnetic resonance imaging: new technique and contrast agents. *Endoscopy* **29**: 504–514.

Snady, H., Cooperman, A. and Siegel, J. (1992). Endoscopic ultrasonography compared with computed tomography with ERCP in patients with obstructive jaundice or small peripancreatic mass. *Gastrointest Endosc* **38**: 27–34.

Stewart, J. and Cuschieri, A. (1994). Adverse consequences of cystic duct closure by clips. *Min Invas Ther* **3**: 153–157.

Zimmerman, H. and Reichen, J. (1998). Hepatectomy: preoperative analysis of hepatic function and postoperative liver failure. *Dig Surg* **15**: 1–11.

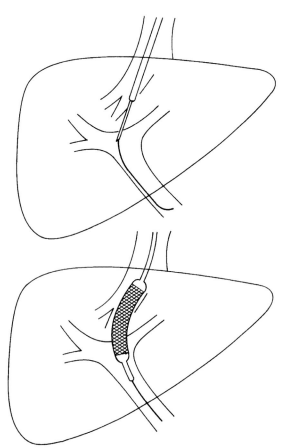

Figure 11.15 Diagrammatic representation of trans internal jugular portasystemic shunt (TIPSS)

Oliguric patients

1 • Obstructive uropathy

2 • Acute renal failure

3 • Renal replacement therapy

4 • Chronic renal failure

5 • Dialysis and haemofiltration

'A reckoning up of the cause often solves the malady'
– Celsus (25 BC–50 AD), De Medicina

Section 12.1 • Obstructive uropathy

Obstructive uropathy is defined as the surgical pathology that causes obstruction to the urinary tract. This can range from congenital obstruction of the pelviureteric junction to phimosis. The abnormalities of renal function associated with obstruction (especially water and salt excretion) are properly termed **obstructive nephropathy**.

Pathophysiology of obstructive nephropathy

Renal damage secondary to obstruction results from an ischaemic injury mediated through a number of well-defined vasoactive hormones including renin, angiotensin, prostaglandins, kinins, endothelin and nitric oxide. The various physiological changes in the kidney secondary to obstruction are shown in Table 12.1.

When the kidney is obstructed glomerular function does not cease, but continues to produce fluid that is reabsorbed by the renal lymphatics and veins. This acts as a safety mechanism so that the acutely obstructed kidney does not necessarily cease to function. Return to useful function is then dependent on:

- the length of time that the kidney is obstructed
- the degree of obstruction
- the presence or absence of infection above the obstruction.

Recovery of renal function after relief of obstruction usually occurs within 2 months but can take up to 6 months. Therefore, renal function 2 months after the relief of renal obstruction reflects the degree of potential renal recovery. After relief of obstruction, tubular function seems to take longer to return to normal than does glomerular filtration rate (GFR). This results in a postobstructive diuresis.

Clinical features

Causes
The causes of obstructive uropathy are shown in Table 12.2.

Clinical presentation
The symptoms and signs vary depending on the level and degree of obstruction. If there is complete and bilateral obstruction the patient will be anuric and serum creatinine will rise. If there is unilateral ureteric obstruction then no detectable change in the

Table 12.1 Pathophysiological changes in the obstructed kidney

Parameter of renal function	Change immediately postobstruction (first few hours)	Change later on in obstructive episode (after first few hours)
Renal pelvis pressure	Increased	Decreased
Renal blood flow	Increased	Decreased
Tubular function	Loss of concentrating ability	Loss of concentrating ability
Glomerular filtration rate	Decreased	Decreased

Table 12.2 Causes of obstructive uropathy

Kidney	Congenital PUJ obstruction
	Stone blocking PUJ
	Tumour blocking PUJ
Ureter	Ureteric tumour
	Ureteric stone
	Blood clot
	Stricture
	Sloughed papilla
	Extrinsic causes, e.g. retroperitoneal tumour, fibrosis, inflammation, haemorrhage
	Prostate cancer blocking the vesicoureteric junction
	Bladder cancer blocking the vesicoureteric junction
Bladder outflow obstruction	Benign prostatic enlargement
	Prostate cancer
	Bladder neck stenosis
Urethra	Stricture
	Carcinoma
	Phimosis

PUJ, pelviureteric junction.

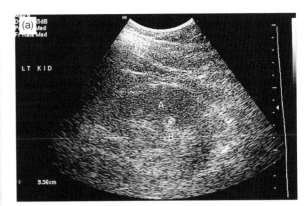

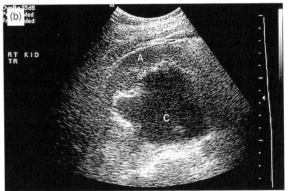

Figure 12.1 Ultrasound of (a) normal kidney; (b) dilated right kidney.

urine output or serum creatinine may be detected. In general, acute obstruction (e.g. ureteric stone) is painful, while chronic obstruction (e.g. a bladder tumour slowly obstructing the lower end of the ureter) is painless. If there is infected urine above the obstruction the clinical features of sepsis may be present as well.

Diagnosis

Ultrasound scanning is a quick, safe and convenient way of diagnosing that urinary tract obstruction is present (Figure 12.1). It generally shows dilatation of the urinary tract proximal to the obstruction. Diagnosing the level and cause of obstruction usually requires further tests (Table 12.3). Other tests are used to confirm that obstruction is present in a dilated urinary tract. An isotope renogram with diuretic can be used to confirm that obstruction is present in a patient with hydronephrosis suspected of having pelviureteric junction obstruction (Figure 12.2). In a patient with a poorly emptying bladder, simultaneous measurements of urine flow rate from the urethra and bladder voiding pressure will indicate whether bladder outflow obstruction is present or not.

Treatment

The treatment of the obstructed urinary tract generally starts with establishing drainage of the urine proximal to the obstruction. This should be performed as soon as possible to prevent ongoing damage to the kidney. The length of time that the kidney is obstructed is one of the factors that determines the degree to which the kidney recovers after relief of the obstruction. If the patient has infected urine proximal to the obstruction (as indicated by a clinically septic patient) or has a sin-

Table 12.3 Diagnosing renal obstruction

Site of obstruction	Findings indicating obstruction	Tests for site/cause of obstruction
Pelvi-ureteric junction	Hydronephrosis on ultrasound (without hydroureter); slow renal drainage on diuretic isotope renogram	Intravenous urogram; retrograde pyelogram
Ureter (intrinsic)	Hydronephrosis on ultrasound, possibly hydroureter, empty bladder if bilateral	Intravenous urogram; retrograde ureterogram; antegrade ureterogram; ureteroscopy
Ureter (extrinsic)	Hydronephrosis on ultrasound, possibly hydroureter, empty bladder if bilateral	Use of the above for site, CT or MRI to show retroperitoneal disease
Urethral and bladder outflow	Large volume of urine in bladder after voiding ± bilateral hydronephrosis	Clinical examination and cystourethroscopy ± urethrography

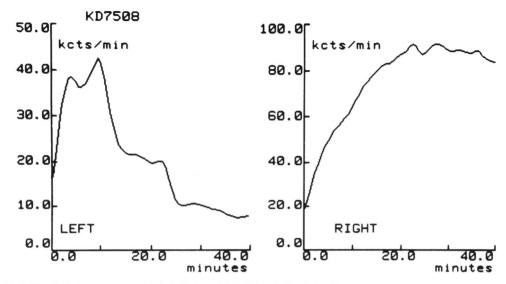

Figure 12.2 Diuretic isotope renogram demonstrating night pelvi-ureteric obstruction.

gle functioning kidney, relief of the obstruction must be undertaken urgently. The ways of draining the urinary tract are shown in Table 12.4.

Once the obstructed urinary tract is drained the situation becomes less urgent and infection and renal failure can be treated before proceeding to definitive treatment (Table 12.5). If drainage of the obstructed urinary tract in the presence of renal failure does not result in an improvement in the renal function then severe renal damage must be assumed. In this situation, referral to the nephrology team for dialysis is necessary.

After relief of bilateral obstruction a **postobstructive diuresis** may occur. The cause of this is not fully understood but probably reflects an imbalance between glomerular function and tubular integrity. In this event it is very important to monitor fluid balance carefully, otherwise the patient can become hypovolaemic and hypotensive with further renal damage occurring. Water and sodium balance is closely monitored and after 24 h potassium balance is also monitored. Sodium and potassium conservation usually return after 48–72 h but concentrating ability can take up to 7–12 days to return to normal. These postobstructive changes do not occur to any great extent when one normal kidney remains unobstructed and retains its normal homeostatic responses.

Section 12.2 • Acute renal failure

Definition

Acute renal failure (ARF) may be defined as the rapid onset of renal impairment that results in accumulation of nitrogenous waste products, most notably urea and creatinine, within the body. The process is often potentially reversible but is not in a minority of cases because either there is pre-existing renal damage (acute on chronic renal failure), the mechanism of damage is irreversible or, in some cases, treatment is delayed. In common usage ARF is often equated to acute tubular necrosis (ATN), where there is intrinsic but reversible damage to the kidney. There are, however, good reasons for attempting to classify ARF according to aetiology. If used clinically this can facilitate rapid diagnosis and, hence, early and appropriate treatment.

Prerenal acute renal failure

Prerenal ARF relates to a problem with the supply of adequate nutrition to the kidney rather than intrinsic dysfunction. This poverty of supply is most often due to acute changes affecting blood supply to the kidney, causes of which are shown in Table 12.6. Clinically, such patients are shocked, with hypotension and tachycardia. When related to sepsis there is peripheral vasodi-

Table 12.4 Immediate treatment of the obstructed urinary tract

PUJ obstruction	Retrograde placement of JJ stent **or** percutaneous placement of a nephrostomy tube
Ureteric obstruction	Retrograde placement of JJ stent **or** percutaneous placement of a nephrostomy tube
Bladder outflow obstruction	Urethral catheterization: usually possible with prostatic obstruction Suprapubic catheter if urethral stricture may not allow urethral catheter to pass

PUJ, pelvi-ureteric junction.

Table 12.5 Definitive treatment of the obstructed urinary tract

Congenital PUJ obstruction	Pyeloplasty **or** endoscopic incision of PUJ
Stone, PUJ	ESWL **or** percutaneous nephrolithotomy
Stone, upper ureter	ESWL *in situ* or after pushing stone back to kidney
Stone, mid ureter	ESWL after pushing stone back to kidney **or** ureteroscopic disintegration/extraction of stone
Stone, lower ureter	Ureteroscopic disintegration/extraction of stone
Tumour, PUJ/ureter	Nephroureterectomy (conservative surgery sometimes possible in a single, well-differentiated and well-localized tumour)
Tumour, bladder	Transurethral resection of tumour If tumour is muscle invasive on histology, radiotherapy or cystectomy may be advised
Tumour, prostate	Transurethral resection of prostate to relieve obstruction Androgen deprivation may be used to prevent/delay regrowth of prostate tumour If prostate cancer has invaded under the bladder trigone to obstruct both lower ureters, then androgen deprivation will cause tumour shrinkage and relief of obstruction in most patients
Tumour, urethra (rare)	Local cystoscopic control of tumour Sometimes requires excision
Bladder outflow	BPE: transurethral resection of prostate Bladder neck stenosis: transurethral incision of bladder neck Urethral stricture: optical urethrotomy Phimosis: circumcision Retroperitoneal disease: depends on cause; long-term stenting can maintain renal function

ESWL, extracorporeal shock wave lithotripsy; BPE, benign prostatic enlargement; PUJ, pelvi-ureteric junction.

latation due the effect of bacterial toxins but in the dehydrated and cardiac compromised patient there is peripheral vasoconstriction.

The vascular disease causes of prerenal failure are rarer and may present without evidence of hypotension or tachycardia. Renal artery thrombosis occurs in hypercoagulable states and large vessel vasculitis, and may occur after aortography or renal arteriography. It is also a rare complication of acute pancreatitis. An increasingly common problem is the presentation of patients with acute deterioration of renal function after introduction of an angiotensin-converting enzyme (ACE) inhibitor. These patients may have unsuspected renal artery stenosis, but such a decline in renal func-

tion can occur in the absence of main artery stenosis and is thought to reflect an ACE inhibitor-mediated deterioration of an already poor intrarenal circulation. Despite this, ACE inhibitors have been shown to improve renal survival in chronic renal failure (CRF) and are being used more frequently in renal disease.

Renal artery embolism is extremely uncommon but is associated with cardiac mural thrombi or valvular vegetations. Renal vein thrombosis differs from other prerenal failure in that the patient, often a vomiting, dehydrated child, may present with renal pain, hypertension and frank haematuria. In adults this rare condition may be associated with use of the oral contraceptive pill or thrombophilic states.

Table 12.6 Causes of prerenal acute renal failure

Reduced cardiac output	Depleted circulating volume	Depleted extracellular fluid	Vascular disease
Acute myocardial infarction	Sepsis	Loss from gastrointestinal tract with diarrhoea, vomiting	Renal artery embolism
Cardiac arrest	Haemorrhage	Loss from urinary tract due to excessive diuresis	Renal artery thrombosis
Cardiac failure	Hypoalbuminaemia	Loss from skin/body surface associated with sweating and burns	Significant valvular disease
Cardiac tamponade			

Table 12.7 Causes of intrinsic acute renal failure

Ischaemia	All prenal causes of acute renal failure	
Ischaemia and toxin	Hypercalcaemia Hepatorenal syndrome	
Toxins	Primary ATN	Aminoglycosides, cephalosporins, paracetamol, salicylates, paraquat, heavy metals, e.g. platinum, arsenic, mercury
	Tubular obstruction	Light-chain deposition in myeloma
	Myoglobinuria	Muscle injury, snakebite, heroin, barbiturates
	Haemoglobinuria	Mismatched blood, nitrofurantoin
Acute interstitial nephritis	Antibiotics	e.g. penicillin, cephalosporins, co-trimoxazole, vancomycin, rifampicin
	NSAIDs	e.g. mefanamic acid, indomethacin, ibuprofen
	Diuretics	e.g. thiazides, frusemide
	Other drugs	e.g. sulfasalazine, allopurinol, gold, phenytoin
	Infections	e.g. infectious mononucleosis, measles, Legionnaire's disease, leptospirosis, brucellosis
Vascular (endothelial damage) hypertension	Vasculitis, haemolytic uraemic syndrome, disseminated intravascular coagulation, accelerated	
Rapidly progressive glomerulonephritis (see Table 12.8)		

Causes of postrenal acute renal failure
Ureteric obstruction	Calculi, blood clot, tumour, e.g. cervical carcinoma, retroperitoneal fibrosis
Urethral obstruction	Prostatic hypertrophy or carcinoma

Intrinsic acute renal failure

The major causes of intrinsic renal failure are shown in Table 12.7. It should be noted that all causes of prerenal ARF could progress to ATN if the underlying cause of the prerenal ARF is not addressed and treated rapidly. In two special circumstances the diminution of perfusion is accentuated by direct toxicity; in hypercalcaemia the associated polyuria and vomiting lead to depletion of extracellular fluid and the calcium itself is directly toxic to tubules, whereas in hepatorenal syndrome hyperbilirubinaemia has a toxic effect on the tubules and liver disease decreases renal perfusion in association with active renal vasoconstriction.

The group of patients with rapidly progressive glomerulonephritis needs to be identified separately (Table 12.8). This type of ARF is associated with an immune attack on the kidney and has to be recognized and, when appropriate, immunomodulatory treatment commenced as soon as possible if there is to be any chance of recovery of renal function. All of the diseases shown in Table 12.8 may present with rapidly progressive glomerulonephritis and, clinically, the patient is found to be suffering from progressive oliguria, hypertension and haematuria with or without proteinuria. If there is coexistent pulmonary haemorrhage Goodpasture's syndrome [antiglomerular basement membrane (anti-GBM) nephritis] may be present but Wegener's granulomatosis or other vasculitides should be included in the differential diagnosis.

In these situations, immunosuppression with or without plasmapheresis is the treatment of choice. Investigation including renal biopsy should be expedited as quickly as possible for the patient in whom any of these diagnoses might be considered.

Another important group of patients with ARF comprises those who are demonstrated to have acute interstitial nephritis (AIN). This condition is often precipitated by certain categories of drugs, including antibiotics and non-steroidal anti-inflammatory drugs (NSAIDs), but may also be associated with infection (Table 12.7). The presentation of this group of patients may be indistinguishable from presentation with ATN, but arthralgia, rashes and eosinophilia are more common in patients with AIN. Treatment for this group of patients is to remove the precipitating factor and, otherwise, is generally supportive as for ATN. If a renal biopsy demonstrates an aggressive inflammatory infiltrate some clinicians treat the patients with steroids, but the evidence for the efficacy of such treatment is equivocal.

Table 12.8 Causes of rapidly progressive glomerulonephritis

Primary glomerulonephritis
Acute idiopathic crescentic glomerulonephritis
Anti-GBM nephritis (Goodpasture's syndrome)
Membranoproliferative glomerulonephritis
Endocapillary glomerulonephritis (e.g. severe post-streptococcal glomerulonephritis)

Renal involvement secondary to systemic disease
Infection	Bacterial endocarditis
	'Shunt' nephritis (usually associated with ventriculoatrial shunts)
	Hepatitis B-associated nephritis
Vasculitis	Henoch–Schönlein purpura
	Systemic lupus erythematosus
	Polyarteritis nodosa
	Wegener's granulomatosis

GBM, glomerular basement membrane.

Postrenal acute renal failure

Postrenal ARF is most commonly applied to obvious anatomical causes of obstruction to the urinary outflow tract (Table 12.7; see Section 1). Some, however, also include pathologies that cause primary tubular obstruction. In this case the deposition of myeloma proteins in the kidney may be included in this category. Although patients with outflow tract obstruction often present with anuria the presence of a seemingly adequate urine flow does not exclude the presence of a significant obstruction. This is because the increase in back pressure associated with obstruction can cause renal dysfunction at the level of the collecting ducts, with a resultant impaired urinary concentrating ability. These patients also often complain of haematuria and back pain that radiates to the groin.

The patient with deteriorating renal function

When faced with a patient with deteriorating renal function assessment should include an adequate history and clinical examination, supported by laboratory, and possibly radiological, investigation. Intervention will be based on the results of all of these, but should be prompt because delay can allow the renal insult to intensify and cause excessive, and potentially irreversible, intrinsic renal damage to occur.

The clinical history will obviously cover the major organ systems but it should be remembered that even over-the-counter medication, e.g. ibuprofen, have been implicated in the aetiology of ARF, as noted above.

At clinical examination an assessment of intravascular hydration should be made. If low, this may be reflected by low blood pressure and tachycardia, signs of cardiac failure, signs of blood loss or signs of sepsis. However, even the patient with sacral and ankle oedema and pleural effusions may have a low circulating volume if the oedema is related to hypoalbuminaemia. Clinical examination of the patient should be completed to include all major systems but specifically to include observation for signs of vasculitis, e.g. skin rash, joint pain and swelling, and examination for causes of renal obstruction, including both abdominal and rectal examinations. It should be remembered that the clinical presentations of renal failure can affect all systems, although the consequences of impaired fluid balance, poor acid–base balance and retention of nitrogenous waste products may be most apparent, with tachycardia, tachypnoea and impaired mental function being prominent signs.

Insertion of central venous lines

Assessment of hydration state based purely on clinical examination may be inaccurate. In the acutely unwell patient more invasive forms of monitoring are vital. This should include insertion of a central venous line but, if this is thought to be an inadequate indicator of left ventricular filling pressure, pulmonary artery catheterization may be necessary. Pulmonary artery pressure monitoring itself has been the subject of recent controversy. Further research is necessary to determine the most appropriate use of these catheters. If a central venous line is to be inserted then the internal jugular route in experienced hands is the safest and success in cannulation of the vein can be improved by the use of small ultrasound probes, e.g. Siterite, to localize the vein.

Low central venous pressure

The response to a low central venous pressure should be to replace the type of fluid that the patient is lacking. If there is evidence of blood loss, replacement by blood is mandatory, although initial resuscitation may include the use of colloid volume expanders, e.g. haemaccel and, in the rapidly bleeding patient, group O Rhesus-negative blood. If there is evidence of sepsis or dehydration, volume expanders are an appropriate agent to improve the CVP but subsequent intravenous replacement can be maintained by crystalloid solutions. In many patients with ARF serum potassium concentrations will be high; therefore, avoidance of the use of Hartmann's solution or other potassium-containing crystalloids is recommended. CVP measurement can be undertaken by electronic transduction, if available, or by regular measurement by trained nursing staff.

High central venous pressure

If the CVP is high an echocardiogram should be sought to distinguish between cardiac failure and other causes of a high CVP, e.g. tricuspid regurgitation, fluid retention or constrictive pericarditis. If left ventricular dysfunction is diagnosed, help from a cardiologist should be sought and the patient treated with inotropic agents such as dobutamine and dopamine if thought appropriate. The latter has been used as a renal protective agent at doses of 2–5 g/kg/min in patients with declining urinary output, but should not be commenced until the patient's intravascular volume is replete. If dopamine is commenced when the patient has a low circulating volume it can further compromise the already ischaemic tubules and this could cause damage to the kidneys. Even when dopamine is used in the fluid-replete patient the benefit that accrues in promoting renal perfusion and function has been questioned and there are no convincing data on the efficacy of this treatment in preventing renal failure.

Urinary catheterization

Close observation of the urinary output is necessary to help with determining fluid replacement and to help with assessment of the patient's response to treatment. This is most accurately done after insertion of a urinary catheter, after which hourly urine volumes are measured. The prescription for intravenous fluid, therefore, can be determined using a combination of the CVP and the previous hour's urinary output. If the CVP reading is satisfactory and insensible fluid loss is unlikely to be excessive, the hourly intravenous input could approximate to the previous hour's urine volume plus 30 ml. For the unstable patient this prescription

Table 12.9 Urinary investigation and interpretation

Differentiation of prerenal ARF and established ARF

	Prerenal	Established
Urinary Na$^+$ (mmol/l)	< 10	> 20
Urinary urea (mmol/l)	> 150	< 150
Urine/plasma osmolarity	> 1.1	< 1.1
Urine/plasma urea	> 8	< 3
Fractional excretion of Na$^+$	< 1	> 1
Fractional excretion of Na$^+$ = (urinary sodium × plasma creatinine)/(urinary creatinine × plasma sodium) × 100)		

Urinary sediment
Red cells of glomerular origin are crenated and deformed
Red cells released from rest of urinary tract have normal morphology
White cells occur in inflammation including infection
Sterile pyuria occurs in tuberculosis, stones and analgesic nephropathy
Hyaline casts have no pathological significance
Granular casts occur in acute tubular necrosis and acute nephritis
Red cell casts indicate haematuria of renal origin, e.g. nephritis

Urinalysis

Multistix analysis can detect	Positive in presence of
Blood	Infection, nephritis, tumour
Bilirubin	Jaundice
Ketones	Fasting state, diabetic ketoacidosis
Glucose	Diabetes mellitus, abnormal renal threshold
Protein	Nephritis, diabetic nephropathy, infection
pH	Indication of H ion excretion
Specific gravity	Indication of concentrating ability
Nitrites	Infection
Leucocytes	Inflammation, infection

Sample of urine should be sent to the laboratory for Bence Jones protein if myeloma is clinically suspected.

would have to be modified and regularly updated. Catheterization also facilitates urinary collection and investigation of the urine (Table 12.9).

Investigation
In addition to the measures outlined above (including investigation of the patient's urine), blood from patients with ARF should be sent for serological analysis as shown in Table 12.10. Furthermore, imaging should include renal ultrasound to demonstrate size and scarring, and to exclude hydronephrosis caused, perhaps, by an obstructing lesion. This investigation will also be useful in excluding the presence of persistent intra-abdominal sepsis, e.g. subphrenic abscess. Technetium–

Table 12.10 Serological investigations of acute renal failure

Immunologically based investigation

Investigation	Positive in
pANCA	Polyarteritis, other vasculitides, SBE
cANCA	Wegener's granulomatosis
ANA	SLE
Anti-DNA antibody	
Complement C3, C4	Membranoproliferative glomerulonephritis type II (decreased C3)
Antiglomerular basement membrane antibody	Goodpasture's syndrome
Immunoglobulin A	Elevated in IgA nephropathy and Henoch–Schönlein purpura
VDRL	Syphilis-associated nephritis
Serum antistreptolysin O titre (ASO)	Post-streptococcal glomerulonephritis
Hepatitis B and C status	Always check before entry to dialysis unit

Biochemical analysis

Creatine kinase and lactate dehydrogenase	High serum levels in rhabdomyolysis
Serum protein electrophoresis	Paraprotein present in myeloma

99m (^{99m}Tc)-DTPA renography or colour flow Doppler ultrasound can be used to demonstrate renal perfusion, although if these investigations are equivocal or delayed digital subtraction angiography may be required. This is necessary because renal perfusion is usually well maintained in ATN but not when the renal artery has been occluded. Early intervention after renal artery thrombosis or embolism can lead to a return of renal function. Straight abdominal X-rays may reveal urinary calculi.

Established acute renal failure

The pathological changes that occur in the development of ATN after an ischaemic or toxic injury have been investigated and precisely defined. The following four major factors are the most important in the initiation and maintenance of ARF.

- **Decrease in glomerular capillary permeability**: the mechanism of this is not well defined, although endothelial swelling has been described.
- **Back-leak of glomerular filtrate**: this mechanism has been well established in animal models and in humans using studies into the differential excretion of dextran and inulin in subjects with ARF. The lower molecular weight inulin was cleared from the circulation less successfully than dextran, suggesting leakage of inulin across the damaged tubular membrane.
- **Tubular obstruction**: tubular cell injury can occur as a response to ischaemia or toxins and results in a release of debris into the tubular lumen. This binds with tubular proteins and casts are created that cause a mechanical obstruction to flow, back-pressure and loss of glomerular filtration. Most tubular cells react in a sublethal way to the insult with movement of the Na/K-ATPase to the apical domain of the cell, loss of renal epithelium attachment to its matrix, loss of the barrier function that normally stops free movement of solute and water across the epithelium, detachment of tubular cells from the basement membrane and abnormal adherence of cells to each other in the tubular lumen. Some cells, however, undergo necrosis or apoptosis. The mechanisms underlying necrosis are highly variable and difficult to target. In apoptosis, however, there are defined mechanisms including loss of cell survival factors, e.g. deficiency of renal growth factors, impaired cell-matrix adhesion and loss of cell–cell adhesion. The development of agents that inhibit apoptosis in the setting of incipient ARF may provide a new way to protect the transiently ischaemic kidney.
- **Changes in renal blood flow and intrarenal vasoconstriction**: the reduction in total renal blood flow in ARF is well established but is of questionable significance. The distribution of blood within the kidney is, however, much more

important. The medulla is chronically hypoxic even in normal individuals. In ARF the medullary blood flow is reduced and the hypoxia accentuated. This reduction results from physical congestion in the medullary capillaries. The congestion relates to ischaemia of the kidney, which causes the local release of cytokines. This results in activation of leucocyte adhesion molecules and expression of the corresponding ligands on endothelial cells. Endothelial injury follows and red cells, platelets and leucocytes are caught in the damaged capillaries. The importance of these mechanisms has been demonstrated in mice that lack intercellular adhesion molecule-1 (ICAM-1). These mice do not develop ARF after ischaemic injury. Endothelial damage causes a shift in balance between endothelin and endothelium-derived nitric oxide (EDNO), with production of the latter being decreased. This change increases leucocyte adherence to endothelial cells. The relative increase in endothelin also causes increasing intrarenal vasoconstriction that further exacerbates the local hypoxia. Reduction of EDNO has been demonstrated particularly in ARF associated with myoglobin and cyclosporin.

Treatment of the cause of acute renal failure

Identification of the cause of ARF is necessary to target the precise treatment required to remove any precipitating cause of the renal failure. The management of fluid balance and correction of dehydration are important, but if there is any evidence of sepsis this must be dealt with promptly. Avoidance of aminoglycosides that can cause renal failure in the patients who has renal impairment seems logical. If it is felt that this type of drug, e.g. gentamicin, cannot be avoided, the side-effects of these drugs are minimized by single daily dose regimes and close monitoring of the serum concentrations is essential. Adherence to local antibiotic protocols, which have been developed to take account of antibiotic sensitivities of the predominant local organisms, is the most appropriate course of action to determine the antibiotics that should be used for the septic patient. For many nephrologists, however, third-generation cephalosporins are thought to be appropriate first-line antibiotics either singly or in combination for septicaemia of unknown origin, intra-abdominal sepsis and severe urinary tract infection.

For the oliguric patient who has an adequate circulating volume it is appropriate to try and promote urine flow by use of an intravenous diuretic. This may promote a diuresis and, even if the renal failure is not reversed, high output failure is associated with a better prognosis than if the patient is anuric.

For the patient with an obstructive cause for ARF the management must be directed to removal of the obstruction if possible. For urethral obstruction this may simply require bladder catheterization but may also require surgical intervention, e.g. for a calculus obstructing a single kidney. For the patient in whom there is ureteric obstruction that cannot be relieved immediately, intervention by nephrostomy may be necessary. This course of action can remove completely the need for consideration of dialysis and, therefore, should be actively pursued.

Conservative management

The conservative management of ARF is only possible when the patient's condition is not so severe that dialysis treatment is indicated immediately. If possible, however, this might include restriction of first-class protein to 30 g/day to minimize symptoms of uraemia such as nausea and anorexia, although too stringent restriction promotes endogenous protein catabolism and results in increased serum urea concentration. Other measures include restriction of potassium intake to 20 mmol/day to minimize the risk of hyperkalaemia, tight control of fluid intake so that it relates appropriately to fluid loss, and maintenance of adequate nutrition including consideration of parenteral nutrition, if required, at an early stage.

Treatment of haematological and biochemical abnormalities

Patients presenting with ARF are unlikely to have developed the anaemia associated with renal failure and so, if anaemia is present, other causes should be sought. Any acutely unwell patient is dependent, however, on adequate oxygen delivery to vital organs for recovery to progress. Therefore, significant anaemia (< 100 g/l) should be corrected by blood transfusion when the patient's fluid balance permits. It should be remembered that patients with ARF are at increased risk of developing gastrointestinal haemorrhage and many centres prescribe antacid treatment (including H_2 antagonists or proton pump inhibitors) for all patients with ARF.

Hyperkalaemia is the most worrying biochemical abnormality associated with ARF because it can cause cardiac dysrhythmias and is associated with sudden death. It is mandatory, therefore, that this particular biochemical abnormality is sought in all patients with renal dysfunction and, if present, treated promptly. Treatment of hyperkalaemia is outlined in Table 12.11.

Nutrition

Nutrition for patients with ARF is extremely important. All patients with dialysis-dependent ARF have higher nutritional requirements than normal but this is especially true in the patient who develops renal failure as a complication of other severe illness. The metabolic and nutritional consequences of ARF in this category of patients have to be recognized to permit adequate treatment. Hormonally, the patients have a relatively insulin-resistant state, a low T_3 syndrome and a decrease in testosterone levels. Energy expenditure is increased to 20–30% above expected resting levels. Hyperglycaemia associated with insulin resistance is not uncommon and glucose oxidation is a smaller component of total energy consumption than is found in normal subjects. Lipid and protein metabolism is also affected, with an increase in plasma triglycerides, a decrease in cholesterol and apoprotein A and a large increase in protein catabolism. Renal replacement therapy (RRT) further complicates the nutritional state. Glucose in haemofiltration replacement fluids can provide a large number of calories but amino acids are lost during RRT. The volume state of the patient may complicate the ability to supply the patient's nutritional requirements adequately and the electrolyte composition of parenteral nutrition may have to be modified. In general, patients with ARF have the same requirements as other acutely sick patients, i.e. a caloric intake of 35 kcal/kg body weight/day and nitrogen 1.2 g/kg body weight/day, with the ratio between glucose and lipid in the non-protein part of energy being 70:30. Some groups have proposed the specific addition to parenteral nutrition solutions of glutamine, which has an important role in the metabolic responses to stress and infection. Dietetic advice is very important to ensure the best management of the complex nutritional demands of patients with ARF.

The diuretic phase

As ARF resolves there is often a diuretic phase that occurs when the concentrating ability of the recovering tubules is not yet re-established. In this situation the patient must not be allowed to become dehydrated. The excessive fluid loss of the diuretic phase must be replaced until the renal tubules are able to concentrate the urine. This often requires intravenous fluid replacement because the fluid losses can be as high as 20 l/day. High urinary volumes such as these are unlikely to persist for more than a few days. The diuretic phase of renal failure may take many weeks to months to become established, but is usually shorter if the patients do not become anuric or severely oliguric.

Prognosis

The prognosis of ARF is dependent on the underlying aetiology. In general, however, the overall mortality of

---

Table 12.11 Treatment of hyperkalaemia

1. 10–20 ml of 10% calcium gluconate or chloride i.v.
   This has no effect on the serum potassium concentration but stabilizes the myocardial membrane
2. 50 ml of 50% dextrose i.v. with 10 units of soluble insulin
   This will drive potassium into the cells and should be started directly after step 1
3. 200–300 ml 1.4% sodium bicarbonate i.v.
   This drives potassium into cells and helps to correct the acidosis of acute renal failure. The fluid load necessary, however, makes use of this agent less desirable in hyperkalaemic acute renal failure
4. Calcium resonium 15 g three times daily orally or by enema
   This binds potassium in the gut and releases calcium in exchange. Unlike the other actions listed this can control the serum potassium for hours to days
5. Dialysis should be implemented if there is severe hyperkalaemia and/or the patient requires dialysis for other reasons, e.g. fluid overload

ARF has not improved in the last three decades. This may reflect the increasing age, associated comorbidity and differing aetiologies of present-day ARF, but the overall mortality remains at 50%. This figure obscures the fact that the mortality rate associated with ARF has improved for certain categories of patients. For instance, patients with ARF associated with trauma are more likely to do well now compared with 30 years ago and obstetric causes of ARF are now associated with a relatively low mortality rate of 10–20%

Coexistent morbidities will affect the mortality rates associated with ARF. Studies have shown that in the setting of an intensive care unit (ICU) ARF has an overall mortality of 70%, whereas ARF in other areas of care has an overall mortality of 30%. This reflects the associated comorbidity of patients in the ICU setting. For all patients, if there is associated failure of one other system the overall patient survival is reduced to less than 30% and failure of two systems reduces survival further, to less than 10%. Not unexpectedly, increasing age of the patient impacts adversely on survival rates.

Section 12.3 • **Renal replacement therapy**

Abnormalities of potassium, calcium and phosphate can be corrected by the various forms of RRT noted below, using dialysate or replacement solutions that are appropriately constituted. Indications for RRT in ARF include:

- uraemia, i.e. significant retention of nitrogenous waste products with associated clinical signs
- metabolic acidosis
- hyperkalaemia, and
- significant fluid overload.

Type of renal replacement therapy

When RRT is required there are choices that must be made regarding the precise type of treatment to be used. Emergency peritoneal dialysis is rarely used in adults with ARF because of the slow removal of all types of molecules and the risk of dialysis-associated peritonitis. Treatment for the majority of patients with ARF, therefore, requires that adequate vascular access be achieved. This is most commonly achieved using the internal jugular, subclavian or femoral approach. The internal jugular line is the preferred method of access when possible; use of the subclavian route has an increased incidence of complications, both immediate, e.g. pneumothorax, and later, e.g. venous stenosis. The femoral route is only satisfactory for a short time because of the high infection rate associated with the use of this site.

If the episode of ARF is likely to be prolonged, temporary lines should be replaced by more permanent venous access using devices such as the Permcath. The use of these devices in this situation is associated with lower rates of infection and lower long-term complications. The use of Scribner AV shunts for vascular access is now uncommon.

Temporary lines may have either a single, double or triple lumen. The double- and triple-lumen lines are associated with improved clearances of uraemic toxins and the triple-lumen line allows administration of intravenous therapy without interfering with the RRT.

The choice of haemodialysis, haemofiltration or haemodiafiltration as a form of therapy is normally decided by the renal physicians and intensivists. Haemodialysis is based on diffusion, exhibits high efficiency with regard to small molecule and volume removal and is cost effective, but relies on well-trained personnel; haemofiltration relies on convection to remove larger molecules and volume with high efficiency, but removes smaller molecules, e.g. potassium, less well. The combination of these two techniques is called haemodiafiltration. This technique requires specialized machines and is much less cost effective.

Filtration techniques require at least a double-lumen venous line and rely on a pumped system to create a gradient across the filter and, hence, a filtrate from the patient. This is venovenous haemofiltration (VVH). It is possible to use an arterial and venous line to create the pressure gradient across the filter line (AVH). This removes the need for a pumped system in the patient with an adequate blood pressure but is much less satisfactory if the patient is hypotensive. This filtrate contains uraemic poisons and the excess electrolytes that accumulate in renal failure, and the fluid is replaced by an appropriately constituted and usually commercially available solution. Some of the fluid removed can be replaced by parenteral fluid solutions.

Haemodialysis, haemofiltration and haemodiafiltration can all be performed on an intermittent or continuous basis. There are no good data that demonstrate which type of therapy is associated with the best outcome. 'Uncomplicated' ARF patients in whom cardiovascular instability is not a problem are possibly best treated with intermittent techniques, whereas the more unstable patients, in whom fluid removal is more difficult, benefit from continuous therapies. In continuous haemofiltration (e.g. CVVH or CAVH) the 24-h filtrate may average at 12 litres or higher. Monitoring the filtrate volume and prescribing appropriate volumes of replacement fluid can control fluid balance very precisely. Continuous techniques of RRT are especially useful for patients with cerebral oedema or hypoxia. Intermittent haemodialysis is probably the treatment of choice when there is a need for emergency removal of water-soluble substances, including potassium, myoglobin and drugs.

In all of these forms of therapy a way of stopping the blood from clotting in the extracorporeal circuit is necessary. Usually, systemic heparin is used but in the patient who has suffered from abnormal bleeding prostacyclin can be utilized. In an attempt to use the anticoagulant properties of heparin but minimize the risk to the patient, some centres have coated the dialysis, or filter, membranes with heparin. This has met with variable success. It is possible to use low molecular weight heparin as a single bolus before a dialysis session rather than a continuous intravenous infusion of conventional heparin to maintain anticoagulation.

Section 12.4 • Chronic renal failure

CRF is an important condition, which is increasingly recognized and treated. Although dialysis technology has been improving over four decades, until recently many patients died without such treatment because of limited dialysis availability. However, selection criteria for RRT are now less rigorous and advanced age, diabetes and other medical problems are no longer regarded as contraindications to treatment. In addition, effective strategies for retarding and even preventing deterioration in renal function as well as mitigating complications of CRF have been developed. As a consequence, many people now enjoy good quality of life despite significant renal disease.

Definition

- CRF results from diseases of the kidney that cause progressive loss of nephrons. Unlike ARF, it is irreversible, although the rate at which function is lost is variable and dependent on a number of factors. However, a general principle is that once a significant proportion of renal tissue is scarred, progression to end-stage renal failure becomes inevitable, regardless of the underlying disease. There is no widely accepted definition of the point at which CRF becomes established, although Table 12.12 gives a guide to degrees of severity.
- It is recommended that all patients who appear to have progressive renal insufficiency and a plasma creatinine above 150 µmol/l are referred to a nephrology service for assessment and follow-up (Renal Association, 1997). However, it should be remembered that plasma creatinine is a poor measure of renal function.

Diagnosis

Biochemical measurements

Measurement of renal function is crucial in the diagnosis of renal failure, and to differentiate between ARF and CRF it is helpful to have a series of measurements over time.

- **Serum or plasma creatinine**, which varies inversely with the GFR, is the simplest and most

commonly used measurement. Creatinine is derived from muscle creatine breakdown and excreted by the kidneys. Therefore, plasma creatinine levels will reflect total muscle mass and to a lesser extent muscle protein ingestion. However, the value of this measurement is limited by a wide range of normality, and considerable renal damage (with over 50% nephron loss) can occur before the plasma creatinine exceeds the upper limit of the normal range.

- **Creatinine clearance**, calculated from plasma creatinine and measurement of 24-h urinary creatinine, improves the sensitivity, but underestimates renal function if the urine collection is incomplete.
- **Radioisotope clearance** methods of determining GFR are accurate, reproducible and safe, although time-consuming for the patient. Plasma clearance over 4 h of $[^{51}Cr]EDTA$ and $[^{99m}Tc]DTPA$ are the techniques most commonly employed. If $[^{99m}Tc]DTPA$ injection is combined with gamma imaging, useful information on relative renal function as well as overall function is obtained.

Imaging of the kidneys

In assessing the cause of renal failure, it is essential to define renal size and shape. The finding of hydronephrosis secondary to obstruction (see Section 1) or small kidneys, an indication of advanced and irreversible chronic renal disease, will determine the nature of further investigations and treatment.

- **Renal ultrasound** is the first choice in renal imaging. It is simple, non-invasive and widely available and will detect renal size, scarring, cysts and tumours. Hydronephrosis is easily recognized, but stones may be more difficult to identify. Ultrasound can be combined with pulse wave **Doppler** to detect renal blood flow, which is valuable in the serial assessment of renal transplants for acute rejection. However, Doppler study of blood flow in the main renal artery of the native kidney is more difficult to perform and is not routinely used, except in a few centres of expertise.
- **Plain radiography** of the kidneys, ureters and bladder (KUB) allows radio-opaque renal calculi and calcification of the urinary tract to be identified.
- **Intravenous urography** (IVU) is the investigation of choice for obstructing urinary tract stones or tumours, but is no longer used in the routine investigation of renal disease. Even modern low osmolality contrast agents are nephrotoxic and in the presence of significant renal failure and impaired concentrating mechanisms, the quality of image is reduced.
- **Nuclear imaging** can be employed, not only to provide a functional renal assessment ($[^{99m}Tc]DTPA$), but also to determine the relative

Table 12.12 Chronic renal failure: degrees of severity

	GFR (ml/min)
Moderate	20–40
Severe	10–19
End-stage	< 10

contribution from each kidney and to identify areas of renal scarring ([^{99m}Tc]DMSA). Delay in excretion is often evaluated by giving a diuretic with the radioisotope, and the ACE inhibitor captopril can be administered beforehand to screen for renovascular disease. However, this technique can be unreliable, particularly if renal function is reduced or arterial disease is bilateral.

- **Renal arteriography** is the usual investigation for diagnosing renovascular disease. It is recommended for patients who have been found to have unequal renal size or uneven split renal function on nuclear imaging. However, symmetrical renal size or function does not exclude bilateral renal artery stenoses and therefore renal arteriography should be considered for patients with renal impairment who, in addition, have multiple cardiovascular risk factors or vascular disease elsewhere and for patients whose hypertension becomes more difficult to control. Renal arteriography is also useful for diagnosing renal tumours, although with the advent of high-resolution contrast computed tomographic (CT) scanning, it is less frequently employed. CT and magnetic resonance imaging (MRI) are now superseding invasive angiography, at least in the preliminary assessment of renal arterial disease.

- **Computed tomographic scanning** permits detailed renal resolution and with contrast is valuable in the diagnosis of complex renal cysts and tumours. **Spiral CT** is proving valuable in the detection of renovascular disease, but is of limited use in the presence of severely atheromatous or calcified vessels, stented arteries and ostial lesions.

- **Magnetic resonance imaging** allows detailed anatomical study of renal parenchyma and vasculature and, where available, is an important diagnostic aid.

Further renal investigations

In a patient with renal dysfunction, various other investigations assist in reaching a diagnosis.

- **Urinalysis** by means of proprietary dipsticks is essential and should be supplemented by **urine culture** and **microscopy**. Haematuria can be characterized as glomerular (dysmorphic or crenated red cells) or non-glomerular (normal red cell morphology) in origin using phase-contrast microscopy. This helps to direct further investigation towards a nephrological or urological cause. Similarly, identification of white cells, crystals or casts can provide clues to the cause of renal impairment. Protein on dipstick testing often signifies underlying renal disease and should be quantified by means of a **24-h urine** collection. If tuberculosis of the urinary tract is a possibility, three early-morning urine specimens should be sent for appropriate culture.

- **Additional biochemical tests** can occasionally point to the underlying diagnosis. Hypercalcaemia associated with a raised ACE level suggests sarcoidosis, or with a monoclonal band on plasma immunoelectrophoresis, multiple myeloma. However, 20% of patients with myeloma produce only light chains and if urinary electrophoresis is not performed to identify characteristic Bence Jones proteins, the diagnosis will be missed. An elevated serum immunoglobulin A (IgA) level is sometimes found in IgA nephropathy.

- **Immunopathology** is often a guide to the presence of immunologically mediated renal disease, although is rarely sufficient to define diagnosis or prognosis. The tests that are routinely performed in patients presenting with haematuria, proteinuria or impaired renal function are shown in Table 12.13, and if positive are usually investigated further by means of renal biopsy.

- **Renal biopsy** is the best method of diagnosing renal parenchymal disease. Biopsy is performed percutaneously, ideally under ultrasound control, providing coagulation and blood pressure are normal and urine culture is negative. As there is a small but significant risk of bleeding, bed rest is recommended for at least 6 h. Rarely (1:3000 biopsies), bleeding is severe or persistent enough to require selective embolization of the vessel or even nephrectomy, and it is therefore advisable to ensure there are two functioning kidneys before biopsy is

Table 12.13 Immunopathology in renal disease

Antinuclear antibody (ANF)	Systemic lupus erythematosus
Rheumatoid factor (RF)	Rheumatoid disease, but often a feature in other immune complex mediated disease
Immune complexes (IC)	Non-specific, present in endocarditis-associated GN, cryoglobulinaemia
Antinuclear cytoplasmic antibody (ANCA)	Marker of systemic vasculitis
pANCA	Antibody to lysosomal myeloperoxidase, present in microscopic polyarteritis
cANCA	Antibody to serine proteinase 3, present in Wegener's granulomatosis
Anti-GBM antibody	Marker of Goodpasture's syndrome, in which antibody is directed against type IV collagen of the glomerular basement membrane
Complement	C3 reduced in types of GN (lupus, endocarditis, measangiocapillary)
Antistreptolysin O (ASO)	High titre suggests post-streptococcal GN

GBM, glomerular basement membrane; GN, glomerulonephritis.

undertaken. There is little point in performing biopsy of small kidneys, because the risk of complication and failure is greater and the biopsy will show only end-stage scarring (glomerulosclerosis) rather than the pathological features of the causal disease. Furthermore, by this stage there is no effective therapy for reversing renal dysfunction.

Presentation of chronic renal disease

Symptoms are often a late feature of CRF and therefore clues to the presence of renal disease are frequently detected as a coincidental finding.

- **Asymptomatic microscopic haematuria and/or proteinuria** can be detected at routine medical examinations for employment or joining a new general practice. The current Scottish recommendations (SIGN Guidelines) are that patients with **microscopic haematuria** on dipstick testing (and/or ≥ 5 red cells per high-power field on urine microscopy) on two or more occasions should be referred for further investigation. In younger patients, nephrological causes tend to predominate, while in older patients the cause is more often urological. **Persistent proteinuria** of + or more on dipstick testing should be quantified and further evaluated by clinical examination and blood analysis for urea, electrolytes, creatinine and glucose. If the proteinuria is greater than 500 mg/l (or 250 mg/l with an elevated creatinine or blood pressure) the patient should be referred to a nephrologist.
- **Asymptomatic elevation of creatinine** above 150 μmol/l that is persisting requires further follow-up by a nephrology service.
- **Pregnancy** is a time when healthy women come to medical attention, and elevation of blood pressure (particularly before the last trimester), proteinuria or raised plasma creatinine can all indicate underlying renal disease. Hypertension should be treated and the woman referred, but full renal investigation usually has to be deferred until the postpartum period.
- **Hypertension** in most of cases will be essential. However, elevation of blood pressure secondary to renal disease should be suspected if it is accompanied by proteinuria, haematuria or elevated serum creatinine. Severe hypertension associated with bilateral retinal haemorrhages, exudates and/or papilloedema (i.e. grade 3 or 4 hypertensive retinopathy) is more likely to be secondary. In vasculopathic hypertensives, the presence of renal artery disease should always also be considered.

Renal disease can also present with symptoms.

- **Macroscopic haematuria** is frequently the pointer to the presence of IgA nephritis. The history is often of intermittent haematuria, particularly during episodes of respiratory infection. The urine is sometimes reported to be 'smoky' and reduced in volume in acute nephritic syndromes (see below), owing to post-streptococcal glomerulonephritis or rapidly progressive glomerulonephritis. However, red or dark urine can also be caused by drugs (rifampicin, phenytoin), vegetable dyes (beetroot, paprika), haemoglobin, myoglobin and rare metabolic disorders (porphyria, alkaptonuria).
- **Disorders of micturition** such as frequency and dysuria often arise as a result of bladder, urethral or prostatic disease (see Urology section), rather than chronic renal disease.
- **Disorders of urine volume** tend to be renal in origin. **Nocturia** is of special importance, because it may indicate impaired concentrating capacity from advanced renal disease. Defective urinary concentration due to medullary disorders such as analgesic nephropathy and nephrocalcinosis can also present with **polyuria**. The differential diagnosis of polyuria should include cranial and renal diabetes insipidus from diminished antidiuretic hormone production or renal responsiveness, respectively.
- **Pain** in the renal angle is an unusual feature of renal disease, although it can occur in association with macroscopic or microscopic haematuria. In the absence of renal biopsy changes of glomerulonephritis or thin basement membrane disease, loin pain haematuria syndrome is recognized.
- **Oedema** is a common presenting symptom of renal disease and can be the result of hypoproteinaemia (see Nephrotic syndrome below) or salt and water retention in CRF.

There are two well-recognized modes of presentation of renal disease, the **nephrotic and nephritic syndromes.** Both are associated with many different renal diseases, so identification of the characteristic clinical picture is a guide to the need for further investigation, rather than to the underlying cause.

The nephrotic syndrome comprises:

- proteinuria > 3 g/24 h
- hypoalbuminaemia < 30 g/l
- oedema.

Patients with these problems are also at greatly increased risk of venous thrombosis and infection and are almost always hypercholesterolaemic. Nephrotic syndrome is a typical presentation of minimal change and membranous glomerulonephritis, renal amyloidosis and diabetic nephropathy. Renal biopsy is required to define the cause.

The nephritic syndrome comprises:

- haematuria, often microscopic
- proteinuria, usually < 3 g/24 h
- hypertension
- oedema
- oliguria
- impaired renal function.

This is the usual presentation of acute nephritis, including rapidly progressive glomerulonephritis, but is also seen in infective endocarditis and haemolytic uraemic syndrome. Further investigation is mandatory.

Around 30% of patients with CRF present for the first time with advanced renal disease when it is too late to treat by means other than dialysis. **Chronic renal failure** causes non-specific symptoms including fatigue, anorexia, nausea and itch. Occasionally, musculoskeletal complications, such as proximal myopathy or bone pain from renal osteodystrophy, are the presenting features. Severe uraemia can lead to pericarditis, hyperkalaemia causing cardiac dysrhythmias and/or myopathy and, in very advanced cases, neuromuscular twitching and coma (Table 12.14).

History and chronic renal disease

Obtaining a detailed history from patients with symptoms suggestive of renal disease often helps to establish whether the problem is chronic. It is useful to determine whether the patient has had urinary infection (especially in very early life) or major, but undefined childhood illness. Non-specific symptoms or early enuresis are occasionally the only reported problems in people who have suffered renal damage as a consequence of reflux nephropathy.

A history of nocturia should always be sought which, in the absence of occlusive prostatic disease, congestive cardiac failure or diuretic therapy, is a very reliable symptom of significant chronic renal impairment. In some conditions such as adult polycystic kidney disease, Alports syndrome and reflux nephropathy, there may be a family history of renal disease, but even hypertension in the family, premature unexplained death or the need for dialysis in distant relatives can be pertinent.

Recent drug ingestion from prescribed and proprietary sources is also relevant, particularly NSAIDs (oral and topical), ACE inhibitors and excessive analgesics. A past history of exposure to cis-platinum, lithium or high-dose aminoglycoside therapy can also be associated with drug-induced renal damage. The drug kardex of hospital inpatients should always be examined, as nephrotoxic agents can contribute to declining renal function in patients with background chronic renal disease.

An occupational history should be taken to rule out any chronic exposure to organic solvents, lead or cadmium, all of which have been implicated as causes of renal disease. Smokers are at increased risk of renal disease, such as renovascular disease, nephropathy if diabetic, tumours of the uroepithelium and kidney, and end-stage renal failure.

It is most helpful to know whether there has been any previous urinalysis, blood pressure or urea and electrolyte measurement, and old inpatient and outpatient notes, including obstetric records, should be consulted. The GP is often a valuable source of information.

Clinical examination and chronic renal disease

General examination can assist in the diagnosis of CRF, although many of the signs are non-specific and late. Nevertheless, a vasculitic rash will alert the clinician to the need for urgent investigation. Dry skin, excoriation due to pruritus and rarely corneal calcification are signs of advanced CRF. Oedema is an important finding when present, and if accompanied by leuconychia is highly likely to be due to hypoalbuminaemia. Accurate assessment of fluid balance by means of skin turgor, jugular venous pressure, and lying and standing blood pressure is essential.

Finding evidence of hypertensive end-organ damage such as a displaced or 'heaving' apex beat from left ventricular hypertrophy (LVH) or retinopathy often lends weight to the diagnosis of significant hypertension and supports the prescription of antihypertensive therapy. All hypertensive patients should also be examined for the presence of radiofemoral delay (aortic coarctation), peripheral pulses and abdominal bruits (renovascular disease). Palpable kidneys are a feature of adult polycystic kidney disease and occasionally hydronephrosis. Rectal and vaginal examinations should be performed if urinary tract obstruction is suspected.

Incidence and causes of chronic renal failure

The development of national and international registries of patients with end-stage renal disease has permitted accurate and comprehensive data collection, including the incidence and causes of CRF. The number of patients starting RRT in Scotland has been increasing steadily over the past 35 years (Figure 12.3).

The leading causes of end-stage renal disease in patients registered with the Scottish Renal Registry have changed, reflecting the broadening criteria for selection of patients for chronic dialysis treatment (Figure 12.4).

Diabetes has now overtaken glomerulonephritis as the most common single cause of end-stage renal disease, but in a large proportion of patients it is impossible to define the cause of CRF (unknown group), usually because of late presentation and reduced renal size. The current leading causes of end-stage renal failure in Scotland are shown in Table 12.15.

Table 12.14 Symptoms and signs of late chronic renal failure

Cardiovascular	Hypertension, left ventricular hypertrophy, dysrhythmias, pericarditis, dyslipidaemia, calcific vascular and valvular disease
Gastrointestinal	Anorexia, nausea, vomiting
Haematological	Anaemia, platelet dysfunction
Musculoskeletal	Renal osteodystrophy, muscle weakness, amyloid arthropathy (β_2 microglobulin), retarded growth and rickets in children
Neurological	Peripheral neuropathy, restless legs, myoclonic twitching, convulsions, coma
Respiratory	Kussmaul's respirations (acidosis)
Endocrine	Loss of libido, oligomenorrhoea, subfertility (women), insulin resistance
Dermatological	Itch, rash (phosphate retention)

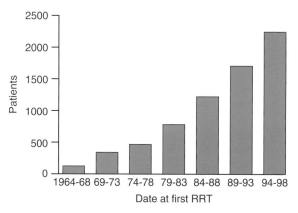

Figure 12.3 Incidence of new patients receiving renal replacement therapy in Scotland (1963–1998).

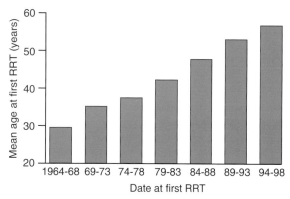

Figure 12.5 Mean age of patients at time of first renal replacement therapy session in Scotland (1963–1998).

Acceptance of older patients for dialysis in part explains the change in prevalence of the various causes of CRF (Figure 12.5) and has important implications because of greater comorbidity in an elderly dialysis population.

Treatment of chronic renal failure in the predialysis phase

Considerable effort has been directed towards slowing the rate of progression of renal disease and preventing and treating the complications of CRF.

Progression of renal disease

In many chronic kidney disorders, a relentless deterioration in renal function is seen. Previously this was thought to be due to continuing renal damage from the primary renal disease, and in some conditions such as

adult polycystic kidney disease this may be the case. However, it is now recognized that other factors (particularly proteinuria and hypertension), which are associated with the renal pathology, but not the disease itself, also play a role. Furthermore, evidence is now emerging that treatment directed at these secondary injurious factors can delay the development of end-stage renal failure.

Regardless of the primary renal disease, the pathological picture in an 'end-stage kidney' is of widespread glomerulosclerosis, vascular sclerosis and tubulointerstitial scarring. While the precise mechanisms of injury are not fully understood, a number of hypotheses has been proposed.

The study of animals subjected to five-sixths nephrectomy has shown that mere reduction in nephron number, without additional renal insult, results in progressive glomerulosclerosis and end-stage renal disease. It has been suggested that extensive renal ablation leads to hyperperfusion of, and hyperfiltration in the remaining intact glomeruli and adaptive glomerular hypertrophy. As a consequence of intraglomerular hypertension, the glomerular capillary wall is stretched

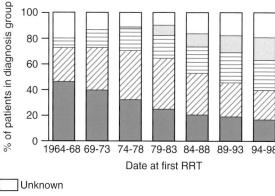

Unknown

Diabetes — *Types 1 & 2*

Multisystem — *Includes renovascular disease, Wegeners granulomatosis myeloma and others*

Interstitial — *Includes pyelonephritis drug-induced interstitial nephritis polycystic kidney disease familial nephritis*

Glomerulonephritis

Figure 12.4 Primary renal diagnoses of patients starting renal replacement therapy in Scotland (1963–1998).

Table 12.15 Causes of end-stage renal disease in Scotland

Primary renal disease	Percentage of patients
Unknown	23.5
Diabetes	16.1
Glomerulonephritis	13.1
Pyelonephritis/obstruction	12.4
Atherosclerotic renal artery disease	9.2
Polycystic kidney disease	7.5
Hypertensive renal disease	3.4
Multiple myeloma	2.4
Other causes (including vasculitis)	12.4

(From the Scottish Renal Registry, Arms Study of new patients presenting between 1.10.97 and 1.9.98, with permission.)

and endothelial and epithelial cells are damaged. Proteins and other macromolecules escape into the mesangium, while platelet aggregates and microthrombi in the glomerular capillaries compound the ischaemic injury. Progressive proteinuria and further loss of glomeruli and renal function ensue.

- **Systemic hypertension** results from loss of functioning renal tissue and exacerbates renal damage by adding to the intraglomerular pressure. Patients with hypertension at the onset of their renal disease are more likely to develop CRF, and those with poorly controlled blood pressure progress more rapidly.
- **Proteinuria** is another adverse prognostic feature in renal disease and may contribute to both the initiation and progression of glomerular damage. Although proteinuria is not entirely independent of the underlying disease process, its attenuation by dietary or pharmacological means is associated with a better outcome. This supports the view that urinary protein is toxic to renal tubular epithelium.
- **Lipids**, too, have been implicated in the pathogenesis and progression of renal disease, possibly because of toxic effects of oxidized lipoproteins on the renal tubules.
- **Genetic factors** undoubtedly play a role in determining susceptibility not only to renal disease, but also to renal scarring. For example, patients with diabetes mellitus or IgA nephropathy who carry the DD ACE gene polymorphism are more likely to progress.
- **Male gender** confers an increased risk of progression in a number of primary renal diseases.
- **Increasing age** also predisposes to more rapid progression of various renal conditions.

There are clear parallels between the pathophysiology of glomerulosclerosis and atherosclerosis and the approach to CRF is constantly evolving, with increasing attention to risk-factor management.

Therapeutic approaches to chronic renal failure

The most important method of preserving renal function in patients with chronic renal disease is to achieve good blood-pressure control.

- **Antihypertensive therapy** slows the inevitable deterioration of function in CRF, thus delaying the need for dialysis. Recently, **ACE inhibitors** have been shown to be superior to other drugs for lowering blood pressure in patients with renal diseases associated with proteinuria (they have been known to be particularly effective in diabetic nephropathy for some time). These are now the first-line agents for patients with systemic hypertension and proteinuria, providing they are used with caution and there is no contraindication such as renovascular disease (see module on ARF and ACE inhibitors). Often, it is necessary to use more than one antihypertensive drug to achieve good blood-pressure control, although there is debate

about what an optimum blood pressure is. Target blood pressures have been falling and it is reasonable to aim for 130/90 or less, providing the patient does not have symptomatic hypotension. A reduction in salt intake can also assist blood-pressure control.

- **Dietary manipulation** used to be the main treatment for patients with progressive renal disease. For many years **protein restriction** has been employed in the belief that it can improve uraemic symptoms, as well as reduce glomerular hyperfiltration and thus slow the rate of decline in renal function. However, the cost of a very low-protein diet is protein malnutrition, and hypoalbuminaemia is a major risk factor for mortality in renal failure. Current guidelines advise against a high protein intake of over 1 g/kg/day in the predialysis phase. Modulation of lipids by **hydroxymethylglutaryl-coenzyme A reductase inhibitors (statins)** may be of potential benefit, though conclusive evidence is awaited.
- **Specific therapies** for renal diseases are sometimes useful, but for the majority of renal diseases treatment is non-specific. The exceptions include systemic vasculitis and crescentic glomerulonephritis for which immunosuppression, usually in the form of steroids, cyclophosphamide and, in severe cases, plasma exchange, are used. Several immunosuppressive regimes have also been reported to be of benefit in progressive membranous nephritis. Omega-3 fish oils have been tried in IgA nephropathy with varying success.
- **Revascularization** by means of **renal angioplasty** is now recommended in patients with reasonably sized kidneys, declining renal function and bilateral renovascular disease (even if only one side is amenable to stretching), as it has been shown to delay deterioration in renal function and postpone or avert the need for dialysis. Angioplasty with stenting is more effective in ostial lesions and revascularization of occluded arteries.
- **Diabetic nephropathy** should be treated vigorously from the earliest stages of abnormal microalbuminuria by means of rigorous blood pressure control with an **ACE inhibitor** and **tight glucose regulation**. Both of these measures help to limit the progression of diabetic renal disease (see section on 'Diabetes mellitus' in Module 20).

Management of other complications of chronic renal failure

Patients with deteriorating renal function are at risk of developing a number of complications: hyperparathyroidism and renal bone disease, acidosis, hyperkalaemia, hyperuricaemia, anaemia, hyperlipidaemia and cardiovascular problems, all of which should be addressed.

Hyperparathyroidism and renal bone disease

Secondary hyperparathyroidism in renal failure is multifactorial in origin. Chronic renal disease results in impaired one-alpha hydroxylation of vitamin D_3 (25-hydroxyvitamin D_3) in the proximal renal tubule and hence inadequate levels of the active form of vitamin D_3 (1,25-dihydroxyvitamin D_3 or calcitriol). Calcitriol's normal inhibitory effects on parathyroid hormone (PTH) secretion are attenuated and the PTH concentration rises. Increased PTH levels can be detected even in mild degrees of CRF (GFR 60–80 ml/min) and have the effect of increasing osteoclast number, thereby causing bony resorption and a rise in serum calcium. Hyperparathyroidism is thus initiated, but as renal failure progresses it is sustained by different mechanisms.

In established CRF, normal vitamin D_3-dependent intestinal calcium uptake is reduced and the serum calcium level falls, which in turn stimulates PTH biosynthesis and secretion. As renal function declines, phosphate is retained and this too can stimulate parathyroid activity. Hyperphosphataemia can also potentiate hypocalcaemia through the formation of insoluble calcium-phosphate complexes.

Prolonged hyperparathyroidism leads to renal bone disease, known as osteitis fibrosis cystica. This is characterized radiologically by bone demineralization, subperiosteal resorption of the lateral clavicles and distal phalanges and bone cysts. Patients suffer bone pain, increased susceptibility to fracture and a characteristic proximal myopathy.

Another serious consequence of altered calcium and phosphate metabolism is metastatic calcification from calcium-phosphate deposition in soft tissues, viscera and, most importantly, arteries. Patients with elevated phosphate and calcium levels are at greatest risk of vascular calcification, a major contributor to the excessively high prevalence of cardiovascular disease in CRF.

All of these complications can be prevented by early dietary and therapeutic manipulation. The aims of treatment are to correct calcitriol deficiency and maintain calcium and phosphate levels within the normal ranges (Table 12.16). When irreversible hyperparathyroidism has developed, such that PTH secretion can no longer be suppressed by exogenous vitamin D, surgical parathyroidectomy is indicated.

TAAcidosis

Metabolic acidosis develops when the kidney's ability to excrete an acid load through generation of ammonium is exceeded. Tubular ammonium excretion usually becomes impaired at a GFR of around 40 ml/min, with the result that acid load is retained. Some hydrogen ions are buffered by bicarbonate, leading to a fall in plasma bicarbonate. However, much of the retained acid is buffered by alkaline salts originating from bone, with consequent bone demineralization.

Metabolic acidosis has the potential both to aggravate renal bone disease and to interfere with normal protein metabolism. It should be corrected by the administration of oral sodium bicarbonate in the predialysis phase, providing the patient does not have fluid overload or uncontrolled hypertension. Acidosis also inhibits cellular uptake of potassium and predisposes to hyperkalaemia.

Hyperkalaemia

Significant potassium retention does not usually develop in chronic renal disease until an advanced stage, because of functional adaptations within the nephron and increased losses from the gastrointestinal tract. However, administration of potassium-sparing diuretics or ACE inhibitors in renal failure can result in significant hyperkalaemia. Modification of the prescription or dietary potassium restriction may be required to restore safe potassium levels.

Hyperuricaemia

Although plasma urate rises in parallel with plasma creatinine in patients with mild to moderate CRF, symptomatic gout is unusual. Diuretic therapy, however, increases the risk and so hyperuricaemia in this context should be treated with allopurinol in a reduced dose.

Anaemia

The leading cause of anaemia in CRF is relative erythropoietin deficiency. However, it is important to exclude other reasons for anaemia such as iron, vitamin B_{12} or folate deficiency and blood loss. If no additional cause can be found and the patient has symptoms or

Table 12.16 Prevention of hyperparathyroidism and renal bone disease

Vitamin D analogues	When calcium reduced, PTH rising or alkaline phosphatase elevated, i.e. early (ensure phosphate level is normal first)
1α-Hydroxycholecalciferol	Alfacalcidol
1,25-Dihydroxycholecalciferol	Calcitriol
Diet	When phosphate > 1.7 mmol/l, reduced phosphate diet and phosphate binders employed
Phosphate binders	When phosphate rises above 1.7 mmol/l
	Administered before food, adjusting dose until phosphate < 1.7 or calcium > 2.6 mmol/l limits dose increase
Calcium carbonate	Monitor for hypercalcaemia
Calcium acetate (aluminium hydroxide)	Rarely used because of aluminium toxicity to brain and bone
Surgical parathyroidectomy	When hyperparathyroidism cannot be controlled by above measures, and hypercalcaemia and hyperphosphataemia are problematic

PTH, parathyroid hormone.

a haemoglobin of less than 10 g/dl, treatment with recombinant human erythropoietin should be considered. Usually, additional iron supplementation is necessary to meet the demands of increased erythropoiesis.

Many patients now benefit from erythropoietin therapy in the predialysis period. Although treatment can result in hypertension and an increased requirement for antihypertensive medication, initial concerns that it might accelerate the rate of deterioration in renal function have not been confirmed. Conversely, the correction of symptomatic anaemia has been shown to enhance quality of life, by improving effort capacity and physical and psychological well-being.

Lipid abnormalities

The lipid profile of patients with chronic renal disease is often abnormal, even in the absence of frank nephrotic syndrome. Proteinuria and declining renal function predispose to a more atherogenic milieu with elevated levels of cholesterol, low-density lipoprotein cholesterol, lipoprotein-*a* and triglycerides in many patients. Although concrete evidence of benefit is not yet available, use of lipid-lowering agents should be considered because of the high incidence and prevalence of vascular disease in patients approaching or receiving dialysis.

Vascular disease

Angina, myocardial infarction, stroke and peripheral vascular insufficiency all contribute to the high morbidity and mortality rates of patients with CRF. Cardiovascular complications now account for over half of all deaths of dialysis and transplanted patients. However, the increased susceptibility to such problems probably begins much earlier in the course of the renal disease. Age, male gender, glucose intolerance and hypertension are known associations, but the role of other conventional cardiovascular risk factors such as smoking and hyperlipidaemia is less certain. Vascular calcification confers additional risk in this population.

Left ventricular hypertrophy

LVH is common in chronic renal disease and by the time of RRT is almost universal. It may, in part, be due to poorly controlled hypertension, but other factors such as anaemia, fluid overload and hyperparathyroidism might also predispose to its development. As LVH has been identified as an independent determinant of survival in end-stage renal disease, strategies for preventing and reversing it are now being explored.

Preparation for dialysis and renal transplantation

Patients with chronic renal disease who have received dialysis counselling well before the time of starting RRT have a better long-term outcome than those who are referred for treatment with advanced end-stage disease. Adequate preparation not only permits creation of permanent vascular access for haemodialy-sis or timely placement of a peritoneal dialysis catheter, but also allows for better psychological adjustment. Some patients even receive a renal transplant without the need for any dialysis, if pre-emptive live donation is planned or the recipient has had a short wait on a cadaveric transplant list.

However, over one-third of patients with end-stage renal disease presents late and requires emergency haemodialysis via a temporary line. These individuals tend to have a higher incidence of complications, require longer hospital admissions at greater cost and have an increased mortality compared with patients referred earlier. Dialysis is sometimes commenced inappropriately because of insufficient background and diagnostic information (see section on 'Selection for dialysis').

Section 12.4 • Dialysis and haemofiltration

Patients with end-stage CRF (i.e. GFR less than 10 ml/min) will require RRT. The ideal in management would be renal transplantation, but a lack of donor kidneys has led to increasing reliance on long-term dialysis therapy, particularly in the elderly. In western Europe, the incidence of dialysis was approaching 120 per million of population in 1998, leading to steadily increasing numbers of patients being maintained on this relatively very expensive treatment.

Regular dialysis is successful and many patients have been treated for many years, but clearance of small solutes and water can only be a small part of the management of the uraemic syndrome and a variety of additional treatments exists for complications including anaemia, renal osteodystrophy and malnutrition. There are two generic types of dialysis: haemodialysis (HD) and peritoneal dialysis (PD).

Haemodialysis

In its basic form, haemodialysis removes solute from the patient by diffusion across a semipermeable membrane, porous in increasing proportion to molecules of less than 500 mol. wt. Blood and dialysing fluid are pumped separately on either side of the membrane, which is usually made from modified cellulose, a natural product, or synthetic alternatives, of which poly-sulfone is one of the most commonly used examples. The choice of membrane for a given patient will depend on a variety of factors, including the degree of permeability to water and solute required, the degree of biocompatibility with the formed elements of blood and the cost. The higher the permeability, the greater the ultrafiltration of water, leading to increasing technical difficulties in controlling the dialysis.

Basic haemodialysis relies on diffusion for solute clearance coupled with ultrafiltration for water removal. The degree of ultrafiltration is proportional to the transmembrane pressure, a hydraulic pressure positive on the blood side of the membrane and negative on the dialysate side. The dialysis membrane is usually configured as thousands of hollow fibres opening out on to plastic plates at either end of the dialyser contained inside a solid plastic cylinder (hollow fibre dialyser). Blood is pumped on to the top of the plates and circulates down inside the fibres, while dialysing fluid is pumped round the outside of the fibres from the bottom to the top of the dialyser. Dialysing fluid is generated from concentrates (acid and base separated to prevent precipitation of bicarbonate) diluted with ultrapure water prepared from tap water by filtration and deionization. The blood and dialysate pumps, together with the dialysate generation system and various alarms (e.g. monitoring blood and dialysate pressures and temperatures, sodium concentration and an air detector), constitutes the kidney machine, which is now a compact structure. A dialysis circuit is illustrated in Figure 12.6 and the formula of a typical dialysis fluid is shown in Table 12.17. A small amount of glucose can be added to the dialysate to prevent hypoglycaemia and

many patients utilize higher dialysate sodium concentrations in the first half of a dialysis treatment to facilitate water removal without hypotension, and a lower concentration in the second half, which reduces serum hyperosmolality after dialysis, lessening thirst and resultant rapid weight gain.

Haemofiltration

Haemofiltration uses a highly permeable (usually synthetic) membrane and negative pressure in the dialysate compartment of the dialyser without dialysate flowing. In this way, up to 80 litres of fluid are removed from the patient in a 4-h session. Solute removal occurs by 'convection', or passive flow of solute with water. The desired proportion of the filtrate is replaced by infusion before or after the dialyser, either from previously prepared sterile bags of replacement fluid (expensive) or by using newly generated dialysis fluid as replacement. The quality of this fluid must be carefully monitored (see Figure 12.6 for circuit).

Compared with diffusion, convection allows greater removal of solutes in the 'middle molecular' range (110–500 mol. wt) but is less efficient at the smaller weight end of the spectrum, which contains most of the life-threatening compounds.

Haemodiafiltration

The benefits of diffusion and convection can be combined where a dialysis circuit similar in every way to that used for haemofiltration is employed (Figure 12.6) but with dialysis fluid being pumped round the dialysate circuit. The intravenous replacement fluid is produced in the same way as for haemofiltration. Using this technology, very high-efficiency dialysis can be performed.

Choice of technique

Techniques that employ convection tend to result in smoother fluid removal and increased haemodynamic stability. Thus haemofiltration and haemodiafiltration are of great value in unstable patients with ARF and in the elderly with cardiac failure and severe arteriosclerosis. In ARF, haemofiltration can be performed slowly and continuously over many hours with the ability to set hourly fluid removal and replacement rates. Extra space can be created for feeding and intravenous drugs. In haemofiltration using prebagged sterile replacement fluid, the buffer is often lactate (rather than bicarbonate) because of its stability in solution, which may lead to complications in severely ill acute patients with lactic acidosis.

High-volume haemofiltration and haemodiafiltration lead to high-efficiency dialysis with superior middle molecule clearances, but although many toxic effects have been attributed to these molecules, the additional benefits of this type of treatment over conventional haemodialysis have yet to be proven conclusively. The synthetic membranes and replacement fluids employed are inherently too expensive for most physicians to justify their use other than in the special cases mentioned above.

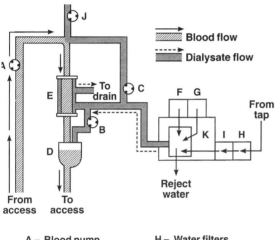

A – Blood pump
B&C – Online dialysate/ filtration fluid pumps
D – Air trap
E – Dialyser
F&G – Acidic, basic concentrates

H – Water filters
I – Reverse osmosis
J – Pre-prepared haemofiltration fluid pump
K – Dialysate/water proportional unit

Figure 12.6 Dialysis circuit.

Table 12.17 Typical composition of haemodialysis fluid

Solute	Concentration (mmol/l)
Na	140
K	0–2[a]
Ca	1.25–1.75[a]
HCO$_3$	35
Mg	0.5
Glucose	0–5[a]

[a]Varying practice, depending on local factors.

Adequacy of treatment

Most patients on haemodialysis have traditionally received approximately 12 h/week divided into three equal doses. Assessing adequacy of dialysis can be difficult using serum urea or creatinine or by clinical assessment alone. A relationship exists between total urea removal during dialysis (the product of the clearance of the dialyser, K, in ml/min and the treatment time, t) and long-term outcome of treatment. Kt is usually expressed as a ratio of the total body water volume, V, and the Kt/V for a dialysis session should normally exceed 1.2 including a component to reflect any residual renal function. A given Kt/V can be achieved in less than the traditional 4 h if blood and dialysate flows are optimized and a dialyser with adequate clearance characteristics is used. To remove adequate quantities of middle molecules and achieve smooth ultrafiltration, a higher flux membrane is used. Although this practice of prescribing a dialysis dose has strong advocates, current majority opinion is that there will ultimately be more cardiovascular complications because of the stress of rapid fluid removal.

Vascular access

Successful haemodialysis requires a blood flow of at least 250 ml/min through the dialyser and many dialysis prescriptions assume a blood flow of 400 ml/min. In acute situations, the required blood flow can be obtained from a central venous catheter, ideally placed in the superior vena cava through the right internal jugular vein. Access can also be obtained via the subclavian veins but there is an unacceptable incidence of later stenosis. The femoral veins, although also frequently used, can make it difficult to mobilize the patient and femoral lines have a high risk of becoming contaminated. Many catheters are dual lumen, allowing a single pump to circulate blood round the dialysis circuit, but single-lumen catheters can also be used with one or two pumps and appropriate capacitance chambers to allow maintenance of flow. A successful central venous catheter, if aseptically placed and adequately cared for, can last for many weeks. Complications include infection (septicaemia) and clotting of the lumen. Subcutaneous tunnelled subclavian or jugular lines can provide permanent access.

For chronic haemodialysis, some form of arteriovenous fistula is created, leading to the development of arterialized veins, which will allow the insertion of large-bore needles for access to the circulation. Brachiocephalic or radiocephalic anastomoses are most commonly used and take 6 weeks to develop enough to allow cannulation (Figure 12.7). As an alternative to the fistula, a length of vein (usually saphenous) or synthetic graft can be looped subcutaneously from artery to vein, allowing enough length for cannulation. The forearm and thigh are common sites. Vein or synthetic loops are usually reserved for situations where fistula creation is deemed difficult or has failed.

Complications of fistulae and loops include primary non-function related to early thrombosis and inade-

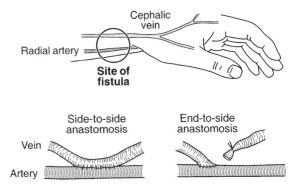

Figure 12.7 Dialysis arteriovenous fistula.

quate achieved flow. Especially in elderly patients, cardiac failure can be precipitated if the blood flow through the arteriovenous shunt is too great.

Peritoneal dialysis

The visceral and parietal peritoneum can act as a semipermeable membrane with characteristics not unlike those of a high-flux haemodialysis membrane. The potential space between the visceral and parietal membranes will accommodate up to 3 litres of dialysis fluid introduced via an implanted silicone rubber tube tunnelled subcutaneously in its extraperitoneal portion and held in place by two woolly Dacron cuffs. One of these cuffs is situated just outside the peritoneal cavity and the other a few millimetres from the cutaneous exit site (Figure 12.8). The straight peritoneal catheter described above is the most widely used, but many variants exist. In some designs, the intraperitoneal portion is coiled to lessen adhesions and in others the extraperitoneal section is U-shaped or swan-necked to ensure that the exit site points laterally or downwards to prevent accumulation of secretions with the attendant risk of infection. Peritoneal catheters can be inserted in theatre by means of a surgical operation, but can also be placed aseptically under local anaesthetic by the physician in the ward. Exact positioning of the catheter is essential: the cutaneous exit site should point downwards, and should be punched out to exactly the correct diameter to allow healing without exudation or the development of granulation tissue, both of which can predispose to exit site infection. This, in turn, can result in subcutaneous tunnel infection and peritonitis requiring catheter removal.

The peritoneal membrane is a complex structure consisting of mesothelial cells on interstitial tissue in which is embedded a rich capillary network. The physiology of peritoneal function is complex, but mathematically, the multilayered structure behaves in a similar manner to a synthetic membrane. Peritoneal lymphatics also play an independent role. Long-term peritoneal dialysis disorganizes the structure of the peritoneum and shrinks the mesothelial cells. After an episode of peritonitis, the mesothelial lining layer is completely denuded and can take many weeks to recover. The dial-

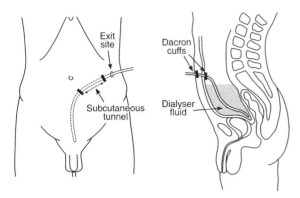

Figure 12.8 Peritoneal access.

ysis fluid used in peritoneal dialysis is similar to that used in haemodialysis, the main difference being that ultrafiltration is achieved osmotically. The fluid is rendered hyperosmolar compared to plasma with the addition of glucose in three concentrations: 1.36%, 2.27% and 3.86%. The very hyperosmolar 3.86% solution can be expected to remove considerable amounts of water. Although widely used, glucose is not the ideal osmotic agent as it is an irritant and will cause glycosylation of various proteins in the long term. Substantial quantities are also absorbed systemically. Many attempts have been made to find a suitable non-toxic, non-absorbable, cheap alternative, but so far only glycerol and amino acid solutions have been studied, with no particular advantages, although the latter may have nutritional benefit in some patients.

Experience is growing with a seven-unit polymeric glucose solution, which is not absorbed and has few of the side-effects of glucose. Although promising as an osmotic agent equivalent to 2.27% glucose, it is metabolized in part to maltose, a glucose dimer that accumulates unchanged in humans, and at best can only be used as part of a daily prescription to allow 'ordinary' glucose dialysis fluid to remove the accumulated maltose. The buffer in most peritoneal dialysis fluid is lactate, although increasing use is being made of the more physiological bicarbonate as methods have been devised to mix the buffer with the rest of the dialysis fluid just prior to use to prevent precipitation of calcium.

Various forms of peritoneal dialysis exist, as follows.

Continuous ambulatory peritoneal dialysis

In continuous ambulatory peritoneal dialysis (CAPD), 1–3 litres of peritoneal dialysis solution are instilled into the peritoneal cavity and allowed to dwell for around 6 h, by which time the fluid will have fully equilibrated with small solutes in plasma and enough glucose should remain to allow net ultrafiltration. The spent dialysate is drained by the patient and replaced using an aseptic technique. Equipment has been designed to facilitate this process and resist the ingress of infection. The most widely used is a Y-system, where a full 2-litre bag of new dialysis fluid and an empty bag

are joined in a Y-shape. The stem of the 'Y' is connected to the peritoneal catheter extension set and the patient drains into the empty bag, flushes a small amount of new fluid into the drain bag to clear the tubing and then drains the new fluid into the peritoneum. The whole Y-system is then disconnected and discarded. This entire cycle takes about 20 min and is ideally suited to home use, but quite compatible with travelling.

Automated peritoneal dialysis

Automated peritoneal dialysis (APD) is used as an alternative to CAPD for convenience, where the patient is unable to perform bag changes or to allow dialysis during periods of sleep. There are several types.

- **Continuous cyclic peritoneal dialysis (CCPD):** an automated cycler performs several exchanges of dialysate during the night and there is a long daytime dwell. This is essentially the reverse of CAPD.
- **Intermittent peritoneal dialysis (IPD)** consists of periods of automated bag changing lasting for 12 h or more (not usually more than 24 h) with a dry peritoneum between dialysis sessions.
- **Nightly intermittent peritoneal dialysis (NIPD)** consists of a number of overnight cycles with a dry day. Because of the short dialysis time, it is relatively inefficient.
- **Tidal peritoneal dialysis (TPD):** a reservoir of several hundred millilitres of dialysate is left in the abdominal cavity and a tidal volume of up to 1 litre is cycled frequently in and out over and above this. By removing the requirement for complete drainage, the cycles are completed quickly, but large volumes of dialysate are required, making the procedure unacceptably expensive in all but a few cases.

Adequacy of peritoneal dialysis

Peritoneal dialysis has lower small solute clearances than haemodialysis and relies on its long duration to achieve adequate dialysis. The technique is most successful in lighter (less than 80 kg) patients and where there is a small but significant level of residual renal function to augment it. The permeability of the peritoneum can be assessed by measuring dialysate:plasma ratios of solutes including creatinine and glucose at regular intervals during a timed cycle. In a high-permeability peritoneum, because of the rapid absorption of glucose, more hypertonic cycles may be required and the efficiency of dialysis can be improved by cycling greater volumes of dialysate, perhaps using APD. In a low-permeability peritoneum, longer dwell times are required, but good ultrafiltration is easier to achieve.

As with haemodialysis, Kt/V can be calculated as a measure of adequacy, and figures in excess of 2.0 should be aimed for. Creatinine clearance is also useful and values in excess of 60 litres per week are required for long-term success. Protein losses in dialysate can be considerable and the technique is associated with greater morbidity and mortality if the serum albumin decreases to less than three-quarters of normal and cannot be corrected by increased dietary intake.

The choice of type of peritoneal dialysis will depend on the preference of the patient and physician and the availability of equipment. In most patients in the normal permeability range, prescriptions can be generated for any type, but at either end of the spectrum, choice will be limited, and in the low-permeability peritoneum with no residual renal function, haemodialysis may be the only option compatible with long-term survival.

Complications of dialysis

Many of the complications of uraemia are not or only partially corrected by dialysis. These are discussed generically and the differing impacts of PD and HD considered under these headings.

Anaemia

The anaemia of CRF is improved by both types of dialysis, especially PD, the mechanism being removal of toxins that suppress blood production or accelerate peripheral red cell destruction. In HD, where there is greater blood loss than in PD, the anaemia can be more marked. The major factor contributing to anaemia is erythropoietin deficiency, and recombinant human erythropoietin is widely used in three-quarters of all dialysis patients. It is administered subcutaneously twice or three times weekly and the target haemoglobin should be 10–11 g/dl, enough to improve quality of life and cardiac function without thrombotic or hypertensive complications. It is essential to ensure adequate iron stores and functional or absolute iron deficiency should be prevented by aggressive supplementation intravenously in haemodialysis and orally or intravenously in peritoneal dialysis.

Renal osteodystrophy

Dialysis does little to improve renal osteodystrophy. Phosphate is poorly removed and accumulates, requiring the continued use of oral phosphate binders, most commonly calcium carbonate. Low ionized calcium and elevated serum parathormone can be corrected by oral or intravenous vitamin D analogues. In a small proportion of poorly dialysed patients or in patients non-compliant with phosphate binders, secondary or tertiary hyperparathyroidism will develop and subtotal parathyroidectomy will be required. Certain haemodialysis membranes such as Hemophan have intrinsically greater phosphate clearances, although not good enough to dispense with the requirement for phosphate binders.

Fluid balance

Assessment of dry or ideal weight in dialysis patients can be very difficult. If the water removal required during dialysis is underestimated, chronic fluid overload can result, causing pulmonary oedema and heart fail-

ure. Overestimation leads to hypotension and cramps, especially in haemodialysis. The dry weight is set by a combination of clinical assessment of fluid balance, blood pressure and cardiac status, and on-line monitoring of haematocrit during dialysis can be used to verify the prediction. Haemodiafiltration and/or dialysate sodium variation(see above) leads to a smoother removal of fluid from intracellular and interstitial compartments than standard haemodialysis.

Cardiovascular complications

Hypertension, hypercholesterolaemia, atherosclerosis and arteriosclerosis are all part of the uraemic syndrome and lead to a higher incidence of myocardial infarction, left ventricular hypertrophy, cardiac failure and cerebrovascular accidents. Although a variety of measures, including obsessive control of blood pressure (with drugs and achievement of an adequate dry weight), fluid balance, cholesterol and hyperparathyroidism can reduce the severity of cardiovascular complications, dialysis patients have a reduced life expectancy.

Haemodiafiltration techniques involving prescription of shorter treatment times may ultimately be counterproductive because of the extra cardiovascular stresses involved in the rapid removal of large quantities of fluid, especially in patients unable to adhere to fluid restrictions.

Nutrition

Malnutrition is a risk in both haemodialysis and peritoneal dialysis patients. It is important to ensure adequate dialysis as described previously, together with prevention of excessive acidosis. Urea generation and protein catabolic rates can be calculated and the effect of dialysis and diet assessed. In peritoneal dialysis, there is often excessive protein loss in the dialysate and chronic hypoalbuminaemia has been associated with a poor prognosis. A protein intake of 1–1.5 g/kg is aimed for in peritoneal dialysis and over 30% of the patients will require energy supplements. In haemodialysis, because of its intermittent nature, potassium and excessive fluid accumulation can occur and must be prevented, making the diet more restrictive. A dietary protein intake of 1–1.2 g/kg is the target in haemodialysis and a significant proportion of patients require energy supplements. Regular dietary and anthropometric assessment are vital in both types of dialysis patient.

Infection

The immune system is globally suppressed in uraemia and dialysis does not fully correct this. Dialysis patients often handle infection poorly and take longer to recover than normal individuals. Increased catabolism during infection necessitates increased dialysis requirements and the response to recombinant erythropoietin is blunted. It may take weeks for the serum albumin to recover. Two special cases are worthy of mention: central line infection and peritonitis in PD.

- **Central venous access infection.** At any one time, up to 20% of the haemodialysis population are dialysed through central lines, usually until permanent access is available or as temporary access in ARF. Gram-positive infections are not uncommon, and both septicaemia and exit site infection should be treated vigorously with parenteral antibiotics and removal of the line. Prophylactic measures are vital and should include insertion of lines using full aseptic technique and rigorous policies for care of exit sites and opening lines for connection to the dialysis machine.

- **Peritonitis in peritoneal dialysis.** Modern fluid delivery systems and connectors have been designed to resist entry of bacteria during bag changing and the incidence of peritonitis is consequently dropping. When it occurs, peritonitis can range in severity from vague abdominal pain to life-threatening septicaemia. The source of infection can be transluminal from the bowel, often in the presence of diverticular disease, but the most common source is during bag changing or from the catheter exit site, along the subcutaneous tunnel. Diagnosis is symptomatic and by examination of dialysis fluid after a 6-h dwell, when the white cell count is greater than 100×10^6/l. Organisms are seen in around 50% of cases and are subsequently cultured in more than 80%. Treatment should continue for around 10 days with intraperitoneal antibiotics.

Recurrent Gram-positive infections with *Staphylococcus epidermidis* may indicate the formation of biofilm on the silicone rubber of the peritoneal catheter and will necessitate changing the catheter. If serious Gram-negative infection occurs in the presence of bowel pathology, peritoneal dialysis will have to be discontinued permanently.

Coagulation system

Uraemic patients have a number of mild clotting abnormalities, especially abnormal platelet function due to uraemic toxins. In peritoneal dialysis, fibrinogen in the dialysate may coagulate on drainage and cause flow problems. It can be prevented in susceptible patients by the use of intraperitoneal heparin injected into the dialysate prior to infusion. Haemoperitoneum is not uncommon in female patients due to ovulation or menstrual retroflow, and may also occur in both genders after prolonged vomiting or coughing.

In haemodialysis, anticoagulation is required to prevent clotting of blood in the dialyser or the tubing. Heparin is the most commonly used because it is cheap and easily monitored, but bleeding complications are not uncommon and clotting times must be regularly checked. Heparinoids and prostacyclin are alternatives but are expensive and used only where problems have been encountered with heparin. Aspirin and warfarin have been used to prevent clotting of arteriovenous fistulae or synthetic grafts.

Selection of patients for dialysis and choice of modality

Although dialysis treatment is now widely available, effective and safe, it is expensive and there has been a tendency to undertreat certain patient groups, including the elderly and patients with concomitant other severe pathologies such as diabetes mellitus, malignancy or cardiovascular disease. The decision to treat must be individual, but there are no absolute contraindications to starting dialysis.

The choice of technique depends on a variety of factors including availability. The only major contraindications to peritoneal dialysis are pre-existing abdominal problems such as colostomies or adhesions after abdominal surgery. Severe chest disease, obesity or social problems may also practically limit its use. It may also be difficult to maintain adequate clearances in overweight patients with no intrinsic renal function.

Contraindications to the use of haemodialysis include inability to establish adequate vascular access and to maintain cardiovascular stability during the dialysis process. In some centres where there are no isolation facilities, human immunodeficiency virus and hepatitis (B or C) infection or carriage would be indications for choosing peritoneal dialysis (see Tables 12.18 and 12.19). Figure 12.9 illustrates the rapid growth of dialysis and shows that, in Scotland, around 60% of patients are maintained on HD. The percentage is higher in Europe and the USA.

Starting dialysis treatment

The timing of initiating regular dialysis treatment depends on a number of factors, including availability of facilities. In general, treatment should be started when GFR falls below 10 ml/min, although evidence is accumulating that an earlier start may preserve endogenous renal function for longer and is associated

Table 12.18 Advantages and disadvantages of haemodialysis

Advantages	Disadvantages
Efficient and controllable	Expensive
No treatment between dialysis sessions	More restricted diet and fluid intake than peritoneal dialysis
	Hypertension and fluid overload must be controlled

Table 12.19 Advantages and disadvantages of peritoneal dialysis

Advantages	Disadvantages
Home based	Requires some endogenous renal function
Free fluid intake	Peritonitis
Relatively unrestricted diet	Body image
Cheaper than haemodialysis	Nutritional problems where high protein and calorie intake impossible

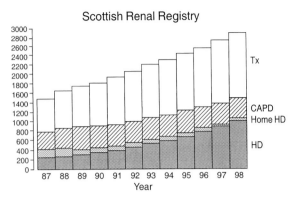

Figure 12.9 Increasing dialysis population. (From the Scottish Renal Registry, with permission.)

with a better long-term outcome. The threshold for a given patient to become symptomatic is variable and treatment should start before this point. It may become difficult to control fluid overload, espe-cially in patients with a degree of heart failure, and dialysis may have to be started in the presence of an otherwise acceptable GFR. It is not tenable to make a decision to start dialysis based on serum creatinine level alone.

Guide to further reading

Blandy, J. and Fowler, C., eds (1996). *Urology*, 2nd edn, Blackwell Science, Oxford.

Emberton, M. and Anson, K. (1999). Acute retention in men: an age old problem. *BMJ* **318**: 921–924.

Investigation of Asymptomatic Microscopic Haematuria in Adults (1997). Sign Publication 17, Scottish Intercollegiate Guidelines Network (SIGN).

Investigation of Asymptomatic Proteinuria in Adults (1997). Sign Publication 18, Scottish Intercollegiate Guidelines Network (SIGN).

Renal Association (1997). *Treatment of Adult Patients with Renal Failure. Recommended Standards and Audit Measures*, 2nd edn, Royal College of Physicians of London.

Patients with pulmonary insufficiency

1 • Normal respiration (ventilation)

2 • Respiratory failure

3 • Chronic lung disease and respiratory insufficiency

4 • Aspiration syndromes, pneumonias and lung abscesses

5 • Acute disorders of the pleura

'Illness is in part what the world has done to a victim, but in a large part it is what the victim has done with his world, and with himself' – Karl Menninger

Section 13.1 • Normal respiration (ventilation)

Normal respiration results in the exchange of oxygen (O_2) and carbon dioxide (CO_2) within the lungs. It has four components:

▪ transport of O_2 and CO_2 by the circulation
▪ gas exchange across the alveolar–capillary membrane
▪ mechanics of breathing required to produce an effective inspiration and expiration
▪ nervous and chemical control of the respiratory centre (drive).

Transport of O_2 and CO_2

At both alveolar and tissue levels, the exchange of O_2 and CO_2 within the blood occurs by simple diffusion and is dependent on adequate concentration gradients. As 98% of the oxygen is carried as oxyhaemoglobin, it is the amount of haemoglobin (Hb) that determines the capacity of the blood to carry oxygen, and this is reduced in severe anaemia. In contrast, the degree of saturation is independent of the Hb concentration, being determined by the oxygen tension gradients in the lungs and the tissues. Thus 15 g of Hb with a saturation of 97% will carry 20 vol. percent while 7.5 g of Hb with the same saturation will carry only 10 vol. percent.

The relationship between the oxygen tension and Hb saturation is defined by the oxygen dissociation curve (Figure 13.1). The sigmoid nature of this curve is a crucial factor in the smooth exchange of oxygen within the lungs and tissues. At rest the arterial (97%) to venous (75%) saturation difference is around 25% but this hides a 60% change in oxygen tensions, i.e. 13 kPa (98 mmHg) arterial to 5.3 kPa (40 mmHg)

venous. Thus the oxygen tensions of about 5.3 kPa in tissues, 13 kPa in the arterial blood, 5.3 kPa in the pulmonary venous blood and 13.3 kPa (100 mmHg) in the alveolar gas result in a pressure gradient of 8 kPa (60 mmHg) at both sites to ensure oxygenation.

On exercise there is an increase in the concentration of both hydrogen ions and CO_2 and a rise in temperature within the tissues, each of which shifts the oxygen dissociation curve to the right, leading to release of more oxygen in the tissues for a given oxygen tension. As more oxygen is utilized, the tissue oxygen tension falls, increasing the blood to tissue oxygen gradient, thereby facilitating oxygen transfer. The resulting lower oxygen saturation and tension in the venous blood increase the oxygen gradient at alveolar level, enhancing pulmonary oxygenation of the venous blood.

By contrast, the oxygen dissociation curve is shifted to the left when there is a fall in hydrogen ion concentration, a drop in the CO_2 tension or in body temperature making it more difficult for oxygen to be released from the blood to the tissues. The shift to the left of the oxygen dissociation curve is also encountered following exposure to carbon monoxide and in the presence of abnormal haemoglobins.

The greater solubility of CO_2 means that a 6 mm difference between arterial (5.3 kPa, 40 mmHg) and venous (6 kPa, 46 mmHg) is sufficient to permit adequate uptake from the tissues and elimination in the lungs. In the tissues, CO_2 rapidly enters the red cells, where some combines with haemoglobin to form carbamino-haemoglobin and the rest forms carbonic acid under the influence of carbonic anhydrase. Although carbamino-haemoglobin accounts for only 6–7% of the total CO_2 content of venous blood, it carries 20–30% of the CO_2 delivered to the alveolar gas. Within the red blood cells (RBCs), the carbonic acid dissociates into hydrogen ion that is taken by the

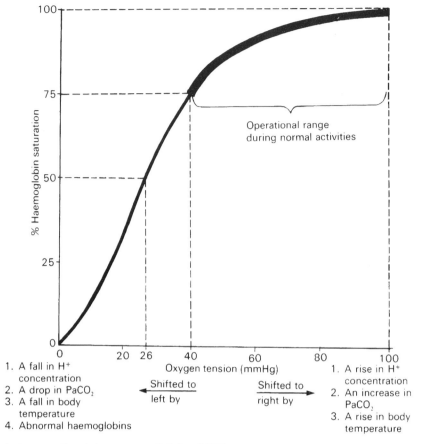

1. A fall in H⁺ concentration
2. A drop in PaCO₂
3. A fall in body temperature
4. Abnormal haemoglobins

Shifted to left by ←

Shifted to right by →

1. A rise in H⁺ concentration
2. An increase in PaCO₂
3. A rise in body temperature

Figure 13.1 Standard oxygen dissociation curve at pH 7.4 and 37°C.

reduced haemoglobin and bicarbonate, which diffuses back into the plasma. The lower alveolar gas tension favours the release of CO_2. This essentially occurs through a reversal of the chemical processes described above.

Gas exchange

The features of alveolar gas exchange under resting conditions are shown in Figure 13.2. During quiet breathing each red cell takes approximately 0.75 s to pass through the pulmonary capillaries (transit time), during which time gas exchange is completed. Ideally, each alveolus should receive its appropriate share of the inspired air and pulmonary circulation, the respiratory rate being adjusted to keep the alveolar tensions of O_2 at 13.3 kPa and CO_2 at 5.3 kPa. Factors that depress the respiratory centre (anaesthetic agents, hypnotics, analgesics) or impair the respiratory movement (severe kyphoscoliosis, morbid obesity, poliomyelitis, myasthenia gravis) may reduce overall alveolar ventilation to such a degree that the alveolar tension of CO_2 rises and that of oxygen falls, leading to hypercarbia and hypoxia.

Even in healthy subjects there is a degree of mismatch of ventilation and perfusion, some alveoli being well ventilated but poorly perfused and vice versa. In the erect posture, the ratio of ventilation to perfusion varies from the apex to the basal segments of the lungs.

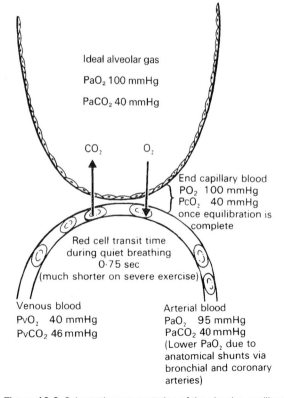

Ideal alveolar gas
PaO₂ 100 mmHg
PaCO₂ 40 mmHg

CO₂   O₂

End capillary blood
PO₂ 100 mmHg
PcO₂ 40 mmHg
once equilibration is complete

Red cell transit time during quiet breathing
0.75 sec
(much shorter on severe exercise)

Venous blood
PvO₂ 40 mmHg
PvCO₂ 46 mmHg

Arterial blood
PaO₂ 95 mmHg
PaCO₂ 40 mmHg
(Lower PaO₂ due to anatomical shunts via bronchial and coronary arteries)

Figure 13.2 Schematic representation of the alveolar–capillary gas exchange.

A change of posture, e.g. supine, alters the pattern of ventilation and perfusion in the lungs due in part to the redistribution of blood flow to the dependent areas. This mismatch of ventilation and perfusion becomes more evident in disease and is a major factor underlying functional abnormalities encountered in chronic bronchitis and emphysema.

The movement of air from mouth to alveolus is made up of two components:

- *transport* involving flow of air through the bronchial tree as far as the alveolar ducts and
- *gas mixing*, by which gas diffuses into the alveoli from the alveolar ducts.

Maldistribution of the inspired air may result from disorders of either component. Bronchial obstruction by mucosal oedema, muscle spasm, secretion or fibrosis as occurs in chronic bronchitis, may impede air flow to some areas, while marked dilatation of the air spaces as seen in emphysema will interfere with gas mixing. Perfusion of poorly ventilated areas in chronic bronchitis and emphysema increases the degree of venous shunting leading to a fall in the oxygen tension. However, the inevitable slight rise in CO_2 tension results in sufficient hyperventilation to reduce the arterial CO_2 to normal levels. In the presence of severe ventilation perfusion imbalance encountered during an acute exacerbation of chronic bronchitis, this mechanism fails and an elevated arterial CO_2 accompanies the hypoxia.

Embolism or thrombosis of the pulmonary arteries is associated with well-ventilated but poorly perfused alveoli but unless the area involved is large (massive pulmonary embolism), this has little effect on the blood gases.

The arterial oxygen tension is a little lower than that at the end of the pulmonary capillaries due to the drainage of blood from the coronary and bronchial systems directly into the left atrium, usually accounting for about 6% of the cardiac output. This percentage is increased:

- in the presence of a right to left anatomical shunt due to congenital heart disease
- by the passage of blood through non-ventilated pulmonary parenchyma, e.g. lobar pneumonia or pulmonary collapse (physiological shunt).

Both mechanisms cause hypoxia but have little effect on the CO_2 tension.

Given the normal oxygen tension gradient between alveolar air and capillary blood, equilibrium occurs across the membrane even if the transit time is considerably reduced, as in severe exercise. Thickening of the membrane by alveolar fluids, oedema or proliferation of alveolar cells as may occur in left ventricular failure, fibrosing alveolitis, sarcoidosis or paraquat poisoning impairs the transport of oxygen resulting in hypoxia, initially with exercise, but subsequently at rest. Hyperventilation and the more rapid diffusion of CO_2 ensure normal or reduced arterial tension of this gas.

Mechanics of breathing

During quiet breathing, only inspiration is associated with active muscular contraction, expiration being the result of the elastic recoil of the lungs and chest wall. The main respiratory muscles are the diaphragm and the intercostal muscles, which are augmented during forced inspiration or forced expiration by the accessory muscles of respiration. These include the neck, shoulder girdle and abdominal muscles. The descent of the diaphragm in quiet breathing by 1.5 cm (increasing to 10 cm on deep inspiration) increases the longitudinal thoracic diameter, which accounts for most of quiet inspiration. This action is impaired in severe emphysema, where movement of the low, flat diaphragm is limited, and indeed, traction by a flat diaphragm may result in indrawing of the lower costal margin during inspiration, which may further embarrass ventilation. Patients who have paralysed intercostal muscles, e.g. following poliomyelitis, depend on diaphragmatic respiration, in which case an acute abdomen or abdominal surgery is associated with severe respiratory difficulties.

During inspiration, the intercostal muscles rotate the ribs upwards and outwards along the axis through the sternal and vertebral connections, increasing the anteroposterior and transverse diameters of the thoracic cavity, and raising the manubrium by up to 5 cm. At the same time, there is a dynamic lengthening of the thoracic vertebral column. When ankylosing spondylitis involves the joints of the thorax or kyphoscoliosis alters the shape of the rib cage, this expansion of the chest cavity is considerably restricted with impairment of lung function.

During forced inspiration the upper ribs are stabilized by the action of the accessory muscles of the neck, while in forced expiration the lower ribs are fixed through contraction of the rectus muscles, making the movement of the other ribs more efficient.

The energy expended in moving air within the respiratory tract depends on the combined resistance of the abdominal contents and the elastic and viscous forces of the chest wall and lungs. Elastic recoil causes the lungs to collapse and the chest wall to expand when a hemithorax is opened at thoracotomy. These two opposing forces are most nearly balanced at the end of quiet expiration.

The distensibility or compliance of the chest wall and lungs refers to the force required to produce a given change in their volume, the relationship for both being linear over the range of ventilation (normally 0.2l/1.5l kPa for each). The lower the compliance the greater the force required. Therefore, factors that reduce the compliance of either the chest wall (obesity, thoracoplasty or kyphoscoliosis) or of the lung (pneumonia, pulmonary collapse, oedema, fibrosis, pulmonary resection and some anaesthetic agents) will increase the work of breathing.

Air flow within the bronchial tree is independent of the compliance, being proportional to the pressure gradient between the alveoli and the atmosphere and the total cross-sectional area of the bronchial tree at any given level. Any narrowing of the respiratory tract, e.g. laryngeal spasm, secretions, bronchospasm, fibrosis, mucosal oedema or tumour, will impede air flow and increase the work of breathing. During quiet breathing 90% of air flow is laminar; however the flow becomes progressively more turbulent the faster the rate of respiration, thereby greatly enhancing the effort required.

Nervous and chemical control of respiration
Breathing is controlled by the respiratory centre (RC), a loosely knit collection of neurones within the reticular formation of the medulla oblongata, which is influenced by several reflex and chemical mechanisms. The depression of brain stem activity by hypnotics, anaesthetic agents, sleep or vascular disorders reduces ventilation. During quiet breathing, the inspiratory component of the RC initiates respiration. Vagal afferent impulses (Hering–Breuer reflex) from the distending lung reach the expiratory component of the RC, which then inhibits further inspiration. This mechanism has been documented in animals but has yet to be confirmed in man.

Activation of the lung receptors following a pneumothorax reflexly stimulates the inspiratory centre, leading to a tachypnoea. Distension of the pulmonary vascular bed, e.g. left ventricular failure or multiple small pulmonary emboli, induces rapid shallow breathing through similar vagally mediated reflexes. Impulses arising from (i) the higher cerebral centres during speaking, crying or laughing; (ii) hypothalamic temperature control centre during pyrexia and (iii) local sensory endings during swallowing, coughing or sneezing, all act on the RC to modify ventilation. Increased ventilation during exercise is initiated by afferent impulses arising in the muscles and joints involved.

In the normal subject, the CO_2 and O_2 tensions and the hydrogen ion concentration of arterial blood are kept within narrow limits through constant monitoring by central and peripheral chemosensitive systems that reflexly act on the RC modifying ventilation. The major sites for chemical regulation are the chemosensitive areas on the anterolateral surfaces of the medulla oblongata that respond to changes in the hydrogen ion concentration within the CSF. Changes in CO_2 tension may act directly on the chemoreceptors, as well as by altering the hydrogen ion concentration within the CSF. An increase in the hydrogen ion concentration or a rise in the arterial PCO_2 above 5.3 kPa both stimulate the RC, increasing the respiratory rate. At altitude, hypoxia stimulates respiration and with acclimatization the RC becomes adjusted to a lower trigger threshold for CO_2 tension.

The peripheral chemoreceptors of the carotid and aortic bodies account for about 20% of the respiratory drive. These areas respond to changes in arterial oxygen tension, although in normal subjects a fall in the inspired oxygen concentration to below 16% (atmospheric 20.89%) is required before there is any significant increase in ventilation. While responding to variations in the hydrogen ion concentration and CO_2 tension within the arterial blood, the peripheral receptors are less sensitive than the brain stem chemoreceptors to these changes.

The reduced oxygen and elevated CO_2 tensions associated with either alveolar hypoventilation, e.g. drug overdose, or significant ventilation–perfusion imbalance from chronic bronchitis, stimulate respiration by activating the chemoreceptors. In severe hypoxia, if the CO_2 tension rises above 70 mmHg, the chemoreceptors become less sensitive to this stimulus, allowing the hypoxic drive to predominate. **Under these circumstances, the injudicious use of high inspired oxygen concentrations without adequate monitoring of the blood gases may cause respiratory depression (vide infra).**

Section 13.2 • Respiratory failure

Respiratory failure is defined as an arterial oxygen tension (PaO_2) at sea level of less than 8.0 kPa, i.e. hypoxia due to inadequate gas exchange within the lung. A PaO_2 of 8 kPa was included in the definition because it lies close to the critical point on the oxygen dissociation curve below which further small changes in the PaO_2 are associated with large falls in the arterial oxygen tension and hence significant reduction in the oxygen available to the tissues.

Respiratory failure can occur in clinical situations where it may be overlooked or inappropriately treated, e.g. immediate recovery period from a general anaesthetic, patients with chronic lung disease, in broncho- and lobar pneumonias, bronchial asthma, pulmonary thromboembolism, fat embolism, pulmonary collapse, tension pneumothorax and left ventricular failure. Respiratory failure may become rapidly worse in patients with chronic failure, e.g. infective exacerbation of chronic bronchitis in the postoperative period. The main causes of respiratory failure are shown in Figure 13.3.

The arterial $PaCO_2$ (arterial CO_2 tension) is used to subdivide respiratory failure into:

- **Type I** – where the $PaCO_2$ is less than 6.6 kPa (50 mmHg), i.e. hypoxia with normal or low $PaCO_2$
- **Type II** – with a $PaCO_2$ greater than 6.6 kPa, i.e. hypoxia with hypercapnia.

However, during the course of an illness, the patient may pass from type I to type II failure and vice versa.

In general type I respiratory failure is associated with pulmonary and cardiac causes where *alveolar hyperventilation* occurs maintaining a normal or low PCO_2, whereas type II is linked to disorders of the central and peripheral nervous system and skeletal abnormalities where *alveolar hypoventilation* predominates. Chronic obstructive pulmonary disease may present as either type I or type II failure, in which case *ventilation perfusion (V/Q) imbalance* rather than alveolar hypoventilation accounts for the type II failure.

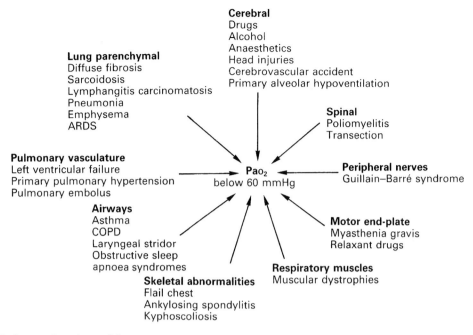

Figure 13.3 Causes of respiratory failure.

Type I respiratory failure
Three mechanisms underline the development of type I respiratory failure:

- ventilation perfusion imbalance
- physiological venous shunting, and
- alveolar capillary block.

Even in normal lungs, ventilation and perfusion of individual alveoli are not perfectly matched, with a varying ratio from the apex to the base of the lungs. This imbalance becomes more marked as a result of most lung disorders, with some alveoli being well ventilated and poorly perfused, while others are poorly ventilated but well perfused. In the blood leaving poorly ventilated parts of the lungs, the $PaCO_2$ is raised by up to 8 kPa, giving levels similar to that in venous blood. The accumulation of CO_2 stimulates the brain stem chemoreceptors, increasing the rate of ventilation leading to the expulsion of CO_2 from well-ventilated areas, thus maintaining a normal or low PCO_2 in the arterial blood. Hyperventilation cannot increase the extraction of oxygen by the pulmonary capillary blood in other alveoli, as the maximum oxygen tension in the best ventilated alveoli breathing air cannot exceed 13.3 kPa. Thus the maximum PaO_2 from well-ventilated areas is 13.3 kPa and this will be diluted by blood from the poorly ventilated areas, thereby reducing the overall arterial oxygen tension. The greater the imbalance, the lower the PaO_2.

In pneumonia or left ventricular failure many alveoli may continue to be perfused but the presence of alveolar fluid prevents ventilation. In these circumstances, venous blood from the right ventricle passes directly through these areas to the left atrium, adding the effect of a physiological shunt to any anatomical shunting already present. Any rise in the $PaCO_2$ would stimulate the respiratory centre leading to hyperventilation expelling the excess CO_2 but having no effect on the PaO_2. In principle, any thickening of the alveolar–capillary membrane as occurs in fibrosing alveolitis, sarcoidosis, and so on, should impair the diffusion of oxygen from the alveolar space to the capillary blood. In practice, this is rarely sufficient in itself to produce hypoxia but becomes significant with concomitant ventilation perfusion imbalance.

If the $PaCO_2$ remains normal or low, type I respiratory failure should be treated with high concentrations of O_2 by appropriate mask or high flow oxygen through a tent, thereby increasing the oxygen tension in the well-ventilated and perfused alveoli and thus raising the overall arterial PO_2.

Type II respiratory failure
In many cases of type II respiratory failure, alveolar hypoventilation is responsible for the breakdown in adequate gas exchange within the lung. The main causes are depression of the neurological respiratory drive and increased impedance. As the lungs themselves are usually normal, the term extra-pulmonary ventilatory failure (EPVF) is sometimes used for the group caused by increased impedance. The causes of type II respiratory failure due to increased impedance are:

- morbid obesity
- chest trauma with large haemo/pneumothorax or tension pneumothorax
- ruptured diaphragm with extensive herniation of abdominal contents

- massive pleural effusion
- massive ascites
- ankylosing spondylitis
- kyphoscoliosis.

In the acute situation oxygen therapy alone is insufficient and ventilatory support by intermittent positive pressure ventilation is usually needed at an early stage. In surgical practice, morbid obesity is the most common cause of EPVF after surgery. In the chronic situation home positive pressure ventilation by nasal face mask is useful, e.g. in ankylosing spondylitis.

Type II respiratory failure can occur in patients with chronic obstructive airways disease when it is caused by gross ventilation perfusion imbalance. However, brain stem chemoreceptor insensitivity to arterial $PaCO_2$ and hydrogen ion concentration may play a part in some patients who are then dependent on stimulation from the aortic and carotid oxygen chemoreceptors for their respiratory drive (hypoxic drive). Even at their best, these patients have a PO_2 set at much lower levels (9.3 kPa) than normal individuals. In the presence of an acute postoperative exacerbation, the PaO_2 may fall to 6 kPa. In patients dependent on a hypoxic drive efforts to raise the PaO_2 to levels above 9.3 kPa are counterproductive since the patient may stop breathing with a rapid increase in the $PaCO_2$ and hydrogen ion concentration, leading to coma and death. Thus careful control of the inspired oxygen (FiO_2) is essential, the exact concentration of which is determined by repeat blood gases. Thus, in these patients controlled oxygen therapy is usually administered by a Venturi-type mask in a concentration that must not exceed 24% and blood gases monitored 1 h later. If the $PaCO_2$ rise is small < 1.3 kPa (10 mmHg) and is below 10 kPa (75 mmHg), the FiO_2 may be increased to 30%. If the $PaCO_2$ increases in spite of these measures, a Doxapram drip is administered in an effort to stimulate the brain stem chemoreceptors. Failure to maintain adequate PaO_2 without a rising $PaCO_2$ or hydrogen ion concentration is an indication for respiratory support by intermittent positive pressure ventilation through a cuffed endotracheal tube.

Acute respiratory distress syndrome
This condition used to be referred to as adult respiratory distress syndrome (ARDs) or shock lung. The new terminology is more appropriate, since the condition may occur in children and the nature of this life-threatening disorder is that of an acute lung injury that may result from a variety of causes, the most common of which are:

- shock
- pneumonia
- severe sepsis
- severe pancreatitis
- major trauma
- aspiration
- drug overdosage
- near drowning.

ARDS may also be caused by massive blood transfusion, although with blood warming and modern transfusion practice, this is less common nowadays. It may complicate cardiopulmonary bypass and is common in fat and air embolism, smoke inhalation, poisoning (Paraquat and other inhaled toxins) and oxygen toxicity.

The reported incidence of ARDS varies from 1.5 to 4 per 100 000 inhabitants in Western countries. The pathogenesis of the acute lung injury is now thought to result from excess sequestration and activation of neutrophils in the lung following activation of the complement system. The neutrophils induce parenchymal damage by release of reactive oxygen species, proteolytic enzymes especially elastase and eicosanoids (thromboxane, leukotrienes and prostaglandins) that cause extensive damage to both the endothelium of the pulmonary capillaries and to the epithelium of the alveolar membrane. This results in increased permeability of the alveolar–capillary membrane with the development of gross non-cardiogenic pulmonary oedema (in the first instance) and impaired gas exchange. The aerated lung volume is reduced to less than one-half of the total lung volume. A proliferation of the alveolar epithelial cells occurs as a result of the injury and this is accompanied by increased fibroblastic activity and collagen formation in the interstitial tissues of the lung. Thus, the pulmonary compliance is greatly reduced.

The onset of ARDS is sudden, with the typical picture being established within 12–72 h of the triggering event. Initially, the physical signs in the chest are minimal despite obvious tachypnoea and hypoxaemia, and the chest X-ray may be normal or show an interstitial infiltrate. As the disease progresses, diffuse bilateral infiltrates causing a 'white-out' (Figure 13.4) become evident. The cardiac output is normal at the onset of ARDS but subsequently falls with progression of the disease. The blood gases show changes of type I respiratory failure: hypoxaemia with a low or normal $PaCO_2$ and a low pH due to mixed respiratory alkalosis and metabolic acidosis. All patients with ARDS

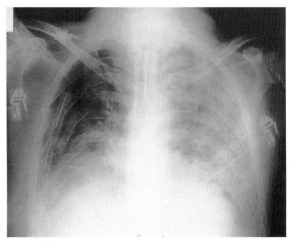

Figure 13.4 PA chest X-ray in a patient with adult respiratory distress syndrome (ARDs).

require ventilatory support and intensive care. The hypoxaemia is often refractory to high FiO$_2$ due to intrapulmonary shunting [**Module 19, Vol. I**]. The recovery from ARDS is dependent on correction of the underling condition and good intensive care with pulmonary and cardiac support. Infection control is very important but prophylactic use of antibiotics is not indicated. Extracorporeal lung assistance (ECLA) is used in some centres but controlled clinical trials have not demonstrated a survival advantage with ECLA over conventional management. There is no evidence that corticosteroids are useful.

Death (overall mortality of 50–60%) usually occurs within 2–4 weeks of onset of the disease, either from infection or multiorgan failure. Surviving patients usually achieve good pulmonary function although weaning from ventilatory support may be prolonged. Some however sustain permanent pulmonary dysfunction.

Fat embolism
This is a rare cause of respiratory insufficiency including full-blown ARDS and is encountered most commonly after major orthopaedic trauma but has been documented as a complication of pancreatitis, parenteral nutrition, cardiac massage, liposuction and bone marrow transplantation. The fat globules are thought to arise from the bone marrow and adipose tissue. These enter the venous circulation and cause occlusion of the pulmonary capillaries, although some pass through into the systemic circulation to embolize in the skin (causing petechial haemorrhages), kidney, brain and retinal capillaries (where they can sometimes be detected by ophthalmoscopy). Within the lung, the globules of neutral fat (large unstable chylomicrons) are hydrolysed by lung lipase producing highly toxic free fatty acids, which are responsible for the acute lung damage and loss of surfactant activity. The triad, mental confusion, respiratory failure and petechial skin haemorrhages should suggest the diagnosis, which may be difficult to confirm. Treatment is supportive.

Tracheostomy
Surgical trachesotomy has been largely replaced by percutaneous systems using the Seldinger wire tech-

nique and this is usually performed by the anaesthetists. Likewise, cricothyroidotomy (incision of the cricothyroid membrane followed by insertion of tube) is rarely practised nowadays. However, the indications for tracheostomy irrespective of technique (surgical, percutaneous, minitracheostomy) remain unchanged and include:

- to bypass a life-threatening obstruction of the upper airway
- to provide access for tracheal toilet
- to protect patients at risk from aspiration
- to enable prolonged ventilatory support.

Irrespective of its nature, every tracheostomy must be presented with well-humidified air or oxygen for both spontaneous breathing or assisted ventilation [**Thoracic Surgery, Vol. II**].

Section 13.3 • Chronic lung disease and respiratory insufficiency

Primary chronic pulmonary disease falls into three main categories:

- **Restrictive**, e.g. fibrosing alveolitis, where there is progressive loss of the alveolar parenchyma by fibrosis ending in respiratory insufficiency usually requiring lung transplantation for survival
- **Infective**, e.g. pulmonary tuberculosis, fungal infections
- **Chronic obstructive airways/pulmonary disease (COAD/COPD)**, e.g. chronic bronchitis and emphysema – this is by far the most common pulmonary disorder encountered in surgical practice.

The changes in the pulmonary function tests in obstructive and restrictive chronic lung disease are shown in Table 13.1.

COAD/COPD is defined as reduced expiratory airflow with reduction of the respiratory reserve. It is caused by chronic bronchitis and emphysema, and bronchial asthma. Overall, due to chronic bronchitis and emphysema, COAD affects 5% of the population in Western countries. The mechanism

Table 13.1 Changes in the pulmonary function tests in obstructive and restrictive chronic lung disease

	FVC	FEV	FEV1/FVC	TLC	RV	RV/TLC	Tco
Obstructive airways disease							
Chronic bronchitis	↓	↓↓	↓	N or ↑	N or ↑	↑	↓
Emphysema	↓↓	↓↓↓	↓↓	↑↑	↑↑↑	↑↑	↓↓
Asthma	↓	↓↓	↓	N or ↑	N or ↑	↑	N or ↑
Restrictive lung disease							
Fibrosing alveolitis	↓↓	↓↓	N	↓	N or ↓	N or ↑	↓↓
Sarcoidosis	N or ↓	N or ↓	N	N	N	N	↓

N = normal, ↑ = raised, ↓ = reduced.
[Module 16, Vol. I for pulmonary function tests]

responsible for the reduced expiratory flow is a combination of increased airway resistance from mucosal swelling, bronchospasm, and turbulence due to tortuosity of the airway in combination with reduced lung recoil caused by the loss of pulmonary elastin and destruction of alveolar walls.

Chronic bronchitis and emphysema are essentially components of one disease, with chronic bronchitis dominating the picture of early COAD and emphysema the advanced stage of the disease, although there are patients where emphysema dominates the clinical picture from the start (primary emphysema).

Chronic bronchitis starts as a bronchiolitis (involving the small bronchioles). It is commonly encountered in smokers but only 15% of regular smokers develop the disease and the generally held view is that these individuals have a genetic predisposition. The clinical picture of chronic bronchitis is dominated by chronic productive cough, wheezing and fluctuating dyspnoea and V/Q mismatch. Chronic bronchitics are prone to hypercarbia, polycythaemia, pulmonary hypertension and cor pulmonale (blue bloaters). Severe hypoxic episodes occurring at night by causing pulmonary hypertension have been implicated in the development of the right heart failure in these patients and nocturnal oxygen therapy is now recommended for this reason.

In emphysema, the air spaces distal to the terminal bronchioles are dilated from over-inflation, destruction of the alveolar walls or both. As the air spaces enlarge, they form blebs or bullae and even large cysts. These may burst, resulting in pneumothorax and pulmonary collapse on the affected side. From an aetiological viewpoint, emphysema is classified as:

- *destructive* – most common, associated with chronic bronchitis but may be primary. A rare cause is α_1-antrypsin deficiency
- *over-inflation* – senile, compensatory, fibrotic scarring
- *atrophy or hypoplasia* – lung agenesis, e.g. MacLeod's syndrome (unilateral emphysema from arrested lung development).

Patients with emphysema have constant dyspnoea from loss of the pulmonary alveolar parenchyma and less cough, sputum and wheezing. As they have less shunting they are able to normalize their blood gases to some extent by increased ventilation (pink puffers). As a consequence of the alveolar damage, there is a progressive loss in the pulmonary capillary bed and this, together with the vasoconstriction of the pulmonary artery induced by the chronic hypoxia, results in pulmonary hypertension and eventually in right heart failure. There is in addition extensive V/Q mismatching aggravating the hypoxaemia and leading to secondary polycythaemia. This shunting may also contribute to the hypercarbia, although this is initially controlled by increasing the minute ventilation. As the expiratory efforts are incomplete, air trapping with permanent hyperinflation of the lung occurs with increase in the total lung capacity (TLC) and residual volume (RV) and the development of emphysematous bullae that can rupture, causing pneumothorax with lung collapse and acute respiratory failure. As emphysema progresses, the respiratory muscles become less efficient and unable to cope with the ventilatory requirements when hypercarbia ensues. Thus raised $PaCO_2$ is a late feature in COAD, with forced expiratory volume in first second (FEV_1) < 1.0 litre.

While 'pink puffers' and 'blue bloaters' form distinct clinical entities within the spectrum of COAD, many patients present a mixed picture and exhibit some improvement in respiratory function following inhalation of a bronchodilator. Before elective surgery every patient with significant COAD should undergo respiratory function tests together with an exercise test. An FEV_1 below 1.0 litre that cannot be improved by bronchodilator therapy or an RV/TLC ratio over 70% are regarded as contraindications to surgery. Blood gases indicate the preoperative status and give a baseline in the event of postoperative problems. Maximum respiratory function should be achieved preoperatively using brochodilators, physiotherapy, antibiotics and occasionally short courses of high-dose steroids.

Acute respiratory failure can occur in patients with COAD and carries a high mortality. It is often precipitated by:

- acute bronchitis or pneumonia most commonly caused by *Streptococcus pneumoniae* or *Haemophilus influenzae*
- sputum retention in the postoperative period due to impaired coughing and increased secretion of viscid mucus
- left ventricular failure – ischaemic or secondary to right heart failure
- pneumothorax/pulmonary collapse caused by rupture of emphysematous bulla.

Section 13.4 • Aspiration syndromes, pneumonias and lung abscesses

Aspiration syndromes

The aspiration of liquids or solids into the tracheobronchial tree is always serious and may have a fatal outcome. Although aspiration can occur in any individual, the risk are significantly increased in the presence of:

- *impaired conscious level from any cause* – anaesthesia, head injury, hypoxia and hypercarbia, drug overdose, alcohol intoxication cerebrovascular accidents, etc.
- *impaired protective reflexes (cough and gag)* – immediately after extubation of endotracheal tube, neurological disease, e.g. myasthenia, motor neurone disease, etc., facial neck and pharyngeal injury/surgery

■ *in the presence of disease/conditions* that result in passive regurgitation of gastric contents – gastro-oesophageal reflux, nasogastric tube, achalasia, intestinal obstruction, oesophageal obstruction and after oesophagectomy.

Aspiration of liquids

The outcome depends on:

■ nature of fluid – pH, corrosive nature and bacterial content
■ amount aspirated.

Overall aspiration accounts for 25% of ARDS. The most severe injury to the respiratory epithelium is caused by an acid aspirate with very high mortality approaching 100% if the pH is < 2.0. Aspiration of acidic fluid (usually gastric contents, when it is referred to as Mendelson's syndrome) is immediately followed by a vagally-mediated marked and diffuse bronchospasm that precedes the loss of surfactant function and the direct corrosive damage to the respiratory epithelium. This results in fluid and protein leakage into the alveolar space causing pulmonary oedema within 1 hour of the aspiration. This almost invariably progresses to ARDS.

Aspiration of neutral fluid such as blood or isotonic solutions, is much less harmful to the respiratory epithelium, unless the volume aspirated is large when 'the near drowning' effect results in severe pulmonary dysfunction with loss of surfactant function, alveolar collapse with pulmonary oedema and shunting.

Aspiration of infected liquid/secretions following colonization of the oropharynx by gram-negative organisms is the underlying cause for *hospital acquired-pneumonia* and is an increasing problem especially in patients treated in intensive care units (ICU), where it is referred to as *ventilator-associated pneumonia.*

Aspiration of solids

The clinical picture and pathology depend on the nature of the foreign body (FB) and the level and degree of occlusion of the airway. The group at greatest risk of asphyxia and accidental death from aspiration of solid foreign bodies are infants. However, major life-threatening upper airway obstruction (mouth to carina) from this cause is also encountered in adults, especially the elderly and individuals with dentures, the accident usually occurring during eating or sucking. Complete upper airway obstruction results in inability to breath, cough and articulate. The patient becomes agitated and rapidly cyanotic. The vigorous attempts at breathing by the victim result in paradoxical chest wall movements with indrawing of the intercostal spaces. Unrelieved, the acute hypoxia causes rapid loss of consciousness, bradycardia and death within minutes. The Heimlich manoeuvre aimed at dislodging the FB may be life saving in this situation. This consists of gripping the victim from behind with the right fist clasped by the left hand over the upper abdomen. Vigorous inward and upper thrusts are applied to raise the intrabronchial pressure in an effort to dislodge the FG. If dislodgment of the FB proves unsuccessful, life-saving measures include:

■ direct laryngoscopy with suction of oropharynx and manual dislodgment of any supraglottic FB
■ orotracheal intubation and ventilation
■ immediate cricothyroidotomy or trans-tracheal jet ventilation if orotracheal intubation fails.

Smaller objects cause partial obstruction with choking and spluttering. If not expectorated they lead to obstruction of distal bronchi/bronchioles with lobar/segmental collapse, consolidation, abscess formation and ultimately bronchiectasis. A particularly severe inflammatory reaction is produced in the collapsed segment by meat and vegetable FBs.

Pneumonias

Pneumonia can be acquired in the community or subsequent to admission to hospital (*hospital acquired pneumonias*). There are important differences between the two, especially with regard to the infecting organisms. Hospital-acquired pneumonia is now defined as infective consolidation, developing more than 3 days after admission to hospital for any reason. It affects approximately 2–5% of patients postoperatively and shows the highest incidence in patients admitted to ICU. When the condition develops in patients on mechanical ventilation, it is often referred to as *ventilator-associated pneumonia.*

The patients at risk are:

■ smokers
■ patients with chronic pulmonary disease (obstructive and restrictive)
■ immunocompromised patients
■ patients on mechanical ventilation
■ patients with subclinical heart failure.

Whereas community-acquired pneumonia is most commonly caused by *Streptococcus pneumonia, Haemophilus influenza*, influenza virus, etc., hospital-acquired pneumonia is due to infection by Gram-negative organisms, for example *Pseudomonas aeruginosa, Enterobacter* spp., *Klebsiella pneumonia* and *Proteus mirabilis* following colonization of the oropharynx by these organisms. The most common bacteria responsible for ventilator-associated pneumonia are *Pseudomonas* and *Acinetobacter* spp.

Pneumonia causes both respiratory and systemic symptoms. The respiratory manifestations include dyspnoea, cough, sputum, pleuritic chest pain, tachypnoea, bronchial breathing, inspiratory crackles and pulmonary infiltrates on the chest X-ray. The systemic signs include fever, rigors, leucocytosis dehydration and hypoxaemia. When severe, pneumonia is accompanied by bacteraemia with hypotension and evidence of renal impairment that may progress to acute tubular necrosis. The hypoxaemia often results in mental confusion or reduced level of consciousness.

The treatment consists of:

- intravenous fluids to correct dehydration
- appropriate antibiotics [Module 5, Vol. I]
- oxygen therapy
- mechanical ventilation if PaO_2 is < 8kPa (60 mmHg) despite oxygen therapy.

Lung abscesses

Any process that causes lung suppuration may produce an abscess, although the term is usually restricted to cavitating lesions caused by pyogenic organisms and thus excluding tuberculosis, fungal infections and cavitating tumours. The incidence of lung abscess has fallen since the introduction of antibiotics. The main causes of lung abscess formation are shown in Table 13.2.

Nowadays, the most common cause of lung abscess is occlusion by a bronchial carcinoma.

Table 13.2 Causes and pathology of lung abscesses

Cause	Pathology
Aspiration	Infected material
Bronchial obstruction	To a major bronchus by tumour, FB or glands
Suppurative pneumonias	Particularly *Staphylococci* and *Klebsiella* infections
Infected infarcts	Resulting from septic emboli or secondary infection of a pulmonary infarct
Chest trauma	Implantation of infected material or secondary infection of lung haematoma
Transdiaphragmatic spread	From hepatic or subphrenic sepsis
Lung cysts or bullae	That become secondarily infected

Aspiration lung abscesses are more common on the right side because the right bronchus is more in line with the trachea. The typical position is in the apical segment of the right lower lobe (Figure 13.5). The initial symptoms, fever, rigors and malaise are non-specific and may be modified by antibiotic therapy. Later, cough, haemoptysis, deep-seated pain and pleurisy may develop. Intrabronchial rupture results in the expectoration of large quantities of foul-smelling pus. Rupture into the pleura with empyema may also occur and may be associated with a persistent bronchopleural fistula. The majority of aspiration lung abscesses respond to postural drainage, physiotherapy and antibiotics (initially benzylpenicillin in large intramuscular doses). Medical treatment may need to be continued for 2–3 months. Healing usually occurs, leaving a fibrous scar. Surgical treatment is required if resolution does not occur with medical treatment. This often entails resection of the involved bronchopulmonary segment.

The suppurative pulmonary infections due to infection by *Klebsiella* and *Staphylococcus* can cause pulmonary abscess formation. Staphylococcal bronchopneumonia occurs predominantly in the elderly and may follow influenza when it carries a high mortality. There are multiple small peribronchial abscesses from which the inflammation rapidly spreads, causing considerable lung destruction with residual fibrosis if the patient survives. Children develop a Staphylococcal lobar pneumonia with abscess formation. These abscess cavities become inflated during coughing and crying, resulting in tension pneumatocoeles through a check-

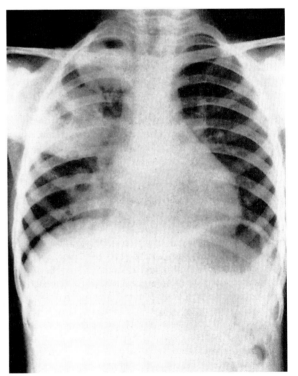

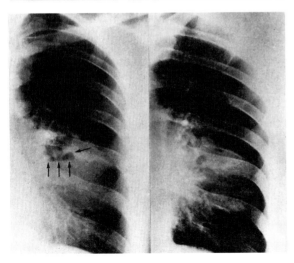

Figure 13.5 Aspiration lung abscess in the apical segment of the right lower lobe.

Figure 13.6 Multiple staphylococcal abscesses of the right lung in a child.

valve mechanism (Figure 13.6). As these expand, they may compress the lung causing respiratory embarrassment or rupture into the pleural space, forming a tension pyo-pneumothorax.

Suppurative Klebsiella pneumonias usually start in the right upper lobe and unless treated aggressively with the appropriate antibiotics, they rapidly spread to the remaining lung producing extensive destruction, abscess formation and fibrosis. Elderly males are principally affected. If the destroyed lobes become the site of persistent or recurrent infection, resection may be necessary.

Section 13.5 • Acute disorders of the pleura

The pleural membranes are normally kept moist by a thin layer of fluid (up to 15 ml) that is constantly being formed and reabsorbed with an hourly turnover of 500 ml. The moistening creates a surface tension which, together with the negative intrapleural space, ensures expansion of the lungs as the chest cavity expands during inspiration. This mechanism breaks down or is impaired to a varying extent if fluid, air or blood accumulates between the visceral and parietal layers.

Pleural effusions

A pleural effusion exists when there is an abnormal amount of fluid within the pleural space detectable on clinical or radiological examination. A collection >100 ml is detected radiologically but for clinical detection the collection has to exceed 500 ml. The mechanisms involved in the formation of pleural effusions are:

- **increased capillary hydrostatic pressure** – left heart failure, congestive heart failure, constrictive pericarditis
- **decreased colloid osmotic pressure** – hypoproteinaemia, e.g. nephrotic syndrome, chronic liver disease
- **increased capillary permeability due to inflammation of the pleura**, e.g. pneumonia, pulmonary infarction, pulmonary tuberculosis. When the primary focus of infection/inflammation is in the subphrenic region, the term *sympathetic effusion* is often used, e.g. acute necrotizing pancreatitis
- **impaired lymphatic drainage** – blockage of the lymphatics by lymph node infiltration by tumour. Damage to the thoracic duct during oesophagectomy or spontaneous rupture from malignant occlusion may result in accumulation of pure lymph in the thorax (chylothorax).

The physical findings of a significant pleural effusion are diminished expansion, stony dullness, reduced or absent breath sounds and diminished focal fremitus and resonance over the affected side. A pleural friction rub

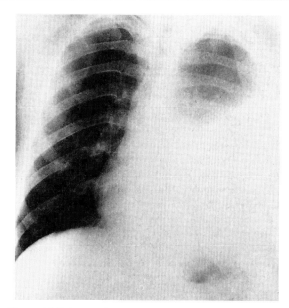

Figure 13.7 Large left pleural effusion with mediatinal shift to the right.

may be audible at the top of a pleural effusion. Radiologically, blunting of the costophrenic angle may be the only finding in small effusions. Large effusions exhibit the characteristic axillary tail with a concave upper border. If massive, the hemithorax may appear opaque, with the mediastinum shifted to the opposite side (Figure 13.7).

Aspiration of a little fluid from an area of maximal dullness confirms the diagnosis and the macroscopic appearance often gives a clue to the probable diagnosis:

- **clear light straw-coloured fluid that does not clot (transudate)** – heart failure, hypoproteinaemia, etc.
- **dark yellow fluid that clots on standing (exudate)** – local pulmonary cause such as tumour or infection
- **blood stained (old/altered blood)** – malignancy, pulmonary infarction, tuberculosis, necrotizing pancreatitis
- **frank blood** – haemothorax from chest trauma
- **turbid** – pneumonic effusions
- **frank pus** – empyema
- **milky white** – chylothorax due to malignant involvement/iatrogenic damage to large lymphatic ducts.

Further conclusive information is obtained by cytology, culture and biochemical analysis of the pleural aspirate.

Empyema

This is defined as infection of the pleural space. The resulting pleural inflammation causes an outpouring of fluid rich in protein and polymorphs and bacteria (pus), which accumulates between the visceral and parietal layers. Empyema is always secondary to:

- **pulmonary infections** – pneumonia, lung abscess, bronchiectasis, fungal infections, tuberculosis
- **surgery and trauma** – leakage from oesophageal anastomosis, spontaneous or iatrogenic perforation of the oesophagus, chest trauma
- **trans-diaphragmatic spread** – subphrenic abscess, hepatic amoebiasis
- **osteomyelitis** – of ribs and vertebrae
- **septicaemia** – multiple small lung abscesses.

The empyema may lie free in the pleural space or be encapsulated by fibrinous pleural adhesions that arise as a local defence mechanism and are encouraged by antibiotic therapy. Continued accumulation of pus compresses the lung with shift of the mediastinum to the opposite side. Fibrin is continually deposited on the pleural surfaces producing a thickening rind, the deeper layers of which become fibrotic and avascular (permitting easy stripping during surgical decortication). Adequate treatment at this stage will produce full expansion of the lung and gradual resolution with no functional impairment.

The transition from acute to chronic empyema is arbitrary; periods of 6–12 weeks have been suggested. Chronic empyema most commonly follows inadequate treatment of the acute phase. Less commonly, it results from (i) persistent bronchopleural fistula, (ii) retained foreign body or (iii) insidious chronic infection, e.g. tuberculosis, actinomycosis, fungal infection. The continued formation and fibrosis of the pleural rind progressively restricts chest wall and diaphragmatic movement, eventually producing a shrunken, flattened, immobile hemithorax with overlapping ribs and scoliosis to the affected side. In addition, there is considerable subpleural alveolar destruction and fibrosis leading to permanent functional impairment, even if lung expansion is achieved by surgical decortication.

The term pyo-pneumothorax refers to the situation where there is air and pus within the pleural space. This may occur:

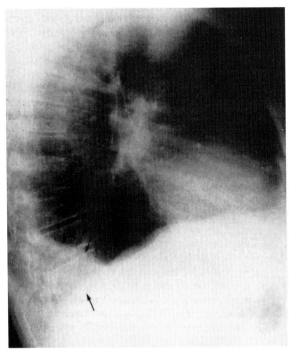

Figure 13.8 Empyema right base posteriorly. Triangular outline.

- if the empyema discharges into a bronchus forming a bronchopleural fistula
- if the empyema results from rupture of a lung abscess again with the formation of a bronchopleural fistula
- if the empyema is due to leakage/perforation of the oesophagus
- following pleural aspiration if the lung is unable to expand
- if the empyema contains gas-forming organisms, e.g. Clostridial species.

The diagnosis of acute empyema is made on the basis of the clinical background, general manifestations and chest signs, chest aspiration and radiology. As a rule, patients with acute empyema are ill with obvious signs of sepsis. Radiologically, a free-lying empyema resembles a pleural effusion. PA and lateral films and

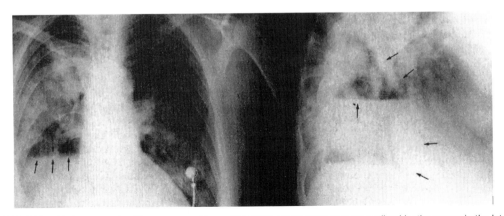

Figure 13.9 Right-sided pneumonia with pyo-pneumothorax. The limits of the empyema are outlined by the arrows in the lateral film.

ultrasound/CT scanning are necessary to localize encapsulated lesions that have different features depending on site (Figures 13.8 and 13.9).

The features of chronic empyema include toxaemia, malaise, anorexia, weight loss, intermittent pyrexia and gnawing chest pain. A persistent cough productive of sputum, particularly when lying on the contralateral side or aspiration pneumonia in the unaffected lung indicate the presence of a bronchopleural fistula. A normochromic normocytic anaemia develops and amyloidosis may supervene. Radiologically, there is dense pleural opacification, elevation of the hemi-diaphragm, with scoliosis to the affected side. Fluid levels occur with bronchopleural fistulas or after aspiration (see Figures 13.10 and 13.11).

Pneumothorax

Pneumothorax is defined as air in the pleural space and results from a defect/injury of the pulmonary parenchyma and the overlying vis-ceral **pleural**. It may be localized, when the volume of air and extent of lung collapse is limited by pleural adhesions, or generalized, when the whole lung recoils towards the hilum. The pneumothorax may be *traumatic* following trauma or surgery or may arise spontaneously – *spontaneous* pneumothorax. From a mechanical standpoint, a pneumothorax may be:

- **closed** – the defect that caused the air leakage has closed preventing further escape of air
- **open** – when air continues to pass freely between the lung and the pleural space, or between the atmosphere and the hemithorax (open chest wound)
- **valvular** – where air freely enters the pleural space during inspiration but becomes trapped during expiration due to closure of the leak.

A *tension pneumothorax* develops from the valvular type when its rapid progressive enlargement causes displacement of the mediastinum, kinking of the great vessels and increasing respiratory and cardiovascular stress. This condition requires

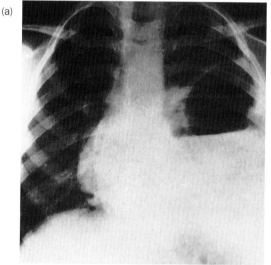

(a)

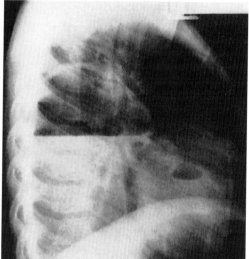

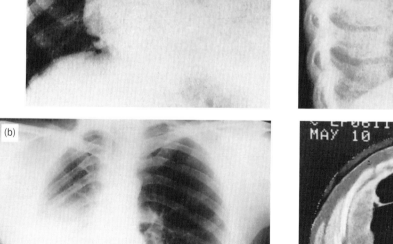

(b)

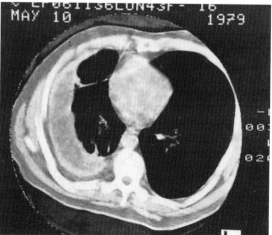

Figure 13.10 Chronic empyema. (a) PA and lateral view of the chest showing a large cavity containing pus. Note the fluid level and the thickness of the cavity wall. (b) PA radiograph and CT scan of a patient with chronic empyema and a contracted hemithorax.

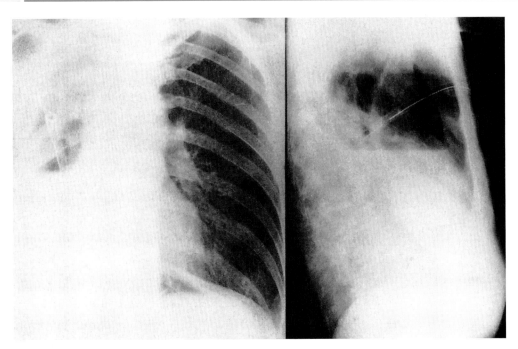

Figure 13.11 Right post-pneumonectomy chronic empyema.

immediate recognition and insertion of a large bore needle or cannula for survival.

Spontaneous pneumothorax is usually caused by rupture of apical blebs in otherwise fit young adults. These are the result of air leakage from minor defects in the alveolar walls during lung development. The air tracks to the apices of the lungs forming subpleural blebs (Figure 13.12), which are frequently bilateral. Spontaneous pneumothorax may also develop in patients with COAD (Figure 13.13) and patients suffering from α_1-antitrpsin deficiency. It may complicate hyperinflation of the lungs during positive pressure ventilation, especially with PEEP (positive end expiratory pressure). Rarely, it results from progressive dilatation and rupture of congenital cysts (Figure

13.14), the pneumatocoeles of childhood Staphylococcal pneumonias, or cysts that may develop in tuberculosis, bronchial carcinoma and pneumoconiosis.

A small closed pneumothorax (1.0–1.5 cm) may be safely observed without active intervention. Some advocate oxygen therapy in the belief that it aids resolution. Simple aspiration of a moderate closed spontaneous pneumothorax with a wide bore needle is practised by some and is reported to be successful in

Figure 13.12 Thoracoscopic view of apical blebs in a young adult patient with spontaneous pneumothorax. The condition is often bilateral.

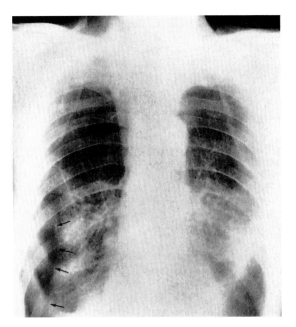

Figure 13.13 Right localized pneumothorax in a patient with chronic obstructive airways disease (COAD).

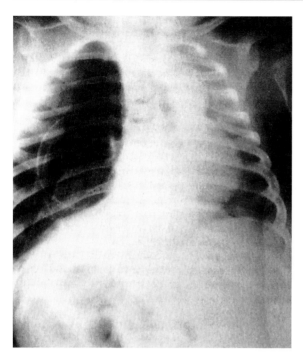

Figure 13.14 Tension cyst in a child with an associated tension right pneumothorax causing mediastinal shift to the left side.

75%. However, the orthodox management of moderate to large pneumothoraces is with insertion of an intercostal tube either in the second space along the midclavicular line anteriorly or preferably in the axilla (fourth and fifth space) between the anterior and posterior axillary folds. When the drain is inserted and connected to the underwater seal system, there should be an immediate stream of bubbles as the lung inflates. This will continue until full inflation is obtained. The drain is left in situ until there is no further leak, even when the patient coughs. Persistent leakage beyond 7–10 days is an indication for surgical treatment.

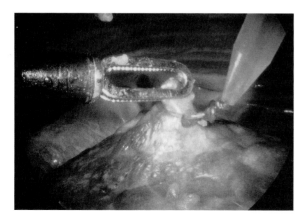

Figure 13.15 Thoracoscopic ligature of small apical blebs in a patient with spontaneous pneumothorax. If the collection of blebs is large, endostaplers are used to occlude and excise the area. In either event some form of pleurodesis or pleurectomy is performed as part of the surgical treatment.

Surgical treatment is also needed for patients with recurrent spontaneous pneumothorax. There is some debate as to how many recurrences (1–3) should be treated conservatively before surgical treatment is advisable. The fact is that a recurrence is likely to be followed by further episodes. The treatment consists of closure/obliteration of the blebs with pleurodesis, which may be effected by parietal pleurectomy, abrasion by gauze swab, coagulation preferably by the argon beamer, painting with irritant agents such as tetracycline, bethidine, etc. Nowadays, the surgical treatment is conducted by the thoracoscopic approach, avoiding the need for a posterolateral thoracotomy (Figure 13.15). This is especially important in patients with underlying lung disease such as COAD.

Haemothorax

The accumulation of blood in the pleural space (haemothorax) is a frequent result of either blunt or penetrating trauma. A plain radiograph of the chest should be obtained as early as possible in the resuscitation of the injured patient. The chest radiograph is examined carefully for abnormalities of the bony thorax, the soft tissues of the chest wall and mediastinum, as well as the lung parenchyma. The presence of rib fractures, pneumothorax, or haemothorax provides information necessary to direct the resuscitation and subsequent management.

Despite the diverse nature of chest injuries, many of these patients present initially with either haemothorax or pneumothorax or both. Treatment of haemothorax or pneumothorax is often the sole intervention required in patients with chest trauma, and aggressive early intervention is critical in achieving the optimal outcome.

The bleeding may range from minimal to massive life-threatening haemorrhage depending on the nature of the injury. The presenting symptoms may also vary widely depending on the degree of haemorrhage. Initial treatment of haemothorax requires placement of a chest tube that is large enough to ensure evacuation of the accumulated blood. In general, this requires a 36 Fr or larger tube. The majority of lacerations to the pulmonary parenchyma involve low-pressure vessels of the pulmonary circulation. Such bleeding can be expected to stop after placement of the chest tube and re-expansion of the lung. Injuries to systemic arteries, including the intercostal arteries and the internal mammary arteries, can lead to massive haemorrhage, especially if the vessels are only partially transected.

Most cases of haemothorax can be treated by intercostal tube drainage alone. In situations of massive initial haemorrhage or significant ongoing haemorrhage, thoracotomy is required for control of the bleeding. The decision for thoracotomy must be individualized. In general, an initial return of 1000–1500 ml or significant continued bleeding in excess of 200–300 ml/h over a period of time should alert one to the possible need for thoracotomy and surgical control of the bleeding.

Increasingly, thoracoscopy is used instead of thoracotomy in these patients. Bleeding from intercostal vessels can be easily controlled by this approach. More serious bleeding injuries require conversion to thoracotomy.

Guide to further reading

Repin, J. E. and Beehler, C. J. (1991). Neutrophils and adult respiratory distress syndrome: two interlocking perspectives. *Am Rev Respi Dis* **144**: 251–252.

Bernard, G. R., Artigas, A., Brigham, K. L. *et al.* (1994). Report of the American-European consensus conference on ARDS: definitions, mechanisms, relevant outcomes and clinical trial coordination. *Intens Care Med* **20**: 225–232.

Scheld, W. M. (1991). Developments in the pathogenesis, diagnosis and treatment of noscomial pneumonia. *Surg Gynec Obstet* **172**(suppl): 42–53.

Dal Nogare, A. R. (1994). Nosocomial pneumonia in the medical and surgical patient. *Med Clin North Am* **78**: 1081–1090.

Arms, R., Dines, D. and Tinstman, T. (1997). Aspiration pneumonia. *Chest* **65**: 136–139.

Elpern, E., Scott, M., Petro, L. and Ries, M. (1994). Pulmonary aspiration in mechanically ventilated patients with tracheostomies. *Chest* **105**: 563–566.

Patients with head injuries

1 • Nature and causes of loss of consciousness

2 • Head injuries and their management

'Your prayer must be for a sound mind in a sound body' – Decimus Junius Juvenalis, 60–130 AD

Section 14.1 • Nature and causes of loss of consciousness

Causes and mechanisms of altered consciousness

Philosophers regard altered consciousness as an elusive concept, but clinicians see it in more concrete terms as a clinically useful measure of global brain activity, which responds quickly to clinical changes and thus provides a mirror of how well or badly the patient is doing.

The neurophysiological basis of consciousness
There is still debate about which neural circuits are mainly involved in determining consciousness, but the reticular system in the brainstem certainly plays a crucial role. An altered balance of electrical activity in its excitatory and inhibitory circuits 'switches off' the tonic discharges that maintain awareness. Recent magnetic resonance imaging (MRI) studies of brain-injured patients suggest that deep lesions of the cerebral hemispheres can initiate coma by suppressing the normal brainstem arousal mechanisms.

What conditions lead to altered consciousness?
Altered consciousness results from mechanical or metabolic damage, temporary or permanent, to these key neurons and their synaptic connections. It can also be produced by abnormal patterns of electrochemical activity in the brain, as in an epileptic fit.

Mechanical injury can be a sudden event or a more gradual process. Sudden energy transfer to the brain, e.g. at the time of a serious head injury or when a cerebral aneurysm bursts, causes structural damage. This may be mild and capable of repair, or severe and destroy much brain tissue. The most severe cases prove immediately fatal.

Raised intracranial pressure (ICP) causes mechanical damage more gradually, e.g. as an expanding intracranial haematoma or other 'space-occupying' lesion distorts and compresses brain tissue. It also reduces cerebral perfusion pressure (CPP) and therefore cerebral blood flow and oxygen delivery, illustrating how a single pathological process within the brain can cause harm through more than one mechanism.

Disordered neuronal metabolism is an important cause of altered conscious level in surgical patients, and reduced oxygen delivery to the brain is the most common reason. This can be due to systemic hypoxaemia from an obstructed airway or inadequate ventilation, or to shock from blood loss or sepsis, or to raised ICP. High carbon monoxide levels – seen in burned patients who have inhaled smoke – cause hypoxia by binding preferentially to haemoglobin and reducing cerebral oxygen delivery. As well as oxygen the brain needs glucose and is therefore damaged by severe or prolonged hypoglycaemia, as in diabetics who take excess insulin. In untreated diabetes the neurons are also starved of glucose by inhibition of membrane transport. A wide variety of prescribed or misused drugs can depress neuronal function and alter conscious level.

Disordered patterns of electrochemical activity within the brain in response to a variety of stimuli cause various types of epileptic fit, often involving a loss or alteration of consciousness as part of the clinical syndrome.

Assessment of altered consciousness

For 25 years the Glasgow Coma Scale (GCS) has been used throughout the world to measure consciousness level in patients with brain injury or illness. It makes no assumptions about the nature of the pathological process, requires no hi-tech equipment, is quick and easy to use after basic training, has good validity and reliability (intraobserver and interobserver), and has proved a useful tool for measuring conscious level and monitoring its trend over time.

The GCS defines consciousness in terms of three aspects of the patient's responsiveness to defined stimuli: the eye opening response, the best motor response in the upper limbs and the best verbal response (Figure 14.1). Each aspect is graded from best to worst and described in words that have been carefully chosen for their lack of ambiguity, to form a hierarchy of responsiveness. For example, a

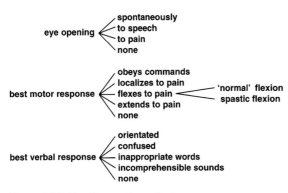

Figure 14.1 The Glasgow Coma Scale.

patient's conscious level may be described as 'eye opening to pain, localizing to pain, and making incomprehensible sounds'.

Measuring the patient's conscious level

The **eye opening response** is quite straightforward. The eyes may already be open spontaneously on starting the assessment. They may be closed at first but open either to **speech** or to the stimulus of **pain**. Finally, there may be **no eye opening** to any stimulus at all.

To test the **motor response**, the patient is asked to **obey commands** using a series of (simple) instructions: 'squeeze my fingers; put out your tongue; lift up your hand'. With a drowsy patient it may be necessary to repeat the commands or to shout them. If there is no response, a painful stimulus is applied to the head (earlobe, supraorbital ridge, or cheek) to see if the patient will **localize** to this stimulus by lifting up one or both arms above the level of the clavicles in its direction. Failing this, a painful stimulus is applied to the finger nail bed to see what response is evoked at the elbow: a rapid and co-ordinated **withdrawal** from the stimulus, **flexion** (often with abnormal movement patterns), **extension** (the 'decerebrate' response), or **no motor response** at all. Many observation charts do not try to distinguish between withdrawal and flexion, and there may be elements of both in a particular response.

Testing the **verbal response** begins by seeing whether the patient is **orientated** by asking about recent events and about time, place and person. Even an apparently well patient may prove to be **confused**, and this should raise concern when it develops in a surgical or trauma patient, as it can be the earliest sign of deteriorating brain function. Some patients only make **inappropriate words** or **incomprehensible sounds**, and others have **no verbal response**.

There are often circumstances where one or more parts of the GCS cannot be assessed, e.g. when both eyes are closed by swelling, or the patient is intubated, or in a young child or someone with learning difficulties. However, the other components can still be assessed.

Using the Glasgow Coma Scale data

The GCS quantifies the altered consciousness level, which is crucial in making triage decisions about the facilities and personnel needed by the patient. For example, coma is defined in terms of the GCS as a state in which the patient does not eye open to any stimulus, does not obey commands and does not speak – clearly a state requiring urgent and skilled attention.

A single set of GCS observations gives only a snapshot of overall brain function. This should be repeated as often as clinically appropriate to establish and monitor the trend, recording the data on the patient's neurological observation chart. For example, a seriously head-injured patient in the resuscitation room might need observations every 10–15 min to detect change as soon as possible, whereas a patient who remains well 24 h after uncomplicated intracranial surgery might merit recordings only every 6–8 h.

Numbers rather than words can be assigned to the components of the GCS, and added to form a GCS score. However, these numbers were only introduced to ease data handling during research on large numbers of head-injured patients, and it is recommended that they are not used for individual patient assessment. Wrong numbers may be assigned to particular responses and the mistake is then passed on down the clinical line. Except at the extremes of the GCS there is always more than one way to add up three numbers to form a GCS score, introducing unwanted ambiguity when the aim is for clarity of communication. If part of the GCS is untestable (as described above), assessment can only be made by words, not numbers.

The level of consciousness should be monitored from an early stage in a patient in whom it is clearly abnormal, or in whom there is a significant risk of deterioration (e.g. after a head injury or when sedative medication has been given). As well as making the measurements and recording them on a chart, it is crucial to respond to any changes that they show, especially deterioration. This is discussed in more detail in the next section.

Emergency management of altered consciousness

The management of a patient with altered consciousness must always begin with the basics. The ABC (airway, breathing and circulation) system of priorities is used to assess and if necessary resuscitate vital functions before any neurological assessment is made. The airway is assessed, cleared if obstructed, and then protected from further hazard. High-flow oxygen is given and the blood oxygen saturation is monitored by pulse oximetry until arterial blood gas levels are known. In an injured patient the cervical spine must be protected throughout all airway manoeuvres. The adequacy of respiratory effort is assessed, and supported if needed, treating any complication such as a pneumothorax. The circulating volume is assessed by simple clinical means, and if there is evidence of shock, vigorous fluid resuscitation is begun, blood is cross-matched, and the cause of the shock (e.g. traumatic haemorrhage, major sepsis) is identified and treated. The early management of the head-injured patient is described elsewhere [**see Module 4, Vol. I**], as is the management of the surgical patient in a collapsed condition [**see Module 6, Vol. I**].

Only when these first steps have been taken is any assessment made of conscious level and other neurological features (e.g. pupil size and reaction, limb asymmetry) to establish the extent to which brain function has been disordered by the disease process. This order of priorities emphasizes the vulnerability of the brain to hypoxia and ischaemia after major pathological events such as a head injury.

Beyond this and the assessment of neurological function using the GCS and other simple measures, the management of the patient with altered consciousness is largely about managing the underlying disease process or injury. The effectiveness or otherwise of treatment is often mirrored in the trend of the consciousness level.

Section 14.2 • Head injuries and their management

Serious head injury, either in isolation or as part of multisystem injury, is a common surgical condition, responsible each year in the UK for over 100 000 admissions to hospital and 10 000 transfers to neurosurgical units. Almost a million others with minor injuries go home from the accident and emergency (A&E) department after assessment and first-aid treatment.

Not surprisingly, most interest centres on the 1% with the most serious injuries, whose mean age is 25–30 years, and who are usually the victims of road traffic accidents, falls or assaults. They inevitably pass through the hands of doctors in several specialties, who must understand the clinical chain of management and the need for good communication. Potentially lethal complications can develop quickly, and while the outcome may depend on getting the patient to the neurosurgeon quickly, sound assessment and management principles must be applied from the start in all cases of severe head injury.

Pathophysiology of traumatic brain injury

Primary and secondary brain damage
Brain damage from head injury is either immediate (primary) or delayed (secondary). Primary brain damage (impact injury) is irreversible, underlining the importance of prevention (e.g. seat belts, alcohol laws). Secondary brain damage (the second insult) is, by definition, the result of complications that occur at some stage after injury, and the aim of treatment from start to finish is to pre-empt or at least to limit their effect. Often what is needed is relatively simple, but it may need to be done quickly.

Primary brain damage
At the moment of injury energy is transferred to the brain and damages neurons (especially their axons) and small blood vessels. The amount of energy determines the amount of damage and the clinical picture ranges from brief concussion to instant death. The term diffuse axonal injury is sometimes used to describe these effects, but some areas (e.g. brainstem, corpus callosum) seem particularly vulnerable. MRI shows local changes in brain water of maximal damage, but practical considerations limit its use in the acute management of head injury.

Secondary brain damage
This can be due to intracranial or extracranial factors, which often interact (Figure 14.2). **The final common pathway is a reduced oxygen supply to the injured neurons, which are highly vulnerable to this further insult and can be damaged beyond hope of recovery.** Not only do they lack a key metabolic fuel but the reduced oxygen supply leads to a hostile microenvironment rich in free radicals and metabolic end-products, which further damages them. It is impossible to overstate the importance of maintaining adequate cerebral perfusion and oxygenation after head injury.

Systemic hypoxaemia and hypercarbia are most often caused by airway compromise or inadequate respiration. These common complications can occur insidiously at any stage after injury and continuing vigilance is needed to detect them.

Normal ICP is 5–15 mmHg, mean arterial blood pressure (MAP) is 80–90 mmHg and the cerebral perfusion pressure (CPP) is the difference between them. After brain injury, autoregulatory mechanisms are lost and the blood flow to the brain then varies in a linear way with CPP. Cerebral perfusion (and hence oxygenation) therefore falls when ICP rises (e.g. haematoma) or MAP falls (e.g. systemic shock).

The skull is a rigid box of bone with little room, and ICP soon rises dramatically with vascular engorgement from hypercarbia, or as an expanding haematoma grows larger (Figure 14.3), or as large areas of contused brain swell as water follows ions and molecules through the

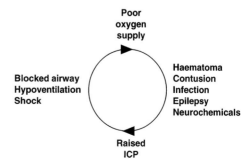

Figure 14.2 Secondary brain damage: continuing damage to neurons.

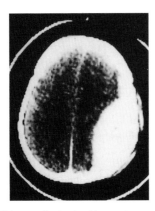

Figure 14.3 CT scan of extradural haematoma.

damaged blood–brain barrier into the interstitial spaces and across cell membranes damaged by trauma or hypoxia.

At the very time that its oxygen supply is most vulnerable, the brain's metabolic requirement for oxygen can be raised by the consequences of injury, e.g. seizures and intracranial infection. Neurotransmitters and free radicals in the 'neurochemical soup' around injured neurons can further damage them by squandering their energy stores or by damaging the integrity of the cell membrane. There is current interest in developing drugs to protect neurons against this.

The following examples illustrate how extracranial and intracranial factors interact to cause secondary brain damage.

▪ When airway obstruction or a pneumothorax causes hypoxaemia and hypercarbia, the injured and hypoxic brain swells, ICP rises, and cerebral perfusion and oxygenation fall. Preventing secondary damage requires attention to the airway and breathing.

▪ A similar sequence of events is seen when extracranial blood loss lowers the CPP; control of haemorrhage and fluid resuscitation then become crucial.

▪ An intracranial haematoma compresses the brain, raises ICP, lowers conscious level, and compromises the airway and breathing. Preventing secondary damage requires not only support of the airway and respiration but also timely intracranial surgery.

Clinical and radiological assessment

Initial assessment and resuscitation: ABC

The priority in every seriously injured patient is to support the oxygenation and perfusion of vital organs, including the brain. The widely used ATLS course teaches a system in which the airway (A), breathing (B) and circulation (C) are assessed and if necessary treated, **in that order**, even in the most obviously head-injured patient. Only then does assessment turn to 'D

for disability' (the neurological assessment) and consideration of the actual head injuries, the need for further investigation and the decision whether to discharge, observe in hospital or refer for a neurosurgical opinion.

Assessing and managing the airway, breathing, and circulation in the injured patient are discussed in **Modules 4 and 19, Vol. I**. Only points specific to head injury will be considered here.

Airway, breathing and circulation
When assessing and securing the airway, care must be taken to protect the cervical spine, to minimize the risk of further harm during airway manoeuvres such as intubation, which is particularly important in those too obtunded to report pain from spinal trauma. There should be no hesitation in intubating a head-injured patient if that is needed to maintain a patent airway and oxygenate the patient, but a decision to intubate is also a decision to ventilate, using short-acting sedative and muscle-relaxant drugs as necessary.

The coincidence of severe head and chest injuries has a treacherous reputation precisely because severe hypoxaemia and hypercarbia can then threaten secondary brain damage.

Fluid resuscitation and control of haemorrhage are both important to preserve cerebral perfusion. The current vogue for hypovolaemic resuscitation after penetrating trunk injury is less relevant to the more usual UK scenario of multisystem blunt injury, and fluid resuscitation should be vigorous and prompt. In the early hours after injury the concern is not about waterlogging the brain but about adequately replacing blood loss.

An isolated head injury virtually never causes shock, so a clinical diagnosis of shock should prompt a thorough search for extracranial sources of blood loss. External bleeding is usually obvious and can be controlled by pressure, but internal haemorrhage needs a high index of suspicion and careful clinical and radiological assessment, especially in the unconscious patient. The mechanism of injury may be suggestive, e.g. pedestrian road accident, fall from a height. Exsanguinating injuries must be dealt with as a priority: laparotomy or external pelvic fixation takes precedence over craniotomy.

Neurological assessment

There is no need for lengthy or detailed neurological assessment. A mini-neurological examination of conscious level, pupils and limb movements is enough to measure the effects of the head injury and guide decisions about investigation and treatment priorities. Assessments must be repeated at frequent intervals, to monitor progress and provide early warning of neurological deterioration so that appropriate action can be taken.

Conscious level
The GCS is a simple yet powerful clinical tool for measuring consciousness level in any condition. It is as useful for doctors and nurses in A&E departments,

surgical wards and intensive care units (ICUs) as for those who work in neurosurgical units.

The GCS score out of 15 at the time of first assessment can be used to determine the seriousness of a head injury:

- **minor** (15)
- **mild** (13–14)
- **moderate** (9–12)
- **severe** (<8).

As well as providing a snapshot of the patient's global brain function, the GCS is used to monitor progress over time. If the recordings are getting worse, so is the patient and the cause needs to be found quickly. Observations are therefore repeated at appropriate intervals to establish a trend, and the information is charted graphically. In a deteriorating patient conscious level almost always changes before focal signs develop, so the GCS is a valuable early-warning system.

Pupil and limb responses
There are many reasons other than a head injury why a patient might have pupils of unequal size or response to light (e.g. local trauma to the eye, previous eye disease or surgery), but after head injury the worst must be assumed and acted upon. Limb responses should be elicited by equal stimuli (verbal in a conscious patient, painful in an unconscious one) to the two sides. As with the pupils, any asymmetry should be ascribed to the head injury and appropriate action taken.

Clinical assessment of injuries
A detailed clinical examination of the head should be made, looking for external evidence of injury. A boggy haematoma or full-thickness laceration of the scalp suggests an underlying skull fracture. Extensive scalp wounds (e.g. degloving injuries) can cause serious blood loss and need to be dealt with under 'C for circulation'. External pressure controls nearly all scalp bleeding, allowing surgical repair to be deferred to a convenient time. Beware the unimpressive scalp injury that might have been caused by a sharp object; the brain may also have been penetrated.

Some skull fractures can be diagnosed clinically. The force needed to fracture the skull base also tears adjacent mucous membranes, and the result is a periorbital haematoma, haemotympanum (seen on auroscopy), mastoid haematoma (Battle's sign) or leak of cerebrospinal fluid (CSF) from the nose or ear. A piece of skull broken off and displaced inwards by a hard object such as a hammer constitutes a depressed fracture, and the overlying scalp wound may contain visible bone fragments or even brain tissue.

Radiology: which investigation for which patient?
Head-injured patients at real risk of intracranial complications need to be urgently identified and treated. There is good evidence that pre-emptive investigation gives better results than awaiting clinical deterioration.

Table 14.1 Risks of intracranial haematoma according to clinical and X-ray features

GCS	Risk	Other features	Risk
15	1:3615	None	1:31 300
		Post-traumatic amnesia (PTA)	1:6700
		Skull fracture	1:81
		Skull fracture and PTA	1:29
9–14	1:51	No fracture	1:180
		Skull fracture	1:5
3–8	1: 7	No fracture	1:27
		Skull fracture	1:4

The risk of haematoma can be stratified by the conscious level and/or skull film appearances (Table 14.1), but the threshold for computed tomographic (CT) scanning continues to fall.

Skull films: showing a fracture
Plain skull films have no added value when a clinical decision has already been made that the patient should have a CT scan, but a skull series (anteroposterior, lateral and Towne's view) is still a useful triage tool in small or remote hospitals, and in some larger hospitals outside normal working hours. It is crucial to demonstrate a fracture in a conscious patient who would otherwise be discharged from the A&E department, and who should instead be admitted for close observation or sent for a CT scan. The factors determining the need for skull films include the mechanism of injury, the amount of scalp injury and the neurological findings.

A skull fracture can be missed because the clinician who reads it is inexperienced, the film is blurred owing to patient movement during the exposure or too few views have been taken. A linear fracture forms a sharp-edged straight line across the skull vault where no markings should be seen. A depressed fracture causes a 'double density' as the bone fragment is seen through the skull vault, and is best seen on a tangential view. Occasionally, a stab wound is seen as a 'slot' fracture on plain films, but this is easy to miss if the history is misleading or the entry wound apparently trivial.

Computed tomographic scanning: imaging the brain
CT scanning reveals haematomas and areas of contused and swollen brain, which have different radiodensity from normal intracranial structures. Its chief value is as a means of distinguishing patients at high and low risk of deterioration from intracranial causes, so that they can be sent to the most appropriate facility.

An extradural haematoma forms when a fracture tears the middle meningeal artery, releasing blood under arterial pressure into the potential space between the skull and the dura to form a rapidly expanding lens-shaped haematoma, which compresses and distorts

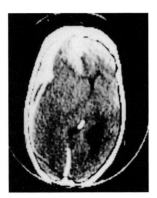

Figure 14.4 Subdural haematoma associated with intracerebral damage.

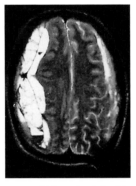

Figure 14.5 MRI scan of bilateral subdural haematomas. Note septa in the subdural space and the different colour suggesting different ages of clot.

the brain (Figure 14.4). An acute subdural haematoma results from a tear of a bridging vein from the cerebral cortex to the superior sagittal sinus, and the clot often extends over and compresses the whole surface of a cerebral hemisphere (Figure 14.5). Trauma to small brain vessels causes an intracerebral haematoma, usually in a frontal or temporal lobe, often forming a 'burst lobe' with disrupted brain tissue (Figure 14.6). Less extensive disruption of local anatomy produces a cerebral contusion of variable size and effects, whose patchy signal change on CT scan reflects the mixture of blood and damaged brain tissue.

Planning a course of action

Severe head injury

Severe head injury is defined in terms of a GCS score of <8, an intracranial haematoma needing surgery or a penetrating injury. Only 1% of head-injured patients have had a severe head injury, but the obvious threat to their life and well-being demands attention. Surgeons must be involved in assessing and treating these patients from an early stage.

Actual or potential complications must be identified promptly and treated effectively. As described previously, immediate and continuing support is needed, to protect cerebral perfusion and oxygenation during assessment, treatment and transfer.

Clinical priorities

A severe head injury may be isolated or form a part of multisystem injury. Determining the best order of treatment priorities is crucial and is defined by the ABCDE system. Securing the airway always comes first in order to guarantee cerebral oxygenation. Stopping major haemorrhage is always a higher surgical priority than opening the head, or else the patient will suffer irreparable ischaemic brain damage before the neurosurgeon can intervene to correct the intracranial pathology. Senior surgical specialists should be involved at an early stage in making these clinical decisions.

Emergency computed tomographic scan

After initial assessment and resuscitation every severely head-injured patient should have a CT scan as soon as possible, to define whether they need intracranial surgery and if so how urgently. Until recently, this almost always involved transfer to a neurosurgical unit, but nowadays it can often be done in the general hospital and this helps to shape decisions about the need for (and the timing of) transfer to neurosurgical care.

A patient with an intracranial haematoma can deteriorate quickly and the outcome is best when it is surgically removed before this happens. Time is clearly of the essence and the best policy is pre-emptive CT scanning of patients at significant risk of a haematoma

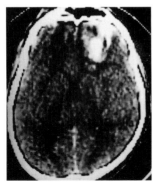

Figure 14.6 Traumatic intracerebral haematoma.

Table 14.2 Clinical features that warrant admission to hospital after head injury

- A history of loss of consciousness
- Persistent post-traumatic amnesia
- A seizure
- Irritability or altered behaviour
- Nausea and vomiting
- Anything that makes it difficult to assess the pupils or limb function
- A suspected full-thickness scalp wound
- Clinical evidence of a skull fracture

(Table 14.1) followed by speedy surgery in positive cases. Repeated neurological assessment is essential to monitor progress in these ill patients.

Clearly, part of this process is contact with the neurosurgical unit. The need for transfer should be discussed with a neurosurgeon:

- when a CT scan in a general hospital shows a recent intracranial lesion (image transfer facilities can be useful)
- when CT scanning should be carried out, but cannot be done in reasonable time
- when clinical features give cause for concern that urgent neurosurgical assessment or treatment may be required, e.g.
    - (i) GCS score deteriorating after admission
    - (ii) persisting coma (GCS score 8 or less) after initial resuscitation
    - (iii) progressive focal neurological signs
    - (iv) a seizure
    - (v) confusion, which persists for more than 6–8 h
    - (vi) compound depressed skull fracture
    - (vii) definite or suspected penetrating injury
    - (viii) a CSF leak.

Whether or not referral actually leads to transfer depends on the individual clinical details, what the scan shows (if one has been done) and the neurosurgical unit's policy on how to manage patients with a severe brain injury not needing operation. Transfer and management at the neurosurgical unit are dealt with later.

Moderate and mild head injury

For every patient with a severe head injury 100 with a much less serious one are seen at hospital. Most do not need sophisticated imaging or transfer to a neurosurgical centre, but none should be lightly dismissed. A few are destined to develop serious complications and a reliable way is needed to detect these in time to allow intervention. The key issues are who to admit, how to monitor them, how to recognize and respond to deterioration, and when to discharge the vast majority who make uneventful progress.

Deciding on admission

Every head-injured patient should have a mini-neurological examination in the A&E department. Those with an altered consciousness level or other neurological features (Table 14.2) should then undergo a period of observation in hospital, so that any symptoms or signs of increasing ICP or delayed intracranial infection can be detected and treated early. Admission to hospital may also be needed if there is no reliable history or if there are other medical or social problems, e.g. extracranial injuries, Warfarin therapy, alcohol misuse or concern about lack of supervision at home.

Clinical observation in hospital

After the patient is admitted to the surgical ward or short-stay unit, repeated assessments should be carried out by staff familiar with the care of head-injured patients, who understand the need to seek help early if deterioration occurs. High standards of verbal and written communication are essential.

Nurses should monitor conscious level by the GCS, using a modified scale for children aged under 5 years to reflect their developmental immaturity. They should also measure and record pupil size and reaction to light, limb movements, respiratory rate, pulse rate, blood pressure and temperature. The frequency of assessments is tailored to the estimated risk of intracranial damage, taking account of time elapsed since injury, GCS score, neurological progress, evidence of skull fracture and special risk factors such as anticoagulant therapy. Patients with an initial GCS score less than 13 or a skull fracture should be assessed at least every 15 min until conscious level becomes normal, then hourly. Those with an isolated mild head injury but an abnormal CT scan should be assessed at 30-min intervals in A&E, on admission, then hourly for at least 12 h.

Patients thought to be under the influence of alcohol or other drugs need very careful observation. The assumption that the drug is the cause of deterioration or failure to improve must be resisted. If the alcohol level is below 200 mg% (43.5 mmol/l), persistent confusion and inability to obey commands warrants an urgent CT scan.

Recognizing deterioration

The GCS gives the earliest warning of neurological deterioration. Urgent reappraisal by an experienced doctor is needed if there is any fall in the GCS (other than the normal diurnal variation in eye opening), increasing headache, persistent vomiting, new neurological symptoms, or a new neurological sign such as limb or facial asymmetry or pupil inequality. The immediate management of deterioration is discussed below.

Even if the patient remains well, a doctor should carry out an assessment at least once in the first 24 h after admission, looking at consciousness level, limb power, signs of skull base fracture, cranial nerves, speech and cognitive function.

Planning discharge

Before discharge a patient with mild or moderate head injury must be assessed by an experienced doctor, to establish that all necessary criteria have been met (Table 14.3).

Every patient sent home should be given a Head Injury Instruction Card, and a friend or relative must take responsibility for continuing to monitor further progress and reporting persistent or deteriorating symptoms. Enquiries about general health and home circumstances are important in the elderly, whose medication may also have contributed to a fall. A referral to the geriatric service may be appropriate for further assessment and management before discharge, and to reduce the future risk of injury. The possibility of

Table 14.3 Checklist for safe discharge after a mild or moderate head injury

- The GCS score has been 15 for at least 12 h
- The patient is eating normally and not vomiting
- All neurological symptoms/signs have resolved, or are resolving and minor, e.g.
  - mild localized headache relieved by simple analgesia
  - anosmia from olfactory nerve damage
  - momentary positional vertigo due to vestibular disturbance
- The patient is mobile and self-caring, or going to a safe and supported environment
- There is no skull fracture or CT abnormality that warrants further observation
- Extracranial injury has been excluded or treated

child abuse should be considered in injured young children when the findings are not consistent with the explanation given or the family is known to be on the 'at-risk' register. The duty social worker should be consulted to allow early investigation while observation continues on a paediatric ward.

Safe transfer to definitive care

Even a short journey is potentially risky for a seriously head-injured patient, and must be taken seriously. It must not begin until all life-threatening injuries have been identified and stabilized.

A seriously head-injured patient should be intubated and ventilated before transfer, to ensure a clear and protected airway, adequate oxygen delivery, adequate ventilation and prevention of hypercarbia. Cardiovascular care requires reliable intravenous access, adequate fluid resuscitation and the same minimum standards of monitoring as in an operating theatre (electrocardiography, invasive blood pressure monitoring, pulse oximetry).

Every seriously head-injured patient must be accompanied by a doctor able to guarantee the airway – anaesthetic skills and training are obviously desirable – assisted by a trained nurse or paramedic. They are professionally responsible for the patient's care during transfer and for ensuring a proper handover to the neurosurgical team.

Management at the neurosurgical unit

Ideally, a patient with severe diffuse brain injury is admitted to an ICU under joint neurosurgical and neuroanaesthetic care. Some neurosurgeons believe that patients who do not need operative intervention should not be exposed to the potential hazards of transfer to a neurosurgical ICU, but the best results in these patients are likely to be obtained by clinicians with an adequate caseload and an interest in this difficult and common problem. The hazards of transfer can certainly be overcome.

Intracranial pressure monitoring

Continuous measurement of ICP over several days can be helpful in:

- patients with borderline haematomas on the CT scan, which may need surgical evacuation if the ICP is shown to be high or rising
- patients with no focal lesion on the initial scan who will be ventilated with sedative and relaxant drugs, as some will develop delayed brain lesions.

Its clinical value is greatly enhanced when the data are linked to other information, e.g. MAP, cerebral blood flow velocity and cerebral oxygen extraction. The details of neurointensive care after head injury are beyond the scope of this chapter.

Craniotomy for the evacuation of traumatic intracranial haematomas

The decision as to whether or not to operate is based on the patient's clinical condition and the type, size and position of the haematoma as revealed by CT scanning. The details of intracranial surgery are beyond the scope of this chapter [**see Neurosurgery, Vol. II**]. Small haematomas or contusions are monitored at the neurosurgical unit by serial CT scans and/or ICP monitoring, and the minority, which cause or threaten delayed deterioration, are removed.

Compound and penetrating injuries

Some types of head injury cause actual or potential penetration of the brain (Figure 14.7). As with closed injuries the patient can suffer primary brain damage or develop a haematoma, but a special risk is secondary brain damage from delayed intracranial infection. Depressed fractures and penetrating brain injuries also carry a high risk of post-traumatic epilepsy, even when early care has been excellent.

Dealing with early crises

Early deterioration after head injury is common and can frighten the inexperienced. The correct response is to apply the same principles used during initial assessment and resuscitation, and to call for skilled help early.

If consciousness level falls, a new neurological symptom or sign appears, or severe vomiting or headache develops, the first step is to ensure a clear airway and high-flow oxygen. Breathing problems may be due to a new tension pneumothorax. Clinical signs of shock in a head-injured patient should be assumed to be due to hypovolaemia from extracranial injuries. Electrolyte imbalance and hypoglycaemia should also be considered. Resuscitation continues while anaesthetic help and neurosurgical advice are sought.

Fits

Most fits do not call for emergency drug treatment. The patient should be protected from the risk of further injury from convulsive movements, the airway secured if not already done, and high-flow oxygen given to prevent secondary brain damage.

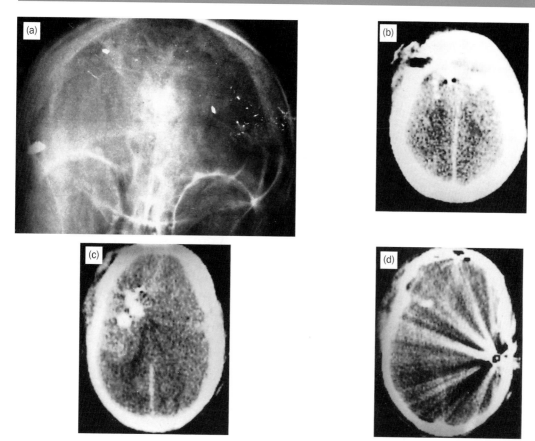

Figure 14.7 (a) Side-to-side gunshot wound with entrance in the left frontotemporal area. Metallic fragments spread intracranially. (b–d) CT scans of the same patient showing the extent of injury from the right frontotemporal to the left parietal regions. The metallic fragments cause the sun-ray appearance.

Restlessness

Restlessness is a symptom, not a diagnosis. It may be due to pain or hypoxia, and these should be treated. Controlled doses of opiates can be used to relieve pain, titrating the dose against the clinical response and recording the amount and timing of all doses. A thrashing patient should not be pinned to the trolley or bed, as this only worsens restlessness and increases the risk of cervical spine injury. A semirigid cervical collar is used on its own until the cause of the restlessness can be identified and corrected.

Conclusion

Most head-injured patients make an uneventful recovery. For those with a more serious injury the quality of the long-term outcome depends heavily on the quality of early care. Many of them have sequelae for long afterwards, and sometimes for life. Although it is not the responsibility of the surgeon to deal with these, we should never forget that head-injury care does not end at the operating theatre or on discharge from the surgical ward.

The patient with cancer

In the vast majority of the common cancers, surgery remains the definitive treatment and offers the only realistic chance of cure. Nevertheless, it is now clear that optimal cancer treatment requires multidisciplinary working, where the surgeon co-operates with colleagues in other disciplines. In this module, the biology and treatment of cancer are covered, and although organ-specific examples are given where appropriate, emphasis is placed on generic principles. Non-surgical approaches to cancer are given some prominence and their implications for the surgeon are highlighted.

The term 'tumour' refers to any swelling in the body, although by common usage it has come to mean neoplasia, benign or malignant. Neoplasia in turn can be defined as an abnormal mass of tissue where the rate of cellular growth exceeds and is no longer co-ordinated with that of the normal tissue from which it has arisen. Oncology, derived from the word *oncos* (Greek: a mass) is the study of tumours, and clinicians who deal exclusively with cancer patients are known as oncologists. Confusingly, a clinical oncologist delivers both radiotherapy, and chemotherapy while a medical oncologist specializes in chemotherapy alone. Surgical oncology is a rather misleading term, as no surgeon would be expected to deal with every type of tumour, and surgeons whose practice embraces cancer will also treat patients with benign disease within their specialty. Nevertheless, surgical oncology has become an important academic discipline, as the principles of cancer surgery are largely universal and transcend specialty barriers.

The term 'cancer' (Latin: a crab) refers specifically to malignant tumours that are characterized by their propensity to infiltrate locally, often giving rise to a spiculated, crab-like shape, and to metastasize. Usually, the distinction between malignant and benign tumours is easy to make both histologically and clinically. However, there are a few situations where this is not the case. Some rare tumours, particularly sarcomas, can be difficult to classify as benign or malignant at a histological level. Some other tumours (basal cell carcinoma is a good example) invade locally but do not metastasize, and malignant tumours of the brain do not metastasize outside the central nervous system.

Dysplasia is characterized by increased cell proliferation and abnormalities in cell size, configuration and orientation. There is, in addition, an increase in the nucleocytoplasmic ratio, loss of polarity, pseudo-stratification and reduction in mucus secretion. Dysplasia is graded histopathologically into mild, moderate and severe. Severe dysplasia is essentially synonymous with in situ cancer. Both differ from intramucosal cancer in one respect only, that the process has not invaded the basement membrane. The risk of invasive cancer is small for mild and moderate dysplasia but is very high for severe dysplasia/*in situ* cancer. Thus, once confirmed by histology, severe dysplasia, irrespective of site always requires urgent treatment. Metaplasia is a change in the type of surface epithelium and is exemplified by the columnar cell change encountered in Barrett's oesophagus. The risk of malignancy in metaplastic epithelium becomes appreciable only when it undergoes dysplastic change. There are many other established premalignant conditions, e.g. atypical mammary hyperplasia and cervical dysplasia.

The patient with a tumour will present in may different ways depending on the site of the tumour and its extent. The patient with a breast tumour will usually notice the lump itself, whereas the patient with gastrointestinal cancer will have symptoms related to disturbance of normal gastrointestinal function such as vomiting, jaundice or change of bowel habit, and the patient with an intracranial tumour will have headache or a neurological deficit. Unfortunately, many patients present not with their primary tumour, but with the effects of metastatic disease, especially when symptoms have been ignored or neglected for a significant period.

In this module, a summary of the biology of neoplastic tumours is followed by sections on investigation, staging and treatment. Screening and early diagnosis are also considered, and the module ends with an appraisal of the role of supportive and palliative care.

Section 15.1 • Tumour biology

Carcinogenesis

In its widest sense, the term carcinogen implies any external influence that can be shown to cause cancer. Classically, carcinogenesis was divided into two steps: **initiation**, in which the cells were transformed into a state capable of producing a tumour, and **promotion**, which stimulated the initiated cells to form a neoplasm. It is now recognized that carcinogenesis is a multistep process and this model, although still relevant for some systems, has been largely abandoned.

The history of carcinogenesis started in 1761 when John Hill in London suggested that snuff might be responsible for nasal cancer. A few years later Percival Pott observed a high incidence of cancer of the scrotum in chimney sweeps and attributed this to exposure to soot. Little further progress was made until, in the late nineteenth century, it was recognized that exposure to industrial agents such as mining dust, paraffin oils and analine dyes were associated with cancer, and it soon became clear that X-rays and, to a lesser extent, sunlight were also hazardous. These epidemiological observations were backed up by experimental studies; Clunet in 1908 showed that X-rays could induce skin cancer in rats, and Yamagiwa in 1915 demonstrated a similar effect of coal tar applied to the ears of rabbits and the backs of mice.

Many carcinogens that affect humans have now been identified, and one of the most important is the polycylic aromatic hydrocarbon (PAH) group, which includes benzo(a)pyrene and 3-methylcholanthrene, both of which are found in tobacco smoke. The epidemiological evidence that smoking is by far the major cause of lung cancer is now incontrovertible, and this ties in well with the observed effect of the above compounds in experimental systems. A list of chemical and physical carcinogens is given in Table 15.1.

A competing theory of carcinogenesis focused on viruses. At the end of the nineteenth century, the 'germ' theory of disease was prevalent thanks to the work of Pasteur and others, and it was thought that

Table 15.2 Some viruses implicated in human cancer

Virus	Organ affected
Papillomavirus	Uterine cervix
Epstein–Barr virus	Nasopharynx, bone marrow
Hepatitis B and C viruses	Liver
Human T-cell leukaemia virus	Thymus, spleen

cancer could be caused by microorganisms. This was given impetus by the work of Peyton Rous, who showed that a virus could induce sarcomas in chickens, and there followed evidence that a number of viruses could cause tumours in animals. Of particular note are the Shope papilloma virus in rabbits, the mammary carcinoma and leukaemia viruses of mice, and the papovaviruses SV 40 and polyoma.

In humans, there is good evidence to link certain types of cancer to viruses, in particular cancer of the uterine cervix, Burkitt's lymphoma, nasopharyngeal cancer, hepatocellular cancer, T-cell leukaemia and Kaposi's sarcoma (Table 15.2). However, most human cancers lack the characteristic features of a transmissible, contagious disease, and it is possible that they do not involve viruses at all. Alternatively, it is possible that viruses may initiate tumorigenesis, but progression requires extra cofactors. If this were the case, there would be very little epidemiological evidence of transmissible disease.

It is now recognized that the basic underlying defect in the cancer cell is genetic, i.e. genes that are important in the regulation of cellular growth and proliferation are damaged or mutated. This provides a unifying theme for the carcinogenic properties of both physicochemical and viral agents. It is known that viruses can transform cells by introducing new genetic material that confers malignant properties on to the cell, and such material is known as an oncogene. As explained in the next section, it is now known that oncogenes are mutated normal genes; transforming viruses pick up these genes from previously infected malignant host cells and by carrying them to new host cells transfer the malignant phenotype. Physicochemical agents, however, may damage the appropriate genes *in situ*.

This is a rather simplistic view of carcinogenesis. The mutagenic activity of a substance can be measured using the 'Ames' test, in which a strain of *Salmonella typhimurium* is exposed to a potential mutagen, and then grown in the absence of an essential nutrient, histidine. In order to activate promutagens, which are only activated by mammalian metabolic systems, extracts of liver cells are added to the bacterial plates. A bacterium with a mutation in an enzyme that degrades histidine will have enough endogenous amino acid to grow, so the number of colonies that forms in the absence of exogenous histidine gives a quantitative measure of a substance's mutagenicity. Evidence that this is valid comes from striking correlations between the muta-

Table 15.1 Some well-recognized chemical and physical carcinogens implicated in human cancer

Carcinogen	Organ affected	Putative mechanism
UV light	Skin	Mutagenesis
X-rays	Bone marrow	Mutagenesis
Alcohol	Lung, oesophagus	Cytotoxicity
Aflatoxin	Liver	Mutagenesis
Asbestos	Lung, pleura	Cytotoxicity
Tobacco smoke	Lung, oesophagus	Mutagenesis
Oestrogen	Breast, endometrium	Stimulation of cell growth

genicity of compounds in the Ames test and their carcinogenic potential in animal systems.

However, many carcinogens are not mutagenic, and this has given rise to the concept of direct and indirect mutagenesis. Thus, some carcinogens damage DNA directly, whereas others are mutagenic because they place more cells at risk of mutagenesis by increasing the rate of DNA synthesis. It is also possible that carcinogens act by activating endogenous mutagens. Oxidants produced by cellular metabolism can damage DNA, and the rate at which these metabolic products are formed can be modulated by exogenous agents or inflammation.

The enzyme cyclo-oxygenase-2 (COX-2) is thought to be one of the central factors in the process of carcinogenesis mediated by oxidants. This enzyme can lead to genetic mutations or increased stability of mutations by virtue of prostaglandin synthesis and the production of free radicals. It is known to be overexpressed by many cancers, and its effects can be abrogated by antioxidants such as vitamins E and C. It is also interesting to note that non-steroidal anti-inflammatory drugs (NSAIDs), which inhibit COX-2, can prevent the formation of colorectal polyps and possibly cancer.

Diet is believed to have an important influence on cancer rates, and there is some evidence of dietary direct mutagens playing a significant role. Cooked meat contains heterocyclic amines, which have been shown to be highly mutagenic, but these can be inactivated by drug metabolizing enzymes that have evolved to protect the organism from the harmful effects of environmental chemicals. Thus, the genetic potential to express these enzymes is important in an individual's susceptibility to cancer. Furthermore, other environmental factors may modulate the expression of these enzymes, and as yet unidentified dietary factors may be important here.

Cancer rates tend to be inversely correlated with the intake of fruit and vegetables, and these foodstuffs are rich in antioxidants that may account for a protective effect. In addition, it is thought that certain vegetables can increase the expression of beneficial drug metabolizing enzymes. Energy intake may also play a role, as calorie restriction decreases the mitotic rate in many tissues and has been shown to reduce tumour incidence in animal studies. Thus, diet may influence tumour rates by exposing the organism to mutagens, by providing antioxidants to counteract mutagenic effects, not only of environmental mutagens but also of normal or modified cell metabolism, and by affecting the rate of cellular proliferation.

Molecular genetics of cancer

The development of cancer is now seen as a complex, multistep process which depends on both external carcinogenic influences and genetic defects. The genetic defects may be caused directly by mutagenic carcinogens, but may be inherited or may occur sporadically (perhaps induced by background radiation). Indeed, as outlined above, not all carcinogenic stimuli cause mutations; they may merely enhance cellular proliferation or survival so that the likelihood of a dangerous mutation occurring and persisting is increased. It is generally accepted, however, that genetic mutations are necessary before cancer can arise.

The genes associated with the development of malignancy when dysfunctional are broadly categorized as oncogenes or tumour suppressor genes, and although this classification may be imperfect, it is still a useful means of thinking about the genetic basis of cancer.

Oncogenes

Oncogenes were first identified when it was realized that the tumorigenicity of many retroviruses could be attributed to specific genes, and the first of these to be cloned was v-src from the Rous sarcoma virus, which causes sarcomas in chickens. It was then discovered that chicken deoxyribose nucleic acid (DNA) contains a very close relative of v-src, and that similar versions of the same gene are present in the DNA of other vertebrates. Thus, it was realized that the retroviral genes that can transform normal cells into cancer cells (i.e. oncogenes) are actually derived from normal cellular genes. These normal genes are now known as proto-oncogenes, and may become oncogenes either by incorporation into the genetic material of a retrovirus or, more commonly, by mutation at their normal site of residence within the cellular DNA.

Because, by definition, an oncogene confers malignant properties on to a cell, mutation of a proto-oncogene generally results in gain of function; this may occur by amplification where the affected gene overproduces a protein that drives cell proliferation or enhances survival, or it may occur by production of a mutant protein that escapes control mechanisms that normally constrain its proliferative activity. It follows that proto-oncogenes encode proteins that stimulate cellular growth or survival, and these can be broadly categorized as growth factors, growth factor receptors, intracellular signal transducers (that transmit the signal from an activated receptor to the nucleus) and transcription factors [which induce protein synthesis by stimulating the DNA in the nucleus to produce messenger ribonucleic acid (mRNA)].

An oncogene (i.e. a mutated proto-oncogene) typically acts as a dominant gene, and so a mutation in one allele will be sufficient for it to become manifest. However, with few exceptions, oncogenes are not inherited, and usually contribute to the pathogenesis of cancer by somatic mutations within the cells of the target tissues. A list of oncogenes commonly implicated in human cancer is given in Table 15.3.

Tumour suppressor genes

In contrast to oncogenes, tumour suppressor genes, in their normal state, encode proteins that act to maintain cell numbers by suppressing proliferation or promoting loss. These genes become involved in the tumorigenic

Table 15.3 Some oncogenes commonly implicated in human cancer

Affected gene	Protein properties	Tumour types
K-ras	P21 GTPase	Colorectal, pancreatic and lung carcinomas; leukaemia
EGFR (erb-b)	Growth factor receptor	Many carcinomas, gliomas
neu (erb-b2)	Growth factor receptor	Breast, ovarian and other carcinomas
myc	Transcription factor	Burkitt's lymphoma, small-cell lung cancer, other carcinomas
CYCD1	Cyclin D	Breast and other carcinomas, B-cell lymphoma
ret	Receptor tyrosine kinase	Thyroid cancer
trk	Receptor tyrosine kinase	Colorectal cancer
hst	Growth factor	Gastric cancer
mdm2	P53 binding	Sarcomas

process when they sustain mutations that result in loss of function. In this case the normal gene tends to act in a dominant fashion, and only when both alleles are damaged will the effect of the mutant gene surface. Because of this, mutations in single alleles of tumour suppressor genes may be passed through the germ line, and virtually all of the genes that have been identified as being responsible for inherited cancer belong to this category. Sporadic loss of tumour suppressor function in a genetically normal individual can and does occur, but as this requires both alleles in a single cell to malfunction because of either mutation or deletion (loss), it occurs much less frequently than in an individual who has an inherited defect in all cells. The common human tumour suppressor genes are given in Table 15.4.

One of the most important tumour suppressor genes is the p53 gene. The product of this gene is a nuclear phosphoprotein (called p53 because of its molecular weight), which appears to occupy a pivotal role in deciding the fate of cells that have been stressed. It is activated by DNA damage, among other stimuli, and in turn activates cellular processes that culminate either in cell-cycle arrest or apoptosis (programmed cell death) (Figure 15.1). Thus, elimination of cells that have sustained genetic damage depends on functional p53, and damage to the p53 gene itself may allow cells bearing other mutant genes to proliferate unchecked.

Inherited cancer

Given that genetic mutations are central to the development of cancer it is hardly surprising that the occurrence of many cancers displays a familial tendency. Thus, the risk of developing colorectal cancer can be estimated on the basis of the number of affected first-degree relatives (Table 15.5). However, several hereditary forms of cancer are caused by a germ-line mutation of a gene which, as described above, is nearly always a tumour suppressor gene.

Colorectal cancer can be inherited, and one of the best known cancer family syndromes is familial adenomatous polyposis (FAP). This condition, which is inherited in an autosomal dominant fashion, is due to mutation of the APC (adenomatous polyposis coli) gene on chromosome 5 and presents as multiple adenomatous polyps in the colon and rectum. These usually appear in late teenage years and lead inevitably to the development of invasive colorectal cancer within one to three decades. It is therefore important to keep the first-degree relatives of affected individuals under close surveillance with flexible endoscopy, and to

Table 15.4 Some common tumour suppressor genes

Affected gene	Protein properties	Tumour types
p53	Stress response	Colorectal, breast, gastric and many other cancers
p16	Inhibition of cyclin-dependent kinases	Melanoma, glioblastoma, bladder cancer
WT1	Transcriptional repressor	Wilm's tumour
Rb-1	Transcriptional regulator	Retinoblastoma, osteosarcoma
APC	Unknown	Colorectal cancer
DCC	Cell adhesion	Colorectal cancer
hMSH2	DNA mismatch repair	Colorectal cancer
hMLH1	DNA mismatch repair	Colorectal cancer
hPMS1	DNA mismatch repair	Colorectal cancer
hPMS2	DNA mismatch repair	Colorectal cancer
BRCA1	Unknown	Breast and ovarian cancer
BRCA2	Unknown	Breast cancer

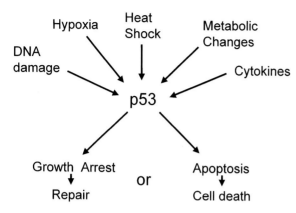

Figure 15.1 The p53 pathway.

Table 15.5 Risk of colorectal cancer and family history

Relatives affected	Lifetime risk of colorectal cancer
None	1/30
One first degree	1/17
One first and one second degree	1/10
One first degree under 45 years	1/8
Two first degree	1/3
Three first degree	1/2

carry out prophylactic proctocolectomy when the polyps appear. However, with the advent of mutation analysis it is now possible to look for the specific mutation in relatives, which will be a useful tool in the future.

Another dominantly inherited form of colorectal cancer is hereditary non-polyposis colorectal cancer (HNPCC), which is attributable to mutations in the DNA mismatch repair genes. This is more difficult to recognize in families than FAP as it lacks the characteristic premalignant phenotype, but it should be suspected when there are multiple cancers in a family or where there is a patient who has developed colorectal cancer at an unusually young age. FAP and HNPCC are covered in detail in Volume II [see Gastrointestinal Surgery, Vol. II].

Other forms of hereditary cancer include the rare eye cancer retinoblastoma, which occurs in childhood as a result of the transmission of an abnormal gene located on chromosome 13, and xeroderma pigmentosa, a condition brought about by failure of DNA repair mechanisms, which results in abnormal sensitivity of the skin to ultraviolet irradiation such that skin cancer is inevitable. Multiple endocrine neoplasia (MEN) types 1 and 2 are associated with abnormalities on chromosomes 11 and 10, respectively, and give rise to tumours of the thyroid and adrenal glands. A selection of well-established hereditary cancer syndromes is given in Table 15.6.

Tumour kinetics

Before considering tumour kinetics, it is very important to stress that a tumour is not entirely composed of cancer cells, and in some cases up to 50% of the tumour mass may be made up of non-malignant components or stroma. The stroma consists of fibrous tissue, fibroblasts, blood vessels, macrophages, lymphocytes, leucocytes, etc., and there is now good evidence that the stromal elements of a tumour are essential for its growth (see section on 'Invasion and metastases').

In addition to this heterogeneity, the cancer cells themselves differ within a single tumour, and it is conventional to divide them into three compartments:

Table 15.6 Hereditary cancer syndromes

Syndrome	Gene	Chromosomal location	Phenotypic expression
Breast/ovarian cancer syndrome	BRCA 1	17q12	Breast and ovarian cancer
FAP	APC	5q21	Colorectal cancer
Gardner's syndrome	APC	5q21	Colorectal cancer and osteomas, dermoids, tumours of the adrenal and thyroid glands
HNPCC	MLH1	3p21	Colorectal cancer
	MSH2	2p21	
Li Fraumeni syndrome	p53	17p13	Sarcomas, breast cancer, brain tumours
MEN 2 (Sipple's syndrome)	ret	10q11	Tumours of the thyroid and parathyroid, pheochromocytoma
MEN 1 (Wermer's syndrome)	?	11q13	Tumours of pancreas, parathyroid, pituitary, adrenals
Retinoblastoma	Rb	13q14	Tumour of the eye
Wilm's tumour	WT-1	11p13	Embryonal renal tumour
Xeroderma pigmentosa	Multiple		Skin cancer
von Hippel–Lindau syndrome	VHL		Tumours of kidney, brain, retina and pheochromocytoma

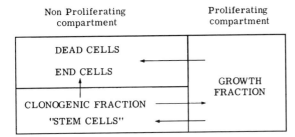

Figure 15.2 Cellular compartments in a malignant tumour.

the growth fraction, the clonogenic fraction and the end cell fraction (Figure 15.2). The growth fraction is composed of cells that are actively dividing, and it is this compartment that is responsible for the growth of the tumour. The clonogenic fraction is made up of non-proliferating cells that retain the capacity to divide if subjected to appropriate stimuli. This fraction is of considerable importance as, if the growth fraction is eliminated, e.g. by chemotherapy, which targets actively dividing cells, it is the clonogenic fraction that can repopulate the tumour by transferring cells into the depleted growth fraction. The end-cell fraction consists of cells that have lost all capacity to divide, and that are destined to die.

Cell death in tumours, as in normal tissue, is largely by apoptosis (Figure 15.3). This process, named after the Greek term for the shedding of leaves from trees, is a physiological process, which involves a series of genetically controlled steps including chromatin condensation and fragmentation and cell shrinkage. The resultant material is then engulfed by neighbouring cells without provoking an inflammatory response. In some tumours, however, a proportion of the cells die by lysis, which involves the inflammatory reaction, and areas of necrosis result.

Whatever the mechanism, cell death is extremely important in tumour biology and kinetics. The inability of certain tumour cell types to undergo apoptosis contributes to perpetuation of genetic instability, resistance to radiotherapy and chemotherapy, and rate of growth. In normal tissues, growth control is a balance between cellular proliferation and loss, and for many solid tumours, the rate of cell division may be less than the normal tissue counterpart. The growth of the tumour is therefore as likely to be due to a decrease in the rate of cell loss as to an increase in the rate of cell division, and the fact that cancer cells may divide more slowly than normal cells has considerable practical implications for the use of cytotoxic chemotherapy.

During the process of cell division, the cell goes through several distinct phases, known as G1 (first gap phase), S (synthetic phase), G2 (second gap phase) and mitosis (Figure 15.4). In G1, the cell synthesizes tissue proteins, which are necessary for the normal functioning of the cell. It then moves into the S phase, in which DNA replication takes place. There follows the second gap phase (G2), and the cell then goes into mitosis. Resting, or clonogenic, cells, which have withdrawn from the cell cycle, are said to be in G0 (Figure 15.4), and in normal cells this is usually induced by withdrawal of growth factors. In malignant cells, in contrast, growth factor deprivation rarely induces G0.

In order to ensure ordered cell replication, the cell cycle is tightly regulated so that one phase of the cycle is completed correctly before the next starts, and the mechanisms that ensure that this happens are known as checkpoint controls. For example, it is important that DNA replication is complete before mitosis starts, and if DNA is damaged, the cell will either go into cell cycle arrest until the damage is repaired or it will self-destruct by means of apoptosis. As outlined above, functional p53 protein is necessary for this checkpoint control to operate, and defects in the p53 system may account for a high proportion of cancers by promoting genetic instability. Another important checkpoint monitors the correct assembly of the mitotic spindle, which is important in maintaining the fidelity of chromosome transmission at mitosis, and failures of this checkpoint may account for the chromosomal instability observed in many human tumours.

Recently, there have been major advances in our understanding of the molecular mechanisms that drive the cell cycle, and there appear to be two types of protein of central importance. One is the **cyclin** family, so called because levels of these proteins vary throughout the cell cycle, and the other is a group of protein kinases which are regulated by the cyclins and are therefore known as **cyclin-dependent kinases**. These proteins regulate the different cell cycle transitions and may be influenced by signals from outside the cell; for example, growth factors activate the expression of cyclins which are necessary for the G1/S transition, and

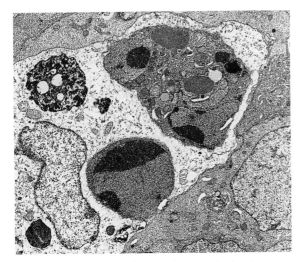

Figure 15.3 Electron micrograph of apoptosis showing apoptotic bodies in a macrophage.

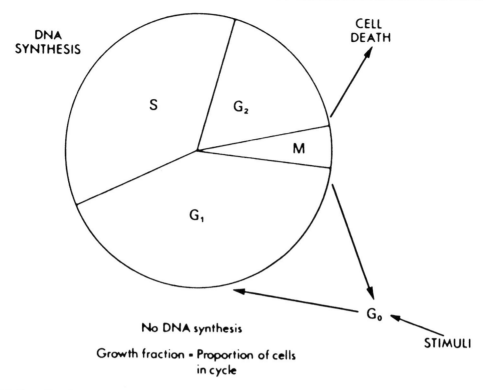

Figure 15.4 The cell cycle.

they can also regulate the expression of proteins which inhibit the activity of cyclin-dependent kinases. Defects in the cell cycle regulatory system and the way that it responds to external stimuli may be important in neoplasia, and genes which encode proteins that inhibit cyclin-dependent kinases are mutated in many cancers.

Thus, tumour development and progression are influenced by many factors, but once a tumour is established, it follows a fairly predictable growth pattern. Instead of expanding in a linear fashion with time, a tumour will normally follow a Gompertzian pattern, i.e. a small tumour grows rapidly, but as it increases in size its rate of growth decreases (Figure 15.5). This is due to a number of factors, including decreased blood supply, nutrition, necrosis and pressure effects. In addition, small tumours have large growth fractions, whereas larger tumours have correspondingly smaller growth fractions. Thus, it follows that a small tumour will be more susceptible to chemotherapy or radiotherapy than will a large tumour, which has important implications for adjuvant therapy and surgical debulking (see sections on 'Surgery' and 'Adjuvant therapy').

Invasion and metastases

The two characteristics of malignant tumours that define their behaviour are local invasion of surrounding tissues and metastatic spread to distant sites.

Invasion

Invasion is thought to occur by three main mechanisms:

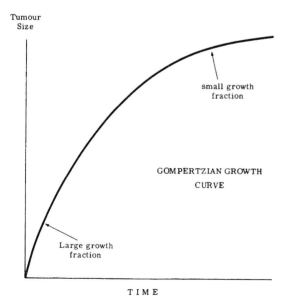

Figure 15.5 Gompertzian curve.

- mechanical pressure caused by rapid cellular proliferation

- increased or altered motility of the malignant cells
- breakdown of the extracellular matrix by proteolytic enzymes.

Although not universal, an increased rate of cellular proliferation is a common feature of malignancy, and this may occur as a consequence of abnormal expression of growth factors or their receptors as part of the malignant transformation. These mechanisms may also act in a paracrine manner to influence the non-tumour cell proliferation of fibroblasts, macrophages and other inflammatory cells that make up the stromal reaction associated with tumours. It must be stressed, however, that invasion can occur without a significant element of proliferation, and so the other mechanisms must come into play.

Tumour cells can dissociate from one another, and this has been shown both *in vitro* and *in vivo*. Such dissociation can be attributed to loss of cellular adhesion, and this is a common finding in all malignant or transformed cells. The mechanism whereby this loss of adhesion occurs appears, in part at least, to be due to the loss of cell membrane receptors for extracellular proteins that mediate adhesion, such as fibronectin and laminin. These receptors are part of a large family of cell surface receptors known as **integrins**, which are important for the attachment of cells to the extracellular matrix, and it is possible that loss of this ability allows migration of cells. In some tumour cells, however, integrins are overexpressed, for example melanoma cells express the $\alpha_v\beta_3$ integrin, and this may assist in the process of metastasis (see below). Altered cell adhesion can also be attributed to failure of production of the extracellular matrix glycoproteins.

Another widely observed aspect of malignant cells is increased motility, and abnormalities of the actin cytoskeleton have been implicated here. Disruption of the actin cytoskeleton is frequently observed in malignant cells, and it is both a target for modulation by certain oncogenes and susceptible to cell-surface proteolysis.

It is now widely accepted that proteolytic enzymes have an important role in the process of invasion, both at the point where a carcinoma *in situ* cell starts the process by transgressing the basement membrane, and later in the process, where a locally advanced tumour is infiltrating widely. Cathepsins and plasminogen activators have both been implicated, but the most important enzymes seem to be the metalloproteinases.

The metalloproteinases make up a family of at least 16 enzymes, the main function of which appears to be degradation of the extracellular matrix. Although some seem to be produced by tumour cells, most are actually synthesized by stromal cells in inactive forms, which are activated by factors on the surface of tumour cells, one of the most important of which appears to be a membrane-bound metalloproteinase. The metalloproteinases are overexpressed in nearly all invasive tumours, and play a crucial role in both invasion and metastasis.

Metastases

The process of metastasis is one of the prime features of malignancy, and implies the breaking off of cells or clumps of cells from the primary tumour, spread to a distant site and growth of secondary tumour at that site. Metastases can be disseminated by the blood, lymphatic system or they may spread throughout the pleural or peritoneal cavities. Malignant tumours of the central nervous system (CNS) do not metastasize in the conventional sense (i.e. to other parts of the body as above), but they spread through the cerebrospinal fluid.

Metastasis is a multistep process, and for it to occur, tumour cells must:

- proliferate
- invade
- enter the blood or lymphatic system
- survive and be transported in a viable form to a new (metastatic) site
- extravasate and proliferate at this new site.

Both experimental studies and those based on *in vivo* human tumours suggest that the formation of metastases is a selective event. Not all cells that enter the blood necessarily have the capacity to form metastases. Although this might in part be due to the destruction of circulating tumour cells by mechanical or immunological mechanisms, it seems that tumour cells are heterogeneous in this respect. This is borne out by the elegant studies of Fidler on the B16 melanoma cells, in which it was shown that only specific clones within a tumour were able to establish metastatic deposits.

The features of a malignant tumour that allow it to invade are also thought to be crucial for metastasis. Metastatic cells have been shown to be able to induce retraction of endothelial cells and thus allow entry into and extravasation from blood vessels, and it is thought that proteolytic enzymes, such as the metalloproteinases, are important in this process. Proteolysis contributes to loss of cell adhesion in the primary site of growth, and it is interesting that blood contains inhibitors of proteolysis, which may thus promote cell adhesion at a distant site. Once the cells have adhered to blood vessels at the site of metastatic growth, their proteolytic activity then facilitates extravasation into the organ and subsequent growth and invasion.

One consistent observation is that, although metastases can occur anywhere, some organs favour metastatic growth more than others. In addition, the site of the primary tumour has some bearing on the likelihood of metastatic spread to certain organs. The reasons underlying these phenomena are not clear, although the frequency of hepatic metastases from gastrointestinal tumours can be explained, at least in part, by the anatomy of the portal circulation. Liver, lung and bone are the most common metastatic sites and the predominant sites of tumours leading to disease in these organs are shown in Figure 15.6.

It used to be thought that carcinomas spread first to the local lymphatics, and only then entered the blood

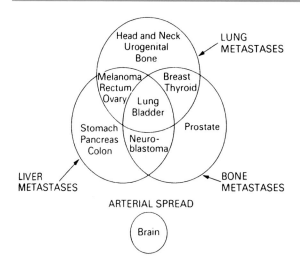

Figure 15.6 Predominant sites of tumours metastasizing to liver, lung and bone.

stream, but there is now abundant evidence that this theory is false. Although unusual, it is perfectly possible for blood-borne metastases to arise without demonstrable lymph-node involvement, and it has been shown that there are many connections between the lymphatic and venous systems and that cells can move freely between the two. In addition, randomized trials in breast cancer have shown that radical lymph-node dissection has no effect on the development of distant metastases, which would have been expected if metastatic spread had been an orderly progression from the lymphatic system to the circulation.

The central role of oncogenes and tumour suppressor genes has generated a great deal of interest in a possible metastasis gene which, when mutated, might confer metastatic potential on to a tumour. However, although some studies have shown that certain oncogenes are associated with a poor prognosis or advanced disease (e.g. ras oncogenes in breast and stomach cancer, and erb-β in breast cancer), there is no clear association with specific gene mutations and metastatic spread. This is perhaps not surprising as the properties that make a tumour invasive presumably also confer the ability to metastasize. There are however, oncogene transfection studies in animals that have been shown to permit metastasis in experimental situations, and it is possible that certain oncogene and tumour suppressor patterns are necessary before metastasis takes place.

To summarize, the factors that contribute to invasion and metastasis are illustrated in Figure 15.7.

Section 15.2 • Investigation and staging

When a patient is suspected of having cancer, it is likely that a series of investigations will be necessary, and if the diagnosis is correct, the tumour will be required to be staged in order to estimate prognosis and to plan treatment. In this section, the following subheadings will be considered:

- blood tests
- radiology
- endoscopy
- biopsy
- histological grading
- staging.

Blood tests

A full blood count is of the utmost importance in any patient suspected of cancer, as anaemia can occur as a result of blood loss (occult or otherwise), marrow infiltration by tumour or merely as a consequence of chronic disease. A hypochromic microcytic anaemia is highly suggestive of gastrointestinal malignancy, and in the absence of other symptoms a caecal carcinoma is the most likely.

Routine biochemistry is also important. Plasma urea and electrolyte estimations are necessary in any patient with acute or chronic illness who might require surgery, and in patients with advanced tumours there are special indications for these tests. For example, the patients with a large villous adenoma or carcinoma of the rectum may be potassium depleted because of mucous discharge, the patient with intestinal obstruction or pyloric stenosis may be dehydrated and potassium depleted, and the patient with ureteric obstruction from a pelvic tumour may have renal failure. Liver function tests should also be routine for the majority of cancer patients, as abnormalities, particularly in the alkaline phosphatase or gamma glutamyl transpeptidase, may indicate liver metastases. Alkaline phosphatase may also be elevated with bone metastases, and if there is any dubiety over a raised alkaline phosphatase, isoenzyme studies can determine whether the elevated enzyme is of liver or bone origin.

The most specific blood tests in cancer, however, are tumour markers. These are substances produced by the tumour that can be detected in the plasma, and they are useful for two reasons. Firstly, they may be helpful in diagnosis. Unfortunately, none of the common tumours have sufficiently sensitive and specific markers to be useful in screening, but the detection of a marker may focus investigation in a symptomatic patient. Secondly, they can be helpful in assessing response to treatment. If a tumour marker disappears after surgery, this is a good indication that there is no gross residual disease. Conversely, if a marker reappears and rises during follow-up this invariably points to recurrence. Tumour marker levels are also used in advanced disease as a surrogate index of response to chemotherapy, and this is particularly useful in phase I trials of new agents.

The most obvious markers are hormones secreted either by a tumour of endocrine origin or by a tumour which is an ectopic hormone producer. In this group, perhaps the most useful marker is the secretion of chorionic gonadotrophin by choriocarcinoma, as the amount of hormone secreted is directly related to the tumour mass.

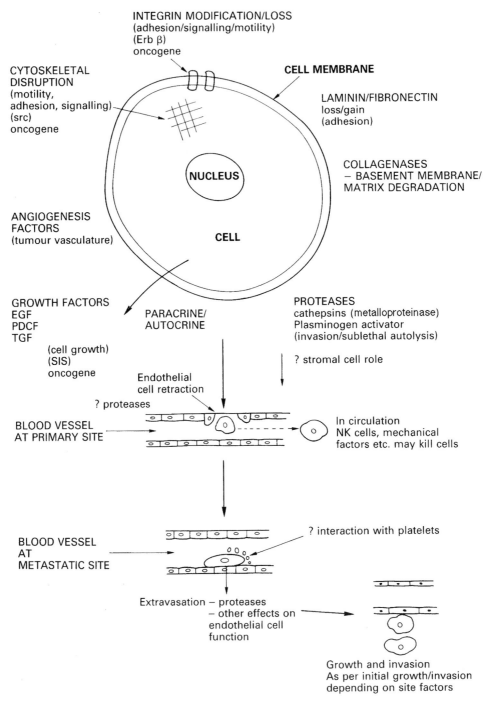

INTEGRIN MODIFICATION/LOSS
(adhesion/signalling/motility)
(Erb β)
oncogene

CELL MEMBRANE

CYTOSKELETAL
DISRUPTION
(motility,
adhesion, signalling)
(src)
oncogene

LAMININ/FIBRONECTIN
loss/gain
(adhesion)

NUCLEUS

COLLAGENASES
– BASEMENT MEMBRANE/
MATRIX DEGRADATION

ANGIOGENESIS
FACTORS
(tumour vasculature)

CELL

GROWTH FACTORS
EGF
PDCF
TGF
(cell growth)
(SIS)
oncogene

PARACRINE/
AUTOCRINE

PROTEASES
cathepsins (metalloproteinase)
Plasminogen activator
(invasion/sublethal autolysis)

? stromal cell role

Endothelial
cell retraction

? proteases

BLOOD VESSEL
AT PRIMARY SITE

In circulation
NK cells, mechanical
factors etc. may kill cells

BLOOD VESSEL
AT
METASTATIC SITE

? interaction with platelets

Extravasation – proteases
– other effects on
endothelial cell
function

Growth and invasion
As per initial growth/invasion
depending on site factors

Figure 15.7 Diagrammatic representation of events associated with invasion and metastasis.

Another type of tumour marker is the oncofetal proteins, glycoproteins so called because of their presence in fetal tissues. Carcinoembryonic antigen (CEA) was one of the first tumour markers to become widely available, and initially it was thought to be associated with colorectal carcinoma. However, it was subsequently shown that, although commonly elevated in this condition, CEA was not specific for large bowel cancer, and could also be raised in a variety of other cancers including pancreatic and breast carcinoma (and, indeed, in a number of benign conditions such as cirrhosis of the liver, viral hepatitis and cigarette smoking). Thus, CEA is of little value in diagnosis and its use is restricted to detection of recurrence and response to therapy.

Another oncofetal protein is α-fetoprotein (AFP), which is elevated in both hepatocellular cancer and testicular teratoma. Other useful markers are Ca 9–19 in gastrointestinal cancer, Ca 72.4 in gastric cancer and Ca

Table 15.7 Commonly used tumour markers

Tumour site	Marker
Colorectum	CEA
Gastrointestinal tract	Ca 9–19
Stomach	Ca 72.4
Ovary	Ca 125
Testis (teratoma)	AFP, βHCG
Prostate	PSA

125 in ovarian cancer. In prostate cancer, prostatic acid phosphatase was widely used, but this has be superseded by prostate-specific antigen (PSA). Commonly used tumour markers are summarized in Table 15.7.

Radiology

Radiological investigations have crucial roles in both the diagnosis and the staging of cancer, and can be considered under the subheadings of plain radiographs, contrast studies, cross-sectional imaging and radionuclide scanning.

Plain radiographs

The two situations where plain radiography is important diagnostically are assessment of the lung fields and in the detection of bone metastases. The posteroanterior and lateral chest X-rays are used to detect both primary bronchogenic carcinoma and pulmonary metastases. Skeletal radiographs display both osteolytic (Figure 15.8) and osteogenic bone metastases and are used to confirm suspected disease on isotope bone scans. They are also used in the diagnosis of primary bone tumours.

Contrast studies

Barium is used to image the whole of the gastrointestinal tract. A barium swallow is a useful means of assessing an oesophageal tumour and a barium meal may be used to diagnose gastric cancer. Both of these investigations have, however, been largely superseded by endoscopy, which has the advantage of allowing biopsy to confirm the diagnosis. Under certain circumstances, however, barium studies may be useful [see Vol. II]. The small bowel can be visualized by means of a follow-through examination or a small bowel enema, and the large bowel by a barium enema. The large bowel enema remains a vital diagnostic tool, particularly in countries (including the UK) where colonoscopy facilities are limited, and it should always be done as a double-contrast examination (i.e. barium and air) to allow scrutiny of mucosal detail (Figure 15.9).

Other situations where contrast is employed in cancer diagnosis include the intravenous urogram for delineating tumours of the urinary tract, and vascular contrast radiology to assess the blood supply in certain tumours. The uses of these modalities are limited, how-

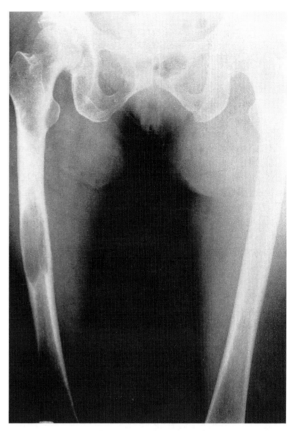

Figure 15.8 Osteolytic bone metastasis (from breast cancer).

ever, and replaced mostly by cross-sectional imaging or endoscopy. Biliary and pancreatic tumours can be studied by contrast, usually introduced directly by means of retrograde cannulation (see below) or by transhepatic puncture.

Cross-sectional imaging

The three cross-sectional imaging modalities used in cancer diagnosis and staging are ultrasound, computed tomography (CT) and magnetic resonance imaging (MRI).

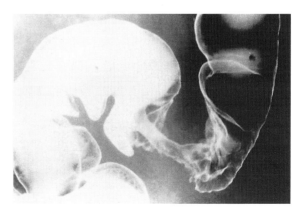

Figure 15.9 Barium enema showing typical 'apple core deformity' of colonic cancer.

Ultrasound

The principle of ultrasound imaging depends on differential reflection and attenuation of ultrasound waves by tissues. Fluid transmits ultrasound, producing a hypoechoic area, whereas tissue–fluid interfaces reflect. Both bone and gas reflect completely, and thus act as a barrier to ultrasound and limit the usefulness of the technique. In terms of cancer, ultrasound is useful in detecting liver metastases, and in obstructive jaundice, dilated intrahepatic ducts will be seen. Unfortunately, however, because of gas in the duodenum the head of the pancreas is often not well seen, and thus the diagnosis of pancreatic cancer can be difficult to make. Intra-abdominal masses can be evaluated, and the pelvic organs are clearly seen, making it a useful means of detecting ovarian cancer. Transvaginal ultrasound is better than transabdominal examination for the latter, and intraluminal ultrasound is also used to assess rectal and oesophageal tumours.

Intraoperative ultrasound (Figure 15.10) is being increasingly used for assessing liver metastases, and this can be done laparoscopically as well as at open surgery. Outside the abdomen, ultrasound can be used to distinguish between cysts and solid tumours in the breast and thyroid gland.

Ultrasound provides a real-time image during the examination, and the plane that is seen in cross-section depends on the angle at which the probe is held. It must be emphasized that, although a hard copy is usually obtained for records, the procedure is highly operator dependent, and a great deal of expertise is required for consistently good results.

Computed tomography

CT has a major role in cancer diagnosis. In CT the X-ray source and corresponding detectors rotate around the patient, and the computer software calculates the attenuation of the X-ray beam at each point within the part of the patient being scanned. This attenuation is expressed in arbitrary Hounsfield units (after one of the developers of CT), and the image produced when these units are reconstructed displays a cross-section of the patient's anatomy (Figure 15.11). The earlier machines built up a picture by carrying out individual sequential

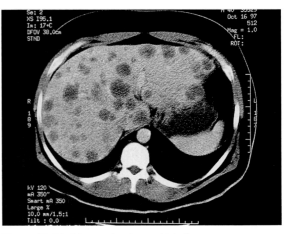

Figure 15.11 CT scan showing multiple liver metastases.

scans at variable intervals along the patient's body. This is now done as a continuous process by the latest spiral CT scanners, which are much faster, and although the image is usually still presented as a series of slices, it is now possible to build up three-dimensional images of the organs to be examined (Figure 15.12).

The information provided by CT scan can be improved by the use of contrast media. For abdominal scans the bowel is normally demonstrated by oral contrast, and this allows lymph nodes and peritoneal or pelvic tumour masses to be distinguished from loops of bowel. Intravenous contrast may be used to demonstrate the relationship between blood vessels and tumours, and certain contrast media can enhance tumours, especially in the liver or brain.

CT has the major advantage of demonstrating fine-detail anatomy of all structures irrespective of their tissue density or relationship to gas. Its disadvantages relate to its cost, the high radiation dose (equivalent to barium examinations) and difficulty in obtaining scans in anything other than a transverse plane.

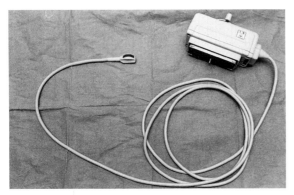

Figure 15.10 Intraoperative ultrasound probe.

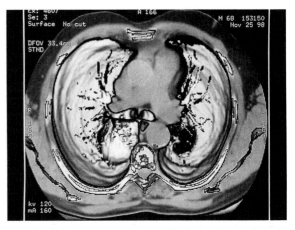

Figure 15.12 Three-dimensional CT image of the thoracic cavity showing tumours on the right.

Magnetic resonance imaging

As with CT, MRI is used to produce cross-sectional images. The principle is based on the fact that a strong magnetic field will align the axes of precession (or 'wobble') of protons in tissues, most of which are found in body water. Pulsed radiofrequency electromagnetic radiation is then applied to change the movement of the protons so that their axes are at right angles to the magnetic field. This holds the protons in a high energy state, and when the radiofrequency pulse ends, the protons revert to their original position and emit energy in the form of photons or radiowaves. The intensity of the emitted radiation is related to the concentration of proton (and thus water), and the rate at which it decays is dependent on the arrangement of proteins in which the water is held. Variations in the pulsed radiofrequency are used to produce different characteristics for imaging different tissues. In addition, contrast enhancement is feasible using gadolinium, which incorporates paramagnetic ions to augment the magnetic field.

MRI is superior to CT in that images can be produced in any plane, i.e. sagittal, coronal and oblique, in addition to transverse or axial (Figure 15.13), and it does not involve the use of ionizing radiation. It is particularly useful in tumours of the brain, spinal column, soft tissues and the pelvis. However, the image acquisition time is considerably slower than that of CT, and this limits its usefulness in terms of both breathing artefact and the efficient use of scanning time.

Radionuclide scanning

Also termed scintigraphy, this technique is based on the administration of radiopharmaceuticals labelled with γ-radiation-emitting radionuclides. The emission of this radiation from the patient's body can then be detected by means of a gamma camera. The use of this technique for detecting liver metastases as filling defects has been superseded by cross-sectional imaging, but bone

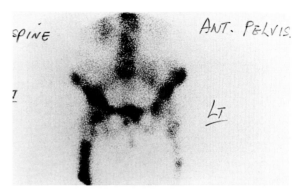

Figure 15.14 Bone scan showing a metastasis on the right femur.

scanning is still used to carry out a skeletal survey to look for metastatic disease. In the latter case, metastases show up as 'hot spots' as the label is taken up by active osteoclasts at the periphery of the lesion (Figure 15.14).

Endoscopy

Endoscopy is the process of inspecting both internal body cavities and the lumens of epithelium-lined organs by means of either rigid or flexible instruments, and in its many forms this has become an essential discipline for the diagnosis and staging of cancer. The flexible instrument is based on fibreoptic technology, although the most modern instruments incorporate a chip camera at the tip of the endoscope instead of relying on a coherent fibreoptic bundle to transmit the image to the endoscopist. Different types of endoscopy are listed below, along with the types of cancer that may be diagnosed. Details of endoscopic equipment and techniques are found in the appropriate sections of Volume II.

Upper gastrointestinal endoscopy: although often called gastroscopy, upper gastrointestinal endoscopy and oesophagogastroduodenoscopy (OGD) are better terms for this procedure. This is the investigation of choice when oesophageal or gastric cancer is suspected, although some surgeons prefer a barium swallow as the first-line investigation for dysphagia.

Endoscopic retrograde pancreatography (ERCP): this involves the use of a side-viewing duodenoscope through which a cannula can be passed into both the pancreatic and common bile ducts to allow contrast radiology of these structures. This is most useful in diagnosing tumours of the head of the pancreas or the bile ducts (Figure 15.15), and allows the palliation of such tumours by the placement of stents to relieve obstructive jaundice.

Lower gastrointestinal endoscopy: depending on its extent, flexible lower gastrointestinal endoscopy is called either flexible sigmoidoscopy or colonoscopy. Colonoscopy is the most accurate means of diagnosing colorectal cancer, and allows removal of polyps by endoscopic snare diathermy (Figure 15.16). Rigid sigmoidoscopy is only really useful for examining the rectum, but affords an opportunity to assess the mobility

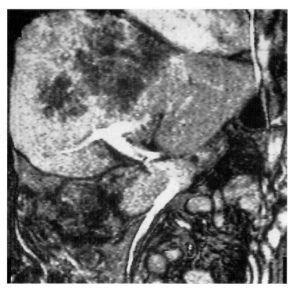

Figure 15.13 MRI, showing a hepatocellular carcinoma.

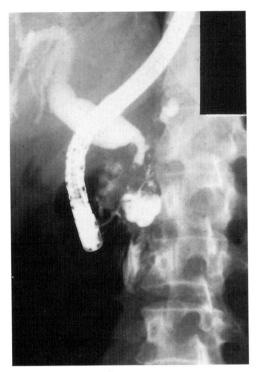

Figure 15.15 ERCP showing malignant stricture in the head of the pancreas.

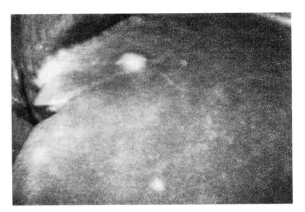

Figure 15.17 Laparoscopic view of peritoneal tumour deposits on the surfaces of the liver.

Bronchoscopy: examination of the larynx, trachea and bronchi is now usually done using a flexible instrument. As visualization is possible down to the level of subsegmental bronchi, most bronchogenic carcinomas can be biopsied at bronchoscopy.

Thoracoscopy: where appropriate, lung biopsies and pulmonary wedge resections can be carried out under direct vision by means of a telescope introduced into the thoracic cavity.

Mediastinoscopy: endoscopic examination of the mediastinum is useful for staging bronchogenic carcinoma, and particularly for assessing operability.

Cystoscopy: examination of the urethra and bladder by means of a rigid telescope allows diagnosis and treatment of both bladder and prostatic carcinoma. For diagnosis alone, flexible instruments can be used.

Brain endoscopy: by gaining access via a burr hole, endoscopy of the ventricles can now be performed, and this has a limited role in the diagnosis of brain tumours.

Biopsy

Biopsy can be divided into incisional, excisional, endoscopic, core needle and needle aspiration. These techniques are central to diagnosis in oncology, as tissue diagnosis is mandatory in most circumstances. With colonic, small bowel, liver and pancreatic cancer diagnosed radiologically, it is common practice formally to excise a tumour and obtain a histological diagnosis postoperatively, but for most other tumours, preoperative biopsy is usual practice.

Incisional biopsy implies removal of a wedge of tumour at open surgery, and care should be taken to obtain a sample from the edge of the lesion and not from its necrotic centre, which may not yield material suitable for histological diagnosis. This is most appropriate for confirming the diagnosis when metastases are suspected, e.g. of the liver or the peritoneal cavity.

Excisional biopsy implies complete excision of the suspected tumour, and this is particularly appropriate for small skin lesions. In other situations,

and position of a tumour; this is not so satisfactory with the flexible instrument.

Enteroscopy: the small bowel can be examined to a greater or lesser extent by flexible endoscopy, but has little role in cancer diagnosis.

Laparoscopy: examination of the abdominal cavity by means of a rigid telescope is an important diagnostic and staging technique. It is widely used in preoperative staging of gastric and oesophageal cancer, and this is greatly enhanced by the use of laparoscopic ultrasound. It is also useful in the diagnosis of malignant ascites (Figure 15.17).

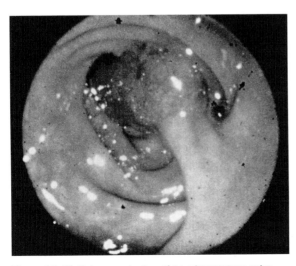

Figure 15.16 Colonoscopic view of an adenomatous polyp.

it is critical to ensure that the site of the biopsy is carefully recorded so that definitive surgery can be planned.

Endoscopic biopsy can be carried out via both rigid and flexible endoscopes by means of specially designed biopsy forceps. The use of a rigid instrument (e.g. a rigid sigmoidoscope) provides larger biopsies, but the flexible instrument allows access to more remote tumours (see 'Endoscopy' section above). Cytological samples can also be obtained endoscopically by brushings or washings.

Core needle biopsy is usually done by a tru-cut needle (Figure 15.18), which obtains a core of tissue 2–3 mm in diameter, thereby allowing definitive histological diagnosis. This can be done percutaneously in situations such as breast masses, or intraoperatively for liver tumours or transduodenal biopsy of a pancreatic mass. Percutaneous needle biopsy can also be used for relatively inaccessible tumours under CT or ultrasound guidance.

Fine needle aspiration is used to obtain cells from tumours for cytological diagnosis. This can be performed on palpable masses (e.g. breast tumours) (Figure 15.19) or on non-palpable lesions under X-ray, CT or ultrasound control. The advantages of cytology include minimal trauma in obtaining the tissue and the opportunity for rapid diagnosis. The disadvantages are that a negative cytology cannot rule out malignancy and that certain tumours (lymphomas and sarcomas in particular) cannot be reliably diagnosed by this technique.

Histological grading

When the pathologist examines a biopsy or a resection specimen at a microscopic level, the histological appearances are used not only to confirm the diagnosis of cancer, but also to grade the tumour in terms of its degree of differentiation (Figure 15.20). The first issue is to determine whether or not there has been invasion of the basement membrane, as this will define a tumour as an invasive malignancy with the potential to invade locally and metastasize. If there is no invasion of the basement membrane and yet the cells are cytologically

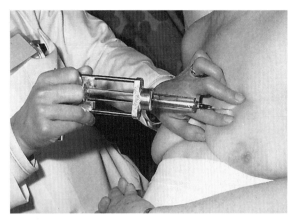

Figure 15.19 Breast FNAB.

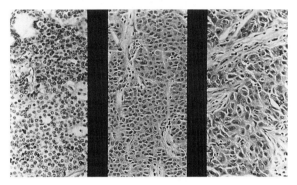

Figure 15.20 Three breast carcinomas showing differing degrees of histological differentiation. Left: well differentiated, Middle: moderately differentiated, Right: poorly differentiated.

indistinguishable from cancer cells this is termed *in situ* cancer. When invasion has occurred, the tumour can be classified according to the pleomorphism of the cells and, in the case of adenocarcinoma, attempts at gland formation. This is termed differentiation, and a tumour can be described as well, moderately or poorly differentiated.

Staging

Staging is the process whereby the extent of a tumour, in terms of both its local and metastatic spread, is estimated, and although this can be classified as either clinical or pathological staging, in practice, staging is achieved by means of a combination of clinical examination, radiological investigations and histopathological examination of resected specimens. The importance of clinicopathological staging can be summarized as follows:

- it allows estimation of prognosis
- it is often useful in treatment planning
- it allows for case-mix when evaluating the outcome of treatment
- it allows comparative trials in patients from different centres.

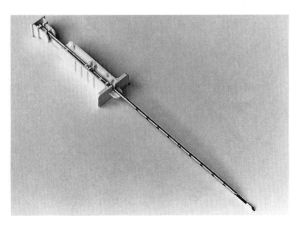

Figure 15.18 Tru-cut needle.

There are many different staging systems for different cancer types, but the most universal is the TNM system adopted by the UICC (Union Internationale Contre le Cancer). TNM stands for tumour, nodes and metastases, and it is based on assessment of:

- the extent of the primary tumour (T)
- the degree of spread to the regional lymph nodes (N)
- the absence or presence of distant metastases (M).

Each category is subdivided, and T1, T2, T3 or T4 indicates the increasing extent of the primary tumour in terms of either size (maximum dimension) or degree of penetration of the affected organ. Additional subdivisions consist of T0, where there is no evidence of a primary tumour despite the presence of metastatic disease, Tx, where it is impossible to assess the extent of the primary tumour, and Tis, which indicates carcinoma *in situ*. Lymph-node status is similarly described as N1, N2, N3, etc., and is based on increasingly distant sites of lymph-node involvement and/or increasing numbers of involved nodes. Each tumour site has specific definitions for the different T or N stage, which is dependent on the anatomy of the primary site and its lymph-node drainage.

The term M0 indicates that there is no evidence of distant metastases (excluding lymph-node deposits), whereas M1 indicates that metastatic disease has been detected, either clinically or radiologically. Mx denotes inability to assess distant spread.

Strictly, the TNM staging system is based on either clinical assessment or histopathology, and when the latter is used the prefix 'p' should be employed (e.g. pT3, pN1). In practice, however, staging is usually a result of combining clinical assessment and histopathology.

Section 15.3 • Principles of cancer treatment

The main modalities for the treatment of cancer are surgery, radiotherapy and chemotherapy. Hormone treatment is important for some tumours, and promising novel therapies are being developed. It must be remembered, however, that the patient also needs expert diagnosis in the form of radiology and/or endoscopy, and that the pathologist has a vital role not only in diagnosis but also in treatment planning. The patient will also need careful counselling, expert nursing care and, in a proportion of cases, compassionate and expert palliative care.

From the above, it is clear that the management of the cancer patient requires a multidisciplinary approach, and for the common cancers at least, surgeons, oncologists and pathologists with a special interest in the site-specific cancer must work together as a multidisciplinary team, and involve appropriate

radiologists, endoscopists, nurses and palliative care specialists (Figure 15.21). The role of the nurse in this respect has many facets, and includes nurses in the wards, theatre, oncology departments and diagnostic facilities. It also includes specialist care nurses, palliative care nurses and nurses in the community, all of whom have a vital part to play.

The days of the surgeon treating cancer in isolation are over, and all surgeons whose practice embraces any sort of cancer must work with their colleagues in the type of team described above. This is particularly true now that adjuvant therapy is so important in many cancer types, and that valuable palliation can be achieved by non-surgical interventions. We must not, however, lose sight of the fact that in the solid tumours, surgery still offers the best chance of cure, and as such remains the definitive treatment in many cancers.

Surgery

In solid tumours, the principal aim of surgery is to gain local control. Clearly, if this is achieved before metastatic spread has taken place, then cure will result, but the main aim must be adequate local removal of the primary cancer. There are other aspects of surgery in cancer, and its different roles can be classified as follows:

- diagnostic
- curative: primary disease
- curative: metastatic disease
- palliative
- preventive
- reconstructive.

Diagnostic

In many cases surgery is required to make a diagnosis. This is the case when a radiological abnormality is seen (e.g. a stricture on a barium enema, or a mass in the

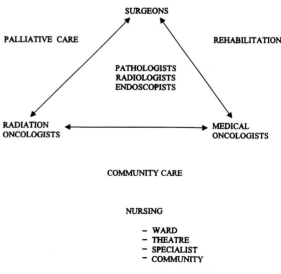

Figure 15.21 The multidisciplinary cancer care team.

head of the pancreas seen on CT scan) but this is, of course, synonymous with the definitive surgery. In other cases, the surgery is primarily a diagnostic procedure, for example where biopsy of a pathological lymph node is required to establish a diagnosis of lymphoma, or where orchidectomy is performed to confirm the presence of a testicular cancer prior to planning chemotherapy and radiotherapy.

Laparoscopy has developed as a useful method of diagnosing the source and extent of intra-abdominal malignancy, and is useful in deciding whether or not surgical excision is feasible. With the advent of laparoscopic ultrasound, it has become a very useful staging procedure, particularly in upper gastrointestinal cancer, where not only can the local extent of the disease be assessed, but liver metastases can be detected. It is also indicated in the diagnosis of malignant ascites, where biopsies of peritoneal tumour nodules can be carried out. Laparotomy used to be widely used for staging lymphoma, but with improvements in cross-sectional imaging and the much wider use of chemotherapy in this condition, it is now hardly ever required.

Curative: primary disease

Traditional cancer surgery is based on the concept of removing the whole tumour and as much of the surrounding tissue as possible in order to maximize the chance of cure. The extent of the surgery needed, however, has varied over the years. At the beginning of the twentieth century, Halstead advocated ultraradical surgery for breast cancer, based on the premise that lymph-node metastases represented a stage of spread that preceded blood-borne metastases, but this concept is now recognized as flawed. It is neither true that all cases with node involvement will eventually develop overt distant metastases, nor that all patients free of nodal disease will be cured by surgery. In addition, in breast cancer at least, randomized trials have been unable to demonstrate any advantage in terms of survival associated with radical lymph-node dissection.

Curative: metastatic disease

Under certain circumstances, surgery may be appropriate for metastatic disease. This is particularly true for isolated metastases that are resectable, and the most common indication is liver metastases from colorectal cancer. It must be stressed that the majority of such lesions are not amenable to surgical treatment, but there is good evidence that hepatic resection for disease limited to one lobe can prolong survival and effect a cure in a small proportion of tumours. Another example where surgery may be effective in metastatic disease is the isolated lung deposit from renal carcinoma.

Palliative

While surgery cannot be expected to be curative, in advanced cancer, it can play a significant role in the relief of symptoms. There are areas where the definitions of cure and palliation become blurred, and an apparently curative operation for a colonic cancer may prove to be palliative when occult metastases grow at a later date. Therefore, many of the excisional operations that are undertaken with cure in view prove to be palliative.

When it is established that the primary disease is either too advanced to eradicate surgically or the patient has specific problems such as bowel obstruction, bleeding, pain or obstructive jaundice, then surgery may play a substantial role in palliation. This can be through excision of the obstructing or bleeding lesion or, in some cases, bypassing. For example, a bypass procedure can be performed to alleviate the symptoms of obstructive jaundice associated with non-removable carcinoma of the head of the pancreas, by anastomosing the gallbladder or bile duct to the jejunum or duodenum.

Prevention

Surgery can be performed prophylactically in the prevention of cancer in premalignant conditions, such as in colectomy for FAP, and for patients with longstanding and extensive ulcerative colitis. There are areas of controversy, such as ductal carcinoma *in situ* of the breast and Barrett's change in the lower oesophagus, where there may be a role for excisional surgery in the prevention of cancer. The morbidity and mortality of surgery must not, however, exceed the risk of cancer in these patients.

Reconstruction

Finally, in the therapy of cancer, surgery can play a role in reconstruction following surgical excision. Examples include reconstruction following head and neck cancer surgery, and breast reconstruction following mastectomy, particularly in patients for whom the original surgery has produced psychological morbidity. In gastrointestinal cancer, reconstruction of the gastrointestinal tract after tumour excision is a crucial part of the operation, and its success will determine the outcome in terms of quality of life at least as much as the ablative aspect of the procedure.

Radiotherapy

The therapeutic use of ionizing radiation is known as radiotherapy, and although there are limited indications for its use in benign disease, it is largely employed in the treatment of malignant conditions.

Radiotherapy delivery systems

Most radiotherapy is delivered in the form of megavoltage X-rays or γ-rays using beams that have a peak generating energy greater than 1×10^6 V. There are four principal advantages to this approach.

- The penetration of the beam is such that deep-seated tumour can be treated.
- Because of the high energy of the beams, secondary electrons generated by interaction

with skin are scattered predominantly in a forward direction so that the radiation dose builds up under the skin, minimizing severe skin reactions.

- This forward scattering allows the radiation beams to be modified in shape to allow more precise targeting.
- The energy transfer is independent of the tissue composition so that absorption of radiation is similar in all tissues. With earlier low-voltage therapy, bone absorbed more energy, resulting in radiation osteitis.

Superficial X-rays (100 kV) and contact sources (50 kV) are used to treat skin cancers, and orthovoltage X-rays (200/300 kV) may be used for palliative treatment, although the latter are being replaced by caesium-137 (^{137}Cs) or cobalt-60 (^{60}Co) teletherapy. Interstitial implantation is sometimes used for superficial cancers such as cancers of the breast, tongue, oropharynx, anal canal and prostate. This is done by using wires, needles or seed of iridium-192, gold-198, iodine-125 or ^{137}Cs.

Intracavitary radionuclide treatments (brachytherapy) are used routinely for cancers of the uterine cervix or corpus and for vaginal cancer. There is also interest in treating oesophageal and rectal cancers in this way. The radioactive sources are usually ^{137}Cs or ^{60}Co, which provide low dose-rate applications, but high-intensity ^{60}Co sources are also available, and these can be preferable because of the short treatment times. Brachytherapy is usually delivered using afterloading methods, whereby the radioactive source is loaded into an applicator after it has been inserted into the patient. This can be done remotely, reducing the radiation hazard to staff. Unsealed radionuclides are used to treat a variety of tumours, e.g. iodine-131 for some thyroid cancers.

Physicochemical effects of ionizing radiation
When ionizing radiation interacts with tissues it does so in two ways: (i) direct action, or the primary ionization of important macromolecules in the target tissue; and (ii) indirect action, or the production of reactive species from the radiolysis of water, which then go on to damage macromolecules.

As water is so important in biological systems, the most important process in radiation damage is the radiolysis of water. When an electron is ejected from water by radiation $H_2O^{+\bullet}$ is formed (• represents an unpaired electron). This unstable free radical ion can form free radicals or uncharged molecules with an unpaired electron in the orbit, thus: $H_2O^{+\bullet} \rightarrow H^+ + OH^{\bullet}$. Although the hydroxyl radical ($OH^{\bullet}$) is more stable, it is still reactive and both the free radical ions and the free radicals disrupt molecules, including DNA.

Oxygen enhances the biological effect of radiation, as it increases the yield of free radicals which are damaging. The reaction of oxygen with the free radicals e_{aq}^- (aqueous electron) and $H^{\bullet}$ produces the relatively stable $HO_2^{\bullet}$ and H_2O_2 (hydrogen peroxide), both of which are highly toxic.

Radiation dosage and radiobiology
When a dose of radiotherapy is prescribed, the following must be defined:

- the energy and type of radiation
- the total dose
- the number of fractions
- the time over which the treatment is to be given
- the therapeutic gain.

The modern SI unit of radiotherapy for the absorbed dose is the gray (Gy), and this is defined as the absorption of 1 J of radiation energy by 1 kg of tissue (1 J/kg). The dose from a single source is prescribed either at the skin surface as an incident plane dose (IPD) or at a given depth. When two identical treatment sources are used on opposite sides of the patient (a parallel opposed pair), the prescribed dose is defined as the mid-plane dose (MPD), and when multiple sources are required to provide a homogeneous dose distribution throughout the tumour it is prescribed as a tumour dose (TD). The TD may be defined as maximum dose, minimum dose or average or 'modal' dose, but the aim is to produce a uniform dose across the tumour with no more than 5–10% variation. Administration of a radiotherapy course in terms of the absorbed dose, the number of fractions and the time course is dependent on four factors: repair, repopulation, redistribution and reoxygenation (the 'four Rs').

Repair
Two types of cellular repair are described after radiation damage: sublethal damage (SLD) repair and potentially lethal damage (PLD) repair. SLD repair takes about 4–6 h after a fraction of radiotherapy has been delivered, and can be demonstrated by the increase in survival of cells when a dose of radiation is split into two fractions separated by several hours, compared with survival when the same dose is given as a single fraction. PLD repair is that which can be accomplished if the cells do not divide within the first 6 h of a fraction of treatment, so that it can be modified by manipulation of the postirradiation conditions.

Repopulation
The killing of tumour cells by radiotherapy provides an opportunity and stimulus for cells in the clonogenic fraction that have survived and retained their reproductive capacity to proliferate. This can happen as a tumour seems to be shrinking, as the overall cell loss during treatment will hide this effect. Shortening of overall treatment times tends to overcome this effect of tumour cell repopulation, e.g. by giving 54 Gy in 16 fractions over 21 days as opposed to 60 Gy in 30

fractions over 42 days. Lower overall doses are required to keep acute reactions and late complications at acceptable levels because of the shorter time course and larger doses per fraction.

Redistribution

Redistribution of the proportions of cells in a tumour that are in different phases of the cell cycle (see Figure 15.4) can be of therapeutic benefit. Cells in late S phase (when DNA is being synthesized) are relatively radioresistant compared with those in G2 or M phases. Thus, synchronization of cells in G2 and M may increase the sensitivity of a tumour to radiotherapy.

Reoxygenation

Tumours contain hypoxic cells because of poor blood supply, and these cells have oxygen levels sufficient for viability but low enough to be radioresistant. The hypoxic fraction of cells is usually in the region of 10%, and reoxygenation is the process whereby cells that were hypoxic at the time of irradiation become oxygenated afterwards and thus susceptible to further radiotherapy. The rate of reoxygenation is variable, but probably takes about 24 h. Thus, fractionation of a course of radiotherapy can minimize the effects of hypoxia by allowing reoxygenation. In addition, oxygen is a powerful radiosensitizer, and the use of hyperbaric oxygen has been advocated. However, technical difficulties with the oxygen administration and impaired blood flow to tumour tissue have led to this approach being largely abandoned.

These four Rs underlie the rationale for fractionation of radiotherapy. Dividing the total dose into a series of fractions lessens the effect on normal tissues because of the repair of sublethal damage and cellular repopulation between fractions. Similarly, fractionation increases tumour damage by means of reoxygenation and redistribution of cells in radiosensitive phases of the cell cycle.

Tumour control and the therapeutic ratio

The therapeutic ratio is the probability of local contr/ol of a tumour compared with the chance of producing serious late adverse effects in normal tissue. For the lower doses of irradiation, a rapidly increasing probability is associated with relatively little increase in normal tissue effects. However, a point is reached where this relationship changes, and increases in the probability of tumour cure are associated with unacceptable increases in morbidity caused by damage to normal tissue. This is illustrated in Figure 15.22. For practical purposes, an acceptable complication rate must be decided on, and from the curve a total derived. For example, in Figure 15.23 a complication rate of around 10% will result in an 80% tumour control rate. The response curve of normal tissues must always lie to the right of the curve for tumour tissue for there to be a favourable therapeutic ratio, and increasing tumour cell killing in direct proportion to normal tissue damage will be of no therapeutic benefit.

Treatment policies
Radical radiotherapy

Radical radiotherapy is used for relatively confined tumours in fit patients where there is a reasonable chance of cure. The dose is normally high, e.g. 60 Gy in 30 fractions over 6 weeks, and side-effects such as diarrhoea, dysuria or mucositis are inevitable.

Radical radiotherapy can be used as sole therapy as in early lymphoma, plasmacytoma, and carcinoma of the cervix, vagina and nasopharynx. In addition, early carcinoma of the head and neck, skin, oesophagus, bladder, prostate and penis may be suitable. In early carcinoma of the larynx, radiotherapy is slightly less effective than laryngectomy, but as it preserves the voice it tends to be used as first-line therapy, reserving surgery for treatment failures.

Radiotherapy may also be used for cure in conjunction with chemotherapy, especially for advanced

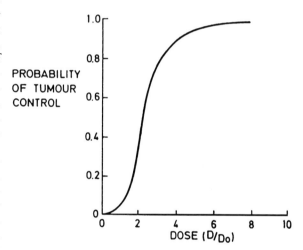

Figure 15.22 Relationship between tumour control probability and radiation dose.

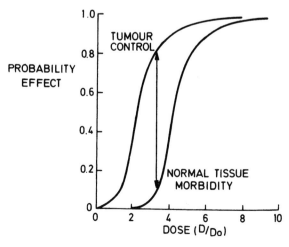

Figure 15.23 Dose–response curves for tumour and normal tissue, indicating the therapeutic ratio.

lymphoma, myeloma, some testicular cancers, certain sarcomas, early paediatric solid tumours, carcinoma of the anal canal and small-cell lung cancer. In many tumours chemotherapy is the primary treatment, but radiotherapy is required to deal with residual tumour. In acute lymphocytic leukaemia, radiotherapy is used for 'sanctuary' sites, such as the meninges, which are unaffected by drugs.

Radiotherapy is also used in conjunction with surgery in order to improve local control, and this is known as adjuvant radiotherapy. This is given either preoperatively or postoperatively in carcinoma of the breast, oesophagus, rectum and many others. Although many of these tumours are not particularly radiosensitive, preoperative radiotherapy can devitalize tumour tissue at the periphery of the main tumour, and postoperative treatment can kill tumour cells left behind after surgery. This approach allows more conservative surgery in many cases. Indications for radical radiotherapy are given in Table 15.8.

Palliative radiotherapy
Palliative radiotherapy is appropriate when the tumour is beyond cure, but where there are symptoms that can be alleviated by radiotherapy. As life expectancy is short, the course of radiotherapy should be correspondingly short. Typical regimes include 10 Gy in a single fraction and 25 Gy in five fractions. Care should be taken to plan the treatment with a view to minimizing side-effects. The main situations falling into this category are pain, obstruction, bleeding, ulceration, pathological fracture, neurological deficits and systemic symptoms.

- **Pain**: the pain from bone metastases from myeloma or carcinoma of the breast, lung or prostate responds well to short courses of radiotherapy. Headache from intracerebral tumour deposits also responds well.
- **Obstruction**: visceral obstruction, e.g. of the oesophagus or bronchus, may be relieved by radio-

therapy. Other examples are superior vena caval obstruction from bronchial carcinoma, ureteric obstruction from carcinoma of the bladder or cervix, and gastric outlet obstruction from lymphoma.

- **Bleeding**: radiotherapy can be useful in relieving bleeding from advanced cancers, especially of the cervix, uterus, pharynx, oral cavity, bronchus and bladder. It can also be helpful in reducing bleeding and mucus discharge from inoperable rectal cancer.
- **Ulceration**: this is a feature of advanced disease in breast and rectal cancer. It causes foul odour and pain, both of which can be ameliorated by radiotherapy.
- **Pathological fracture**: radiotherapy to a large, bony metastasis may prevent a pathological fracture. Once this has occurred, it is necessary to fix the fracture surgically prior to radiotherapy. Occasionally, prophylactic fixation may be appropriate before commencing radiotherapy.
- **Neurological deficits**: spinal cord compression from metastatic deposits may be relieved by radiotherapy, although surgical decompression is often indicated first. Symptoms from intracranial deposits may also respond.
- **Systemic symptoms**: symptoms such as night sweats from lymphoma, neuropathy or myopathy from small-cell lung cancer and myasthenia gravis from thymic tumours may all respond to treating the tumour with palliative radiotherapy.

Factors influencing the success of radiotherapy
The factors deciding the effectiveness of a course of radiotherapy are related to the tumour that is being treated and the surrounding normal tissues that are irradiated as part of the treatment.

Tumour factors
Tumour factors of importance include radiosensitivity, tumour volume and the site of the tumour.

- **Radiosensitivity**: this is an inherent property of tumour cells and varies considerably according to the site-specific cancer. Seminoma and lymphoma are the most radiosensitive, whereas gliomas and soft-tissue sarcomas in adults are highly radioresistant. In both instances, however, radiotherapy may be of value in the adjuvant setting to minimize recurrence after surgery. A list of common tumours in descending order of sensitivity is given in Table 15.9.
- **Tumour volume**: as large tumours have more and higher proportions of hypoxic and noncycling (G0) cells, radiation is more effective against small tumours.
- **Tumour site**: the anatomical location of a tumour will determine the permissible dosage, as the sensitivity of the surrounding normal tissues has to be taken into account. This is dealt with in detail below.

Table 15.8 Indications for radical radiotherapy

I. Primary elective management

Operable lesions	(a) Optimum control rates
	(b) Preservation of form and function
Inoperable lesions	(a) Local extension
	(b) General unfitness for surgery

II. Primary combined management

Adjuvant to surgery	(a) Local residual disease
	(b) Lymph-node metastases
	(c) Other metastases
Adjuvant to chemotherapy	(a) Local residual disease
	(b) Protected organs (sanctuary sites)

III. Secondary management

After elective surgery	(a) Local recurrence
	(b) Lymph-node metastases

Table 15.9 Common tumours in decreasing order of radiosensitivity

- Seminoma
- Lymphocytic lymphoma
- Other lymphomas, leukaemia, myeloma
- Small-cell lung cancer
- Choriocarcinoma
- Ewing's sarcoma
- Squamous cell carcinoma
- Breast cancer
- Rectal cancer
- Bladder cancer
- Hepatoma
- Melanoma
- Glioma
- Other sarcomas

Normal tissue factors

The ability to treat a tumour with radiotherapy depends crucially on the reaction of the surrounding normal tissue, which is inevitably irradiated. The bone marrow, gonads, the lens of the eye and gut mucosa are the most sensitive tissues. The walls of the gut, skin, nervous tissue, lung, kidney and liver are less sensitive, and bone, connective tissue and muscle are relatively insensitive.

- **Bone marrow**: the haemopoetic tissues are extremely sensitive, and a single whole-body dose of 4 Gy is sufficient to cause fatal myelosuppression in 50% of patients. This has been overcome by the use of allogeneic bone marrow transplantation, which can allow whole-body irradiation of up to 10 Gy in the treatment of various malignancies such as acute leukaemia.
- **Gonads**: both the ovaries and testes are sensitive; in the testis oligospermia is caused by doses of between 100 and 200 cGy. In the ovary, doses of around 10 Gy cause amenorrhoea. Secondary sex characteristics are not greatly affected in men owing to the radioresistance of the Ledig cells, but they can be affected in women.
- **Eye**: the main structures that can be damaged by radiotherapy are the lens, the eyelashes and the lachrymal glands. Cataract may follow very small doses, although it probably requires in the region of 20 Gy to produce visual impairment.
- **Gastrointestinal tract**: the mucosa of the gastrointestinal tract is highly sensitive, and the acute effects of nausea, vomiting and diarrhoea are very common wherever the gastrointestinal tract is affected. Late effects include malabsorption and bleeding. Radiation damage to the wall of the gut leads to stricture formation and fistula formation.
- **Skin**: small doses of irradiation will merely cause erythema, similar to sunburn. As the dose increases, however, dry then moist desquamation occurs, followed by epilation and loss of both sebaceous and sweat gland function. Later effects include pigmentation, fibrosis and telangiectasia.
- **Nervous tissue**: using conventional fractionation, the maximum tolerable dose of radiotherapy for the brain and spinal cord is around 50 Gy. Radiation myelitis of the spinal cord will result in hemiplegia or paraplegia, with sensory signs, Brown–Sequard syndrome and sphincter dysfunction.
- **Lung**: 5 Gy in a single fraction or 20 Gy in 10 fractions may cause radiation pneumonitis, which manifests itself as cough, dyspnoea and fever, and leads to pulmonary fibrosis in the longer term. Steroid therapy may be used to good effect in the acute phase. This complication is seen after treatment of lung, breast or oesophageal cancer.
- **Kidney**: acute radiation nephritis followed by chronic radiation nephropathy with proteinuria, anaemia hypertension and renal failure can result from doses in the region of 25 Gy over 10 fractions.
- **Liver**: the liver can only tolerate around 30 Gy in 15 fractions; above this, liver dysfunction is seen.
- **Bone**: avascular necrosis is seen after large doses, especially in the head of the humerus or femur, and radiotherapy to the vertebrae can lead to kyphoscoliosis. In children, irradiation of the epiphyseal plate may stunt growth.

Other late sequelae of radiotherapy

There is no doubt that irradiation can cause cancer. Studies of patients and radiologists exposed to inappropriately high doses of X-rays in the early days of diagnostic radiology, and the experience from the atomic weapons used in Japan have shown this conclusively. The role of therapeutic irradiation in carcinogenesis is less clear, as most patients are elderly, and many have limited life expectancy. However, there is a well-documented risk of malignancy in various sites after treatment of carcinoma of the cervix. Radiotherapy may also cause mutations in germ cells, posing the risk of fetal death or abnormality. This is rare, however, as it is thought that few germ cell mutations caused by ionizing radiation are viable. Teratogenesis is another major risk, and for this reason irradiation of a pregnant woman is contraindicated.

Treatment planning

Given the importance of achieving an optimum therapeutic ratio, careful treatment planning is central to the practice of radiotherapy. The first aim is to deliver a homogeneous dose to the tumour, but tumours rarely occupy a compact, easily definable area. Rather, a tumour will infiltrate normal tissue, and will often occupy an asymmetrical space. It must be appreciated that if even a small part of the tumour receives inadequate dosing the treatment will fail, but if too much normal tissue is irradiated the unwanted effects may represent a price that is too high to pay, even for tumour eradication. The two crucial factors in planning are the volume to be treated and the dosage.

Volume

The main aim in delivering a dose of radiotherapy is to treat as small a volume as possible and yet treat every tumour cell. In order to develop the concept of this problem, five different volumes have been defined (Figure 15.24). The **gross tumour volume** (GTV) encompasses the demonstrable tumour, whereas the **clinical target volume** (CTV) also includes the volume that contains suspected but undetectable tumour cells (i.e. the infiltrating margin around the GTV and the regional lymph nodes). The **planning target volume** (PTV) consists of the CTV and a margin to accommodate variations in the shape of the tumour and its position relative to the treatment beams. When the treatment is delivered, however, it is practically impossible to confine irradiation to the PTV; the volume receiving a dose within the range considered sufficient for tumour control is termed the **treated volume** and the volume that receives a dose considered significant in terms of normal tissue tolerance is called the **irradiated volume**.

As micrometastases involve smaller numbers of cells than the main bulk of a tumour, it is possible to use relatively small doses of radiotherapy at the periphery of a tumour. Thus, it is possible to tailor treatment to an individual tumour in a more sophisticated way than can be achieved by using a single target volume. This involves the definition of an initial, large target volume, which encompasses all the possible sites of tumour infiltration and local spread. When a specific dose has been given to this volume, a further dose is given to a reduced volume, which corresponds more closely to the GTV. This allows a larger than usual volume to be treated in the knowledge that normal tissue tolerance will be preserved owing to the lower dose to the initial volume, and it also permits a higher dose to be delivered to the second or 'cone-down' volume, which will target the more radioresistant tumour core. This process is known as shrinking volumes.

Dosage

The term dosage includes not only the overall dose expressed in Gy, but also the number of fractions, the overall time of treatment and the structure of fractions within the overall time (e.g. it is sometimes advantageous to have split-course therapy). With brachytherapy, an important additional variable is the dose rate as there are different clinical responses per unit dose at a high rate (10–100 cGy/min) compared with a low rate (0.1–1.0 cGy/min).

Dosage schedules are therefore variable, but the following categories are recognized:

- **normal fractionation**: four to six daily fractions per week over 3–6 weeks. Note that the main reason that seven daily fractions per week are not normally given is that radiotherapy units tend to close at weekends. There is now evidence that treatment may be enhanced if weekend breaks are omitted
- **hypofractionation**: fewer than four daily fractions per week
- **hyperfractionation**: two or more fractions of reduced size per day given over the same period as normal fractionation
- **accelerated hyperfractionation**: two or more fractions of normal size per day given over a reduced period
- **split-course schedule**: two or more abbreviated courses of normal fractionation separated by a rest period of 1 or 2 weeks' duration.

The actual dosages used have been determined by clinical experience and will depend on the tumour type, the size of the tumour and its anatomical location. Typical dosages are 60 Gy in 30 fractions over 6 weeks (popular in the USA) or 50 Gy in 15 fractions over 3 weeks (popular in the UK), but there is a considerable range. Of course, the dose will also depend on the type of normal tissue to be irradiated as part of the treatment, and the tolerance doses (the dose associated with a 5% chance of significant damage) are highly variable.

Field arrangement

In order to ensure the highest and most homogeneous dose to the tumour and the lowest dose to tissues outside the target volume, it is usually necessary to use more than one field. In order to plan the treatment a planning computer is now regarded as indispensable, and CT scanning is often employed to define the extent of the tumour. Increasingly, there is interest in CT-generated three-dimensional images for planning.

As it is the simplest arrangement, a single field is used where possible, but this should only be done when it

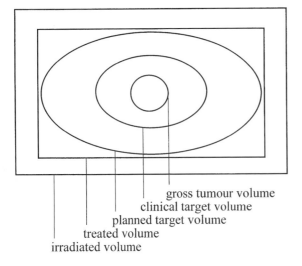

gross tumour volume
clinical target volume
planned target volume
treated volume
irradiated volume

Figure 15.24 Diagrammatic representation of the different volumes to be taken into account in radiotherapy.

delivers optimal treatment. It must be remembered that a megavoltage beam delivers its maximum dose at a level below the surface of the skin, so if it is necessary to treat the surface it is necessary to apply a tissue equivalent (e.g. wet gauze or wax) of a thickness that is equivalent to the build-up depth for the radiation energy.

Parallel opposed fields are often used for the simpler clinical situations, e.g. tumours of the head and neck and some pelvic tumours, but for deep-seated tumour sites such as oesophagus, bladder, prostate, cervix and rectum, three or four-field plans are commonly used. Shielding blocks, usually made of lead, are used when an important sensitive organ lies within or close to the treatment volume. These shields may block transmission either completely or partially, according to their thickness.

Combined modality treatment

In many circumstances, combined modality treatment is employed. Often, radiotherapy may be used in conjunction with surgery, and this is covered in the section on adjuvant therapy. However, the combined use of radiotherapy and chemotherapy is increasing for two reasons.

Firstly, it is recognized that although radiotherapy may be effective for treatment of the primary tumour, it is also necessary to treat micrometastases, and this approach is commonly employed for childhood cancers. In some cases, and in acute lymphocytic leukaemia in particular, chemotherapy is the primary treatment, and radiotherapy is reserved for sanctuary sites such as the CNS.

Secondly, there is evidence that radiotherapy and chemotherapy may act synergistically, i.e. the tumour response from both modalities is greater than would be expected from simple summation of the predicted effects of the modalities alone. It has to be borne in mind, however, that the normal tissue toxicity may also be greater when combination therapy (or radio-chemotherapy) is used.

Different modalities of radiotherapy may also be used in combination, and external beam therapy and brachytherapy may be used together. For example, cancer of the cervix may be treated with external beam for the parametria and pelvic nodes with intracavitary treatment to the cervix itself. Another example is carcinoma of the tongue, which is frequently treated with initial external beam therapy followed by an extra dose to the primary tumour area.

Chemotherapy

During the 1980s and 1990s there have been major changes in the role of drug therapy in the treatment of cancer. This is partly because of the development of new drugs, but also because of the introduction of combination chemotherapy in which several active drugs are used in treatment. The ideal drug, or drug combination, has not yet been found, yet the improvements made in the treatment of some forms of cancer make it necessary to consider the integration of chemotherapy into the management of many of the cancers regularly seen by surgeons.

At present there are over 40 drugs shown to have activity against many forms of cancer. If two or three drug combinations are considered then the number of potential interactions is enormous. Many of the active drugs have been discovered by chance, although it has been possible to design some of these using the basic principles of biochemical pharmacology. The screening for new drugs is a costly and time-consuming exercise, yet it is necessary to identify new agents of clinical value.

Clinical trials

Following initial evaluation, potentially useful drugs are introduced into clinical practice through three levels of trial.

- **Phase I studies** assess the maximum tolerated dose of a drug, within a given schedule and route of administration, and identify the toxicity profile. These studies involve small numbers of patients with advanced disease.
- **Phase II studies** determine the spectrum of activity of the drug in the dose range already established. These studies involve patients with advanced specific types of cancer, when conventional approaches have failed. Further toxicity information is acquired.
- **Phase III studies** compare the drug with established methods of treatment, and should be randomized. Patients are recruited for these studies at an earlier stage than in phases I and II. Again, toxicity has to be carefully recorded. Phase III trials may be large scale and multicentre, particularly when the drug is to be used in an adjuvant role. Patients must be randomized into treatment groups, and must be carefully monitored to the end-point of the trial, which may be some years later.

Classification of chemotherapeutic agents

The mechanism of action of chemotherapeutic agents can be described in many ways, and is linked to chemical structure, biochemical function or site of action on the cell cycle. Each method of classification has its own advantages and disadvantages. A limitation of all methods of classification, however, is that they focus attention on one method or mode of action, while the drug itself may have several. One classification commonly used is that based on the mechanism of action on the biochemical pathways leading to DNA synthesis or replication. Drugs may therefore be classified as follows.

Alkylating agents
These drugs (e.g. cyclophosphamide, nitrogen mustard, chlorambucil, melphalan) are highly reactive agents that

are able to bind to important biological molecules such as proteins or DNA. By binding to these molecules they inhibit or restrict their function.

Antimetabolites
These drugs (e.g. 5-fluorouracil, methotrexate, cytosine arabinoside, 6-mercaptopurine) act by inhibiting specific metabolic pathways, usually those of DNA synthesis, thus preventing cell replication and inducing cell death.

Vinca alkaloids
These drugs (vincristine, vinblastine, vindesine) act specifically by inhibiting or arresting cells in mitosis, thus functioning as spindle poisons.

Antibiotics
Many such compounds are now available including adriamycin, bleomycin, streptozocin, actinomycin D and mitomycin C. Their mechanism of action is complex but it is likely that they interact with the double-stranded DNA molecule, preventing its replication.

Miscellaneous agents
It is naturally impossible to classify all cytotoxic drugs in the ways described above. Indeed, several of these drugs may act in more than one way to produce their cytotoxic effect. For some drugs, however, the mechanism of action is by no means clear.

Mechanism of action in relation to the cell cycle
As described previously, the cell cycle may be divided into a number of phases and it is possible to classify chemotherapeutic agents on the basis of their site of action on the cell cycle. In general, most drugs have no effect if the cell is not in cycle.

Using animal models drugs can be divided into:

- **cycle non-specific**: these drugs are active at all phases of the cell cycle and include cyclophosphamide, the nitrosoureas and adriamycin
- **cycle specific or phase specific**: these drugs act only at certain parts of the cycle, e.g. mitosis vincristine, bleomycin, S phase cytosine arabinoside, hydroxyurea and methotrexate.

A knowledge of the kinetics of drug action may be useful in the design of drug combinations.

Mechanisms of selectivity and drug resistance

The problems of selectivity and resistance are central to an understanding of the use of drugs in clinical practice. All cytotoxic drugs are effective against cancer cells if given in large enough doses. However, the therapeutic ratio of most of the drugs used (that is the ratio of the maximum tolerated dose to the minimum effective dose) is often very small. This means that toxicity and effectiveness are closely related. Thus, no matter how effective the drug may be, it may not be able to be used in an appropriate combination because of toxicity. Great care must therefore be exercised in the use of these drugs.

Resistance to cytotoxic agents
It may be useful to distinguish between intrinsic resistance to drug action and acquired resistance, which arises after several exposures to the drug. Acquired resistance may result from the selection of resistant mutant cells by destruction of the sensitive cell population or by a biochemical modification of the initially sensitive cells. These modifications may include:

- altered cell kinetics
- inaccessibility of the cells to drug action, e.g. fibrosis
- altered immune responses to cancer cell antigens
- impaired transport through the cell membrane
- various biochemical changes, e.g. increased level of drug catabolizing enzymes, decreased levels of activating enzymes, deletion of specific cell-binding proteins necessary for cytostatic activity of the drug, and inactive stress–response pathways.

In an attempt to overcome drug resistance, cytotoxic drugs are administered in combination in order to delay the emergence of drug resistance. However, it seems that many tumours are still able to overcome the impact of separated metabolic insults. It is likely that insufficient attention has been paid in the past to the effect of combination therapy on the immune response and altered antigenicity, which permits emergence of the resistant strain.

Effect of drugs on the growth kinetics of the tumour
As described earlier, tumours are composed of different growth compartments and in general chemotherapeutic agents act only on the growth fraction. Even with a very effective agent, which would reduce the growth fraction almost completely, there would still be recruitment of cells from the non-dividing clonogenic compartment. This is one of the major reasons for giving chemotherapeutic agents over a prolonged period.

It is usual nowadays to administer drugs intermittently. In this way, side-effects can often be minimized and efficacy improved. From a kinetic point of view it may also explain why in some instances a drug is effective and in others it is not. In Figure 15.25 drug treatment is given with reduction in tumour size, but at the same time marrow toxicity occurs and the drug has been discontinued. Thus, although the cancer was sensitive to the drug, host toxicity has prevented repeated drug administration. This is in contrast to Figure 15.26, where the cancer is responsive to the agent and where the host tissues have been able to recover more rapidly than the tumour, allowing selectivity of cytotoxicity. Tumour resistance may also result in tumour growth (Figure 15.27).

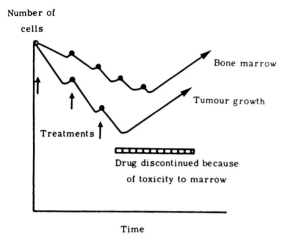

Number of
cells

Bone marrow

Tumour growth

Treatments

Drug discontinued because
of toxicity to marrow

Time

Figure 15.25 Effect of marrow toxicity on the drug response. Repeated treatments have resulted in bone marrow toxicity. The drug is discontinued and the tumour grows.

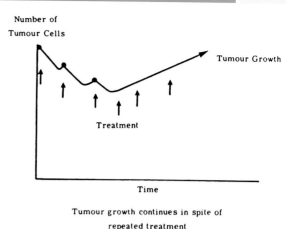

Number of
Tumour Cells

Tumour Growth

Treatment

Time

Tumour growth continues in spite of
repeated treatment

Figure 15.27 Effect of drug resistance on tumour growth. Although drug treatment is initially effective, resistance develops and the tumour grows despite repeated treatment.

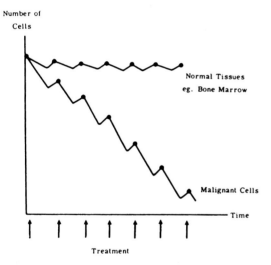

Number of
Cells

Normal Tissues
eg. Bone Marrow

Malignant Cells

Time

Treatment

Figure 15.26 Differential effect of treatment on normal and malignant cells. The drug is administered, the bone marrow is not damaged and the tumour shrinks.

Combination chemotherapy

One of the most important advances in the use of drug therapy in the treatment of cancer has been the introduction of drug combinations. In almost all types of cancer, with some important exceptions, combinations of drugs are superior to single agents.

Combinations of drugs have been designed in a variety of ways, although some of the most effective combinations have been discovered by chance. Combinations may be based on known biochemical synergisms or kinetic differences. The principles of combination chemotherapy are usually stated as follows:

- drugs used should be active as single agents against the particular cancer to be treated

- drugs with similar toxicities should be avoided
- drugs with different mechanisms of action or different sites of action should be used together
- drugs used in combination should be used in doses as near as possible to their maximum doses when used as single agents.

Design of combination chemotherapy for clinical use
As with the overall management of the patient with cancer, it is useful to have a plan for the selection of use of drug combinations (Figure 15.28).

As before, the patient must be considered as an individual and prior to the commencement of chemotherapy the aims of treatment and possible side-effects should be reviewed. The choice of chemotherapy will depend on the diagnosis, and site and histology of the tumour and the condition of the patient. The individual drugs are then considered in the light of their effect as single agents, possible combinations and kinetic parameters. On the basis of this information, a tentative treatment protocol is drawn up. The administration of this protocol is then considered in two ways. The first is the relationship to other forms of treatment, possible drug interactions, the pharmacology of the drugs and their kinetics. The second relates to where, and by whom, the drugs are to be administered.

This will vary from protocol to protocol but it is essential that it is considered at an early stage. Finally, it is paramount that the treatment protocol is evaluated and its results accurately recorded and reported. In some instances these drugs will be given as part of a clinical trial and the importance of such trials in the future management of the cancer patient cannot be overemphasized.

Role of chemotherapy in the treatment of cancer

Although the most successful use of cytotoxic agents has occurred in the management of leukaemia and

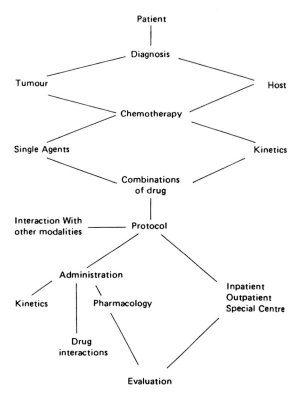

Figure 15.28 Chemotherapy treatment plan.

lymphoma, there is the ever-present hope that it will ultimately prove possible to combine the modalities of surgery, radiotherapy and chemotherapy in therapeutic programmes capable of altering the natural history of common solid tumours. In fact, such developments have either been established, e.g. certain childhood embryonal cancers and carcinoma, or are nearly evaluated, e.g. testicular cancer and soft-tissue sarcomas. Other tumours such as breast and ovarian cancer are often responsive to cytotoxic treatment and this can play a significant role if applied at the correct time in the course of the patient's illness.

Surprisingly, it looks as though some tumours are more sensitive than normal tissues to the action of drugs, although this is not usually the case. Furthermore, it is known that some normal tissues affected by cytotoxic drugs are usually capable of proliferating more rapidly than neoplastic tissue and repair drug-induced damage before tumour cells can do so. Despite these encouraging observations, cytotoxic drug therapy has not yet significantly assisted cancer control of most solid tumours.

Recently, there has been a revival of interest in local infusion (or regional) chemotherapy. This is largely because of new developments in implantable or miniaturized external pumps, rather than a breakthrough in drug design. As malignant tissue develops a neocirculation drawn from the local arterial supply, it is possible to deliver high concentrations of drug in small volumes to the tumour provided that a single arterial supply is

present. Because total drug doses are lower and spillover into the general circulation is reduced, there may be less systemic toxicity. Furthermore, it is quite often possible to provide continuous delivery of the drug, which is useful when administering cell cycle active agents such as fluorouracil and floxuridine. Implantation of catheters into the common hepatic artery is currently of great interest. A response rate of 50% is normally achieved but the median survival of patients with metastatic disease is still only 1 year and it has not yet been demonstrated that improved survival occurs over matched controls. It remains to be shown that arterial infusion of cytotoxic drugs is advantageous but with the availability of totally implantable, refillable and rechargeable pumps there is an added stimulus to investigate new drug schedules and means of increasing the potency of established drugs.

The use of drugs in the management of cancer is a rapidly changing field. It is therefore only possible to give an overall view of its role, recognizing that this might change at any time. Tumour-specific treatment is covered in Volume II and is summarized in Table 15.10. Chemotherapy is now an established part of cancer management and its role is likely to develop in the future.

Complications of chemotherapy

As has been mentioned, the therapeutic index for anticancer drugs is small. Toxicity is therefore a major problem and in some cases can be severe enough to be life threatening. If they are used properly then the side-effects can be minimized, but there is a need to exercise great care in their use and, in some instances, administration should be restricted to special centres.

A wide variety of non-specific complications is associated with chemotherapeutic agents. These include nausea, vomiting and mucositis. This latter problem, affecting mainly the mouth, throat and gastrointestinal tract, can be especially difficult to deal with, particularly if complicated by superinfection. Alopecia occurs fairly frequently, particularly if certain drugs, such as adriamycin, are used. Haematological problems, leucopenia and thrombocytopenia occur, and may be an accepted part of management if treatment is aggressive. Active haematological support must be given in this instance, with the use of prophylactic antibiotics to prevent infection, together with leucocyte and platelet support. If the patient is severely immunosuppressed, reverse barrier nursing or the use of protected environments may be required. Where indicated, white cell transfusions may be necessary, although this is rare. Wherever possible the drugs used should be administered in doses that do not cause severe leucopenia. It should be remembered that this risk is compounded by previous or concurrent radiotherapy.

Chemotherapeutic agents induce a variety of hormonal changes and affect endocrine organ function. Of particular importance is the effect on testicular and ovarian activity. In the premenopausal

Table 15.10 Cancer chemotherapy

Cancers in which drugs have been responsible for some patients achieving a normal life span	
Acute leukaemia in children	Ewing's sarcoma
Hodgkin's disease	Wilm's tumour
Histiocytic lymphoma	Burkitt's lymphoma
Skin cancer	Retinoblastoma
Testicular carcinoma	Choriocarcinoma
Embryonal rhabdomyosarcoma	
Cancers in which responders to chemotherapy have had demonstrated improvement in survival	
Ovarian carcinoma	Lymphocytic lymphomas
Breast carcinoma	Neuroblastoma
Adult acute leukaemia	Oat cell lung cancer
Multiple myeloma	Malignant insulinoma
Endometrial carcinoma	Gastrointestinal cancer
Prostatic cancer	Osteogenic sarcomas
Cancers responsive to drugs for which clinically useful improvement in survival of responders has not been clearly demonstrated	
Head and neck cancers	Malignant carcinoid tumours
Central nervous system cancer	Soft-tissue sarcomas
Endocrine gland tumours	
Cancers only marginally responsive or unresponsive to chemotherapeutic agents	
Hypernephroma	Pancreatic carcinoma
Bladder carcinoma	Hepatocellular carcinoma
Cancer of the oesophagus	Thyroid carcinoma
Epidermoid carcinoma of the lung	Malignant melanoma

woman menstruation may cease, and following termination of therapy, infertility may occur. This is also found in relation to testicular function, although in this instance sperm banking may be used, prior to treatment, in case infertility occurs. There is no evidence that the offspring of individuals who have had chemotherapy have any greater chance of developing birth defects or genetic abnormalities.

However, it would appear that the incidence of second tumours arising in patients who have had chemotherapy is higher than would be expected. Although the risk is not great it is certainly real, and must constantly be remembered, particularly when drugs are being used in an adjuvant setting, in fit patients, and over a long period.

In addition to the non-specific toxicities described above, certain specific complications are known. These include the cardiotoxicity associated with the use of adriamycin, the lung toxicity with bleomycin and busulphan, the renal toxicity with methotrexate and cis-platinum, and the bladder toxicity with cyclophosphamide. These side-effects may become so severe as to be life threatening. However, with careful pretreatment assessment and attention to detail these can be avoided in most instances.

Hormonal therapy

Hormonal methods of treatment have a role to play in the management of certain types of cancer, both as therapy in their own right and as methods for symptom control and general support of the patient. Steroid hormones exert their effect through binding to cytoplasmic receptors. The hormone-receptor complexes are transferred to the nucleus, where they play a role in influencing transcriptional events. Peptide hormones, in contrast, bind to cell membrane receptors and set off a chain of events involving the activation of 'second messengers', which transmit information to the nucleus. Hormone-sensitive tumours bear receptors that are often overexpressed.

Receptor levels can be assayed for a number of hormone receptors including those for oestrogen, progesterone, glucocorticoid and several peptide hormones and growth factors. Levels of oestrogen receptor (ER) in breast cancer tissue have been correlated with a better prognosis, and conversely high levels of epidermal growth factor receptor (EGFR) have been correlated with a poor prognosis. How they may interrelate is not clear. The two may simply be reflections of cellular functional (de)differentiation. Certain oncogenes such as the myc family and erbA act as nuclear transcriptional factors, in a way similar to the steroid receptors, and interact with steroid hormones. Alteration of the function of steroids and their receptors has been postulated as an effect of such oncogene activity.

Uses of hormones in the treatment of cancer
Hormonal therapy is employed in the following ways:

- **ablative procedures**, e.g. oophorectomy and adrenalectomy in the treatment of breast cancer, and orchidectomy in the treatment of prostatic cancer. In these cases the major sources of appropriate hormones are removed
- **added hormones**, e.g. prednisolone, progestagens, oestrogens and androgens. In these instances, the hormones are given at doses well above their

physiological level. In some cases the effect will be direct. In others, the effect is due at least in part to suppression of androgenic hormones

- **hormone antagonists**, e.g. tamoxifen, which binds competitively to the oestrogen receptor and is believed to exert its effect through this, cyproterone acetate, which competes with testosterone for binding to its receptor, and goserilin (Zoladex), which is a luteinizing hormone-releasing hormone (LHRH) analogue, and thereby acts as an antagonist
- **drugs that interfere with hormone synthesis or release**, e.g. aminoglutethamide, which has two modes of action. It is an adrenal inhibitor through inhibition of the desmolase enzyme system (a mediator of the initial stages of steroid hormone synthesis in the adrenal glands). In addition it is an aromatase inhibitor, inhibiting the peripheral conversion of androstendione to oestrogen, the major source of oestrogen in postmenopausal women. The second mode of action is currently believed to be the more significant.

Hormonal therapy has been used to treat male and female breast cancer, prostatic cancer and endometrial cancer. Corticosteroids can induce a brief response in a number of haematological malignancies, and are used in combination regimens in the primary treatment of leukaemias and lymphomas. Recently, a great deal of work has been carried out on gastrin and its receptor in gastrointestinal malignancy, but this has yet to be translated into effective therapy.

Other uses of steroid hormones

Steroids have a place in the management of some other aspects of cancer care. Anorexia may respond to small doses of prednisolone, and as part of the overall management of hypercalcaemia, corticosteroids may be of benefit. Dexamethasone is well known for its action in reducing the effects of cerebral oedema associated with intracranial malignant neoplasms.

Adjuvant therapy

In addition to surgery to control localized disease, radiotherapy, chemotherapy and hormonal therapy can be given as additional measures to attempt to improve disease control and survival. This therapy 'in addition to' surgery has been termed surgical adjuvant therapy, and is generally given in cases where there is considered to be a significant risk of residual disease after surgery or the development of metastatic disease as a result of micrometastases present at the time of initial presentation. It is anticipated that this additional therapy might eradicate both residual local disease and micrometastatic disease and thereby improve long-term survival.

In evaluating the role of adjuvant therapy, the following basic points need to be considered.

- It should not be given to patients for whom it is unlikely to be of any benefit, e.g. patients with Dukes A carcinoma of the rectum would have a small chance of either local recurrence or micrometastatic disease. Clearly, it is inappropriate in patients with advanced disease that cannot be completely excised by surgery, because of either extensive local disease or established metastases. In this instance, any non-surgical therapy would be termed palliative rather than adjuvant.
- The adjuvant therapy should ideally be demonstrated to have a survival benefit for the patient. The benefit gained from adjuvant therapy may be marginal. For example, surgery for colorectal cancer produces a 5-year 'cure' rate of 40%. Present adjuvant therapy appears likely to have the capacity to improve the survival to 45%. Any benefit of adjuvant therapy therefore needs to be clearly demonstrated by well-organized clinical trials before being widely applied.

Randomized clinical trials of adjuvant therapy continue to be the major instrument by which the effectiveness of any new therapy can be established. It is important not to subject patients unnecessarily to toxic adjuvant therapy if no benefit in terms of survival (or disease-free survival in some instances) can be obtained. In addition, the cost of adjuvant therapy needs to be balanced against the potential benefits.

Adjuvant therapy has been shown to be beneficial in breast and colorectal cancer. Adjuvant therapy with tamoxifen has been demonstrated to improve survival in premenopausal and postmenopausal women with breast cancer, more significantly so in postmenopausal patients. Combination chemotherapy has been shown to produce a survival benefit in premenopausal women with lymph-node involvement at the time of surgery. In colorectal cancer 5-fluorouracil in combination with folinic acid may be of benefit in patients with Dukes C cancer.

Radiotherapy is commonly used in an adjuvant role for rectal cancer, and may be given preoperatively or postoperatively. Preoperative treatment is favoured in the UK and the rest of northern Europe, whereas postoperative irradiation, often in combination with chemotherapy, is recommended in the USA. There is good evidence that these approaches confer benefit in reducing the incidence of local recurrence, and improved survival has been demonstrated with preoperative radiotherapy.

Preoperative chemoirradiation (chemotherapy and radiotherapy) is currently being evaluated in gastric and oesophageal neoplasms. Significant down-staging and objective regression is observed in 20% of cases at the time of excisional surgery, although improved survival has yet to be demonstrated.

Immunotherapy

The role of the immune system in the aetiology and treatment of cancer has remained one of continued investigation. Paul Ehrlich, in 1906, observed that, on transplantation from one animal to another, cancers failed to grow, suggesting an immune mechanism, although this phenomenon proved to be part of the general phenomenon of transplant rejection rather than a tumour-specific event. Historical attempts to modulate immunity to act against tumours have included specific immunotherapy using tumour extracts and passive therapy using (anti)serum, to limited, if any, effect.

Although many virally and chemically induced cancers will induce a strong rejection response, there are many others in which the immune response is minimal. The lack of an immune response may be due to lack of tumour cell antigenicity or lack of host immune responsiveness. In this latter area there may be host genetic influences via Ir (immune response) genes. The Ir genes are located in chromosome 6 in the human and are responsible for the production of molecules that appear to be associated with the immune response. These gene products have been designated DS, DR and S11, molecules that are present on macrophages, B-cells, some T-cells, dendritic cells and Langerhans cells. The functional role of these gene products is under further investigation.

Immunotherapy has been directed either through the concept that cancers might have specific antigenicity or through the concept that the immune response is diminished in cancer.

Monoclonal antibodies

The discovery of tumour-specific and tumour-associated antigens has suggested the basis for altered cell functions, which might be the target for specific immunotherapy. This enthusiasm was enhanced with the advent of monoclonal antibodies, which, it was conceived, might permit the specific targeting of tumour cells. Although a number of tumour-associated antigens has been recognized, there is presently little ground for belief that human tumours present specific identifying antigenic features. Therapy using monoclonal antibodies to tumour-associated antigens has been applied, mainly using the antibodies conjugated to toxic molecules (drugs, radioisotopes, toxins). Two major problems have made this potential therapy relatively unrewarding to date.

- The antibodies are not sufficiently specific for therapy to be selectively effective.
- The monoclonal antibodies (being murine in origin for the most part) are immunogenic themselves, and are attacked by the host.

Research therefore continues with the aim of producing relatively more tumour-specific antibodies, better toxic conjugates and reduced antibody-directed host response.

Cytokines

An alternative view in immunotherapy is to enhance the host response, on the assumption that the cancer has either elicited a suboptimal response or specifically suppressed the immune response. Initial attempts to enhance the immune response were directed towards non-specific mechanisms, such as bacille Calmette-Guérin (BCG), corynebacterium and levamisole. Randomized prospective trials of such therapies in the 1980s failed to demonstrate any significant effects of such therapies.

The cytokines are a group of active polypeptides, originally identified from lymphocytes, and thereby initially called lymphokines. Some of the cytokines have been demonstrated to have an anticancer effect, but have yet to be used to clinical effect.

Interferons

Interferons were initially identified as antiviral agents. α-, β- and γ-interferons have been identified, and to date the α-interferons are the only ones of clinical use in cancer. α-Interferons are effective in the uncommon leukaemia and hairy cell leukaemia, and some activity has been demonstrated in renal cell carcinoma, some lymphomas and chronic leukaemias, myeloma, malignant carcinoid and malignant melanoma, although their use is still being evaluated. Side-effects of anorexia, nausea, tiredness, malaise, myelosuppression, disturbance of liver function tests and neurotoxicity occur.

Interleukin-2

Although lymphocytes are detected in a variety of tumours, they are not normally considered active. It is postulated that there may be a relative inability to generate cytokines in the tumour environment. Interleukin-2 (IL-2) has the ability to activate a subpopulation of T-lymphocytes, which then demonstrate the capacity to destroy tumour cells, known as lymphokine-activated killer cells (LAK cells). IL-2 has substantial side-effects when given systemically, and initial *ex vivo* stimulation of lymphocytes by IL-2 may be more effective. Activity has been demonstrated in relation to renal cell carcinoma and melanoma. Currently, the therapy involves *ex vivo* stimulation of the patient's lymphocytes by IL-2 followed by their reinfusion and the systemic administration of IL-2. The therapy is more effective when the lymphocytes are harvested from the tumour itself, tumour infiltrating lymphocytes (TILs).

Tumour necrosis factor

Tumour necrosis factor (TNF) is released by mononuclear phagocytes following exposure to endotoxin. TNF is also produced by monocytes, macrophages, endothelial cells, large granular lymphocytes and neutrophils. It is a peptide hormone with the capacity for:

- direct toxicity for cancer cells
- stimulation of procoagulant activity by vascular endothelial cells
- activation of neutrophil adherence and phagocytosis
- induction of fever by direct effect on the thermoregulatory centre.

TNF has been produced by genetic engineering and its clinical use is being evaluated. It appears to be a major effector molecule for macrophage-mediated cytotoxicity, and it plays a central role in the pathogenesis of endotoxic shock. Since it is not tumour specific, an alternative term, cachectin, has been used.

Anti-idiotypic antibodies

These are antibodies raised against specific antibodies, which thus mimic the original antigens. In cancer, such antibodies have been used in an attempt to immunize the patient against a tumour-associated antigen. Initial work indicated that this did indeed provoke an immunological reaction to human cancer, but clinical trials have been disappointing to date.

Novel treatments

There are various novel treatment under investigation and in clinical trials, which do not fall into any of the categories of cancer treatment described above. Perhaps two of the most exciting at present are the metalloproteinase inhibitors and gene therapy.

Metalloproteinase inhibitors

The metalloproteinases, of which there are at least 16 subtypes, are proteolytic enzymes, which are universally overexpressed by human cancers. They are thought to be crucial for the processes of invasion and metastasis, and hence the development of synthetic inhibitors of these substances has been heralded as a major therapeutic innovation. To date, phase I and phase II trials have indicated that they may have a role in halting or slowing tumour progression, but they cause quite significant reversible arthropathy. This may be related to the broad spectrum of activity of existing drugs, and work is underway to identify which enzymes are important in human cancer, and to develop specific inhibitors.

Gene therapy

Gene therapy is the treatment of disease by transferring genes into patients. It was introduced initially as treatment of genetic disorders and was first applied by Michael Blaese as replacement therapy for adenosine deaminase deficiency. Cancer has now become the major target of this treatment and considerable research on gene therapy for cancer is being conducted worldwide. Several approaches have been explored and these include:

- genetic immunomodulation by introducing genes for specific cytokines into cancer cells or lymphocytes
- suicide gene transfer, e.g. herpes simplex virus thymidine kinase (HSV-TK) followed by antiviral drugs such as ganciclovir
- gene transfer to protect normal tissue against chemotherapy
- antisense oligodeoxynucleotide transfer
- gene replacement with tumour suppressor genes, e.g. p53, the stress response protein, the function of

which was described earlier in this chapter. As the p53 gene is the most commonly mutated gene in human cancer, restoration of p53 function has attracted considerable attention.

Transfection of the gene into cells requires a vector, and this is most commonly a retrovirus or adenovirus. Such anticancer gene–vector combinations have been studied in both experimental systems and human cancer patients. Although initial results have shown promise, gene therapy is still in its infancy. The key factors that will determine success are (i) an effective methodology for targeting cancer cells and tissues, and (ii) high-efficiency gene transfer. Currently both are suboptimal and, for this reason, it is difficult to repair or destroy all malignant cells by gene transfer. Thus, the advance of gene therapy for cancer will depend as much on advances in molecular oncology as in technology and delivery systems to overcome the current limitations. It may prove impossible to kill all cancer cells in an established tumour by gene therapy, and initial surgical removal of the primary or *in situ* ablation followed by gene therapy for residual disease and micrometastases is a more realistic expectation.

Section 15.4 • Early diagnosis, screening and epidemiology

Early diagnosis

It seems self-evident that early diagnosis is beneficial in cancer, and this stems from the consistent finding that early tumours have a better prognosis than late tumours. In a clinical context, an early tumour is one which is at a favourable stage, i.e. small size, limited local invasion, no lymph-node or distant metastases. However, whether this is related more to the duration of the malignant process or to the biological behaviour of the individual tumour is open to question. The strongest evidence that early detection increases the chance of cure comes from the randomized trials of screening described below. However, there is also evidence that survival after diagnosis is related to duration of symptoms, and this has led to public-awareness campaigns to persuade individuals to seek advice regarding suspicious symptoms at an early stage. There is, however, no evidence as yet that this strategy can improve survival.

Screening

Screening is the application of a test in order to detect a disease while it is still asymptomatic. For this to be effective at a population level, certain criteria must be met by the disease to be screened for, the screening test and the screening programme. These are outlined below.

The disease
- its natural history must be well understood
- it must have a recognizable early stage

- treatment at an early stage must be more effective than at a later stage
- it must be sufficiently common in the target population to warrant screening.

The test
- it must be sensitive
- it must be specific
- it must be acceptable to the population to be screened
- it must be safe
- it must be inexpensive.

The programme
- there must be adequate facilities for diagnosis in those with a positive test
- the quality of treatment for screen-detected disease must be very high
- screening should be repeated at intervals if the disease is of insidious onset
- benefit must outweigh physical and psychological harm
- benefit must justify the cost.

The issue of whether or not treatment of the disease to be screened for at an early stage is more effective than at a later stage is central to screening theory. To support a screening programme it is insufficient merely to compare the outcome of screen-detected disease with that of disease that has presented with symptoms. The reason for this is that three biases operate in favour of screen-detected disease: lead time bias, length bias and selection bias.

Lead-time bias is illustrated in Figure 15.29. In essence, this arises from the fact that if early diagnosis advances the time of diagnosis of a disease, then the period from diagnosis to death will lengthen irrespective of whether of not treatment has altered the natural history of the disease. Only if treatment can shift the survival curve (Figure 15.30) will screening be of any value.

Length bias operates as slow-growing tumours are more likely to be detected by screening tests than are fast-growing tumours, which are more likely to present

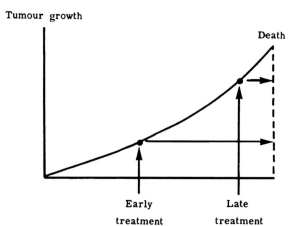

Figure 15.29 Lead time bias.

with symptoms before a screening test can be applied. Thus, screen-detected tumours will tend to be less aggressive and to be associated with a relatively good prognosis.

Selection bias results from the type of individual who will accept an invitation to be screened. Such a person is more likely to be health conscious than one who refuses or ignores screening, and is therefore more likely to survive longer irrespective of the disease process.

These three biases combine to make patients with screen-detected tumours **appear** to do better than those whose tumours present with symptoms. For the true value of screening to be uncovered, screening research must take these biases into account and eliminate them. The only way to do this is to carry out randomized, controlled trials in which the disease-specific mortality in a complete population **offered** screening (including those who present with symptoms before screening can take place and those who refuse to be screened) with that in a population **not** offered screening. In cancer, such trials have been carried out in breast and colorectal cancer (see below and in appropriate chapters in Volume II).

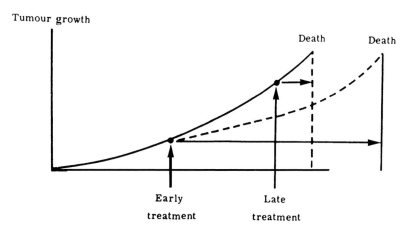

Figure 15.30 Effect of early or late treatment on survival where early treatment is truly beneficial and therefore associated with a change in the survival curve.

In screening it is also important to have a target population so that large numbers of fruitless tests are not conducted. This is particularly true in the common cancers, where the incidence is highly age dependent, and for cancer screening it important to establish an age range in which the disease is relatively common, and in which the patients are likely to be fit enough for treatment. There are other high-risk groups, however, and family history is becoming very important in this respect, particularly as it is now possible to detect specific genetic mutations from blood samples and use these to screen close relatives. These conditions are dealt with in the sections on breast and colorectal cancer in Volume II.

When a screening test is being developed, it is clearly important that it must be acceptable and safe so that it will be adopted by the target population. It must also be accurate, and accuracy is usually described in terms of sensitivity and specificity. Sensitivity is expressed as the proportion of individuals with the disease who have a positive test, and specificity as the proportion of individuals without the disease who have a negative test (Figure 15.31). Thus, the ideal test would be acceptable to the whole population, have no associated morbidity or mortality and have both a sensitivity and a specificity of 100%. Unfortunately, this ideal has never been realized, and any screening test represents a compromise between these factors.

When a screening programme is established, it is important to ensure that the diagnostic facilities are adequate, and this inevitably requires additional funding. It is also very important that the diagnosis is of the highest quality to avoid the patient dissatisfaction and litigation that stem from missed disease. Likewise, treatment of early disease must be associated with minimal morbidity and mortality.

Finally, it must be remembered that screening creates a certain amount of psychological morbidity, and along with any physical morbidity caused by investigation and treatment, this represents part of the cost of screening. It must be firmly established that the benefit gained outweighs such morbidity, and society must make a decision as to whether or not the health gain justifies the financial cost.

Epidemiology of cancer

Epidemiology is an extremely important discipline in cancer and it is useful to the surgeon in the following ways.

- **Definition of the size of the problem**: the extent of a cancer in a community is described in terms of its **incidence**, which indicates the rate of development of new cases in a defined period as a proportion of the whole population, and its **prevalence**, which constitutes the number of cases in the population at any one time. This is important in order to allocate resources to deal with the problem.
- **Identification of high-risk groups** is useful in developing strategies for early detection and prevention. Again, by ensuring that only appropriate groups are targeted, it is a guide to resource allocation
- **Identification of poor prognostic groups** by using variable characteristics of the tumour and the patient will allow logical planning of treatment for an individual case.
- **Indication of aetiological factors**: epidemiological studies have been particularly useful in determining the causes of many cancers, and especially in leading to the positive identification of carcinogens. Smoking as a cause of lung cancer is perhaps the best example, but extensive studies on diet and infective agents are now bearing fruit.

Section 15.5 • Quality of life, palliation and hospice care

Although the prime objective in the treatment of patients with cancer may be to cure, it has to be accepted that in many cases any treatment will ultimately be

DIAGNOSIS

TEST		Disease present	Disease absent
	Positive	True positive (a)	False positive (c)
	Negative	False negative (b)	True negative (d)

$$\text{SENSITIVITY} = \frac{a}{a+b}$$ $$\text{SPECIFICITY} = \frac{d}{d+c}$$

Figure 15.31 Sensitivity and specificity.

palliative. This may be obvious in the patient with established metastatic disease at the time of presentation, but may be less obvious when the initial surgical procedure has been considered curative. Attempts have been made to evaluate objectively the effectiveness of therapy to the patient, the best-known assessment being the Karnofsky index.

Karnofsky index

10. Normal
9. Minor signs or symptoms
8. Normal activity with effort
7. Unable to continue normal activity, but cares for self
6. Requires occasional assistance with personal needs
5. Disabled
4. Requires considerable assistance and medical care
3. Severely disabled and in hospital
2. Very sick; active supportive treatment necessary
1. Moribund

Once it is established that treatment may not be curative, then all therapy might be considered palliative. It should be recognized that many patients who have undergone a clinically palliative procedure may continue to have an excellent quality of life, and that it may not be in their best interests to be identified as undergoing palliative therapy until their clinical condition deteriorates.

Palliative medicine has developed as a specialty and might be defined as the study and management of patients with active, progressive, far-advanced disease, for whom the prognosis is limited and the focus of care is the quality of life.

Hospices have evolved following pioneering work by Dame Cicely Saunders in the 1950s and 1960s. Hospices provide a special environment for individuals with advanced cancer, providing home-care services, hospital support and inpatient hospice care. The aim of the hospice service is to provide the best quality of life for the terminally ill. This is orientated around:

- relief of symptoms such as pain and nausea
- psychological support to patient and relatives
- inpatient hospice care for terminal care, where necessary, and respite care when the burden of care on relatives requires temporary relief.

Guide to further reading

Berman, C. G., Brodsky, N. J. and Clark, R. F. (1998). *Oncologic Imaging*, McGraw-Hill, New York.

Bishop, J. M. and Weinberg, R. A. (1996). *Molecular Oncology*, Scientific American, New York.

Dunlop, R. (1998). *Cancer: Palliative Care*, Springer, New York.

Eremin, O. and Sewell, H. (1992). *The Immunological Basis of Surgical Science and Practice*, Oxford University Press, Oxford.

McKenna, R. J. and Murphy, G. P. (1994). *Cancer Surgery*, J.B. Lippincott, Philadelphia.

Price, P. and Sikora, K. (1995). *Treatment of Cancer*, 3rd edn, Chapman & Hall Medical, London.

UICC (1987). *TNM Classification of Malignant Tumours*, Springer, New York.

Patients undergoing elective surgery

'Surgery is a legalized and controlled assault on a human being with a therapeutic intent, and with consent obtained under duress imposed by pain, suffering or fear of death'

There is some truth in this cynical statement, as it emphasizes the inevitable physical and mental trauma to the patient inflicted by an operation. Good surgery minimizes this traumatic component and enhances the therapeutic benefit. Even so, to operate on a human being must be considered a privilege. This module deals with the management of patients undergoing surgery on an elective basis. By definition, these patients should carry the lowest risk commensurate with the nature of the disease and the magnitude of the intervention [see Module 3, Vol. I].

Section 16.1 • Elective surgery

Elective surgery is defined as a surgical intervention that is planned for a given date to suit both patient and surgeon, following the appropriate work-up and preparation of the patient for the operation. It involves admission to a surgical ward (inpatient surgery) or 5-day ward (short-stay surgery) or to a day-case unit (day-case surgery, DCS). In most situations, patients are admitted from the waiting list after completing their preoperative investigations and assessment as out-patients. For those undergoing inpatient surgery, the severity of the operation and the presence of comorbid disease [see Module 3, Vol. I] determine the need or otherwise for high-dependency or intensive care after operation, and the availability of such must be established before the intervention proceeds on the intended date. The ultimate objective is to ensure that the patient is in the best possible mental and physical state for the intervention and is fully aware of the nature of the operation for which consent is given.

Aside from psychological support, special considera-tions apply to patients undergoing elective surgery for cancer. In the first instance, surgical intervention is often part of a management strategy that involves other specialties and the operation may be followed by some form of adjuvant therapy, or indeed may have been preceded by chemotherapy or chemoirradiation [see Module 15, Vol. I]. The patient thus encounters more than one specialist during the treatment of the disease and it is important that the surgeon, chemotherapist and radiation oncologist 'sing from the same hymn sheet'. Increasingly, case discussion in the relevant disease-related treatment group is recognized as the best option to deal with this aspect and to formulate the treatment plan in the individual patient. When, it comes to surgery for cancer, considerable confusion exists between the terms 'operability' and 'resectability', which are often used interchangeably.

Operability refers to the patient's general con-dition (fitness for surgery and anaesthesia) and disease stage. A patient is considered inoperable if his or her condition or disease stage rules out any benefit from a surgical intervention, i.e. this decision precludes surgical intervention. **By contrast, resectability is an intraoperative verdict that qualifies whether the primary disease can be removed or not, i.e. resectable or non-resectable**. At the end of the operation, the resection may be considered potentially curative or non-curative (palliative). The 'potentially curative' verdict may need to be qualified by the detailed pathology report of the resected specimen. Reduction of the number of patients who are found to have non-resectable disease at operation to a minimum is an index of good clinical assessment of these unfortunate patients.

Section 16.2 • Scope and nature of investigations

Scope of preoperative investigations

Investigations are performed preoperatively in order to:

- confirm or establish diagnosis
- perform routine preoperative tests
- stage patients with cancer
- assess risk for surgery.

Tests to confirm diagnosis

A good clinical history and physical examination often indicate the nature of the condition and for some common conditions, such as external hernia, the findings on clinical examination are confirmatory and no diagnostic tests are needed. In disorders affecting the internal organs, confirmatory investigations are a necessary component of the preoperative work-up of the patient. In this respect, for the majority of surgical disorders affecting internal organs, there is usually one (rarely more) that will confirm the suspected disease. This is referred to as the **key investigation (or investigations)**, which may be endoscopic, radiological or biochemical. Some examples are shown in Table 16.1. It is obvious that the key investigation is performed before others. Often, the initial key investigation suggests the need for other tests to obtain more information on the disease, e.g. in a jaundiced patient, dilated bile ducts and a mass in the head of the pancreas are further investigated by computed tomography (CT) and will require a laparoscopy [see Hepatobiliary and Pancreatic Surgery, Vol. II].

Routine preoperative tests

These are discussed elsewhere [see Module 3, Vol. I]

Staging tests for patients with cancer

All patients with cancer undergo staging tests to determine resectability and potential curability. Patients considered inoperable may need palliative therapy that may include resection of the primary, surgical bypass or some form of radiological or endoscopic stenting. The results of the staging tests together with the clinical findings determine the clinical TNM (tumour, node, metastasis) stage of the disease. This may be altered by the results of the pathological examination of the resected specimen when the pTNM of a particular cancer is defined [see Module 15, Vol. I].

Radiological and radionuclide investigations

These include:

- plain radiology
- contrast radiology: oral and intravascular
- ultrasound examination: external, endoscopic and laparoscopic
- CT scanning
- magnetic resonance imaging (MRI)
- radionuclide studies: oral or i.v. administration of radionuclides with external counting and imaging by a gamma camera.

The various investigations that fall within these major categories of radiological investigations are considered in various modules in Volumes I and II. The present account covers the principles behind these investigations and their general applicability and usefulness in assessment of patients undergoing elective surgery.

Radiation risk with radiology and radionuclide studies

There is insufficient appreciation of the radiation hazard of these investigations, especially when repeated over a period in the same patient. These investigations must be used sparingly and only when strictly indicated. The effective dose is defined by the Royal College of Radiologists as 'a weighted sum of equivalent doses (in milliSieverts) to a number of body tissues where the weighting used depends upon the relative risk of fatal malignancy or severe hereditary effect for low radiation

Table 16.1 Some key investigations

Peptic ulcer disease and reflux oesophagitis	Upper gastrointestinal endoscopy
Oesophageal and gastric cancer	Upper gastrointestinal endoscopy
Gallstone disease	Abdominal ultrasound of biliary tract, ERCP
Jaundice	Ultrasound of liver, biliary tract and pancreas
Pancreatic neoplasm	CT/MRI
Hepatic tumours	CT/MRI
Small bowel disease	Barium follow-through or small bowel enema
Inflammatory bowel disease	Barium enema or colonoscopy
Colonic cancer	Barium enema or colonoscopy
Rectal cancer	Sigmoidoscopy
Haematuria	Cystoscopy + ultrasound examination of kidneys
Thyrotoxicosis	Thyroid function tests

Table 16.2 Relative doses of common radiological investigations and their equivalent natural radiation period

Examination	Effective dose (mSv)	Equivalent no. of chest X-rays	Equivalent period of natural background radiation
Chest (single PA) film	0.02	1	1.5 days
Skull	0.1	5	2 weeks
Lumbar spine	2.4	120	14 months
Pelvis	1.0	50	6 months
Abdomen	1.5	75	9 months
Barium studies:			
Oesophagus	2.0	100	1 year
Stomach	5.0	250	2.5 years
Small bowel	6.0	300	3 years
Large bowel	9.0	450	4.5 years
CT chest or abdomen	8.0	400	4 years
Lung ventilation scan	0.1	5	2 weeks
Lung perfusion scan	1.0	50	6 months
Thyroid scan	1.0	50	6 months

doses'. Examples of relative doses and their equivalent natural radiation period are shown in Table 16.2.

Radiological investigations in non–urgent patients

Aside from chest X-ray in selected groups, plain radiology of the abdomen is seldom indicated in patients undergoing elective surgery. Plain films of the abdomen for the detection of gallstones and oral cholecystography for gallstones have been superseded by abdominal external ultrasound scanning.

For disorders of the upper gastrointestinal tract (oesophagus, stomach and duodenum), contrast radiology has been largely replaced by flexible endoscopy as the initial investigation, but it is used selectively in some of these patients to provide more information on the pathological anatomy and site of the lesion before surgical treatment.

Barium meal and follow-through and enteroclysis (small bowel enema) are, however, the first investigation used in the diagnosis of small bowel disease. Currently, small bowel enteroscopy is reserved for problematic cases [see Gastrointestinal Disorders, Vol. II].

There have been few comparative studies between barium meal and follow-through and small bowel enema. The available evidence indicates that enteroclysis is superior except in Crohn's disease, where the follow-through can be more accurate. In one study, 12 out of 18 follow-through examinations were negative in patients with primary malignant neoplasms of the small intestines as opposed to two out of 20 patients examined with enteroclysis. Barium follow-through is of little use in the diagnosis of partial or intermittent intestinal obstruction. Enteroclysis yields more diagnostic information and is superior to CT in these cases. However, CT is accurate in showing site and cause in patients with established high-grade obstruction. Enteroclysis is superior to barium follow-through and even better than radionuclide studies in the diagnosis of Meckel's diverticulum.

Barium enema preceded by sigmoidoscopy remains the standard initial investigation in patients with suspected colorectal disease. A significant percentage of patients with colonic disease, including all those with inflammatory bowel disease, will require a colonoscopy for complete evaluation. Colonoscopy is difficult and is attended by increased risk in patients with diverticular disease.

In general, the radiation dose imparted by the standard radionuclide investigations compares favourably with those of other imaging modalities but there are exceptions, e.g. thallium-201 scanning myocardial perfusion study. Useful radionuclide investigations include:

- bone scintigraphy for femoral neck fractures (not visible on the initial X-ray film) and tumour deposits
- localization of septic foci and in the assessment of inflammatory bowel disease [see Module 17, Vol. I; Gastrointestinal Disease, Vol. II]
- location of obscure gastrointestinal bleeding
- provision of functional data: isotope renography, ejection fraction of the left ventricle, distribution of blood flow to the cerebral cortex, etc.
- location of ectopic tissue: Meckel's diverticulum
- detection of specific tumours or deposits: radio-labelled octreotide scan for insulinomas, sentinel node biopsy (melanoma and breast cancer), CEA-labelled antibody for colonic cancer, etc.

Technetium-99m (^{99m}Tc) hepatic scans for metastatic disease of the liver should no longer be used in view of their limited diagnostic yield compared with CT and MRI.

Ultrasonography

Basic principles of ultrasound

Audible sound waves have a frequency of 20–20 000 Hz (1 Hz = 1 cycle/s). Ultrasound waves have a much higher frequency (1–30 MHz) and are produced by vibration of piezoelectric crystals. These change shape and vibrate when electrically pulsed. Vice versa, piezoelectric crystals generate electric voltage when deformed [see Module 2, Vol. I].

The propagation of ultrasound waves depends on the number of molecules present in the medium. Thus, ultrasound waves do not travel in a vacuum and propagate poorly in gas (hence the need for acoustic coupling with gel between probe and skin). Propagation is better in liquids but is best in solids. The propagation speed of ultrasound waves through biological tissues is 1500 m/s (similar to water). Ultrasound waves are absorbed by bone, fat and gas, i.e. ultrasound scanning is useless for bones or in the presence of gaseous distension and gives poor results in obese patients.

Ultrasound scanning is based on the pulse echo principle, which deploys the following components.

- The piezoelectric crystal in the transducer head vibrates and emits ultrasound waves that propagate through the tissues. Some of the ultrasound waves are reflected back by tissues, depending on density (acoustic impedance) as 'echoes'.
- The reflected returning echoes reach the piezoelectric crystal of the transducer.
- The crystal vibrates again when the echo received generates electric voltage that is equivalent to strength of returning echo. The strength of the echo is related to the angle at which the propagated ultrasound waves strike at the acoustic interface, with maximal intensity being achieved when this is perpendicular. It also depends on differences in acoustic impedance between component tissues.

The equipment used consists of the transducer probe with an integral cable that docks into the ultrasound machine (image processing unit), which elaborates the ultrasound signals as images (in various modes) displayed on a monitor. Each ultrasound probe operates at a set frequency, i.e. the number of times that the ultrasound pulse is repeated per second (Hz). Increasing frequency improves resolution but decreases penetration. The range of transducer frequencies used for external ultrasound scanning is usually 2.5–5.0 MHz. Frequencies for contact (operative) and endosonography vary from 5 to 10 MHz. Each transducer has a focal zone (depth of sound beam where resolution is highest), although most modern transducers have electronic focusing, i.e. the transducer can be focused at varying depths.

Modern ultrasound probes

Modern ultrasound probes are either mechanically steered (rotary or sector) or electronically steered. The latter are of three types:

- **linear arrays**: a series of transducer elements (multiples of 64) pulsing sequentially in groups producing a rectangular image

- **phased arrays**: a series of 32 or more transducer elements electronically co-ordinated to produce a wedge-shaped picture that can be varied in size
- **annular arrays**: crystals of the same frequency mounted in a circle.

Elaboration of ultrasound images

Several types of display can be obtained from the ultrasound signals:

- **A-mode**: amplitude modulation; unidimensional image with amplitude (vertical) and distance (horizontal) axes
- **B-mode:** brightness modulation; two-dimensional (2D) image; brightness dots on the screen corresponding to the reflector point positions in the scanned region
- **M-mode:** time–motion screening of returning echo signals (e.g. echocardiography)
- **real-time:** immediate imaging and real-time motion.

Ultrasound Doppler

The Doppler effect refers to the change in sound frequency after reflection from a moving column, such as the red blood cell (RBC) mass in the centre of the blood stream:

- **continuous wave Doppler**: sound continuously emitted by one transducer and continuously received by a second transducer
- **pulsed Doppler**: sound transmitted and received intermittently by one transducer
- **duplex scanning**: pulsed Doppler alternates with real-time imaging
- **colour flow Doppler**: velocity frequency change is given a colour code. Varying shades of red are used for flow towards the transducer, and blue away from the transducer.

Value of ultrasound scanning in surgical practice

The common and important applications of diagnostic ultrasound are shown in Table 16.3. There is no question that ultrasound imaging has had a major impact on surgical practice across the specialties. It has been described as 'the surgical electronic stethoscope'. Although in many centres it is still regarded as 'a radiological investigation', clinicians, and in particular surgeons should learn how to use and interpret ultrasound images. Surgeons, by virtue of their knowledge of anatomy, are in a unique position to acquire this skill. In many European hospitals ultrasound scanning by the surgical registrar is an integral part of the clinical assessment in emergency and urgent situations, e.g. acute abdomen, blunt abdominal injury or suspicion of postoperative intra-abdominal collection.

Computed tomography

Conventional CT provides detailed high-resolution images of the transverse sectional anatomy (axial slices).

Table 16.3 Use of ultrasound imaging in surgical practice

- **External ultrasonography**
  Standard preoperative work-up: detection of gallstones, hepatic tumours, cysts and fluid collections, abscesses, etc.
     Clinical assessment of patients: acute abdomen and abdominal trauma, obstructive uropathy, etc.
     Guided percutaneous interventions: drainage of abscesses, fluid collections, etc.
     Ultrasound guided biopsy of breast lesions: impalpable lesions identified on screening for breast cancer

- **Endoluminal ultrasonography (endoscopic ultrasound)**
  Tumour staging and assessment of anatomy: most sensitive and accurate system for staging for upper gastrointestinal, proximal pancreatic and rectal cancers. Endoanal ultrasound essential for accurate assessment of sphincter integrity

- **Intraoperative contact ultrasonography**
  Open surgery: hepatic and pancreatic resections
     Laparoscopy: staging of pancreatic cancer, detection of islet cell tumours
     In situ ablation: laparoscopic ultrasound-guided in situ ablation of hepatic tumours

- **Vascular surgery**
  Non-invasive vascular assessment of peripheral limb ischaemia
     Detection of abdominal aortic aneurysms
     Duplex scanning: carotid artery stenosis

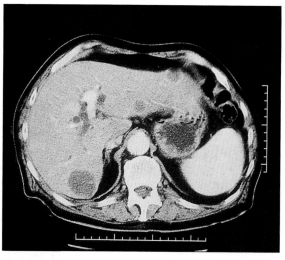

Figure 16.1 Spiral angio-CT of the liver showing non-enhancing tumour deposits from a primary pancreatic carcinoma.

permits discontinuous axial images that are acquired during separate intervals of breath holding. There is a dramatic reduction in the scanning time; for example, it is possible to scan the entire abdomen in less than 1 min. The fast scanning time allows more precise and complete studies following intravascular injection of contrast agents (Figure 16.1). Several types of helical CT scan can be performed on the liver **[see Hepatobiliary and Pancreatic Disorders, Vol. II]**.

Magnetic resonance imaging

MRI has two unique advantages: it does not carry any radiation hazard and it can provide multiplanar (sagittal, coronal, oblique) images (Figures 16.2–16.4). It has

In contrast to ultrasound, it provides good anatomical detail in obese patients as fat provides good contrast with structures of soft-tissue density (measured in Hounsfield units). For the same reason, it is less rewarding in very thin patients and children, where ultrasound is preferable. CT is now established as the optimal investigation for clinical problems within the chest and abdomen, despite its radiation risks: preoperative information of complex masses, evaluation of blunt abdominal trauma, detection of postoperative complications such as fluid collections and masses. CT has revolutionized the diagnosis and management of intracranial disorders and injuries. It is now the standard method of staging for the majority of malignant disorders including lymphomas, and allows accurate guidance for percutaneous drainage and biopsy procedures.

The more recent scanners are faster and scan round the patient in a spiral fashion (spiral or helical CT), thus producing volumetric data sets that provide greater definition and can be image processed to provide a three-dimensional (3D) reconstruction of the surface of the anatomy and of the inside of hollow organs. The latter is an exciting new image-processing technique referred to as virtual endoscopy (see below). Spiral CT scanning is obtained by moving the patient at a constant rate through a rotating gantry equipped with a third-generation scanner that takes about 1 s for each 360° rotation. The images are therefore obtained without any interscan delay during a single breath hold, as distinct from conventional CT, which only

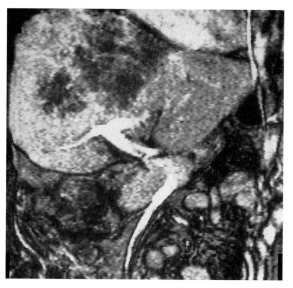

Figure 16.2 Oblique coronal MR of liver with i.v. gadolinium contrast showing a large hepatoma extending from the right lobe into segment IV but clearly separable from the portal vein and its main branches.

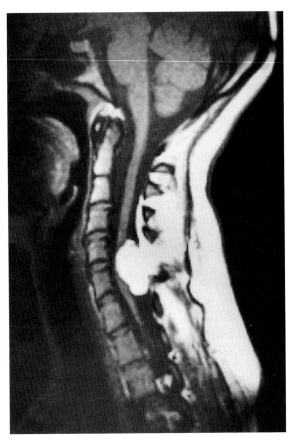

Figure 16.3 Mid-line sagittal MRI of the cervical spine showing cord compression by a posterior tumour: diagnosis – lipoma.

largely replaced CT in the investigation of patients with neurological disorders except for head injury, where CT is still the mainstay for diagnosis of intracranial haemorrhage.

The principle of MRI involves the application of a strong magnetic field (measured in Tesla), which aligns the protons in the tissues (mostly found in water). With the patient in this magnetic field, the alignment of the protons can be disturbed momentarily with pulsed radiofrequency electromagnetic radiation. On realignment, the protons emit a characteristic radiation and these signals can be detected and form the basis for the imaging. This involves fast computer image-processing algorithms of the signals. Variations in the pulsed radiofrequency (echo sequences) are used to produce diverse characteristics for imaging of different tissues. Contrast enhancement is possible by using contrast agents that incorporate paramagnetic ions and thus augment the magnetic field, e.g. gadolinium-DTPA and Endorem (superparamagnetic iron oxide).

MRI cannot be used in patients with cardiac pacemakers and metal heart valves. Diagnostic MRI machines have a closed tunnel magnet into which the trolley carrying the patient is moved. This closed, confined system and the noise generated during scanning can be awesome and claustrophobic to some patients, and indeed a few patients find the procedure intolerable. A two-way communication between the operator and the patient is standard in all machines, so that the procedure can be interrupted if the patient feels unwell or panics.

Magnetic resonance cholangiopancreatography (MRCP) will probably replace diagnostic endoscopic retrograde cholangiopancreatography (ERCP) in the future because it is completely non-invasive and does not need contrast injection. Although techniques of MRCP are still evolving, the basic principle is based on heavily T2-weighted 2D or 3D echo-train spin echo sequences, which produce a very high signal intensity in stationary fluids (bile, pancreatic juice) compared with the surrounding liver, pancreas and flowing blood

Figure 16.4 Sagittal MRI through the thorax showing the vessels: diagnosis – coarctation of the aorta.

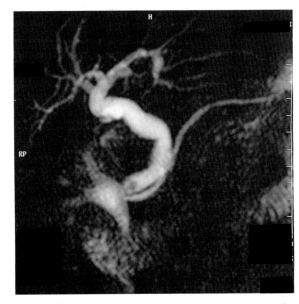

Figure 16.5 Magnetic resonance cholangiopancreatography (MRCP).

(Figure 16.5). Reports including prospective comparisons have shown that MRCP provides equivalent diagnostic information to ERCP.

Flexible endoscopy

Upper gastrointestinal endoscopy, flexible sigmoidoscopy and colonoscopy form an essential part of the diagnostic armamentarium of medical and surgical gastroenterology. Small bowel enteroscopy is a specialized investigation for small bowel disorders, e.g. obscure bleeding and tumours [Gastrointestinal surgery, Vol. II]. ERCP (Figure 16.6) and choledochoscopy are invaluable in pancreaticobiliary disorders [see Hepato-pancreatico-biliary disorders, Vol. II].

Virtual endoscopy

The availability of imaging techniques that enable the acquisition of volumetric data sets from patients (spiral CT and MRI) has led to the development of virtual endoscopy in the mid 1990s. Virtual endoscopy is essentially a 3D computer reconstruction (virtual reality) by a process of segmentation and image post-processing algorithms of both the surface and, in the case of hollow organs, the inside appearances of an organ under scrutiny. The various techniques are not as yet established, but virtual endoscopy holds great promise and will undoubtedly be used extensively in the future to obtain more anatomical information from the MRI and spiral CT images obtained from patients needing these investigations. Virtual-reality 3D reconstructions will materially influence screening for colon cancer and treatment planning. The most studied to date is virtual colonoscopy, which has been shown to identify tumours as small as 1.0 cm (Figure 16.7).

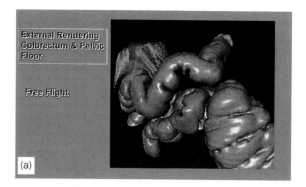

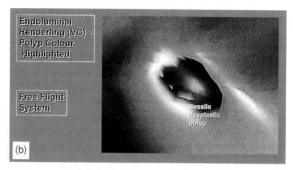

Figure 16.7 Virtual colonoscopy derived from spiral CT volumetric data set: (a) surface rendered appearance; (b) internal appearance showing a small sessile polyp.

Tests of cardiac function

Patients with moderate cardiac risk factors [see Module 3, Vol. I] and poor functional capacity require tests of cardiac function, e.g. stress electrocardiogram (ECG), 24-h Holter monitoring for ST depression and myocardial perfusion scanning, or invasive tests such as coronary angiography before the decision to proceed with surgery is taken [see Module 20, Vol. I]. Patients in the high-risk category may need coronary revascularization or angioplasty before the general surgical intervention. However, as there have been no prospective studies to document the benefit of coronary revascularization prior to general surgical operations, the decision is not easy and each case has to be assessed individually with expert cardiological advice.

Tests of respiratory function

These are indicated in patients with chronic respiratory disease (obstructive and restrictive) requiring surgical treatment. The simplest tests (e.g. exercise tolerance), while being clinically valuable, are relatively insensitive, i.e. they require significant functional impairment before changes can be detected. More sophisticated tests detect impairment earlier but require the co-operation and active participation of the patient.

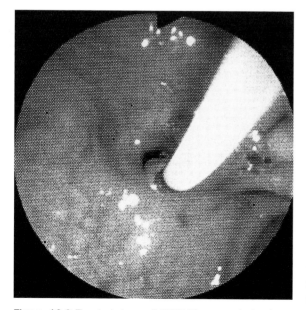

Figure 16.6 The technique of ERCP. The cannula is shown being placed within the ampula.

Lung function tests are useful in:

- confirming the diagnosis of respiratory disease
- assessing its severity
- predicting the response to treatment, including surgery.

Exercise tolerance can give useful information on the overall respiratory reserve, bearing in mind that the results may be influenced by the patient's cardiovascular and locomotor state and their general fitness. Standard tests based on metabolic equivalents (METs) record, for example, the number of stairs climbed or the distance walked within a set time, usually 6 or 12 min [see Module 20, Vol. I].

Measurement of ventilatory function

These tests are performed using a spirometer (vitalograph) or a peak flow meter or gauge. Spirometry measures the total volume and the rate of flow of air during a forced expiration immediately after a maximum inspiration where two measurements are made:

- forced vital capacity (FVC): total amount of expired air in litres
- forced expiratory volume in one second (FEV_1).

The ratio FEV_1/FVC is a useful indicator of functional impairment. The results are compared with predicted values that take into account the height, age and gender of the patient. Two patterns of abnormality are detected by spirometry:

- obstructive airways disease
- restrictive lung disease.

In obstructive airways disease (chronic bronchitis, emphysema, asthma) both the FVC and the FEV_1 are reduced but the deterioration of the latter is more marked, causing a fall in the FEV_1/FVC ratio. In restrictive lung disease (fibrosing alveolitis, sarcoidosis, pulmonary oedema) there is an equal reduction in both the FVC and FEV_1 so that the FEV_1/FVC ratio is unchanged.

The peak flow meter or gauge records the maximum rate in litres/min at which air can be expired following a full inspiration: the peak expiratory flow rate (PEFR). This is reduced in airway obstruction but may be normal in restrictive lung disease. The peak flow meter or gauge is portable and thus permits serial measurements in the wards and at home. It is used extensively in assessing the response to treatment in asthmatic patients.

Static lung volumes

These are measured by rebreathing air containing a known concentration of an inert gas (usually helium) until equilibrium is reached between the gas in the spirometer and that in the lungs. The most important measurements are:

- total lung capacity (TLC): the amount of air in the lungs in litres at the end of a full inspiration
- residual volume (RV): the volume of air in litres remaining after a maximal expiration.

The RV may be expressed as a percentage of the TLC, the RV/TLC ratio. This gives a measure of the amount of air trapped in the lungs at the end of expiration. Predicted values for each of these parameters are available taking into account height, weight and age. Both the TLC and the RV are raised in obstructive airways disease but the RV is elevated to a greater extent, thus producing a high RV/TLC ratio that exceeds 70% in severe cases. In restrictive lung disease the TLC is reduced, while the RV may be normal or reduced.

Transfer factor

The transfer factor (T_{CO}) is an index of the rate in ml/min/mmHg at which carbon monoxide passes from the atmosphere into the red blood cells. The important factors that influence this transfer are:

- airflow obstruction: alters gas movements from mouth to the terminal bronchioles
- distance between the terminal bronchioles and the alveoli: increased in emphysema
- thickness of the alveolar–capillary membrane: increased in fibrosing alveolitis and sarcoidosis
- total available area of the alveolar–capillary membrane: reduced in emphysema and after pulmonary resection
- amount and type of haemoglobin: reduced in anaemia
- cardiac output.

T_{CO} is influenced by lung size. This is overcome by the use of the Krogh transfer coefficient (K_{CO}), which is obtained by dividing the T_{CO} by the alveolar volume.

Table 16.4 Changes in pulmonary function tests in obstructive and restrictive lung disorders

	FVC	FEV_1	FEV_1/FVC	TLC	RV	RV/TLC	T_{CO}
1. Obstructive airways disease							
Chronic bronchitis	↓	↓↓	↓	N or ↑	N or ↑	↑	↓
Emphysema	↓↓	↓↓↓	↓↓	↑↑	↑↑↑	↑↑	↓↓
Asthma	↓	↓↓	↓	N or ↑	N or ↑	↑	N or ↑
2. Restrictive lung disease							
Fibrosing alveolitis	↓↓	↓↓	N	↓	N or ↓	N or ↑	↓↓
Sarcoidosis	N or ↓	N or ↓	N	N	N	N	↓

↓, reduced; ↑, increased; N, normal.

Measurement of T_{CO} and K_{CO} is useful in the assessment of the severity of interstitial lung disease. The patterns of ventilatory function, static lung volumes and transfer factor encountered in the main types of respiratory disorders are summarized in Table 16.4.

Blood gas analysis

Some patients with established chronic bronchitis (blue bloaters) have reduced oxygen tension (P_{O_2}) and raised carbon dioxide tension (P_{CO_2}) at rest, even at their best. The management of these patients after surgery requires repeated blood gas analyses as the inspired oxygen given by a Ventimask will depend on the arterial pH and the P_{CO_2}. In contrast, patients with primary emphysema (pink puffers) have a normal P_{O_2} but reduced P_{CO_2}.

Section 16.3 • Preoperative care

Preoperative care entails:

- assessment of operative risks [Module 3, Vol. I]
- adequate explanation of the nature of the operation and procurement of informed consent [Module 23, Vol. I]
- correction of nutritional [Module 8, Vol. I], blood volume [Module 6, Vol. I], fluid and electrolyte deficiencies [Module 7, Vol. I]
- institution of prophylactic measures against common postoperative complications
- general preparation of patient for surgery
- reasoned estimate of the amount of blood required to cover the operation (blood tariff)
- assessment of the likely immediate postoperative course and thus the need for high-dependency or intensive-care support [see Module 19, Vol. I].

Certain general principles are so self-evident that they are infrequently reiterated and remembered only in sad retrospection following the occurrence of avoidable tragedies. Good nursing care, safe prescription and administration of drugs, error-proof methods of patient identification, reassurance of the patient and an adequate explanation of the intended treatment to relieve anxiety, marking the operative site, the maintenance of essential replacement therapy, etc., whenever abused or misused may directly or indirectly led to disastrous consequences. Avoidable deaths in surgical practice are rarely the result of one 'front-line' surgical error, but follow a sequence of minor, apparently inconsequential latent errors that build up to form a trajectory for disaster. The ultimate prophylaxis against avoidable deaths in surgical practice is an obsession to check and double check.

Risk management

This has been broadly defined as 'the reduction of harm to the organization by the identification and, as far as is possible, the elimination of risk'. The concept adopted from industry was primarily introduced within the National Health Service (NHS) to control litigation and reduce the cost of malpractice to the various Trust Hospitals. As clinicians, however, surgeons should adopt this policy primarily to improve the quality of care and reduce risk or harm to the patients. This is referred to as **clinical risk management**, which has been defined as 'a particular approach designed to improve the quality of care and which places special emphasis on occasions on which patients are harmed or disturbed by their treatment'. Nowhere in surgical practice is clinical risk management more applicable than in patients undergoing operations.

Prophylactic measures

Several specific prophylactic measures are indicated not routinely but selectively in some patients owing to the presence of risk factors, which predispose to certain complications. The important ones are:

- prevention of infective endocarditis
- chemoprophylaxis against surgical infections
- prophylaxis against deep vein thrombosis (DVT)
- prevention of renal failure.

Prevention of infective endocarditis

The findings of the survey conducted by the British Cardiac Society showed that 43% of patients who develop infective endocarditis either had normal hearts or a previously unrecognized cardiac abnormality before the onset of the disease, stressing the fact that **valves of normal hearts can be infected and destroyed in severe bacteraemic episodes**. In this respect, the patients at risk include elderly patients, diabetics, alcoholics, the immunosuppressed and drug addicts. Streptococci are the most common responsible organisms for infective endocarditis (*Streptococcus viridans* in 48%, other streptococci in 15%), followed by staphylococci (19%), enteric bacteria (14%) and a wide variety of other organisms.

Aside from dental work, the invasive procedures that may result in bacteraemic episodes include all common gastrointestinal and genitourinary operations, endoscopic procedures, liver biopsy and percutaneous transhepatic cholangiography, blood donation, phlebography, haemodialysis, fractures and cardiac catheterization. In a recent study, bacteraemia was reported in 17–20% of patients after nasotracheal intubation.

The recommendations of the British Society for Antimicrobial Chemotherapy for patients at risk because of cardiac lesions are: **intravenous amoxycillin; vancomycin or teicoplanin or clindamycin for those allergic to penicillin; and a combination of amoxycillin and gentamicin against bowel organisms in patients with artificial valves or who have had endocarditis**. The provision of antibiotic cover in elderly patients with apparently normal hearts is not settled but the consensus view is that such a policy is not without risk in view of the large number of patients above the age of 60 years undergoing surgical, investigative and dental procedures.

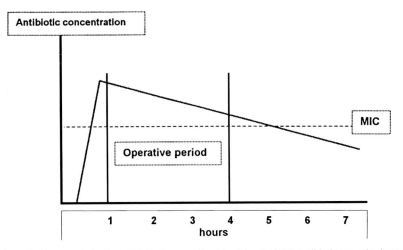

Figure 16.8 Principle underlying prophylactic antibiotic therapy: the blood level of the antibiotic must be kept above its minimum inhibitory concentration (MIC).

Chemoprophylaxis against surgical infections

In the UK National Survey of Hospital Infections, a total of 19% of patients was found to have infections. In 9%, the infection was acquired in hospital and wound infection accounted for 20% of these. Postoperative wound infections have been shown to occur in about 40% of patients after colorectal surgery where antibiotic prophylaxis was not used. A meta-analysis of 26 randomized trials has confirmed that chemoprophylaxis in patients undergoing colorectal surgery not only halves the postoperative infection rate but also reduces significantly the postoperative mortality (from 11.2% in the no antibiotic group to 4.5% in patients receiving antibiotic prophylaxis).

Antibiotic prophylaxis is not an alternative to good surgical practice including strict aseptic technique, and is indicated when the risk of infection is high (clean–contaminated and dirty operations) or the results of infection (if it occurs) are serious. The situations in surgical practice where antibiotic prophylaxis is

indicated because of proven benefit (evidence-based policy) are shown in Table 16.5. The antibiotics recommended in this table reflect general consensus but may indeed vary from hospital to hospital.

The principles governing safe and effective antibiotic prophylaxis in surgical practice are well established and include the following.

- Therapeutic tissue concentrations of the antibiotic (minimum inhibitory concentration, MIC) must be present at the time of the skin incision and maintained throughout the operation (repeated dosing during prolonged operations). In this respect the pharmacokinetics (half-life and protein binding) are important (Figure 16.8). Thus, the MIC of the antibiotic must be maintained throughout the duration of the operation. This entails repeated dosing if the half-life of the antibiotic (or combination) used is shorter than the duration of the operation.
- The antibiotic should, whenever possible, be bactericidal in nature with high tissue penetration ability and low toxicity.
- The choice of agent(s) depends on the pathogens most likely to be encountered in a given situation.
- Topical antibiotics are less effective and do not provide protection against intra-abdominal abscesses and bacteraemia.

A single dose administered either intramuscularly 2 h before the operation or intravenously at induction is sufficient. The recent report commissioned by the NHS Health Technology Assessment concluded that a single dose or short-term use (less than 24 h after operation) is as efficacious as long-term postoperative use of antibiotic prophylaxis, and may be associated with less toxicity, fewer adverse events, reduced risk of bacterial resistance and lower overall costs. Short-term use involves further injections at 12 and 23 h after surgery.

Antibiotic prophylaxis should not be used (as a routine) in clean operations. There is no evidence that it

Table 16.5 Chemoprophylaxis against surgical infections

Clinical condition/ situation	Antibiotic regimen
Breast surgery	i.v. Co-amoxiclav or i.v. erythromycin
Gastro-oesophageal surgery	i.v. Co-amoxiclav or i.v. cephalosporin (or gentamicin) + i.v. metronidazole
Biliary surgery	i.v. Cephalosporin or Co-amoxiclav
Colorectal surgery	i.v. Gentamicin (or cephalosporin) + metronidazole
Acute appendicitis	Intrarectal metronidazole (suppositories) or i.v. Co-amoxiclav
Orthopaedic surgery	i.v. Cephalosporin
Endoscopic urological surgery	i.v. Gentamicin
Vascular surgery	i.v Co-amoxiclav or cephalosporin

prevents postoperative chest infections even in patients with tracheostomies or endotracheal tubes. The exception to this is where prosthetic material (vascular grafts, mesh repair of hernia, etc.) is used. Gelatin-bonded fluorinated polyester vascular prostheses enable antibiotic bonding (rifampicin) to the graft immediately prior to insertion. The prosthesis is soaked in rifampicin solution for 15 min prior to use, when the antibiotic binds to the gelatin coating. These antibiotic-bonded grafts are used in high-risk areas by some vascular surgeons. More recently, the same material has become available as mesh for the repair of large incisional hernias. Experience with this type of mesh hernioplasty is limited and its efficacy in reducing infection remains to be confirmed by prospective studies.

Prophylaxis against deep venous thromboembolism

The importance of this is stressed by the report of a major UK study that 0.9% of patients admitted to general hospitals die from pulmonary embolism (PE), with most fatal emboli resulting from deep vein thrombosis in the lower limb. The estimated cost of DVT/PE to the NHS in 1993 exceeded £200 million and the Office of Health Economics concluded that if all patients at high risk of developing postsurgical DVT had received prophylaxis, the NHS would have saved between £33 and £81 million. The Thromoembolic Risk Factors (THRiFT) Consensus Group now **recommends that prophylaxis should be given to patients according to the degree of risk, at least until discharge from hospital**. This recommendation is accepted and practised in all surgical specialties with the exception of orthopaedics. There exists considerable debate amongst orthopaedic surgeons on the benefits of DVT heparin prophylaxis versus the complications and cost, and many prefer mechanical methods such as foot impulse technology (FIT) and intermittent pneumatic compression (IPC). As yet, direct randomized comparisons between heparin and mechanical measures have not been conducted.

The risk factors for DVT are covered elsewhere [see Module 19, Vol. I]. It is useful to divide patients into three categories depending on their risk of DVT, proximal venous thrombosis (VT) and fatal PE. These are outlined in Table 16.6.

The recommended THRiFT policy for the three groups is as follows:

■ **low-risk patients: graduated compression stockings (GCS) and early mobilization**
■ **moderate- to high-risk patients: GCS, early mobilization, mechanical prophylaxis (FIT or IPC), unfractionated heparin (UFH)/low molecular weight heparin (LMWH) and establishment of specific local prophylaxis protocol.**

Local protocols

Local protocols are recommended for the moderate- and high-risk groups of patients to accommodate specific local factors and informed clinical preference. Each surgical specialty should develop its own protocol in accordance with recognized guidelines. Aside from risk assessment, these protocols should take into account the nature of the operation, the incidence of thromboembolic disease after specific operations, the risk of bleeding (pertinent to joint replacement surgery especially of the knee) and surgical preference.

Chemical prophylaxis
Subcutaneous low-dose heparin: the therapeutic intent is to reduce thrombin formation and thus the initiation and extension of fibrin-rich venous thrombi without full anticoagulation of the patient. UFH is administered in a dose of 5000 units 2 h before

Table 16.6 Thromboembolic disease: risk level, risk rates and patient groups

Risk level	DVT	Risk rates (%) Proximal VT	Fatal PE	Patient group
Low	< 10	< 1	0.01	Minor surgery, no risk factors other than age Major surgery, age < 40 years, no other risk factors Minor trauma or medical illness
Moderate	10–40	1–10	0.1–1	Major general, urological, gynaecological, cardiothoracic, vascular or neurological surgery, age > 40 years or other risk factor Major medical illness: heart or lung disease, cancer, inflammatory bowel disease Major trauma or burns Minor surgery, trauma or illness in patients with previous deep vein thrombosis, pulmonary embolism or thrombophilia Orthopaedic surgery or amputation of lower limb Lower limb paralysis
High	40–80	10–30	1–10	Major pelvic or abdominal surgery for cancer Major surgery, trauma or illness in patients with previous deep vein thrombosis, pulmonary embolism or thrombophilia Full limb paralysis Major limb amputation

operation and then every 8 or 12 h until discharge from hospital. The 8-hourly regimen is associated with a significant increase in the incidence of wound haematoma. LMWH is an alternative to UFH and may have some advantages, although the matter remains unresolved. Thus, data from individual studies suggest that LMWH is no more effective than UFH in preventing postoperative thromboembolism, while a meta-analysis of 32 separate investigations indicated that LMWH may be slightly more effective. There is some evidence that LMWH may have a lower incidence of bleeding. Obvious major advantages of LMWH are convenience and cost savings, since the same level of prophylaxis is obtained with one single daily injection. Subcutaneous heparin (UFH or LMWH) is the mainstay of prophylaxis in both moderate- and high-risk patients, and **must be administered in all these patients together with mechanical methods in accordance with local protocols**. Even so, protection in high-risk groups may not be complete, particularly in those with a history of recent venous thrombosis, and various chemical combinations have been advocated, e.g. low-dose heparin + dihydroergotamine. Some advocate intravenous heparin administered with a calibrated infusion pump in these patients. The heparin is started before surgery and adjusted to maintain a heparin level in the blood of 0.1 unit/ml. This is gradually increased to 0.2 unit/ml in the postoperative period. Extended prophylaxis with LMWH after discharge from hospital and up to 35 days postsurgery has been recommended in high-risk patients after certain major operations, although the efficacy of this approach remains unproven.

Heparin chemoprophylaxis is not used in neurosurgery because of the risk of postoperative intracranial haemorrhage. Likewise, it is not administered routinely in urology except in patients undergoing extensive pelvic surgery for invasive carcinoma of the pelvic organs, where it is usually combined with mechanical methods.

Concern has been expressed on the use of subcutaneous heparin in patients receiving epidural analgesia for postoperative pain relief. In fact, there have been very few cases where epidural haematoma has occurred in patients on subcutaneous heparin and the majority has been obstetric cases. It appears that the risk of epidural haematoma is not increased significantly from that observed in patients not receiving any anticoagulants. There is a consensus view amongst the majority of anaesthetists that heparin prophylaxis with LMWH is commenced after the epidural catheter has been placed. This seems a sensible precaution, although there is no evidence that it reduces the risk. Heparin is attended by specific problems in pregnant women, e.g. allergic reactions, thrombocytopenia and heparin-induced osteoporosis. The risk of thrombosis in pregnant women requiring surgery must be balanced against the risk of heparin.

Oral anticoagulants: these are administered in doses that result in prolongation of the prothrombin time to between 1.5 and two times the control value. The major disadvantage of this regimen is increased risk of perioperative bleeding. A modified approach whereby the treatment is commenced 2–3 days after operation reduces the risk of bleeding to acceptable levels. The reported literature on oral anticoagulant prophylaxis for thromboembolic disease is scanty and, in general, these agents are confined to the treatment of established disease.

Dextran 70: prophylaxis with Dextran 70 is as effective as low-dose heparin in the prevention of fatal PE after general surgical operations. The dextran solution is administered in a volume of 500 ml at the time of surgery and repeated once daily for the first 2–5 days. Its disadvantages include hypersensitivity reactions, circulatory overload in the elderly and a slight risk of bleeding when commenced at the time of surgery. Dextran prophylaxis is used extensively in orthopaedics, especially in patients undergoing elective hip surgery. Dextran is contraindicated in pregnant females (anaphylactoid reactions that cause fetal distress, perinatal death or severe neurological damage).

Other agents: antiplatelet drugs such as aspirin and hydroxycholoroquine have a demonstrable but limited efficacy in preventing deep vein thrombosis. There are ongoing studies to determine the effect of aspirin on PE and mortality in patients with hip fracture, but these results are still awaited. Drugs that stimulate endogenous fibrinolysis such as anabolic steroids have been shown to have some activity in preventing DVT.

Mechanical methods of prophylaxis against thromboembolic disease
These include:

- graduated compression stockings (GCS)
- intermittent pneumatic compression (IPC)
- foot impulse technology (FIT).

GCS are the most commonly used mechanical method, either alone or in combination with chemoprophylaxis. The reported studies indicate that GCS reduce the risk of DVT in patients undergoing general surgical operations by 68%. IPC is an effective method of prophylaxis in general surgical, urological and neurosurgical patients, provided the intermittent compression is started at operation and continued throughout the postoperative period until the patient is fully ambulant. IPC is currently being investigated in patients undergoing laparoscopic surgery, where it has the added benefit of reducing the adverse cardiovascular effects of the positive pressure pneumoperitoneum [see Module 21, Vol. I].

Prevention of renal failure
The cause of renal failure in the postoperative period is often multifactorial. Damage may result from hypoxia, sustained hypovolaemia with hypotension, the accumulation of endogenous nephrotoxic substances (e.g. free haemoglobin, myoglobin, endotoxin or excess bilirubin) or drug-induced nephrotoxicity (most commonly

non-steroidal anti-inflammatory drugs, NSAIDs). The high-risk groups include:

- patients undergoing cardiopulmonary bypass and aortic surgery
- jaundiced patients
- patients with significant hypovolaemia from blood loss or severe fluid and electrolyte deficits.

Apart from avoiding known precipitating factors, effective prophylaxis is based on the maintenance of an adequate renal perfusion and oxygenation. Specific prophylaxis of renal failure in these high-risk groups is based on the proven observation that if sodium absorption is inhibited, the hypoxic damage due to a fall in the renal blood flow is reduced. This natriuresis is achieved by a loop diuretic (frusemide) or an osmotic diuretic (mannitol). As the resulting diuresis causes dehydration, these patients have to be well hydrated by intravenous crystalloids and 5% dextrose for at least 12 h before surgery.

In patients with jaundice due to large bile duct obstruction, the preoperative oral administration of bile salts (Na^+ cholate) reduces the risk of postoperative renal failure by blocking the absorption of endotoxin produced by the gut microflora. Another prospective trial showed that oral lactulose in a dose of 30 ml three times a day also protects patients with obstructive jaundice from postoperative renal failure.

Maximum surgical blood order tariff

Recurrent shortages of blood are becoming increasingly common in surgical practice. To some extent, this is the result of wastage of red cell units through outdating as a result of the widespread practice of ordering more blood to cover operations than is actually needed. Several audit surveys in the UK and USA have shown an excessively high ratio of blood cross-matched to that transfused. Wastage is enhanced when, as often happens, the blood transfusion department is not informed soon enough that some or all of the blood has not been used. Re-cross-matching of the blood that has not been transfused is therefore delayed

Table 16.7 Maximum surgical blood order tariff

Operation	Routine tariff group and screening procedure (G + S) no. units cross-matched	Blood requirements	
		Increased tariff due to clinical considerations	Indication leading to increased tariff
General surgery			
Abdominoperineal resection	4		
Bowel resection	3		
Breast biopsy/lumpectomy	G + S		
Cholecystectomy	G + S		
Partial gastrectomy	G + S		
Total gastrectomy	3	4	Thoracotomy
Haemorrhoidectomy	G + S		
Hernia repair	G + S		
Ileostomy	G + S		
Laparotomy	G + S	2	Malignancy
Liver biopsy	G + S		
Radical mastectomy	2		
Simple mastectomy	G + S		
Splenectomy (elective)	2		
Thyroidectomy	G + S		
Vagotomy (truncal, HSV)	G + S		
Varicose vein operations	G + S		
Urology			
Partial cystectomy	2		
Total cystectomy	4		
Transurethral resection of bladder lesions	G + S	2	Larger tumours
Nephrectomy	2		
Nephrolithotomy	2		
Prostatectomy	2		
Thoracic surgery			
Oesophagogastrectomy	4		
Hiatus hernia	G + S		
Pneumothorax	G + S		
Thoracotomy for pulmonary resection	3	4	Reoperation
Mediastinoscopy	2		
Arterial surgery			
Aortic aneurysm	6	10–12	Ruptured
Femoropopliteal bypass	3		

(After Napier, J. A. F., et al. (1985). *BMJ* **291**: 799–801, by courtesy of the Editor.)

to the extent that it cannot be used for other patients. This unsatisfactory situation has led to the formulation of 'tariffs' (maximum order schedules) by regional blood transfusion centres. These maximum order tariffs indicate the appropriate amount of blood to be cross-matched for the various operations (Table 16.7). The use of these blood tariffs is combined with a policy of blood grouping and antibody screen only in those patients undergoing operations that do not usually require blood. The tariff for any given operation may be increased by virtue of certain clinical considerations, such as anaemia, malignancy, previous radiotherapy and reoperation. The tariff policy has been validated by a number of studies that have demonstrated its safety and efficacy in terms of substantial reduction in the amount of unused and wasted blood.

General preparation of patients for surgery

Nursing procedures

Routine measures include bathing the patient, application of identification bracelets, removal of dentures and other items such as jewellery and prostheses, administration of the premedication at the specified time, and total starvation for 4–6 h before surgery. Whole-body disinfection by 4% chlorhexidine gluconate soap showers on the preoperative day, the preoperative evening and the morning of the operative day is widely practised in Sweden but recent trials have failed to show any significant reduction in the incidence of postoperative wound infections.

The patient should be requested to empty the bladder on the morning of the operation. Although still widely used, shaving enhances the incidence of wound infection, especially if performed several hours before the operation. It causes a myriad of tiny wounds in the skin that encourage bacterial growth. The use of depilatory creams is preferable in this respect, although repeated application may result in allergic skin reactions.

Gastrointestinal preparation

There is little doubt that adequate preparation reduces both the morbidity and mortality following surgery on the gastrointestinal tract. In the emergency situation, the insertion of a nasogastric tube to evacuate the gastric contents is mandatory and its routine use has reduced the incidence of aspiration during induction **[see Modules 13 and 17, Vol. I]**. However, the situation is different in elective surgery. Patients with pyloric stenosis may require frequent gastric washes via a nasogastric tube with isotonic saline. However, the routine insertion of a nasogastric tube in patients undergoing elective abdominal surgery is inappropriate, causes unnecessary discomfort to most patients and incurs a certain morbidity with a higher incidence of chest infection, oesophagitis and sore throat. The only indication for nasogastric suction in elective surgical practice is after subtotal oesophagectomy with gastric pull-through and a cervical anastomosis since these patients are at risk of aspiration, particularly if the laryngeal nerves have been damaged. In this situation, the standard Ryle's tube is inadequate and a Salem sump tube attached to a suction machine is necessary to ensure that the intrathoracic stomach is kept empty.

Adequate bowel preparation is necessary for procedures on the intestinal tract and is particularly relevant to colorectal surgery. Both mechanical preparation and bowel sterilization (or systemic antibiotics) are important as they reduce infection and leakage rates. Traditional mechanical cleansing of the colon entails a liquid low-residue diet, purgation and colonic washouts with tap water or phosphate enema. Increasingly, mechanical bowel preparation is achieved by osmotic oral purgation with balanced crystalloid solutions of polyethylene glycol (PEG) such as Golytely and KleanPrep. About 2 litres of orange-flavoured PEG solution achieves very satisfactory mechanical cleansing of the bowel. The whole-gut isotonic saline irrigation technique, although very effective, has been abandoned because it is poorly tolerated, particularly by the elderly and induces distressing colic in patients with stenotic lesions.

Mechanical preparation of the colon is often incomplete in the presence of a distal stenosing lesion, and the proximal colon may have to be cleared of faecal matter at the time of surgery. There are two techniques for achieving this safely. The first method (retrograde) uses a special tube (Muir's) that is introduced via a colotomy proximal to the stenosing lesion. The second technique (prograde) involves an appendicectomy with insertion of a DePezzer/Malecot catheter through the appendix stump into the caecum. Alternatively, the tube is inserted through a small stab incision in the terminal ileum through the ileocaecal valve into the caecum (Figure 16.9).

Mechanical bowel preparation has no effect on the bacterial counts in the colon. Effective reduction of the colonic bacterial population can be achieved by oral administration of neomycin and erythromycin or neomycin and metronidazole on the day prior to operation. However, the majority of surgeons has abandoned bowel sterilization for systemic antibiotic prophylaxis.

Catheterization of the urinary bladder

The urinary bladder should be catheterized in all patients undergoing operations in the pelvis, in patients at risk from renal failure and in those who require prolonged intravenous fluid therapy.

Nutrition

This is covered elsewhere **[see Module 8, Vol. I]**. A period of parenteral or enteral nutrition (if the gastrointestinal tract is functioning) may be needed in patients with protein calorie malnutrition prior to major surgery. If considered necessary, parenteral nutrition should be maintained for a minimum of 2 weeks to impart any real benefit. The central line for parenteral nutrition should be inserted in theatre with full aseptic precautions.

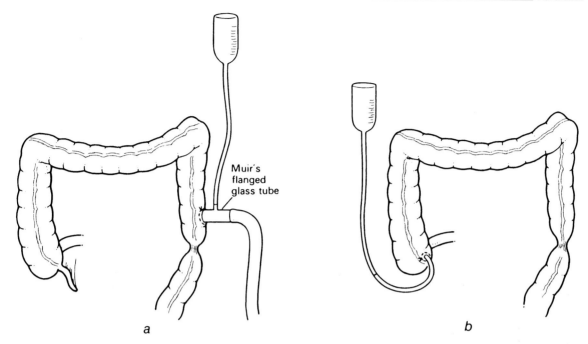

Muir's
flanged
glass tube

a   *b*

Figure 16.9 (a) Diagrammatic representation of the use of Muir's technique for cleaning the colon of faecal matter proximal to a stenosing lesion at operation (retrograde technique). The Muir's tube is introduced in to the colon proximal to the lesion and held in place by a tight purse-string suture. The Paul's tubing attached to the exit end of the Muir's tube is clamped and 1–1.5 l of detergent solution is run into the colon, which is then kneaded to break down the faecal concretions. On release of the clamp, the colonic contents are discharged via the Paul's tubing into a bucket containing antiseptic solution. (b) Prograde method of dealing with faecal impaction of the colon proximal to a stenotic lesion at operation. An appendicectomy is performed and a Malecot or DePezzer catheter (size 24–26) is introduced into the caecum and held in place by a purse-string suture. The detergent solution is then run into the colon and the catheter is clamped. The colon is massaged to break down the faecal concretions. Thereafter, the tubing is unclamped and the colonic contents siphoned off. Alternatively, the catheter is introduced into the caecum via a stab wound in the terminal ileum.

Consent for operation

The onus for this rests with the surgeon or an experienced member of the junior staff. Consent must be informed with a clear explanation of the nature of the operation [**see Module 23, Vol. I**]. Most disputes have arisen in the context of alleged non-disclosure of the risks involved in a particular treatment.

Premedication

In the past, the scope of premedication was to ensure the smooth induction and maintenance of anaesthesia by reducing salivation and secretions, raising the threshold of pain and producing euphoria. Since the advent of intravenous induction, the primary goal has been to relieve the anxiety that is present in the majority of patients before surgery.

Often the patients cannot explain why they are anxious, although some may have had previous unfortunate experiences with inhalational anaesthesia and surgical complications. Children who have had repeated operations are often frightened.

Drug premedication does not absolve the surgeon and anaesthetist from reassuring the patient and providing him or her with an adequate explanation of the intended operation. **Narcotics** (opiates) have become less popular as premedicating agents. In the first instance, timing of the injection is crucial since their effects wear off after 1 h. This becomes an important consideration when the operation is delayed. Secondly, they have undesirable side-effects, e.g. postoperative nausea and vomiting (PONV) and respiratory depression. **Barbiturates** are seldom used nowadays. **Phenothiazines** produce sedation and antiemesis at the expense of increased restlessness, tachycardia and hypotension. However, promethazine + pethidine is popular with some anaesthetists as the promethazine enhances the sedative effect of pethidine and reduces its emetic effect.

Table 16.8 Benzodiazepines used for sedation

Drug	Mean elimination half-life (h)	Dose and route of administration
Diazepam	33	0.1 mg/kg i.v.
	32	10 mg b.m.
Lorazepam	13	5 mg i.v.
	14	5 mg b.m.
Oxazepam	8	45 mg b.m.
Nitrazepam	30	5 mg b.m.
Temazepam	8	20 mg b.m.
Triazolam	4	0.25 mg b.m.

The **benzodiazepines** are the most popular premedicating agents nowadays. They have anxiolytic and hypnotic effects and act on receptors in the cerebral cortex and limbic system, in addition to facilitating gamma-aminobutyric acid (GABA) transmission. Their main advantages include minimal cardiorespiratory depression and high blood levels after oral administration. They are effective within 1 h of oral administration and their action lasts for 2–4 h. The amnesia produced by benzodiazepines is particularly helpful in patients undergoing endoscopy and operations under local anaesthesia. Some of the commonly used benzodiazepines are shown in Table 16.8.

Section 16.4 • Operative care

Good operative care militates against the occurrence of accidental hazards to the patient and attending staff. Furthermore, it ensures the safe execution and completion of the surgical treatment. The design of modern operating theatres, although conducive towards the attainment of these goals, in no way absolves the staff from the strict observation of fundamental surgical principles governing the safe execution of surgical procedures: strict aseptic ritual, reduction of human traffic to the bare minimum possible, exclusion of infected individuals from the theatre and a relaxed but prepared atmosphere.

Operating theatres (rooms)

Hospitals are nowadays equipped with operating theatre suites (OTS) with reception and recovery wards serving several operating theatres, each with its own anaesthetic/induction, immediate recovery and scrub rooms. The layout of the OTS is designed to facilitate traffic and communication with essential services such as the theatre sterile supply unit (TSSU), blood transfusion, pathology and microbiology departments, surgical wards, high-dependency unit and intensive care. Other features include positive-pressure filtered-air ventilation with frequent air changes (20/min) to reduce bacterial airborne infection, piped services for anaesthetic gases, electric power cables, monitoring and suction, ducting of escaped anaesthetic gases, monitoring and imaging equipment. Standard safety features are incorporated to prevent electrical mishaps from stray discharges and static electricity: waterproof sockets, careful siting of electrical sockets well above floor level, antistatic floors, etc.

Sterilization facilities

Almost all sterile items and instruments are supplied to each OTS by the TSSU and the standard method of sterilization used is autoclaving. Ethylene oxide sterilization is used for items that are damaged by autoclaving. This requires a long turnaround (5–7 days) as time is required for the gas to leach out following the sterilization. There are items that need to be sterilized in

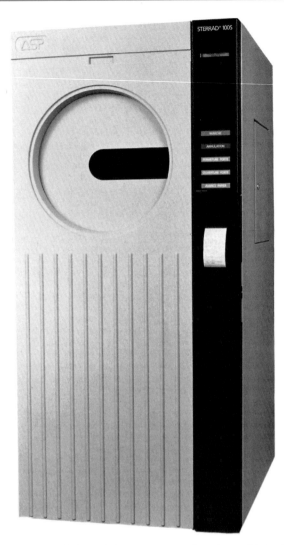

Figure 16.10 Sterrad: low-temperature ion plasma (derived from H_2O_2) sterilization system.

the operating suites, e.g. dropped instruments, operating ultrasound probes and endoscopes. Some theatres have small autoclave units for metal instruments. The majority of OTS have until recently relied on chemical sterilization with glutaraldehyde or equivalent disinfectants. Problems have been encountered with this practice, including chest problems from fume inhalation, skin irritation and conjunctivitis amongst the nursing staff undertaking the sterilization and disinfection. Considerable research has been undertaken in recent years to develop a substitute, effective and quick method of sterilization of small heat-sensitive equipment such as endoscopes and ultrasound probes. The most promising technique that has been introduced in a number of hospitals is H_2O_2-plasma sterilization, e.g. Sterrad, Ethicon (Figure 16.10). Essentially, this is a sealed cabinet through which an electric current is generated that converts the H_2O_2 to free radicles that act as the bactericidal and sporicidal agents. It is extremely likely that this system of sterilization will replace chemical disinfection in all theatre suites.

High-tech operating theatres

There is little doubt that the current design of operating theatres and essential components, including the operating table, is unsuitable for the conduct of minimal access surgery. The large number of freestanding unconnected devices used, with a myriad of floor-trailing cables leading to the sterile area and foot switches, amounts to a situation bordering on ergonomic chaos and is intrinsically unsafe (e.g. accidental activation). The surgeons have to adopt unusual and strenuous postures to undertake the surgical manipulations. The patient has often to be placed in extreme positions on a standard pedestal-operating table that was not designed for this purpose. Some interventions require sophisticated imaging during the intervention, best achieved by open (operating) MRI units. These considerations stress the need for the development of specific high-tech operating theatres for minimal access and image-guided surgical interventions [see Module 21, Vol. I].

Skin preparation

The skin bacteria comprise a resident and transient group of organisms (Table 16.9). The resident flora may change, particularly in patients who have been hospitalized for long periods. As it is not possible to sterilize the skin, the term 'preparation' is used. The aim of this is to reduce the resident flora by the application of antiseptic solutions. The various preparations in common usage are shown in Table 16.10. In general, their efficacy in terms of reduction of the skin sample counts of viable bacteria is improved by repeated use. All available antiseptics have limitations, e.g. chlorhexidine is not sporicidal.

Intra-abdominal packs soaked in antiseptic solution are used by some surgeons during gastrointestinal operations. If this practice is adopted, the antiseptic used must not be toxic locally and after absorption into the blood stream. A fire hazard is well documented when electrocautery is used close to packs soaked in alcohol-based antiseptic.

Gowns and drapes

Traditionally, surgical drapes and gowns have been manufactured from cotton textiles or mixed cotton–polyester fabrics. Although these have a number of advantages including comfort, drapability, tensile strength and steam permeability and sterilizability, they do not meet the recent mandatory European Standard for 'Surgical Clothing and Drapes'. This stipulates that fabrics used for surgical drapes and gowns must meet certain requirements that ensure:

- resistance to microbial penetration
- resistance to liquid penetration
- minimal release of particles.

Thus, cotton gowns and drapes will be replaced by reusable items made from different materials or quality, single-use, disposable products. Two types of material are likely to be used: microfilament yarns and laminates.

Microfilament yarns

These microfilament materials consist of densely woven fine polyester filaments that release virtually no particles during use. They exhibit high resistance to tearing and abrasion and have high tensile strength. The weave incorporates conductive carbon fibres, which ensures absence of a static charge. The fabrics have a durable liquid-repellent finish and are lightweight. Their disadvantage lies in the reduction of the bacterial barrier property with each laundry cycle unless subjected to hydrophobic treatment.

Laminates

Trilaminates provide the best protection during long and complex surgical procedures. They consist of three layers made from a microporous membrane that is bonded between two layers of endless polyester fibres. The pore size is such that bacteria, viruses or liquid cannot penetrate the laminate, yet the material is permeable to water vapour molecules.

Care of the anaesthetized patient during surgery

This is undertaken by the anaesthetist but a close rapport is needed between the surgeon and the anaesthetist. The main components of intraoperative care are:

Table 16.9 Skin bacterial flora

Resident flora	*Staphylococcus aureus* (some patients)
	Staphylococcus spp.
	Diphtheroids
	Micrococci
	Gram-negative bacilli
Transient flora	*Staphylococcus aureus*
	Pseudomonas spp.
	Other Gram-negative organisms
	Clostridial spores

Table 16.10 Antiseptic solutions used for the preoperative preparation of the skin

Preparation	Mean % reduction in skin-viable bacterial count	
	After one treatment	After six treatments
Chlorhexidine 4%	86.7	99.2
Povidone–iodine 10%	68	99.7
Hexachlorophane 3%	46.3	91.9
Irgasan DP 300 2%	11.2	95.8
Chlorhexidine 0.5%, in 95% ethanol	97.9	99.7
Phenolic 0.1%, in 95% ethanol	91.8	99.5
Chlorhexidine 0.5%, in water	65.1	91.8

[Modified from Lowbury, E. J. L. (1982). Special problems in hospital antiseptics. In: *Principles and Practice of Disinfection, Preservation and Sterilization* (A. O. Russell, ed.), Blackwell Scientific Publications, Oxford, pp. 262–284.]

- monitoring
- replacement of fluid and blood losses
- maintenance of body temperature
- protection of patient against damage
- special measures.

Monitoring

In general surgery, this has two components: (i) anaesthetic and respiratory, and (ii) cardiovascular.

Anaesthetic and respiratory
This entails:

- **basic monitoring**: supply pressure gauges, flow meters, reservoir bag tension, anaesthetic breathing connections
- **reservoir bag excursions**, chest-wall movement and respiratory pattern (precordial stethoscope in small children and babies)
- **oxygen failure alarm**
- **inspired oxygen concentration analyser and alarm**
- **pulse oximetry**: display of arterial oxygen saturation
- **airway pressure alarms:** overpressure or disconnection
- **capnography**: end-tidal CO_2
- **exhaled gas spirometry**: expired minute volume.

Cardiovascular
This is aimed at ensuring a stable cardiovascular state and adequate perfusion to the essential organs. The extent of the monitoring depends on the patient's condition (comorbid disease) and the magnitude of the operation being performed.

- **basic**: skin colour, peripheral perfusion, pulse rate/volume, blood pressure, electrocardiographic monitoring, temperature and central venous pressure (CVP)
- **urine output**: if cardiovascular state is compromised and for major or long interventions
- **arterial (radial) cannulation** in patients undergoing high-risk procedures: continuous display of the arterial blood pressure and its wave form
- **balloon flotation catheter** in patients with cardiac disease: to measure the pulmonary wedge pressure and filling pressure of the left ventricle
- **cerebral functioning monitoring**: when the circulation to the brain is at risk.

Replacement of fluid and blood losses
Intravenous fluid replacement is carried out with crystalloids, which are now preferred to colloid solutions [see Module 6, Vol. I]. The volume of blood lost during surgery is estimated by weighing the swabs (before drying) and adding this to the measured amount in the reservoir of the suction device. An extra 25% is added to this cumulative total to account for other losses such as that on the surgical drapes. Blood transfusion is only necessary when 20% or more of the blood vol-

ume has been lost [see Module 6, Vol. I]. After major intraoperative blood loss when the patient has sustained a period of shock, myocardial contractility may be depressed (ischaemic damage, circulating depressant substances, metabolic factors) and, for this reason, adequate cardiac output may not return immediately after the blood volume has been restored. This is indicated by a rising CVP with continued hypotension. These patients often require inotropic support.

Maintenance of body temperature
Considerable heat loss occurs in the anaesthetized patient. This is particularly important during long procedures and in children. Several mechanisms are involved. In the first instance, anaesthesia depresses the thermoregulatory centre in the hypothalamus. Shivering is abolished by the neuromuscular blocking agents, and direct losses occur by evaporation from the exposed body cavities and from the respiratory epithelium. In addition, the patient is usually lightly clad. Hypothermia is thus a problem unless body heat is conserved during surgery.

The environmental temperature within the operating theatre must never be less than 24°C. The temperature should be higher for high-risk adults (28°C) and children (30°C). The measures adopted to reduce heat loss in patients during surgery are:

- active warming blankets below or above the patient
- covering all exposed parts with soft insulating material
- warming intravenous fluids
- warm humidification of the inspired gases.

Protection against damage
This includes protection against mishaps and injuries (see below) and measures to prevent venous stasis and damage to the vascular intima of the calf veins. The use of soft rubber mattresses and careful positioning of the patient minimize but do not abolish prolonged calf vein compression during prolonged surgical procedures. The situation is aggravated in patients undergoing laparoscopic surgery with positive pressure pneumoperitoneum, where the venous return from the lower limbs is markedly reduced. It is now customary practice for all patients to wear graduated compression stockings during all operative interventions. Patients at risk and those undergoing major operations or prolonged laparoscopic operations benefit from IPC or FIT to stimulate the calf muscles during the operation.

Special measures
Examples include controlled haemodilution, often used in cardiac surgery, hypotensive and hypertensive medication, e.g. in patients undergoing resection of pheochromocytomas [see Adrenal Gland, Vol. II]. In patients undergoing major hepatic resections, in addition to inflow occlusion (portal vein and hepatic artery), reduction of the CVP (between 2 and 5 cmH$_2$O) is an important factor in reducing operative

blood loss. This is achieved by avoiding fluid volume loading at operation and a glyceryl trinitrate infusion, which is commenced at the start of the hepatic resection. It is important, however, that a negative CVP is avoided as this can lead to air embolism through small or unrecognized lacerations of the hepatic veins.

Prevention of mishaps and injuries to patients

Mishaps and accidents

The avoidable mishaps that usually lead to litigation are:

- operating on the wrong patient or site
- anoxic cerebral damage during anaesthesia
- drug interaction or misuse
- compression or traction injuries
- high-frequency electrosurgical burns **[see Module 2, Vol. I]**
- retention of swabs, instruments and needles.

These accidents are all preventable by attention to detail and by a practice that involves in-built safety checks designed to attain the ALARP region, i.e. the risk is As Low As is Reasonably Possible.

Patient identification

This process starts with the salutary practice of the surgeon or one of the staff having a brief chat with the patient before induction. Apart from being a source of reassurance to the patient, this occasion provides an opportunity for a final check on the identification of the patient with cross-reference to the identification bracelets, case notes, marked operation site (e.g. unilateral hernia repair) and relevant radiographs, which should always be put up on the viewing box within the operating theatre before the start of the operation.

Drug reactions

This is largely the responsibility of the anaesthetist and covers the intravenous administration of fluids and drugs during the surgical procedure. Adverse drug interaction, abnormal reaction to drugs and anaesthetic agents can be avoided or envisaged by adequate preoperative assessment, including detailed drug and anaesthetic histories of the patient. The choice of prophylactic antibiotic (when indicated) is made by the surgeon in consultation with the anaesthetist.

Nerve injuries

These neuropraxic injuries, although recoverable, are a source of anxiety and prolonged disability to the patient. They arise from faulty positioning of the patient and are due to compression or traction of nerve trunks, especially during prolonged operation. The most common positions of the patient that predispose to these injuries include the Trendelenburg tilt, the left or right thoracic position, hyperabduction of the arm and lithotomy. An increase in the incidence of traction injuries has been observed in minimal access surgery. This is due to the exaggerated tilt that is often needed to achieve an optimal endoscopic view of the operative site. This results in gradual slipping of the patient on the operating table.

The nerves most commonly injured are the popliteal, brachial plexus, radial and ulnar nerves. Adequate positioning and strapping of the patient with use of padding for protection constitute essential safeguards.

Intraoperative hypoxia

Although instances of fatal hypoxia have occurred during surgery as a result of oxygen supply failure, this eventuality is extremely rare with the current basic monitoring that is considered mandatory, including oxygen supply alarm failure, inspired oxygen concentration analyser with alarms, pulse oximetry, and disconnection and overpressure alarms. Hypoxia may arise during the course of an operation if the endotracheal tube becomes displaced as the patient slides up or down on the operating table with extreme head-down or head-up tilts. Another cause of hypoxia is tension pneumothorax that can develop during laparoscopic surgery with positive pressure pneumoperitoneum, e.g. laparoscopic antireflux surgery or laparoscopic cardiomyotomy.

Retained items

It is universal practice nowadays to have three counts for swabs and instruments, the first two being taken before closure and the final count before the patient is reversed. The most frequent cause for concern nowadays is a small needle, usually from an atraumatic pop-off suture. A radiograph of the area is undertaken if after a thorough search and recount, the needle is still missing. There has been an increasing number of successful litigations against surgeons and hospitals for retained needles in patients after laparoscopic surgery.

Laparoscopic surgery poses special problems with regard to retained items. The first relates to detachable instruments that are inserted and applied within the abdomen and then released from their applicator, e.g. detachable intestinal clamps. These have been developed to reduce the number of ports needed. Unless some mechanism is in place to remind the surgeon and scrub nurse that such a clamp has been deployed within the closed abdomen, there is a real risk that such an item may be overlooked. The second situation that has been well documented is lost gallstones during laparoscopic cholecystectomy. This arises when the gallbladder is perforated during either the dissection or extraction of the organ. Every effort should be made to retrieve such spilt stones as a significant number of these patients subsequently develop intra-abdominal abscesses and other complications. Currently, the consensus of opinion is that conversion to open laparotomy is not necessary if the stone cannot be found and retrieved laparoscopically, but the patient should be informed and followed up by ultrasound examination for at least 6 months since most complications declare themselves within this time frame.

Cardiovascular collapse during surgery

This is the surgeon and anaesthetist's nightmare. Its occurrence may be expected and the cause obvious, e.g. massive blood loss, but often the cardiovascular collapse is sudden and without any warning signs. It is important to consider the common causes of cardiovascular collapse and to have a preset strategic plan of action.

The common causes are:

- **myocardial events**: infarction, severe arrhythmias, etc.
- **bleeding**: this may not be obvious, especially if retroperitoneal, a situation encountered in laparoscopic surgery as a result of injury to the aorta and major retroperitoneal vessels inflicted during the creation of a closed pneumoperitoneum.

Less common causes are:

- **tension pneumothorax**
- **air/gas embolism.**

Essential initial monitoring of the situation includes:

- **ECG**: cardiac problems
- **CVP**: raised/normal (cardiac, air embolism, tension pneumothorax) or low (blood loss)
- **auscultation of heart and lungs**: tension pneumothorax and air/gas embolism.

The action plan depends on the exact cause (Figure 16.11). Arrest of bleeding is a priority and the method depends on whether the **territorial distribution of the bleeding vessel** is known or not, e.g. bleeding from distal aorta into the retroperitoneum needs a proximal aortic clamp, whereas bleeding from the hepatic artery is readily controlled by Pringle's manoeuvre. **If the territorial distribution of the bleeding cannot be readily determined, packing with manual compression is applied. Compression with hand or packs or both is also necessary if vascular clamps are not immediately available**. Once bleeding is controlled, the surgeon should wait until the anaesthetist has made up the volume deficit and a reasonable blood pressure has been restored.

Cardiac problems require the necessary measures and inotropic support and the services of a cardiologist should be sought if possible. Tension pneumothorax is remedied immediately by a chest drain. Air/gas embolism causing an outflow block of the right ventricle is treated in the first instance by posture.

Use of drains

There are few more controversial issues in operative surgical practice than the use of drains. Some surgeons insert drains routinely, others selectively and an increasing cohort only when they have to, as in the drainage of abscess cavities. Drains come in various shapes and sizes and are referred to by a confusing array of eponymous names.

The major factor that determines the performance of drains is the tissue reaction to the material composition of the drain. **Latex rubber** is soft but excites a profound inflammatory reaction within 24 h, which encases the drain, rendering it ineffective. **Polyvinyl chloride (PVC)** is much less reactive and thus more effective. It is, however, firm and unyielding and tends to harden and split with prolonged use, especially when in contact with bile. The best drain material is **silicon**, which is the least reactive and the most pliable, and shows no tendency to harden with prolonged use.

There is no doubt that drainage is essential after certain surgical procedures. Often, however, there is no reason for drain insertion other than habit. The use of drains must be selective and should be tempered by the realization that drains cause a definite morbidity that includes pain, increased incidence of wound infection, impaired healing, pressure necrosis of oedematous hollow organs, restricted mobility and delayed convalescence.

Drainage systems

Various systems are used and they are best discussed separately.

Open (static) drainage
The drain (Penrose, multitubular, corrugated, Ragnall, etc.) is exteriorized either through the operation wound or via a separate stab wound. It is stitched to the skin or held in place by a safety pin, and then covered with a gauze pad. **This type of drain contributes to wound infection and to general dissemination of bacteria in surgical wards, including methicillin-resistant *Staphylococcus aureus* (MRSA), in a substantial way.**

Closed siphon drainage
In this system, tube drains of PVC or silicon are connected to drainage bags equipped with a one-way valve at the entrance to the bag, which has an emptying tap at the other end. This allows daily emptying without disruption of the connection between the drain and

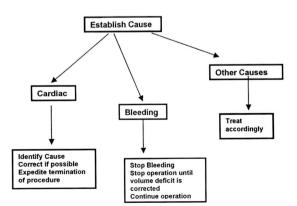

Figure 16.11 Action plan in the event of intraoperative cardiovascular collapse.

the collecting bag. Some systems incorporate bacteriological filters as an added precaution against infection via the drain path.

Closed suction drainage
Firm polyethylene tubes with multiple perforations are connected to portable and disposable suction flasks. Some use a low-pressure vacuum (−100 to −150 mmHg) such as the Portovac and the Reliavac systems. Others employ a higher negative pressure (−300 to −500 mmHg), e.g. Redivac and Sterimed. Closed suction drains are of proven efficacy, particularly in the drainage of the parieties. There is little to choose between the various types in terms of efficiency.

Sump suction drainage
This is the most efficient system of drainage and is especially suited to the collection of irritant discharges or those that contain activated digestive enzymes (high small bowel and pancreatic fistulae). The drain has a parallel air vent that prevents the adjacent soft tissues from being sucked into the lumen of the drain when the negative pressure is applied. Some of the available sump suction drains incorporate a bacteriological filter inside the air vent to prevent contamination of the cavity with airborne bacteria. Most are made of PVC but silicon sump drains are also available.

Underwater seal drainage
This is essential for drainage of the pleural space. The drains are straight or angulated near the tip and are constructed from PVC or silicon.

Indications

The present position regarding the use of drains can be summarized as follows.

Conditions in which the use of drains is a life-saving measure
The only disorder that comes into this category is tension pneumothorax, where the rapid insertion of an apical drain is the sole factor affecting the immediate survival of the patient. There is an increased incidence of tension pneumothorax in patients on positive-pressure ventilation and the prophylactic use of chest drains in these patients has been advocated, although this policy is not practised widely.

Conditions in which drainage imparts undoubted therapeutic benefit or constitutes a safe prophylactic measure
These include:

- chest drainage: haem/pneumoperitoneum, empyema
- thoracotomy, cardiothoracic procedures, oesophageal resections and perforation
- drainage of abscesses and infected cysts
- sump suction drainage of gastrointestinal, biliary and pancreatic fistulae
- closed suction drainage after extensive dissections and elevation of skin flaps

- after operations for injuries to solid organs and partial excision of these organs
- after pancreatic necrosectomy.

Conditions where drainage is generally advocated but its value remains unproven
Either routine or selective drainage is carried out in the following:

- supraduodenal direct exploration of the common bile duct
- duodenal stump after Polya gastrectomy and gastroduodenal anastomosis
- anterior resection, particularly of the low variety
- pancreatic resections.

Conditions where drainage is counterproductive
There is good evidence that drainage can be harmful, either by introducing infection within the peritoneal cavity or by increasing the incidence of wound infection. In one trial, it appeared to nullify the beneficial effects of prophylactic antibiotics on wound infection. The conditions where drainage is not recommended routinely are:

- peritonitis due to perforation of a hollow organ: the use of drains is certainly no substitute for adequate peritoneal toilet and lavage
- acute appendicitis.

Prevention of transmission of infectious disease

Surgeons, nurses and other health-care workers are at risk of contracting serious, at times fatal, viral infections. These include viral hepatitis, cytomegalovirus infections and acquired immunodeficiency syndrome (AIDS) [see Module 5, Vol. I]. Special precautions are necessary to avoid viral transmission to other patients. The transmission of viral disease from the medical staff to patients can also occur but is rare. Most frequently, patients contract viral infections from the transfusion of blood and blood products [see Module 6, Vol. I]. The prevalence of hepatitis B and C and human immunodeficiency virus (HIV) positive status amongst medical staff is not known. If a surgeon is HIV positive or an infectious carrier after contracting hepatitis B or C, he or she is duty bound to inform the relevant hospital infectious disease specialist and cease operating until the matter is clarified [see Module 5, Vol. I].

Measures for the prevention of spread of viral disease

Transmission of viral disease to members of staff may result from:

- direct percutaneous inoculation of infected blood, e.g. accidental needle pricks or scalpel wounds
- spillage of infected blood on the skin may introduce infection through minute skin abrasions

contamination of mucosal surfaces by infected blood, e.g. accidental splashing of eyes

transfer of infected material via fomites, e.g. blood-contaminated equipment.

In addition, there is some concern of the transmission of viral particles in the CO_2 gas effluent from infected patients undergoing laparoscopic surgery, although to date, this mode of transmission has not been confirmed.

Special procedures during care of infected patients

These involve:

identification of the patient's infectivity: by appropriate serological tests

special accommodation and nursing

precautions by the operating team

treatment of used disposable items and clinical waste material

treatment of used non-disposable equipment

disposal of the deceased.

Accommodation and nursing

These patients should be admitted and kept in single-room accommodation (preferably with *en suite* toilet facilities) and barrier nursing. All staff involved with the patient or handling specimens from the patient should be aware of the diagnosis. Long-sleeve gowns and masks should be worn by all staff. Additional isolation techniques, e.g. gloves, plastic aprons and eye protection, are necessary when invasive procedures are undertaken. Room cleaning should include daily floor mopping and damp dusting with hypochlorite (Chloros diluted 1:100 giving 1000 ppm available chlorine).

Precautions by the operating team

All members of the operating team should wear disposable plastic aprons beneath laminate-type disposable gowns, double gloves and eye goggles. Drapes should also be disposable. Extra care is taken to prevent accidental injuries (sharps), blood spurting and spilling. **In particular, hand-to-hand transfer of sharp instruments between the scrub nurse and surgeon should not take place. Instead 'a place and pick' routine is used, whereby the exchange is through an intermediate repository.**

All external surfaces and equipment, trolleys, etc., within the theatre and the floor are wiped with Chloros or glutaraldehyde at the end of the procedure.

Treatment of used disposable items and clinical waste material

Soft disposables should be double bagged and incinerated. Disposable equipment, including needles, is placed in an impervious container of metal or thick cardboard before incineration.

Treatment of used non-disposable equipment

Whenever possible, these should be sterilized by heat (autoclaving); otherwise, chemical disinfection is carried out by soaking for at least 1 h in either 2% glutaraldehyde or a 10% dilution of formaldehyde solution BP. Chemical sterilization is less satisfactory than autoclaving.

Disposal of the deceased

In the event of death, the corpse is inserted in a polythene cadaver bag before coffining and the undertaker should be informed.

Section 16.5 • Postoperative care

Following surgery, reversal and extubation, the patient is either transferred to the recovery ward or, in the case of major surgery, directly to the intensive care unit. At the end of the period of observation in the recovery ward, if the patient's condition is considered stable, transfer to the ward or high-dependency unit takes place. Detailed postoperative instructions are written down and the drug therapy is prescribed in the hospital prescription sheet. The operation notes should be dictated soon after the operation when details are still fresh in the surgeon's mind; meanwhile, a brief note is entered in the case notes on the essential findings and the nature of the procedure.

Immediate recovery phase

This is conducted in the recovery ward within the theatre suite. The advantages of a recovery ward are:

close observation of the patient during the immediate recovery phase by qualified nurses under supervision by an anaesthetist. This, together with monitoring of vital signs, enables the early recognition of physiological derangements

immediate availability of staff, equipment and essential services to deal with any life-threatening complication

immediate access to the operating theatre in the event of a complication, such as haemorrhage, that requires re-operation.

During the immediate recovery phase, the patient regains consciousness, with the normal respiratory drive and muscle activity that enable adequate pulmonary ventilation through a patent airway that is guarded by vital protective reflexes. In the early stages, attention is directed primarily to the airway. **The patient is nursed in the lateral position with the jaw held forward and must not be left unattended until he or she (i) is capable of protecting the airway and (ii) responds to simple commands.**

Maintenance of airway

The problems related to the airway that can occur at this stage are:

obstruction

irritability

vomiting and aspiration.

Obstruction of the airway

The most common cause is decreased muscle tone of the pharyngeal muscles leading to supraglottic flaccidity. It is remedied by pulling the chin up and extending the head, or more effectively, by pulling the mandible forward from behind the angles while the mouth is kept open. An oropharyngeal or nasopharyngeal airway solves the problem. Fortunately, laryngeal oedema is rare and is usually the result of a specific deficiency of C1 esterase inhibitor. This and other causes of oedema necessitate immediate tracheostomy.

Other monitoring and assessment in recovery ward

The extent of monitoring and clinical assessment depends on the patient's ASA status and the magnitude of the operation. The standard monitoring and assessment in the recovery ward after major surgery include:

- conscious level
- ECG
- CVP, blood pressure, pulse rate and temperature
- pulse oximetry: oxygen saturation
- urine output
- output from any drain
- pain control (see below).

Oxygen therapy

The factors that may cause abnormal gas exchange in the postoperative period are:

- reduction in the tone of the muscles of the chest wall
- changes in the bronchomotor and vascular tone
- diaphragmatic splinting (pain, abdominal distension)
- retained bronchial secretions.

These result in a reduction of the pulmonary functional residual capacity and collapse in the dependent segments of the lung. Functionally, these changes cause increased arteriovenous shunting and ventilation–perfusion mismatch leading to hypoxaemia, especially if the mixed venous oxygen content is low as a result of inadequate cardiac output or increased oxygen consumption.

Oxygen should be administered routinely until the patient is fully awake and extended beyond this to 24 h or more after major surgery and in patients with comorbid cardiac or respiratory disease.

Oxygen can be administered by a variable-performance mask (*c.* 35–60%), e.g. Hudson (5 l/min), or by nasal catheter (4 l/min). Toxicity is unlikely if the concentration of inspired oxygen is less than 60%. Fixed-performance high air flow oxygen (HAFOE) masks, e.g. Ventimask, are essential in patients with chronic lung disease who have lost the normal ventilatory control and depend on moderate hypoxaemia to stimulate respiration. When prolonged oxygen therapy is needed, humidification of the inspired oxygen/air mixture is essential to avoid drying of the bronchial mucosa and encrustation of secretions. In surgical wards, this is best achieved by use of the Venturi-type nebulizing humidifiers.

Ward management

In essence, ward management is based on the principle of progressive care with frequent clinical assessment/monitoring during the first 24 h. After abdominal operations, a period of adynamic ileus is inevitable but this should resolve in the majority of patients by 48 h after surgery. The objectives of postoperative ward management are:

- early detection of complications [**Module 18, Vol. I**]
- adequate pain relief
- maintenance of fluid and electrolyte balance with fluid balance charts [**Modules 6, 7, Vol. I**]
- continuation of prophylactic measures
- wound care
- early ambulation
- planning further treatment/follow-up visits after discharge.

Minor ailments such as insomnia, restlessness, anxiety and hiccups, which are very important to the patient, must not be overlooked.

In cancer patients, a full discussion of the prognosis and any need for further treatment is best delayed until the pathology report of the resected specimen is received. If adjuvant therapy is needed, the patient is best seen by the respective specialist before discharge from hospital, even if the treatment is not scheduled to start until after discharge from hospital.

Follow-up visits at the outpatient clinic are arranged before discharge. It is good practice for the general practitioner to be informed by phone when the patient is discharged from hospital, as usually a delay is incurred before receipt of the discharge letter. Special arrangements may be needed for elderly patients who are no longer able to lead an independent life. Some may require admission to nursing homes or sheltered care or home help, depending on the results of assessment of the individual case. Terminal cancer patients are best managed by hospice care.

The problem of multidrug resistant bacteria

This has arisen from misuse of antibiotics. It has been estimated that between 20 and 50% of hospital prescriptions for antibiotics are unnecessary. The most important is MRSA. This constitutes an increasing problem in surgical wards. Although MRSA are no more pathogenic than ordinary antibiotic-sensitive *S. aureus*, some strains of MRSA can spread rapidly in wards, colonizing the nose and skin of patients and staff. The most frequent sources of MRSA are sputum, pus and effluent from open drains. If a patient becomes infected (rather than colonized), the infection is difficult to treat because the range of antibiotics that can be used is very limited (vancomycin).

MRSA infection is usually spread from one patient to another on the hands of medical, nursing and paraclinical staff. Patients whose skin is heavily colonized with MRSA include those with eczema, pressure sores and leg ulcers. These patients shed large numbers of bacteria into their immediate environment. As most strains of MRSA can survive drying in dust for several days, the potential for widespread infection is significant and may have serious consequences, particularly in orthopaedic wards, neurosurgical and intensive care units. Hand washing by the staff with detergent soap is the most important method of prevention of spread of infection from patient to patient.

When a patient is colonized or infected by MRSA, special precautions are necessary. The patient should be treated in a single room, preferably with its own washing and toilet facilities. Plastic aprons should be worn when in contact with the patient and before entering the room. Gloves should be used when bed making, dressing wounds, attending to intravenous infusions, changing drainage bags and providing the patients with bedpans and urinals. Thereafter, the gloves are removed and the hands washed thoroughly with detergent soap (Hibiscrub) before leaving the room. On no account must bar soap be used for washing. Disposal of waste and linen should conform to the hospital policy for infected materials. Should the patient require transfer to another ward or unit, the transferring ward is responsible for providing the receiving unit with details of the MRSA problem and for reporting the situation to the infection control nurse.

Strains of multidrug resistant *Streptococcus pneumonia*, *Escherichia coli* and *Mycobacterium tuberculosis* have caused serious community-acquired infections.

Section 16.6 • Postoperative pain relief

Pathophysiology and classification

Pain has been defined as 'an unpleasant sensory and emotional experience associated with actual or potential tissue damage'. This definition is important since it recognizes the group of patients who experience pain (usually chronic) for which no physical cause can be established and where psychological factors are operative. The main categories of pain are nociceptive, neuropathic and pain due to psychological factors.

- **Nociceptive pain** is produced by stimulation of normal nerve fibres by thermal, chemical or physical injury and is further subdivided into somatic (peripheral nerves), e.g. postoperative wound and joint inflammation, or visceral (splanchnic nerves), e.g. biliary colic.
- **Neuropathic pain** is the result of diseased or damaged components of the nervous system with pain arising in the absence of any peripheral stimulation. Several aetiologies are recognized:
  - mononeuropathies: post-traumatic and post-herpetic neuralgias
  - polyneuropathies: diabetic neuropathy
  - deafferentation pain: following brachial plexus avulsion
  - reflex sympathetic dystrophy.
- **Pain due to psychological factors**: important component in chronic pain.

From a clinical standpoint, pain is categorized into **acute** and **chronic** or **intractable** pain. **Pain in malignant disease** is distinguished from both and is a mixture of acute and chronic pain, often with nociceptive, neuropathic and psychological components. It is now recognized that there are no specific pain pathways in the CNS. Instead, the pain pathways change and the peripheral, CNS and autonomic nervous systems, with various peptide neurotransmitters, inhibitory and facilitatory mechanisms, are involved. The gate theory was introduced in 1950 in an attempt to explain the perception of pain, i.e. transmission of pain impulses from the dorsal horns of the spinal cord to higher cerebral centres. The gate is opened or closed depending on relative activities of C and A β-fibres.

Acute pain

This is usually nociceptive in origin and self-limiting. Postoperative pain falls into this category. However, acute pain can progress to chronic pain, as exemplified by the deafferentation pain after thoracotomy, phantom limb pain after amputation and reflex sympathetic dystrophy after trauma. Psychological components are also important and explain the variable threshold of pain by patients. Pain in trauma victims falls into the category of acute pain. Again, the extent of pain suffered does not correlate closely with the extent of the injury, especially prior to resuscitation. Many patients have surprisingly little pain immediately after major trauma but suffer severe pain after resuscitation. The extreme example of this is battle analgesia, well documented in warfare, when a very seriously injured soldier experiences little or no pain.

Chronic pain

The pathophysiology of chronic intractable pain is poorly understood, although clinically it presents a major problem and has led to the establishment of pain clinics. In the majority, neuropathic and psychological factors operate, although in some cases a definite nociceptive component can be identified, e.g. chronic pancreatitis or spondylosis. In the absence of a nociceptive component, chronic pain is the most difficult to treat and requires expert management in pain clinics [see Module 20, Vol. I].

Principles of management of pain

Practice has changed in the 1980s and 1990s and this has resulted in substantial improvements in the management of both acute and chronic pain. In the first instance, the policy of **pre-emptive analgesia**, i.e. pain prevention by administration of analgesics before surgery, has been introduced. This is particularly rele-

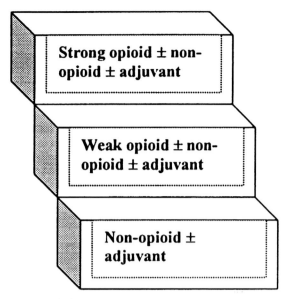

Figure 16.12 The WHO analgesic ladder.

Aside from the inhumanity, painful postoperative periods have adverse psychological effects on patients. In this respect, patients who have had good postoperative pain relief in the past react positively to the prospect of further surgical intervention, as opposed to those who experienced poor relief. With the establishment of acute pain services, the situation of inadequate control of postoperative pain should not arise. The methods available for postoperative analgesia are:

- intramuscular opioids
- patient-controlled analgesia (PCA)
- constant-rate intravenous infusion of opioids
- subcutaneous opioids
- transdermal opioids
- oral and rectal opioids
- epidural analgesia: opioids, local anaesthetics
- peripheral local anaesthetic block
- pre-emptive analgesia: day-case and ambulatory surgery
- others: cryoanalgesia and acupuncture.

Bolus intramuscular opioids

This traditional method has fallen out of favour because of the variable plasma concentrations and individual requirements, in addition to concerns over the adverse effects such as respiratory depression, sedation, hypoxaemia, drug dependency, nausea and vomiting. This resulted in both underprescribing by doctors and infrequent administration by nurses. In many hospitals, intramuscular opioids have been replaced by PCA. None the less, with care, satisfactory, safe analgesia can be obtained. Small intravenous injections producing a peak some 20 min later should be given to gain control of pain in the early stages. The standard dose of morphine is 0.1–0.2 mg/kg and it normally acts within 15–30 min, with a peak effect at 45–90 min. If the circulation is poor, both the onset of pain relief and its peak are delayed. The average duration of action is 4 h. Injections may be needed more often than this by some patients. **All patients on intramuscular opioids must be checked by the nurses at regular intervals for signs of respiratory depression, excessive drowsiness and the need for further analgesia.**

Patient-controlled analgesia

Here, the opioid is contained in a sterile delivery system that administers a preset bolus dose intravenously when the button is pressed by the patient. Thus, within the permissible maximal dose, the delivery is controlled by the patient. The system incorporates certain intrinsic safety features designed to prevent overdosing: bolus dose, lockout interval, background infusion and maximal dose dosage. All of these are preset for a given patient before the system is used. The bolus dose is the dose that the machine delivers each time the patient presses the button. The lockout time is the period after a given dose during which any further demands by the patient are ignored

vant to day-case or ambulatory surgery (see below). Secondly, **balanced or combination analgesia** is practised. This entails the use of more than one type of analgesic drug, e.g. opioid + NSAID. Following the report of the Royal College of Surgeons of England, **acute pain services** have been established in many of the hospitals to manage acute pain, and **pain clinics** have been set up by anaesthetists to deal with the problem of chronic intractable pain.

The World Health Organization (WHO) introduced the concept of the **analgesic ladder** (Figure 16.12), initially for the relief of cancer pain. However, the principle of this is now applied to other types of pain. Newer techniques and modalities including acupuncture have been introduced or are being evaluated in the quest for better pain control with minimum morbidity. Acupuncture works by the release of endorphins and stimulation of inhibitory mechanisms in the spinal cord.

Relief of postoperative pain

Satisfactory pain relief is an essential component of good postoperative care. It is conducive to good respiratory exchange and effective coughing, and ensures sleep and early mobilization. Although the response to surgery is not abolished by good analgesia, its severity may be reduced, particularly when effective methods are employed to achieve pain control. Adequate analgesia in patients with comorbid cardiac disease has been shown to decrease the incidence of postoperative myocardial ischaemic episodes. Yet, despite general agreement on these issues, several studies have shown that a significant percentage of patients (20–75%) experiences an unacceptable level of pain after surgery, especially when this is managed by intermittent intramuscular opioid therapy.

by the system. The background infusion relates to a continuous infusion of opioid by the machine, which is delivered throughout the period and is additional to the bolus injections activated by the patient's commands. The maximal dose is the total dose (boluses and continuous infusion) that the system will deliver during a 24-h period.

PCA undoubtedly results in good postoperative analgesia in the majority of patients and is safe, although on rare occasions respiratory depression can occur. It is not advisable in frail, elderly patients, who either forget to press, simply refrain from pressing the button or become upset when the PCA system is taken down. PCA is useless in patients with confusion, dementia or mental impairment.

Constant-rate intravenous infusion of opioids

This guarantees delivery of the opioid and hence pain control but has several disadvantages that preclude its routine use. In the first instance, it takes a long time for the opioid to reach a steady state concentration in the blood (approximately four times the half-life of the opioid). Thus, toxicity may develop several hours after the start of the infusion. Obstructive sleep apnoea and severe episodic hypoxaemia can occur. Respiratory depression is significantly more common with constant-rate opioid intravenous infusion than with PCA. The use of the regimen thus requires a low patient:nurse ratio and pulse oximetry.

Subcutaneous opioids

The continuous subcutaneous infusion of more soluble opioids such as diamorphine is attended by a reduced risk of respiratory depression compared with intravenous infusion and is useful in some patients, including children. It does, however, carry similar problems to those encountered with intramuscular opioids.

Transdermal opioids

This method uses a patch containing the fat-soluble synthetic opioid fentanyl. This simple and safe technique can be quite effective

Oral and rectal opioids

Oral opioids are contraindicated in the immediate postoperative period but may have a place when gastrointestinal function has been fully restored towards the end of the postoperative period. Rectal formulations of opioid preparations are available, which result in reasonable blood levels following administration as suppositories. They are useful in children.

Epidural (extradural) analgesia

Undoubtedly, this gives the best postoperative pain relief, but in view of risks, its use is restricted to patients undergoing major thoracic, abdominal, vascular and orthopaedic operations. Local anaesthetics (bupivacaine) or opioids (morphine, fentanyl) can be administered via a catheter introduced before the operation in

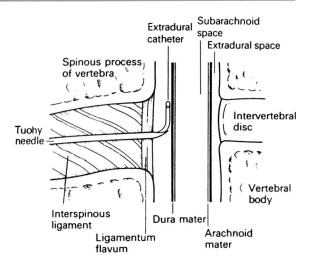

Figure 16.13 Use of a Tuohy needle to introduce an extradural catheter.

the epidural space via a Tuohy needle (Figure 16.13). However, because of the real risk of severe respiratory depression after epidural opioids, bupivacaine (continuous infusion or top-up boluses) is preferred and is the standard technique used nowadays. Epidural analgesia has advantages in that it:

- produces intense segmental analgesia that is continued from surgery into the postoperative period
- reduces the need for opioids and their side-effects
- is not patient dependent like PCA
- is good for confused patients
- increases the blood flow in lower limbs and thus reduces incidence of DVT
- provides lower limb vasodilatation after peripheral vascular operations.

Patients on epidural analgesia must be nursed in high-dependency units because of the risk of hypotension (sympathetic block), especially in the presence of even mild hypovolaemia. Thus, blood-pressure monitoring is essential in all patients on epidural analgesia.

The serious complications of epidural analgesia are inadvertent intravascular injection (toxic manifestations) and intrathecal (subarachnoid) misplacement of the epidural catheter when the large volume of local anaesthetic solution causes total spinal block with cardiovascular collapse, loss of consciousness and respiratory arrest requiring immediate intensive inotropic and ventilatory support.

Peripheral local anaesthetic blocks

These provide excellent analgesia and are used extensively in DCS (see below). The techniques include local infiltration of the operative site and blockade of specific nerves, e.g. 12th thoracic, iliohypogastric and ilioinguinal nerves for repair of inguinal hernia. Intrapleural bupivacaine produces reasonable analgesia after thoracic surgery.

Other techniques
These include cryoanalgesia and acupuncture. Cryoanalgesia involves freezing of sensory nerves, such as the intercostal nerves during thoracotomy, by a liquid nitrogen probe. Although it reduces the amount of opioid administration needed in the postoperative period, its effects are variable and the recovery of nerve function (numbness) takes several weeks to months. The place of acupuncture in postoperative pain has not been evaluated in the West. Acupuncture works by inducing the release of endogenous opioids (endorphins) and by stimulating the inhibitory mechanisms in the spinal cord.

Section 16.7 • Day-case surgery

Elective surgery can be undertaken through the following surgical services:

- inpatient stay surgery: admission and care in surgical wards
- inpatient short-stay surgery: 5-day wards (closed at weekends)
- ambulatory surgery
- day-case surgery (DCS)
- outpatient surgery.

In the first instance DCS must be distinguished from outpatient surgery where no facilities are required for the patient to recover. In the UK a surgical day case is defined as 'a patient who is admitted for investigation or operation on a planned non-residential basis but none the less requires facilities to recover'. By definition, DCS excludes an overnight stay. This is in contrast to ambulatory surgery practised in North America, which involves surgical treatment in 23-h units that may include an overnight stay. This distinction is important since ambulatory care units are able to cope with a wider spectrum of surgical disorders and patients than DCS, where the patient is treated surgically and discharged the same day.

Ideally, DCS should be conducted in purpose-designed day surgery units (DSU), but this objective is currently achieved in only 67% of DCS in the UK and 33% of patients are admitted to surgical wards. The reasons for the latter include (i) lack of day-case facilities, (ii) remote location of the day-case unit in relation to the surgical speciality concerned, and (iii) consultants' preference for mixed lists (inpatients and DCS patients on the same list) or to operate in their designated theatres, as these are more appropriately equipped.

The need for expansion of DCS is now recognized world-wide and stems from the increased number of elective admissions for surgery, which have risen significantly more quickly than emergency surgical admissions to hospitals. DCS releases resources and increases the total number of patients treated. The benefits of DCS include cost containment without jeopardizing clinical outcome. Cost of surgical treatment has two components: direct and indirect. Direct costs are incurred only when a patient is treated and concern the expenditure involved in patient care, consumables, etc. Indirect costs are incurred regardless of clinical activity (treatment), e.g. cost of building, equipment and maintenance. Greater utilization (efficiency) lowers the unit costs (cost per patient). The average unit cost of DCS is 50% of inpatient costs for the same type of operation. This saving is real, as there is no evidence that DCS adds significantly to the community health costs. In other words, the saving obtained from DCS does not result in any significant transfer of expenditure from the hospital to the primary health-care sector.

DCS is unquestionably safe, with a reported mortality of 4/257 000 (0.00002%) from myocardial infarction, pulmonary embolus, respiratory failure and stroke. However, it does carry a recognizable minor morbidity rate at 24 h after surgery. [see Module 18, Vol. I].

Day-case units

Nature
The ideal is a dedicated DSU. This is a self-contained unit with its own admission/reception area, day unit office, staff rooms, stores, ward, twin theatres suite and recovery ward. An open-plan type ward of 20 beds or trolley-spaces has become the norm and with an 80% occupancy, this enables an annual turnover of approximately 6000 patients. The recovery ward is equipped and staffed as a high-dependency area (piped services, resuscitation and monitoring and ventilation equipment). The DSU has its own administrative and management structure. The DSU is closed at night and weekends and operates efficiently through a bookable system: beds are booked in advance and never blocked by emergencies.

Less satisfactory is a day-case ward (DCW), with patients being treated in the main operating theatre suite of the hospital, where lists are made up entirely of day cases. In some cases, day-case operations are included in routine inpatient lists (mixed lists). This is less satisfactory from the viewpoint of both the ward and the patients.

Provision of day cases within standard general surgical wards is considered totally unsatisfactory since this arrangement nullifies the advantages offered by the DSU.

Selection of patients for day-case surgery
In general, DCS is ideal for patients undergoing operations that require a relatively short general anaesthetic and which do not carry a risk of postoperative complications. The suitability for day surgery is usually assessed at the time of outpatient consultation when the patient is put on the waiting list. The following are usually considered unsuitable:

- obese patients: BMI > 30
- elderly patients: upper age limit of 65–70 years

Table 16.11 Examples of appropriate operations for day-case surgery

General surgery	Orthopaedics	Urology
Minor operations on skin and subcutaneous tissues	Joint manipulation	Diagnostic urethrocystoscopy
Hernia repair	Epidural injections	Biopsy of bladder mucosa and tumour
Anal fissure: sphincterotomy	Removal of pins, plates and screws	Diathermy of bladder lesion
Removal of anal warts	Excision of ganglia and synovial cysts	Urethral dilatation and hydrostatic dilatation of the bladder
Rectal polypectomy	Decompression of carpal tunnel	Circumcision
Laparoscopy	De Quervain's release	Vasectomy
Needle biopsy of liver	Removal of superficial neuroma	Excision of scrotal lesions
Oesophageal dilatation	Amputation of fingers and toes	Testicular puncture biopsy for infertility
Breast biopsy	Ingrowing toe-nail surgery	Percutaneous nephrostomy
Biopsy lesions of the mouth	Tenotomy	Extracorporeal shock wave lithotripsy
Removal of salivary calculus	Excision of exostoses	
Varicose veins: ligation and avulsion	Interphalangeal fusion of the toes	
Varicocoele	Release of trigger finger	
Biopsy of lymph nodes	Removal of external fixator	
Excision of thyroglossal cyst	Excision of palmar fascia: Duputyren's contracture	
Excision of branchial sinus	Scar revision	
Vasectomy	Small free skin grafts	
	Arthroscopic procedures	

- patients with ASA status > II if a general anaesthetic is required
- home conditions/personal circumstances: those who live alone or have no home telephone, or home is more than a 1-h journey from hospital.

Examples of operations currently undertaken as day cases in three surgical specialities are shown in Table 16.11.

Management structure and operational policy

The DSU is run by a senior consultant clinician who acts as the overall director, but the day-to-day running is conducted by a nurse manager. The unit must have a forum for views of the consultants from the various specialties using the facility.

The unit operates:

- an efficient patient booking, reminder and confirmation system
- a preadmission assessment programme
- a discharge policy: fitness for the patient to go home (accompanied by a relative or friend)
- a monitoring policy: use of theatre sessions, patient throughput (against preset targets), utilization of beds and theatres, outcomes, non-attendance rates, stay-in rates, readmission rates, levels of DCS conducted outside the unit, cost of running the unit.

Pain management in day-case units

Pain and side-effects attributable to analgesics are the most common problems in DSU patients and at 24 h after discharge. Analgesia must be continued for 2 days after discharge from DSU. Opioids are responsible for postoperative nausea and vomiting (PONV). Because of its half-life (4–6 h), morphine should be reserved for pain that cannot be controlled otherwise. Fentanyl, in small intravenous doses, has a short half-life and provides near instant analgesia. It is ideal for acute management of pain in the DSU recovery area.

The techniques used for obtaining analgesia in DSU patients include:

- **local infiltration anaesthesia**: bupivacaine by infiltration or by nerve blocks
- **balanced analgesia**: if opioids are used as part of this balanced analgesia, those with the shortest half-life (fentanyl and remifentanyl) will cause minimal postoperative side-effects but will not provide any postoperative analgesia. Thus, administration of some other form of analgesia is necessary if postoperative pain is expected. The NSAIDs used commonly for DSU patients are ibuprofen, diclofenac and ketolorac. They control mild to moderate acute postoperative pain and reduce opioid requirements for severe acute pain. Administration is oral (usual), intravenous (ketolorac), intramuscular (ketolorac, diclofenac)

or rectal (diclofenac). Regardless of route, all take 30 min for onset of analgesic action and must be administered early as pre-emptive analgesia or balanced anaesthesia. They are useless for severe acute postoperative pain, when fentanyl is indicated.

It is likely that cyclo-oxygenase-2 inhibitors will replaced current NSAIDs because of the high incidence of side-effects, i.e. gastrointestinal irritation and renal damage (tubular necrosis). NSAIDs should be avoided in elderly patients undergoing DCS and in patients with known renal impairment. Hydration is important in patients on NSAIDs. Use in asthmatics is controversial as some of these patients are made worse with NSAIDs. The current consensus is to avoid them in patients with severe asthma and those with aspirin allergy.

Guide to further reading

Bret, P. M. and Reinhold, C. (1997). Magnetic resonance cholangiopancreatography. *Endoscopy* **29**: 472–486.

Hara, A. K., Johnson, C. D., Reed, J. E. *et al.* (1996). Detection of colorectal polyps by computed tomographic colography: feasibility of a novel technique. *Gastroenterology* **110**: 284–290.

Nolan, D. J. (1997). The true yield of small-intestinal barium study. *Endoscopy* **29**: 447–453.

Royal College of Surgeons of England. Commission on the Provision of Surgical Services (1992). *Guidelines for Day Case Surgery*, Royal College of Surgeons of England, London.

Rubin, G. D., Beaulieu, C. F., Argiro, V. *et al.* (1996). Perspective volume rendering of CT and MR images: applications for endoscopic imaging. *Radiology* **199**: 321–330.

Song, F. and Glenny, A. M. (1998). Antimicrobial prophylaxis in colorectal surgery: a systemic review of randomised controlled trials. *Health Technol Assessment* **2** (7).

Thompson-Fawcett, M. W., Cook, T. A., Baigrie, R. J. and Mortensen, N. J. McC. (1998). What patients think of day case proctology. *Br J Surg* **85**: 1388.

Thromboembolic Risk Factors (THRiFT) Consensus Group (1992). Risk of and prophylaxis for venous thromboembolism in hospital patients. *Br Med J* **305**: 567–574.

Tokunaga, Y., Nakayma, N., Nishitai, R. *et al.* (1998). Effects of closed system drains in surgery: focus on methicillin-resistant *Staphylococcus aureus*. *Dig Surg* **15**: 352–356.

Patients undergoing emergency general surgical operations

1 • Acute abdomen

2 • Peritonitis

3 • Abscesses

4 • Intestinal obstruction

5 • Gastrointestinal haemorrhage

'There are still many who do not appreciate to the full significance of the earlier and less fragrant symptoms of the acute abdomen' – Zachary Cope, 1881–1974

Section 17.1 • Acute abdomen

The term 'acute abdomen' is widely used to denote the rapid onset of abdominal pain severe enough to warrant the patient's admission to hospital. The assessment of such patients and the decision-making process regarding their management is crucial, since some will have life-threatening conditions that require surgical intervention either immediately or soon after resuscitation. Others need a period of observation and conservative management, which may lead to surgery if the condition fails to settle or complications ensue. Diagnostic errors at the initial assessment may at best result in unnecessary surgical intervention, and at worst demise of the patient or a protracted illness due to the development of complications, which could have been avoided by prompt intervention. The acute abdomen also covers patients with intra-abdominal injuries to solid and hollow organs, but this is covered elsewhere [see Module 4, Vol. I].

Aetiology

The aetiology of the acute abdomen is most conveniently summarized by considering the anatomical area in which the underlying disease might occur.

The chest
Myocardium
An inferior myocardial infarct may present with epigastric pain. This may be the only symptom in 0.7% of cases and occurs in 3.3% of all myocardial infarctions. Congestive cardiac failure can also cause acute epigastric pain owing to congestion of the liver and tenderness under the right costal margin may be present.

Pericarditis may cause epigastric pain if the diaphragm is affected and tenderness with guarding may also be present.

Lungs
Lobar pneumonia, particularly if basal and close to the diaphragm, may cause acute abdominal pain, especially in the elderly patient.

The upper abdomen
Liver
Acute hepatitis of viral or alcoholic aetiology may cause abdominal pain owing to swelling of the liver and stretching of Glisson's capsule. Liver tumours, either secondary metastases or primary hepatoma, may become acutely painful owing to haemorrhage or infarction.

Biliary tract
Biliary colic or acute cholecystitis are common causes of acute abdominal pain. Less frequent but more serious is acute cholangitis caused by infection of an obstructed biliary tree, often secondary to common duct stones. This presents with the typical 'Charcot's triad' of pain, jaundice and rigors.

Oesophagus
Reflux oesophagitis may present with acute epigastric pain, although the symptoms of heartburn and dysphagia are usually predominant. Spontaneous rupture of the oesophagus consequent on severe vomiting or retching (Boerhaave's syndrome) presents with very severe epigastric and lower chest pain immediately following an episode of violent vomiting or retching.

Stomach and duodenum
Peptic ulceration of the stomach and duodenum can often present with acute abdominal pain and if

perforation occurs this will be severe, often of sudden onset and will be associated with abdominal rigidity. Acute gastritis, usually induced by alcohol, is another common cause of acute abdominal pain. Very rarely, gastric cancer may present with rapid onset of pain.

Spleen
Very unusually, the spleen may undergo torsion and/or infarction, giving rise to abdominal pain in the left upper quadrant.

The lower abdomen
Small bowel
Obstruction of the small bowel leads to typical acute colicky abdominal pain (see section on 'Intestinal obstruction'). The small bowel can also become ischaemic owing to peripheral vascular disease, embolism, strangulation or vasculitis and may subsequently undergo infarction. Typically, the patient with mesenteric ischaemia has very severe abdominal pain but minimal physical signs on examination. Tenderness only ensues when infarction has become established. Inflammation of a Meckel's diverticulum can mimic acute appendicitis, as can terminal ileitis due to Crohn's disease or *Yersinia* infection.

Large bowel
Large bowel obstruction (see section on 'Intestinal obstruction') and acute diverticulitis are common causes of acute abdominal pain. Occasionally, ulcerative colitis or Crohn's colitis may give rise to pain as a prominent symptom.

Appendix
Acute appendicitis remains the most common reason for intervention in acute abdominal pain. Especially in children, acute Meckelian diverticulitis must be kept in mind, as the clinical picture is indistinguishable from acute appendicitis.

Omentum
Torsion of a portion of the greater omentum leads to infarction and can often mimic acute appendicitis.

The pelvis

Ovaries
Mid-cycle lower abdominal pain can be caused by rupture of the Graafian follicle at ovulation. This is known as Mittelschmerz. Ovarian cysts, both benign and malignant, may undergo torsion or rupture.

Fallopian tubes
An ectopic pregnancy most commonly presents as lower abdominal pain, usually associated with a missed period. More rarely, it can present with sudden abdominal pain and circulatory collapse. The fallopian tubes can also be affected by pelvic inflammatory disease.

Uterus
The endometrium can be affected by pelvic inflammatory disease and occasionally fibroids may undergo torsion or infarction.

The retroperitoneum

Pancreas
Acute pancreatitis, usually secondary to gallstones or alcohol, is a common cause of acute abdominal pain. Chronic pancreatitis may be complicated by acute exacerbations. Very rarely, a pancreatic tumour may present with acute pain.

Renal tract
Ureteric colic caused by stones or a clot from a bleeding lesion in the kidney gives rise to severe pain of sudden onset in a characteristic distribution radiating from the renal angle to the groin. Pain in the kidney itself can be due to acute obstruction of the renal pelvis or to pyelonephritis. Cystitis may present as lower abdominal pain of sudden onset but is usually associated with dysuria or frequency.

Aorta
A ruptured aortic aneurysm can present primarily with abdominal pain but is more commonly associated with back pain and may indeed mimic ureteric colic.

Other causes
Non-specific abdominal pain
Non-specific abdominal pain (NSAP) is a term used to describe acute self-limiting abdominal pain of unknown aetiology. It must be emphasized that NSAP is not a diagnosis but merely a convenient label to describe this category of patients with an acute abdomen.

Infections
A variety of infections can cause acute abdominal pain, and mesenteric adenitis due to *Yersinia pseudotuberculosis* can mimic acute appendicitis. Similarly, infection with campylobacter and cryptosporidium can be accompanied by quite severe abdominal pain.

Diabetic ketoacidosis
Ten per cent of patients with diabetic ketoacidosis complain of acute abdominal pain and in children this may be mistaken for appendicitis. The reason for the pain is unexplained [see Module 20, Vol. I].

Herpes zoster
The pre-eruption stage of herpes zoster produces a severe burning pain and when in the appropriate nerve root distribution can mimic an acute abdomen.

Spinal disorder
Vertebral collapse due to osteoporosis or metastatic deposits and acute disc prolapse can give rise to root pain in the distribution of the lower thoracic nerves, leading to abdominal pain.

Lead poisoning

Lead poisoning can present with episodes of intestinal colic. Other toxic causes of acute abdominal pain include arsenic, chromium, copper, mercury, organophosphates and certain fungi.

Sickle cell disease

Sickle cell anaemia is a hereditary chronic haemolytic anaemia in which erythrocytes become deformed in conditions of hypoxaemia. This gives rise to aggregations of cells, which block the microcirculation and lead to both abdominal pain and tenderness.

Porphyria

Acute intermittent porphyria is caused by an inborn disorder of haem/porphyrin metabolism. When an attack occurs it produces neurovisceral effects including abdominal pain and vomiting. Porphyrin is present in the urine during the attack.

Familial Mediterranean fever

An autosomal recessive condition, familial Mediterranean fever is largely confined to the eastern Mediterranean countries. It is characterized by sudden episodes of severe abdominal pain and vomiting with signs suggesting peritonitis.

These causes of the acute abdomen have been organized in a systematic manner, which does not indicate their relative frequency. In the Western world the most common causes of acute abdominal pain necessitating hospital admission in decreasing order of frequency are shown in Table 17.1.

History in patients with an acute abdomen

When taking a history from a patient with acute abdominal pain, it is important to use a systematic approach in order to avoid missing important information. Although a complete history is essential, it will suffice here to concentrate on those parts of the history that are of specific importance in the acute abdomen. **These are: pain, weight loss, appetite, jaundice, dysphagia, nausea and vomiting, bowel habit, micturition, gynaecological symptoms, past medical history, and drugs and allergies.**

Pain

Questions regarding the pain can be divided into a series of discrete attributes.

Site of pain

In order to establish the site of the pain it is useful to ask the patient to point with one finger to the precise spot. If the pain is diffuse, however, the patient will usually open the hand and rub it over the affected area. It is then important to describe the site of the pain, and this is best done as left upper quadrant, right upper quadrant, left lower quadrant, right lower quadrant, right half, upper half, left half, lower half, central or general (see Figure 17.1).

Shift of pain

It is very important to establish whether or not the pain has shifted in position throughout its duration. This is particularly useful in establishing a diagnosis of acute appendicitis, when the initial visceral pain is usually felt centrally and then shifts to the right lower quadrant when the overlying parietal peritoneum becomes inflamed.

Radiation of the pain

Initially, it is important to ask whether the pain radiates anywhere and, if this is not clear to the patient, to go

Table 17.1 Causes of acute abdominal pain necessitating admission to a surgical ward

Condition	%
NSAP	34
Acute appendicitis	28
Acute cholecystitis	10
Small bowel obstruction	4
Gynaecological conditions	4
Acute pancreatitis	3
Renal colic	3
Perforated peptic ulcer	3
Malignancy	2
Diverticulitis	2
Dyspepsia	1
Miscellaneous	7

After De Dombal (1991). *Diagnosis of Acute Abdominal Pain*, 2nd edn, Churchill Livingstone, Edinburgh.

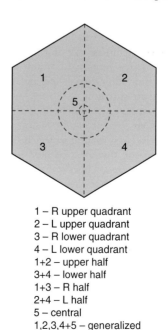

1 – R upper quadrant
2 – L upper quadrant
3 – R lower quadrant
4 – L lower quadrant
1+2 – upper half
3+4 – lower half
1+3 – R half
2+4 – L half
5 – central
1,2,3,4+5 – generalized

Figure 17.1 Diagram illustrating the descriptive regions of the abdomen.

on to prompt, i.e. 'does the pain radiate through to the back or to the shoulder or down to the groin?' Typically, retroperitoneal pain such as acute pancreatitis will radiate to the back, irritation of the diaphragm will radiate to the shoulder and the pain of ureteric colic will radiate from the renal angle into the groin.

Duration of pain
It is clearly important to establish the duration of the present episode of pain but it is also necessary to understand whether the episode is an isolated event or part of a long-standing history of recurrent pain.

Progress of pain
The simple question, 'is the pain getting better, worse or staying the same?' is crucial in the patient's management. The pain that is getting better is likely to resolve, whereas the pain that is getting worse may well require urgent intervention.

Nature of the pain
Classifying pain according to descriptive terms such as burning, stabbing and boring is not useful in terms of reaching a diagnosis. It is, however, important to know whether or not the pain is intermittent. If it is intermittent, it is then important to establish whether it is colicky in nature (i.e. coming and going every few minutes). This is the typical pattern of intestinal colic and should be differentiated from biliary or ureteric colic (see Figure 17.2). In general, episodes of colicky pain reach a crescendo of intensity and make the patient restless.

Severity of pain
The severity of the pain is very difficult to quantify and terms such as mild, moderate and severe are not very helpful. The most useful question to ask is 'is this the worst pain you have ever had?' and if the patient answers yes, the symptom can be taken to be extremely significant. Visual (Figure 17.3) and linear analogue scales are used in clinical trials but are not practical in the routine acute situation.

Aggravating factors
Establishing clear aggravating factors is central to making a diagnosis and the effect of abdominal movement is of particular interest. This can be established by asking the patient whether the pain is made worse by shifting position, coughing or laughing.

Relieving factors
Equally, it is important to ask about factors that make the pain better and in particular lying still, vomiting, food and any particular drugs (especially antacids).

Weight and appetite
Weight loss is a particularly suggestive factor, particularly in the patient with a long-standing history. It is highly indicative of malignancy or a severe chronic inflammatory condition.

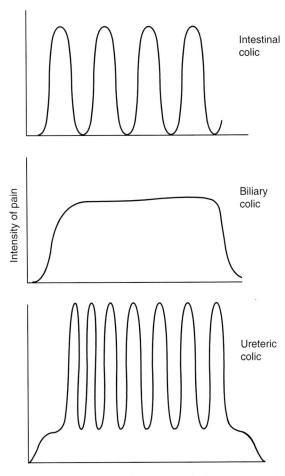

Figure 17.2 Patterns of different types of colic.

Change of appetite is important in the acute situation and recent anorexia is often found with intra-abdominal inflammation. It is best to ask the patient 'are you hungry just now?' and to establish when he or she last had anything to eat or drink. This is also essential information if a general anaesthetic is being considered.

Jaundice
If the patient is jaundiced at the time of interview this will be obvious, but it is useful to find out whether

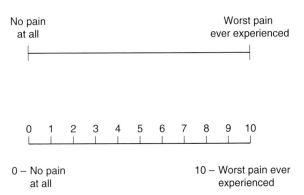

Figure 17.3 Visual and linear analogue scales.

there have been previous episodes of jaundice. It is best to ask whether the patient has noticed any change in the colour of the whites of the eyes and to ask about changes in colour of urine and stool. This is particularly important when suspecting biliary tract disease [see Module 11, Vol. I].

Dysphagia

In the patient with severe oesophagitis or a neoplasm of the lower oesophagus or proximal stomach, dysphagia is a common symptom. It is important to realize, however, that the question 'do you have any difficulties swallowing?' may not in fact elicit a history of dysphagia. To most people, the term swallowing implies the act of deglutition rather than the passage of a bolus of food into the stomach. It is therefore more important to ask, 'does food stick on the way down?'

Nausea and vomiting

These symptoms should be elicited carefully, as the question 'have you been sick?' may mean different things to different people. It must be appreciated that although nausea can occur without vomiting, vomiting may also occur without nausea and this is of diagnostic importance. If the patient has been sick, enquiry should be made as to the nature of the vomit, i.e. blood, bile or unaltered food.

Bowel habit

When asking about bowel habit the most important feature is whether or not this has changed in the recent past. The term constipation is entirely relative to the patient's normal experience and it is well established that 95% of the normal population open their bowels between three times a day and three times a week. If the patient has been having diarrhoea, it should be established whether this is watery or merely loose stool and whether there has been any recognizable blood. A history of melena should also be actively sought.

Micturition

The patient should be asked whether there has been any frequency, dysuria and cloudy or blood-stained urine. This will help in the diagnosis when a urinary tract infection or ureteric colic is suspected.

Gynaecological symptoms

Particularly in the young women with lower abdominal pain, gynaecological symptoms are of the utmost importance. A missed period may indicate pregnancy, ectopic or otherwise, and vaginal discharge may indicate pelvic inflammatory disease. Pain occurring midcycle is suggestive of Mittelschmerz. It is therefore important to ask the date of the last period, whether or not the periods are regular and if there has been any abnormal intermenstrual bleeding or vaginal discharge.

Past medical history

Clearly, a past history of severe illness has implications for the management of the patient with abdominal pain, but as far as the diagnosis is concerned, the most important fact to establish is whether or not there have been previous episodes of similar pain and whether a diagnosis has been made in the past. Previous surgery is also significant and it is important to find out what was done, when it was done and where it was done. Any complications resulting from either the surgery or the anaesthetic should be carefully recorded. If possible, it is ideal to refer to previous operation notes.

Drugs and allergies

An accurate list of current medication is essential, especially when considering surgery. Frequently, a patient may be unable to provide the names of all the drugs and it may be necessary to consult the family doctor. Allergies to medication, particularly antibiotics, must also be established.

Acute abdomen in tropical countries

In tropical countries the spectrum of disease causing acute abdominal pain is very different from that seen in Western countries. For this reason the following conditions will be covered briefly in this section to highlight their importance in the acute abdomen. Details of the specific diseases are covered elsewhere [see Module 5, Vol. I]:

- malaria
- ameobiasis
- schistosomiasis
- typhoid
- abdominal tuberculosis
- abdominal crises of sickle cell disease.

Malaria

Malaria is still the most common communicable disease in the tropics, and nearly one billion people world-wide are at risk. The two most common parasites are *Plasmodium vivax* and *Plasmodium falciparum*. The parasite is transmitted by the anopheline mosquito after ingestion of infected human blood. Sporozoites develop within the mosquito, which are then transmitted to a human host via a bite. These sporozoites develop in the parenchymal cells of the liver to form merozoites, which enter the circulation to infest erythrocytes. The parasitized red blood cells now rupture releasing merozoites, most of which re-enter erythrocytes. In response to an unknown stimulus a number of the merozoites released develop into male and female forms known as gametocytes, which are inert in the human but which provide a reservoir for infection.

Plasmodium vivax and *P. falciparum* can lead to acute abdominal problems as follows.

Plasmodium vivax

Fever is the most constant sign after a brief period of remittent pyrexia. The pattern of intermittent recurring fever every second day is established. The spleen enlarges early in the disease, some degree of anaemia may be present and there is often mild leucopenia. Abdominal pain is not a major feature but the enlarged spleen may rupture, either spontaneously or in response to minor trauma.

Plasmodium falciparum

Here the fever is irregular and occurs daily. Headache, malaise, nausea and vomiting and generalized joint pains may be the only other presenting symptoms of an uncomplicated attack. On examination there may be hepatosplenomegaly and a variable degree of anaemia. Abdominal presentations resembling appendicitis and acute abdominal pain have been described.

Amoebiasis

The only amoeba pathogenic in the gut is *Entamoeba histolytica*. It lives in the large intestine causing ulceration of the mucosa, with consequent diarrhoea. Secondary lesions may occur most commonly in the liver but other tissues can be affected. Ameobiasis has a world-wide distribution but clinical disease occurs most frequently in tropical and subtropical countries. It tends to be found in areas where standards of personal hygiene and environmental sanitation are low.

The classic clinical picture is amoebic dysentery, the symptoms of which appear within a week or two of infection or may be delayed for months to years. The onset is gradual with some looseness of stools for a few days, followed by frequent bloodstained motions. Colic and tenesmus may occur. The attack usually subsides spontaneously and there follows a period of remission, varying from a few days to several months or even years. At any time complications may occur and in fulminating disease there may be severe intestinal haemorrhage or perforation leading to amoebic peritonitis. In addition to sudden perforation of an amoebic ulcer, a form of slow leakage through an extensively diseased bowel may result in peritonitis. In an amoebic liver abscess the patient complains of discomfort and fullness in the liver region, and the liver enlarges and becomes tender. This tenderness is maximal over the site of the abscess, usually in the right intracostal region, latterly over the lower ribcage.

Schistosomiasis

Schistosomiasis is a common infestation and the species that regularly infect humans are *Schistosoma haematobium*, *Schistosoma mansoni* and *Schistosoma japonicum*. It has been estimated that a total of about 200 million people are affected in various parts of the world. *Schistosoma haematobium* occurs in many parts of Africa, parts of the Middle East and in some areas of southern Europe. *Schistosoma mansoni* is found in the Nile Delta, Africa, South America and the Caribbean. *Schistosoma japonicum* occurs in China, Japan, the Philippines and other parts of the Far East.

Schistosomiasis is caused by a trematode worm. The adult worms are found in the veins, *S. haematobium* predominantly in the vesical plexus, *S. mansoni* in the in inferior mesenteric vein and *S. japonicum* most commonly in the superior mesenteric vein. The female lays eggs which pass through the bladder or bowel into the urine and faeces, respectively. The intermediate host is a snail of the appropriate species and within the snail the worm undergoes a process of multiplication to become the infective larval stage. It emerges from the snail and on contact with humans under water, it penetrates the skin and migrates to the usual site for mature adults of that species.

The clinical features depend on the species.

Schistosoma haematobium

Because of the anatomical distribution of the adult worm, the symptoms are related to the urinary tract. Initially, the patient complains of dysuria, frequency and urgency of micturition and when ulceration occurs it is accompanied by suprapubic or perineal pain. Ureteric and renal involvement can give rise to hydroureter, hydronephrosis and pyelonephritis. Calculi can occur in the bladder, ureter, kidneys and urethra and give rise to renal colic.

Schistosoma mansoni and *Schistosoma japonicum*

The onset of egg laying in a first infection is accompanied by bloody diarrhoea. In some cases severe dysentery associated with frank ulceration and massive haemorrhage can occur and may be fatal. Perforation and stricture of the colon occur but are relatively uncommon.

Typhoid

Typhoid fever remains endemic in tropical and subtropical countries. It is caused by *Salmonella typhi* and the terminal ileum in the region of the Peyer's patches is the main site of intestinal infection. A longitudinal ulcerating lesion on the antimesenteric border, situated within 45 cm of the ileocaecal valve, is present in the majority of patients. This ulceration may give rise to frank perforation and severe bleeding. The incidence of perforation varies considerably from one endemic area to another, being especially high in west Africa (15–33%) and low in Cairo and Iran (1–3%). The high incidence in west Africa has been attributed both to late diagnosis and to a particularly virulent strain of the bacterium. The differential diagnosis includes perforated appendicitis.

Abdominal tuberculosis

This includes tuberculous peritonitis and intestinal tuberculosis. The primary variety of gastrointestinal tuberculosis results from the ingestion of milk contaminated by *Mycobacterium bovis*. The secondary type of intestinal tuberculosis is due to swallowing infected sputum (*Mycobacterium tuberculosis*). As a result of tuberculin testing, pasteurization of milk, effective chemotherapy and general improvement in living conditions, abdominal tuberculosis is rare in Western countries. However, it is very common in underprivileged countries, such as the Indian subcontinent and parts of Africa, where tuberculous intestinal obstruction accounts for a significant proportion of emergency hospital admissions.

Tuberculous peritonitis

In the majority of cases, chronic tuberculous peritonitis results from reactivation of a latent primary peritoneal focus and is therefore blood-borne in origin. It causes malaise, ill health, weight loss, fever and ascites. Acute tuberculous peritonitis occurs infrequently as part of miliary disease or follows perforation of an intestinal lesion or rupture of tuberculous mesenteric lymph nodes.

Intestinal tuberculosis

This can be divided into four forms.

- hypertrophic
- ulcerative
- fibrotic
- ulcerofibrotic.

The systemic manifestations of this disease include chronic ill health, anorexia, fever and night sweats, dyspepsia and weight loss. The hypertrophic type predominantly affects the ileocaecal region but can also involve the ascending and transverse colon. The clinical features are of recurrent episodes of subacute intestinal obstruction with colicky abdominal pain and vomiting and occasionally with a mass in the right iliac fossa. The ulcerative type affects mainly the terminal ileum and healing results in multiple strictures, which in turn lead to subacute intestinal obstruction. The fibrotic variety affects the terminal ileum caecum and ascending colon and presentation is again with acute or subacute intestinal obstruction.

Abdominal crisis of sickle cell disease

Sickle cell disease is very common in Africa, where in certain regions up to 40% of the population are heterozygous for the inherited condition. Although the abnormal haemoglobin S is soluble when oxygenated, it polymerizes and crystallizes out when it looses oxygen. As a result, the red cells become elongated, sickle shaped and rigid, leading to increased blood viscosity. The rigid cells block the microcirculation to various organs, inducing episodes of pain and infarction in various organs, including the gastrointestinal tract. Thus, a sickle cell crisis can present with acute abdominal pain and even with perforation and peritonitis.

Examination of the patient with acute abdomen

In the first instance, the patient with acute abdominal pain should be given adequate analgesia, preferably morphine intravenously before the physical examination. Concerns that this may mask physical signs are totally unfounded and have been excluded by clinical trials. Analgesic medication is nowadays considered an integral part of patient resuscitation as it minimizes stress responses and facilitates co-operation during physical examination.

The first part of the examination of the acute abdomen takes place as soon as the interview with the patient begins. This is the stage of general observation when the patient's colour (pallor, jaundice, etc.) is observed and the general level of anxiety and distress is assessed. When it comes to the formal part of the examination, it is essential to assess the patient's circulatory state by feeling the pulse and looking for signs of hypovolaemia or dehydration. It is also extremely important to carry out a thorough examination of the cardiorespiratory system, but here we shall concentrate on the examination of the abdomen itself.

The patient should lie as flat as is reasonably comfortable and the examiner should be positioned level with the patient so that **observation** and palpation are optimal. Firstly, any obvious abnormalities such as distension, visible peristalsis, ecchymosis, visible masses and previous operation scars are noted. The patient should then be asked again to indicate the point of maximum tenderness so that palpation does not start at this point and increase the patient's level of distress. It is convenient at this point to ask the patient to cough and to observe his or her face while this is carried out. The patient with peritonitis will wince on coughing.

Gentle **palpation** then begins, starting distant from the point of maximum tenderness. This is best achieved by keeping the hand and forearm straight and dipping the fingers into the abdomen by flexing at the metacarpophalangeal joints (Figure 17.4). This is performed to delineate the area of tenderness and to assess for guarding or rigidity. It is not necessary to elicit classical rebound tenderness if the cough test has been positive and if guarding or rigidity is found. If it is feasible, then deeper palpation should follow to feel for abdominal masses and to palpate the liver, kidneys and spleen.

Percussion is often useful in assessing the acute abdomen as this will help in the detection of gas-filled loops of bowel (tympanic note) or fluid (dull note). If ascites is suspected then shifting dullness may be demonstrated. Gentle percussion may also be useful in assessing pain due to peritonitis.

Auscultation then follows and with intestinal obstruction, typical high-pitched 'cavernous' sounds will be heard. Definite absence of bowel sounds is less easy to be sure about and auscultation should continue for 3 min before reaching this conclusion.

It is then necessary to examine the groins, particularly for an irreducible hernia, and in the male it is essential to examine the external genitalia, as testicular pathology such as torsion or orchitis may well present as lower abdominal pain.

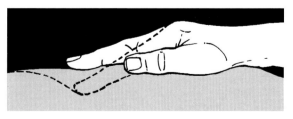

Figure 17.4 Movement of the hand in palpation of the abdomen. (From Jones, P. F., Krukowski, Z. H., Youngson, C. G. (1999). *Emergency Abdominal Surgery*, 3rd edn, Chapman & Hall, with permission.)

Rectal examination is regarded as an integral part of the abdominal examination, although there is now good evidence that it is not always essential to make a diagnosis in the acute abdomen. When there is doubt, however, a rectal examination may provide very useful information. When carrying out this procedure it is very important to palpate the prostate in the male and the cervix in the female. If movement of the cervix causes pain this is in keeping with pelvic inflammatory disease. Pain on exerting pressure on the right side of the rectum may indicate a pelvic appendicitis and abnormal masses in the pelvis should be noted. When the finger is withdrawn it is important to look at the bowel contents to check for blood, mucus or melena.

Investigations

In the acute abdomen the minimum investigations are a full blood count, urea and electrolytes and urinalysis (microscopy, glycosuria, proteinuria). A raised white cell count is useful in making a diagnosis of intra-abdominal inflammation and it is important to have an estimation of the haemoglobin level if surgery is contemplated. Likewise, urea and electrolytes may well be deranged in the patient with acute abdominal pathology and this may require correction prior to operative intervention. Other biochemical investigations and in particular a serum amylase level and liver function tests may be indicated in certain circumstances. While blood is being taken it is often sensible to send a sample for Group and Save in anticipation of operation.

Other investigations that may be indicated are plain radiography, contrast radiography, endoscopy, ultrasound, computed tomographic (CT) scanning and radionuclide scanning.

Plain radiography

Radiography is not always necessary. For example, in the patient with clear-cut appendicitis it will add very little to the diagnostic process. Under most circumstances, however, it is useful to have an erect chest X-ray and a supine abdominal X-ray. An erect chest X-ray will demonstrate gas under the diaphragm and will also provide information on relevant cardiopulmonary pathology.

A plain abdominal radiograph should be scrutinized for:

- dilatation of intestinal loops
- free blood or fluid in the peritoneal cavity
- distortion of the stomach air bubble
- obliteration of the psoas outline
- kidney outlines
- calculi
- calcified wall of an aneurysm or other vessels
- fractures (ribs, spine, pelvis).

An erect abdominal film may also be useful when intestinal obstruction is suspected as this will demonstrate fluid levels. Occasionally, when there is a lot of fluid in the intestinal lumen, the supine film may not demonstrate an intestinal obstruction and this will only be seen on the erect film.

Contrast radiology

A contrast enema is essential in the diagnosis of large bowel obstruction in order to distinguish a mechanical obstruction from pseudo-obstruction. While dilute barium may be used, water-soluble contrast is better as this is easily evacuated from the large bowel. If there is a risk of perforation, e.g. diverticulitis, barium most certainly should not be used as extravasation of barium into the peritoneal cavity can lead to considerable difficulties in peritoneal toilet at the time of operation.

A contrast swallow is indicated where rupture of the oesophagus is suspected and again water-soluble contrast tends to be favoured. Gastrograffin used to be the favoured water-soluble contrast medium, but it is hypertonic and may lead to serious complications including electrolyte imbalance, significant fluid shifts from the vascular compartment and pulmonary oedema if aspirated. For this reason, non-ionic contrast such as Niopam is preferable.

Contrast radiology of the renal tract in the form of an intravenous urogram is necessary for patients with haematuria and renal colic. It may also be necessary at the time of operation when the pathology found necessitates removal of one kidney and the presence of a functioning contralateral kidney must be confirmed. Mesenteric angiography is necessary for the evaluation of massive bleeding from the small or large bowel.

Endoscopy

Upper gastrointestinal endoscopy is useful in the diagnosis of epigastric pain and is essential in the assessment of upper gastrointestinal bleeding. In patients with endoscopically proven varices, an alternative site of bleeding (e.g. an ulcer) is found in 20–40% of cases. In cases of bleeding peptic ulcer, the endoscopic finding of a visible vessel indicates a high risk of rebleeding and the possible need for surgical intervention. Furthermore, upper gastrointestinal endoscopy may be used as a therapeutic modality (injection, sclerotherapy of varices and injection or coagulation of bleeding peptic ulcer).

Colonoscopy has a limited role in the acute abdomen but in the patient with pseudo-obstruction it is a useful means of decompressing the large bowel. Flexible sigmoidoscopy may be used to deflate a sigmoid volvulus and to investigate the nature of a stricture seen on contrast enema and it may also be helpful when inflammatory bowel disease is suspected. However, flexible endoscopy of the large bowel should not be used when there is any perceived risk of perforation. This includes the presence of active inflammation with peritoneal irritation such as toxic megacolon or acute diverticulitis. Rigid sigmoidoscopy or proctoscopy may be helpful in elucidating the cause of rectal or anal bleeding.

Ultrasound scanning

External abdominal ultrasound scanning now has an established place in the investigation of acute intra-abdominal disorders and is routinely used in the following situations:

- suspected cholelithiasis or acute cholecystitis
- acute appendicitis
- detection of intra-abdominal abscesses and fluid collections, e.g. pancreatic pseudocysts or ascites
- obstructive jaundice
- investigation of palpable abdominal masses
- suspected abdominal aortic aneurysm.

Computed tomographic scanning

CT scanning is particularly accurate in the detection of intra-abdominal abscesses and with intravenous contrast (angio-CT) it is the most reliable test for documenting pancreatic necrosis in severe pancreatitis.

Radionuclide scanning

This has a limited role in the diagnosis of the acute abdomen, although in patients with suspected acute cholecystitis E-HIDA scintiscanning is an extremely sensitive test for the diagnosis of cystic duct obstruction. A normal E-HIDA gallbladder scan excludes this condition.

Management of patients with acute abdomen

Resuscitation

Although not required in all cases of acute abdominal pain, it is often necessary to establish intravenous access and to give intravenous fluids (crystalloids) in the patient who has become dehydrated. In order to ensure adequate rehydration, it is important to monitor pulse, blood pressure and urine output. In the elderly or unstable patient, monitoring of central venous pressure is also necessary.

Observation

In many patients with acute abdominal pain the diagnosis is not immediately obvious. If the patient is not at immediate risk of deteriorating, then a period of observation is quite reasonable. This is particularly true of the patient in whom the pain is either static or improving. It is essential, however, that a definite plan for reassessment is made and that this is carried out by the original observer, so that any change in the signs can be observed. Observation entails re-evaluation of the symptoms and physical signs in addition to an hourly pulse, blood pressure and temperature chart.

Laparoscopy

Increasingly, diagnostic laparoscopy is being used in the assessment of the acute abdomen. This is particularly useful for the management of lower abdominal pain in young women and has been shown to reduce the rate of negative appendicectomy in this category of patient. When laparoscopy for lower abdominal pain is carried

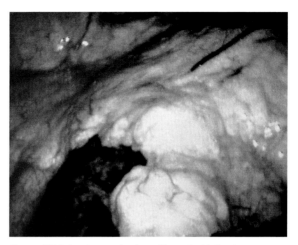
Figure 17.5 Laparoscopic view of intestinal infarction.

out, it is important to view the appendix, the ovaries and the fallopian tubes. It is also important to scan the rest of the abdomen, looking for free fluid or signs of inflammation or infarction (Figure 17.5).

A thorough diagnostic laparoscopy will require the introduction of at least one accessory port in order to introduce a probe or grasper, so that overlying loops of bowel may be displaced. In some centres, the cause of the acute abdomen (e.g. appendicitis or perforated peptic ulcer) may actually be dealt with by means of the laparoscopic approach. Laparoscopic cholecystectomy is now the treatment of choice for acute cholecystitis and is carried out during the same hospital admission on the next available list (early cholecystectomy).

Laparotomy

Laparotomy remains the mainstay of treatment in the acute abdomen. When the diagnosis of acute appendicitis has been made, either laparoscopically or clinically, the muscle splitting, right iliac fossa incision is used routinely. Otherwise, a midline laparotomy incision is favoured by the majority of surgeons, particularly when there is doubt as to the precise aetiology of the underlying condition. In most cases the responsible pathology is immediately evident but when this is not the case, it is important for the surgeon to follow a rigorous routine when performing an exploratory laparotomy. This entails examining the liver, biliary tract, duodenum, stomach, spleen, pancreas, small bowel, large bowel, pelvic organs and retroperitoneum. Only when this has been done can the laparotomy be said to be complete.

Section 17.2 • Peritonitis

Peritonitis is inflammation of the peritoneal cavity and this may be caused by bacteria or by irritation by extravasated secretions. Classification of peritonitis is based on the pathogenesis and the important types are:

- acute secondary bacterial peritonitis
- primary bacterial peritonitis
- acute non-bacterial peritonitis
- chronic bacterial peritonitis (tuberculous)
- chronic non-bacterial peritonitis (granulomatous).

These five categories will be dealt with separately.

Acute secondary bacterial peritonitis

This accounts for the majority of cases. When generalized and severe it still carries an appreciable mortality, which varies from 20 to 60%. It is generally caused by perforation of the gastrointestinal tract, most commonly secondary to the following:

- acute appendicitis
- perforated peptic ulcer
- acute diverticulitis of the colon
- perforation of an intestinal tumour
- inflammatory bowel disease
- intestinal infarction
- acute cholecystitis
- intestinal trauma
- anastomotic dehiscence.

Pathophysiology

The severity of disease depends largely on the site of the perforation. The perforated peptic ulcer leads to mild peritonitis as gastric contents have a low bacterial count. In contrast, peritonitis resulting from a free perforation of the large bowel with faecal contamination is very severe and can lead to death within a few hours.

The acute inflammatory response is exudative, with the outpouring of large amounts of fluid rich in protein, including opsinons and fibrinogen and polymorphonuclear leukocytes. The fibrinogen polymerizes to fibrin and this is involved in the process of localizing the infection. The peritoneum therefore becomes oedematous, hyperaemic and covered with a thick fibrinous exudate that coats the viscera and binds adjacent bowel loops together and to the omentum and parietal peritoneum. At the same time there is complete cessation of peristaltic activity in the gastrointestinal tract. The opsinons, together with the complement system, are necessary for phagocytosis of bacteria by the polymorphonuclear leucocytes.

Toxaemia, bacteraemia, endotoxaemia and shock of varying degrees accompany all cases of acute secondary bacterial peritonitis. The massive outpouring of inflammatory exudate causing hypovolaemia and death is usually due to septic shock. The infection is mixed, with Gram-negative aerobes and anaerobes (*Escherichia coli*, *Klebsiella*, *Proteus*, *Pseudomonas* and *Bacteroides*) and Gram-positive bacteria (*Enterococcus*, *Staphylococcus*, *Streptococcus* and *Clostridia*). Usually, however, only one aerobic and one anaerobic species are recovered from the peritoneal exudate.

Presentation

The main presenting symptom is abdominal pain, usually of rapid onset. This may start as localized pain at the site of the origin of the peritonitis and become generalized. Movement and coughing exacerbate this pain. Abdominal tenderness and rebound tenderness are marked and the area of tenderness reflects the localized or generalized nature of the disease. Reflex spasm of the abdominal muscles with rigidity is seen and the abdominal wall ceases to move with respiration. Extreme board-like rigidity is confined to cases of perforated peptic ulcer. It is important to realize, however, that the reflex spasm of the abdominal musculature is lost during advanced stages of bacterial peritonitis.

The absence of peristaltic activity leads to a quiet abdomen on auscultation. However, in the absence of nasogastric decompression, progressive distension of the flaccid intestine ensues and tinkling sounds can be heard at this stage owing to the passive movement of fluid within these distended loops. It is also important to appreciate that the sequestration of fluid and electrolytes in these dilated loops of small intestine can result in hypovolaemia, dehydration and electrolyte imbalance.

A rising tachycardia is always present and the temperature is elevated initially. Hypothermia may ensue, however, and this is a grave prognostic sign, which indicates advanced irreversible septic shock. Tachypnoea accompanies the pyrexia and can be aggravated by the development of abdominal distension and diaphragmatic splinting. The moribund patient has sunken eyeballs and a drawn, anxious expression (Hippocratic facies, cold clammy skin, hypotension and oliguria or anuria).

On investigation, the full blood count will reveal a polymorphonuclear leucocytosis and biochemistry will often demonstrate a raised blood urea because of dehydration and electrolyte disturbance, usually a hyponatraemia. Jaundice with elevation of the transaminase enzymes may accompany severe acute bacterial peritonitis and may be the result of hepatitis or haemolysis secondary to bacteraemia and endotoxinaemia. The latter may lead to disseminated intravascular coagulation.

Plain abdominal X-rays often demonstrate dilated small intestinal loops, and in some cases free fluid in the peritoneal cavity giving a ground-glass appearance. An erect chest X-ray may show free gas under the diaphragm (Figure 17.6).

Management

The management of patients with acute bacterial peritonitis can be considered under the following headings: supportive measures, antibiotic therapy and laparotomy.

Supportive measures

The relief of pain and neurogenic shock is an essential part of the resuscitation. Supportive measures include nasogastric suction, intravenous fluid to correct the hypovolaemia and electrolyte deficiencies,

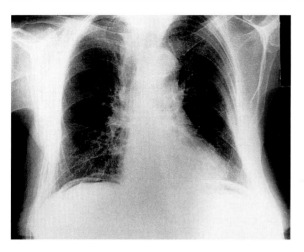

Figure 17.6 Erect chest X-ray demonstrating gas under the diaphragm.

monitoring and prompt and adequate pain relief. Volume expansion is best carried out with crystalloid solutions such as isotonic saline and dextrose or Hartmann's solution. The intravenous fluid therapy is monitored by the central venous pressure and hourly urine output, which must be kept between 30 and 50 ml/h. Blood is administered if the haematocrit is low.

Antibiotic therapy
Secondary bacterial peritonitis is always polymicrobial in origin and combination antibiotic therapy is essential. Several combinations are currently in use but the most favoured is an aminoglycoside or third-generation cephalosporin plus metronidazole regime, which is maintained for 10 days. If continued beyond 2 weeks, this treatment carries a significant risk of fungal infection. Blood levels of the antibiotics are necessary to ensure an adequate therapeutic level and, in the case of aminoglycoside, for the prevention of renal and cranial nerve damage.

Laparotomy
This is most commonly performed through a midline incision. After dealing with the primary lesion, complete removal of the purulent peritoneal exudate and loose fibrinous deposits is carried out. A specimen of pus is obtained for bacteriology (aerobic and anaerobic culture). Thereafter, peritoneal lavage with saline is performed until the peritoneal cavity appears clean and free of debris. The addition of antibiotics to the lavage fluid (tetracycline or cephalosporin) is favoured by some surgeons.

Drainage of the peritoneal cavity is of no value unless postoperative continuous peritoneal lavage is to be carried out. Indeed, drains have been shown to increase the morbidity in these patients by causing wound sepsis and fistulae. In very severe cases, however, it may be helpful to establish continuous peritoneal

lavage. A silicone dialysis catheter (Tenckhoff) is introduced in the immediate subumbilical region together with drainage catheters in the supracolic compartment, the pelvis and in both flanks. After closing the abdomen, lavage is performed with peritoneal dialysate solution containing 1 g of cefoxitin/litre infused through the Tenckhoff catheter at a rate of 250 ml/h while the drainage tubes are spigotted. After 1 litre has been administered, it is left for 30 min and then drained over the next 30 min. This is maintained for 72 h after surgery but it is important that accurate fluid balance charts should be kept and monitoring of the serum, albumen and plasma potassium is essential.

Radical peritoneal debridement (removing all the fibrinous membranes within the peritoneal cavity) has been advocated but prospective studies have shown this to be of no value and to be associated with excessive blood loss. In severe contamination it is sometimes advisable to leave the skin wound open and packed with a gauze soaked in disinfectant such as acriflavine. The wound is inspected and secondary suture performed at 5–7 days if it is clean. In patients with a heavily contaminated abdominal cavity, laparostomy has been advocated by some. Here, the entire abdominal wound is left open, packed with gauze and covered with 'Opsite'. Alternatively, a Marlex mesh with a zip fastener is sutured to the wound edges. This approach allows repeated inspection of the peritoneal cavity but its value has not been fully evaluated by prospective studies and cannot be recommended as a routine measure.

Primary bacterial peritonitis

In this form of bacterial peritonitis there is no intra-abdominal disease or focus responsible for the bacterial invasion of the peritoneal cavity.

Pathophysiology
One type of primary bacterial peritonitis (PBP) is **haematogenous** and occurs predominately in children. It usually follows an acute febrile illness, e.g. chest or urinary tract infection, and the common responsible organisms are *Streptococcus pneumonia* and group A *Streptococcus*. Risk factors include malnutrition, intra-abdominal malignancy, immunosuppression and splenectomy.

Most commonly, however, the disease affects patients with cirrhosis of the liver and the reported prevalence of PBP varies from 18 to 25% in this group of patients. PBP can also occur in patients with other causes of chronic liver disease. The pathogenesis is multifactorial. It is usually encountered in patients who are jaundiced, or have a low serum albumin, varices and impaired clotting. Infection with enteric organisms (*E. coli*, *Streptococcus faecalis*, *Klebsiella*, *Bacteroides*, etc.) occurs via the blood stream. Most of the infections are aerobic and 50–60% of the reported cases are caused by *E. coli*.

As the gut mucosal integrity is impaired and the phagocytic activity of the Kupffer cells is depressed, intestinal bacteria reach the peripheral blood and thus infect the peritoneal cavity. An impaired humoral immunity in the ascitic fluid, due to low levels of complement (C_3), opsonins and fibronectins (due to the excess transudate) is thought to be involved in the increasing susceptibility to infection of the peritoneal cavity. Thus, patients with a low concentration of protein in the ascitic fluid (< 1.0 g/dl) are especially prone to PBP.

Presentation

The disease develops insidiously and localizing signs of peritonitis are often minimal. In cirrhotic patients there is obvious deterioration in the level of consciousness progressing to hepatic coma. This may be accompanied by septic shock. In order to make the diagnosis, it is essential to obtain a specimen of ascitic fluid for bacteriological examination and microscopy for white cells.

Management

In some patients the differentiation between primary and secondary bacterial peritonitis may be difficult. Examination of peritoneal fluid may help, as in secondary bacterial peritonitis; the fluid white cell count and protein concentration is usually high. If, however, doubt remains, laparoscopy or laparotomy should be performed. In patients with hepatic or renal disease, the most favoured antibiotic is Cefoxitin but the antibiotic therapy may need to be changed when the results of bacteriological culture and sensitivity become available. In patients who do not improve within 48 h, repeat paracentesis is performed and if the white cell count has not been reduced by 50%, the antibiotic regimen is changed. Recurrence of PBP in cirrhotic patients occurs in 50% and prophylactic measures include the use of antibiotics, elimination of ascites, absence from alcohol, nutritional support and liver transplantation.

Acute non-bacterial peritonitis

Here, the peritoneal inflammation is due to non-infected irritants escaping into the peritoneal cavity, e.g. gastric juice following perforated peptic ulcer, bile after biliary surgery and urine following trauma to the bladder. In all of these instances, although the peritoneal exudate is initially sterile, it becomes infected within 6–12 h owing to bacterial proliferation. It is therefore important to treat these emergencies promptly.

Chronic bacterial peritonitis

In the majority of these cases the infection is tuberculous in origin but another example is abdominal actinomycosis. Abdominal tuberculosis is a common emergency in India [**see Gastrointestinal disorders, Vol. II**].

Granulomatous peritonitis

The formation of multiple peritoneal granulomas with ascites may be due to sarcoidosis when differentiation from tuberculous can be difficult. Until recently, however, the most common cause of granulomatous peritonitis was starch peritonitis owing to the lubricant used on surgical gloves. The starch granuloma syndrome has a well-recognized clinical picture. It starts 2–6 weeks after abdominal surgery with low-grade fever, anorexia, nausea and vomiting, abdominal distension, cramp-like pain and tenderness. Multiple granulomas develop on both the visceral and parietal peritoneum and there is accumulation of ascitic fluid. The granulomatous nodules consist of collections of lymphocytes, macrophages, polymorphs and eosinophils around starch granules, which have a characteristic Maltese-cross appearance on light microscopy. It is thought to represent either a hypersensitivity reaction to starch or a foreign-body reaction. The diagnosis is best made by laparoscopy with biopsy to confirm the diagnosis. Treatment is conservative and systemic corticosteroids may accelerate progress. Prognosis is generally good and the majority of cases will resolve, but adhesion formation with intestinal obstruction and fistula formation may ensue. This problem has largely been resolved by the introduction of a hydrogel polymer as the lubricant only on the inner surface of gloves ('Biogel'). These gloves are totally starch free and have eliminated the problem.

Section 17.3 • Abscesses

The formation of an abscess is a process whereby infection is localized. It starts as a focal accumulation of neutrophils in an area of liquefactive necrosis around bacteria. When established, it is made up of a localized collection of pus within a pyogenic membrane. Pus consists of necrotic leucocytes and tissue cells; the pyogenic membrane is composed of an inner layer of neutrophils and an outer layer of vascular granulation tissue.

Pathophysiology

Neutrophils are attracted to the focus of infection by chemotaxis and they release proteolytic enzymes as they undergo necrosis. At the periphery of the necrotic tissue and neutrophils some damage occurs to blood vessels. Activated platelets stimulate fibroblasts and together with the blood vessels and neutrophils and monocytes form granulation tissue. More neutrophils and macrophages are drawn into the abscess cavity as it expands.

This process is favoured by the proteolytic breakdown of large molecules within the abscess cavity to form more osmotically active particles. The granulation tissue acts as a barrier to bacteria, thus preventing spreading infection. Unfortunately, it also prevents the entry of antibiotics into the cavity. In addition, most antibiotics are inactivated by different factors in the pus and when the bacteria within the abscess have reached their maximum concentration they become less metabolically active and thus less sensitive to antibiotics.

Eventually, macrophages appear within the fibroblastic zone and these come to be in close proximity to areas of active necrosis. When healing occurs, macrophages replace the neutrophils within the pyogenic membrane, which then becomes less vascular and finally contracts into a scar. When an abscess does not resolve the circulation around the expanding cavity may become compromised by a pressure effect and result in thrombosis and cell death. This may then lead to spontaneous discharge of the abscess or tracking of the abscess along fascial compartments.

Classification

Abscesses may form anywhere in the body and the causative organism varies according to the site of the abscess. Abscesses in specific anatomical sites are dealt with in the appropriate sections [see Vol. II], but some of the more common forms of abscess are described briefly below.

Skin and subcutaneous abscesses

These are the most common types of abscess and normally arise owing to staphylococcal infection of infected sweat glands. They are particularly common on the neck or on the buttock in young adolescents. Occasionally, several such abscesses or boils can become confluent to result in a carbuncle and this can result in extensive destruction of the skin and subcutaneous tissue. These tend to occur in debilitated and diabetic patients.

Perianal abscesses

Perianal abscesses arise from infected anal glands, which are situated between internal and external sphincters in the anal canal. Infection can then track down between the sphincters to present as a perianal abscess or through the external sphincter into the ischiorectal fossa to form an ischiorectal abscess. The organisms tend to originate from the bowel and therefore *E. coli*, *S. faecalis* and *Bacteroides* are common. When these abscesses discharge or are drained, a communication between the skin and the anal canal may persist. This is a fistula-in-ano.

Breast abscesses

Breast abscesses occur predominantly in the female during child-bearing age and are most common during breast feeding. They may, however, occur at other times. *Staphylococcus aureus* infections are the most common. Recurrent periareolar abscesses are a feature of mammary duct ectasia [see Diseases of the breast, Vol. II].

Intra-abdominal abscesses

Intra-abdominal abscesses usually occur as a result of perforation of the gastrointestinal tract (e.g. perforated

peptic ulcer, perforated appendicitis and perforated diverticular disease). These abscesses can be further classified into subphrenic abscess, appendix abscess, intraloop abscess and pelvic abscess.

Subphrenic abscesses
Subphrenic abscesses are situated immediately below the right or left domes of the diaphragm. These may result from perforation of the upper gastrointestinal tract or, more commonly, from infection introduced during laparotomy.

Intraloop abscesses
These abscesses, which are often multiple, result from generalized peritonitis that has not been adequately treated.

Appendix abscess
Although perforated appendicitis may lead to generalized peritonitis; commonly the inflamed appendix is surrounded by omentum and loops of small bowel (inflammatory phlegmon). If the inflammation does not settle this may then develop into an abscess.

Pelvic abscess
A pelvic abscess may arise from a perforated appendicitis, perforated diverticulitis or breakdown of a rectal anastomosis.

Presentation

The clinical presentation of an abscess depends on its location. A superficial abscess such as a boil, a perianal abscess or a breast abscess will present as a tender, hot, red swelling. In the later stages the pain may become severe and throbbing in quality, especially when the pus is under tension.

When an abscess is of any size, there are usually accompanying systemic effects with intermittent pyrexia, general debility, weight loss and a pronounced leucocytosis. In deep-seated abscesses, particularly intra-abdominal, there may be no localizing signs or symptoms. In this case the patient will develop signs of toxicity and a hypercatabolic state, which may progress to multisystem organ failure. With all abscesses there is the ever-present risk of bacteraemia progressing to septic shock. This is especially the case with rupture of an intra-abdominal abscess causing widespread peritonitis.

Management

The diagnosis of a superficial abscess is obvious, but in the patient with a deep-seated, 'silent' intra-abdominal abscess, diagnosis may be problematical. In the patient with suspicious symptoms (rigors and malaise) and signs (rise in pulse rate and intermittent pyrexia) the first investigation should be blood cultures so that appropriate antibiotic therapy can be started as soon as possible. Plain radiographs of the chest and abdomen may be helpful in revealing in a localized ileus soft tissue swelling or sympathetic pleural fusion, but the first investigation of choice is now usually ultrasound examination, which will detect abscesses in about 70% of patients. CT scanning is particularly helpful in difficult areas such as the chest, pelvis or cranium. Radionuclide scanning with indium–labelled autologous leucocytes can also localize pus. However, it does not distinguish between pus and inflammation and although it has an accuracy of up to 80%, it may also produce false-positive results.

Once an abscess has been localized, the mainstay of treatment is drainage. Appropriate antibiotics may be helpful in minimizing the effects of systemic infection but for the reasons discussed above, they are rarely effective in bringing about the resolution of anything but the smallest abscesses. Delay in draining established abscesses is dangerous owing to the potential for septicaemia and local tissue necrosis (synergistic gangrene).

For superficial abscesses drainage is a relatively simple matter of incising over the area of maximum fluctuation and evacuating the pus. Traditionally, the abscess cavity is then left open in order to heal by granulation. However, there has been a recent move towards primary suture after drainage combined with antibiotic therapy and, with breast abscesses in particular, needle aspiration of the abscess along with systemic antibiotic treatment proves successful in the majority of cases.

In deep-seated abscesses, the treatment of choice is by ultrasound or CT-guided percutaneous drainage. With this approach, the drainage catheters may need to remain in place for several days until the abscess cavity collapses around the drainage tube. Where this is not available or when it is unsuccessful, formal surgical drainage may still be necessary. This is particularly the case with multiloculated abscesses containing significant slough.

Section 17.4 • Intestinal obstruction

By convention, the term intestinal obstruction applies to the small and large bowel and does not include obstructive pathology of the oesophagus, stomach or proximal duodenum. The term ileus can be used synonymously with obstruction but it is commonly, although incorrectly, used to denote lack of peristalsis. To avoid confusion the term mechanical obstruction will be used to denote a structural lesion causing obstruction to the bowel and the term paralytic ileus to denote obstruction caused by lack of peristalsis.

Mechanical obstruction is **simple** when the blood supply is intact and **strangulated** when there is direct interference to the intestinal blood supply, most commonly caused by extrinsic compression. Other important definitions are **intussusception**, in which a segment of bowel invaginates itself into an adjacent segment, **volvulus**, which denotes a twist of a bowel loop on its mesenteric pedicle, and **closed loop obstruction**, which can result from a volvulus or from a colonic obstruction in the presence of an intact

ileocaecal valve. The latter leads to a rapid rise in intraluminal pressure within the closed loop, leading to impairment of blood supply necrosis and perforation.

Mechanical obstruction is sometimes further classified as **acute**, **subacute** and **chronic**. These are rather confusing and unhelpful terms but as they are in common usage, they should be defined. In **acute obstruction**, the clinical course is rapid in onset and involves both early vomiting and acute abdominal pain. **Chronic obstruction** is characterized by progressive constipation with late distension and vomiting. In general, acute intestinal obstruction is caused by a small bowel lesion, whereas the chronic form is caused by a large bowel lesion. In practical terms, it is better to refer to small bowel obstruction and large bowel obstruction. The term **subacute obstruction** implies an incomplete obstruction as used for both small and large bowel disease. It is characterized by recurrent episodes of abdominal colicky pain and distension, which are relieved by the passage of liquid or semiformed stool.

Aetiology

The aetiology of intestinal obstruction is best subdivided into mechanical obstruction and paralytic ileus and further subdivided into small bowel and large bowel obstruction.

Mechanical obstruction
When considering mechanical obstruction, it is useful to categorize the aetiology into extramural (extrinsic), intramural and intraluminal. Using this classification, the possible causes of small and large bowel obstruction are given in Table 17.2.

Paralytic ileus
Loss of peristaltic activity may result from the following:

- reflex inhibition of intestinal motility
- metabolic abnormalities
- intraperitoneal sepsis
- mesenteric vascular disease
- various drugs (e.g. tricyclic antidepressants).

Table 17.2 Causes of intestinal obstruction

Extramural	Intramural	Intraluminal
Small bowel		
Adhesions	Crohn's disease	Gallstone
Hernia	Tumour (lymphoma,	(gallstone ileus)
Peritoneal tumour	carcinoma	Food bolus
Volvulus		Foreign body
Large bowel		
Volvulus	Tumour (carcinoma)	Faecal impaction
Peritoneal tumour	Diverticulitis	
Hernia	Crohn's disease	
Adhesions	Ulcerative colitis	

Pathophysiology

Simple mechanical obstruction

Below the point of obstruction, the intestine continues to exhibit normal peristalsis and absorption until it becomes empty. Proximal to the obstruction, however, it dilates and develops altered motility. The initial response consists of strong peristaltic contractions initiated by stimulation of the stretch reflexes. These account for the severe colicky abdominal pain. Several hours after the onset of the obstruction, however, this reflex activity diminishes until inhibition of intestinal motility occurs.

The distension is caused by excess accumulation of fluid and gas in the bowel lumen, and the amount of fluid sequested and dilated into intestinal loops is substantial. In the case of low small bowel obstruction, this may approximate to one-half of the total interstitial fluid. This is because in intestinal obstruction not only is the reabsorption of fluid and salt inhibited but also there is increased secretion of water and electrolytes into the obstructed bowel lumen. The huge increase in intestinal gas seen in obstruction is due to swallowed air and also from gas produced by the marked increase in gut bacteria. In the upper small bowel, the bacterial flora is scanty and consists of a few Gram-positive aerobes. In the distal small bowel, anaerobic bacteroides and coliforms are relatively numerous. When small bowel obstruction intervenes the bacteria count rapidly rises and the normal gradient of organisms from jejunum to the ileum is lost. In large bowel obstruction, anaerobic organisms predominate and this may explain the increased incidence of serious sepsis in these patients compared with those suffering from small bowel obstruction.

Strangulating mechanical obstruction

In this case, in addition to the changes seen in simple intestinal obstruction, the viability of the intestinal wall is threatened because of impairment of the blood supply. This can be caused by compression of the mesenteric blood vessels or from rising intraluminal pressure. In general, the venous return is affected before the arterial supply, and this results in increased capillary pressure and consequent escape of intravascular fluid and red blood cells into the bowel wall. The bowel therefore becomes oedematous and haemorrhagic and both the intestinal contents and peritoneal exudate are heavily blood stained. This leads to haemorrhagic infarction and, concomitant with the decreased viability of the gut wall, transmigration of bacteria takes place. Thus, the haemorrhagic exudate is always heavily infected with intestinal organisms, and there is a risk of bacteraemia and septic shock in all strangulating mechanical obstruction, particularly when the strangulated segment is extensive and lies within the peritoneal cavity.

Paralytic ileus

The most common cause of paralytic ileus is reflex inhibition of intestinal motility, following a variety of conditions including abdominal operations, pneumonia, crush injuries, fractures of the spine and retroperitoneal haemorrhage. It is thought to be the result of increased sympathetic discharge with hyperpolarization of the smooth muscle cells, which become unresponsive to both neural and hormonal stimulation. Absent or diminished peristaltic activity of small intestine may accompany metabolic abnormalities such as hypokalaemia, hyponatraemia, uraemia and diabetic ketoacidosis. The ileus seen in bacterial peritonitis is due to both reflex inhibition of intestinal motility and a direct effect of bacterial toxins on the myenteric nerve plexuses. The most serious form of paralytic ileus results from acute mesenteric infarction.

Presentation of patients with intestinal obstruction

Mechanical obstruction

The clinical features of intestinal obstruction can be divided into the history and the findings on examination. The cardinal features of the history are pain, nausea and vomiting, constipation and distension.

Pain

The pain of simple mechanical obstruction consists of waves of severe pain, which are found to coincide with peristaltic rushes on ausculation of the abdomen. These episodes of pain last for a few minutes at a time and subside completely for a few minutes. This is the typical pattern of intestinal colic and is quite different from the pattern of pain found in biliary or ureteric colic. When the peristaltic activity ceases owing to increasing distension of the bowel, this colicky pain is replaced by a constant diffuse pain, which is not usually very severe. **The development of severe constant pain is very significant as it may indicate the onset of strangulation.**

Nausea and vomiting

Although nausea and vomiting may accompany all forms of intestinal obstruction, the more distal the obstruction the longer the interval between the onset of the obstruction and the appearance of these symptoms. Thus, even though complete obstruction of the distal colon may have been present for several days, vomiting may not occur at all. In contrast, a high small bowel obstruction will lead to nausea and vomiting early in the course of the episode. As intestinal obstruction progresses, the vomitus becomes faeculent owing to bacterial overgrowth in the small intestine. This must be distinguished from true faecal vomiting, which can only occur when there is gastrocolic fistula.

Constipation

Absolute constipation (passage of neither faeces not flatus) is a feature of complete intestinal obstruction. However, many patients may pass faeces or flatus after the onset of the obstruction. This simply reflects the evacuation of the intestine distal to the obstruction and has no particular significance. Partial obstruction is often accompanied by diarrhoea.

Distension
The degree of abdominal distension varies, as does its onset. Distension is minimal or absent in proximal small bowel obstruction and in mesenteric vascular occlusion. It is delayed in colonic obstruction. Severe abdominal distension is usually encountered in low small bowel obstruction, mechanical obstruction of the left colon, volvulus of the sigmoid and Hirschsprung's disease.

Examination
Abdominal examination of the patient with intestinal obstruction typically reveals a distended timpanic abdomen. In simple obstruction tenderness is absent but will be found if there is a loop of strangulated bowel. Masses are not usually felt because of gaseous distension. Although not widely recognized, the patient with long-standing intestinal obstruction with large amounts of fluid and gas in the intestine will exhibit shifting dullness, which can be confused with ascites.

On auscultation of the abdomen the patient with mechanical obstruction will have high-pitched 'plinking' bowel sounds, which have a cavernous resonance. In the late stages of obstruction, however, the abdomen may be silent.

In the patient with intestinal obstruction it is essential to examine the hernial orifices, and in the patient with an irreducible hernia tenderness suggests strangulation. It is also important to assess the patient for dehydration or hypovolaemia caused by loss of extracellular fluid by vomiting or sequestration into distended loops of bowel. This can by achieved simply by examining the pulse, skin turgor and venous filling on the back of the hand.

Paralytic ileus
The clinical course of paralytic ileus is characterized by progressive abdominal distension and effortless vomiting. Intestinal colic is absent but patients usually complain of tight diffuse abdominal discomfort. With the recovery of intestinal motility, intestinal colic, often described as wind pain, is often experienced by the patient. On examination, the abdomen is rarely grossly distended but rather exhibits flaccid distension. Auscultation commonly reveals a silent abdomen although occasional high-pitched sounds may be heard. **There is a real risk of pulmonary aspiration in these patients.**

Investigations

Temperature, pulse rate and blood pressure must always be monitored. Pyrexia may signify the onset of strangulation or the presence of inflammation associated with the obstructing lesion, e.g. an abscess associated with diverticulitis, a localized perforation or inflammatory bowel disease. A tachycardia will also accompany

these complications. Measurement of the pulse and blood pressure is also important in estimating hypovolaemia, which may result from fluid and electrolyte depletion or from septicaemia.

Haematology, urea and electrolytes
Estimation of haemoglobin, packed cell volume (PCV) and white cell count are very important in intestinal obstruction. A low haemoglobin may result from an obstructing lesion that has been causing chronic blood loss. A raised PCV will indicate water and salt depletion and a marked leucocytosis suggests strangulation. Because intestinal obstruction and small bowel obstruction in particular lead to loss of extracellular fluid, both from vomiting and sequestration of fluid and electrolytes in dilated bowel loops, it is very important to estimate the levels of urea and electrolytes. Potassium may be lost, especially if there is excessive vomiting, but a rise in the serum potassium level may accompany the onset of strangulation. It should be noted that elevated levels of serum amylase and lactate dehydrogenase may be observed and marked elevation of both enzymes is often encountered in strangulation.

Radiological investigations
The standard radiological examination in the patient with suspected intestinal obstruction consists of erect and supine abdominal X-rays. The erect film demonstrates fluid levels (Figure 17.7) but these may also be seen in non-obstructing conditions such as inflammatory bowel disease, acute pancreatitis and intra-abdominal abscesses. They may also be observed after the

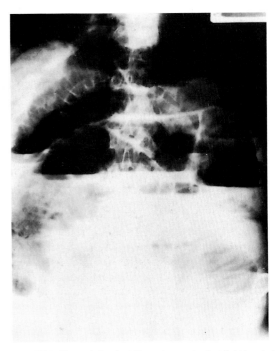

Figure 17.7 Erect abdominal X-ray demonstrating fluid levels in small bowel obstruction.

administration of enemas. However, multiple fluid levels indicate obstruction and, if centrally placed, signify dilated loops of small bowel.

The supine X-ray outlines the distended intestinal loops and gives more information regarding the site of intestinal obstruction. In small bowel obstruction the dilated jejunal and ileal loops are usually arranged transversely in the centre of the abdomen and no gas is seen in the colon (Figure 17.8). Usually, small bowel can be differentiated from large bowel by the presence of circular transverse ridges due to the valvulae conniventes (plicae semilunaris). These are quite different from the colonic haustra, which do not cross the entire distended lumen of the colon (Figure 17.9). In colonic obstruction, the dilatation of the colon, predominantly with gas, can usually be seen easily on the supine films arranged around the periphery of the abdomen in the characteristic anatomical position. The exception to this is volvulus of the sigmoid colon, which produces a grossly dilated loop of bowel, arising from the pelvis and extending obliquely across from the left lower quadrant to the right upper quadrant (Figure 17.10).

It is important to appreciate that mechanical obstruction cannot be differentiated from paralytic ileus on radiological appearances alone, as both may give rise to dilatation of both the small and large intestine. Contrast radiology can be helpful but in the acute situation it is better to use water-soluble contrast. Barium is contraindicated in the presence of the possible perforation of the bowel and when surgery is contemplated it is better not to have large amounts of barium present within the lumen of bowel.

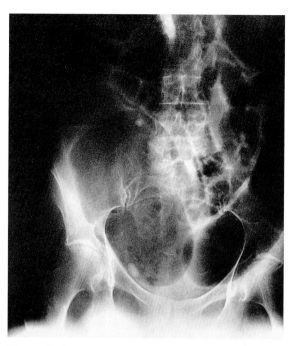

Figure 17.9 Plain abdominal X-ray showing large bowel obstruction.

The most important indication for contrast radiology is an apparent large bowel obstruction; a contrast enema will differentiate between a true mechanical large bowel obstruction and pseudo-obstruction [see **Gastrointestinal Disorders, Vol. II**].

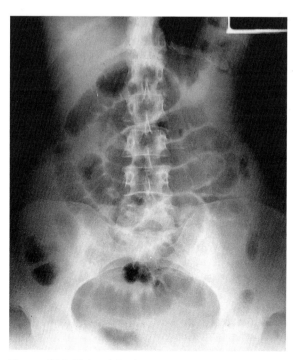

Figure 17.8 Plain abdominal X-ray showing small bowel obstruction.

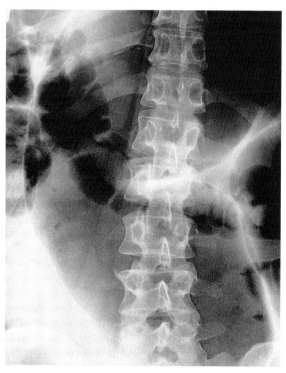

Figure 17.10 Plain abdominal X-ray demonstrating sigmoid volvulus.

Management of patients with intestinal obstruction

The first steps in the management of intestinal obstruction are intestinal decompression by nasogastric aspiration and maintenance of fluid and electrolyte balance using intravenous infusion. Monitoring of pulse, blood pressure and urine output is essential. In some instances (e.g. uncomplicated paralytic ileus, adhesive small bowel obstruction) these measures alone are sufficient. However, surgical intervention is necessary for most cases of mechanical obstruction but this should usually be delayed until fluid and electrolyte deficits have been corrected. Exceptions to this rule include signs of strangulation or peritonitis, where early intervention is necessary.

Supportive management

Nasogastric suction by a non-vented (Ryle) or preferably vented (Salem) tube is the first step. The suction may be applied continuously or intermittently; the Salem tube is less likely to become blocked during suction and is therefore more reliable than the Ryle's tube. This is necessary not only to decompress the intestine but also to make sure that the stomach is empty, thus reducing the hazards of aspiration during induction of anaesthesia where surgical intervention is indicated.

As the basic biochemical abnormality is water and sodium depletion, the appropriate intravenous fluid for replacement is isotonic saline. The amount needed varies and is influenced by the clinical findings (signs of dehydration), urine output and biochemical and haematological parameters. Careful monitoring of the potassium level is necessary to avoid hypokalaemia. Once the fluid and electrolyte deficit has been corrected, maintenance therapy is continued until the return of normal bowel function and motility.

There is a good case for using antibiotics active against both Gram-negative aerobes and anaerobes because of the inevitable bacterial overgrowth in intestinal obstruction. Prophylactic antibiotics are mandatory in all patients requiring resection of small or large intestine.

Stenting

Although the majority of patients with mechanical intestinal obstruction will require surgical intervention, there has recently been a move towards stenting of left-sided colonic lesions. This is done using an expanding nickel–titanium alloy metal (Wall) stent introduced under radiological or endoscopic control (Figure 17.11). When successful, this will relieve the obstruction and allow the patient to be treated in a semielective fashion.

Surgical treatment

The vast majority of patients with mechanical intestinal obstruction will require a laparotomy, although in some selected cases laparoscopic division of adhesions may be appropriate. A long midline incision is usually

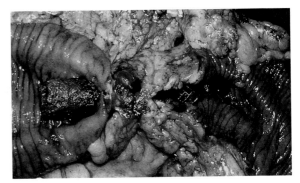

Figure 17.11 Wall stent in place across a malignant colonic stricture.

used and care must be exercised to avoid damaging the dilated loops of bowel, particularly if adhesions are present. Small bowel obstruction is usually due to adhesions and it may be a long, painstaking procedure to trace the small bowel down to the site of the obstruction (junction between proximal dilated and distal collapsed segments).

It is then very important to assess the viability of the intestine. The obviously infarcted bowel with its greyish, green–black appearance is easily distinguished and must be resected. However, there are many circumstances where the viability of the bowel is in doubt, particularly when it is heavily bruised. It is best under these circumstances to wrap the bowel in warm moist packs and to leave it for at least 10 min. If viability is still then in doubt, the choice is between resection or a second-look laparotomy at about 24 h.

When the obstruction has been relieved the small bowel is usually grossly dilated and the abdomen may be difficult to close. Under these circumstances it is possible to milk the intestinal contents back into the stomach. It is essential, however, to ensure that the stomach is completely emptied and if this is not possible by aspiration on the nasogastric tube, it may be necessary to ask the anaesthetist to pass a large stomach tube via the oral route.

In large bowel obstruction, particularly if this is distal, the grossly distended large bowel may make laparotomy difficult. In this case, it is usually easy to decompress the bowel by inserting an 18-gauge needle through one of the taenia and aspirating the gas by attaching the needle to suction. The obstructing lesion (usually a carcinoma) should then be resected if possible and if the patient's general physiological state will allow it. The proximal colon is then usually brought out as an end colostomy and the distal colon is either brought out as a mucus fistula or closed off (Hartmann's procedure). Recently, however, there has been a move towards resection with primary anastomosis after on-table colonic preparation **[see Module 16, Vol. I; Gastrointestinal Disorders, Vol. II]**.

Where the patient is considered to be unfit for a resection, then a proximal loop colostomy through a small incision is appropriate. This will allow the obstruction to settle and provide an opportunity to improve the patient's physiological condition.

Postoperative management
In the postoperative phase, it is very important to pay close attention to fluid and electrolyte balance, as large amounts of extracellular fluid will have been lost as a result of the obstruction. In the patient who has had extensive small bowel resection it is also important to bear in mind the possible nutritional consequences. The exact site of resection and the length of the resection should always be recorded and arrangements for parenteral nutrition made if less than 2 m of the small bowel remain. In patients with 100 cm or less, permanent home parenteral nutrition is likely to be necessary [see Module 8, Vol. I; Gastrointestinal Disorders, Vol. II].

Management of paralytic ileus
Surgical treatment is necessary when the paralytic ileus is secondary to a surgically remediable disorder, e.g. peritonitis or mesenteric vascular occlusion. Otherwise, treatment is conservative with intestinal decompression, intravenous fluids and the correction of metabolic disorders, particularly hypokalaemia. Rarely, paralytic ileus may be the consequence of medical therapy (e.g. tricyclic antidepressants), and withdrawal of the drugs or change to a new medication is necessary. Elimination of the cause and adequate supportive therapy are usually successful in restoring intestinal motility.

Occasionally, medical therapy with an adrenergic blocking agent in association with cholinergic stimulation, e.g. neostigmine (Catchpole regimen), is indicated for resistant cases of ileus, providing that an intraperitoneal cause has been excluded. Recent clinical trials have demonstrated the efficacy of ceruletide compared with metoclopramide or placebo, especially in postoperative ileus. Ceruletide is a synthetic analogue of the naturally occurring peptide caerulein. It stimulates peristaltic contractions and is administered either intramuscularly or as a slow intravenous infusion.

In the special case of colonic pseudo-obstruction, the caecum may become dangerously distended such that it can perforate. Under these circumstances, urgent colonoscopic decompression should be carried out, and this may need to be repeated on several occasions. If this fails, or the patient becomes very tender over the caecum, it may be necessary to establish a tube caecosotomy.

Section 17.5 • Gastrointestinal haemorrhage

The epidemiology, aetiology, presentation and general management of gastrointestinal bleeding are covered elsewhere [see Module 6, Vol. I]. In this section, preoperative preparation, operative principles and postoperative care are covered.

Preoperative preparation

When the patient has been resuscitated and the diagnosis established, usually by endoscopy, preparation of the patient will depend very much on their physiological status. In the patient who is actively bleeding, from either the upper or the lower gastrointestinal tract, rapid transfer to the operating theatre is mandatory. In the patient who has had an endoscopy for profuse upper gastrointestinal bleeding this may already have been done in theatre with cuffed endotracheal intubation.

In any event, as the patient is being prepared in the anaesthetic room the surgeon and the scrub nurse should prepare for the operation. Although it is ideal to have central venous pressure monitoring and intra-arterial pressure monitoring, when a patient is in extremis the anaesthetist must be prepared to induce anaesthesia rapidly and to establish intravascular monitoring intraoperatively. If not already present, a transurethral catheter should be placed into the bladder to monitor urine output.

Clearly, the patient must be cross-matched but in extreme cases it may be necessary to use group-specific or even O-negative blood. When blood is being infused at a rate exceeding 100 ml/min, complications are likely to arise after the delivery of about 6 units. These include potassium toxicity, citrate toxicity and coagulation problems. The citrate toxicity can be avoided by warming the blood to 25°C prior to transfusion or by giving 10 ml of 10% calcium gluconate after the first 6 units. The coagulation problems arise mainly because of the absence of viable platelets in transfused blood, but as total transfusion of 10 units is approached, deficiency of clotting factors is also a problem in the patient who requires a massive transfusion. Therefore, it is advisable to obtain platelets at the outset and to give 2 units of platelet concentrate after each 6 units of rapidly transfused blood. After 10 units, a clotting screen should be performed and 4 units (800 ml) of fresh frozen plasma given if there is an abnormality.

Prophylactic antibiotics should not be forgotten and 500 mg of metronidazole plus 1.5 g of cefuroxime given intravenously at induction of anaesthesia is an appropriate regime that will cover both upper and lower gastrointestinal surgery. Prophylaxis for deep vein thrombosis should not be forgotten either, but few surgeons would wish to use subcutaneous heparin in a patient who already has coagulation problems. TED stockings should be used and consideration should be given to introduction of subcutaneous heparin once the patient is fully stable with a normal coagulation screen.

In the patient who is stable but in whom surgical intervention is deemed necessary, preparation for surgery can be carried out in a more leisurely fashion and full intraoperative monitoring established prior to operation.

Principles of operative management of patients with gastrointestinal haemorrhage

In the vast majority of patients requiring surgery for gastrointestinal haemorrhage, a midline incision is used.

It must be stressed that every attempt should be made to localize the bleeding point preoperatively as this can be difficult to do at laparotomy. In the patient with colonic bleeding, however, if prompt mesenteric angiography is not available this may be impossible.

The operative procedures for the common conditions giving rise to gastrointestinal bleeding are outlined below.

Oesophageal varices

In the rare situation where oesophageal variceal bleeding has not been controlled by endoscopic intervention, the surgical procedure of choice is oesophageal transection. This is now done using a circular end-to-end anastomizing stapler, which simultaneously divides and anastomoses the oesophagus, thus interrupting the flow of blood from the portal to the systemic circulation by way of the varices (Figure 17.12). When the patient comes to theatre for this procedure, there is invariably a Sengstaken–Blakemore tube *in situ*. This should be left in place until the stomach is opened. When the patient is bleeding from gastric varices, these should be underrun through a high gastrostomy.

The role of portosystemic shunting is controversial in acute bleeding. The principle here is to create an anastomosis between the portal and systemic circulations to reduce the portal pressure, and the most commonly performed shunt is now the Warren shunt, which involves anastomosing the splenic vein to the left renal vein with preservation of the spleen and left gastric vein, thus in effect achieving transsplenic decompression without significantly lowering the portal flow to the liver (Figure 17.13). The Warren shunt has the advantage over the more conventional portocaval or H-mesocaval shunts of having a lower incidence of hepatic encephalopathy, but it must be appreciated that results in patients with deranged hepatic function (Child grade C) are poor and the Warren shunt is indicated only in Child A patients. It requires expert surgery, but if carried out expeditiously, it carries the lowest incidence of rebleeding of any treatment. The alternative to surgical shunting is the radiological insertion of the transjugular intrahepatic portosystemic stent shunt (TIPSS). The role of this procedure in acute bleeding, however, is not fully established. TIPSS undoubtedly results in effective decompression in the short term but the thrombosis rate of the shunt is high beyond 6 months. Its main indication is in Child C patients with bleeding from portal hypertension and who are awaiting hepatic transplantation.

Arterial bleeding from oesophagitis

Again a very rare indication for surgical intervention, this may require a thoracoabdominal approach to the lower oesophagus with opening of the oesophagus and underrunning of the bleeding vessel.

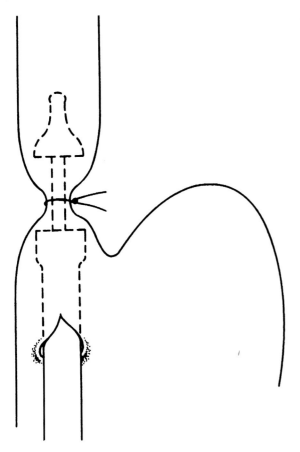

Figure 17.12 Transection of the oesophagus using a circular end-to-end anastomosing stapler.

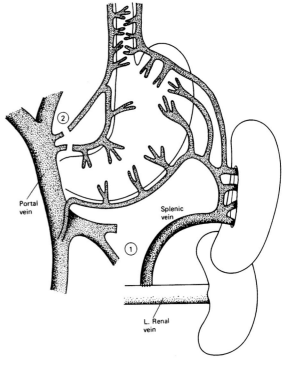

Portal vein

Splenic vein

L. Renal vein

Figure 17.13 The Warren shunt operation.

Gastric ulcer

Traditionally, the surgical treatment of a bleeding gastric ulcer is an appropriate partial gastrectomy. However, simple ulcer excision, particularly when the ulcer is on the lesser curve of the stomach, is a useful and less extensive procedure. It has to be performed with care, however, and involves removing most of the lesser curve of the stomach. Gastrotomy and simple underrunning of a bleeding gastric ulcer carry a high risk of rebleeding. Histological examination of the excised ulcer is essential to exclude malignancy in these patients.

Duodenal ulcer

Most duodenal ulcers requiring surgery are on the posterior wall of the duodenum where they have eroded into the gastroduodenal artery. In this case it is necessary to perform a prompt duodenotomy and to underrun the bleeding ulcer securely. In the past, the duodenotomy would have been converted to a pyloroplasty and truncal vagotomy carried out. This practice has now changed, however, partly owing to the recognition of the role of *Helicobacter pylori* in the pathogenesis of duodenal ulcer and partly owing to a lack of surgical expertise in vagotomy. The role of highly selective vagotomy in the acute situation has always been controversial. Today, simple underrunning of a duodenal ulcer and anatomical closure of the duodenotomy is to be recommended. Occasionally, with a giant duodenal ulcer it will be impossible to close the duodenotomy safely and under these circumstances it will be necessary to carry out a partial gastrectomy with oversewing of the duodenal loop. There are situations when intraduodenal underrunning of the bleeding vessel is not feasible. This is the case when the main gastroduodenal artery is eroded. In this situation, the artery can be suture ligated in continuity extraduodenally, either as it comes off the common hepatic or between the head of the pancreas and the duodenum in the lesser sac.

Diffuse gastritis

Again an unusual cause of gastrointestinal haemorrhage requiring surgery, gastritis can present as a life-threatening emergency. In this case, total gastrectomy will be required.

Bleeding from small bowel lesions (vascular malformation or vascular tumour)

Surgical treatment for these lesions is straightforward and involves a small bowel resection with primary anastomosis. Difficulty can arise in actually locating the lesion, however. Ideally, it is best for the interventional the radiologist to locate the lesion by angiography and then to leave a superselective catheter as close to the lesion as possible. It is then a relatively easy matter for the surgeon to inject a small amount of blue dye through the catheter and this will highlight the area of the small bowel required to be removed.

Bleeding lesion in the colon

The most common underlying pathology in massive bleeding from the colon is diverticular disease, followed by angiodysplasia. Under ideal circumstances, the bleeding lesion will have been identified by mesenteric angiography but this may not be available and even if it is, active bleeding may be intermittent and not demonstrated by the leaking of contrast into the bowel lumen. If the lesion has been identified then an appropriate large bowel resection should be carried out. If, however, the lesion has not been identified, it can be extremely difficult to localize the bleeding point. Some authorities would recommend intubation of the caecum with antegrade colonic lavage with warm saline followed by colonoscopy to try to identify the bleeding point. This is time consuming, however, and in the patient who is bleeding rapidly it may not be feasible. Under these circumstances it is acceptable to carry out a subtotal colectomy with ileorectal anastomosis if the patient is fit or with an ileostomy if this is not the case.

Postoperative management

The postoperative care of patients following surgery for gastrointestinal bleeding is similar to that for all patients who have undergone abdominal surgery for acute abdominal pathology. However, it is important to bear in mind that patients with peptic ulceration must have the underlying disease process treated. Immediately postoperatively, it is standard practice to use acid suppression with an H_2 receptor antagonist such as ranitidine. After 4–6 weeks of treatment, it will then be appropriate to carry out an upper gastrointestinal endoscopy to check for healing and also to take an antral gastric biopsy for *H. pylori* testing. If this is positive (which it usually is) the patient should then be treated with a *H. pylori* eradication regimen. The efficacy of this can then be tested using a urea breath test.

Guide to further reading

Attard, A. R., Corlett, M. J., Kidner, N. J. *et al.* (1992). Safety of early pain relief for acute abdominal pain. *Br Med J* **305**: 554–556.

De Dombal. (1991). *Diagnosis of Acute Abdominal Pain*, 2nd edn, Churchill Livingstone, Edinburgh.

Ducharme, J. (1994). Emergency pain management: a Canadian Association of Emergency Physicians (CAEP) consensus document. *J Emerg Med* **12**: 855–866.

Jones, P. F., Krukowski, Z. H. and Youngson, G. G. (1998). *Emergency Abdominal Surgery*, 3rd edn, Chapman & Hall, London.

Patients with postoperative complications

1 • Postoperative death

2 • Types of complication

3 • Cardiovascular complications

4 • Pulmonary complications

5 • Wound complications

6 • Cerebral, psychological and neuropsychiatric complications

7 • Mortality and morbidity of day-case surgery

'There are some patients whom we cannot help, there are none whom we cannot harm' – Arthur L. Bloomfield, 1888–1962

Postoperative complications (morbidity) account for considerable human suffering, increase the health-care costs and can lead to postoperative death. The increased costs of dealing with even relatively minor complications such as wound infections are substantial on both the primary and secondary heath-care sectors. The costs of treating major complications can be prohibitive as this usually entails remedial surgery, often in a tertiary referral centre, and prolonged hospital stay. It has been estimated, for example, that the cost of dealing with one infected artificial hip joint equals the resource required for treating three such patients. Thus, the health-economic impact of surgical morbidity is such as to reduce the available resource for treating patients within any health-care system irrespective of its nature.

More importantly, the quality of life of the patient and the expected survival may be compromised. The worst consequence of postoperative complications after surgical intervention is death of the patient.

Section 18.1 • Postoperative death

Definition of postoperative death

Postoperative death is variously defined as **death before discharge from hospital, death within 30 days of surgery** and **death within 60 days of surgery**. These definitions result in different mortality rates. Thus reports based on death within 30 days, although they account for the majority, miss those patients (2–5%) who die after a protracted illness, often on a background of sepsis. The complete picture is only obtained by the definition as **death within 60 days**, since this includes patients who die at home from such conditions as pulmonary embolism. In the UK, death occurring during surgery or within 24 h of the intervention has to be reported to the Coroner or Procurator Fiscal.

Location and cause of postoperative death
The data from a UK Audit of three large regions show that 4% of perioperative deaths occur in the operating theatre, 1% in recovery and 1.5% at home, compared with 72% in the wards and 19% in the intensive care unit (ICU). There is, as expected, a correlation with the ASA grade, and deaths in ASA I patients have to be regarded as avoidable in the vast majority of cases.

Perioperative deaths occur because:

- the patient's disease is beyond cure
- the patient sustains a fatal myocardial infarction or cerebrovascular accident
- the patient exsanguinates or the blood loss precipitates a fatal myocardial infarction
- the patient aspirates
- the patient develops major complication(s)
- the patient develops serious sepsis
- the management departs from ideal clinical practice.

Undoubtedly, some postoperative deaths are avoidable and the surgical intervention itself is the primary cause in approximately 7% of postoperative deaths (**surgical failure**) because of:

- **inappropriate preoperative and postoperative management**
- **inappropriate operation: not needed or unlikely to benefit patient**

- inappropriate surgeon: inexperienced or without the specialist expertise
- inappropriate resource: available operating theatre, equipment, etc.

In practice, nearly all avoidable deaths arise when management departs from what is considered ideal practice. Often this relates to inadequate perioperative evaluation, preparation and selection. Lack of suitable prophylaxis, inadequate control of medical disorders such as diabetes, poor fluid and electrolyte management, and inadequate monitoring are also important, as is delay in the recognition of complications and timely intervention.

Section 18.2 • Types of complication

Complications following surgical interventions can be considered under various headings, e.g. technical, medical and system based. To some extent all of these are arbitrary as a major technical complication inevitably leads to a train of medical complications that in themselves may be life threatening. From a practical viewpoint, it is more useful to consider postoperative complications in two main categories:

- **immediate or early**: occurring during the postoperative period or during convalescence (Table 18.1)
- **late**: the consequence of the intervention in the long term (Table 18.2).

Table 18.1 Immediate postoperative complications

Respiratory	Collapse/consolidation, aspiration, etc. [Modules 13, 16 and 18]
Cardiovascular	[Modules 19 and 20]
Thromboembolic	[Modules 16 and 19]
Postoperative haemorrhage	[Modules 2 and 6]
Septic	[Modules 5 and 17]
Gastrointestinal	Intestinal obstruction, anastomotic leakage, intra-abdominal abscess formation, enterocutaneous fistulae, etc. [Modules 5 and 17]
Wound complications	Infections, dehiscence, etc. [Module 18]
Renal	Oliguria, acute renal failure [Modules 12 and 19]
Jaundice and hepatocellular insufficiency	[Modules 11 and 19]
Cerebral, psychological and neuropsychiatric complications	[Modules 18 and 20]
Drug-related morbidity	[Module 20]
Nerve injuries	[Module 16]

Table 18.2 Late postoperative complications

• Wound	Hypertrophic scar, keloid, wound sinus, implantation dermoid, incisional hernia
• Adhesions	Intestinal obstruction, strangulation
• Altered anatomy/ pathophysiology	Short gut syndrome, bacterial overgrowth, postgastric surgery syndromes, etc.
• Susceptibility to other disease	Malabsorption, incidence of cancer, tuberculosis and other disease

Many immediate postoperative complications are covered in other modules and these are indicated in Table 18.1. Whereas the vast majority of immediate complications is preventable, many late complications cannot be prevented as they generally represent the limitations of the procedure and are often the consequences of the traumatic surgical insult or the altered physiology or anatomy following the surgical intervention. Nonetheless, some of these late complications can be avoided or minimized by good long-term follow-up at the primary care level, e.g. administration of B_{12} injections after gastrectomy and ileal resections.

- **Technical complications** arise from surgical execution or procedural errors during the course of an operation such that:
  - **the surgical task quality is inadequate**, e.g. the anastomosis leaks, the resection is incomplete or not radical enough, or vessels are not secured adequately
  - **an important structure is damaged during the operation**, e.g. bile-duct injury, damage to major blood vessels or ureteric damage. These are referred to as iatrogenic injuries and are often the subject of litigation.
  A substantial percentage of iatrogenic injuries is not recognized during surgery and declare themselves with major complications postoperatively. This is particularly the case with injuries to the bile duct and ureters. A special situation arises in relation to laparoscopic surgery, where 60% of bowel injuries (usually caused by collateral damage during energized dissection) are not recognized during the operation. As many of these patients leave hospital within 24–48 h, delayed perforation with peritonitis may develop after discharge [**see Module 21, Vol. I**].
- **Septic complications** form the largest component of surgical morbidity. The most common septic complications are wound, chest and urinary infections. Major intra-abdominal septic complications arise as a result of technical complications, e.g. leaking anastomosis. This illustrates the close relationship between technical and septic complications. Multiorgan failure, usually arising on a background of sepsis, is often not recoverable [**see Module 19, Vol. I**].

■ **Drug-related morbidity** is an ever-increasing problem [see Module 20, Vol. I].

Section 18.3 • Cardiovascular complications

These cover a wide spectrum, such as haemorrhage [see Module 6, Vol. I], thromboembolic disease, myocardial infarction, arrhythmias and heart failure [see Module 20, Vol. I].

Deep vein thrombosis

Despite the well-established risk factors for deep vein thrombosis (DVT) and the efficacy of specific prophylaxis [see Module 16, Vol. I], it has been estimated that fewer than 50% of high-risk surgical patients receive any form of prophylaxis. This aspect of management is particularly prone to be overlooked in the emergency situation. The pathogenesis of DVT was first formulated by Virchow and involves:

■ **reduction of the venous flow from the lower limb** resulting from recumbency, immobility and loss of the muscle pump

■ **damage to the vascular intima** from compression trauma on the veins of the soleal plexus in the calf

■ **changes in the cellular and protein constituents of the blood**: thrombocytosis, increased platelet adhesiveness, margination of white cells and platelets, activation of the clotting cascade with fibrin production at a rate which overwhelms the anticoagulant/fibrinolytic system.

Two clinical groups are recognized: calf vein thrombosis and the more dangerous ileofemoral thrombosis, which is significantly more common on the left side. Calf vein thrombosis is notoriously difficult to diagnose clinically. Thus, many patients with classical symptoms (calf tenderness, mild pyrexia, some ankle oedema and warm leg) may not have the condition on investigation, and calf vein thrombosis is clinically silent in 40% of cases. **In any event, the clinical assessment must not include the performance of Homan's sign (calf pain on dorsiflexion of the foot) as this manoeuvre can dislodge the clot and precipitate pulmonary embolism.**

In contrast to calf vein thrombosis, ileofemoral thrombosis can usually be diagnosed clinically by diffuse pain, swelling and pitting oedema of the lower limb, which also appears blanched initially (phlegmasia alba dolens), but if the thrombosis extends to obstruct all the venous return, the affected limb assumes a bluish discoloration (phlegmasia caerulea dolens). If left untreated, this condition can progress to venous gangrene.

In practice, the diagnosis of DVT is made by investigation by Doppler ultrasound, duplex scanning or bilateral ascending venography (phlebography). ^{125}I-Fibrinogen scanning, although a useful research tool in clinical trials concerned with documenting efficacy of prophylactic regimens, gives so little anatomical information, aside from a 'hot spot' in the calf, as to be useless in the clinical setting, particularly as it cannot detect thrombi in the larger and pelvic veins. The diagnosis of venous obstruction by Doppler ultrasound velocimeter probe is based on the absence of the normal respiratory variation and flow augmentation on compression of the vein distal to the probe. Duplex imaging (combination of Doppler ultrasound velocimetry and B-mode ultrasound imaging) is a more reliable non-invasive test and is particularly useful in the diagnosis of proximal vein thrombosis. Bilateral ascending venography is considered the gold standard as it provides detailed information on the exact site and extent of the thrombus and its adherence or looseness, hence its propensity for embolization. However, it is expensive and invasive. In most centres, duplex scanning is replacing phlebography as the routine investigation for DVT.

Once the diagnosis of DVT is made, treatment is by full anticoagulation with heparin, which is then converted to oral anticoagulation [see Module 20, Vol. I], and this treatment is then continued for about 3 months. Special measures may be needed in patients with phlegmasia caerulea dolens and threatened venous gangrene. The choice is between venous thrombectomy or fibrinolytic therapy with streptokinase or recombinant tissue plasminogen activator [see Module 20, Vol. I].

The consequences of DVT may be:

■ pulmonary thromboembolism

■ complete resolution: recanalization without damage to the valves

■ chronic venous insufficiency: following phlebitic leg, either the vein does not recanalize or the valves are destroyed.

Pulmonary embolism

Pulmonary embolism accounts for 10% of all hospital deaths, many of which are diagnosed only at post mortem. It results from dislodgement and embolism of clots from the leg veins (usually iliofemoral, much less commonly calf vein) to the pulmonary trunk and main pulmonary arteries (central pulmonary embolism) or distal segmental arteries (peripheral pulmonary embolism). Central pulmonary embolism is characterized by sudden collapse with profound hypotension and engorged neck veins. In peripheral embolism, the patient is stable but demonstrates dyspnoea with tachypnoea and/or pleuritic chest pain, although the clinical signs and symptoms are non-specific and this accounts for the overall high misdiagnosis rate (30%). Most patients who develop pulmonary embolism have a major predisposing risk factor, e.g. major surgery or cardiorespiratory disease.

It has been recommended that hospitals should develop their own strategies for diagnosis and management of pulmonary embolism, but these should be formulated on (i) basic investigations for all patients, and (ii) the clinical state of the patient.

Basic investigations

These are undertaken in all patients and include an electrocardiogram (ECG), chest X-ray and arterial blood gases. Although the majority of patients with pulmonary embolism have reduced arterial oxygen tension and increased alveolar–arterial oxygen difference, these values may be normal in patients with clinical manifestations of acute pulmonary embolism. A normal plasma D-dimer measured by an enzyme-linked immunosorbent assay (ELISA) excludes all but 10% of patients with pulmonary embolism, especially if the level of clinical suspicion is low.

Stable patient

The appropriate investigation in the stable patients is a ventilation–perfusion isotope scan. The ventilation scan with krypton-81m or technetium-99m DTPA aerosol with more precise mulitview image is nowadays preferred to the unidimensional view obtained with xenon-133. Most agree that the perfusion part of the scan is the more important. The next investigation in the stable patient is a Doppler ultrasound scan of the leg veins to detect venous thrombosis. If the ultrasound scan is negative, some have argued for the need for pulmonary angiography, although this is debatable. These patients are treated by heparinization followed by oral anticoagulation. Full heparin treatment is started before the diagnosis is confirmed. Bed rest is unnecessary in patients with pulmonary embolism and DVT once therapeutic levels of anticoagulants have been achieved. A follow-up non-invasive study of the legs (e.g. impedance plethysmography, ultrasound, magnetic resonance imaging of the legs) is indicated in patients with a continuing predisposition to pulmonary embolism and DVT.

Unstable patient

In patients with cardiovascular collapse, the first recommended investigation is echocardiography, which can identify large central emboli or evidence of right ventricular hypokinesis and/or ventricular dilatation. Echocardiography may demonstrate another cause for the sudden cardiovascular collapse (ventricular septal rupture, aortic dissection, cardiac tamponade). However, the echocardiogram may show no dysfunction in patients with extensive pulmonary embolism. If the echocardiogram is normal or inconclusive, the next investigation is either spiral computed tomography or pulmonary angiography, depending on local availability and expertise. Spiral tomography is highly sensitive for proximal emboli down to the segmental arteries, and is increasingly preferred to pulmonary angiography since the risk of bleeding with thrombolytic therapy is reduced. Hypotension and continuing hypoxaemia despite high fractions of inspired oxygen (F_{I},O_2) are indications for intervention: intravenous thrombolytic

therapy (most extensively used), pulse spray thrombolytic therapy directly into embolus, open embolectomy, catheter-tip embolectomy or catheter-tip fragmentation (other options depending on local expertise). Intravenous thrombolysis (infusion of 100 mg alteplase over 2 h) is the recommended treatment of choice in patients with large central emboli causing cardiovascular collapse. A pulmonary angiogram is considered necessary by many before intravenous thrombolysis. The indications for a vena caval filter are:

- when anticoagulants are contraindicated
- when pulmonary embolism has recurred despite adequate anticoagulation
- severe pulmonary embolism.

Section 18.4 • Pulmonary complications

During the administration of general anaesthesia, there is an increase in the right-to-left shunting of the pulmonary blood flow and a depression of the ciliary activity of the bronchial mucosa. These changes are temporary and pulmonary function has usually returned to normal within 1 h of surgery and general anaesthesia. None the less, hypoxaemia is extremely common during the first two postoperative days. The hypoxaemia is the result of diaphragmatic elevation, which causes a reduction in functional residual capacity (FRC), and underventilation of the lung bases to which the greater proportion of the pulmonary blood flow is distributed. Elevation and tenting of the diaphragm is due to an increase in the intra-abdominal pressure, usually from gastrointestinal distension, and to pain, particularly from upper abdominal vertical incisions that induce reflex contraction of the abdominal musculature. The importance of pain in the aetiology of postoperative hypoxaemia is demonstrated by its virtual absence in patients with epidural blocks after major abdominal surgery. The raised intra-abdominal pressure after surgery is especially pronounced after reduction and repair of large ventral hernias and in the morbidly obese.

An increased bronchorrhoea is encountered in habitual smokers and in patients with chronic bronchitis. The impaired ciliary activity in these two groups further aggravates the bronchiolar and bronchial obstruction by viscid mucous plugs. The categories of patients at risk of respiratory complications are shown in Table 18.3. The important postoperative pulmonary complications are pulmonary collapse and consolidation, aspiration, pulmonary embolism and respiratory insufficiency.

Pulmonary collapse and consolidation

Although the terms atelectasis and collapse are often used synonymously, atelectasis refers to lung parenchyma that has never been expanded. The correct term for the postoperative condition is therefore pulmonary collapse. This arises from impaired ventilation of the

Table 18.3 Patients at risk of postoperative pulmonary complications

Condition	Mechanism
Obesity	Reduced functional residual capacity
Chronic obstructive airways disease	Secretional airway obstruction, diminished ciliary activity, pneumothorax, especially with emphysema and IPPV
Chronic smokers	Secretional airway obstruction, diminished ciliary activity
Restrictive airways disease	Diminished vital capacity
Elderly patients, subtotal oesophagectomy	Aspiration
Cystic fibrosis	Bronchial obstruction by secretions, pneumothorax
Operative damage to recurrent laryngeal nerve(s)	Ineffective cough, aspiration, respiratory obstruction if bilateral

IPPV, intermittent positive pressure ventilation.

lung bases and accumulation of bronchial secretions. It may be basal, patchy (segmental) or more extensive, i.e. lobar and even total lung collapse. The degree of hypoxaemia is related to the extent of the collapse.

Infection with consolidation often supervenes in the collapsed lobe or segment, the most common organisms responsible being *Haemophilus influenza* and *Streptococcus pneumoniae*, although coliform, pseudomonas and methicillin-resistant *Staphylococcus aureus* (MRSA) are common after abdominal operations. The clinical picture is extremely varied. On the one hand, the patient may experience little inconvenience. Others develop a mild pyrexia and a productive cough, and are rapidly improved with physiotherapy aimed at encouraging deep breathing and expectoration of the bronchial secretions. In the elderly, obese, chronic smokers and patients with pre-existing pulmonary disease, the condition is more severe, with tachypnoea, cyanosis, dullness to percussion over the affected region and bronchial breathing. These patients require antibiotic treatment with amoxycillin in the first instance until a culture report on a sputum sample is obtained. Oxygen is administered with a controlled O_2 therapy mask giving an inspired O_2 concentration of 30–40% with humidification and vigorous physiotherapy. If the chest radiograph shows extensive collapse, urgent fibre-optic bronchoscopy and clearing of the bronchial secretions by suction are necessary. However, some rely initially on nasally introduced endobronchial catheters for this purpose and proceed to bronchoscopy if this method in association with physiotherapy proves unsuccessful. Vigorous physiotherapy is maintained to prevent further collapse and the situation is monitored by daily posteroanterior chest radiographs. All patients with serious chest infections and lung collapse should be monitored by pulse oximetry and have repeated blood gas estimations, and the oxygen saturation should be kept above 90% and the arterial oxygen tension not be allowed to fall below 10 kPa (75 mmHg). If secretional airways obstruction persists, considerable improvement is obtained by the use of a minitracheostomy (Figure 18.1). This disposable device, which permits the insertion of fine suction catheters into the tracheal lumen through the cricothyroid membrane, is very effective in clearing bronchial secretions in patients unable to expectorate effectively despite adequate physiotherapy. In some patients, however, hypoxaemia and difficulty in breathing are not improved as the consolidation, pulmonary congestion and fluid progress. These patients require endotracheal intubation and assisted ventilation [**see Module 13 and 19, Vol. I**].

Other measures can be used in patients at risk of pulmonary complications. The first is the incentive spirometer (Figure 18.2), which greatly improves deep breathing and is of undoubted benefit if the patient is well motivated and uses it. Alternatively, others prefer the Entonox apparatus, which is premixed with 50% nitrous oxide in oxygen to achieve the same objective and administer additional analgesia. More recently, the use of the respiratory stimulant doxapram as an intravenous infusion (1.0–1.5 mg/kg) during the first 2 h of the postoperative period has been reported to improve arterial oxygen during the first two postoperative days. However, this drug is contraindicated in patients with ischaemic heart disease as it is a very powerful myocardial stimulant and may cause severe arrhythmias.

Pulmonary aspiration

Massive aspiration of the gastric contents in the bronchopulmonary tree is a serious complication that often proceeds to cardiorespiratory failure and continues to carry a high mortality. Minor degrees of pulmonary aspiration are common and manifest themselves clinically as postoperative pneumonia and pulmonary abscess. The presence of a cuffed endotracheal tube is not a complete safeguard against minor degrees of aspiration, which is also well documented in patients with a tracheostomy. In this respect, large-volume, low-pressure cuff tubes are said to be more protective than the standard variety, although recent evidence casts doubt on this assumption. Prophylactic nasogastric intubation after elective abdominal surgery increases the risk of aspiration.

Massive aspiration occurs either during induction and endotracheal intubation or during recovery from general anaesthesia, particularly in the elderly and

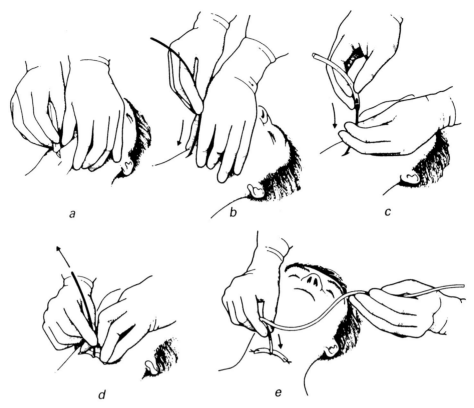

Figure 18.1 Minitracheostomy: (a) small stab incision in skin and cricothyroid membrane; (b) insertion of plastic curved introducer; (c) insertion of PVC tracheostomy tube over introducer; (d) removal of introducer; (e) insertion of endobronchial suction catheter through minitracheostomy.

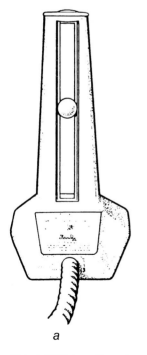

DIAL SETTING

1800	1800	3600	5400	7200	9000	10,800	12,600	14,400	16,200	18,000
1440	1440	2880	4320	5760	7200	8640	10,080	11,520	12,960	14,400
1095	1095	2190	3285	4380	5475	6570	7665	8760	9855	10,950
765	765	1530	2295	3060	3825	4590	5355	6120	6885	7650
505	505	1010	1515	2020	2525	3030	3535	4040	4545	5050
285	285	570	855	1140	1425	1710	1995	2280	2565	2850
145	145	290	435	580	725	870	1015	1160	1305	1450

| | 1 | 2 | 3 | 4 | 5 | 6 | 7 | 8 | 9 | 10 |

SECONDS PATIENT HOLDS BALL AT THE TOP
Figures represent minimum volume in cubic centimetres.

a   *b*

Figure 18.2 Incentive spirometer. (a) The calibrated dial indicates the minimum flow (ml/s) at the various dial settings that are required to be generated by the patient's inspiratory effort to raise the ball to the top of the flow chamber; (b) the chart shows the minimum volume obtained for efforts up to 10 s at various settings.

(a)

(b)

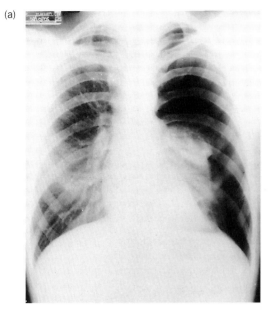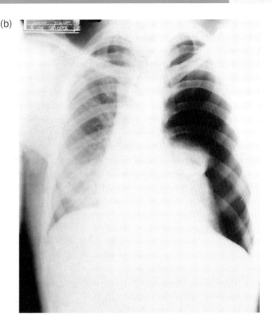

Figure 18.3 Pneumothorax. (a) Large left pneumothorax with (b) mediastinal shift during expiration.

enfeebled. Later on during the postoperative period, the condition may complicate acute gastric dilatation and paralytic ileus. In the emergency situation, a full stomach is a well-recognized hazard and underlies the importance of aspiration of the stomach contents prior to induction of general anaesthesia.

Massive aspiration of gastric contents induces severe bronchospasm and a chemical pneumonitis that is associated with significant fluid shifts from the circulating blood to the pulmonary parenchyma, and circulatory collapse. In addition, the patient becomes markedly cyanosed and tachypnoeic. Moist rales and diminished air entry, particularly over the lung bases, are found on auscultation. The condition often progresses to adult respiratory distress syndrome (ARDS) with myocardial failure requiring ventilatory and inotropic support [**see Modules 13 and 19, Vol. I**]. The treatment entails vigorous suction toilet of the bronchial tree, administration of pure oxygen by intermittent positive pressure ventilation, bronchodilators, methyl-prednisolone and antibiotics.

Other pulmonary complications

These include pneumothorax and pleural effusion. The most common cause of pneumothorax in the postoperative period is insertion of a central venous or feeding line. A chest radiograph is necessary after this procedure to exclude this potential complication (Figure 18.3). There is also an enhanced risk of pneumothorax in patients on positive pressure ventilation, presumably from rupture of pre-existing bullae. Pneumothorax can also complicate laparoscopic antireflux surgery, particularly in patients with an associated large hiatal hernia. It is also encountered in some patients after thoracoscopic sympathectomy and

pulmonary surgery. The insertion of an underwater seal drain is usually followed by rapid expansion of the lung. Negative suction may be applied to the system if the expansion of the lung is delayed or becomes static after initial improvement.

Pleural effusions (Figure 18.4) may be secondary to other pulmonary pathology such as collapse and consolidation, pulmonary infarction and secondary deposits. They may also result from congestive failure or from subdiaphragmatic collections of pus. Pleural effusions may also accompany severe pancreatitis.

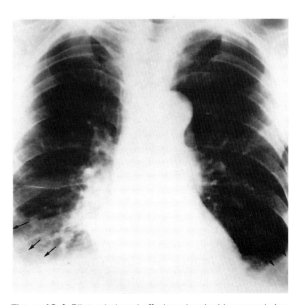

Figure 18.4 Bilateral pleural effusions (marked by arrows) due to cardiac failure. They have a crescentic upper margin and no air–fluid level.

Uncomplicated pleural effusions do not exhibit an air–fluid level. This is encountered in three situations:

- following aspiration when air is introduced in the pleural cavity: artefactual
- bronchial fistula or leak
- oesophageal perforation, rupture or leakage from intrathoracic anastomosis.

Thus, a pleural effusion following an oesophageal resection indicates leakage from the anastomosis and precedes the development of frank empyema. As air, in addition to fluid, leaks into the pleural cavity from the oesophageal lumen, the chest radiograph shows the pathognomonic fluid level (Figure 18.5).

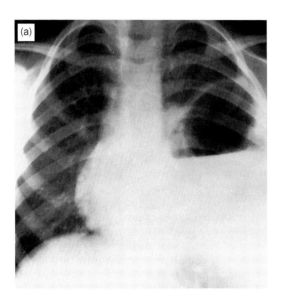

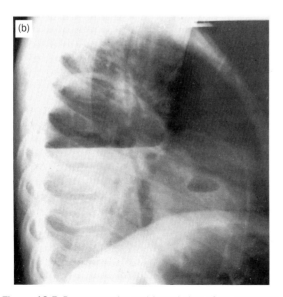

Figure 18.5 Posteroanterior and lateral view of an empyema with air–fluid level on the left side following spontaneous rupture of the lower oesophagus (Boerhaave syndrome).

Section 18.5 • Wound complications

It has been said that the average general surgeon operates on the abdominal wall much more often than on any other region, and yet pays the least attention to this aspect of operative practice. Wound complications are thus common and include infection, dehiscence, haematoma, incisional hernia and ossification.

Postoperative wound infections

These constitute the most common postoperative complication overall. The reported incidence varies widely and is influenced by:

- the nature of the operation
- the definition of wound infection used
- the postoperative time scale used to report wound infections.

Overall, the incidence of wound infection diagnosed when the patient is in hospital averages 5%. The nature of the operation is an important factor and the lowest incidence is encountered after clean procedures [see Modules 2 and 3, Vol. I]. The incidence after the various operation categories is, however, influenced by the definition used. In the past, wound infection was defined as a '**collection of pus, which empties itself spontaneously or after incision**'. This definition is nowadays considered too restrictive and wound infection is said to be present if:

- the wound becomes red and swollen
- the wound requires opening, even partially
- the wound exudes serous fluid or pus
- antibiotics are prescribed because of concern over the wound.

A positive culture is not considered essential for the diagnosis of wound infection. The most accurate method of assessing postoperative wound infection is the ASEPSIS score devised by Wilson *et al*. This involves awarding each wound a score of 0–5 for erythema and serous exudate and a score of 0–10 for purulent exudate and deep tissue separation. In addition, penalty points are awarded for antibiotic treatment, drainage of pus under local anaesthesia, wound debridement, positive culture and an in-hospital stay > 14 days. The ASEPSIS score is used widely in clinical trials but is not practicable for routine purposes.

As mentioned previously, the time course for the development and detection of wound infection determines the rate observed. Nowadays, a period of 4–6 weeks after surgery is considered essential for documenting the true incidence of wound infection. This is at least double the rate of wound infections diagnosed during the patient's hospital stay as at least 50% of wound infections declare themselves after discharge from hospital.

From a clinical standpoint, wound infections exhibit a wide spectrum of severity and may present as:

- cellulitis
- localized abscess around a suture
- non-clostridial cutaneous and subcutaneous gangrene [Module 5, Vol. I]
- clostridial infections, non-gas forming and gas-forming [Module 5, Vol. I].

Wound infections are best prevented by meticulous surgical technique that avoids contamination, gentle handling of tissues, accurate haemostasis and selective use of prophylactic antibiotics. The treatment of established wound infections depends on the nature and severity of the infections. Usually, opening of the wound (in part or whole) with healing by granulation tissue suffices. Life-threatening infections require systemic antibiotics (with advice from a bacteriologist) and an aggressive approach that involves debridement and excision to non-infected regions [see Module 5, Vol. I]. The consequences of wound infection include an ugly pitted scar and incisional hernia formation.

Wound dehiscence

The reported incidence of this complication varies from 0.2 to 3% of abdominal wounds. It is more frequent after emergency surgical procedures than elective interventions. Furthermore, it affects male patients much more frequently than females; the male:female ratio is 4–5:1. The abdominal wall dehiscence may be partial or complete but, by definition, it is normally considered to involve the deeper layers of the wound rather than the skin and subcutaneous tissues. The following patterns of clinical presentation are recognized.

- The patient has an unexpected stormy postoperative period with cardiopulmonary symptoms and a prolonged ileus.
- There is a serosanguinous discharge from the wound after 2 or 3 days.
- There is failure to develop the 'inflammatory' healing ridge over the first 10 postoperative days.
- There is sudden disruption of the wound on removal of the skin sutures with herniation of a knuckle of intestine through the wound.
- There is obvious weakness and bulging on straining in the convalescent period (subclinical incisional hernia).

In essence, wound dehiscence results from increased intra-abdominal pressure and poor healing, although poor closure technique and the use of inappropriate suture material, e.g. catgut, are responsible for some cases. While it is not crucial to close the peritoneal layer of an abdominal wound, and indeed this may be beneficial in reducing adhesion formation, closure of the musculoaponeurotic layer is essential. Nowadays, the preferred technique for this is by mass closure with a continuous strong (1/0) monofilament biodegradable material that has a prolonged tensile strength, or non-absorbable suture. For mechanical reasons, wound dehiscence is more common after longitudinal than transverse incisions. The factors associated with increased intra-abdominal pressure include:

- prolonged postoperative ileus or adhesive obstruction
- repeated retching and vomiting
- persistent hiccup and coughing paroxysms
- ascites.

Wound healing may be impaired for various reasons and several of these are often present in the individual patient [see Module 1, Vol. I]. In the context of wound dehiscence, the important ones are:

- hypotension during surgery
- wound infections
- presence of drains
- obesity
- uraemia
- cachexia
- diabetes
- chronic liver disease
- old age
- drugs: cytotoxic agents and corticosteroids.

The management of wound dehiscence demands urgent action with resuture of the wound as soon as the patient's condition permits. One of two techniques may be used:

- closure with interrupted deep tension sutures
- mass continuous closure taking large bites of the musculoapneurotic layers except the skin: this is favoured in the presence of wound infection.

Patients with a poor healing ridge may be managed by accepting the situation and delaying removal of the sutures for several weeks. The almost certain development of an incisional hernia may be a better option than taking a risk on full disruption in a compromised patient.

Wound haematoma

Most wound haematomas result from accidental damage during closure of vessels within the rectus compartment. If a large vessel is injured, e.g. superior epigastric, musculophrenic or inferior epigastric, the haematoma may be extensive and require evacuation. Otherwise, wound haematomas are self-limiting but may become infected, when they present as deep musculoaponeurotic abscesses. When detected early, needle aspiration may allow resolution. Chronic haematomas and other degenerated tissue within a wound may undergo dystrophic calcification.

Late complications: incisional hernia and ossification

Incisional hernia is the outcome of a poor healing ridge. It occurs predominantly in patients who sustain a postoperative wound infection and in the obese [see

Abdominal wall and herniae, Vol. II]. Rarely, ossification of the wound may occur, probably as a result of active wound fibroblasts that assume osteoblastic function. Ossification is usually encountered in upper midline abdominal wounds. The patient complains of hardness rather than pain. On examination because of the 'infiltrative hardness', the possibility of metastatic disease in patients who have had cancer surgery has to be excluded by a plain radiograph of the abdominal wall.

Section 18.6 • Cerebral, psychological and neuropsychiatric complications

Psychological

There is an insufficient appreciation of the extent and severity of psychological morbidity suffered by patients undergoing surgery and general anaesthesia. Anxiety is inevitable in all patients. This must be allayed by adequate explanation and provision of emotional support rather than prescription of tranquillizers, which are rarely needed.

Major psychological morbidity is incurred following the loss of a body part (altered body image and function), e.g. mastectomy and amputation. These patients need expert professional counselling and support from charitable support groups.

The **post-traumatic stress disorder** (PTSD), previously known as the ICU syndrome or silent psychosis, is characterized by vivid recurring nightmares and flashbacks of the experience or incident. It occurs in patients requiring intensive-care support and has been documented in 10% of patients surviving multiple injuries from road traffic accidents. The disorder is thought to result from sleep deprivation, pain, prolonged drug administration, anxiety and fear. The patient's perception and memory are impaired, with inability to think and to sustain a conversation. Restlessness and apathy are other features. Confusion and delirium may be present in severe cases. Full recovery is the norm, but this may take several weeks to months.

Neuropsychiatric disturbances

These are frequent and cover a wide spectrum of disorders. The most common is mental confusion with agitation and disorientation in the elderly. This may arise against a background of senile dementia but is often precipitated or worsened by the injudicious administration of sedative and hypnotic drugs. A metabolic cause should be excluded in all cases, irrespective of age. Mental confusion, altered sleep rhythm and increasing somnolence may be the result of hepatic encephalopathy in patients with chronic liver disease.

Anxiety and depression are frequent in patients recovering from complicated surgery requiring prolonged hospital stay, and particularly in young to middle-aged patients recovering from surgery for cancer.

Depression and fear of death in these cancer patients can often be changed to hopeful optimism and a positive attitude to life by firm psychological support, the right body language and explanation, with the emphasis on what needs to be done. The feeling of helplessness in these patients is only overcome with the realization that the surgeon and the rest of the oncological team are in control of the disease.

In the postoperative phase three types of acute confusional state or delirium may be encountered: emergence delirium, interval delirium and delirium tremens.

Emergence delirium

This acute confusional state is encountered soon after recovery from anaesthesia and is due to the anticholinergic drugs used in the anaesthetic medication. It is usually short lived and may afflict any age group. If anything, it is more common in the young than in the elderly [**see Module 20, Vol. I**].

Interval delirium

As the name implies, this acute confusional state develops after an interval of 1–7 days following the operation. It is the most common type of delirium encountered in the postoperative period and its incidence rises steadily with age, reaching 10–15% in patients over 65 years old. Interval delirium is usually precipitated by an underlying complication such as infection, especially respiratory (accounting for 30%), cardiac failure (20%), other causes of hypoxia, e.g. sedation, inadequate pain control and fluid/electrolyte imbalance. Correction of the underlying disease or abnormality usually reverses the acute confusional state within a few days but expert psychiatric advice may be needed. Important prophylactic measures include avoidance of sedation and prevention of chest infections by physiotherapy and incentive spirometry.

Delirium tremens: acute alcohol withdrawal syndrome

This can be predicted in most instances from a detailed medical and drinking history. Prodromal symptoms include anxiety and tremors. The fully developed condition is characterized by extreme agitation and overactivity, visual hallucinations, total confusion, pyrexia and, less commonly, convulsions. It leads to rapid dehydration and often to abdominal wound dehiscence. Chlormethiazole 0.8% (heminevrin) is administered as an intravenous infusion of 30–50 ml. The solution is run at 60 drops/min (4 ml/min) until the patient becomes drowsy. Thereafter, the drip rate is decreased to 10–15 drops/min and frequent checks on the level of consciousness are maintained. Oral therapy with chlormethiazole capsules is commenced as soon as possible. Chlormethiazole is contraindicated in acute pulmonary insufficiency. Adequate rehydration and the correction of metabolic alkalosis are important features of the management of these patients. Prevention of delirium tremens in susceptible patients can be achieved by the administration of intravenous alcohol (5% ethanol in 5% dextrose, 150 ml/h) to maintain the blood alcohol level at 2–10 mg/100 ml.

Cerebrovascular accidents

These are often precipitated by sudden hypotension during or after surgery in elderly hypertensive patients with severe atherosclerosis. Postoperative strokes are also a well-documented hazard after carotid endarterectomy and occur in 1–3% of these operations. They may arise from emboli released at or after surgery, ischaemia during the period of carotid clamping and postoperative thrombosis of the internal carotid artery. Cerebrovascular accidents may also complicate open cardiac surgery, although this is less common nowadays as a result of the increased safety and efficiency of modern extracorporeal perfusion systems.

Section 18.7 • Mortality and morbidity of day-case surgery

Day-case surgery (DCS) is unquestionably safe, with a reported mortality of 4:257 000 (0.00002%) from myocardial infarction, pulmonary embolus, respiratory failure and stroke. It does, however, carry a recognizable minor morbidity rate at 24 h after surgery. According to a recent survey in the UK, morbidity in patients undergoing DCS lasts more than 24 h in 42%, 2 days in 28% and 3 days in 14% of patients.

The common complications in order of frequency encountered in these patients are:

- sore throat 28%
- pain 27%
- headache 12%
- drowsiness 11%
- dizziness 10%
- postoperative nausea and vomiting (PONV) 7%
- fever 5%
- venous irritation 2%.

Guide to further reading

Buck, N., Devlin, H. B. and Lunn, J. N. *The Report of a Confidential Enquiry into Perioperative Deaths*. The Nuffield Provincial Hospital Trust, The King's Fund.

ACCP Consensus Committee on Pulmonary Embolism (1996). Opinions regarding the diagnosis and management of venous thromboembolic disease. *Chest* **109**: 233–237.

Polk, H. C. Jr, Simpson, C. J., Simmons, B. P. and Alexander, J. W. (1983). Guidelines for prevention of surgical wound infection. *Arch Surg* **118**: 1213–1217.

Royal College of Surgeons of England and the Royal College of Psychiatrists (1997). *Report of the Working Party on the Psychological Care of Surgical Patients*.

Wilson, A. P. R., Treasure, T., Sturridge, M. F. and Gruneberg, R. N. (1986). A scoring method (ASEPSIS) for postoperative wound infections. *Lancet* **i**: 311–313.

Management of critically ill patients

1 • Sudden loss of consciousness with cardiopulmonary arrest

2 • Pathophysiology of shock

3 • Intensive care management

'Delays have dangerous ends' – William Shakespeare, Henry VI, Part I, Act 3, 1592

Section 19.1 • Sudden loss of consciousness with cardiopulmonary arrest

Sudden loss of consciousness with cardiovascular collapse can occur under varied circumstances and thus the correct approach entails immediate resuscitation that is tailored to the individual case. In the first place, an 'arrest call' does not necessarily mean that the patient has had a cardiac arrest, although this is the most common cause. In essence, sudden unconsciousness can result from:

- **true cardiac arrest: no carotid pulse**
  - ischaemia-induced arrhythmia or heart block
  - pulmonary embolism
  - cardiac tamponade
  - vasovagal faint
  - cardiac rupture
  - intramyocardial (tumour) rupture
- **respiratory arrest alone: carotid pulse initially present**
  - upper airway obstruction from any cause
  - tension pneumothorax
  - loss of respiratory drive, narcotic depression, etc.
- **causes other than cardiac or respiratory arrest: both carotid pulse and respiration initially present**
  - cerebrovascular accident
  - hypoglycaemia
  - drug overdose
  - trauma: head injury
  - rupture of intracranial aneurysm.

Cardiac arrest

This is diagnosed if no carotid pulse is palpable and there is no spontaneous respiration. The most common cause is ischaemia-induced cardiac arrest but it must be remembered that the cause could vary from a massive pulmonary embolism to a simple vasovagal faint.

Management: cardiopulmonary resuscitation

Airway and breathing

The patient is positioned flat. The head is extended, the mouth opened and the jaw pulled forwards for quick inspection of the upper airway, especially for foreign bodies. Artificial ventilation is commenced after insertion of airway with a high-flow oxygen mask and a respirator bag. This is a temporary expedient until trained personnel arrive (anaesthetist), when the patient is intubated and ventilated with 100% oxygen. Adequate ventilation is checked by auscultation of both lungs and to exclude an unsuspected pneumothorax.

Circulation

External cardiac massage is commenced at the approximate rate of five compressions to each lung inflation for a two-person resuscitation or 15 cardiac compressions to two lung inflation for a one-person resuscitation team. The efficacy of chest compression in producing a cardiac output must be checked by finding a palpable carotid or femoral pulse.

Electrocardiography and intravenous access

An electrocardiogram (ECG) is necessary to determine the abnormal rhythm: ventricular fibrillation (VF) or tachycardia, asystole and electromechanical dissociation. It is undertaken once effective chest compression and artificial ventilation have been established. If an ECG cannot be obtained immediately, a precordial thump followed by a single 'blind' direct current (d.c.) shock (160 J) is advocated. The blind d.c. shock is given in case the cardiac arrest is due to VF, since this becomes increasingly difficult to reverse with time.

An intravenous access is needed, preferably in a central vein (jugular, subclavian), for drug administration. Intravenous sodium bicarbonate (8.4%) is given in a dose of 50–100 ml for every 10 min of cardiac arrest, although ideally the amount should be monitored by measurement of arterial blood gases, pH and base deficit.

The specific treatment of VF is:

1. immediate d.c. conversion (220 J), followed by
2. 15 chest compressions, followed by a further 200 J shock
3. a further 15 chest compressions followed by a 360 J shock
4. intravenous adrenaline (10 ml of 1:10 000 sol or 1.0 ml of 1:1000 sol)
5. continuation of chest compression and attempt at further cardioversion (360 J).

Bretylium 400 mg i.v. may be used if VF remains refractory to the above, in which case cardiopulmonary resuscitation (CPR) should be continued for 20–30 min after its administration because of its slow onset of action. Repeated cardioversion may be harmful to the heart, but there is little to lose in refractory VF. If cardioversion is successful, attention is then focused on correction of any predisposing factors, e.g. electrolyte imbalance, acidosis or hypoxaemia. A lignocaine infusion (1–4 mg/min) is indicated if there are frequent ventricular ectopics or runs of ventricular tachycardia (VT).

VT produces a range of clinical responses depending on various factors. At one extreme, the patient is conscious and has an adequate cardiac output; at the other, the patient is unconscious as in the patient with VF. Whereas urgent CPR is needed in the latter situation, the conscious patient with VT requires treatment and monitoring but no precipitate action.

The management of VT is similar to that of VF, except that adrenaline should not be used. In a haemodynamically compromised patient, d.c. conversion is undertaken, after administration of a short-acting anaesthetic. The d.c. conversion is repeated several times before and after lignocaine 100 mg i.v.

In patients with VT and an adequate cardiac output, lignocaine 100 mg i.v. is tried before d.c. cardioversion. If lignocaine and d.c. cardioversion fail to restore a normal rhythm, then other drugs may be tried, e.g. bretylium, disopyramide (50–150 μg i.v.) or amiodarone (5 mg/kg i.v.).

The initial therapy for asystole is:

1. adrenaline 1.0 mg i.v., followed by
2. atropine 2.0 mg i.v.
3. repeating adrenaline and atropine, followed by
4. isoprenaline 1.0–2.0 mg i.v.
5. temporary pacing catheter if the above measures fail.

In electromechanical dissociation, there is a poor cardiac output and low blood pressure despite normal electrical activity on the ECG. It is usually caused by:

- **drug therapy**
- **severe mechanical problems**: tension pneumothorax, pulmonary embolism, cardiac tamponade, myocardial rupture or intramyocardial obstruction by tumour.

The management is directed towards reversing any identifiable cause and administration of adrenaline 1.0 mg i.v. In terms of reversible causes, the only two that can be corrected in the short time available are tension pneumothorax and cardiac tamponade. Thus, these two causes are particularly important to keep in mind.

Use of calcium in cardiopulmonary resuscitation
For many years, calcium was administered with adrenaline in all cardiac arrests. This practice has changed to selective use of this agent. Intravenous calcium chloride (5–10 ml of 10% sol.) is indicated only in the following circumstances:

- in the presence of hyperkalaemia
- for cardiac arrest after a recent blood transfusion
- when the patient had been on high doses of calcium antagonists
- as a last resort.

Post-cardiopulmonary resuscitation management
In general, CPR should be continued for around 30 min, although a decision to abandon further attempts is best taken by a senior doctor who knows the clinical details of the patient. If resuscitation is successful, it is crucial to review possible reversible causes to prevent repetition of the arrest. Blood is taken for full blood count, glucose, electrolytes, arterial pH and gases. A full 12-lead ECG is obtained to exclude myocardial infarction, arrhythmia, heart block or pulmonary embolism. A chest X-ray is needed to exclude pneumothorax, aspiration, tamponade and aortic dissection and to check for the position of the endotracheal tube and any fractures sustained during the CPR.

Section 19.2 • Pathophysiology of shock

The ability to recognize the features of circulatory shock and a basic understanding of the pathophysiology underlying the shock process are crucial in the management of surgical patients, both elective and emergency. In the management of trauma patients, a failure to recognize the presence or extent of blood loss has been identified as an important contributory factor leading to a considerable number of preventable deaths. In established low-output shock, the clinical features are clear-cut and easily recognized, particularly in shock of acute onset:

- hypotension
- tachypnoea
- pallor
- sweating
- cold extremities
- mental confusion
- oliguria.

However, as described below, problems with diagnosis can arise in certain situations, e.g. trauma, sepsis and shock of slow onset. It is important to realize that patients may be in a state of circulatory shock despite a normal heart rate and blood pressure. Furthermore, in sepsis, patients can be significantly shocked in the presence of a cardiac output four or five times normal. Guidelines on the early and accurate diagnosis of shock are given below, under the appropriate headings, for the various broad categories of shock.

Definition and classification of shock

Since the clinical features observed in a patient suffering from shock are extremely variable, it is impossible to define shock in these terms. Regardless of the underlying cause, the shock state is characterized by inadequate cellular perfusion leading to cellular damage and subsequent dysfunction or failure of major organ systems. Shock can be defined as **'a state of inadequate cellular perfusion'**.

Perfusion, in the above definition, describes not only blood flow but also the supply of substrates (including oxygen) and removal of waste products from the cells. The inclusion of the term **inadequate** is also fundamental to the definition, since blood flow and substrate supply may be grossly elevated in hypercatabolic states, such as trauma and sepsis, and yet be inadequate for the metabolic demands of the tissues. Many descriptive clinicopathological terms are used when discussing shock, e.g. haemorrhagic shock, hypovolaemic shock, traumatic shock, burn shock and neurogenic shock. Although some of these terms are in everyday usage they do not help in understanding the basic underlying haemodynamic abnormalities in shock. An understanding of the shock process can be aided by the use of a simple classification of shock (Figure 19.1) and a knowledge of basic pathophysiology (Figure 19.2).

From Figure 19.1 it can be seen that all patients with shock can be considered to have an inadequate cardiac output; not always low, but always inadequate for the metabolic needs of the tissues. There are then only two causes for the inadequacy of cardiac output:

- primary pump failure (including cardiogenic shock and obstructive shock)
- peripheral circulatory failure, due to either loss of circulating volume (true hypovolaemia) or vasodilatation, with an increase in the capacitance of the vascular system (apparent hypovolaemia).

The major categories of shock within these broad groupings are cardiogenic, hypovolaemic and septic, and each of these will be discussed separately. Figure 19.2 shows the basic pathophysiology underlying shock. It represents a gross oversimplification and includes some important omissions, including the fact that following hypovolaemia fluid shifts occur from the interstitial fluid space to the intravascular space as an additional compensatory mechanism. Nevertheless, it illustrates three important points. First, the pathophysiology of shock can be thought of as consisting of several vicious cycles. It illustrates how, in the absence of early and complete resuscitation, shock can be a self-perpetuating process leading to cellular injury, organ dysfunction and death of the organism. Secondly, the diagram depicts several compensatory mechanisms, notably vasoconstriction. These compensatory mechanisms are a normal physiological response to low-output shock and are essential for survival, helping to maintain blood flow and perfusion pressure to vital organs. However, it is these very compensatory mechanisms that initiate the changes that ultimately lead to organ damage.

Vasoconstriction affects different vascular beds to varying degrees and some organs, notably those in the splanchnic circulation, take the brunt of the ischaemic hypoxic injury that can result from regional hypoperfusion. Thirdly, the diagram illustrates how simple haemorrhage (a form of **hypovolaemic** shock) can be complicated by both **cardiogenic** and **septic** factors. For instance, tachycardia occurring as a response to hypovolaemia will lead to an increase in myocardial oxygen demand at a time when coronary blood flow, and thus myocardial oxygen supply, is decreased. This can lead to myocardial impairment, particularly in

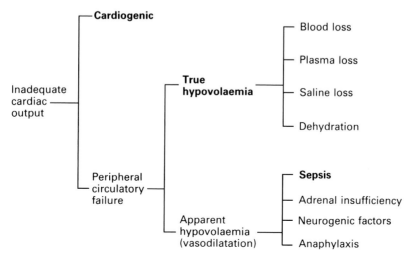

Figure 19.1 Classification of the mechanisms underlying the shock process (those in bold type are discussed in the text).

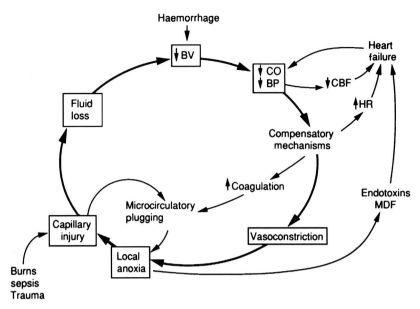

Figure 19.2 Basic pathophysiology: vicious cycles in shock. BV, blood volume; CO, cardiac output; BP, blood pressure; CBF, coronary blood flow; HR, heart rate; MDF, myocardial depressant factors.

patients with coexistent ischaemic heart disease. Splanchnic vasoconstriction occurring in response to hypovolaemia can lead to the release of endotoxin or inflammatory mediators from the gastrointestinal tract and the liberation of myocardial depressant factors from ischaemic splanchnic organs, resulting in severe hypovolaemia and the overlay of features resulting from sepsis syndrome, as well as potentiating the possibility of myocardial impairment. Likewise, sepsis, which is normally characterized by a high cardiac output, can be complicated by hypovolaemia resulting from fluid loss secondary to capillary permeability changes. Thus, in some instances, hypovolaemic and cardiogenic factors can coexist with sepsis in the same patient. This should be borne in mind when reading about descriptions of individual categories of shock. Hypovolaemic shock, cardiogenic shock and sepsis will now be discussed separately. The majority of the details on the monitoring and treatment of shock, most of which are relevant to all three categories, are given in the Hypovolaemic shock section. Discussion in the cardiogenic shock and sepsis sections will concentrate only on details of pathophysiological monitoring and treatment specific for that particular category.

Hypovolaemic shock

Aetiology
Haemorrhage is a common cause of hypovolaemia. Its effects vary with the duration and severity of blood loss, the patient's age and myocardial condition, and with the speed and adequacy of resuscitation. In previously healthy young adults it has been shown that the acute loss of 10% of the total blood volume reduces arterial pressure by 7% and cardiac output by 21%; the acute loss of 20% of the blood volume reduces arterial

pressure by 15% and cardiac output by 41%. In contrast, the gradual loss of 10% of the blood volume frequently results in no change in arterial pressure or heart rate, although cardiac output still falls. The response of an individual to blood loss is remarkably variable. While the above figures give some guidelines, it is certainly possible to lose as much as 25% of circulating volume with no change in arterial blood pressure, particularly in young patients who are capable of mounting intense vasoconstriction in response to volume loss. In contrast, pre-existing ischaemic heart disease or anaemia can also be expected to alter the pattern of response, increasing the risk of a critical reduction in tissue oxygen supply. In an accident victim, the additional insult of **trauma** alters the neuroendocrine and metabolic response. Patients with acute upper gastrointestinal haemorrhage, for example, may exhibit quite different physical signs from patients suffering from trauma, even when the degree of haemorrhage is similar. It has been noted that in trauma patients with mild to moderate volume loss, cardiac output may even be slightly increased initially, and at the time of presentation trauma patients may be hypertensive, normotensive or hypotensive. The heart rate response can also be variable and again trauma patients may exhibit either a tachycardia or a bradycardia at the time of presentation. The reasons for the variability in clinical signs after trauma are currently only partly understood. Certainly, the neuroendocrine response to tissue damage is largely responsible. Trauma victims tend to comprise a younger population than do groups of patients suffering from other causes of haemorrhage. There is no doubt that these varying haemodynamic responses to trauma contribute to deficiencies in trauma care; it is now well recognized that in deaths from trauma that are deemed preventable, an important factor in many cases is a failure to recognize the presence and/or extent of blood loss.

The reduction in blood volume following **thermal injury** results from loss of plasma at the site of burn, and the rate and volume of plasma deficit are roughly proportional to the extent of the area burned. A generalized increase in capillary permeability also occurs and subsequent sequestration of intravascular fluid into the interstitial space occurs. Together, these factors lead to tissue oedema and an increase in haematocrit, with the packed cell volume often reaching 70–80% in situations where fluid replacement is inadequate [see Module 4, Vol. I].

Hypovolaemia may also be due to **dehydration** from either a primary deficit of water or a primary deficit of saline (salt and water). A primary water deficit generally results from reduced intake rather than from increased loss. The most common cause in clinical practice is inability of the patient to acquire an adequate volume of fluid either because of exhaustion or disturbance of consciousness (as in the case of intrinsic brain pathology or the effects of drugs such as sedatives), or because drinking is forbidden (as may be the case following upper gastrointestinal surgery). Increased water loss may result from diabetes insipidus. In contrast, a primary deficit of salt generally arises from increased loss rather than reduced intake. The deficiency may be of salt alone if the patient loses both salt and water and replaces the water by drinking, as may happen in diarrhoea, copious sweating or Addison's disease. A deficiency of both salt and water occurs most commonly when fluid is lost from the gastrointestinal tract as, for instance, in intestinal obstruction, severe diarrhoea and high intestinal fistulae.

The principal features of water and salt depletion are contrasted in Table 19.1. A primary deficit of water leads to cellular dehydration as a result of the increase in tonicity of the extracellular fluid and the metabolic response to stress; thus, circulatory failure from a shrinking blood volume is a late manifestation of this syndrome. By contrast, a primary deficit of salt leads to a reduction in the volume of both interstitial and intravascular fluid, but not to cellular dehydration. This is because sodium is the main positive ion in both extracellular fluid spaces, while potassium is the main positive ion in intracellular fluid.

In a typical patient undergoing elective surgery it can be seen, from the above, that there are many reasons for hypovolaemia to occur. Mechanical bowel preparation is commonly employed prior to colonic surgery. Because of the purgative action of most bowel preparation regimens this results in increased saline loss from the gastrointestinal tract. This is then followed by an overnight fast, which may continue until the afternoon portion of a theatre list, leading to water depletion and dehydration. In theatre, it is standard practice to measure blood loss during surgery, but there are additional insensible losses that may be easily underestimated. Insensible water loss from respiration can be increased by artificial ventilation and in excess of 500 ml of water may be lost by evaporation during a 1 h laparotomy, as a result of the large surface area

Table 19.1 Contrasting features of water depletion and salt depletion

	Water depletion	Salt depletion
Cause	Deficient intake	Excessive loss (especially loss of intestinal secretions)
Dehydration	Cellular	Extracellular
Thirst	+++	Absent
Urine volume	Scanty	Normal (even increased until late)
Lassitude	+	+++
Weakness	Late	Early
Vomiting	Absent	Maybe +++
Plasma volume	Normal until late	Reduced +++
Haemoconcentration	Late and slight	Early and severe
Arterial pressure	Normal until late	Decreased +++
Blood urea	Increased +	Increased +++
Blood sodium	Slight increase	Reduced ++
Blood chloride	Slight increase	Reduced +++
Urine sodium	Reduced + + +	Reduced +++
Urine chloride	Reduced	Absent
Cause of death	Uncertain (increase in intracellular osmotic pressure?)	Peripheral circulatory failure

exposed to the atmosphere. Thus, the typical surgical patient requires replacement of both water (5% dextrose) and salt (saline) in addition to replacement of operative blood loss with colloid and/or red blood cells. These factors make it all too easy to underestimate fluid requirements in surgical patients, potentially leading to perioperative hypovolaemia which, as a result of splanchnic vasoconstriction, has important implications for anastomotic healing in gastrointestinal surgery.

Assessment

A clinical history must always be part of the initial assessment, but may be difficult or impossible to obtain in patients with a disturbed conscious level resulting from head injury, alcohol intake or decreased cerebral perfusion. In cases of trauma, useful information can be obtained indirectly from witnesses to the scene of the accident. In road traffic accidents in particular, knowledge of the degree of disruption of the vehicle structure, and of whether other occupants of the vehicle were injured or killed, can give a useful indication of the magnitude of likely injury.

Physical examination needs to be carried out in a logical sequence in order to avoid serious oversights. In shocked patients, particularly trauma victims, the resuscitation team needs to carry out a rapid initial assessment followed by immediate resuscitation and airway management, before turning to a secondary, and more complete, survey. All doctors likely to be exposed to the management of trauma cases would be well advised to attend an advanced trauma life-support (ATLS) course; such courses are now available in most areas of the country.

Detection of the presence of hypovolaemia would seem a relatively simple task and, in many instances, the combination of overt fluid loss with inadequate replacement (in 24 h) makes it an easy diagnosis. In a proportion of patients, however, the clinical presentation may be less clear-cut; perhaps, as alluded to above, because of multifactorial aetiology or prior, partial resuscitation. Even when the existence of hypovolaemia is not in doubt, accurate quantification of volume deficit is often difficult. Subjective visual estimation of fluid loss is fraught with problems and may be grossly inaccurate. Blood loss may be assessed on the basis that a handful of blood clot represents 500 ml, but this method makes no allowance for losses from major vessel bleeding. In thermal injury, the figure of 4 ml of fluid replacement per kilogram body weight for each per cent of body surface area burned is widely accepted, but in some cases may be a significant underestimate. Clinical features of dehydration are important for diagnostic purposes, but cannot be used to quantify extracellular losses. Thirst is an insensitive measure of water deprivation and becomes obvious only after a deficit of 1.5 litres has occurred. Severe water deprivation may be associated with deficits as high as 10 litres. Salt depletion, associated with lassitude and postural hypotension, implies a deficit of up to 4 litres of isotonic saline.

Direct measurement of blood volume using tracer substances has been performed, and can be accurate in the presence of an intact and a normovolaemic circulation. However, the techniques are less reliable in situations of hypoperfusion or increased capillary permeability, where incomplete mixing and extravascular losses lead to inaccuracies.

For these various reasons, assessment of hypovolaemia is usually made by a combination of a careful history, clinical examination, estimation of apparent or observed losses, and indirect measurements including haematocrit, heart rate and pulse volume, arterial and venous pressures, and indices of tissue perfusion. **In the early assessment and management of a hypovolaemic patient it is these indices of tissue perfusion that are most useful with, for example, peripheral skin temperature or nail bed capillary refill representing skin perfusion, urine output representing renal perfusion and, in the absence of a head injury, conscious level reflecting cerebral perfusion.** In view of factors already alluded to, including variable degrees of vasoconstriction, haemodynamic measurements should always be considered as complementary to this clinical appraisal of clinical perfusion. One should not be misled into thinking that the patient is normally perfused simply because the blood pressure and heart rate are normal. **However, a patient with rapid capillary refill, warm dry skin, a good urine output and a lucid mental state is unlikely to be significantly hypovolaemic.**

Monitoring and invasive instrumentation

Monitoring of the patient with hypovolaemic shock must be simple but adequate. The following are reasonable suggestions for initial management.

- Establish good venous access with a minimum of two large-bore peripheral cannulae.
- Insert a bladder catheter (in the absence of any contraindication due to urethral injury).
- Monitor ECG.
- Insert a central venous catheter for pressure monitoring and blood sampling (in cases where rapid stabilization is not achieved).
- Attach a pulse oximeter using a finger probe.

In addition, in some cases, especially later in the course of resuscitation, it is often appropriate to insert an arterial catheter and a pulmonary artery flotation catheter (PAFC), the latter also being known as a Swan–Ganz catheter.

Initial venous access is normally obtained in the antecubital fossa. If difficulty is encountered in gaining venous access then cut-downs can be performed, either in the antecubital fossa or on to the long saphenous vein in the leg. In severely shocked patients it is appropriate to obtain initial central access by percutaneously cannulating the femoral vein at the groin. In the early resuscitation of an overtly hypovolaemic patient it is inappropriate to take the time to place a central venous catheter. It is extremely difficult to overload a trauma patient with fluid and only where the underlying aetiology of the shock state is in doubt, or in a patient who appears to be requiring inappropriately large volumes of fluid, does central venous pressure (CVP) become useful. A small-bore (18 g) central venous line is adequate for monitoring but quite useless for the rapid infusion of fluid. It is often appropriate to use a PAFC insertion sheath for initial central venous cannulation in the neck, since it allows the rapid infusion of fluid and facilitates subsequent insertion of a PAFC, if required. Whenever possible, central venous catheters should be inserted by a high approach to the internal jugular vein, for two reasons. First, misplacement of the catheter is rare when inserted by this route; it invariably passes into the superior vena cava. Secondly, the alternative subclavian route carries a higher risk of pneumothorax, which in an unstable patient may well potentiate the cardiorespiratory problems.

Monitoring of the ECG is useful for detecting arrhythmias and evidence of myocardial ischaemia. Insertion of a bladder catheter allows measurement of urine output and, in trauma cases, allows early detection of haematuria, which may be indicative of renal trauma. Pulse oximetry using a finger probe is now increasingly used as an adjunct to monitoring in the accident department. In a patient with adequate perfusion the oximeter will estimate arterial oxygen saturation. However, failure of the apparatus to obtain a good signal is indicative of poor tissue perfusion. For this reason an oximeter that displays the pulse plethysmogram is preferable.

Insertion of an arterial catheter allows not only continuous on-line monitoring of intra-arterial pressure but also repeated blood gas analysis. In a severely shocked patient arterial catheterization may be carried out utilizing the femoral artery, although it is more common to use the radial artery. Prior to inserting any catheter into the radial artery it is essential to check that the ulnar artery is patent and also supplying the palmar arch. The incidence of complication from radial artery catheters is exceedingly low and the need for repeated radial stabs for blood gas analysis is obviated.

With the above manoeuvres completed, a series of measurements may be obtained, including:

- conscious level
- heart rate and rhythm
- arterial and venous pressure
- respiratory rate and rhythm, blood gas analysis
- core–peripheral temperature gradient
- urine output
- haemoglobin and haematocrit
- electrolytes and acid–base balance
- chest radiograph
- PAFC to obtain additional information (see below).

The core–peripheral temperature gradient is a useful, non-invasive indicator of peripheral perfusion. In a well-perfused patient, in a warm, ambient temperature, the gradient is a very sensitive indicator of decreased perfusion but is entirely non-specific and cannot be used as a guide to changes in cardiac output. Assessment of respiratory rate is often omitted from initial measurements in the accident department. However, in hypovolaemia, it is a much more useful measurement than assessment of heart rate. Blood gas analysis may signal early development of respiratory complications, particularly when used in conjunction with the inspired oxygen saturation, from which an estimation may be made of the alveolar–arterial oxygen tension gradient.

Tests of haemoconcentration include measurement of haematocrit or the haemoglobin concentration. Haematocrit can be carried out on site using a microcentrifuge. Neither can be relied on to indicate the magnitude of blood loss during the acute stage, but they are important as baseline readings and also for use in judging the effectiveness of blood transfusion during resuscitation. Serum concentrations of sodium and chloride are often measured, but the results can be difficult to interpret. A deficit or excess of sodium concentration tends to lead to either excretion or retention of water and thus relatively little change in the sodium concentration in plasma. Measurement of electrolyte concentrations and osmolality in plasma and urine together allows one to distinguish between prerenal and intrinsic renal failure and also, in the case of the former, the principal deficit (salt or water). In the accident department, in the presence of hypovolaemia, a decreased urine output will always be assumed to be due to prerenal factors. **Subsequently, a urine:plasma osmolality ratio of greater than 1.4 suggests prerenal failure, while a ratio of 1.2 or less suggests intrinsic renal failure**.

Single readings of CVP can often be very misleading, as a guide to hypovolaemia. Classically, marked hypovolaemia will present as low arterial pressure with a low or negative CVP. Partial resuscitation, underlying myocardial ischaemia, chronic lung disease, pericardial tamponade, contusional injury to the myocardium and positive pressure ventilation can all lead to difficulties in interpreting static measurements of CVP. Where CVP values are equivocal the technique of 'fluid challenge' can be useful. **A fluid challenge involves measurement of changes in central venous and arterial pressure in response to the rapid administration of a small volume of colloid (100–200 ml over 2–3 min)**. Figure 19.3 shows diagrammatically two hypothetical cases indicating how a fluid challenge may unmask hypovolaemia in an intensely vasoconstricted patient, or give an early indication of myocardial impairment, without the risk of fluid overloading.

Pulmonary artery flotation catheter

There are many occasions in the resuscitation of shocked patients when catheterization of the pulmonary artery by means of a PAFC is indicated. Any of the situations listed above in which interpretation of static measurement of CVP is inaccurate are relative indications for insertion of a PAFC, particularly if fluid

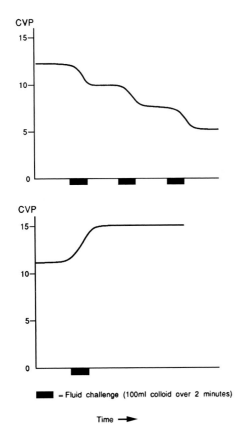

= Fluid challenge (100ml colloid over 2 minutes)

Time →

Figure 19.3 Use of fluid challenges in patients with equivocal CVP values. In the top example, occult hypovolaemia due to intense vasoconstriction in a young trauma patient has been unmasked by a series of fluid challenges. In the lower example a rapid and sustained rise in CVP in response to fluid challenge indicates myocardial impairment, without the risk of seriously overloading the patient with fluid.

arteriole, obstructing pulsatile flow beyond the tip of the catheter. Pressure monitoring through the distal (pulmonary artery) channel with the balloon in the normal (deflated) position gives pulmonary artery systolic and diastolic pressures, while with the balloon inflated a pulmonary capillary wedge pressure (PCWP) is obtained, the latter being an estimate of left atrial filling pressure (a left-sided CVP). An electrical connection to a thermistor at the tip of the catheter also allows calculation of thermodilution cardiac output.

Thus, insertion of the PAFC facilitates the following:

- monitoring of right atrial pressure
- monitoring of pulmonary artery pressure
- monitoring of PCWP
- measurement of thermodilution cardiac output
- sampling of mixed venous blood for blood gas analysis, including oxygen saturation.

From the above, in conjunction with arterial gas analysis, a number of other variables can be calculated, including:

- pulmonary vascular resistance
- systemic vascular resistance
- oxygen extraction ratio (oxygen delivery and consumption)
- systemic oxygen consumption.

Pathophysiology

Hypovolaemia is the most common cause of shock in a general hospital population. It is diagnosed when the clinical features of hypotension, tachycardia, pallor, sweating, peripheral cyanosis, hyperventilation, clouding of consciousness and oliguria are predominantly attributable to diminished venous return. The latter may be the result of overt fluid loss (directly or indirectly) from the circulation or sequestration of fluid within body spaces; examples of such 'third-space' collections include ascites, massive oedema, haemothorax, intestinal obstruction and haemoperitoneum. Myocardial failure and sepsis are, by definition, not of major clinical significance in the early stages of hypovolaemic shock, although both factors will inevitably become important if the shock process is not rapidly reversed.

The onset of hypovolaemic shock may be sudden, for example after major vessel injury, or more gradual, for example in association with inadequate fluid replacement after surgery. In the first example, the diagnosis is not in doubt; the complete package of physiological compensatory mechanisms is immediately called into play, producing the typical features of hypovolaemic shock. Assuming rapid and adequate volume repletion, outcome depends on securing haemostasis. In the second example, the onset is more insidious and the diagnosis may be less obvious, the clinical presentation obscured by additional, time-dependent factors such as compartmental fluid shifts, and the outcome influenced to an extent by shock-related organ dysfunction. Individual patients may

challenges fail to clarify the situation. Patients admitted to the intensive care unit (ICU) and requiring inotropic support should probably all undergo insertion of a PAFC. In particular, patients with sepsis, patients in whom myocardial impairment complicates hypovolaemic shock, and patients suffering from multiple trauma (particularly where thoracic trauma makes myocardial contusion a possibility) are all candidates for insertion of a PAFC, although a recent consensus statement questioned the value of using a PAFC in many of the above-mentioned diagnoses.

A PAFC is a long catheter with two monitoring/sampling channels, one situated in the tip of the catheter, which after insertion lies in the pulmonary artery, and the other (30 cm back from the tip) which lies in the superior vena cava (SVC)/right atrium. In addition, the catheter has a further channel for inflation of a balloon at the tip of the catheter. This balloon is inflated after insertion of the catheter into the SVC and guides the catheter, with the flow of blood, through the right side of the heart and into the pulmonary arterial trunk. Following insertion, if the balloon is inflated, the tip of the catheter moves forward into a wedged position where the balloon impacts in a pulmonary feature anywhere in the spectrum between these two extremes, with age, general health and concomitant illness further contributing to the ultimate clinical presentation.

A critical reduction in oxygen availability to the cell is the final common pathway leading to death from shock of all varieties; reduced substrate supply and accumulation of the products of cell metabolism (some of which can usefully be measured, e.g. lactate) are contributing factors.

Cellular dysfunction
At the cellular level, two important features of cell injury may be considered: altered cell volume regulation and altered energy metabolism. One of the earliest consequences of reduced oxygen availability is a decrease in cellular adenosine triphosphate (ATP) content. High-energy phosphates are required by the cell for many functions. One such function is the fuelling of the ionic exchange pump, present in the plasma membrane of the cell. ATP is normally broken down to adenosine diphosphate (ADP) and phosphate in the presence of ATPase. The absence of the high-energy phosphate bond leads to depression of pump function and cellular swelling, the cells tending to approach Gibbs–Donnan equilibrium with an increase in intracellular sodium, calcium and water content together with a loss of potassium and magnesium (sick cell syndrome). However, membrane dysfunction has been observed in the face of normal tissue ATP concentrations, suggesting that energy depletion is only one of a number of factors involved. When oxygen tension decreases to a critical value within the mitochondria (thought to be in the order of 0.1 kPa) the electron transfer mechanism, which accounts for 90% of the body's oxygen consumption, becomes defective. Oxidative phosphorylation is uncoupled and ATP production gradually ceases. Associated structural changes, visible on light and electron microscopic examination, include mitochondrial swelling and disruption of the lining membrane, initially involving only the outer layer. Eventually, the inner membrane also deteriorates as a result of continued low ATP concentrations. ATP deficiency also contributes to two other metabolic consequences of importance in hypovolaemic shock: abnormalities of calcium flux within the cell and lactic acidosis. Persistence of high intracellular calcium concentrations leads to myocardial cell fatigue, failure and asystolic cardiac arrest. In sepsis, as opposed to hypovolaemia, changes in calcium channel flux are thought to be partly responsible for alterations in vascular adrenoreceptor responsiveness, leading, in some instances, to a relative resistance to therapy with adrenergic agents such as dopamine.

Lactic acidosis, stimulated by increased phosphofructokinase activity, augments calcium slow-channel inhibition at pH less than 6.8, as well as having adverse effects on other enzyme systems. A relationship between poor perfusion and lactic acidosis has been recognized for many years. It has led some authors to describe 'probability of survival' curves based on initial lactate measurements. While the association between lactate and outcome appears to be close in traumatic and simple hypovolaemic shock, some centres report a more complex relationship in sepsis. Serial lactate measurements are better in predicting outcome than single measurements, and failure of blood lactate to fall appropriately during resuscitation usually indicates that the resuscitative manoeuvres have been inadequate. The possibility of washout of lactate from poorly perfused tissues during resuscitation, leading to an early rise in lactate, appears to be more of a theoretical possibility than a true phenomenon. However, it has been reported in some postoperative situations, particularly with hypothermia. One must always remember that blood lactate measurements reflect both production in tissues and extraction, mainly in the liver.

The aforementioned pattern of pathophysiological disturbance occurs in all cells, but the susceptibility of different cells to hypoxia and ischaemia is very variable. Astrocytes, for example, cease to function after seconds, while skeletal muscle will function anaerobically for 30 min and hepatic cells for several hours; increased supplies of glucose are required to maintain this anaerobic glycolysis, which may be a problem in low-flow states. Clearly, in the presence of complete ischaemia the progress of cellular disintegration will be more rapid but, depending on a variety of factors, the kidney and liver, for example, have survival times at 37°C of 1–2 h. The plasma membrane and early mitochondrial changes are readily reversible if the cause of shock is promptly eliminated and rapid, complete resuscitation performed. A number of pharmacological agents has been used in an attempt to attenuate cellular damage in shock, e.g. ATP-MgCl$_2$, glucose–insulin–potassium, calcium channel blockers and steroids. None of these agents is of proven clinical value in this setting.

Neurohumoral response
The sequence of physiological events leading to the fully established clinical presentation of hypovolaemic shock is generally well understood. In shock, the central disturbance is a critical fall in oxygen availability, largely due to changes in the cardiovascular system. However, almost all of the major organ systems play a part in modulating the homeostatic response to shock.

The central nervous system initiates the body's homeostatic responses to acute injury (including fluid loss) by mechanisms, which are complex. Multiple afferent stimuli (arterial and venous pressures and volume, osmolality, pH, hypoxia, pain, anxiety and tissue damage) reach the hypothalamus, where they are integrated and relayed to the sympathetic nervous system and adrenal medulla. Simultaneously, the anterior pituitary initiates the hormonal response characteristic of the metabolic response to injury.

Vasopressin (AVP), also known as antidiuretic hormone, and adrenocorticotrophic hormone (ACTH) are commonly regarded as the principal stress hormones. Increased production of these hormones follows a variety of different stimuli, principally increased osmo-lality (detected by osmoreceptors in the hypothalamus), decreased arterial pressure and volume (detected by volume receptors and relayed via the tractus solitarius) and psychological stress (relayed via the limbic system). ACTH is released into the blood stream in response to corticotrophin-releasing factor, AVP and adrenaline. ACTH stimulates the production of cortisol, which plays a major role in protecting the organism from the effects of hypovolaemia. The importance of cortisol was underlined by the observation that when etomidate (a suppressor of adrenocortical function) was used for sedation in intensive care, it led to an increase in mortality in some patient groups. Another anterior pituitary peptide, β-endorphin (derived from the same precursor as ACTH), is also released during stress and is thought to mediate longer term neuronal and endocrine changes.

The basic endocrine activation in shock involves release of catecholamines and angiotensin, with related later increases in the plasma concentrations of such hormones as cortisol, growth hormone, glucagon, AVP and aldosterone. The combined effect is to mobilize energy reserves and conserve salt and water. In the short term these mechanisms can be regarded as pro-tective, but ultimately they lead to the breakdown of cellular integrity.

Angiotensin II, a most potent vasoconstrictor, is also released into the blood following shock and has been incriminated as a cause of heart failure after prolonged severe haemorrhage. Another extracardiac cause of heart failure is the presence in the blood of myocardial depressant factor (MDF), a circulating peptide released from hypoxic pancreatic acinar cells. The endogenous opiates β-endorphin and met-enkephalin have also been implicated in producing cardiovascular depression in shock. Opiate antagonists, e.g. naloxone, have been used in an attempt to suppress this action, but they have no convincing role to play in the management of shock.

Other substances released into the blood during shock include histamine, plasma kinins, complement components and arachidonic acid metabolites. Hista-mine is a vasodilator substance and there is evidence that endotoxin stimulates the rate of its production by activating histidine decarboxylase. It is unlikely that histamine plays a major role in uncomplicated hypovolaemic shock.

Plasma kinins are vasodilator polypeptides, which increase capillary permeability. They are released by both hypoxia and endotoxaemia from inactive precur-sors (kininogens) present in the α$_2$-globulin fraction of the plasma protein. The initial step appears to be activation of Hageman factor (factor XII), which leads to the conversion of kininogen to kinin by proteolytic enzymes (kallikreins) released from leucocytes and injured tissues. Activation of Hageman factor also pro-motes complement activation, with the subsequent release of a number of pharmacologically active sub-stances, which appear to be responsible for leucocyte aggregation and endothelial cell damage, such as

platelet-activating factor (PAF), intracellular adhesion molecule-1 (ICAM-1) and E-selectin. Putative local mediators of the microvascular injury include the arachidonic acid metabolites, plasma or phagocyte-derived proteases (particularly elastase), fibrinogen degradation products and toxic oxygen radicals released by activated leucocytes. Serotonin and histamine may play a secondary role in the pulmonary vascular response to shock. These various effects are unusual fol-lowing uncomplicated hypovolaemia, but occur in the presence of prolonged shock or when shock is com-pounded by trauma or sepsis.

Hypovolaemia complicated by the presence of trau-ma or sepsis is known to be associated with the pro-duction, from macrophages, of cytokines, such as tumour necrosis factor (TNF) and interleukins. Many of the microcirculatory and metabolic changes in sep-sis are due to these cytokines (see below). Some of the actions of cytokines appear to depend on arachidonic acid metabolism and the coagulation cascade.

Regional and microcirculatory flow disturbances

The early, catecholamine-induced, vasoconstrictor response in hypovolaemic shock is not uniform throughout the body and redistribution of blood flow occurs in favour of certain vital organs, notably the brain and the heart. As a result, the main brunt of the initial microcirculatory changes is in the skin, muscle and gastrointestinal tract. The kidney response varies with the rapidity of onset of hypovolaemia: the slower the onset, the greater the opportunity for auto-regulation and diversion of flow to juxtamedullary glomeruli. The magnitude of reduction in blood flow in some of the non-vital areas is not reflected in any of the routine clinical haemodynamic measurements and this is often not appreciated. For example, a 10% reduc-tion in blood volume occurring gradually over 1 h may produce negligible changes in heart rate and arterial pressure, but a very profound reduction in splanchnic blood flow and oxygen delivery. This decrease in splanchnic blood flow has important implications for liver function, since approximately 70% of hepatic blood flow and 50% of hepatic oxygen delivery nor-mally traverses the portal vein. Placement of oximetric catheters in the hepatic vein has shown that inter-mittent hypoxia can occur in this region, in critically ill patients, even during procedures such as tracheal suc-tion and bronchoscopy. It has been shown that in some situations hypovolaemia can result in an acute ischaemic insult to the gut, leading to gut-barrier failure with hypothetical translocation of endotoxin and organisms or shedding of inflammatory mediators into the portal circulation (more fully discussed in the section on 'Sepsis'). Although hepatocytes themselves are relatively resistant to hypoxia, it is common to see marked rises in the transaminases 36–48 h after a profound hypotensive event. It is also clear from more sensitive tests of liver function, such as indocyanine green clearance, that disturbances in hepatocellular and reticuloendothelial function are demonstrable much earlier. Interaction between these two functions is increasingly recognized to be important in the pathogenesis of multiple organ failure (MOF).

A number of additional factors can complicate the microcirculatory response to shock. Autoregulation may be adversely affected by pathological changes in the blood vessels. In both hypertension and atherosclerosis there tends to be a greater decrease in blood flow for a given decrease in arterial pressure. In addition, the normal vasoconstrictor responses to hypovolaemia may be obtunded during the administration of general anaesthetic, sedative or related agents, causing the already reduced circulating volume to be more widely spread. Maldistribution of tissue perfusion is fundamental in shock, but its pathogenesis remains incompletely understood. It is known that, even when overall flow to an organ or region seems adequate, the flow may be transversing preferred-route capillaries rather than nutrient vessels. In addition, oxygen extraction and utilization or oxygen release at a cellular level may be impaired, particularly in sepsis.

Microcirculatory flow can also be impaired by a number of factors: an increase in red cell and platelet adhesiveness, together with a decrease in red cell deformability; an increased adhesiveness in the neutrophil population with margination, leading in some instances to capillary plugging; endothelial cell swelling leading to partial occlusion of the capillary lumen; and increases in blood viscosity, particularly in hypovolaemia without red cell loss. It has been shown that, in low flow states, a degree of haemodilution (to a haematocrit of around 30%) produces improved oxygen delivery, assuming that arterial oxygen tension and cardiac output are adequate. In uncomplicated hypovolaemic shock a haematocrit of this level has been shown to be the optimum balance between blood viscosity and haemoglobin concentration, leading to the optimum oxygen delivery. The decrease in viscosity helps to prevent rouleaux formation. In practice, during resuscitation of, for instance, a trauma patient, one would aim for a haematocrit between 30 and 35%, in order to allow a margin of safety for further bleeding. Platelet aggregation is enhanced by many factors, including adenosine diphosphate, thrombin, collagen fragments, hydrogen ions, noradrenaline and endotoxin. As already indicated, endotoxaemia can readily occur because of ischaemic gut-barrier failure in response to trauma, pancreatitis, mesenteric occlusion and thermal injury. The severity of the peripheral circulatory failure associated with these latter conditions is, in part, attributable to the effects of endotoxaemia on the complement, coagulation and fibrinolysis cascades. In particular, subclinical or overt disseminated intravascular coagulation (DIC) is known significantly to worsen microcirculatory flow, leading to organ damage.

The microcirculatory response to shock is partially dependent on changes in the interstitial fluid compartment, which is by far the larger of the two extracellular fluid spaces. The fluid volume within the interstitial space is almost four times greater than the plasma vol-

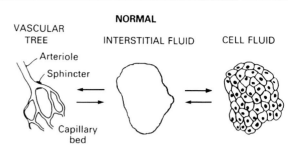

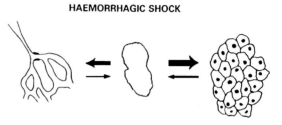

Figure 19.4 Fluid flux and fluid spaces in hypovolaemic shock. (From Shires and Carrico (1966). *Current Problems of Surgery*, March, with permission.)

ume. A simplified diagram of the changes in interstitial volume and fluid flux between the three fluid spaces is shown in Figure 19.4. In the early stage of hypovolaemic shock the decreased intravascular hydrostatic pressure leads to a fluid flux from the interstitial space to the intravascular. Later, as microvascular pressure relationships alter, transport of fluid from the vascular compartment to the interstitium occurs; a proportion of this fluid enters the hypoxic cells, which to a degree is dependent on the severity and duration of the shock, as a result of the breakdown of ATP-dependent membrane pumps. Again, it has been suggested that the gastrointestinal tract may be more vulnerable to these effects than other organ systems.

Hypovolaemic shock may prove fatal during the acute phase if treatment is delayed or the underlying cause cannot be controlled. Recovery from the acute phase is usually consistent with long-term survival, but incomplete recovery, often associated with surgical or septic complications, may lead to single or multiple organ failure. Until recently, the study of MOF tended to focus on changes involving the lung and the kidney, largely because the clinical effects on these organs are obvious. However, it is now thought likely that damage to the gastrointestinal tract, particularly the splanchnic circulation, is of fundamental importance in the pathogenesis of MOF (see below).

Treatment

The prime objective of treatment is to restore adequate oxygen availability for the metabolic requirements of the tissues. The importance of prompt and adequate resuscitation in the early stages of hypovolaemia is clear, and often dictates that therapy begins before the diagnosis can be confirmed. Initial attention to the ABC of resuscitation (airway, breathing and circulation) needs to precede a survey of the patient to look for the underlying causes of the shock process. In practice, this is possible because acute resuscitation of a patient suffering from any form of shock is influenced more by the nature of the associated physiological disturbances than by specific aetiological factors. Success of subsequent treatment, however, is largely dependent on detection and elimination of the underlying cause; for instance, arrest of haemorrhage or drainage of a source of sepsis.

Initial resuscitation

The mainstays of the early treatment of shock are the infusion of fluid and the administration of oxygen. By contrast, pharmacological agents have little role to play in the initial stages of resuscitation. The immediate aims of augmenting intravascular volume and ensuring adequate pulmonary gas exchange are achieved by minimizing further fluid loss, replacing estimated losses with colloid or crystalloid and transfusion with concentrated red cells to a haematocrit of 30–35%, and by the administration of oxygen, together with mechanical ventilation when indicated.

The wise counsel, found in all first-aid manuals, of reducing the risk of further fluid loss in the hypovolaemic patient appears to carry less weight once the patient has crossed the hospital threshold. It should be realized that avoidance of unnecessary movement, immobilization of broken limbs, gentle handing of damaged tissues and maintenance of pressure dressings are just as important in the accident and emergency department, the operating theatre or the intensive therapy unit as they are during prehospital care. The role of antishock trousers (MAST) in prehospital care is uncertain. When applied to the legs at low to moderate pressures, the garment functions as a useful splint and may control venous bleeding and reduce venous pooling, thus aiding venous return to the heart. However, when applied at higher pressures the increase in total peripheral resistance may elevate the systemic pressure while decreasing cardiac output. There is also a worry that inflation of the abdominal bolster may compress the inferior vena cava, impairing venous return to the heart. Thus, the MAST device may be of value as a temporizing device, for instance during transfer of a leaking aneurysm to a centre with vascular specialists. Under normal circumstances the abdominal bolster should not be inflated and, most importantly, use of the device should in no way delay the earliest possible replacement of intravascular volume, which must in any case precede decompression of the MAST device. The practice of tilting a hypovolaemic patient head-down in an attempt to augment venous return is frequently carried out. There is, however, no evidence that this manoeuvre achieves any consistent haemodynamic improvement, and adverse pulmonary and cerebral effects are possible. In the absence of limb injury, raising the legs is an adequate and safe alternative.

Fluid administration

The type of fluid loss in shocked patients has little influence on the choice of initial fluid replacement. Thus, whether the loss is caused by haemorrhagic, burns or gastrointestinal pathology, either colloid or crystalloid solutions, or both, are used in the first instance. Red cell concentrates are given later, preferably after cross-matching, but with the use of non-cross-matched, group O blood being necessary in some extreme situations. Successful initial resuscitation is dependent more on the rapidity and adequacy of fluid replacement than on the composition of the regimen. Dispute as to the selection of non-blood fluid for resuscitation (the 'colloid vs crystalloid' controversy) centres mainly on issues relating to philosophy, side-effects and economics.

The terms 'colloid' and 'crystalloid' were coined by Thomas Graham in 1861 and refer, respectively, to solute particles that are larger or smaller than an arbitrarily determined particle weight, usually taken as 30 000 in the case of body fluid components. In effect, this means that colloid particles, such as albumin, will not pass through semipermeable membranes. The volume of literature on colloids and crystalloids, addressing the question of which type of fluid is superior, gives a clue to the fact that there is little difference between them. The major points made in the arguments can be summarized as follows.

- Crystalloids are sodium-containing solutions and, because of their prompt equilibration with the interstitial fluid space, they need to be infused in amounts exceeding estimated intravascular losses by a factor of three to four times. Crystalloids equilibrate with the interstitial space, because sodium is the main positive ion in both the intravascular and interstitial spaces. It is worthy of note that 5% dextrose is not a crystalloid but merely water rendered isotonic by the addition of glucose. When infused, 5% dextrose equilibrates not only with the interstitial space but with the much larger intracellular space, making it quite useless as a resuscitation fluid. However, 5% dextrose is the ideal fluid for correction of cellular dehydration. Colloid solutions, unlike crystalloids, tend to remain within the intravascular space (although changes in capillary permeability can alter this) and are thus more rapidly effective in correcting losses of circulating volume.

- It has been argued that crystalloids, by reducing the colloid osmotic pressure and thus altering the Starling equation for microvascular fluid flux, should favour the occurrence of pulmonary oedema. This is probably not the case since crystalloids, by virtue of their rapid equilibration with the interstitial space, will also reduce the interstitial osmotic pressure and, in addition, the lung is capable of increasing lymphatic flow, thus protecting against the formation of oedema. There is no doubt, however, that resuscitation with crystalloids alone leads to marked peripheral oedema and this may have detrimental effects in some situations, for instance in the context of wound healing.

- One school of thought, initially popularized by Shires, states that a key problem in shock is shrinkage of the interstitial fluid compartment (Figure 19.4), making replacement with crystalloid more appropriate.
- Crystalloids are free from the risk of occasional anaphylactoid reactions, which can occur with any colloid solution, including plasma protein solutions.
- Crystalloids are considerably cheaper than albumin solutions and, even allowing for the larger volumes required for resuscitation, also tend to be cheaper than most synthetic colloids.
- Crystalloids are also chloride-containing solutions, which were recently shown to be one of the causes of the acidosis frequently seen during shock.

It is likely that the common practice of using crystalloids and colloids in combination is a sensible one, combining the best effects of both types of fluid. Thus, initial resuscitation with a synthetic colloid can achieve rapid restoration of intravascular volume with subsequent administration of red cell concentrates, according to haematocrit, supplemented by a combination of colloid and crystalloid. At all times careful judgement is required in striking the optimum balance between the volume of fluid per unit time needed for adequate tissue perfusion and that which will induce overload; the value of 'fluid challenge' and the occasional need for a PAFC has already been indicated. However, it should be stressed that, in the management of multiple trauma patients, it is exceedingly difficult to overload a patient with fluid during initial resuscitation and harm is much more likely to occur through inadequate fluid replacement.

Some clinicians have expressed enthusiasm for the use of hypertonic saline solutions in the treatment of hypovolaemic shock, including use in severely burned patients. Such solutions act through an osmotic effect, sucking fluid into the intravascular space from the interstitial and intracellular spaces. Thus, while they may be of value in the field, they do not remove the need for later replacement of adequate volume.

Large-volume fluid transfusion tends to lead to a dilutional coagulopathy, which may be compounded by specific effects on the coagulation system with the use of some synthetic colloids, notably dextrans. Dilution of clotting factors (fibrinogen, factors V and VII and platelets) may require replacement with fresh-frozen plasma and/or platelet transfusions, as dictated by coagulation assays. The need for massive fluid transfusions should also dictate the use of blood-warming equipment, both for red cells and for non-blood fluids. Currently, there is no synthetic alternative to red cells as an oxygen-carrying medium, although promising lines of research continue in the development of stroma-free haemoglobin solutions and fluorocarbons.

If hypovolaemic shock proves refractory to fluid repletion, as outlined above, and oxygen administration (see below), the following factors may be responsible:

- **initial underestimate of the degree of hypovolaemia**
- **failure to arrest haemorrhage**
- **cardiac tamponade or tension pneumothorax**
- **underlying sepsis**
- **delayed treatment, leading to secondary cardiovascular effects.**

Oxygenation
In the initial stages of resuscitation, the administration of high concentrations of oxygen to patients with overt shock is to be recommended; fears about oxygen toxicity are inappropriate in this situation. Subsequent oxygen administration will be based on measurement of arterial oxygen tension (Pa,o_2) or on oxygen saturation estimated by a pulse oximeter (Sp,o_2). In patients with hypovolaemic shock, hypoxaemia will vary in degree and is of multifactorial aetiology: patients may have underlying conditions such as chronic obstructive airway disease; hypovolaemia itself can lead to intrapulmonary shunting; trauma patients may suffer direct chest injury and, finally, any shocked patient with obtunded conscious level may be at risk of aspiration of gastric contents or blood.

Ventilatory assistance is required when there is excessive respiratory work or ventilatory inadequacy with hypercapnia. Failure of adequate oxygenation ($Pa,o_2 < 8.7$ kPa) when breathing oxygen 15 l/min through a high flow mask (inspired oxygen concentration approximately 70%) represents a shunt of 20–25% of the cardiac output and calls for the use of positive pressure ventilation. Techniques that increase mean intrathoracic pressure, such as positive end expiratory pressure (PEEP) and continuous positive airway pressure (CPAP), should be used with caution in hypovolaemic patients and continuous monitoring should be used to select the optimum pressure, in order to provide maximum oxygen delivery.

In a traumatized patient, the presence of a significant head injury should prompt the early use of endotracheal intubation, with or without mechanical ventilation, to protect the airway and reduce the risk of a secondary insult to cerebral function.

Adult respiratory distress syndrome (ARDS) or 'shock lung' is not a factor that needs to be considered in the emergency room. However, it is an important cause of later deterioration in gas exchange. ARDS is relatively uncommon in uncomplicated hypovolaemic shock. It is more common in patients suffering from trauma (although in this situation it needs to be distinguished from direct pulmonary contusion) and is very common in patients with sepsis. Although ARDS is often described as a specific entity, it should really be thought of as a lung manifestation of MOF, the latter representing a body-wide endothelial injury. Potential systemic mediators of MOF will be discussed below, in the section on sepsis. In ARDS, an important local mediator is the neutrophil, which marginates and adheres to the endothelium within the pulmonary vasculature. These activated neutrophils then release proteases, including elastase, leading to an increase in capillary permeability. One important factor in this process is damage to basement membrane-associated fibronectin, which is important for endothelial cell adhesion. In addition, increases in the measured pulmonary vascular resistance occur, largely due to changes in the flow characteristics in the postcapillary venule. These two factors, capillary permeability and local increase in hydrostatic pressure, lead, in the early stages of ARDS, to a protein-rich exudate passing into the alveolar interstitium. The diagnosis of ARDS depends on finding changes consistent with pulmonary oedema, in the absence of a raised pulmonary artery capillary occlusion pressure; indeed, in the past it was known as non-cardiogenic pulmonary oedema. The subsequent pathological and physiological changes in ARDS are complex, but lead ultimately, in a surviving patient, to healing by fibrosis. The pulmonary circulation is normally a low-pressure system and, in ARDS, the high pulmonary vascular resistance places a marked afterload on the right ventricle, leading to right ventricular strain and in some cases right ventricular infarction. The potential for such dissociation between left and right ventricular function is another factor that weighs in favour of the insertion of a PAFC.

Pharmacological agents

If the elimination of surgical factors together with restoration of blood volume, red cell mass and adequate oxygenation fails to restore an adequate cardiac output and oxygen delivery, then pharmacological agents may be required. The drugs most commonly used in these circumstances are the inotropic agents (to increase myocardial contractility) with or without the use of vasodilators or vasoconstrictors. Dopamine has proved attractive because of its effects on both cardiac output and urine output. In higher doses, dopamine is also a vasoconstrictor and the physiological response to a given dose of dopamine can be extremely variable in patients with shock, particularly trauma or sepsis. However, as a guide the following dose ranges are commonly quoted: the effects of a dose of 2–5 µg/kg/min are predominantly dopaminergic, leading to improvement in renal and mesenteric blood flow; dose rates of 5–20 µg/kg/min produce predominantly an inotropic effect; when the dose administered exceeds 20 µg/kg/min α-adrenergic effects predominate and a vasoconstrictor response results: this is usually detrimental in uncomplicated hypovolaemia but may be required in severe sepsis, when the systemic vascular resistance is exceedingly low. It must be stressed that in individual patients the above dose responses cannot be assumed and the haemodynamic and oxygen-delivery effects of the administration must be checked.

Dobutamine, acting directly on β_1-adrenergic receptors, has a more pronounced inotropic action on the heart than dopamine, with less marked effects on heart rate, although care must be taken to restore circulating volume fully before administration of dobutamine or any other inotrope. A popular protocol is to use dopamine by low-dose infusion during the early stages of resuscitation to maintain renal perfusion and, if cardiac output needs to be augmented, to add dobutamine, with the aim of achieving the best combination of pharmacological actions. Again, in severe sepsis, an α-adrenergic agonist may be required to elevate blood pressure, in the presence of a low systemic vascular resistance, requiring the use of high-dose dopamine or noradrenaline.

It is imperative that any patient requiring inotropic doses of any of the above agents is fully monitored, including the use of a PAFC. It must be ensured that any change in the dose of drug infusion results in a beneficial effect on tissue perfusion. As already stated, the ultimate aim of resuscitation is to achieve an adequate oxygen delivery to match the metabolic needs of the tissues. In addition, a secondary goal is to maintain an adequate mean arterial pressure.

Specific mention should be made of the role of corticosteroids in shocked patients. A large number of animal experiments has shown beneficial effects from the early administration of corticosteroids. In clinical studies, a variety of beneficial early effects has been noted, but there is no proven benefit in terms of mortality. This may be due to an effect of steroids on the body's immune system, resulting in late infections and infection-related mortality, although data have been inconclusive. There may be a role for the prophylactic administration of a single dose of corticosteroid to high-risk surgical groups, prior to surgery, which is likely to induce hypovolaemia or sepsis. However, the balance of current opinion would not favour their routine use following trauma.

Metabolic control

Acid–base imbalance rarely requires pharmacological correction. Non-respiratory acidosis associated with perfusion failure is rapidly self-correcting once cardiac output is improved and its disappearance may be used as a marker of the adequacy of resuscitation. Occasionally, bicarbonate is required when pre-existing hyperkalaemia is exacerbated by a decreasing extracellular pH as a result of non-respiratory acidosis. Even in this situation, bicarbonate should only be given in the presence of a severe metabolic acidosis (pH < 7.2 and base excess > +10) and sufficient should be given to correct only partially the acidosis. **Overzealous administration of bicarbonate can have deleterious effects by producing a leftwards shift in the oxyhaemoglobin dissociation curve, resulting in a decreased release of oxygen from haemoglobin at tissue levels of oxygen tension.**

Respiratory acidosis demands correction of ventilation to achieve a decrease in arterial carbon dioxide tension (Pa,CO_2). Electrolyte balance is calculated from knowledge of input, serial serum estimations and analysis of 24 h urinary output and other measurable external losses. Diuretics may be required in the later stages of resuscitation, usually to minimize the risk of pulmonary overload; in this context both frusemide and dopamine may be administered by intravenous infusion.

Analgesia

Effective safe analgesia should not be withheld from hypovolaemic, especially injured patients. Despite the availability of a wide range of agents, morphine probably remains the most frequently used. **There is no place for subcutaneous or intramuscular injection of narcotic agents in hypovolaemic shock since, because of impaired blood flow, absorption is unreliable, unpredictable and dangerous. Increments of morphine (e.g. 2 mg) should be administered intravenously every 2–5 min until a satisfactory level of pain control is achieved**. It is rarely necessary to exceed 10 mg in a 70 kg patient. Duration of action by this route is short, however, and the dose may have to be repeated at 30–60 min intervals. All narcotic analgesic drugs are mild peripheral vasodilators but this is of no consequence in a monitored patient undergoing resuscitation. Such careful administration of analgesics should not interfere with assessment of conscious level, reduces anxiety and suffering by the patient, and has the additional benefit of decreasing oxygen consumption.

Analgesic effects equal to those of morphine can be produced by 25–50% nitrous oxide and oxygen. It can be useful for short-term, occasional use, particularly for interhospital or intrahospital transfer of intubated patients. It should, however, be avoided in patients with the potential for air collections in body cavities (e.g. pneumothorax or head injury). Extradural and intrathecal blockade are not recommended during resuscitation from shock, although once the initial resuscitation phase is over, these techniques have their place. They are particularly useful in allowing the early mobilization of an injured patient, avoiding recumbency and reducing the need for prolonged ventilation, both of which have their attendant risks. The infiltration of local analgesic drugs or the production of regional nerve blocks deserves due consideration in the acute situation. For instance, femoral nerve block can be performed rapidly, allowing good pain control in patients suffering from fracture of the femur.

Additional treatment

In general, patients should be adequately resuscitated from shock before surgery. Taken at its simplest, a patient in whom a good diuresis is obtained prior to surgery is less likely to suffer from postoperative renal failure. In some instances full resuscitation prior to surgery is not possible: in a ruptured ectopic pregnancy, for instance, it is often impossible to maintain a normal arterial pressure until bleeding is controlled and blood cleared from the peritoneal cavity; in a leaking aortic aneurysm it is usually best to commence surgery as soon after initiation of resuscitation as possible, lest further major haemorrhage occurs; and in the presence of sepsis, normal cardiovascular function may be difficult to restore until the source is eliminated.

Once haemodynamic stability has been achieved, it is important to take immediate stock of further fluid needs, since even small amounts in excess of requirement will tend to provoke pulmonary oedema, while even mild hypovolaemia may be associated with an increased risk of renal failure.

Cardiogenic shock

A full description of the diagnosis and therapy of cardiogenic shock is beyond the scope of this section. Many of the basic principles are similar to those outlined in the section on 'Hypovolaemia'. **In the simple classification of shock depicted in Figure 19.1, 'cardiogenic shock' is taken to imply any failure of the heart as a pump**. This may be brought about by either primary myocardial dysfunction from myocardial infarction, serious cardiac arrhythmias or myocardial depression from a variety of causes, or a miscellaneous group of causes, including tension pneumothorax, cardiac tamponade, vena caval obstruction and dissecting aneurysm. A more purist use of the term 'cardiogenic shock' would be to indicate a state of inadequate circulatory perfusion caused only by a primary cardiac dysfunction and excluding other causes such as disturbances of cardiac rhythm.

The most common cause of cardiogenic shock is, by far, myocardial infarction. Typical features, also used for the initial diagnosis, are: systolic blood pressure < 90 mmHg, or at least 30 mmHg lower than the previous baseline level, urine output < 30 ml/h, impaired conscious level and peripheral vasoconstriction. These are largely indistinguishable from features seen in other forms of low-output shock, although signs of left or right heart failure may also be seen.

Overall, the mortality from cardiogenic shock remains high but there are subgroups of patients, identified by invasive monitoring, in whom the prognosis is more favourable, when appropriate therapy is given. Initial therapy must include early correction of cardiac arrhythmias, provision of adequate oxygenation and correction of metabolic acidosis. Treatment of metabolic acidosis in this situation often requires the judicious use of bicarbonate, unlike the situation in uncomplicated hypovolaemic shock where correction of circulating volume usually results in prompt reversal of acidosis without the need for bicarbonate.

Monitoring and treatment

All patients should have an ECG monitored continuously to detect any arrhythmias and also to look for evidence of extension of myocardial damage. Insertion of a PAFC is obligatory if therapy is to be sensibly directed. A PAFC allows a wide variety of measurement, as listed in the 'Hypovolaemic shock' section, and is also of special value in patients with cardiogenic shock who have developed a new systolic murmur. During insertion of the PAFC, blood can be sampled from the right atrium and right ventricle and analysed for oxygen saturation, to detect any significant intracardiac left to right shunt, and once inserted monitoring of pulmonary artery occlusion pressure (PAOP) tracing may show giant V-waves. In a patient with a new systolic murmur, these findings would be in keeping with a ventricular septal defect or prolapse of the mitral valve.

Assessment of the PAOP also allows identification of a subgroup of patients who will benefit from volume expansion. If PAOP is < 20 mmHg then it is appropriate to give fluid challenges, monitoring the response of PAOP. An important cause of low left-sided filling pressures is right ventricular infarction which, as stated earlier, can complicate ARDS. In right ventricular infarction the clinical picture is one of distension of the neck veins, elevation of right atrial pressure (CVP) and normal or low left-sided filling pressure (PAOP). When cardiac output does not improve with fluid loading alone then inotropic agents are indicated; dobutamine appears to be the agent of choice in this situation.

Vasodilator therapy may be indicated in some patients. Sodium nitroprusside tends to have a predominantly arterial dilator effect and can be used to reduce afterload, while nitroglycerine has predominantly a venodilator effect and also improves coronary artery perfusion. In many cases, however, arterial hypotension is also present and precludes the use of vasodilator therapy. As outlined in the section on 'Hypovolaemic shock', the impact of any pharmacological intervention on cardiac output and oxygen delivery must be assessed. It is inadequate to look at the response of a single variable such as arterial pressure or CVP.

In a subgroup of patients cardiogenic shock develops following a myocardial infarction because of mechanical defects, and surgery is indicated. Such defects would include rupture of the interventricular septum, and rupture or ischaemic malfunction of a papillary muscle resulting in acute mitral valve dysfunction. Ventricular septal defects most often occur following anteroapical infarcts involving occlusion of the left anterior descending artery, while papillary muscle dysfunction is more usually seen following inferobasilar infarcts. Both of these complications may occur early following infarction but more typically occur 7–10 days later. In patients recovering from significant myocardial infarction, sudden deterioration into cardiogenic shock with pulmonary oedema and the finding of a new systolic murmur should alert the clinician to the possibility of these mechanical complications.

As already mentioned, the diagnosis may be made by the insertion of a PAFC. Blood sampled from the right atrium, right ventricle and pulmonary artery can be analysed for oxygen saturation. The finding of a step-up in oxygen saturation from right atrium to right ventricle would confirm the presence of a left-to-right shunt secondary to a ventricular septal rupture. If

monitoring of the PAOP trace shows large V-waves (analogous to 'cannon' waves on CVP monitoring) this would strongly suggest mitral valve dysfunction.

These patients should be aggressively treated and further investigated using echocardiography and formal cardiac catheterization. Virtually all postinfarction ventricular ruptures and ruptures of papillary muscle should be treated surgically, unless other factors make the patient an inappropriate candidate. However, patients whose mitral insufficiency is due to papillary muscle dysfunction, rather than rupture, need to undergo further assessment, including echocardiographic assessment of ventricular contractility and degree of annuloventricular dilatation.

The third, and largest, group of patients with cardiogenic shock are those who neither respond to volume loading nor have mechanical defects. Such patients have pump failure due to significant loss of functioning left ventricular myocardial mass, either acutely from a single massive infarct or accumulatively from a series of infarcts. At first sight aggressive treatment of such a group of patients would seem inappropriate. Indeed, aggressive treatment is based on the concept that part of the non-functioning myocardium lies in an area of reversible ischaemia. Some of the patients should be assessed and considered for aortocoronary bypass or cardiac transplantation.

In summary, cardiogenic shock occurs in approximately 7% of patients following acute myocardial infarction. In patients presenting to an accident department with circulatory shock, it is essential to recognize early the subgroup of patients with a primary myocardial cause for their shock, thus allowing early transfer to a coronary care unit for further management. During the intensive care management of patients with sepsis and ARDS the possibility of right ventricular infarction should be borne in mind in a patient who deteriorates suddenly, with a high CVP and a normal or low PAOP.

Sepsis

Unlike the situation with hypovolaemia and cardiogenic shock, the pathophysiology of sepsis is currently incompletely understood, although major advances have been made recently and it remains the subject of ongoing research. Sepsis is a very common condition, although because of difficulty with terminology and diagnosis its precise incidence is uncertain. It has been estimated that there are 350 000 cases of 'septic shock' each year in the USA, with up to 150 000 patients dying of the condition. Over the past few decades, the term septic shock has commonly been used to describe the state of circulatory shock associated with Gram-negative bacterial infections, but now the concept of sepsis is extending; in particular, the concept of 'non-bacterial sepsis' has been recognized. The term 'septic shock' is probably inadequate as a description of patients with sepsis, because of the long-standing association between the term and Gram-negative bacter-aemia and also because patients with early sepsis do not exhibit the features of low-output shock (as listed above), and therefore cannot meet the clinical criteria laid down for the diagnosis of septic shock. No single diagnostic term has been described with a definition that covers all patients with sepsis, although the term 'sepsis syndrome' comes close.

Definitions

Although not universally accepted, the following defi-nitions of terms used in the description of patients with sepsis may be useful.

Bacteraemia

This term merely indicates the presence of microorganisms in the bloodstream. For most organisms a single positive blood culture is ade-quate. Further positive blood cultures may be required before bacteraemia can be confidently diagnosed, in situations where *Staphylococcus epidermidis* or other organisms that may be skin commensals are isolated.

Septicaemia

This is to a confusing term, with no discrete meaning, which should be dropped from com-mon usage. It is generally taken to refer to the acute, toxic state produced by microorganisms, their toxins or secondary mediators, in response to an invasive infec-tion. It need not necessarily indicate the presence of bacteraemia.

Systemic inflammatory response syndrome

This term was introduced to describe the clinical features seen in patients exhibiting a systemic toxic response. Since the presence of bacteraemia, or proof of a significant infected source, is not required as part of the diagnosis, systemic inflam-matory response syndrome (SIRS) covers the group of patients suffering from non-bacterial sepsis. The crite-ria used for the definition of SIRS have been described by Bone *et al.* (1992) as follows:

- temperature >38°C or <36°C
- heart rate >90 beats/min
- respiratory rate >20 breaths/min or Pa,CO_2 <32 mmHg
- white blood cell count >12 000/mm^3, <4000/mm^3 or >10% immature forms.

An important factor in this definition is that the patient should be considered to have clinical evidence of infection but need not be proved to be infected. Sepsis can now be defined as SIRS in a patient with a confirmed infection.

Septic shock

A number of different definitions has been used for septic shock in the past. **Currently, it can be defined as sepsis (SIRS + infection) with a systolic blood pressure <90 mmHg or a drop of >30 mmHg.**

Table 19.2 Clinical features of sepsis

Early	Late
Restlessness and slight confusion	Decreased conscious level
Tachypnoea	Tachypnoea
Tachycardia	Tachycardia
CVP maintained	**CVP low**
Low SVR	**High SVR**
High cardiac output	**Low cardiac output**
Systolic BP normal or slightly decreased	**Systolic BP < 90 mmHg**
Oliguria	Oliguria
Elevated blood lactate	Elevated blood lactate
Warm dry suffused extremities	**Cold extremities**

BP, blood pressure; CVP, central venous pressure; SVR, systemic vascular resistance.

Bold type indicates the main differences between early and late features.

Mortality from sepsis

Quoted mortality rates in bacteraemia, sepsis and sep-tic shock are widely different, as would be expected. In septic shock the mortality rate is high, ranging from 40 to 90% in previously published series. In a single large series looking at patients with Gram-negative bacter-aemia, the mortality rate was less than 10% in the absence of shock, whereas in bacteraemic patients with shock (i.e. septic shock) the mortality rate was 47%.

Clinical features of sepsis

The clinical features of sepsis can usefully be consid-ered in two groups, **early** and **late**, as listed in Table 19.2. In fact, the clinical features listed as early and late in Table 19.2 represent opposite ends of a spectrum and, depending on the timing of diagnosis, aggressive-ness of resuscitation and use of vasoconstrictor agents a given patient may, at different stages, exhibit differing features. It should be appreciated that the clinical fea-tures in the early stages of sepsis are rather subtle, mak-ing diagnosis difficult in the absence of invasive monitoring using a PAFC. Such a patient may look remarkably well, owing to the pink, well-perfused extremities. A high index of suspicion is required to diagnose sepsis at an early stage. In the postoperative patient the early diagnosis of sepsis often depends on measurement of blood gases or blood lactate, and it is all too easy for inexperienced personnel to treat restlessness with sedation, rather than appropriate resuscitative manoeuvres.

Changes in core temperature with sepsis are variable. An infected patient may well present with pyrexia. However, in the presence of a cool ambient tempera-ture, peripheral vasodilatation can lead to excessive heat loss and a fall in core temperature. Thus, at the time of presentation, a patient with sepsis may be either hypothermic or hyperthermic. In either situation, monitoring of the core–peripheral temperature gradient can be useful.

In Table 19.2 high SVR and low cardiac output are listed as late clinical features, and this requires further explanation. It is certainly true that in patients who present late, cardiac output tends to be low. However, with aggressive resuscitation, it is virtually always possible to elevate cardiac output, to an above-normal level. It is now recognized that a low cardiac output, in an aggressively resuscitated patient, is a late, end-stage feature, occurring prior to the demise of the patient. In a patient presenting late, it is true that calculated SVR may be higher. This does not mean that vasoconstriction has occurred; it is merely the result of the fall in cardiac output, since the value of SVR is calculated and not measured ($SVR = (MAP–CVP)/CO$).

The early features of sepsis are predominantly due to peripheral vasodilatation and redistribution of blood flow. The low SVR leads to a reflex increase in cardiac output and thus blood pressure is maintained. The later features begin to resemble the features of classical low-output shock (listed above), the change being due either to failure of the heart to maintain an elevated output appropriate to the fall in afterload, or secondary hypovolaemia. Myocardial failure in this situation is relative, since the output may be extremely high, but may be due to either pre-existing coronary artery disease or the release of myocardial depressant substances. Secondary hypovolaemia occurs as a result of fluid losses from the vascular space as a result of increased capillary permeability. These two factors (cardiac decompensation and secondary hypovolaemia) explain the changes from early to late features listed in bold type in Table 19.2.

Pathophysiology

It is generally agreed that the complicated pathophysiology of sepsis is produced by a large number of primary and secondary mediators. It is also now accepted that invasion of microorganisms is only one of a number of possible triggers for mediator release. Mediators that have been implicated as playing a role in the pathophysiology of sepsis include:

- endotoxin
- TNF, PAF, nitric oxide interleukins and other cytokines
- bradykinin and other products of the contact activation system
- cyclo-oxygenase and lipo-oxygenase products (prostaglandins, leukotrienes and thromboxane)
- histamine
- β-endorphins
- myocardial depressant substances
- complement-derived anaphylotoxins (C5a, C3a).

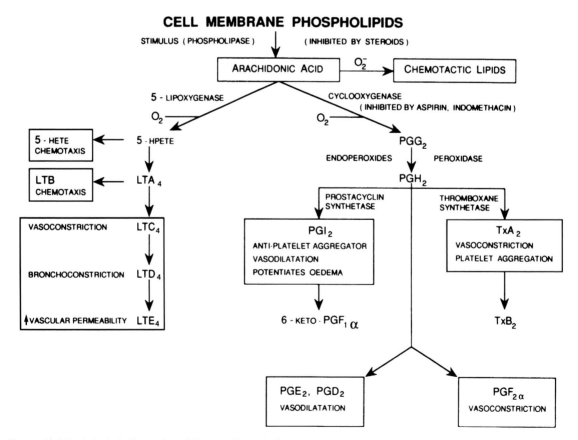

Figure 19.5 Pathological effects of arachidonic acid metabolites.

Although the precise role played by these effector substances is incompletely understood, the resulting haemodynamic changes have been well described. Interest is now focusing on the balance between proinflammatory and anti-inflammatory mediators.

Haemodynamic response to sepsis

The haemodynamic response to sepsis can usefully be considered under the headings peripheral circulatory failure, pulmonary vascular effects and direct myocardial effects.

Peripheral circulation

The primary haemodynamic response to sepsis is a decrease in SVR, with the subsequent change in cardiac output being a direct compensatory response. The fall in SVR appears to be due to loss of vascular tone and vasodilatation, particularly at a precapillary sphincter level, mainly caused by nitric oxide release. In experimental sepsis there is also some evidence of anatomical AV shunting, with blood flow being diverted away from nutrient capillaries. As in all other forms of shock the normal response to a fall in cardiac output and decreased arterial pressure would normally be sympathetic nervous activity and reflex vasoconstriction. It appears that in sepsis the vasodilatation produced by mediator release overrules this normal sympathetic response. The mediators released in sepsis include some that are potent vasoconstrictors and others that are potent vasodilators (e.g. see Figure 19.5) and it would appear that the balance of these mediators in different vascular beds also affects regional responses. Ultimately, blood flow to various organs depends on a balance of the above effects, together with the ability of the heart to maintain a high output. Typically, in human sepsis, it appears that coronary and cerebral circulation are relatively maintained while splanchnic flow is decreased, even in the presence of a hyperdynamic circulation.

In addition to vasodilatation, a number of other microcirculatory factors affects regional blood flow in sepsis: intravascular pooling, probably due to an increase in venous capacitance, microvascular sludging, partly due to a decrease in red blood cell deformability together with an increase in platelet adhesiveness, formation of cellular aggregates leading to microvascular plugging, endothelial cell swelling leading to a decrease in capillary diameter, interstitial oedema, leading to extrinsic capillary compression, due to an increase in microvascular permeability.

The increase in capillary permeability in sepsis can be very marked and generalized soft tissue oedema is often a remarkable clinical feature. When severe there is no doubt that the gross oedema can interfere with oxygen diffusion. The transcapillary escape rate of albumin has been shown to be markedly increased in sepsis. In the absence of ARDS, the lung appears to be relatively resistant to interstitial oedema; pulmonary interstitial albumin can be mobilized and lung lymph flow can increase dramatically to counter the increased transcapillary flux. Nevertheless, in severe sepsis a degree of

ARDS is almost invariable as part of the MOF syndrome.

Pulmonary circulation

As the only organ to be perfused with virtually all of the cardiac output, the lung is probably uniquely vulnerable to the damaging effects of circulating mediators, particularly those of splanchnic origin. Within the pulmonary circulation the most obvious response is an increase in pulmonary vascular resistance. In experimental endotoxaemia this occurs within minutes of the start of endotoxin infusion and endotoxin may have a direct effect on the smooth muscle of the pulmonary vasculature, although it is more likely that secondary mediators are responsible. In terms of injury to the pulmonary vasculature, the relative contribution of leucocytes, platelets, microemboli, neurogenic influences and mediators such as prostaglandins, leukotrienes, alveolar macrophages, oxygen radicals and complement is unclear. It is known that neutrophil aggregation in the lung capillaries is an important mechanism of damage. After this initial aggregation the capillary damage may result from oxygen free radicals released by the activated white cells. These include superoxides and peroxides, which inactivate proteins, cause lipid peroxidation, destroy nucleic acids and kill cells. Proteases, including elastase, are also released and may damage structural proteins and cleave circulating proteins including Hageman factor, fibrinogen, complement and fibronectin. Damage to basement membrane fibronectin, by proteases, will also contribute to permeability changes.

In prolonged sepsis changes in pulmonary vascular resistance leading to high pulmonary artery pressures can place considerable strain on the right ventricle, culminating in some cases in right ventricular infarction.

Direct myocardial effects

Impaired ventricular function is an important factor in fatal cases of sepsis. It may seem inappropriate to talk of cardiac dysfunction in a situation where cardiac output may be up to four or even five times the normal level, but decreases in myocardial contractility have been well demonstrated in sepsis.

In cases of pre-existing coronary artery disease, myocardial impairment may result from the increase in myocardial oxygen demand that occurs as a result of the increase in cardiac output in response to a low SVR. It has been demonstrated that left ventricular dilatation and a decrease in ventricular ejection fraction occur, with a return to normal in patients recovering from sepsis. ARDS and intermittent positive pressure ventilation, particularly with the use of PEEP, can also change ventricular compliance, by altering the volume–pressure relationship of ventricular filling. Increases in capillary permeability have already been stated to lead to generalized peripheral oedema, and myocardial oedema can also contribute to myocardial dysfunction. Finally, myocardial depressant substances can be released from the splanchnic bed during sepsis.

Delivery

In the treatment of sepsis, as with all other forms of shock, the ultimate aim is to restore adequate oxygen delivery to the tissues. Systemic oxygen delivery (Do_2) can be calculated as follows: $Do_2 = CO \times$ arterial content.

The amount of oxygen in whole blood includes that bound to haemoglobin (1.38 ml O_2/g of haemoglobin) and an almost negligible amount dissolved in plasma (0.003 ml/mmHg of oxygen tension). Arterial oxygen content is therefore (1.38 × Hb concentration × Hb saturation) + (0.003 × Pa,o_2). In a clinical situation the second component of this equation is excluded, because of the negligible contribution to the total. Since Do_2 is dependent on cardiac output and arterial oxygen content, one can understand the problems with Do_2 that occur in various forms of shock. In both cardiogenic and hypovolaemic shock the cardiac output is reduced, thus reducing Do_2. In addition, problems with gas exchange may occur as a result of pulmonary oedema or intrapulmonary shunting, respectively, leading to a decrease in arterial oxygen content. Haemorrhage will have a profound effect on both cardiac output and arterial oxygen content, through a decrease in haemoglobin. In sepsis, with a hyperdynamic circulation, Do_2 may be grossly elevated and yet still appear to be inadequate for the demands of the tissues, as evidenced by a high blood lactate. In sepsis, problems with Do_2 may arise in a number of areas: systemically arterial content may be reduced because of ARDS; regionally, there may be marked differences in quantitative blood flow, for instance with relative splanchnic vasoconstriction; in the microcirculation all of the factors previously listed, including microvascular sludging and AV shunting, are important; and there is some evidence of a primary inability of cells to utilize oxygen as a result of changes at a mitochondrial level.

Inadequate oxygen consumption (Vo_2) is present in all forms of shock, but quantification of the inadequacy of Vo_2 in sepsis may be difficult to determine.

Gut failure and sepsis

Until relatively recently it was assumed that all patients with septic shock were suffering from infection, usually Gram-negative bacteraemia. However, it was always recognized that at the time of presentation less than 50% of patients with septic shock had positive blood cultures. In addition, when quantitative endotoxin assays came into use, it was discovered that endotoxin levels in systemic blood bore no relationship to the presence of organisms, and that furthermore, endotoxin was found in patients with Gram-positive bacteraemia, fungaemia and in culture-negative patients, as well as in patients with Gram-negative bacteraemia. It has also been shown that in patients with prolonged severe sepsis who develop MOF, endotoxin levels in the systemic blood correlate with deterioration of hepatic function. These factors, together with other pieces of evidence, have led to the hypothesis that endotoxin translocation

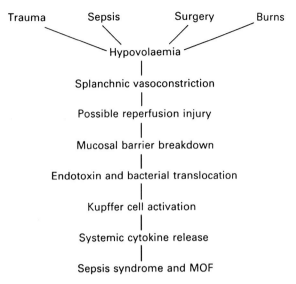

Figure 19.6 Gut-barrier failure and the production of 'non-bacterial' sepsis and MOF: a proposed hypothesis.

from the gastrointestinal tract may play an important role in the triggering of both sepsis syndrome and MOF, as a result of what has become known as gut-barrier failure. In brief, gut-barrier failure represents a breakdown in the mucosal barrier to translocation of both endotoxin and intact organisms from the gastrointestinal tract into the portal circulation or lymphatic system. As detailed above, hypovolaemia can lead to an acute ischaemic–hypoxic gut injury and it has been shown that endotoxin translocation occurs within hours of both haemorrhage and trauma. More chronically, factors such as lack of enteral nutrition can also lead to loss of gut mucosal barrier function. However, translocation of endotoxin was also shown to occur in healthy volunteers and in surgical patients without complications. Recent studies indicate that the release of inflammatory mediators from the ischaemic–reperfused area may be more important than endotoxin.

The hepatic circulation is compromised by the same factors that lead to splanchnic vasoconstriction, since 80% of liver blood flow is comprised of portal venous flow. Hepatic ischaemia, together with other factors such as jaundice, can lead to a failure of hepatic filtration, allowing translocated organisms or endotoxin to spill over into the systemic circulation. Perhaps more importantly, endotoxin and inflammatory mediators in the portal circulation can activate the fixed macrophage population (Kupffer cells) within the liver, leading to systemic cytokine release. Although it remains controversial, it is possible that endotoxin translocation secondary to gut-barrier failure, leading to Kupffer cell activation with cytokine release or direct cytokine release from the gut, is responsible for both the sepsis syndrome and subsequent MOF. A proposed scheme for this hypothesis is illustrated in Figure 19.6.

Treatment of sepsis

Resuscitation and early management of a patient with sepsis follows the same principles as those outlined in the section on hypovolaemia. In addition, patients with sepsis tend to follow a prolonged course, within intensive care, frequently developing MOF and requiring individual organ support. For instance, prolonged mechanical ventilation, enteral or parenteral nutrition, haemofiltration and/or haemodialysis for renal support and inotropic support for the cardiovascular system are all frequently required.

Virtually all patients with sepsis will require insertion of a PAFC, allowing measurement of oxygen delivery and consumption. In a situation where respiratory, cardiac and peripheral circulatory factors can all affect oxygen delivery and consumption, it is imperative to measure the effect of any change in therapy on oxygen transport. For instance, administration of a vasoconstrictor may elevate arterial pressure but adversely affect oxygen delivery and consumption. Addition of PEEP, in a ventilated patient, can improve oxygenation but may adversely affect cardiac output, through an effect on ventricular filling and compliance. It is no longer adequate to resuscitate a patient to normal blood pressure, heart rate and CVP. It is not even acceptable to monitor the effect on cardiac output alone. It is imperative, in such critically ill patients, to obtain some indication of the adequacy of tissue perfusion. Gut tonometry seems to be a useful technique in this regard. The precise levels of oxygen delivery and consumption, which should be aimed for, cannot be defined and vary for individual patients with time. If, on increasing Do_2 levels, blood lactate is also seen to return to normal, then it is likely that Do_2 is adequate for that patient at that time.

Until recently, direct therapy for sepsis consisted of antibiotics and, where possible, surgical eradication of the septic focus. Appropriate antibiotic therapy has been shown to be important in preventing the onset of sepsis in infected patients. However, in patients with fully established septic shock, antibiotics have remarkably little effect on outcome. It has been well demonstrated that in patients in whom a septic focus is found, which is surgically eradicable, outcome will be better than in a group of patients with no identifiable focus or in whom the focus of sepsis is not amenable to surgical treatment (e.g. pneumonia). For this reason it is imperative to make a careful search for any potential focus of infection; this may be particularly difficult in cases of intra-abdominal infection. However, as has already been stressed, not every patient with sepsis will be infected and in that situation therapy is primarily directed at maximizing oxygen transport and minimizing regional deficiencies in perfusion, particularly in the splanchnic circulation. For this latter group, gastric tonometry may be the monitoring tool of choice. Currently, there is a great deal of interest in the development of treatment aimed at reversing the exaggerated inflammatory response during sepsis. Results of trials with single-agent therapies have been dis-appointing, but a future role for these substances may be found in combining multiple agents in the therapy of sepsis. In terms of prevention, it would seem essential, in patients suffering from hypovolaemia or trauma, to concentrate on early and aggressive resuscitation in order to avoid an ischaemic hypoxic insult to the splanchnic bed and thus avoid gut failure.

Summary

Sepsis should be thought of as a state of excessive macrophage activation, with cytokine release and subsequent activation of complex mediator cascades. There is clearly a large number of triggers for this macrophage activation, of which infection is only one. It is now appreciated that endotoxin, perhaps of gut origin, and other mediators released by tissue damage can lead to what has become known as non-bacterial sepsis. A careful search for infection remains essential in all patients presenting with sepsis.

In all forms of shock, cell damage is due to an ischaemic hypoxic injury. The primary aim of resuscitation and therapy is to restore adequate oxygen delivery for tissue needs and to control the initiating factor, whether this be pump failure, hypovolaemia, haemorrhage or infection.

Section 19.3 • Intensive care management

Intensive care owes its origins to the advent of positive pressure ventilation in the treatment of respiratory failure due to poliomyelitis, and subsequently traumatic flail chest. The finding that those patients requiring respiratory support were most effectively managed in a single area of a hospital led to the development of assisted ventilation units, which in time evolved into ICUs. Intensive care is a major integral component in the management of many surgical patients. Successful intensive care management requires the combined efforts of specialist intensivists and surgeons.

Role of the intensive care unit

Hospitals admitting acute medical and surgical patients should have an ICU, the purpose of which is to provide intensive monitoring and support of patients with organ failure or failures. The most commonly supported organ is the lung, but facilities should be provided for the diagnosis, monitoring and treatment of other organ dysfunctions. In smaller hospitals where the volume of workload is insufficient to justify a dedicated ICU, facilities should be available for the transport of critically ill patients to a hospital equipped with an ICU.

Intensive care is appropriate for patients:

- requiring or likely to require advanced respiratory support (ventilation)
- requiring the support of two or more organ systems, e.g. circulatory shock and acute renal failure

Table 19.3 Categories of organ system monitoring and support

1. Advanced respiratory support
- Mechanical ventilatory support (excluding mask continuous positive airways pressure (CPAP) or non-invasive, e.g. mask ventilation)
- The possibility of a sudden, precipitous deterioration in respiratory function requiring immediate endotracheal intubation and mechanical ventilation

2. Basic respiratory monitoring and support
- The need for more than 40% oxygen via a fixed performance mask
- The possibility of progressive deterioration to the point of needing advanced respiratory support (see above)
- The need for physiotherapy to clear secretions at least two-hourly, whether via a tracheostomy or minitracheostomy, or in the absence of an artificial airway
- Patients recently extubated after a prolonged period of intubation and mechanical ventilation
- The need for mask CPAP or non-invasive ventilation
- Patients who are intubated to protect the airway, but needing no ventilatory support and who are otherwise stable

3. Circulatory support
- The need for vasoactive drugs to support arterial pressure or cardiac output
- Support for circulatory instability due to hypovolaemia from any cause and which is unresponsive to modest volume replacement. This will include, but not be limited to, postsurgical or gastrointestinal haemorrhage or haemorrhage related to a coagulopathy
- Patients resuscitated following cardiac arrest where intensive or high-dependency care is considered clinically appropriate

4. Neurological monitoring and support
- Central nervous system depression, from whatever cause, sufficient to prejudice the airway and protective reflexes
- Invasive neurological monitoring

5. Renal support
- The need for acute renal replacement therapy (haemodialysis, haemofiltration or haemodiafiltration)

with chronic impairment of one or more organ systems who also require support for an acute failure of another system.

In the postoperative situation, a patient may require intensive care in the following circumstances:

- when an operation causes major physiological disturbance requiring close monitoring and/or organ support (e.g. major cardiac surgery)
- when an unexpected major medical or surgical complication occurs during surgery, threatening organ dysfunction (e.g. intraoperative haemorrhage or myocardial infarction)
- when previous intercurrent disease compromises physiological reserve (e.g. patient with severe chronic obstructive pulmonary disease undergoes major abdominal surgery).

The critically ill patient is much more dependent on nursing and medical care than are other hospital patients and therefore requires a much higher intensity and standard of care. In general, each patient should have one nurse at the bedside continuously. This requires the employment of about seven full-time equivalents to staff a bed (Intensive Care Society), a major contributor to the cost of intensive care. Medical cover should be provided by a dedicated resident doctor, supported by a designated consultant immediately available 24 h/day.

Role of the high-dependency unit

Many patients undergoing planned major surgery who previously received postoperative intensive care are now treated in the recovery room until airway, breathing and circulation are stable, and subsequently in the high-dependency unit (HDU). This approach often requires an equal or even greater medical input in the form of, for example, epidural analgesia, but is more

Table 19.4 Indications for admission to intensive care and high-dependency units

Intensive care is appropriate for:	High-dependency care is appropriate for:
Patients requiring or likely to require advanced respiratory support alone[a]	Patients requiring support for a single failing organ system, but excluding those needing advanced respiratory support[a]
Patients requiring support of two or more organ systems[a]	Patients who can benefit from more detailed observation or monitoring than can safely be provided on a general ward
Patients with chronic impairment of one or more organ systems sufficient to restrict daily activities (comorbidity) and who require support for an acute reversible failure of another organ system[a]	Patients no longer needing intensive care, but who are not yet well enough to be returned to a general ward
	Postoperative patients who need close monitoring for longer than a few hours

[a]See Table 19.3 for the categories of organ system monitoring and support.

Table 19.5 Definitions

◻ **Sepsis: the systemic response to infection, manifested by two or more of the following as a result of infection:**
- Temperature > 38°C or < 36°C
- Heart rate > 90 bpm
- Respiratory rate > 20 breaths/min or hyperventilation (Pa,co_2 < 4.25 kPa; 32 mmHg)
- WBC > 12×10^9/l or < 4×10^9/l or presence of > 10% immature neutrophils

◻ **Severe sepsis[a]: sepsis (as defined above) plus evidence of inadequate organ perfusion or organ dysfunction: one of the following:**
- Acute alteration in mental status
- Hypoxaemia: Po_2 < 9.5 kPa (overt pulmonary disease not the cause of hypoxaemia)
- Hyperlactataemia
- Oliguria (urine output < 0.5 ml/kg/h)
- Hypotension

◻ **Septic shock: sepsis-induced hypotension (systolic BP < 90 mmHg OR reduction of ≥ 40 mmHg despite adequate fluid resuscitation**

◻ **Systemic inflammatory response syndrome (SIRS): systemic inflammatory response to a variety of severe clinical insults. Two or more of the criteria of sepsis (as defined above)**
In the setting of a known cause of endothelial inflammation such as:
- Infection
- Pancreatitis
- Ischaemia
- Multiple trauma and tissue injury
- Haemorrhagic shock
- Immune-mediated organ injury

◻ **Multiple organ dysfunction syndrome (MODS)[b]: presence of altered organ function in an acutely ill patient such that homeostasis cannot be maintained without intervention**

[a]Previously described as sepsis syndrome.
[b]More generally known as multiple organ failure (MOF).

---

economical in terms of nurse staffing. The HDU generally requires one nurse per two patients, compared with one-to-one nursing in the ICU. In general, ventilation would not be carried out in an HDU, but other support of a single-organ dysfunction could be managed (Tables 19.3 and 19.4).

Systemic inflammatory response syndrome and multiple organ failure

The major causes of morbidity and mortality in critically ill patients who require intensive care are sepsis and SIRS. SIRS, which may be a sequela of major surgery, trauma, shock and hypoxia, is a clinical response indistinguishable from sepsis in the absence of an infecting organism (Table 19.5). The precise aetiology of SIRS is not yet defined, but one likely factor is splanchnic hypoperfusion, resulting in gut ischaemia with mucosal permeability and translocation of organisms from the gastrointestinal tract lumen into the portal venous and lymphatic circulations. The subsequent release of inflammatory mediators, including cytokines (e.g. interleukin-1, TNF) from hepatic Kupffer cells and other macrophages or circulating monocytes, initiates a sequence of events culminating acutely in the clinical signs of sepsis or septic shock, and thereafter in MOF. Factors implicated in the pathogenesis of MOF include inadequate tissue oxygen delivery, sequestration of neutrophils, damage to vascular endothelium and release of vasoactive substances (e.g. nitric oxide, endothelin, prostacyclin, thromboxane), with resultant loss of

microvascular regulation. Cellular dysfunction also results, with failure of oxygen utilization.

Identification of the critically ill patient requiring intensive care management

There is evidence that early recognition and preventive intensive care management is beneficial in terms of patient outcome. It may be that pressure on ICU beds dictates that patients with potential but not yet established organ dysfunction cannot be accommodated in ICU, but they should be managed aggressively to forestall and treat organ dysfunction.

The following situations would indicate a requirement for patients to be assessed for intensive care management.

Cardiovascular system:
◻ cardiac arrest (unless circulation rapidly restored with return of consciousness)
◻ signs of shock: tachycardia and/or hypotension not responsive to volume resuscitation
◻ evidence of tissue hypoperfusion/hypoxia: clinically poor peripheral perfusion; metabolic acidosis, hyperlactataemia
◻ diminished conscious level
◻ poor urine output (< 0.5 ml/kg/h).

Respiratory system:
◻ threatened or obstructed airway, e.g. due to diminished conscious level
◻ respiratory arrest/ respiratory rate < 8 breaths/min

- tachypnoea: respiratory rate > 35 breaths/min; respiratory distress
- Sp,O_2 < 90% on high-flow (> 60%) oxygen
- rising Pa,CO_2 compromising conscious level (generally > 8 kPa or > 2 kPa above the patient's 'normal' level, with respiratory acidosis).

Renal:

- renal failure is a frequent complication of respiratory or cardiovascular failure and its development should dictate early ICU admission for prompt cardiorespiratory resuscitation to restore renal perfusion and oxygen delivery. ICU is also the appropriate setting for renal replacement therapy, generally haemofiltration in patients with MOF.

Neurological:

- threatened or obstructed airway
- absent gag/cough
- failure to maintain normal Pa,O_2 and Pa,CO_2
- failure to obey commands
- management of raised intracranial pressure
- status epilepticus: prolonged/recurrent seizures failing to respond to conventional anticonvulsant therapy.

Referral to the intensive care unit

In general, ICU management is led by a specialist intensive care team. With the development of the specialty of intensive care medicine in many Western countries, this team is led by a consultant trained in the specialty, and in general the patient referred to ICU will be seen by a senior member of the team.

Transfer and admission to the intensive care unit

Following agreement to admit to the ICU, the patient's condition will be assessed with respect to stability for transfer to the ICU. In situations where transfer to another hospital is involved, the assessment, resuscitation, monitoring and transport assume major importance.

Monitoring of ECG, Sp,O_2 and blood pressure should be instituted in the ward, theatre or accident and emergency department where the patient is located. Correction of hypoxaemia to an acceptable level (Pa,O_2 10–12 kPa) with mask (and reservoir bag if necessary) or endotracheal intubation and ventilation is essential before moving the patient. Intubation, while often essential, may be extremely hazardous in the critically ill patient with cardiovascular and respiratory failure. Continuous monitoring, particularly of ECG and blood pressure, preferably with an indwelling arterial cannula prior to intubation, is essential, and resuscitation drugs should be available.

Gross hypovolaemia and hypotension should be immediately corrected and this may require CVP monitoring prior to transport to the ICU. In hypotensive patients not responding to volume resuscitation,

vasoactive therapy (e.g. adrenaline or dopamine infusion) may be required before transfer to the ICU.

Every ICU should have equipment for transfer of the critically ill patient, including a battery-driven monitor (ECG, invasive and non-invasive blood pressure, Sp,O_2, end-tidal PCO_2), transport ventilator driven from an oxygen cylinder, infusion pumps, resuscitation equipment, anaesthetic and resuscitation drugs.

Admission assessment and day-to-day management in the intensive care unit

On arrival in the ICU the patient should have a full assessment, including a review of past medical history and the events leading up to admission. Sometimes stabilization of the patient will take priority (see above). This should follow the basic principles of airway, breathing and circulation. Uncertainty of diagnosis should not impede this process. A management plan should then be formulated and communicated to other staff. Relatives should be kept fully informed as they may be under considerable stress at this time.

Monitoring

Monitoring should be applied as soon as the patient arrives in the ICU and should be continued throughout the stay. Recordings should be made at least hourly. The data are manually entered on to a specially designed 24-h chart, which records all physiological variables, fluid prescription and balance. With advances in information technology the role of computers in gathering and recording this data is increasing. Physiological changes can occur rapidly and may need prompt action or alterations in therapy.

Electrocardiograph: heart rate, rhythm, QRS and ST segment changes.

Direct intra-arterial blood pressure monitoring: an arterial cannula allows continuous accurate blood pressure measurement and arterial blood sampling avoiding frequent venepuncture. It is usually inserted in the radial artery, but in hypotensive patients this can be difficult and valuable time can be saved by inserting a femoral cannula. Brachial cannulation should be avoided since distal ischaemia is a risk. The cannula should be clearly labelled to prevent accidental drug injection. The cannula is connected to a transducer that converts the pressure into an electrical signal. This is amplified and displayed as a continuous trace with numerical values for systolic, mean and diastolic pressures. The transducer and cannula are continuously flushed with normal saline delivered from a bag pressurized to above systolic pressure. Heparin is not usually required. A flow restrictor limits flow to about 3–5 ml/h but a rapid flush can be delivered to clear the line.

Inaccuracies can result if the transducer system is incorrectly damped. Overdamping results from air bubbles or kinks, resulting in a rounded trace with underestimated systolic pressure. With a rigid system underdamping can occur, with a peaked waveform that overestimates systolic pressure.

Non-invasive blood pressure: automated non-invasive blood pressure measurements are the mainstay of HDU monitoring. They can be very accurate but are affected by movement artefact and faulty cuff positioning. They can be very inaccurate with dysrhythmias and there is a tendency to overestimate very low blood pressures, especially in sepsis, with potentially disastrous results. Shocked patients require direct arterial pressure monitoring.

Central venous pressure: a central venous line is inserted into internal jugular or subclavian vein and a pressure transducer is connected. The transducer should be zeroed at the level of the right atrium. The waveform and mean pressure should be displayed on the monitor.

Pulmonary artery catheterization: a pulmonary artery floatation catheter can be used to measure pulmonary artery pressure, pulmonary artery wedge pressure (PAWP) and cardiac output. The catheter has a balloon tip which, after insertion into superior vena cava, is inflated with about 1 ml of air. The distal lumen is used to monitor pressure. During insertion the catheter follows the flow of blood and the distinct waveforms of right atrial, right ventricular and pulmonary artery pressure are seen. Eventually, the balloon wedges in a branch of the pulmonary artery. With the proximal flow occluded the pressure trace changes as the distal lumen of the catheter now communicates with the left atrium via the pulmonary vascular bed. The measured wedge pressure is an indication of left atrial and left ventricular filling pressures, thus avoiding some of the inaccuracies of the CVP for assessment of volume status and left heart function.

The catheter can measure cardiac output by a thermodilution technique. Cold dextrose is injected through a proximal lumen and the fall in temperature is measured by a thermistor at the tip. The shape of the curve is used to compute cardiac output. Continuous thermodilution cardiac output measurements can made using a special pulmonary artery catheter, incorporating a heating element. Mixed venous oxygen saturation (Sv,O_2) can be measured by sampling from the distal lumen or continuously by oximetry catheter.

From the basic measurements many derived cardiovascular and oxygen transport variables can be calculated and used to assist diagnosis and management. Derived measurements of value include **systemic** and **pulmonary vascular resistance**, **left and right ventricular stroke work**, and **global oxygen delivery** and **consumption**. Being invasive, pulmonary artery catheters carry significant risks and must only be used when the potential benefits outweigh risks.

Complications specific to pulmonary artery catheters include:

- **life-threatening dysrhythmias**
- **endocarditis**
- **pulmonary artery rupture**
- **pulmonary infarction.**

Pulse oximetry: pulse oximetry estimates arterial oxygen saturation (Sp,O_2) by calculating relative absorption of light from two light-emitting diodes (LEDs) at different wavelengths. The process is repeated many times a second and the non-pulsatile (non-arterial) component is subtracted. Sp,O_2 is measured continuously in the ICU.

General management

Every patient should have a full daily assessment by the medical staff, which should be recorded in the case notes and which covers the following items:

- review of history
- general examination
- cardiovascular examination, noting haemodynamics, fluids and inotropes
- respiratory examination, noting ventilator settings and blood gases.
- abdomen, noting nutrition and nasogastric aspirates
- neurological examination, noting Glasgow Coma Scale and sedation level
- renal function, urine output, renal support
- fluid balance
- laboratory results
- bacteriology, antibiotic therapy
- drug therapy
- X-rays
- management plan.

Sedation

Most patients require sedation during their stay in the ICU. The main reason for this is to provide relief of anxiety and to allow tolerance of the endotracheal tube, mechanical ventilation and invasive procedures. In addition, surgical patients will usually have pain from the wound and need adequate analgesia. Neurosurgical patients may require deep sedation as part of the control of intracranial pressure. The need for sedation usually declines as the patient's condition improves, and should be reviewed regularly. Oversedation is a common problem and can inadvertently prolong the ICU stay.

The basic principle of sedation is to give a combination of hypnotic and opioid analgesics such as midazolam and morphine. Midazolam is a short-acting, water-soluble benzodiazepine. A typical dose is 1–5 mg/h. It can accumulate in the elderly and those with renal failure, particularly if given by continuous infusion. An alternative is propofol, which is an intravenous, short-acting general anaesthetic agent. Given by infusion it is an excellent sedative, with typical doses of 5–20 ml/h of a 1% solution. Its short duration of action allows rapid titration to effect and it is less prone to accumulation. This advantage is offset by higher cost. The solvent is a lipid emulsion that can result in hyperlipidaemia in higher doses and has calorific value.

The choice of opioid is important. Morphine is inexpensive and suitable for most cases. It provides analgesia with a useful sedative effect. Morphine can be used as a sole agent in a stable, calm, postsurgical patient. It is metabolized to inactive morphine 3-glucuronide and active morphine 6-glucuronide, which are excreted by the kidneys. It should be avoided in renal failure as accumulation of morphine 6-glucuronide can result in prolonged sedation. Alfentanil is a synthetic opioid with a short duration of action and little accumulation suitable for use in renal failure. It is almost devoid of sedative action but provides analgesia and tolerance of the endotracheal tube. Its short duration of action also makes it suitable when rapid recovery is required. These properties make it ideal for neurological cases.

Muscle relaxation (using neuromuscular blockers) is used less frequently than in the past, owing partly to improved sedative agents and partly to the advent of new ventilators that synchronize with the patients' respiratory efforts. Nevertheless, paralysis is still used in certain situations:

- to facilitate endotracheal intubation and initial settling on ventilation
- in patients with critical oxygenation and poor lung compliance
- in patients with raised intracranial pressure where any coughing or straining may be deleterious.

Commonly used neuromuscular blockers are atracurium or vecuronium, generally by infusion.

The level of sedation should be assessed regularly and sedation reduced when appropriate. This will allow the patient to re-establish spontaneous breathing and to be weaned from the ventilator. The patient should be awake at the time of extubation, with intact airway reflexes.

Nutrition

Critical illness is characterized by a catabolic phase in which there is liberation of glycogen-derived glucose, skeletal muscle-derived amino acids and adipose fatty acids. This is mediated by glucocorticoids, glucagon, growth hormone, prolactin and aldosterone and results in insulin resistance. In surgical patients this usually coincides with a period of fasting and gut dysfunction. The result is nutritional stress with wasting of fat and, more importantly, skeletal muscle. This, in turn, can lead to weakness and respiratory muscle fatigue. Much of the liberated amino acid is used for thermogenesis, immune function and wound healing. A well-nourished adult can withstand about 1 week of nutritional stress without feeding, after which immunodeficiency, organ dysfunction, sepsis and death can supervene. Many critically ill patients are already malnourished, accelerating this problem.

Nutrition is therefore of vital importance and should be considered as soon as the patient is haemodynamically stable. It can be given by the enteral or parenteral route. **Enteral nutrition** is less expensive and is associated with less infection than parenteral nutrition, which requires a central venous catheter for administration. In addition, there is evidence that parenteral nutrition is associated with gut mucosal atrophy, bacterial translocation and SIRS. This appears to be prevented by enteral nutrition, which provides a trophic stimulus to the gut. Enteral nutrition is usually given through a nasogastric tube. The greatest single problem in enteral feeding is failure of gastric emptying. The tube should be aspirated regularly to assess residual volume; an aspirate of greater than 200 ml in 4 h suggests gastric stasis. A feeding flow chart can be used by nurses to guide the feeding rate according to gastric residuals. Excess gastric residuals can result in regurgitation and aspiration of feed.

Parenteral nutrition is used if enteral feed is not tolerated or contraindicated. A dedicated central line is required and this should not be used for any other purpose, to reduce the risk of infection. Usually, one lumen of a multilumen catheter is used. Parenteral nutrition is either purchased in prepacked form or made up daily in the pharmacy. A standard daily bag usually has 2000 kcal as glucose and fat, 14 g nitrogen, electrolytes, vitamins and trace elements. These can be altered according to requirements. The infusion can be started at the intended rate without the need for incremental increase. Thus, nutritional targets can be met more rapidly than with enteral nutrition. Hyperglycaemia frequently occurs and some patients need an insulin infusion.

Fluid balance

Accurate information on and tight control of fluid balance is vital in the critically ill. Measurable losses from all sites should be accounted for. Fluid management should be planned on a daily basis, but with alterations on an hour-to-hour basis as circumstances dictate. Most surgical patients require a minimum of about 2000 ml intake/day, which may be nutrition. Insensible losses usually amount to about 500 ml/day, but will be increased by pyrexia, skin loss and gastrointestinal losses. Following surgery, fluid is sequestered in the tissues (third-space losses). This is due to leakage from capillaries into the extravascular space, a process triggered by trauma and sepsis and mediated by cytokines. This excess fluid is effectively lost from the circulation and needs replacement acutely. As the patient recovers the fluid is returned to the circulation and a diuresis occurs. At this time intake should be reduced, otherwise overload can occur.

Cardiovascular failure (circulatory shock)

The pathophysiology and management of shock have been discussed in greater detail elsewhere. In the context of the surgical patient, who is frequently elderly and suffering from pre-existing cardiovascular disease, it should be noted that a number of factors may contribute to the development of shock, complicating accurate diagnosis and management. It is also extremely important to recognize that differing aetiology and differing levels of metabolic demand and physiological reserve may dictate very different therapeutic goals in individual patients.

Shock cannot be absolutely defined by a single level of blood pressure or cardiac output (CO), and indeed may best be defined by the presence of tissue hypoxia, which if uncorrected will lead to MOF. Indicators of tissue hypoxia include a metabolic acidosis, hyper-lactataemia (lactate > 2 mmol/l), evidence of end-organ dysfunction, e.g. oliguria, or more controversially signs of regional hypoperfusion, e.g. gastric intra-mucosal acidosis. Absence or clearance of lactic acidosis does not exclude the presence of shock, but is nevertheless a favourable prognostic sign.

Volume resuscitation

Restoration of circulating volume is a prerequisite to the optimization of CO and hence tissue oxygen delivery (D_{O_2}), but is hard to measure precisely. In the non-septic patient, and even in some septic patients where vasoregulation is intact, lower limb temperature, and in particular the level of interface between warm, well-perfused and cool skin is an excellent guide to venous filling.

The traditional measure of right heart filling, CVP measurement, can be confusing as a measure of circulating volume since it is influenced by:

- venous tone
- right heart function: sepsis and ARDS frequently are associated with pulmonary hypertension and right ventricular dysfunction, with resultant raised CVP even in the presence of hypovolaemia
- raised intrathoracic pressure due to IPPV.

Pulmonary artery catheterization has recently been the subject of critical reappraisal. It nevertheless remains the most practical and reproducible means of measuring CO and hence global D_{O_2}, and also provides a more precise measure of left ventricular filling and function. PAWP allows differentiation between pulmonary oedema caused by LVF or fluid overload and ARDS, but even PAWP may be misleading as an indication of circulating volume, since it may be affected by left ventricular dysfunction and pulmonary vascular tone.

Mixed venous oxygen saturation (Sv_{O_2}), sampled from the distal port of the pulmonary artery catheter or measured by an oximetry catheter, allows assessment of CO in relation to metabolic demand and is useful in managing low cardiac output shock, e.g. cardiogenic shock following myocardial infarction or cardiac surgery. In septic shock, oxygen extraction is impaired owing to microvascular shunting and cellular dysfunction, and the Sv_{O_2} measurement per se is a poor measure of tissue oxygenation.

Choice of fluid for volume restoration in the critically ill is also controversial, with colloids and, in particular, albumin being subject to critical review. Nevertheless, in the profoundly hypovolaemic patient, colloid solutions have a longer half-life in the circulation, and hence are more practical for rapid resuscitation, while in sepsis and ARDS, where capillary leak is prominent, large volumes of colloid may be required to maintain circulating volume and 5% albumin remains one of the mainstays of therapy. There is evidence that high molecular weight hydroxyethyl starch compounds may have benefits in terms of retention in the circulation.

Vasoactive therapy

The role of vasoactive therapy in shock is to correct hypotension and/or restore CO after appropriate optimization of circulating volume. Vasoactive agents can be classified according to receptor binding and physiological action (Table 19.6) and choice is determined by the cardiovascular disturbance.

In cardiogenic shock and left ventricular failure (post-myocardial infarction or neurogenic pulmonary oedema, etc.) an inodilator agent, e.g. dobutamine, is the agent of choice. However, concurrent hypovolaemia may be unmasked by the vasodilatation, with resultant hypotension. In this situation, a pulmonary artery catheter may aid management.

In septic shock varying components of hypovolaemia, vasodilatation and myocardial depression may be present, and combined α- and β-agonist activity is generally required. As first-line therapy, dopamine (which also has a DA_1 agonist activity, of doubtful relevance) is suitable, while if severe hypotension is present, adrenaline is a useful rescue therapy by a small bolus of dilute solution (1:100 000) or infusion. Noradrenaline (predominantly α-agonist; some β activity) is often the ultimate agent of choice to control the vasodilatation of septic shock, but before its introduction adequate volume status should be established clinically or more generally by measuring PAWP and cardiac output.

Table 19.6 Actions of catecholamine vasoactive agents

	Haemodynamic effect			Receptor action			
	Vasoconstriction	Inotrope	Vasodilator	α	β_1	β_2	Dopamine
Methoxamine	+++	−	−	+++	−	−	−
Noradrenaline	+++	+	−	+++	+	−	−
Adrenaline	++	++	+	++	++	+	−
Dopamine	+	++	+	+	++	+	++
Dobutamine	− (+)	+++	++	±	+++	+	−
Dopexamine	−	++	+++	−	+	++	++

Respiratory failure

Respiratory failure may be defined as an impairment of pulmonary gas exchange sufficient to cause hypoxaemia with or without hypercarbia.

This may arise before, during or after surgery. The causes of acute respiratory failure in the surgical patient are:

- ARDS
- postoperative pneumonia
- aspiration pneumonitis
- pulmonary, lobar or basal collapse
- exacerbation of chronic respiratory disease
- acute pulmonary oedema
- neuromuscular disease
- airway obstruction.

Management of respiratory failure

Oxygen therapy

Although mechanical ventilation is the most common form of organ support in the ICU, it is not needed by all patients. The inspired oxygen level should be titrated against the arterial blood gases, aiming for a Pa,o_2 of 10–12 kPa and Sp,o_2 of $> 95\%$. Many patients with SIRS hyperventilate to a low Pa,co_2 in response to a metabolic acidosis. A rising Pa,co_2 may indicate exhaustion and impending respiratory arrest. In patients with coexisting chronic respiratory disease a common mistake is to attribute this to the very rare scenario of dependency on hypoxic drive. A reduction in inspired oxygen concentration at this time can prove fatal.

Mechanical ventilation

The decision to perform tracheal intubation and ventilate is largely based on clinical criteria, rather than particular values of arterial blood gases. The indications for ventilation are:

- $Sp,o_2 < 90\%$ on $> 60\%$ oxygen
- respiratory arrest or rate < 8 breaths/min
- tachypnoea > 35 breaths/min
- sweating, fatigue
- agitation, confusion, refusal of oxygen mask
- diminished conscious level
- airway obstruction or impairment
- rising Pa,co_2
- worsening respiratory acidosis.

Mechanical ventilation requires endotracheal intubation. In the conscious patient this requires induction of anaesthesia and adequate muscle relaxation. In a hypoxic patient this can be very hazardous and needs an experienced operator. Many surgical patients arrive in the ICU from the operating theatre already ventilated.

Ventilatory support usually involves the application of intermittent positive pressure via an endotracheal tube or tracheostomy. Regular aspiration of secretions and physiotherapy is required. The underlying condition needs to be treated while the lung is supported. The endotracheal tube acts as a conduit for infection, and ventilator-associated pneumonia is a common problem.

When the patient recovers from respiratory failure the inspiratory oxygen fraction (Fi,o_2) can be reduced. When it is below 50% weaning from ventilation can be considered. Any muscle relaxants are stopped and sedation is reduced to encourage respiratory effort. After a short period of ventilation it may be possible to convert rapidly to spontaneous breathing and extubate the patient, but usually a process of weaning is required. Respiratory support is gradually reduced until the patient is performing the work of breathing.

Modes of ventilation

With the development of sophisticated electronically controlled ventilators there is an increasing range of modes of ventilation.

- **Controlled mandatory ventilation (CMV)**: this is the most basic and classic form of ventilation. A preset tidal volume is delivered at a preset rate, regardless of any patient effort. The patient may 'fight' the ventilator and require deep sedation or muscle relaxation. Traditionally, tidal volumes of 10 ml/kg are used and patients are ventilated to normocarbia. There is now an increasing awareness of the potential of ventilator damage to the lung (barotrauma) in those patients with severe respiratory failure (see below).
- **Synchronized intermittent mandatory ventilation (SIMV)**: a preset tidal volume is delivered synchronized with the patients' respiratory effort, usually detected as a small negative or 'trigger' pressure. In the absence of effort the breath is given after a set time lapse known as the SIMV period. In between mandatory breaths the patient is free to breathe, but through the ventilator circuit. It is often combined with inspiratory pressure support. SIMV can be used as a weaning mode, with the number of mandatory breaths being reduced as the patient's respiratory effort recovers.
- **Pressure support**: when patient effort is detected the machine applies a preset pressure to the airway, thus assisting inspiration. As the lungs fill, the flow decreases and the inspiratory phase is terminated. In the absence of patient effort no ventilation occurs at all, so this is only suitable for patients with adequate respiratory drive. Pressure support is an excellent mode for weaning from ventilation and can be combined with SIMV. As the patient recovers the preset pressure is reduced, titrating against tidal volume and respiratory rate.
- **Pressure control ventilation**: positive airway pressure is applied with a fixed rate. Unlike pressure support, patient effort is not required or sensed. The tidal volume depends on the resistance and compliance of the tubing, airways and lungs, and therefore needs to be observed carefully. Pressure control ventilation is used in paediatric practice to compensate for variable leaks around uncuffed endotracheal tubes and in severe respiratory failure (see below) to limit barotrauma.

Positive end expired pressure (PEEP): this is an adjunct to positive pressure ventilation. The airway pressure is never allowed to fall to zero, thus splinting the alveoli open in expiration. This aids recruitment of lung and improves matching of ventilation and perfusion. Typical values are 5–10 cmH$_2$O. This is useful in any condition where the alveoli are prone to collapse, such as in ARDS. Excessive PEEP can reduce cardiac output and blood pressure by raising intrathoracic pressure.

Continuous positive airways pressure (CPAP): this is effectively PEEP without positive pressure ventilation. The patient breathes spontaneously without assistance, but gains the benefit of airway splinting. It is used in two different situations: (i) via an endotracheal tube, when the patient has been weaned from ventilatory support but is not ready for extubation; (ii) via a tight-fitting face-mask as an alternative or a precursor to intubation and ventilation. When delivered via a ventilator it can be combined with pressure support.

Severe respiratory failure

In some cases high $Fi_{,O_2}$ does not reverse hypoxaemia owing to intrapulmonary shunting. This is typically seen in ARDS. Various strategies can be employed.

PEEP should be applied to optimize lung compliance and gas exchange, without compromising cardiac output.

Pressure control inverse ratio ventilation (PCIRV): the normal ratio of inspiration to expiration time is altered from 1:2 to 2:1. This increases mean airway pressure, thus aiding recruitment of lung units. Pressure control is used to limit peak airway pressure and small tidal volumes are used (5–7 ml/kg). This prevents barotrauma but may result in a higher $Pa_{,CO_2}$ (permissive hypercarbia), which is not usually harmful. There is some evidence that this strategy is beneficial in severe ARDS.

Prone ventilation: placing the patient prone often improves oxygenation, by redistributing blood flow to better ventilated areas. The manoeuvre can be hazardous in the unstable patient but the beneficial effects can be dramatic.

Inhaled nitric oxide: nitric oxide is a very short-acting pulmonary vasodilator. Delivered to the airway in concentrations of 1–20 parts per million, it improves blood flow to ventilated alveoli, thus improving ventilation–perfusion ratios. Significant increases in $Pa_{,O_2}$ can be achieved in some patients, although there is no evidence as yet for improvement in outcome.

Tracheostomy

A tracheostomy is often performed for long-term ventilation (> 7–10 days), although there is no set time limit. A tracheostomy has a number of advantages over an oral endotracheal tube:

- increased patient comfort
- reduced sedation requirement
- reduced dead space
- reduced resistance
- ease of access for tracheal toilet
- reduced chance of accidental extubation.

A formal surgical or percutaneous dilatational tracheostomy (PDT) can be performed. The percutaneous method is being used increasingly as it is a bedside technique, avoiding the need for transfer to the operating theatre, and can be performed by the intensivist. A needle is inserted into the trachea and a track dilated around a guidewire until it is wide enough for the tracheostomy tube. Performance of PDT under bronchoscopic control ensures correct placement.

Renal failure

In the ICU, acute renal failure is generally the result of persistent and uncorrected hypoxic, hypotensive or ischaemic insult, i.e. it complicates respiratory and/or cardiovascular failure. In the presence of pre-existing chronic renal impairment, acute renal failure may result from relatively minor ischaemia or hypotension.

The pathogenesis and treatment of acute renal failure are described elsewhere [see Module 12, Vol. I]. In the context of the ICU, the presence of oliguria, whether prerenal or renal failure, necessitates early intervention to correct hypoxaemia, hypovolaemia, hypotension and renal hypoperfusion. Invasive haemodynamic monitoring (arterial, CVP, pulmonary artery catheters) is generally indicated. There is little evidence that specific renoprotective treatments, such as low-dose dopamine, frusemide or mannitol, have additional beneficial value in restoring renal function, over and above aggressive haemodynamic resuscitation to achieve normovolaemia, normotension and an appropriate cardiac output.

Sepsis is generally implicated in acute renal failure through either global haemodynamic effects, i.e. septic shock, or local microvascular effects; for example, due to DIC or intrarenal vasoconstriction. It is essential that sepsis is adequately treated if renal function is to be restored.

Obstruction of the renal tract should always be excluded by abdominal ultrasound examination, particularly where potential obstructing lesions such as pelvic tumours may be present. If obstruction is present it should be relieved. In cases of ureteric obstruction, this will require a percutaneous nephrostomy. If renal function cannot be restored following resuscitation, renal replacement therapy needs to be instituted in the following situations:

- fluid overload, notably where pulmonary oedema threatens oxygenation
- hyperkalaemia: K > 6 mmol/l despite treatment
- uraemia: urea > 35–40 mmol/l
- severe acidosis, although this can be controlled by sodium bicarbonate.

While evidence of benefit in terms of outcome is lacking, the choice of renal replacement therapy in the ICU is pumped venovenous haemofiltration. This is associated with fewer osmotic fluid shifts and hence greater haemodynamic stability than haemodialysis, and is carried out using a double-lumen central venous catheter placed percutaneously, avoiding previous problems with vascular access. Haemofiltration should initially be continuous or semicontinuous, changing to intermittent treatments once the patient is haemodynamically stable. Outcome from MOF including acute renal failure is around 50% survival to ICU discharge, with 40% survival to discharge home. Most survivors regain renal function.

Hepatic dysfunction

Hepatic dysfunction is a common accompaniment of critical illness, being a component of MOF. Its effects contribute to the cardiovascular picture of septic shock (vasodilatation, capillary permeability) and frequently predispose to acute renal failure, ARDS and coagulopathy.

Two distinctive hepatic dysfunction syndromes present in the critically ill.

■ **Shock liver or ischaemic hepatitis** results from extreme hepatic tissue hypoxia due to either ischaemia or hypoxaemia. It is characterized histologically by centrilobular hepatocellular necrosis and may occur in severe traumatic, hypovolaemic or cardiogenic shock. Transaminase levels are often massively raised (> 1000–5000 IU/l) at an early stage, often in the first 24 h, followed by moderate hyperbilirubinaemia. There is often associated hypoglycaemia, coagulopathy and lactic acidosis. Following successful resuscitation, hepatic function generally returns to normal.
■ **Hyperbilirubinaemia (ICU jaundice)** is a frequent later accompaniment of critical illness following sepsis or trauma. It results from the failure of bilirubin transport within the liver, with a histological appearance of intrahepatic cholestasis in most cases. The bilirubin level is generally around 150–300 μmol/l (mainly conjugated) and there is a normal or only mildly elevated transaminase level. The presence and degree of jaundice appear to be associated with an increased mortality. There is no specific therapy other

than prompt resuscitation and meticulous intensive care, with emphasis on optimal multisystem support and the early institution of enteral feeding.

It is very important to exclude other causes of hepatic dysfunction, e.g. drugs and extrahepatic cholestasis. The latter should be suspected when an elevated bilirubin is accompanied by raised alkaline phosphatase. Abdominal ultrasound can aid diagnosis.

Neurological disease

A diverse range of neurological conditions require management in the ICU. In broad terms, these can be classified as:

■ **acute brain injury of diverse aetiology**: trauma, aneurysmal subarachnoid haemorrhage, ischaemic or haemorrhagic stroke, infection, vasculitis or demyelination), with resultant loss of consciousness, loss of airway reflexes and disturbance of central respiratory control
■ **peripheral neuromuscular disorders**, with consequent respiratory muscle weakness, ventilatory failure and loss of bulbar function.

Important elements of neurological intensive care include:

■ endotracheal intubation for airway protection
■ maintenance of normal Pa,O_2 and low normal Pa,CO_2 (4–4.5 kPa)
■ maintenance of cerebral perfusion pressure to maintain cerebral oxygen delivery. This demands adequate volume resuscitation and where appropriate vasoactive therapy.
■ monitoring and control of intracranial pressure.

Guide to further reading

Bone, R. C., Fisher, C. J., Clemmer, T. P. et al. (1989). Sepsis syndrome: a valid clinical entity. *Crit Care Med* **17**: 389–393.

Bone, R. C., Balk, R. A., Cerra, F. B. et al. (1992). Definitions for sepsis and organ failure and guidelines for the use of innovative therapies in sepsis. *Chest* **101**: 1644–1655.

Hinds, C. J. and Watson, J. D., eds (1995). *Intensive Care: A Concise Textbook*, 2nd edn, W.B. Saunders, Philadelphia, PA.

Oh, T. E., ed. (1996). *Intensive Care Manual*, 4th edn, Butterworth-Heinemann, Oxford.

Webb, A. R. et al., eds (1998). *Textbook of Critical Care*, Oxford University Press, Oxford.

MODULE 20

Management of patients with medical disorders

1 • Hypertension

2 • Myocardial ischaemia

3 • Arrhythmias

4 • Diabetes mellitus

5 • Hyperlipidaemia

6 • Bleeding disorders

7 • Thrombotic disorders: thrombophilia

8 • Adverse drug reactions

9 • Drug-induced disorders

10 • Drugs commonly used in surgical practice

11 • Acute psychiatric states

'I haven't asked you to make me young again. All I want is to go on getting older' – Konrad Adenauer (1876–1967)

Section 20.1 • Hypertension

Hypertension in general

Hypertension is a very common problem in the population. Precise definitions of hypertension vary from one country to another, but blood pressure values above 140–160/90–95 mmHg would generally be considered hypertension.

In the vast majority of patients, the hypertension is **essential**, but there are a few **secondary** causes, e.g. phaeochromocytoma, coarctation of aorta, hyperaldosteronism, Cushing's disease and renal artery stenosis (Table 20.1). It is important to detect these when present, as specific therapy can cure the hypertension for life, whereas for most patients antihypertensive drugs only exert lifelong containment. Antihypertensive therapy is now known to reduce the incidence of complications such as myocardial infarction, cerebrovascular accident (stroke), heart failure and renal failure. The four classes of drugs commonly used are:

- thiazide diuretics
- β-blockers
- calcium antagonists
- angiotensin converting enzyme (ACE) inhibitors.

A new class of drugs called the angiotensin II receptor antagonists is now being used more widely for the treatment of essential hypertension.

Hypertension in the surgical patient

In surgical practice hypertension is encountered in three circumstances:

- high blood pressure is discovered during routine physical examination for a surgical disorder
- patients on medical treatment for essential hypertension may develop a surgical condition that requires treatment
- surgical treatment is required for a disorder causing secondary hypertension.

Table 20.1 Types and aetiology of secondary hypertension

Cerebral	Brain tumour[a]
Endocrine	Primary aldosteronism (Conn's syndrome)[a]
	Phaeochromocytoma[a]
	Cushing's syndrome[a]
	Hyperparathyroidism[a]
Renal	Renal artery stenosis[a]
	Acute/chronic glomerulonephritis
	Pyelonephritis
	Polycystic kidneys
	Diabetes mellitus
	Polyarteritis nodosa
Vascular	Coarctation of the aorta[a]
	Porphyria
	Polycythaemia rubra vera

[a]Surgical treatment necessary or considered.

The importance of hypertension in a surgical patient mainly relates to the fact that the hypertensive patient is at higher than normal risk of having coronary artery disease. However, the risk of undeclared coronary disease is relatively low, such that even uncontrolled systemic hypertension is considered by the American College of Cardiology and the American Heart Association (ACC/AHA) Task Force as being only a low-risk clinical predictor. As discussed in the section on Myocardial Ischaemia (see below), what this means in practical terms is that only if such a patient was undergoing a high-risk surgical procedure **and** had a low functional capacity (< 4 MET) would it be desirable to carry out extra investigations before surgery. MET indicates metabolic equivalent (i.e. energy expenditure possible) and is used in estimating the activity status index (Table 20.2). These extra investigations would be the non-invasive tests of an exercise electrocardiogram (ECG) or a myocardial perfusion scan. Only if these tests gave very abnormal results would it be necessary to proceed to coronary angiography which, if very abnormal, would indicate the desirability of preoperative coronary revacularization.

Despite this, patients with preoperative hypertension are known to be more likely to show exaggerated fluctuations in blood pressure during surgery, often associated with ECG evidence of myocardial ischaemia. These blood-pressure fluctuations could be important, since intraoperative myocardial ischaemia correlates with postoperative cardiac morbidity. It follows therefore that control of blood pressure preoperatively should help to reduce the tendency to blood-pressure fluctuations during surgery and to perioperative myocardial ischaemia. This is the rationale behind ensuring that the resting blood pressure is controlled adequately prior to surgery. In some cases, this may require surgery to be delayed until blood-pressure control can be achieved.

Table 20.2 Estimated energy requirements (functional status)

Energy (MET)	Examples
> 10	Participate in strenuous sports, e.g. swimming, singles tennis, football
1–4	Can take care of oneself: eat, dress, use toilet
	Walk indoors/around house
	Walk a block or two on level ground at 3–5 km/h (2–3 mph)
	Do light work around the house, e.g. dusting, dish washing
4–10	Climb a flight of stairs or walk up a hill. Walk on level ground at 6.4 km/h (4 mph). Run a short distance
	Do heavy work around the house, e.g. scrubbing floors, lifting/moving heavy furniture
	Participate in moderate recreational activities, e.g. golf, bowling, dancing, doubles tennis

MET, metabolic equivalent.

Clinical assessment of preoperative hypertension

For this and other reasons, it is desirable that the hypertensive patient undergoes a full clinical assessment prior to surgery. This should focus on three issues. The first is a careful review of whether existing medications are controlling the blood pressure and, when necessary, additional therapy is instituted. The second key issue is to determine whether the hypertension has produced any target organ damage, especially with regard to checking the ECG changes in left ventricular hypertrophy and renal function (hypertensive renal damage). Any target organ damage increases the operative risks. The third issue is to exclude rare secondary causes of hypertension, the principal one being a phaeochromocytoma that could lead to enormous problems during surgery if it was not diagnosed beforehand. Phaeochromocytoma is not common but if it is a serious possibility in an individual patient, surgery should be delayed to ensure its exclusion. Other clues as to secondary causes of hypertension are hypokalaemia, which would alert the surgeon to the possibility of Conn's syndrome, a radial to femoral artery delay indicative of coarctation and an abdominal bruit, which might suggest renal artery stenosis.

Antihypertensive medication should be continued through the perioperative period in order to maintain control of blood pressure and prevent rebound hypertension. In particular, β-blocker therapy should not be withdrawn, even if this requires the use of parenteral β-blocker in patients unable to take oral medications. Although clonidine is rarely used nowadays, it is worth stressing that clonidine must not be stopped suddenly because rebound sympathetic activation on its withdrawal is a major problem even for a resting, unstressed individual, and it would be very dangerous for a patient to undergo surgery at the same time as clonidine withdrawal.

If blood pressure needs to be controlled more before surgery, then some manipulation of the patient's oral therapy can normally be undertaken with a successful result in a few days and hence surgery does not need to be delayed unduly. If surgery is required more urgently, rapidly acting agents, especially β-blockers, can be used to control blood pressure in a few minutes or hours.

Intraoperative management

There is an interesting paradox here in that patients with preoperative hypertension are more likely to develop intraoperative hypotension than patients who were normotensive preoperatively. The reasons for this are unclear but it could be related to the fact that many antihypertensive drugs interfere with baroreflex mechanisms that stabilize the blood pressure. Alternatively, hypertensive patients may have less inherent baroreflex activity. Whatever the mechanism, this intraoperative hypotension can be associated with perioperative cardiac events. What is difficult to know is which is the chicken and which is the egg. In other words, does intraoperative hypotension cause myocardial ischaemia or does ischaemia cause intraoperative hypotension? Thus, although intraoperative hypotension can be a problem in hypertensive patients, this is not a reason for relaxing blood-pressure control preoperatively, especially since the intraoperative hypotension may be a consequence of intraoperative ischaemia rather than the primary event.

In summary, the hypertensive patient requires careful preoperative assessment to make sure that the blood pressure is controlled and to exclude secondary causes, especially phaeochromocytoma. These may require surgery to be delayed somewhat but hypertension itself seldom causes anything more than a slight delay to surgery.

Section 20.2 • Myocardial ischaemia

Risk assessment

When it comes to operating on patients with myocardial ischaemia, the surgeon has to balance the need for the surgery against the risks of the surgery in that particular individual. Emergency surgery is undoubtedly far more risky than elective surgery because emergency surgery is, by definition, necessary irrespective of the risks. Indeed, cardiac complications are two to five times more likely to occur with emergency surgery than with elective surgery.

In balancing the risks versus the benefits of elective surgery, standardized methods should be applied. To this end, *Circulation* has recently published guidelines for perioperative cardiovascular evaluation in non-cardiac surgery. These guidelines were prepared by a joint task force of the ACC/AHA. These guidelines not only review the literature extensively but also make precise recommendations, which are directly applicable to individual patients. The original article (see 'Guide to further reading') contains a detailed literature review for readers who wish to investigate the rationale behind the guidelines below. **The risk relates to the likelihood of a serious perioperative cardiac event: myocardial infarction, heart failure or death**.

The guidelines basically divide the risk of the surgical procedure into three levels and also categorize the patients into three groups based on their individual risk factors. Table 20.3 shows which surgical procedures can be considered to have high, intermediate and low cardiac risk. This pattern follows common sense. Table 20.4 shows the clinical predictors that would be considered high, intermediate and low risk for individual patients.

The high-risk patient

Patients with high-risk clinical predictors should usually have their surgery cancelled or delayed until the cardiac problem has been investigated and appropriately treated. Investigation will often

Table 20.3 Cardiac risk stratification for non-cardiac surgical procedures

High risk	(i)	Emergency major operations, especially in the elderly
	(ii)	Aortic, peripheral and major vascular surgery
	(iii)	Anticipated prolonged surgical procedures associated with blood loss and large fluid shifts
Intermediate risk	(i)	Carotid endarterectomy
	(ii)	Intraperitoneal and intrathoracic surgery
	(iii)	Head and neck surgery
	(iv)	Orthopaedic surgery
	(v)	Prostate surgery
Low risk	(i)	Endoscopic procedures
	(ii)	Cataract surgery
	(iii)	Breast surgery
	(vi)	Superficial procedures.

Table 20.4 Clinical predictors of increased perioperative cardiovascular risks (myocardial infarction, congestive heat failure, death)

Major
Unstable coronary syndromes:
  Recent myocardial infarction[a] with evidence of important ischaemic risk by clinical symtoms or noninvasive study
  Unstable or severe angina (Canadian Class III or IV)[b]
Decompensated congestive heart failure
Significant arrythmias:
  High grade atrioventricular block
  Symptomatic ventricular arrythmias in the presence of underlying heart disease
  Supraventricular arrythmias with uncontrolled ventricular rate
Severe valvular disease

Intermediate
Mild angina pectoris (Canadian Class I and II)
Prior myocardial infraction by history or pathological Q waves
Compensated or prior congestive heart failure
Diabetes mellitus

Minor
Advanced age
Abnormal ECG (left ventricular hypertrophy, left bundle branch block, ST-T abnormalities)
Rhythm other than sinus
Low exercise capacity
History of stroke
Uncontrolled hypertension

[a]Recent MI = greater than 7 days but less than 30 days.
[b]May include patient with stable angina who are unusually sedentary.

mean coronary angiography, depending on the precise circumstances. Exactly what happens thereafter will be dictated by the findings of the cardiac investigations. It may require optimization of the patient's medical management prior to the surgery, or in certain circumstances it might necessitate coronary angioplasty or a coronary artery bypass procedure prior to the non-cardiac elective surgical procedure. Surgery in such patients is a daunting procedure and it would be appropriate to review with the patient the risks and benefits of the proposed surgery, so that he or she is fully aware, since it is only really the patient who knows how troublesome the symptoms are.

Intermediate-risk patients

For patients with medium-risk clinical predictors, it can be useful to subdivide them further on the basis of their functional capacity. The dividing line for functional capacity is at about 4 MET, which is equivalent to the ability to climb one flight of stairs or to do light housework such as washing dishes or dusting. If a patient is unable to do each of these activities, or is borderline, then it is best to perform non-invasive cardiac tests to risk stratify that particular individual further. Such non-invasive cardiac tests should also be performed if a patient with intermediate-risk clinical predictors is about to undergo a high-risk surgical procedure. For other patients with medium-risk clinical predictors but good functional capacity, non-invasive cardiac tests are not necessary as a routine.

Non-invasive cardiac testing usually refers to the performance of an exercise ECG test, which is able to assess the patient's functional capacity in more detail as well as to detect the presence of myocardial ischaemia from the ST segment changes that develop on exercise. In patients with pre-existing ST segment abnormalities that would make an exercise test difficult to interpret, or in patients unable to exercise, a myocardial perfusion scan is an alternative. Echocardiography is useful in estimating left ventricular function in angina and pressure gradients across valves in mitral and aortic valve disease. If these tests signify high risk then coronary angioplasty may be appropriate. The subsequent care of the patient will depend on the results obtained. In some cases, cancellation of the original proposed surgery will be appropriate, while in other cases, coronary revascularization or optimization of medical therapy should precede the proposed surgical procedure. In many cases, however, the more detailed cardiac tests will be reassuring and surgery can then proceed.

The low-risk patient

If patients have either low-risk or even no clinical risk predictors then it is still worth performing non-invasive cardiac tests if the patient has poor functional capacity and is due to undergo a high-risk surgical procedure. The non-invasive cardiac tests are not worthwhile if the low-risk patient is due to undergo either a low-risk or an intermediate-risk surgical procedure.

The above procedure constitutes a standardized approach to match each patient's inherent risk with the risk associated with each surgical procedure. In many clinical situations, it will be very obvious that the risk:benefit ratio of performing a certain surgical procedure in a certain patient is either very high or very low and appropriate action can be taken. When this is not the case, and the balance of risk and benefit is borderline, then detailed discussions should take place with the patient, who is the best person to make this judgement, once appraised of the facts by the surgeon.

Monitoring of the patient

When surgery is undertaken in a patient with known myocardial ischaemia, then careful surveillance should be undertaken during the perioperative period. A recent study has suggested that major benefits accrue with the use of β-blockers during the perioperative period in patients with an adverse risk profile for angina. On this basis, a strong case can be made for initiating and continuing β-blockers through the perioperative period in patients with myocardial ischaemia, assuming that there is no contraindication to β-blockade such as asthma or cardiac failure.

Several studies have shown that ST segment changes that develop during routine surgery are often missed. Computerized ST segment trend analysis is therefore extremely valuable. In addition, retrospective data have shown that perioperative ST segment changes indicative of myocardial ischaemia are the strongest independent predictor of perioperative cardiac events in high-risk surgical patients. Postoperative ST segment changes have also been shown to predict worse long-term survival in high-risk surgical patients. Therefore, the AHA/ACC Task Force recommends that computerized ST segment analysis provides increased sensitivity to detect perioperative myocardial ischaemia and may therefore identify patients who would benefit from postoperative investigations and interventions to improve their long-term prognosis. However, further research is required to establish the cost-effectiveness of computerized ST segment analysis in the reduction of perioperative morbidity.

It is also wise for high-risk surgical candidates to undergo surveillance for perioperative myocardial infarction. This should be at least an ECG at baseline, an ECG immediately after the surgical procedure and an ECG daily on the first 2 days postoperatively. Measurement of cardiac enzymes and troponins is best reserved for patients at high risk or those who demonstrate ECG or haemodynamic evidence of cardiovascular dysfunction.

Thus, multidisciplinary teamwork is required for the patient with myocardial ischaemia who is undergoing surgery. This should involve the surgeon, the anaesthetist and often a cardiologist or physician. Investigations should be tailored according to the patient's inherent cardiac risk, the risk of the surgical procedure and the necessity for the surgical procedure in the first place. In some patients, the balance of risk and benefits is fine but in the majority of patients, the balance of risk and benefit is clearly in one direction. If surgery proceeds in such high-risk patients, surveillance during the perioperative period should be intensified.

Section 20.3 • Arrhythmias

Arrhythmias in general

The important arrhythmias to the surgeon are atrial fibrillation (AF), heart block ventricular extrasystoles, ventricular tachycardia (VT) and ventricular fibrillation. Probably the most common arrhythmia is AF, which is found in 11% of elderly patients compared with a 1% incidence of complete heart block. There is a substantial risk of intracardiac emboli with AF, such that warfarin is generally indicated as prophylaxis in patients with either paroxysmal or sustained AF. It is desirable where possible to convert the rhythm back from AF to sinus rhythm. This can be achieved by d.c. cardioversion, β-blockade, amiodarone or virtually any antiarrhythmic drug (but not digoxin).

If sinus rhythm cannot be achieved, the next best option is to control the ventricular rate. AF normally produces a fast ventricular rate, which does not give the left ventricle enough time to fill and empty. Indeed, the dyspnoea and haemodynamic upset seen with AF is usually due to the fast ventricular rate and the patient feels much better if the ventricular rate is reduced to 60–100 beats/min, even if the underlying rhythm remains as AF. In order to reduce the ventricular rate, one can use digoxin, β-blockade, verapamil, diltiazem or amiodarone. Several drugs such as β-blockers and amiodarone have dual effects in that they can both convert the rhythm back to sinus rhythm and help to control the ventricular responses, even if the patient stays in AF. Other treatments will only achieve one of these aims, i.e. d.c. conversion will help to revert the AF patient back to sinus rhythm, whereas digoxin will only reduce the ventricular rate.

A common mistake is for a fast rhythm on an ECG to be misinterpreted as being sinus tachycardia when it is really fast AF or supraventricular tachycardia (SVT). A careful search should be undertaken during any tachycardia for the presence or absence of P-waves, which are present in sinus tachycardia but absent in AF. Aberrant P-waves may be present in supraventricular tachycardia but the clue to differentiating sinus tachycardia from SVT is mainly the heart rate, which is usually < 160 beats/min in sinus tachycardia. Differentiating sinus tachycardia from fast AF or SVT is crucial, since the treatment of fast AF and SVT is to slow down the heart (and change the rhythm where possible), whereas sinus tachycardia is usually a manifestation of a separate underlying problem such as pulmonary oedema or fever, and the therapy must be directed against the underlying cause rather than the sinus tachycardia. Indeed, sinus tachycardia itself should almost never be treated by drugs, which are designed to alter the heart rate. **It is very dangerous to slow down the heart rate in sinus tachycardia, but slowing the heart rate is the aim of therapy in fast AF or SVT.** Differentiation of sinus tachycardia from SVT and from AF can be difficult but is absolutely essential before

embarking on treatment. Expert advice is also essential if there is any doubt, since the wrong therapy can have dire consequences in this situation.

Ventricular extrasystoles are very common even in normal individuals, and often require no action except to double check that no cardiac structural abnormalities exist, and no metabolic abnormalities, e.g. hypokalaemia, or drug toxicity, e.g. digoxin toxicity, are present.

VT is much more serious, especially since it can degenerate into ventricular fibrillation. It is usually divided into non-sustained VT and sustained VT, the latter being the main concern. However, it is odd that even sustained VT can cause a wide range of clinical pictures, from the patient being occasionally asymptomatic or mildly dizzy to the patient being grossly hypotensive and semiconscious. In the latter case, immediate d.c. cardioversion is necessary. In the former case, one could elect for intravenous lignocaine or for d.c. cardioversion. A short-acting anaesthetic is required prior to the d.c. cardioversion if the patient is awake.

Preoperative arrhythmias in surgical patients

Cardiac arrhythmias are common even in surgical patients. Ventricular and supraventricular arrhythmias are independent risk factors for perioperative cardiac events but this is often because they are a manifestation of underlying and unsuspected serious cardiopulmonary disease. Therefore, the presence of arrhythmias in a preoperative patient should stimulate three main considerations. The first is how serious the arrhythmia is, since this has a major effect on whether extra cardiac investigations are required before surgery is undertaken. The second consideration is whether the arrhythmia is a pointer towards serious but unsuspected cardiopulmonary disease. The third consideration is whether there is some easily reversible cause of the arrhythmia, e.g. a metabolic derangement such as diuretic-induced hypokalaemia or toxicity due to a drug such as digoxin. Clearly, any such reversible factor should be corrected before surgery is contemplated.

In the ACC/AHA Task Force guidelines, a rhythm other than sinus is considered a minor clinical risk predictor, while 'significant arrhythmias' is considered a major clinical predictor of risk. The approach to a patient with arrhythmias should therefore follow the guidelines discussed in the section on 'Myocardial ischaemia'. In patients with significant arrhythmias, it may be wise to perform coronary angiography prior to

Table 20.5 Significant arrhythmias which constitute high surgical risk

- Symptomatic ventricular arrhythmias
- Supraventricular arrhythmias with an uncontrolled ventricular rate
- High-grade atrioventricular block

surgery in order to exclude severe coronary disease. The crucial question is how to define significant arrhythmias. These include patients with symptomatic ventricular arrhythmias, patients with supraventricular arrhythmias with an uncontrolled ventricular rate and patients with high-grade atrioventricular (AV) block (Table 20.5). Such patients are certainly high risk and a detailed assessment is required as to whether the original planned surgery is warranted.

At the other extreme, asymptomatic arrhythmias would constitute low risk and further non-invasive cardiac testing would only be warranted if the patient was undergoing a high-risk surgical procedure and had a low functional capacity (< 4 MET). At this mild end of the spectrum, patients with ventricular ectopy or even non-sustained VT do not need any specific therapy on their own, as these conditions are usually benign in the absence of underlying myocardial ischaemia or underlying left ventricular dysfunction. If cardiopulmonary disease is present, then the surgical risks are increased according to the underlying disease. Patients with arrhythmias therefore represent a wide spectrum of risk and each patient needs to be assessed as an individual, taking into account not only what the rhythm is but also whether the rhythm produces symptomatic or haemodynamic upset.

Another high-risk situation is the patient with high-grade conduction abnormalities such as complete heart block, which considerably increases operative risk and requires temporary or permanent transvenous pacing. At the other extreme, patients with intraventricular conduction delays in the absence of symptoms or a past history of worse AV blockade have a fairly benign prognosis.

In conclusion, careful preoperative assessment is essential to grade the risk of the arrhythmia in the individual patient undergoing a particular operation. If arrhythmias occur during the operative or postoperative period, a definite diagnosis of the abnormal rhythm is essential before embarking on any treatment. Differentiating sinus tachycardia from AF or SVT can be difficult but is crucial and may require expert assistance where there is any doubt.

Section 20.4 • Diabetes mellitus

Diabetes mellitus (DM) is a common endocrine disorder that affects at least 1% of the population in the West, although the prevalence of undiagnosed diabetes is high and many patients have evidence of complications at the time of diagnosis. Both the classification and the diagnostic criteria for DM have been modified recently by the American Diabetes Association and the World Health Organization (WHO). The disease is now diagnosed in individuals with classic symptoms who have a random plasma glucose concentration of ≥ 11.1 mmol/l, preferably repeated or confirmed by a raised fasting glucose value on a separate day. A fasting glucose ≥ 7.0 mmol/l is now regarded as diagnostic (it used to be ≥ 6.0 mmol/l).

The new classification recommended by WHO is as follows.

- Type I includes immune-mediated and idiopathic forms of β-cell dysfunction that lead to absolute insulin deficiency.
- Type II is disease of adult onset that may originate from insulin resistance and relative insulin deficiency, or from a secretory defect.
- Type III covers a wide range of specific types of diabetes, including the various genetic defects of β-cell function, genetic defects in insulin action and diseases of the exocrine pancreas including pancreatectomy.
- Type IV is gestational diabetes.

In addition, carbohydrate intolerance is commonly found in Cushing's syndrome, in individuals suffering from phaeochromocytoma and the rare glucagonoma syndrome. Drug-induced diabetes is encountered in patients on glucocorticoid or adrenocorticotropic hormone (ACTH) therapy and has been reported during treatment with benzothiazide diuretics and thyroxine.

The disease is of interest to the surgeon, largely because of its complications. It causes an individual to be more sensitive to protein depletion, disturbances of carbohydrate intake and to water and electrolyte changes associated with surgical intervention. The main metabolic danger of undiagnosed or poorly controlled DM is the development of a severe ketoacidosis during the course of an acute illness. Furthermore, diabetic ketoacidosis may be a cause of severe abdominal pain, thus mimicking an acute abdomen.

While a well-controlled young diabetic patient is at no greater danger of infection than a normal individual, uncontrolled DM is accompanied by a greater incidence of infection. Although a normal polymorphonuclear leucocytosis occurs in a diabetic in the presence of infection, the phagocytic activity of the leucocytes is impaired. There is also a tendency for an overgrowth of microorganisms in uncontrolled DM, resulting in an increased incidence of non-clostridial gas-forming wound infections. In diabetic ketoacidosis precipitated by surgical infection, granulocyte mobilization is impaired, adding to the reduced phagocytic activity. Furthermore, antibody formation is depressed.

Small vessel disease in the form of non-specific thickening of the basement membrane occurs in the ageing diabetic, in addition to the ordinary changes of atherosclerosis in the major vessels. The resulting peripheral ischaemia and neuropathy lead to an increased frequency of infection by both anaerobic and microaerophilic organisms, and trophic ulcers of the feet follow repeated trauma. Diabetic nephropathy in the form of glomerulosclerosis, usually accompanied by retinopathy, complicates the disease in 15% of patients who have been diabetic for 20 years or more. Whereas coronary heart disease (CHD) is more common in the diabetic than in the general population and is the single most common cause of death in these patients, there is no firm evidence for an increased incidence of cerebrovascular accidents in diabetic individuals.

Neuropathy is related to the duration rather than the severity of the disease and is therefore encountered usually in the elderly. The most common type is sensory loss associated with paraesthesia in the legs and feet, and absent ankle jerks. The development of Charcot's type of arthropathy and trophic ulceration is common in this condition. Other types of neuropathy encountered in DM include mixed subacute sensory and motor neuropathy causing impotence, diarrhoea and an atonic bladder.

Actions of insulin

The severity of the diabetic state is determined by the degree of insulin deficiency caused by the β-cell hypofunction. Insulin consists of two chains (A, B) linked by disulfide bonds and, like other polypeptide hormones, it interacts with highly specific receptors (glycoproteins) located in the cell membranes of target tissues. The binding of insulin with its receptors is an essential first step in the *in vivo* activity of this hormone, the effects of which can be conveniently described as **rapid** and **long-term**. The rapid actions of insulin are:

- increased glucose uptake and metabolism by muscle and adipose tissue
- increased glycogen formation within the liver
- increased synthesis of proteins, especially in muscles
- decreased release of fatty acids from the adipose tissue stores.

The long-term actions of insulin are:

- enhancement of the activity of enzymes concerned with glucose metabolism
- depression of enzymes involved in gluconeogenesis.

Insulin release is chiefly governed by elevations in the blood glucose but certain amino acids, such as arginine, also promote insulin release. Thus, a protein-rich meal raises the blood levels of insulin. The sulfonylurea drugs are used therapeutically in some cases of maturity-onset diabetes (type II) to promote release of the hormone by the β-cells of the endocrine pancreas. Hormones that antagonize the actions of insulin include glucagon, adrenaline, growth hormone, adrenal steroids and ACTH. Specific insulin antagonists have been identified in some patients with DM.

Clinical features

The two main types of DM are insulin-dependent (juvenile-onset, ketosis-prone, type I) and non-insulin-dependent diabetes (maturity-onset, ketosis non-prone, type II). The inherited tendency is stronger in type II, which is three times as common in children of diabetic parents than in the offspring of non-diabetic individuals. In type I disease, a genetic predisposition is associated with certain human lymphocyte antigen (HLA) types, e.g. B_8, B_{15}, B_{12}, but the action of a non-genetic factor, e.g. pancreatotropic viral infection, is required to promote the disease. The region of the sixth human chromosome where the HLA loci are located is in close proximity to the D locus, which is concerned with the immune response. The hypothesis is that type I DM is the consequence of an immune disorder that results either in failure to eradicate a pancreatotropic virus or in an autoimmune reaction to the islet tissue. Both a seasonal incidence of type I disease and high titres of antibodies to Coxsackie virus have been reported in these patients. Furthermore, islet-cell antibodies are found in 60–80% of newly diagnosed type I disease.

Diabetes may occur in chronic pancreatitis (type III) or follow resection of the gland. These patients have a particular tendency to hypoglycaemia because of the absence or reduction of the α-cells and therefore glucagon production that normally antagonizes the action of insulin. Haemochromatosis, otherwise known as bronze diabetes, is associated with the development of DM in 75% of cases. This disorder is much more common in males than females, and is characterized by skin pigmentation, hepatosplenomegaly (cirrhosis), absence of body hair, chondrocalcinosis and arthritis. The primary defect is an accumulation of abnormal amounts of iron in the tissues from excessive absorption.

The classical symptoms of DM include thirst, polyuria, tiredness and weight loss. The clinical differences between type I and type II disease are shown in Table 20.6. The raised blood glucose is accompanied by a glycosuria (hence the polyuria). More elaborate tests such as the oral glucose tolerance test (GTT) and its modifications are only required in patients with borderline values of random and fasting blood glucose.

Treatment of uncomplicated disease

Type I: insulin-dependent diabetes

These patients always require replacement therapy. Until a few years ago porcine and bovine insulins were used. Both were antigenic to humans because of minor differences in the amino-acid sequence from the human hormone and from contaminants such as proinsulin and

Table 20.6 Clinical differences between type I and type II diabetes mellitus

Clinical features	Insulin-dependent	Non-insulin-dependent
Gender ratio	Males = females	Females > males
Age	Children and adolescents	Middle age and elderly
Onset	Usually acute	Gradual
Weight loss	Often marked	Usually absent, often obese
Ketoacidosis	Common	Rare and mild
Plasma insulin level	Low or absent	Normal or reduced
Response to insulin	Sensitive	Relatively insensitive
Effects of hypoglycaemic agents	None	Responsive

pancreatic peptides. These insulin antibodies that developed in patients caused lipoatrophy at the site of injection and, more importantly, led to insulin resistance.

The development of monocomponent (single-peak) neutral insulins of porcine origin significantly reduced the problem of antibody production. The semisynthetic enzyme-modified porcine (emp) insulin was introduced as a further safeguard against the development of insulin antibodies. It has the human amino-acid sequence. Human insulin synthesized by recombinant DNA technology using bacteria containing the genetically engineered plasmids is now used clinically. It is designated by the suffix 'crb' (chain recombinant DNA bacteria). Insulin-crb was the first genetically engineered product used in humans. Its activity is similar to that of highly purified monocomponent and human emp-insulin but it is absorbed more quickly after subcutaneous injection and its duration of action is shorter. Insulin-crb is now administered to newly diagnosed diabetics, to diabetic pregnant mothers and to those individuals needing short-term or intermittent treatment.

Soluble insulin (short-acting) starts to act within 1 h, and has a maximum effect for 2–3 h and a total duration of about 8 h. Various complexes and combinations are available in order to prolong its action (intermediate-acting and long-acting insulins).

Type II diabetes

In the first instance, management depends on whether the patient is overweight or not. Overweight patients are treated initially by carbohydrate restriction alone. An oral antidiabetic drug of the sulfonylurea group, e.g. glipizide or gliclazide, is added if the control is not achieved by carbohydrate restriction alone. These act by promoting the release of endogenous insulin and by decreasing hepatic glucose output. The biguanide metformin is used if persistent hyperglycaemia cannot be controlled by one of the sulfonylurea drugs. The action of biguanides is not dependent on the presence of functional islet cell tissue. They increase the glucose uptake by peripheral tissues and enhance the insulin sensitivity. Metformin is contraindicated in renal failure owing to the risk of lactic acidosis.

Insulin therapy is only considered in type II DM when therapy with diet and oral antidiabetic drugs has failed to achieve control of the diabetic state.

Diabetic coma

This is commonly due to diabetic ketoacidosis, but coma may occur in the absence of ketosis (aketotic diabetic coma, hyperosmolar coma).

Diabetic ketoacidosis

This is consequent on insulin lack and is characterized by hyperglycaemia and ketosis. The precipitating causes include the omission of insulin and acute infections. Not infrequently, diabetic ketoacidosis may be the presenting feature of a previously undiagnosed diabetic. The severe glycosuria and the resulting osmotic diuresis cause severe dehydration from loss of water and electrolytes, with the development of haemoconcentration, hypovolaemia and shock. The ketosis is produced by the increased breakdown of fat, resulting in profound acidosis, hyperventilation and vomiting, the latter aggravating the dehydration. The vomiting is frequently accompanied by generalized abdominal pain. If no treatment is given, the patient becomes increasingly drowsy and unconscious, and finally dies in deep coma.

Apart from signs of dehydration, shock and mental confusion or coma, the face is flushed and the breath has a characteristic sweet smell due to the acetone content. The abdominal signs that may be present include guarding, distension, absent bowel sounds and a succussion splash due to paralytic ileus that is thought to be due to intracellular hypokalaemia.

The biochemical changes associated with diabetic ketoacidosis include hyperglycaemia, ketonuria, low pH and low plasma bicarbonate (base deficit). The level of blood glucose is not a reliable guide to the severity of the illness. The serum electrolytes are commonly normal, although the K^+ concentration may be raised. The blood urea is always elevated and reflects the severity. Leucocytosis is common, even in the absence of infection.

Treatment
The treatment of diabetic ketoacidosis involves the following measures.

- Soluble insulin is administered together with replacement of fluid and electrolyte losses. In an adult, soluble insulin is administered by intravenous infusion at a rate of 5 units (U)/h, by a constant infusion pump. In children under the age of 10 years, the dose is reduced to 2–3 U/h. Insulin therapy is maintained until a satisfactory and consistent response is obtained, which usually takes place between 4 and 8 h after commencing treatment. It is monitored by blood glucose and electrolyte estimations performed 2-hourly until control is achieved.

- The intravenous fluid therapy consists of rapid administration of isotonic saline initially at the rate of 1 l/h, reducing to 1 l/3 h as the dehydration and hyperventilation improve. **As the blood glucose falls in response to treatment, K^+ re-enters the cell and hypokalaemia can develop.** If at any stage the serum K^+ falls below 4.0 mmol/l, 1–2 g KCl (13–26 mmol) is administered hourly via the saline drip throughout the duration of the insulin therapy. $NaHCO_3$ may be necessary to correct the metabolic acidosis, the exact requirements being calculated from the base deficit.

- In addition to the above measures, nasogastric suction is instituted and a broad-spectrum antibiotic administered if there is any evidence of infection. Oxygen therapy is used to correct the hypoxaemia and to prevent the development of cardiac arrhythmias.

Aketotic diabetic coma

This condition differs from diabetic ketoacidosis in that the dehydration is not accompanied by overt ketosis and hyperventilation is absent. This complication is more frequently found in previously undiagnosed diabetics and appears to be more common amongst certain ethnic groups, such as the West Indians. It is characterized by marked elevation of the blood glucose level and plasma osmolality. Although the level of ketones in the plasma is elevated, acidosis is not marked and the plasma bicarbonate level is only slightly reduced. The condition carries a significant mortality of between 10 and 20%, and because of the severe hyperosmolar state, arterial thrombotic episodes are common.

Treatment

Because these patients are usually rather sensitive to insulin, only 3 U/h of soluble insulin should be administered via a constant infusion pump. Fluid therapy consists of large amounts of isotonic or 0.45% saline, depending on the plasma osmolality. Intravenous K^+ is required during the insulin therapy, and heparin is administered either intravenously or subcutaneously in view of the considerable risk of thrombosis.

Management of diabetic patients before and after surgery

This depends on the magnitude of the operation and the severity of the diabetes. Diabetic patients should be placed first on the operating list.

No special preoperative treatment is required for operations performed under local anaesthesia.

Type II diabetic patients undergoing general anaesthesia can be managed without special care but require close postoperative observation. The clinical state should be monitored together with the blood glucose level and the presence of glycosuria confirmed. Soluble insulin by 4-hourly injections or low-dose continuous infusion giving 1–3 U/h is administered if there is significant loss of control of the diabetes.

The management of patients with type I DM undergoing surgery has been considerably simplified by the adoption of GKI infusion bags, which contain 500 ml of 10% glucose, 10 mmol KCl and added insulin determined by the blood glucose range (Table 20.7). One GKI bag is administered every 5 h. The GKI infusion is commenced at the time when the first dose of insulin is usually taken by the patient. The blood glucose is checked 2-hourly by BM Stix. The urea and electrolytes are checked during the afternoon of the operation and then daily. The potassium is omitted from the infusion if there is any renal impairment (creatinine > 150 mmol/l).

The GKI infusion is continued postoperatively up to and including the first light meal. If the first light meal is tolerated by the patient, the normal dose of insulin is

Table 20.7 Insulin dose in GKI infusion

Blood glucose (mmol/l)	Insulin units in bag
4–7	10
7–13 (target range)	15
13–17	20

NB. Expert diabetic advice sought if level of glucose gets < 4 or > 17. Each dose change requires a new GKI bag.

given at the beginning of the next day. The GKI infusion is maintained for 1 h after the second meal and then discontinued.

Hypoglycaemia

This is the most common complication of insulin therapy, and must be distinguished from spontaneous hypoglycaemia that may be caused by islet cell tumours. It is more commonly reactive (functional) in origin, when it results from an exaggerated response to a rise in the blood glucose, and is commonly encountered after gastric surgery.

Hypoglycaemia is especially likely to occur in type III diabetes (after pancreatectomy or severe chronic pancreatitis). The time of onset of exogenous insulin-induced hypoglycaemia depends on the time of injection and the type of insulin used. Patients with moderate to high levels of insulin antibodies show a delay in the recovery from exogenous insulin-induced hypoglycaemia. Hypoglycaemia may also complicate therapy with sulfonylurea compounds but not with the biguanide drugs.

Symptoms and signs

These are produced when the blood glucose falls below 2 mmol/l and include hunger, sweating palpitations, tremor, tingling sensations and mental changes such as slow cerebration, fainting, aggressive behaviour, epileptiform convulsions and coma.

The patient is observed to be pale with tachycardia (catecholamine response), although the blood pressure and the respiratory rate remain normal. Signs in the central nervous system (CNS) include monoplegia or hemiplegia, uncoordinated eye movements and extensor plantar responses. The mental state varies from drowsiness to aggressive behaviour or coma.

Treatment

Hypoglycaemic attacks are best prevented by ensuring adequate buffer carbohydrate meals at suitable time intervals depending on the nature of the hypoglycaemic agents used. Diabetic patients should carry cards in addition to carbohydrate foods such as Hypostop gel (a convenient form of oral glucose). The treatment of established hypoglycaemia is by subcutaneous glucagon in the first instance, but if this is not effective in 15 min, intravenous glucose is administered.

Table 20.8　Hyperlipidaemias

Type	Incidence	Plasma lipid profile
I	Rare	Cholesterol$^+$, chylomicron^{++}, TG^{++}, LDL-, VLDL^n
IIa	Common	Cholesterol^{++}, LDL$^+$, VLDL^n
IIb	Common	Cholesterol^{++}, LDL$^+$, TG$^+$, VLDL$^+$
III	Uncommon	Cholesterol^{++}, LDL$^-$, TG^{++}, remnants^{++}
IV	Common	Cholesterol$^+$, LDLn, TG^{++}, VLDL$^+$
V	Uncommon	Cholesterol+, chylomicron+, TG^{++}, TG^{++}, LDL$^-$, VLDL^{++}

$^+$Moderate elevation; $^{++}$marked increase; $^-$decreased; ^{n}normal. LDL, low-density lipoprotein; VLDL, very low-density lipoprotein; TG, triglycerides.

Section 20.5 • Hyperlipidaemia

There is undoubted evidence that hyperlipidaemia, together with smoking, hypertension and insufficient physical exercise, is an important risk factor in coronary heart disease (CHD). Hyerlipidaemia may be primary or secondary (hypothyroidism, diabetes and alcohol misuse). The main types of hyperlipidaemia are shown in Table 20.8. The particular individuals at risk of hyperlipidaemia and who therefore require screening and surveillance are those with:

- a family history of CHD, especially below 50 years of age
- a familial history of hyperlipidaemia
- the presence of xanthoma, xanthelasma or arcus senilis below 40 years of age
- obesity
- DM and hypertension.

The initial screening test is random plasma total cholesterol (TC). If this exceeds 6.6 mmol/l, a detailed plasma lipid profile is obtained. The elevation of low-density lipoprotein-cholesterol (LDL-C) strongly correlates with the development of CHD. By contrast, the high-density lipoprotein-cholesterol (HDL-C) level is inversely related to the risk.

Most patients can be effectively treated by diet alone. If this proves ineffective, therapy is usually with an anion-exchange resin (cholestyramine or colestipol) with or without nicotinic acid. In severe mixed hyperlipidaemia (especially type III), treatment with fibric acid drugs (clofibrate, bezafibrate, gemfibrozil) is recommended.

Section 20.6 • Bleeding disorders

Bleeding disorders may be **inherited** or **acquired**. The former, although rare, are important in surgical practice because special measures are needed to cover surgical intervention. In addition, the recurrent spontaneous bleeding episodes lead to organic disease that may require surgical treatment, e.g. severe joint disease and treatment of intracranial haematoma. Acquired bleeding disorders are much more commonly encountered and are secondary to disease or drug therapy.

Hereditary bleeding disorders

Inherited bleeding disorders may affect all components of the haemostatic process: **vascular** and **coagulative** aspects, **platelet function** and the **fibrinolytic system**. All are rare and the important group to surgeons is that comprised by the genetically determined defects of coagulation: haemophilia A, haemophilia B and von Willebrand's disease. The UK incidence of haemophilia A is 5:100 000, as opposed to 1:100 000 for haemophilia B and 2.5:100 000 for von Willebrand's disease. Very rare hereditary coagulation disorders include afibrinogenaemia, dysfibrinogenaemia and other specific deficiencies (factors II, V, VII, XII, XIII).

The inherited vascular and connective tissue disorders include hereditary haemorrhagic telangiectasia (Osler Weber Rendu syndrome), the Ehlers–Danlos syndrome, Marfan's syndrome and osteogenesis imperfecta. Hereditary haemorrhagic telangiectasia is the most common.

Inherited disorders of platelet function fall into two categories:

- absence of specific surface glycoproteins, e.g. Glanzmann's thrombasthenia
- defects in secretory granules, e.g. Grey platelet syndrome, Wiscott Aldrich disease.

The most common of these rare disorders is Glanzmann's thrombasthenia. In this disease, the absence of membrane glycoproteins, GpIIb and GpIIIa, results in a markedly defective platelet aggregation. Affected individuals exhibit a prolonged bleeding time but have a normal coagulation screen. These patients are liable to spontaneous bleeding and require platelet transfusion. Regrettably, repeated platelet transfusions lead to alloimmunization with a rapid decline in efficacy of the transfused platelets. HLA-matched platelet packs minimize this problem. The only patient encountered by the author in 35 years of practice eventually died aged 50 years of massive and uncontrollable gastrointestinal haemorrhage.

Haemophilia A and B (Christmas disease)

These disorders have similar clinical features. Haemophilia A is the result of a deficiency of the procoagulant portion of factor VIII (FVIII Act), whereas haemophilia B is due to the lack of factor IX. Both factors are crucial to the intrinsic system of blood coagulation and are located on the X-chromosome. This explains the recessive sex-linked inheritance, whereby males are affected and females acts as carriers. Although this is largely true in the sense that clinical problems are largely confined to males, some female carriers may have a bleeding tendency that becomes obvious only when major surgery is undertaken.

Aside from family and genetic history, both conditions are diagnosed by documentation of prolonged activated partial thromboplastin time (APTT), a normal prothrombin time (PT) and assays of factors VIII and IX. In both disorders the deficiency can be mild (5–20% of normal level of the respective clotting factor), moderate (1–5% of normal activity) or severe (< 1% of normal).

The clinical picture is dominated by recurrent bleeds, most commonly in the muscles and joints (haemarthroses), especially in toddlers and children, although neonatal bleeding is not uncommon. Haematuria is fairly frequent and intracranial bleeding (intracerebral, subarachnoid, subdural) may be fatal. Gastrointestinal haemorrhage is usually secondary to disease such as peptic ulceration and may be precipitated by non-steroidal anti-inflammatory drugs (NSAIDs), which are contraindicated in these patients. The most common chronic disability is severe arthropathy from recurrent intra-articular bleeds and this often requires orthopaedic treatment (synovectomy, arthrodesis, arthroplasty).

Replacement therapy with clotting factors is required for the management of active bleeding episodes and to cover surgical treatment or dental extraction. It consists of the intravenous infusion of plasma-derived factor VIII concentrates for haemophilia A and factor IX concentrates for haemophilia B. Factor VIII concentrates are heat treated to inactivate human immunodeficiency virus (HIV) and other viruses, and are available as lyophilized powder in vials containing 250 IU, which is reconstituted with 10 ml of water for injection. Factor IX concentrates also contain prothrombin and factor X. They are heat treated against HIV and other viruses, and packaged in vials containing 300 IU. Cryoprecipitate, which is rich in factor VIII (100 IU/pack), fibrinogen and fibronectin can be used as an alternative to factor VIII concentrates in haemophilia A. Cryoprecipitate is simpler to produce and requires a small donor pool. However, as it does not contain factor IX, cryoprecipitate is ineffective in haemophilia B.

The dose of the respective concentrate needed in the individual patient depends on:

- the severity of the defect
- the nature of the intended operation
- the presence of acquired coagulation inhibitors (antibodies that develop in some patients).

The formula for calculating the dose of factor VIII or factor IX is shown in Table 20.9. As the half-life of factor VIII is only 8–12 h, twice-daily administration is necessary to maintain therapeutic levels in haemophilia A. By contrast, in haemophilia B single daily dosing is usually sufficient, as the half-life of factor IX is 18–24 h. Elective surgery in haemophilia A and B patients must be planned several weeks beforehand and requires that adequate notice be given to the blood transfusion or haemophilia centre. The preoperative work-up must include a coagulation–inhibition screen

Table 20.9 Formula for the calculation of the dose of factor VIII or factor IX

$$\text{Dose in units} = \frac{\% \text{ rise desired} \times \text{weight in kg}}{K}$$

where K = 1.5 for factor VIII concentrates
1.5 for cryoprecipitate
0.7 for factor IX concentrates
2.0 for fresh-frozen plasma (ml)

Desired factor level in patient's blood (range)

Minor bleed	10–20%
Major bleed/dental extraction	20–70%
Major surgery or trauma	70–100%

test. The first dose is administered 1 h before surgery and is followed by an assay of the factor level in a sample of the patient's blood taken 30 min later. Postoperative factor assays are also performed and replacement therapy continued to maintain a level > 40% for the first 10 postoperative days. **Patients with haemophilia A and B must never receive intramuscular injections of any sort.**

The complications of clotting factor therapy include urticarial reactions, which are common, severe anaphylactoid reactions (rare), viral disease and the development of antibodies to factor VIII. Until recently, the vast majority of patients developed hepatitis C. This and hepatitis B should be rare nowadays because of strict donor screening and heat activation. The tragedy of the HIV-contaminated clotting factor concentrates enacted in the early 1980s resulted in widespread seroconversion, especially in patients who received factor VIII concentrates. At one time 40% of UK haemophiliacs were HIV positive, although the number has since declined as many of these unfortunate patients have died of acquired immunodeficiency syndrome (AIDS).

Isoantibodies develop in some 6–12% of patients with haemophilia A. They impose great difficulty in replacement therapy, and these patients must be managed in specialist centres. The present options include large doses of factor VIII, or the use of porcine VIII or activated prothrombin concentrates. Other therapeutic options include immunosuppressive therapy, plasmapheresis (to reduce antibody levels) and the induction of immunological tolerance. Although isoantibodies may develop to factor IX, these instances are rare.

Von Willebrand's disease

This familial bleeding disorder was first described by von Willebrand in the inhabitants of the Åland Islands in the Baltic Sea. The disease is inherited as an autosomal dominant trait and therefore appears in consecutive generations affecting both males and females equally. It is caused by the deficiency of von Willebrand factor (vWF), normally produced by the endothelial cells and the megakaryocytes, and present in both plasma and platelets as high molecular weight multimeric molecules of varying sizes. vWF is essential for platelet adhesion to subendothelial tissues following vascular injury and as a carrier molecule for factor VIII, which it stabilizes (factor VIII/vWF complex). Several variants of the disorder are recognized but the classical disease is characterized by prolongation of the skin bleeding time and APTT with a normal PT, reduced FVIII Act, vWF Ag (vWF antigen) and vWFRCo (*in vitro* cofactor activity for platelet aggregation induced by ristocetin).

Von Willebrand's disease is characterized by bleeding mainly from skin and mucous membranes, and often presents as bleeding after surgical intervention (particularly ear, nose and throat operations) or dental extraction. In women, menorrhagia is a common feature. In contrast to haemophilia A and haemophilia B, haemarthroses are rare. Fresh-frozen plasma (FFP), cryoprecipitate and some intermediate purity factor VIII concentrates will restore the bleeding time and the coagulation defect to normal. Following infusion of any of these products, there is an immediate rise in FVIII Act followed by a secondary peak 18–24 h later due to the release of endogenous factor VIII in response to the administered vWF. Preparation of patients for surgery is essentially along the same lines as that previously described for haemophilia A and B. In some cases (type I disease) intravenous infusion of deamino-D-arginine vasopressin (DDAVP, desmopressin) will increase the plasma FVIII Act and vWF levels, and is therefore used as an alternative to replacement therapy in these patients to cover dental extractions and minor operations. As desmopressin also stimulates the release of plasminogen activator, it is administered in conjunction with an antifibrinolytic agent such as tranexamic acid.

Acquired bleeding disorders

Acquired bleeding disorders are common and often involve more than one function of the haemostatic response (Table 20.10). The most common abnormality

Table 20.10 Acquired bleeding disorders

Impaired haemostatic function	Aetiology
Thrombocytopenia	ITP, hepatic disease, tumours, drugs, blood transfusion, DIC (sepsis)
Defective platelet adhesion	Uraemia, drugs
Defective platelet aggregation	Uraemia, hepatic disease, extracorporeal circulation, drugs, leukaemias
Defective coagulation	Hepatic disease, DIC, tumours, anticoagulation, massive transfusion
Coagulation inhibitors	Heparin, lymphomas
Excess fibrinolysis	DIC, drugs

encountered in clinical practice is bleeding caused by oral anticoagulant therapy. In some patients with malignant tumours, impaired platelet function may lead to purpuric bruising but major disturbances of coagulation are rare, although some neoplasms may release products and cytokines that activate the coagulation cascade and lead to disseminated intravascular coagulation (DIC).

The major acquired bleeding problems usually arise on a background of acute or chronic liver disease. The bleeding diathesis in this situation reflects a complex picture due to defective synthesis of clotting factors (II, VII, X and the vitamin K-dependent factors), with the exception of factor VIII, which is elevated, abnormal (hypocarboxylated or acarboxylated) clotting factors, abnormal fibrinogen (excess sialic acid that impairs polymerization), increased fibrinolysis and thrombocytopenia. In patients with jaundice due to large bile duct obstruction, the defective synthesis of the vitamin K-dependent factors is rapidly reversed by parenteral vitamin K analogue. Lack of response with persistence of the prolonged PT despite vitamin K therapy indicates severe hepatocyte malfunction.

Disseminated intravascular coagulation

This syndrome arises from the intravascular activation of procoagulant factors, chiefly thrombin, and platelet aggregation and adhesion leading to widespread thrombosis of the microcirculation of several organs, a consumptive coagulopathy and a secondary activation of plasminogen to plasmin causing a concurrent fibrinolysis. The net result is multiple organ damage/failure (adult respiratory distress syndrome, acute renal failure, hepatic insufficiency and CNS changes) owing to occlusion of the microcirculation of any or all the organs by **microclots**. This is accompanied by a bleeding tendency manifested by petechiae, ecchymosis and bleeding from the mucous membranes (gastrointestinal haemorrhage, haematuria, epistaxis, etc.). The important causes are shown in Table 20.11.

Role of endotoxin
In surgical practice, the most common causes are sepsis and trauma. In sepsis, the orthodox view has been that the pathological sequence is initiated by endotoxin (lipopolysaccharide associated with the cell membrane of Gram-negative microorganisms). The lipid A portion of endotoxin induces expression of cytokine genes and hence a cytokine/inflammatory agents cascade [tumour necrosis factor (TNF), platelet activating factor, interleukin-1 (IL-1), IL-6 and IL-8, arachidonic acid metabolites, erythropoietin and endothelin, etc.]. These induce a widespread inflammatory change and its deleterious consequences, hence the alternative term for septic shock, systemic inflammatory response syndrome (SIRS). The endothelial cells are damaged directly by neutrophil–endothelial cell interaction (various mechanisms may be involved, e.g. expression of adhesion molecules, excess local nitric oxide production with direct oxidant damage) with exposure of the

Table 20.11 Causes of disseminated intravascular coagulation

Condition	Cause
Tissue trauma	Exposure, release of inner cell wall aminophospholipid
Sepsis	Endotoxin/inflammatory agent-induced endothelial cell damage
Peritoneovenous shunting	Cellular debris/cellular aminophospholipid
Obstetric complications: abruptio placentae, amniotic fluid embolism, dead fetus syndrome	Cellular debris/aminophospholipid
Immune reactions	Antigen–antibody complex-mediated endothelial cell damage, and complement-mediated intravascular coagulation
Extracorporeal circulation: cardiopulmonary bypass, artificial heart, haemodialysis	RBC/leucocyte damage
Blood disorders: haemolysis, sickling, paroxysmal nocturnal haemoglobinuria	ADP and RBC aminophospholipids activate procoagulants and platelet aggregation
Advanced cancer	Bronchial, pancreatic, ovarian and prostatic cancer, acute leukaemia. Predominantly thrombotic manifestations

subendothelial collagen and activation of factor VII, initiating intrinsic coagulation. In addition, endotoxin activates circulating monocytes, which then release cytokines such as TNF and IL-1. These cause the activation of T-lymphocytes (IL-1) and polymorphs (TNF), which then adhere to and damage the endothelial cells, causing the release of tissue thromboplastin, thereby activating the extrinsic coagulation cascade.

It is now considered that the endotoxin–inflammatory cascade theory is unlikely to be the cause, or at least the only pathway for DIC and septic shock (essentially the same thing), for two reasons. In the first instance, the assumption that endotoxin contributes to the mortality of Gram-negative infections has never been proved. The only experimental observation that has been interpreted as evidence that endotoxin is the primary agent in septic shock is the shock-like state it induces when injected into experimental animals in doses that far exceed those encountered in human sepsis. Secondly, the failure of various anti-inflammatory therapies, and lack of consistent benefit by monoclonal antibodies to TNF and endotoxin casts doubts on the endotoxin–inflammatory cascade theory.

Cell-wall aminophospholipids: shock toxin and autotoxin
The concept of a shock toxin was first proposed in World War I, when shock was attributed to a toxin released from damaged or dying tissue. It is well documented that shock and DIC can occur in pathological states that do not have an infection component, e.g. traumatic shock, amniotic fluid embolism, peritoneovenous shunting for ascitis, abruptio placentae and incompatible blood transfusion. It has been demonstrated recently that translocation of the aminophospholipids from the inner to the outer leaflet of cell membranes activates intravascular thrombosis (documented in sickling and paroxysmal nocturnal haemoglobinuria). Small amounts of this inner-wall aminophospholipid (exposed by trauma) have been shown to activate both intravascular coagulation and the kinin system. Recent experiments involving trauma to thighs of anaesthetized pigs have added considerable weight to the involvement of cell-wall aminophospholipid as a cause of DIC and shock, especially when accompanied by hypovolaemia. More importantly, treatment with a fibrinolytic agent (urokinase) prevented the development of multiple organ failure and reduced mortality significantly. Early phase I and II studies in patients with tissue plasminogen activator (tPA) have yielded promising results.

Haematological findings in disseminated intravascular coagulation
The consumptive coagulopathy leads to a multifactorial deficiency with prolongation of the prothrombin and kaolin–cephalin times. The fibrin-split products are elevated and thrombocytopenia is present and may be severe (< 50 000). The level of antithrombin III (AT-III) is reduced as it is also consumed by the excessive thrombin and clot formation. The level of AT-III is a good guide to prognosis and recovery from the disease.

Treatment
In the first instance, the initiating cause must be treated vigorously. This is particularly important in relation to sepsis. Hypovolaemia is corrected by fresh blood collected in heparin. Active bleeding is reversed by use of FFP or cryoprecipitate and platelet transfusion if the platelet count is below 50 000. Some advocate the use of heparin but this approach is suspect in view of the low levels of AT-III in this condition (heparin acts by enhancing the inhibition by AT-III of thrombin). Low molecular weight heparins (LMWH) may be better as they possess greater anti-factor Xa activity. In any event, heparin therapy is contraindicated in the presence of open wounds and overt active bleeding. The administration of concentrates of AT-III is a much better and safer option than heparinization. More recently, treatment with tPA has yielded promising results and if these are confirmed by larger studies, this may well become the mainstay of therapy of the established condition.

Section 20.7 • Thrombotic disorders: thrombophilia

These disorders, although rare, are important because of they predispose to venous thromboembolism. They are caused by a deficiency or inactivity of certain key proteins that normally regulate activation of blood coagulation, hence the tendency to venous occlusive episodes. The important ones are:

- antithrombin III
- protein C
- protein S.

AT-III is the most important antithrombin in the plasma and provides a protective mechanism against activation of intravascular coagulation. Deficiency of AT-III is found in approximately 1:4000 of the population and may be familial. It usually presents with recurrent deep venous thrombosis in the lower limbs dating from the late teens. The diagnosis is established by measurement of AT-III. These patients require lifelong oral anticoagulation.

Proteins C and S are vitamin K-dependent factors synthesized in the liver. Protein C in its activated form C(a) inhibits factors V and VIIIc. Low levels of C(a) are associated with a tendency to recurrent venous thrombosis. Extensive acute skin necrosis due to thrombosis of the cutaneous vessels ensues if patients with protein C deficiency are given warfarin, since this reduces the protein C activity further. Protein S serves as a cofactor for protein C(a) but exerts a regulatory effect on coagulation in its own right.

Section 20.8 • Adverse drug reactions

Adverse drug reactions are an ever-increasing problem, and account for a sizeable morbidity and mortality that can be minimized by careful selection of drug therapy and vigilance. A substantial majority of middle-aged and elderly patients requiring surgical care arrive in hospital with a variety of medications, the nature of which is usually unknown to the patient. It often transpires that some are unnecessary and others may be detrimental, particularly hypnotics as these tend to cause confusion in the aged. **The exact chemical formulation must be ascertained as some of the drugs may interact with specific therapy started during the hospital stay.** Rarely, specific bizarre surgical syndromes may follow drug treatment.

In 1969 the Committee of the World Health Organization (WHO) defined an adverse drug reaction as 'one which is noxious, unintended and occurs at doses normally used in man for prophylaxis, diagnosis and therapy'. This definition therefore excludes the effects of both intentional and accidental overdose. Drug reactions fall into five broad categories:

- dose-related
- non-dose-related
- long-term
- teratogenic
- drug interactions.

Dose-related adverse reactions

These may be produced by an excessive therapeutic response, e.g. bleeding from recent surgical wounds due to use of anticoagulants, hypoglycaemia from exogenous insulin, or by the development of side-effects that may be pharmacological, e.g. blurred vision following propantheline administration, or toxic. The latter include vestibular damage by gentamicin, especially in patients suffering from renal failure, marrow depression from cytotoxic drugs, etc. Other dose-related adverse drug reactions may be caused by secondary effects, e.g. superinfection of the gastrointestinal tract following the administration of antibiotics, a specific example of which is *Clostridium difficile* pseudomembranous colitis. Reactivation of tuberculosis can occur in patients on immunosuppressive drug therapy.

The difference between the dose required to produce a therapeutic effect by a drug and the dose that produces toxic effects is referred to as the **therapeutic ratio**. This is obviously an important determining factor in the development of toxic side-effects.

Non-dose-related adverse reactions

These include idiosyncrasy to a particular drug. This is usually genetically determined and predisposes the individual to an abnormal reaction following the administration of certain drugs. Examples of this type of response include the haemolysis caused by sulfonamides or aspirin in patients with G-6-PD deficiency. Drug allergy is not related to dose, and although sensitization to a drug may be produced by any route of administration, it is most commonly encountered after topical applications.

Long-term reactions

Long-term effects may be produced as a result of prolonged treatment, e.g. chronic interstitial nephritis and papillary necrosis may follow long-term administration of analgesic mixtures containing phenacetin, aspirin or amidopyrone. They may also be delayed, the adverse effects occurring months or years after the cessation of treatment, e.g. the hypothyroidism that follows iodine-133 therapy for thyrotoxicosis, or lymphoma and leukaemia that may develop some time after immunosuppressive or cytotoxic therapy.

Teratogenic reactions

Thalidomide, apart from causing incalculable human suffering, created formidable surgical problems. All new drugs must now undergo rigorous testing for teratogenecity in animals before being tested in humans in phase II studies.

Risk factors for adverse drug reactions

The risk is greater with the following:

- administration of drugs with a narrow therapeutic ratio, e.g. digoxin, warfarin, antihypertensive drugs
- elderly patients
- patients with hepatic and or renal disease
- multiple prescriptions.

The risk increases with the number of drugs prescribed to the patient. Often, proprietary (trade) names are used without the clinician being fully aware of the exact chemical formulation. This is especially hazardous as many of the proprietary preparations contain more than one drug.

Drug interactions

These may result in **antagonism** causing loss of the therapeutic effect of a particular drug; **potentiation** leading to an excessive therapeutic effect, **increased toxicity** or the development of an **unusual** reaction that does not occur with either drug alone. In addition, chemical and physical interaction between drugs may result in their **inactivation** when they are used in combination. In this respect, the addition of drugs to intravenous fluids carries a definite risk. Thus, heparin is completely inactivated and frusemide is precipitated by dextrose solutions. Calcium salts precipitate in sodium bicarbonate. Dextrose saline/isotonic saline solution affects the stability of many antibiotics, which results in a substantial loss of their activity. Examples include benzylpenicillin, ampicillin, methicillin and gentamicin. Certain antibiotic combinations are manifestly incompatible when added to intravenous fluids. The Na^+ and K^+ salts of benzylpenicillin and the semisynthetic penicillins inactivate gentamicin and precipitate the tetracyclines; carbenicillin inactivates colistin and gentamicin itself is inactivated by kanamycin. Many other drug incompatibilities in intravenous fluid have been documented and, therefore, **one should avoid mixing drugs in intravenous fluids whenever possible.**

The mechanisms involved in *in vivo* drug interactions include effect on transport to the site of action due to changes in the absorption and/or protein binding. Thus, phenylbutazone displaces warfarin from the binding sites and thereby potentiates its anticoagulant effect. Intracellular transport may also be altered. For example, the antihypertensive effect of guanethidine is inhibited by the concomitant administration of tricyclic antidepressants and sympathomimetic amines, both of which block the active transport mechanism necessary for guanethidine to enter the cell.

Drug interaction may also cause alterations in the renal excretion of certain agents, e.g. phenylbutazone interferes with the excretion of chlorpropamide causing hypoglycaemia. Drug metabolism may also be altered owing either to enzyme induction, as occurs when warfarin metabolism is stimulated by barbiturates, or by enzyme inhibition, e.g. anticholinesterase

drugs that potentiate the action of suxamethonium and may cause prolonged apnoea. Monoamine oxidase inhibitors potentiate the actions of sympathomimetic amines.

Drug interactions may result from competition at specific receptor sites or from an additive physiological effect. Thus, sedatives, tranquillizers and antidepressants may induce severe hypotension in patients on antihypertensive drugs. Potentiation of tubocurarine may be produced by drugs with neuromuscular blocking activity such as the aminoglycosides.

Electrolyte abnormalities induced by drugs may be of sufficient magnitude to cause significant side-effects. Thus, carbenexolone, loop diuretics or steroid therapy may induce hypokalaemia and enhance digoxin toxicity, and hyponatraemia caused by excessive administration of diuretics increases the hypotensive effects of sedatives and tranquillizers.

The mechanisms of many types of drug interactions are not fully understood, and thus the clinician should take this factor into consideration when unexplained or unexpected deterioration of the condition of the patient occurs.

Section 20.9 • Drug-induced disorders

The disorder may develop during the drug treatment or some time (months to years) after its withdrawal. The changes may or may not be reversible and often result in significant morbidity. Several categories are recognized and many are important in surgical practice. Disorders caused by antibiotic therapy are discussed elsewhere [**see Module 5, Vol. I**].

Fibrotic disorders

These are outlined in Table 20.12. Some are now of historical interest as the precipitant drug has been withdrawn from clinical practice, but others such cytotoxic agents and metalloproteinase inhibitors, e.g. marimistat, introduced recently as novel anticancer agents are of great relevance in oncological practice [**see Module 15, Vol. I**].

Oculomucocutaneous syndrome
This consists of a sclerosing peritonitis and pathological changes in other sites: eyes, skin, ears, pleura and pericardium. It was induced by the β-blocker practolol, introduced in 1970. Significant side-effects were recognized shortly after its introduction. At first, these appeared to be restricted to the skin, eyes and ears. A large variety of skin lesions were described and the eye lesions resulted in the development of the dry-eye syndrome, with keratinization, symblepharon, corneal thinning, opacification and ulceration. Deafness and tinnitus occurred from involvement of the auditory nerve.

A sclerosing peritonitis was described later. This differed from retroperitoneal fibrosis and occurred 2–3 years after treatment with normal doses of prac-

Table 20.12 Drug-induced fibrotic disorders

Disorder	Drug responsible
Dupuytren's contracture	Phenobarbitone, metalloproteinase inhibitors
Myocardial ventricular extrasystoles fibrosis and constrictive pericarditis	Methysergide
Pulmonary fibrosis	Bleomycin, busulfan, melphalan, cyclophospamide, methotrexate, nitrosoureas, amiodarone, nitrofurantoin, methysergide
Oculomucocutaneous syndrome	Practolol
Retroperitoneal fibrosis	Methysergide, phenacetin, methyldopa
Carpal tunnel syndrome	Oral contraceptives, high-dose progesterone, thalidomide, disulpuran, metalloproteinase inhibitors

tolol. The condition presented as one of acute or acute-on-chronic small bowel obstruction. At laparotomy, the visceral and parietal peritoneal surfaces were covered by a greyish-white pseudomembrane that invested the small intestine like a capsule or cocoon. In some patients, the anterior and lateral parietal peritoneum was also involved, resulting in complete obliteration of the peritoneal cavity. The pseudomembrane was avascular and could be peeled from the underlying bowel without excessive bleeding. Histological examination of the membrane showed a mesothelial lining, below which were prominent lamellar layers of collagen with a collection of lymphocytes and macrophages separating the deeper aspect from the serosa of the bowel. Although other β-blockers (propranolol, oxprenolol, timolol, metoprolol, atenolol) have been suggested rarely to induce a similar condition, there is no firm evidence to link these with the development of sclerosing peritonitis since this condition may occur, albeit rarely, spontaneously.

Retroperitoneal fibrosis
Usually this condition is idiopathic. In addition to the retroperitoneal fibrosis that often causes an obstructive uropathy, there may be involvement of the mediastinum, aorta, myocardium, pericardium, heart valves (fibrosis, valve regurgitation, constrictive pericarditis), thyroid gland, orbit and the gallbladder. The disorder presents with weight loss, anorexia, abdominal and back pain radiating to the thighs and testes, and a raised erythrocyte sedimentation rate. Continuous long-term administration of methysergide may induce the condition. Other drugs have also been implicated (phenacetin, methyldopa, etc.), but without confirmation.

Pulmonary fibrosis
This is most commonly the result of cytotoxic therapy, especially with bleomycin and busulfan. The condition

is usually irreversible and often fatal, although prednisolone therapy has been reported to be effective in reversing the signs of pulmonary toxicity in some cases. The pathological picture consists of fibrosing alveolitis, interstitial fibrosis, alveolar squamous metaplasia and hyalinization. The onset is variable, from days to several months after the initiation of therapy. The clinical manifestations of the disorder include fever, cough and progressive dyspnoea.

Carpal tunnel syndrome
Although included in the fibrotic category, drug-induced carpal tunnel syndrome is more often the result of either oedema (oral contraceptives, high-dose progesterone therapy), a neuropathy (thalidomide, disulfuran) or synovitis induced by injecting diazepam intravenously on the anterolateral aspect of the wrist.

Gastrointestinal and hepatobiliary disorders

Some of the common drug-induced disorders are shown in Table 20.13. Drug-induced cholestatic jaundice and hepatitis are covered elsewhere [**see Hepatobiliary and Pancreatic Disorders, Vol. II**].

Gastrointestinal bleeding and ulceration
The peptic ulceration and bleeding problem associated with aspirin and other NSAIDs is covered elsewhere [**see Module 6, Vol. I**].

The thiazide diuretics induce a hypokalaemia that is particularly dangerous because it intensifies the action of digoxin on the myocardium. To obviate this problem, a combined entero-coated tablet containing the diuretic and a core of potassium chloride was

Table 20.13 Drug-induced gastrointestinal and hepatobiliary disorders

Disorder	Drug
Ulcers and haemorrhage	Aspirin and non-aspirin NSAIDs
Strictures	Potassium chloride
Pseudo-obstruction	Tricyclic antidepressants, monoamine oxidase inhibitors, narcotic analgesics, excess purgation
Cholestatic jaundice and hepatitis	[Hepatobiliary and Pancreatic Disorders, Vol. II]
Peliosis hepatis	Androgens, oestrogens, methotrexate
Focal nodular hyperplasia and hepatic adenomas	Oral contraceptives, androgens
Hepatocellular carcinoma	Androgens, oral contraceptives
Reye's syndrome	Aspirin in children
Acute cholecystitis	Diuretics, parenteral nutrition?

introduced. The use of this formulation led to the development of ulceration in the small bowel presenting with haemorrhage, perforation or intestinal obstruction due to stricture formation. This complication was caused by the rapid release of potassium chloride over a short segment of small intestine. The high concentration of potassium chloride produced focal mucosal necrosis with a varying degree of submucosal erosion and an acute-on-chronic inflammatory reaction. Since then, the formulation of the tablet has been altered such that the solubility of the potassium chloride was lowered by coating the crystals with an inert wax–sugar combination. This results in a much slower release of potassium over a period of several hours. Since the advent of small bowel enteroscopy, small bowel ulceration causing obscure bleeding has been documented following the oral administration of a variety of drugs, including NSAIDs.

Liver tumours

The vast majority of both benign and malignant liver tumours is not the consequence of drug administration. However, a definite association between the development of both liver-cell adenoma and hepatocellular carcinoma and oral contraceptive use and androgen intake has been established.

The association between oral contraceptives and focal nodular hyperplasia is less certain and disputed by some. Focal nodular hyperplasia is an entirely benign condition that resembles regenerative nodules of cirrhosis on histological examination. It is difficult to diagnose on needle biopsy of the liver and often requires an excision biopsy for confirmation, preferably by the laparoscopic approach.

Liver-cell adenoma complicating oral contraception and androgen administration is very rare. The lesion usually measures 10 cm or more at the time of diagnosis. The tumour, although benign, is very vascular and presents acutely with rupture and bleeding in some 30% of cases. The progression to hepatocellular carcinoma is debatable. Regression of the tumour may occur on withdrawal of oral contraception and androgen treatment.

There are some notable differences between the hepatocellular carcinomas that complicate oral contraception and androgen treatment, and those arising *de novo*. In the first instance, the steroid-associated tumours are more vascular and exhibit no vessel encasement on hepatic arteriography. This accounts for their common presentation with bleeding and rupture, which occur in 55% of cases. Furthermore, these malignant tumours are not accompanied by an elevation of the serum α-fetoprotein level.

Cholecystitis

The administration of thiazide diuretics predisposes to the development of acute cholecystitis in patients who harbour gallstones. An association between prolonged parenteral nutrition and the development of both biliary sludge/gallstones and acute acalculous cholecystitis

has been reported. It is, as yet, unclear whether the prolonged fasting or the underlying illness rather than the parenteral nutrition is responsible for the development of acute acalculous cholecystitis in these patients.

Reye's syndrome

This frequently fatal condition, consisting of encephalopathy and liver failure due to yellow atrophy, occurs in children who are given aspirin, usually for chicken pox. There is some evidence that the condition results from the release of TNF from macrophages brought about by the aspirin.

Endocrine and metabolic disorders

Drug-induced endocrine disorders are common and cover a wide spectrum (Table 20.14). Both hyperactivity and hypoactivity may be induced by medication, usually over long periods.

Hyperprolactinaemia

The manifestations of hyperprolactinaemia include galactorrhoea, oligomenorrhoea, amenorrhoea, loss of libido and infertility in females; and impotence, gynaecomastia and decreased libido in males. It is produced by drugs that either deplete the hypothalamic stores of cathecolamines or block dopamine receptors, as prolactin secretion is normally under the inhibitory control of hypothalamic dopamine. Examples of drugs

Table 20.14 Drug-induced endocrine and metabolic disorders

Disorder	Drug
Hyperprolactinaemia	Phenothiazines, benzodiazepines, monoamine oxidase inhibitors, metoclopramide, butyrophenones
Growth retardation	Corticosteroids, androgens
Hyperthyroidism	Iodide preparations, amiodarone, lithium
Hypothyroidism	Sulfonylureas, phenylbutazone, aminoglutethimide, amiodarone, pentazocine, cyclophosphamide, ethionamide, lithium
Adrenal insufficiency	Steroids, metyrapone, aminoglutethimide, trilostane, ketoconazole, etomidate, oral anticoagulants
Gonadal dysfunction	Combination chemotherapy
Gynaecomastia	Oestrogens, spironolactone, digitalis, cimetidine, isoniazid, ethionamide, griseofulvin
Dilutional hyponatraemia	Chlorpropamide, carbamazepine, vincristine, cyclophosphamide, cisplatin
Partial nephrogenic diabetes insipidus	Lithium, demeclocycline
Osteoporosis	Steroids

that cause this abnormality include phenothiazines, butyrophenones, monoamine oxidase inhibitors, metoclopramide, tricyclic antidepressants and cimetidine.

Growth retardation

This is encountered in prepubertal children following long-term administration of corticosteroids that reduce the release of growth hormone and delay bone maturation. Androgens cause premature fusion of the epiphyses and thereby stunt growth, despite an early temporary acceleration of linear growth. Drug-induced hypothyroidism may also be a cause of retardation of growth in children.

Thyroid dysfunction

Both hyperthyroidism and hypothyroidism may be encountered. The most common cause of drug-induced hyperthyroidism is the administration of iodine-containing preparations in areas of endemic iodine deficiency. Rarely, hyperthyroidism may be caused by other drugs including lithium and the antiarrhythmic agent, amiodarone.

Drug-induced hypothyroidism is more common than hyperactivity. It may follow prolonged iodide administration. The precipitant drugs either interfere with the trapping of iodide or block its organification (aminogluthetemide, phenylbutazone, sulfonylureas, etc.). The exact mechanisms responsible for the hypothyroidism encountered with other drugs (lithium, amiodarone) are not known.

Adrenal insufficiency

Suppression of the hypothalamic–pituitary–adrenal axis results from the continued administration of cortisone and synthetic glucocorticoids in a dose exceeding daily physiological requirements (20–30 mg hydrocortisone or equivalent/day). The suppression of corticotrophin (ACTH) secretion may persist for several months after slow withdrawal of therapy, and may even be permanent. These patients therefore require replacement steroids during stress periods, including surgical operations. Adrenal insufficiency due to suppression of corticotrophin release can also occur as a result of prolonged therapy with cyproterone acetate (an antiandrogen), which is often used in the treatment of hirsutism.

Gonadal dysfunction

This is frequently encountered in patients undergoing systemic chemotherapy, especially in males, who may even develop permanent azospermia following combination chemotherapy. In most young females recovery of ovarian function is usual after cessation of chemotherapy, although permanent ovarian failure is often encountered in older women.

Metabolic abnormalities

These are wide-ranging and constitute one of the most common side-effects of drug medication. A dilutional hyponatraemia is caused by a variety of drugs that reduce the excretion of free water as a result of increased release of vasopressin from the neurohypophysis, in addition to a direct antidiuretic action on the renal tubule, e.g. chlorpropamide and carbamazepime, and some cytotoxic agents (vincristine, cisplatin, cyclophosphamide) that induce an inappropriate antidiuresis. The recognition of this dilutional hyponatraemia is important as excessive saline administration may precipitate circulatory overload in these patients.

One of the most important consequences of prolonged high-dose steroid therapy is osteoporosis, which leads to considerable disability from back pain and pathological fractures.

Genitourinary disorders

Many drugs are nephrotoxic. Some of the commonly implicated drugs are outlined in Table 20.15. Whenever possible, nephrotoxic drugs should be avoided in patients with known renal impairment. In addition, drugs that are excreted by the kidneys should be administered in a reduced dosage and blood levels obtained to prevent toxic levels.

The most common drugs responsible for precipitating retention of urine in surgical practice are narcotic analgesics, anticholinergics and loop diuretics. Epididymitis can occur as a complication of amiodarone therapy.

Haematological disorders

The important drug-induced haematological disorders in surgical practice are myelosuppression varying from neutropenia to complete agranulocytosis, and bleeding disorders that most commonly arise as a result of drug interactions during warfarin therapy, particularly in patients who require long-term oral anticoagulation.

In surgical practice myelosuppression is usually due to cytotoxic therapy, hence the need for regular blood counts to detect the onset of this complication. Reduction of the dosage or complete withdrawal, depending on the severity of the blood picture, is indicated. This often results in haematological improvement. In patients with severe bone marrow depression, blood transfusions and cell component therapy (e.g.

Table 20.15 Drug-induced genitourinary disorders

Disorder	Drug
Papillary necrosis	Phenacetin, amidopyrine, etc.
Renal failure	Neomycin, cephaloridine, cephalothin, colistin, vancomycin, amphotericin, cisplatin, penicillamine, cyclosporin, anti-inflammatory drugs, etc.
Retention of urine	Anticholinergic drugs, narcotic analgesics, diuretics
Epididymitis	Amiodarone

Table 20.16 Drug-induced haematological disorders

Disorder	Drug
Myelosuppression	Cytotoxic agents, carbimazole, sulfonamides, etc.
Bleeding tendency: potentiation of warfarin	NSAIDs, co-trimoxazole, metronidazole, latamoxef, cephamandole, erythromycin, neomycin, ketoconazole, miconazole, alcohol, danazol, clofibrate, cimetidine, anabolic steroids, etc.
Haemolysis	Salazopyrine, sulfonamides, aspirin, etc.
Thrombosis	Oral contraceptives

platelets) may be required as supportive measures in addition to treatment with corticosteroids or anabolic steroids (oxymetholone) and marrow rescue with recombinant colony-stimulating factors.

Potentiation of warfarin is the result of a reduction in its metabolism by concomitantly administered drugs, some of which are shown in Table 20.16. It is important to realize that some drugs have the opposite effect. They reduce the anticoagulant effect of warfarin, usually by enzyme induction, e.g. barbiturates, rifampicin and dischloralphenazone.

Neuromuscular disorders

The surgically important disorders in this category are shown in Table 20.17. Neuromuscular blockade can result from:

- presynaptic inhibition
- postsynaptic blockade of acetylcholine receptors
- combined presynaptic and postsynaptic effect
- inhibition of ionic conductance across the muscle membrane such that an end-plate potential cannot be generated.

Postoperative peripheral (as opposed to central) respiratory depression may be due to either drug interaction leading to potentiation of the effects and duration of the muscle relaxants, or to the occurrence of suxam-

Table 20.17 Drug-induced neuromuscular disorders

Disorder	Drug
Postoperative respiratory depression	Aminoglycosides, polymyxins, tetracyclines, lincomycin, clindamycin, chloroquine
Suxamethonium apnoea	Phenelzine, ecothiopate, aprotinin, ketamine, procaine, promazine, lignocaine, clindamycin, lincomycin, lithium
Aggravation of myasthenia gravis	Aminoglycosides, procainamide, β-blockers, chloroquine, phenytoin, lithium, etc.
Myasthenic syndrome	Aminoglycosides, polymixins, anticonvulsants, β-blockers

ethonium apnoea. This is usually an inherited disorder that is characterized by an abnormal pseudo-cholinesterase, which is incapable of inactivating suxamethonium. An acquired form may be the result of hepatic disease or drug interaction.

Certain drugs can aggravate or unmask latent myasthenia gravis. This is distinguished from the drug-induced myasthenic syndrome by the demonstration of antibodies to acetylcholine receptors in the plasma (AChR–ab). The drug-induced syndrome is very rare. It is encountered in elderly patients and individuals with renal impairment if the blood levels of the precipitant drugs are high and hypocalcaemia or hyperkalaemia is present.

Section 20.10 • Drugs commonly used in surgical practice

These include antibiotics [see Module 5, Vol. I], analgesics [Module 16, Vol. I], cytotoxic agents [Module 15, Vol. I], anticoagulants, diuretics, steroids and inotropic agents.

Anticoagulants and related drugs

Unfractionated heparin

Heparin produces immediate anticoagulation and is given parenterally as it is inactivated by mouth. Heparin is a mixture of glycosaminoglycans and acts by forming a complex with AT-III, thereby inactivating several clotting factors including activated factor II (IIa), factor X (Xa). It also potentiates the naturally occurring factor Xa. For therapeutic purposes, heparin is administered intravenously, preferably by constant infusion pump as its action is short lived. For this reason, when heparin is given by intermittent intravenous injection, the time interval between the doses should not exceed 6 h. Lower doses are usually indicated in the elderly, in patients with low serum albumin and those with impaired hepatic or renal function.

Usually, oral anticoagulation is started at the same time and heparin is withdrawn on the third day. If oral anticoagulants cannot be administered, anticoagulation is continued with heparin when the dose is adjusted by the estimation of the partial thromboplastin time. When used for the prophylaxis of deep vein thrombosis, unfractionated heparin (UFH) is administered subcutaneously in a dose of 5000 U 8 hourly.

Side-effects include hypersensitivity reactions, acute thrombocytopenia, haemorrhage and bruising, raised transaminases, osteoporosis and alopecia. Hypersensitivity reactions are rare. The symptoms and signs include fever, lacrimation, urticaria and conjunctival itching. Acute thrombocytopenia is usually reversible on withdrawal of heparin. Rarely, the thrombocytopenia is severe and complicated by venous or arterial thrombotic episodes. For this reason, platelet counts should be measured in patients under heparin therapy for longer than 5 days. Bruising at or around the site of subcutaneous injection is common when UFH is used for prophylaxis of thromboembolic disease. Osteoporosis and alopecia have been reported in patients on prolonged heparin therapy exceeding several months.

Overt haemorrhage is due to overdosage. It requires immediate withdrawal of the drug. If rapid reversal is required, this is achieved by protamine sulfate, administered as a slow intravenous infusion. One milligram of protamine sulfate inhibits 100 U of heparin. The maximum permissible dose of protamine sulfate is 50 mg and this dose should not be exceeded as in larger doses, protamine sulfate has an anticoagulant effect.

Low molecular weight heparins

UFH includes a series of mucopolysaccharides of varying chain length and composition. The fractionated heparins are, by contrast, individual low molecular weight mucopolysaccharides produced by filtration or fractionation. Examples include dalteparin, fragmin and enoxaparin. They provide more effective anticoagulation. Thus, LMWH have a Xa:antithrombin ratio ranging from 2:1 to 4:1 compared with 1:1 of UFH. In addition, LMWH have other therapeutic advantages: higher bioavailability when administered by subcutaneous injection, longer half-life and reduced risk of thrombocytopenia. The risk of haemorrhagic complications is reduced as LMWH have a lower affinity for vWF, a weaker inhibitory effect on platelets and a smaller tendency to increase vascular permeability. Thus, they are less likely to produce bleeding and their action lasts longer. Results of controlled studies have shown equal efficacy between LMWH and UFH in terms of prevention of thromboembolic disease but a reduction in the incidence of haemorrhage. The other practical advantage of LMWH is that only a single daily subcutaneous administration is needed for effective prophylaxis against thromboembolic disease. In addition, they can be used to achieve full anticoagulation in patients with established thromboembolic disease and for managing patients with unstable angina, thus dispensing with the need for heparin infusion pumps.

Ancrod (Arvin)

This is an effective parenteral anticoagulant. It acts by producing controlled therapeutic defibrination. It is used mainly in the treatment of established thromboembolic disease, where it is administered intravenously, and in its prophylaxis, especially for orthopaedic procedures in the elderly, e.g. fractures of the femur and hip joint replacement. The main advantage of ancrod in the treatment of thromboembolic disease is the absence of a rebound hypercoagulability when treatment is stopped. Haemorrhage may occur during therapy. This can be managed either with reconstituted freeze-dried fibrinogen or the administration of ancrod antivenom. The other complication is anaphylaxis, which is treated with adrenaline and hydrocortisone.

Oral anticoagulants

These consist of dicoumarol and warfarin, which have an identical mode of action. In the UK, warfarin is preferred in view of its more rapid action and the smaller doses needed. Oral anticoagulants are used for both short-term and long-term therapy. They antagonize vitamin K by inhibiting the action of the enzyme responsible for the carboxylation of factors II, VII, IX and X. The anticoagulant effect is not achieved until 36–48 h after initiation of therapy, which is monitored by the estimation of the PT. Bleeding during therapy with oral anticoagulants requires cessation of the drug, estimation of the PT, administration of phytomenadione (vitamin K_1) and FFP, together with the investigation of the cause, which is usually either overdosage or potentiation by other drugs.

Patients who are kept on long-term anticoagulant therapy, e.g. prosthetic heart valves, should carry anticoagulant cards.

Antiplatelet drugs

These agents reduce platelet adhesiveness and thereby inhibit thrombus formation, predominantly on the arterial side of the circulation. They are ineffective in the treatment of established venous thrombosis. They include aspirin, dipyridamole (Persantin) and sulfinpyrazone (Anturan). Aspirin is being investigated in the prophylaxis of thromboembolic disease in patients after hip fracture. Antiplatelet agents are used in combination with oral anticoagulants in patients with prosthetic heart valves. Other indications include coronary artery disease, after cardiac transplantation, transient cerebral ischaemic attacks, diabetic retinopathy and thrombocythaemia following splenectomy.

Fibrinolytic agents

Fibrinolytic agents are used to activate the plasmin system responsible for fibrinolysis in order to lyse intravascular thrombi and embolized clots:

- major deep vein thrombosis
- pulmonary embolism
- rethrombosis after arterial surgery
- clotting of AV shunts
- myocardial thrombosis
- more recently for DIC and adult respiratory distress syndrome (ARDS).

Three agents are available: streptokinase, urokinase and recombinant tPA. Streptokinase is of bacterial origin and is therefore strongly antigenic, whereas urokinase is extracted from human male urine and is non-antigenic.

To date, streptokinase is the agent that has been used most extensively in the treatment of thromboembolic disease and acute arterial thrombosis. It acts by activating the proactivator to form the activator of plasminogen, which is then converted to active plasmin. Streptokinase is infused intravenously in isotonic saline, 5% dextrose or Haemaccel (100 000 U in 100 ml) in a loading dose of 250 000–500 000 U over 30–60 min. This loading dose neutralizes antibodies to streptokinase commonly found in humans due to prior exposure to streptococci. The maintenance dose consists of 100 000 U/h for 72 h for deep vein thrombosis and 24 h for pulmonary embolism. In arterial thrombosis, the duration of treatment varies from 24 to 72 h. Therapy, which is monitored by the thrombin time, results in a decrease in the plasminogen and fibrinogen levels with an increase in the level of fibrin degradation products (FDPs). Heparin therapy, as a constant infusion, is started 3–4 h after the end of the streptokinase infusion, when the thrombin time has decreased to less than twice the control value, to prevent recurrence of the thrombosis. In view of its marked antigenicity, streptokinase therapy should be covered routinely with intravenous hydrocortisone (100 mg), which is given prior to the loading dose. The other important complication is haemorrhage. This requires immediate cessation of therapy and the administration of an antifibrinolytic agent (tranexamic acid, 10 mg/kg). Because of the inevitable rise in the antistreptokinase titre, repeated therapy is contraindicated within 3–6 months.

Urokinase acts by activating plasminogen directly to form plasmin. In surgical practice, urokinase has been restricted to recanalization of clotted AV shunts when 5000–25 000 U in 2–3 ml is instilled into the affected shunt, which is then clamped off for 2–4 h.

Recombinant tPA is likely to replace either agent in fibrinolytic therapy since it provides more controlled therapeutic fibrinolysis as it binds strongly to fibrin and, unlike streptokinase, is much more active when bound to fibrin. Furthermore, it is not antigenic. In practice, there are fewer problems with the use of tPA but the therapeutic margin is still narrow and bleeding remains a significant problem.

Problems with fibrinolytic therapy
Contrary to the physiological degradation of fibrin, where the reactants are bound to the fibrin in the clot with minimal activation of the free circulating plasmin, in fibrinolytic therapy large doses have to be administered, high enough to overcome the naturally occurring plasma inhibitors before a therapeutic effect on the clot can be achieved. This high plasma concentration has adverse consequences by inducing the proteolysis of coagulation factors and fibrinogen. The resulting degradation products interfere with platelet function, inhibit thrombin and disturb fibrin polymerization. Thus, fibrinolytic therapy has an inherent risk of severe bleeding that may be difficult to control, especially in patients after surgery with recent healing wounds.

Diuretics
The commonly used diuretics in surgical practice are:

- **thiazide**: chlorotiazide, bendrofluazide
- **loop**: frusemide, ethacrynic acid
- **osmotic**: mannitol
- **potassium-sparing**: triamterene
- **aldosterone antagonist**: spironolactone.

The thiazide diuretics are usually administered as chronic medications in patients with oedema due to heart disease. They act directly on the kidney tubules and increase the excretion of sodium, chloride, bicarbonate and potassium. As the excretion of chloride is proportionately greater than bicarbonate, prolonged therapy may be followed by hypochloraemia alkalosis in addition to hypokalaemia. They should thus be used with extreme caution in patients with liver disease as they may precipitate encephalopathy.

The loop diuretics are more powerful and are often used in surgical practice in oliguric patients after adequate hydration has been achieved. They act primarily on the ascending limb of Henle and on both the proximal and distal tubules, inhibiting the reabsorption of sodium and chloride through the entire length of the renal tubule. They act within 15 min of an intravenous bolus injection. Usually, frusemide in a dose of 40 mg is administered, but some advocate much larger doses (100–200 mg) in oliguric patients, although the enhanced efficacy of these large doses is unproven. Loop diuretics cause hypokalaemia and may precipitate encephalopathy in patients with chronic liver disease.

Mannitol is used extensively in surgical practice. Its common indications include:

- renal shutdown (oliguria) following hypovolaemia and subsequent to volume replacement. The alternative here is low-dose dopamine
- to reduce intracranial pressure in neurosurgery
- as a prophylaxis against renal failure in jaundiced patients undergoing surgical intervention.

Mannitol is a sugar that is only marginally metabolized by the liver and readily excreted through the glomerular membrane. It therefore expands the plasma volume and exerts its diuretic activity by increasing the osmotic pressure of the glomerular filtrate. This results in impaired reabsorption of water and solutes (sodium, chloride, potassium, calcium, phosphorus, magnesium, urea, etc.). Aside from electrolyte disturbances, pulmonary oedema and congestive heart failure may be induced by mannitol therapy, especially in patients with severe renal disease and diminished cardiac reserve. It is thus contraindicated in anuric patients and in individuals with known cardiac disease or pre-existing pulmonary congestion. It is administered as a 20% solution in a dose of 1.5–2.0 g/kg over a period of 30–60 min. It is important to stress that any hypovolaemia must be corrected before mannitol infusion in oliguric patients and in the prophylaxis against renal failure in jaundiced patients.

Spironolactone inhibits aldosterone-mediated reabsorption of sodium and is used in patients with ascites due to chronic liver disease, either alone or in combination with a loop diuretic. It does not cause hypokalaemia, which is an important consideration in cirrhotic patients. It is active by mouth. The initial dose is 25 mg three times daily, but this may be increased to 200–300 mg daily, if necessary, to obtain a diuresis.

Inotropic drugs

Inotropic drugs are cardiac stimulants and include the cardiac glycosides, β_1-adrenoreceptor drugs and methyl xanthines.

Cardiac glycosides

The positive inotropic activity of digoxin and other cardiac glycosides is mediated via an action on Na^+ and K^+-ATPase. The principal indication for their use is congestive cardiac failure associated with atrial fibrillation. They are no longer used as chronic medication in mild heart failure, especially in the elderly. As potassium and digoxin share the same myocardial binding sites, hypokalaemia exaggerates the toxic effects of cardiac glycosides. These are cardiac and extracardiac. The cardiac side-effects precede the extracardiac ones and include ventricular bigeminy, multifocal ventricular extrasystoles, VT and heart block.

β_1-Adrenoreceptor drugs

The β_1-receptors are situated in the myocardial muscle fibres and their stimulation by these drugs results in an increased activity of the adenylate cyclase system and enhanced Ca^{2+} uptake by the sarcoplasmic reticulum of the myocardium. They also stimulate the peripheral α- or β_2-receptors to a varying extent. The resulting peripheral vasoconstriction and the oxygen-wasting tachycardia are undesirable in patients with cardiac decompensation (e.g. adrenaline, noradrenaline, isoprenaline).

The most widely used drug of this category in intensive care is dopamine (Intropin), which exerts its beneficial effects by acting on different receptors at various dose ranges as follows.

- **In small doses** (1–5 μg/kg/min), dopamine dilates the renal and mesenteric vascular beds by its unique action on dopaminergic receptors. The effects on the kidneys result in an increase in the renal blood flow, glomerular filtration rate, sodium excretion and urine output. Hence, its use in prerenal shutdown.
- **At a higher dose range** (5–20 μg/kg/min), dopamine has a direct inotropic action on the myocardium by its action on the β_1-receptors, causing a dose-related increase in the cardiac output with a minimal increase in the heart rate. The blood pressure rises as a consequence of the enhanced cardiac output.
- **In high doses** (20 μg/kg/min or above), dopamine, in addition to increasing the cardiac output further, stimulates the α-receptors on the peripheral blood vessels, causing a systemic vasoconstriction and a further rise in the blood pressure. Despite this, the renal blood flow is maintained at a high level.

The most frequently reported reactions to dopamine are ectopic beats, tachycardia, anginal pain, palpitations, dyspnoea, nausea and vomiting. Dopamine is contraindicated in uncorrected tachyarrhythmias and in patients with phaeochromocytomas.

Dobutamine is also a selective stimulant of the β_1-receptors of the myocardium. It is also used in cardiogenic shock but has no advantage over dopamine and no selective action on the renal blood flow **[see Module 19, Vol. I]**.

Steroids

As treatment with steroid hormones and their synthetic analogues is both complex and attended by a significant morbidity, it should never be undertaken lightly.

Corticosteroids

These include a wide range of substances synthesized by the adrenal cortex with a 21-carbon steroid nucleus. The basic physiological actions that are shared to a varying extent by all the adrenal corticosteroid hormones are:

- retention of sodium by the kidney and its excretion of osmotically free water
- deposition of glycogen in the liver
- increased protein breakdown
- stabilization of cell membranes and anti-inflammatory effect
- mobilization of fat in response to adrenaline.

Adrenal corticosteroids, such as cortisol and cortisone, with a predominant effect on carbohydrate metabolism and usually with an associated anti-inflammatory action, are referred to as **glucocorticoids**, whereas aldosterone, which has a marked action on sodium retention and potassium excretion, is known as a **mineralocorticoid**.

The synthetic analogues may possess either action (Table 20.18). The selective action of these synthetic derivatives allows a more favourable therapeutic ratio than the naturally occurring hormones. Cortisone is no longer used for replacement therapy in adrenal insufficiency. Instead, hydrocortisone is used in the acute situation and hydrocortisone + fludrocortisone (mineralocorticoid) for chronic insufficiency, e.g. Addison's disease. Prednisolone is the glucocorticoid

Table 20.18 Relative potencies of some corticosteroids using hydrocortisone as the reference compound

Steroid	Anti-inflammatory effect	Relative Na^+ retaining action
Hydrocortisone	1.0	1.0
Cortisone	0.8	0.8
Prednisone	4.0	0.8
Prednisolone	4.0	0.8
Methyl prednisolone	5.0	0.5
Fludrocortisone	10.0	125.0
Triamcinolone	5.0	0
Betamethasone	25.0	0
Dexamethasone	25.0	0

most commonly used for long-term administration. Prednisone is only active after conversion to prednisolone in the body. Dexamethasone is mainly used when mineralocorticoid activity is not desirable, e.g. cerebral oedema, and is effective in reducing opioid-induced nausea.

Therapeutic uses of corticosteroids

Topical steroid applications are often attended by side-effects. Secondary infection is common, including folliculitis, boils and fungal infections, due to local suppression of the inflammatory response. Allergy causing a contact eczema occurs very frequently following topical applications of steroids, particularly when these are combined with antibiotics. Prolonged topical steroid applications lead to atrophy of the skin due to loss of dermal collagen. Absorption through the skin into the blood stream with suppression of the pituitary–adrenal axis occurs to a significant extent in children with the more potent corticosteroid applications, and in adults if more than 30 g daily is used. Topical steroids should not be used:

- **in the presence of cutaneous infection**
- **when a definite diagnosis has not been made**
- **in gravitational ulcers where they cause delayed healing due to inhibition of collagen formation**.

Systemic corticosteroid therapy may be essential, as in Addison's disease and hypopituitarism. More commonly, systemic corticosteroids are used (i) in emergency life-threatening states and (ii) for long-term suppression of inflammation and the immune response.

Systemic corticosteroids are used in the following acute situations:

- acute adrenal insufficiency
- organ transplantation
- severe exacerbations of inflammatory bowel disease
- acute exacerbations of connective-tissue disorders and vasculitides
- raised intracranial pressure from cerebral oedema caused by tumours and infarcts
- status asthmaticus
- pulmonary aspiration
- anaphylactic reactions
- blood-transfusion reactions.

Their use in ARDS and septic shock remains controversial, without any definite evidence of benefit. Dexamethasone is ineffective in the cerebral oedema that complicates liver failure and is contraindicated in acute pancreatitis. Whereas corticosteroids do not impart any benefit in acute fulminant liver failure, they significantly improve survival in subacute hepatic necrosis, chronic active hepatitis and non-alcoholic cirrhosis in the female.

Systemic steroids are now used less frequently and more selectively to suppress the inflammatory response. The principles of long-term suppression include a short period (1–2 weeks) of high-dose therapy to achieve a maximal response, followed by a gradual reduction until either the drug, usually prednisolone, is withdrawn or a small maintenance dose is continued. Rapid steroid withdrawal is harmful because, apart from the risk of flare-up, it may precipitate acute adrenal insufficiency. **If the maintenance dose necessary to suppress the disease is greater than 20 mg of prednisolone or its equivalent, serious complications will develop within 12 months.** The disorders for which systemic corticosteroids are used in selected cases are:

- rheumatoid arthritis
- rheumatic carditis
- the nephrotic syndrome in childhood
- connective tissue disorders and vasculitides
- malignant conditions, e.g. advanced breast cancer, acute lymphocytic leukaemias
- autoimmune haemolytic anaemias
- inflammatory bowel disease
- neurological disorders, e.g. multiple sclerosis, Bell's palsy
- bronchial asthma of the severe chronic non-allergic type
- certain skin disorders, e.g. pemphigus
- sarcoidosis.

All patients on long-term corticosteroid therapy should carry steroid cards.

The contraindications to systemic corticosteroid therapy are:

- tuberculosis
- local and systemic infections (unless controlled)
- heart failure
- hypertension
- peptic ulceration
- psychosis
- renal dysfunction
- diabetes mellitus
- glaucoma
- myasthenia gravis
- thromboembolic disease
- pregnancy.

Adverse reactions to systemic corticosteroid therapy

A number of side-effects is inevitable after prolonged use of these agents. These include increased protein breakdown, which is associated with atrophy of dermal collagen, striae, bruising, muscle wasting; myopathy and osteoporosis, the latter leading to pathological fractures; the development of hirsutism and the cushinoid habitus with the typical moon face, buffalo hump, supraclavicular fat pads, central obesity and acne; fluid and electrolyte disturbances, e.g. hypokalaemic alkalosis and oedema; hyperglycaemia and glycosuria; diminished resistance to both acute and chronic bacterial infections; adrenal suppression and inability to respond to stress, including surgical intervention; immunosuppression and elevation of the blood urea.

Other sporadic complications include peptic ulceration with perforation and bleeding, cardiac failure, psychoses and behavioural changes, precipitation/aggravation of DM, hypertension, growth stunting in children, posterior subcapsular cataracts and amenorrhoea.

The adverse reactions that may develop on withdrawal of the steroid therapy include reactivation of the disease, a withdrawal syndrome (fever, myalgia, arthralgia, malaise), adrenal insufficiency and peripheral neuropathy.

Adrenocorticotropic hormone

ACTH is used in preference to systemic corticosteroids in children, in whom prolonged steroid therapy may result in growth inhibition. A number of disorders seems to respond more readily to ACTH than to systemic corticosteroids. These include multiple sclerosis and some acute allergic conditions. The main indications for the administration of ACTH in clinical practice are in the diagnosis of adrenal function and its reserve capacity, and for adrenal suppression consequent on steroid withdrawal.

Androgens and anabolic steroids

The most powerful naturally occurring androgenic hormone is testosterone. Derivatives of testosterone with a pronounced anabolic and reduced androgenic effect include ethylestrenol (taken orally), stanozolol (oral and intramuscular), nandrolone and nandrolone phenylproprionate, the last two being administered as depot intramuscular injection. None of the currently available anabolic steroids is entirely free of androgenic effects. In general, anabolic steroids have proved disappointing in those conditions characterized by muscle and tissue wasting, e.g. osteoporosis, chronic debilitating conditions and protein breakdown after major surgery, trauma or sepsis. They are used in the treatment of some aplastic anaemias and in advanced breast cancer.

The only indications for androgen treatment are hypogonadism and hypopituitarism (in conjunction with chorionic gonadotrophin and menotrophin). Neither androgens nor anabolic steroids should be administered for delayed puberty and allied growth disorders since, despite an initial acceleration of linear growth, they lead to premature fusion of the epiphyses and result in short stature. Androgens and some of the anabolic steroids are known to cause hepatic tumours in humans after prolonged therapy. The other adverse reactions to anabolic steroids and androgens are cholestatic jaundice, fluid and salt retention, hirsutism and masculinization in some females.

Oestrogens

The primary oestrogens produced by the ovaries are oestrone and oestradiol-17β. Oestriol, which is a metabolite of oestradiol, is much less potent than either oestrone or oestradiol. Several synthetic oestrogens are available. The most commonly used non-steroidal synthetic oestrogen is stilboestrol, whereas the most powerful synthetic steroidal derivative is ethinyloestradiol.

Oestrogens are used in the treatment of some patients with prostatic cancer. Their use in advanced or recurrent breast cancer has been largely replaced by the antioestrogen tamoxifen.

The important adverse responses to oestrogens are the stimulation of the breast parenchyma, cervical and uterine cancers and thromboembolic disease, especially in postoperative patients, in individuals suffering from varicose veins and in obese and diabetic women. Other females also complain of dyspepsia and withdrawal vaginal bleeding.

Progestogens

These compounds act on tissues that are sensitized by oestrogens. Progestogens fall into two categories: nortestosterone analogues (ethisterone, norethisterone) and progesterone and its derivatives (allyloestrenol, dihydrogesterone, hydroxyprogesterone, medroxyprogesterone). The nortestosterone analogues are partially metabolized to potent oestrogens in the body and, therefore, have oestrogenic as well as progesterone-like effects. The progestogens are used for oral contraception in conjunction with oestrogens and in certain gynaecological disorders. They can also be effective in endometrial, renal and breast cancers. The progestogens that are used in malignancy are norethisterone, hydroxyprogesterone, medroxyprogesterone and megestrol. In advanced breast cancer, they are administered in high dosage in patients who relapse after a remission obtained with tamoxifen. Overall, a 30% objective response rate is obtained in these patients. Progestogens do not have any serious side-effects.

Section 20.11 • Acute psychiatric states

A degree of psychological disturbance is inevitably associated with physical illness. Severity varies from transient, self-limiting anxiety and apprehension to more prolonged and debilitating conditions, such as depression, which may require specialist treatment. An individual diagnosed with organic disease faces several psychological as well as physical challenges. Often a sense of helplessness and uncertainty about the future can present as passivity, irritability or demanding behaviour. This may compromise treatment and the patient is at risk of being labelled inappropriately as 'difficult to manage' and thus alienated. A sense of injustice or loss of control is often prominent, especially in conditions that develop without evidence of obvious risk factors, e.g. some forms of malignancy. Patients may struggle to attach meaning to their illness, and if the disease cannot be conceptualized as having a likely physical cause, inappropriate self-blame may emerge. Feelings of guilt and failure can undermine self-esteem and act as risk factors for the development of depressive illness in vulnerable individuals.

Physical illness can also change the way an individual is treated by others. Myths and stigmata exist about particular conditions. For example, beliefs that cancer is somehow transmissible by direct contact may result in patients becoming isolated from their friends and family. This distancing erodes further the likelihood of emotional support being available when most needed.

An awareness of likely psychological difficulties is important when treating physically unwell patients, and good-quality surgical care should seek to address their emotional needs. Patients derive much benefit from empathic management and considered, jargon-free information given in a spirit of collaboration. Concerns and anxieties should not be dismissed as inconsequential or inevitable. It is only when they are acknowledged that patients may feel able to disclose other concerns and attempt to make adjustments to their new situation.

Psychiatric disorders

Psychiatric disorders occur two to three times more commonly in hospital settings than in the general population, with rates of 13–61% reported for inpatients and 14–52% for those attending outpatient clinics. Conditions most commonly encountered are depression, adjustment and anxiety disorders, drug and alcohol problems, somatization, delirium and dementia, but despite their high prevalence, detection rates of below 50% are reported. There are several possible reasons for this.

- Training of medical and nursing staff in the recognition of psychiatric symptoms is generally inadequate.
- There is reluctance to enquire explicitly about psychological issues. Interview techniques do not, in general, facilitate disclosure of emotional problems and all too often dialogue becomes irretrievably caught up in details about physical complaints and treatment.
- The importance of psychological issues is often lost as management becomes focused on technologically advanced investigations and treatment.
- Staff may believe that psychological problems are inevitable in response to physical illness, and that they will resolve spontaneously, do not constitute psychiatric illness or warrant treatment.
- Patients may be reluctant to disclose psychological problems, fearing that this would indicate emotional frailty or failure to cope in adversity. They often feel protective towards the surgical team and do not wish to burden staff, whom they perceive as generally very busy, with anything other than somatic symptoms.

Failure to identify psychological disturbance is, however, associated with many adverse consequences, which include increased morbidity and mortality, impaired psychosocial functioning, delay in discharge, excessive use of medical resources and abnormal illness behaviour. It is thus essential to be able to recognize and, if appropriate, introduce treatment for psycho-

logical problems when they present in surgical practice. The most common and significant conditions relevant to surgical practice are described here.

Delirium

Delirium (acute confusional state) is a common condition. It often occurs during the immediate postoperative period and affects at least 10% of patients admitted to hospital with acute illness. It is associated with prolonged hospitalization and increased mortality. The fundamental change in delirium is reduced level of consciousness and this is the essential differentiating feature from dementia where, despite memory impairment and confusion, full consciousness is maintained.

The syndrome is produced by disturbed brain function secondary to an extensive range of possible underlying conditions, many of which arise outside the CNS (Table 20.19).

Whatever the cause, the clinical features of delirium are remarkably consistent and consist of:

- **Clouding of consciousness**: the degree of impairment can vary from mild disturbance, through progressive drowsiness, to coma. It can be difficult to detect subtle changes in conscious level. There may be problems holding the patient's attention, disorientation to time, apprehension, impaired ability to self-care, episodic incontinence and disturbances of the sleep–wake cycle with distressing dreams, daytime drowsiness, nocturnal excitability and insomnia. The onset of delirium is often rapid and its severity fluctuates throughout the day, with lucid periods and characteristic exacerbation at night.
- **Thinking**: loss of clarity and direction in thought processes becomes manifest as disjointed, rambling and chaotic speech, which is difficult to understand. Comprehension of external events is lost and the boundaries between reality and fantasy become blurred. Poorly elaborated, fleeting persecutory delusions often develop and loss of insight is generally an early feature.
- **Memory impairment**: this is invariably present with impairment of immediate recall and short-term memory. Remote memories may remain initially intact but, with progressive deterioration in conscious level, also become affected. There is amnesia for the period of delirium on recovery.
- **Perceptual abnormalities**: distortions may occur in any sensory modality but are most often visual, with objects appearing misshapen or changed in size. Misidentification of individuals is common and may lead to suspicion or hostility. Visual hallucinations, which can be vivid and frightening, are often evident.
- **Emotional disturbance**: this is highly variable and may change unpredictably during the course of delirium. Fear is common and anxiety, suspicion, depression, apathy or perplexity may also colour the clinical presentation.

Table 20.19 Causes of delirium

Hypoxia	Respiratory disease, heart failure, cardiac dysrhythmia, carbon monoxide poisoning, postoperative	
Trauma	Head injury	
Infection	Intracranial:	Meningitis
		Encephalitis
		Meningovascular syphilis
	Extracranial:	Septicaemia
		Bronchopneumonia
		Urinary tract infection
Neoplasia	Primary or metastatic cerebral tumours	
Vitamin deficiency	Thiamine (Wernicke's encephalopathy)	
	Nicotinic acid (pellagra)	
	B_{12} deficiency	
Endocrine	Hypopituitarism	
	Myxoedema	
	Thyrotoxicosis	
	Cushing's syndrome	
	Addisonion crisis	
	Hypoparathyroidism and hyperparathyroidism	
	Diabetes mellitus	
Degenerative	Dementia with associated physical disorder, e.g. anoxia, sepsis	
Vascular	Stroke	
	Transient cerebral ischaemia	
	Hypertensive encephalopathy	
	Systemic lupus erythematosus	
Epilepsy	Generalized seizures	
	Postictal states	
Toxic	Drugs:	Alcohol
		Barbiturates and other sedatives or hypnotics
		Amphetamines
		Hallucinogens
		Opiates
		Cocaine
		Tricyclic antidepressants
		Lithium
		Anticholinergics
		Neuroleptics
		Steroids
	Industrial metals:	Lead, mercury compounds, arsenic
Metabolic	Uraemia, hepatic failure, electrolyte disturbance	
	Acute intermittent porphyria	
	Alkalosis	
	Acidosis	
	Hypercapnia	

■ **Psychomotor disturbance**: mental sluggishness and apathy usually develop as consciousness becomes progressively impaired, but overactivity can also occur, with restlessness and disordered, unpredictable behaviour.

Outcome and treatment

Recovery from delirium depends on the rapid diagnosis and treatment of its underlying cause. Full resolution often occurs within a week. In a minority of cases the acute symptoms may clear to reveal cognitive impairment caused by the original brain insult. Mortality is directly related to the severity of the precipitating condition, and death occurs in 10–30% of patients.

Nursing input requires consistency in an evenly lit room, and tranquillization (see below) may help to allay restlessness and prevent injury.

Dementia

Dementia is a syndrome of progressive global cognitive impairment with memory dysfunction as a prominent feature, accompanied by disorders of language (the dysphasias), praxis and perceptual function (agnosia). Dementia must be distinguished from delirium, although the syndromes may coexist. Differentiating factors include rate of onset (delirium acute, dementia insidious), course (delirium fluctuating, dementia progressive), level of consciousness (lowered in delirium, unimpaired in dementia), and the presence of hallucinations and delusions (more common in delirium, less so in dementia).

The syndrome has many causes, and although generally progressive, some forms of dementia are reversible. These include hypothyroidism, nutritional deficiencies, alcoholism and normal pressure hydrocephalus. The most common form of the disorder is Alzheimer's disease, followed by the vascular dementias. Other causes include Lewy body dementia, Parkinson's disease, and other neurodegenerative disorders such as Pick's disease and Huntington's disease.

Memory failure, personality disintegration and behavioural abnormalities may make demented patients vulnerable and difficult to manage in surgical settings, while loss of capacity to give informed consent may raise practical ethical issues. Specialist referral is recommended in such circumstances.

Depression

Studies suggest that between 10 and 50% of hospitalized patients suffer from depression. The elderly are at particular risk and depression is more commonly found in association with severe, chronic, debilitating and painful conditions such as cancer, neurological disorders, arthritis and stroke. Surgical procedures associated with altered body image or function, such as mastectomy or colostomy formation, carry a high psychiatric morbidity, most often taking the form of an anxiety or depressive disorder. Depression may also precede the onset of physical illness. For example, depressive features may declare the presence of an otherwise occult neoplasm in the absence of any physical signs. Physical illness and comorbid depression has been shown to be associated with prolonged hospitalization and greater utilization of health resources after discharge. Depressed patients often describe physical complaints in an exaggerated way, and their threshold for pain may be reduced.

Table 20.20 Features of depressive illness

- Low mood which may be worse in the morning
- Feelings of inappropriate worthlessness or guilt
- Pessimism and hopelessness about the future
- Recurrent thoughts of death, self-harm or suicide
- Lowered self-esteem or self-confidence
- Agitation and irritability
- Loss of interest and pleasure in usual activities
- Lack of energy, fatigue and apathy
- Disturbed sleep, often with early-morning waking
- Impoverished appetite and weight loss
- Poor concentration with associated memory difficulties
- Problems in decision making
- Loss of libido

Presentation is variable, but an appreciation of common depressive features is important (Table 20.20). Part of the difficulty in identifying depression in hospital settings is that some somatic symptoms, such as fatigue, sleep disturbance, anorexia and weight loss may develop as part of a physical illness. Specific self-rating scales have been developed to help identify mood disorders in hospital populations and of these the Hospital Anxiety and Depression Scale has widespread utility.

Chemical antidepressants are highly effective, even in the face of clear precipitants to the disorder, such as serious physical illness. Care must be taken to ensure that sufficient doses are used, and that potential interactions with other medication, or physical illness (e.g. liver disease, cardiac disorders) are identified.

Reactions to stress and anxiety disorders

Anxiety, stress and fear are common, indeed almost inevitable, accompaniments to the investigation and treatment of physical illness. The physical manifestations of anxiety, caused by increased sympathetic autonomic activity, affect most systems and may mimic a wide range of disorders. Common symptoms may include subjective breathlessness and hyperventilation with attendant hypocapnia and consequent neurological symptoms, chest pain and palpitations, tremor and sweating, gastrointestinal upset with nausea and diarrhoea, urinary frequency, and sexual dysfunction. Such physical symptoms may worsen the anxiety state, become amplified and lead to a vicious circle of escalating distress. In most cases, anxiety is self-limiting, with simple reassurance and explanation being all that is necessary, although practitioners need to set aside time to recognize, assess and deal appropriately with affected patients. Good communication skills are essential, with careful history taking and selective investigation sometimes necessary to differentiate anxiety states from other illnesses, such as pain of cardiac origin, thyroid disease and phaeochromocytoma.

Acute stress reaction

Individuals vary greatly in response to stress. Following severely stressful events, some patients will display behavioural reactions in which they appear dazed, confused and perplexed. They may not appear to understand what is happening around them, be withdrawn or agitated, and have difficulty in giving a coherent history or in following instructions. This acute state usually subsides within hours or days once the stressful situation has resolved.

Adjustment disorder

Less severe events, commonly those necessitating lifestyle changes (including surgical treatment), may be followed by a period of low mood, worry, irritability and anxiety in the absence of prominent depressive symptoms. Such adjustment reactions are also self-limiting, generally within 6 months, but require appropriate reassurance, explanation and support.

Post-traumatic stress disorder

Post-traumatic stress disorder (PTSD) is characterized by repetitive, intrusive and distressing thoughts, nightmares or memories (flashbacks) of previous trauma with emotional numbing, social withdrawal, autonomic overarousal, anxiety, depression, insomnia and irritability. Situations that evoke memories of the traumatic experience are avoided and the use of alcohol or drugs may complicate the clinical picture. Although described in relation to trauma of exceptional severity, such as natural disasters and warfare, PTSD can occur following less catastrophic experiences, e.g. road traffic accidents or assault. Suggested predisposing factors include a marked acute stress response to the original trauma, neurotic personality traits, poverty, unemployment, childhood behavioural problems, parental divorce and physical abuse. Recent trials suggest that psychological treatments (especially cognitive behaviour therapy) are useful in reducing symptom intensity and may be augmented by various drugs including antidepressants (selective serotonin reuptake inhibitors), carbamazepine or lithium.

Generalized anxiety disorder, panic disorder and phobias

More severe anxiety disorders may be classified in terms of their time course. In generalized anxiety disorder the psychological and physical symptoms of anxiety tend to be continuous and are often long-standing, while in panic disorder acute attacks of severe anxiety occur in episodic form, with physical symptoms prominent. Attacks can last from minutes to hours and may be so severe that sufferers fear they will die. Anxiety symptoms may be spontaneous or triggered by certain situations. Highly specific fears, such as fear of snakes or needles, are known as phobias; more general stimuli, such as public places (agoraphobia = fear of the market place) or social situations (social phobia), may result in disabling avoidance behaviour. As a result, patients may be unable to attend clinics or comply effectively with treatment.

Treatment of anxiety

Minor tranquillizers, such as the benzodiazepines, will effectively and safely attenuate anxiety in the short term, but symptoms are likely to recur when the drugs are withdrawn and prolonged use is associated with the development of tolerance and dependence. β-Blockers are occasionally helpful where physical symptoms are marked, while antidepressants are particularly useful in panic disorder. Specialist psychological treatments, such as systematic desensitization for phobias, or cognitive behavioural therapy for generalized anxiety disorder, may be indicated. Depression and anxiety often co-exist, and depressive disorder should always be considered when evaluating anxious patients.

Somatization

Somatization is the process by which psychological disturbance is expressed as physical complaints, often referred to as functional or medically unexplained symptoms. It does not constitute a specific disease entity, is commonly associated with psychiatric disorders such as depression and anxiety, and is the seminal feature in a group of conditions known as the somatoform disorders. Somatization may occur in the presence or absence of organic pathology; when physical disease is present, symptoms are generally described in a florid, exaggerated and persistent way.

Unexplained medical symptoms are among the most common reasons for requesting a psychiatric opinion in the general hospital and are frequently encountered in certain specialist settings such as gastroenterology, cardiology, neurology and pain clinics. The course of a somatized illness is variable. It is often transient, mild and self-limiting, but in a minority of cases symptoms may become chronic and profoundly debilitating, and require specialist treatment.

Preoccupation with physical complaints is often accompanied by persistent requests for medical investigations. This can become a prolonged, unnecessary and expensive process in which the patient is placed at risk of developing iatrogenic illness. In addition, the compliant doctor reinforces the patient's already tenaciously held belief that his or her symptoms result from undetected physical illness.

Negative test results often fail to reassure the patient that there is no evidence of organic disease and there may be a resultant breakdown in the doctor–patient relationship, with medical staff distancing themselves from patients whom they come to perceive as management problems. Mutual hostility develops, patient dissatisfaction mounts and there may be threats of litigation or requests for referral to other specialists.

This relentless pursuit for causes and cures can produce profound physical and social disabilities. The individual may be unable to work and there is increasing reliance on the medical profession, social services and family for support. In extreme cases, such exaggerated and maladaptive behaviour can result in the patient becoming bed or wheelchair bound.

Somatoform disorders

Hypochondriasis

The essential feature of this condition is a preoccupation with the possibility of having a serious and progressive disease. This belief is often based on misinterpretation of benign bodily sensations and persists despite multiple negative investigations and reassurance. Anxiety and depression often coexist.

Body dysmorphic disorder

Also referred to as dysmorphophobia, persistent complaints about an imagined defect in appearance are the hallmark of this condition. In cases where a minor abnormality does exist, the individual's focus on it is excessive, with extreme distress, anxiety and social withdrawal. Facial asymmetry and minor skin blemishes are common preoccupations. Careful assessment is required, for dysmorphophobia can be a feature of developing psychiatric illness such as schizophrenia or depression. It is often associated with severe personality disorder and obsessional traits; the suicide risk is increased.

Many affected patients embark on a relentless quest for cosmetic surgery or dermatological treatments, but such requests should be treated with extreme caution. The prevalence of body dysmorphic disorder is unknown, but it is thought to affect up to 5% of patients attending cosmetic surgery clinics and it is thus important to be aware of presentation differences between this group of patients and others for whom surgical correction may confer significant psychological benefit. In body dysmorphic disorder there is likely to be marked dysfunction and preoccupation with the perceived deformity, concern about multiple defects and objective disagreement about the extent of deformity. Expectations are often unrealistic and if corrective procedures are undertaken, the individual is likely to re-present with different, but equally insignificant aesthetic concerns. Psychiatric opinion should be sought.

Somatization disorder (Briquet's syndrome)
This is a chronic condition found almost exclusively in women. It fluctuates in severity over many years and is characterized by a convoluted history of multiple contacts with the medical profession for a variety of different symptoms. It generally begins in early adult life and is associated with disruption of personal relationships and work difficulties. Medical overinvestigation is common and misuse of medication may be seen. Depression or anxiety are often associated features. Symptoms can affect any bodily system and often include gastrointestinal upset with diarrhoea, nausea and vomiting, pain, dyspnoea, palpitations, amnesia, seizures, paraesthesia, loss of visual acuity, impotence or dysparenuia and dysmenorrhoea. The importance of the condition lies in its chronicity, associated profound debilities and the drain that it places on both medical and financial resources. Psychological treatment may produce improvement and there are studies demonstrating that psychiatric involvement in management can reduce subsequent health-care costs.

Chronic pain
The investigation and management of chronic pain consumes vast resources and can be frustrating for both patient and clinician. Up to 95% of patients seen in pain clinics have concurrent psychological difficulties, most commonly depressive, anxiety and personality disorders. Successful treatment of comorbid depression may relieve pain, while in cases without an obvious mood component some antidepressants (e.g. tricyclic drugs) may have useful adjuvant analgesic properties. It is, however, important to appreciate that other forms of psychological disturbance, not readily classified as mental disorder, may also produce or exacerbate pain. In such circumstances cure may be difficult to find and helping the patient to cope represents a more realistic therapeutic goal.

The term somatoform (psychogenic) pain disorder may be used to describe chronic, unremitting pain, which cannot be explained fully in terms of organic pathology and which may vary in response to changing psychological stress. Examples include psychogenic backache, atypical facial pain syndromes and non-specific abdominal pain.

Facticious disorders and malingering

Central to this group of conditions is the intentional production of signs or symptoms to suggest either mental disorder or physical illness, i.e. the patient has a need to assume the sick role. Various presentations may be seen:

Facticious disorder (Munchausen's syndrome)
Symptoms are fabricated to secure admission to numerous different hospitals. Such individuals tend to be itinerant, aliases are often employed to avoid detection and symptoms are usually described floridly, but inconsistently. Medical knowledge may be extensive and symptoms tend to evolve and change during the course of an admission, to avoid discharge. Presenting complaints are limited only by the individual's imagination and commonly include self-induced fevers and infections, bleeding, pain syndromes, haemoptysis, diarrhoea, collapse and various skin eruptions. Extreme methods are often employed to produce physical signs. Self-mutilation, ingestion of toxic chemicals and injection of irritants to produce skin eruptions and abscesses result in significant morbidity and mortality. There is no obvious external gain in this behaviour and predisposing factors are complex. These may include grievances against the medical profession, perhaps as a result of perceived mismanagement during a past episode of illness, extensive hospitalization in childhood and previous employment in paramedical settings. Management is difficult but joint confrontation by surgical and psychiatric staff can be helpful. The patient may react with hostility and leave hospital, but if he or she can be engaged in a collaborative relationship, psychological treatment may be of some benefit.

Munchausen's syndrome by proxy
This is a serious condition that constitutes child abuse. The victim of the disorder is a young child who is presented to different doctors with a multitude of physical signs and symptoms, fabricated by the parent, usually the mother. She often appears overattentive towards the child and wishes to stay by the bedside during any periods of hospitalization or investigation. A nursing background has been found in up to 50% of mothers implicated in such cases, with approximately one-fifth suffering from Munchausen's syndrome themselves.

Malingering
Unlike facticious disorders, malingering is associated with the intentional feigning of symptoms driven by

obvious external incentives, such as evading prosecution, securing accommodation, seeking sanctuary or obtaining drugs.

Alcohol misuse

In the UK, more than 90% of adults drink alcohol and misuse is commonly identified in hospitalized patients. It has been estimated that approximately 25% of male inpatients have alcohol-related problems and many will have been admitted with a condition directly linked to alcohol misuse. To improve detection rates, an alcohol history should be part of every patient interview and, in this regard, the use of screening instruments such as the CAGE questionnaire or the Michigan Alcoholism Screening Test (MAST) may be helpful.

Presentation of alcohol misuse

Alcohol intoxication

This is a common occurrence in accident and emergency departments and is important because of its association with complex psychosocial problems, deliberate self-harm (DSH), physical injury and disturbed or violent behaviour.

Dependence syndrome

This syndrome may develop after the prolonged use of alcohol. Sufferers experience a compulsion to drink, and while the desire for more alcohol is recognized as irrational and damaging, it is poorly resisted and intense craving makes drinking inevitable. Despite evidence of harmful consequences such as health, relationship and financial problems, drinking continues to dominate the individual's life. Alternative pleasures and interests are increasingly neglected, and the ability to moderate alcohol intake in various social situations is lost while drinking to excess becomes habitual. Repeated withdrawal symptoms are experienced (Table 20.21) when heavy drinking is stopped completely or significantly reduced. Onset is usually 6–12 h after the last drink and resolution is complete within 24 h.

Table 20.21 Features of alcohol withdrawal

- Anxiety
- Irritability
- Depression and fear
- Tremor
- Autonomic hyperactivity with sweating, elevated blood pressure and tachycardia
- Sleep disturbance, often with vivid nightmares
- Nausea, vomiting and flu-like symptoms
- Hyperacusis, tinnitus, itching and muscle cramps
- Transient, poorly formed hallucinations or perceptual distortions occurring in both visual and auditory modalities

To avoid withdrawal, alcohol intake is maintained throughout the day, often beginning first thing in the morning. Tolerance to alcohol becomes evident, as more and more alcohol has to be taken to produce intoxication. In the later stages of dependence, tolerance may be lost suddenly.

Alcoholic convulsions

Withdrawal may be complicated by seizures, with approximately 10% of alcohol-misusing patients having experienced convulsions. Fits are usually generalized, occur within 12–48 h of abstinence and, in approximately one-third of cases, herald the onset of delirium tremens.

Delirium tremens

This is the most florid form of alcohol withdrawal, occurring in approximately 5% of patients hospitalized with alcohol dependence. It is rare when alcohol consumption is less than approximately 15 units per day. It may be associated with a concurrent illness or injury that has reduced or stopped alcohol intake. Features include delirium (see above), vivid hallucinations (most commonly visual), marked tremor, delusions, instability of mood (ranging from terror to elation) and insomnia. Autonomic overactivity with elevated pulse, sweating, mild pyrexia, flushing or pallor and dilated pupils is common.

Mortality is up to 5% and is due to associated infection, commonly pneumonia, hyperthermia or cardiovascular insufficiency. After approximately 3 or 4 days the patient may fall into a deep and prolonged sleep from which he or she emerges fully recovered. Rarely, however, once delirium clears, there may be residual memory impairment characteristic of Korsakoff's psychosis (see below).

Alcoholic hallucinosis

This term refers to auditory hallucinations occurring alone in alcohol-dependent patients, usually within 12–48 h of abstinence or a substantial reduction in intake. There is no associated clouding of consciousness and in a minority of cases symptoms develop while the patient continues to drink. Hallucinations usually begin as simple sounds or noises, which later evolve into persecutory, critical voices. These may address the patient by name or discuss him or her in the third person. Rarely, they direct the individual to act against his will with resultant disordered behaviour or attempts at self-harm. Secondary delusional interpretation of persistent hallucinations may follow, with the clinical picture resembling acute paranoid schizophrenia. Other diagnostic features of schizophrenia such as loss of insight, distorted thinking or disturbances of volition are, however, absent. Management usually involves hospital admission for alcohol detoxification, during which the symptoms most often resolve within a week. A minority of patients goes on to develop chronic hallucinations, which require treatment with antipsychotic agents.

Management of alcohol withdrawal

Mild cases may only require advice, reassurance and support but where symptoms are more severe, a reducing regime of long-acting benzodiazepines may offer partial symptomatic relief. The aim is to maintain adequate sedation during withdrawal and medication should be titrated to achieve this. Chlordiazepoxide, introduced at a daily maximum of 60–80 mg and gradually tapered off, is an appropriate treatment for adequately supported patients in the community. Inpatient detoxification should be considered in the following situations:

- history of severe withdrawal symptoms, seizures or delirium tremens
- malnutrition (risk of Wernicke's encephalopathy; see below)
- significant comorbid psychiatric or physical problems.

For hospitalized patients, chlordiazepoxide 50 mg orally every 2 h, up to a maximum of 400 mg in a 24-h period, may be required. Diazepam equivalents can also be used as an alternative. Caution should be exercised when treating patients with severe liver damage since this impairs benzodiazepine metabolism and increases the risk of respiratory depression. Chlormethiazole is an alternative to benzodiazepines, but its use is discouraged because of possible dependence with prolonged treatment and potentially fatal respiratory depression in combination with alcohol. Antipsychotics, although sedative, are not recommended as they may lower the seizure threshold.

Thiamine deficiency, as part of a general vitamin B complex depletion, is common in alcohol misuse and arises from poor diet, impaired absorption, increased requirements, reduced storage and disordered utilization. In well-nourished individuals with mild withdrawal features, oral thiamine should be given at a dose of 300–600 mg/day for 3 weeks.

In patients experiencing withdrawal who develop confusion and disorientation, ataxia, hypotension, hypothermia or ophthalmoplegia, Wernicke's encephalopathy should be suspected and parental thiamine replacement given. Thiamine 500 mg i.v. should be given three times daily for 2 days and if improvement is noted, one vial should be given daily for a further 5 days. To minimize the relatively rare risk of anaphylaxis with parenteral thiamine preparations, thiamine should be diluted in normal saline and given as an infusion over a period of 15–30 min. Resuscitation facilities must be available. Oral supplementation should continue once the acute features have resolved. Mortality is up to 20%, with approximately 85% of survivors developing the chronic, largely irreversible form of the syndrome, Korsakoff's psychosis.

Management of delirium tremens

Hospital management is mandatory. Sedation must be adequate. If oral medication is not tolerated then diazepam given by slow intravenous injection (5 mg/min) at a dosage of up to 10 mg every 4 h is useful in gaining control in very disturbed patients. When sedation is satisfactory, it can be maintained using oral preparations. Maintenance of adequate fluid intake is essential and electrolyte abnormalities such as hypomagnesaemia, hypokalaemia and hypoglycaemia must be excluded. Consistent nursing input with frequent orientation in an evenly lit room reduces the likelihood of perceptual distortions. Vitamin B_1 supplementation is essential to avoid the development of the Wernicke–Korsakoff syndrome, as described above.

Hepatic encephalopathy

Psychiatric symptoms can be the presenting feature of liver disease and may occur even before there is biochemical evidence of hepatocellular dysfunction. Whatever the underlying hepatic condition, the features of hepatic encephalopathy are due to the accumulation of nitrogenous compounds in the systemic circulation. Clinical presentation (see Table 20.22) is variable and may follow a deteriorating, chronic course or be characterized by exacerbation and remissions, possibly occurring over years.

During periods of remission there may be evidence of personality change with loss of insight, unwarranted cheerfulness, aggressive outbursts, paranoia, impulsivity, impaired self-care and disregard for social protocol. Treatment of the underlying liver condition is usually associated with an improvement of the acute psychiatric symptoms, but this is largely dependent on the degree of hepatocellular damage. In severe cases, neuronal degeneration may be evident at autopsy.

Psychiatric syndromes associated with drug misuse

Benzodiazepines

Since the height of their popularity in the 1970s, when they were prescribed for the treatment of insomnia and anxiety disorders, benzodiazepines are now dispensed with more circumspection. It is generally agreed that to minimize the risk of dependence, their use beyond 4 weeks should be discouraged. During withdrawal in a dependent individual, an abstinence or a discontinuation syndrome develops (Table 20.23).

Table 20.22 Clinical features of hepatic encephalopathy

- Fluctuating conscious level with profound confusion during exacerbations. This may progress to coma
- Visual hallucinations
- Mood lability with anxiety, depression or elation
- Characteristic flapping tremor affecting the hands
- Increased muscle tone, clonus and hyperreflexia
- Rest tremor, dysarthria and ataxia
- Ophthalmic disturbances including nystagmus, diplopia or blurring of vision

Table 20.23 Features of benzodiazepine withdrawal

- Sleep disturbance with insomnia, nightmares and drowsiness
- Fatigue, lethargy and flu-like symptoms
- Anxiety with tremor, agitation, concentration difficulties, sweating, palpitations and panic attacks
- Depression
- Gastrointestinal symptoms with nausea, anorexia and weight loss
- Muscle twitching and ataxia
- Increased sensitivity to light, sound, taste or smell

Convulsions are rare during slow withdrawal from therapeutic doses of benzodiazepines, but may occur if there is abrupt discontinuation of short-acting preparations, associated alcohol dependence or the concurrent administration of drugs that reduce seizure threshold, e.g. neuroleptics or antidepressants. Following abstinence, withdrawal features emerge between the second and fifth days, increase in severity until about day 10 and then persist at this plateau for a further month before settling gradually.

In preparation for reduction, patients taking short-acting benzodiazepines should be established on an equivalent dose of a more slowly eliminated drug such as diazepam or chlordiazepoxide. Gradual withdrawal can then proceed with a 25% reduction in daily dose introduced at intervals of a week or a fortnight. The process may take months to complete. If necessary, the coadministration of a β-blocker may help to alleviate rebound anxiety.

Cannabis

Cannabis is the most commonly used illicit drug in the UK. Cannabis resin (hashish, charas), oil or dried leaves (marijuana, grass, pot) are usually mixed with tobacco and smoked, although the drug can also be taken orally, often added to foodstuffs. In common with many other illicit substances and alcohol, the effects of cannabis are dependent on the environment and coloured by the user's mood and expectations.

Adverse effects are generally dose related and transient, and resolve spontaneously:

- acute anxiety reactions with panic, depersonalization, agitation and paranoid ideas
- delirium with confusion, memory impairment and hallucinations
- acute, transient psychotic episodes occurring in clear consciousness and resembling schizophrenia or mood disorders. Such episodes are not sustained and resolve within a few days
- transient depression.

There is no specific physical withdrawal syndrome associated with cannabis use at normal levels, but abrupt abstinence from very high doses may be associated with anxiety, irritability, sleep disturbance and anorexia. No causal link has been proven between cannabis use and the development of schizophrenia, although in predisposed individuals, use of the drug may precipitate or exacerbate an episode of psychotic illness. The concept of a specific amotivational syndrome linked to personality deterioration secondary to prolonged cannabis use is poorly substantiated, but habitual users can become apathetic and lethargic.

Cocaine

The acute stimulant effects of cocaine are related to dose, method of use and the presence of other drugs that may have been taken in combination. Pupils are dilated, accompanied by tachycardia and hypertension. Mood is elated, often with loss of judgement, while fatigue is reduced. Persecutory delusions leading to aggression and hostility, and hallucinations may occur. These take the form of voices, twinkling lights or a sensation of insects felt moving under the skin (formication). Resolution is normally complete within a few days of abstinence. Delirium with disorientation and violent behaviour may follow heavy use.

Once acute intoxication has resolved, mood may crash with agitated depression, suicide risk and an intense craving for more stimulants. This usually settles within 24 h after a period of prolonged sleep, but may persist for weeks in dependent individuals. Possible adverse complications are seizures, strokes, myocardial ischaemia or infarction, and cardiac arrhythmias. Treatment is symptomatic and may require benzodiazepines or neuroleptics if psychotic features are prominent.

Amphetamines

Amphetamines are the most widely used stimulants in the UK. They include methylphenidate, fenfluramine, methamphetamine, methylamphetamine and diethylproprion. They are taken either intravenously or intranasally as performance enhancers and euphoriants. Amphetamine-like drugs have a much longer half-life than cocaine and do not need to be taken with the same frequency to sustain their effects. The features found in amphetamine intoxication, withdrawal, delirium and psychosis are indistinguishable from similar states precipitated by cocaine use (described above).

Opiates

Many opiates are used illicitly in the UK, with local trends being dictated by black-market availability. Popular drugs include Diconal (dipipanone and cyclizine mixture), Temgesic (buprenorphine), methadone and heroin. Injecting behaviour carries a risk of cross-infection, most significantly with hepatitis B and C and HIV.

Opiates may be smoked, ingested or injected. Effects include euphoria (typically a rush followed by sedation and apathy), pupillary constriction, and drowsiness with slurred speech and mental clouding. Tolerance, which develops to all opiates, is lost rapidly when the drug is

Table 20.24 Features of opiate withdrawal

- Abdominal cramps, nausea and diarrhoea
- Intense craving for opiate drugs
- Irritability and anxiety
- Muscle aches
- Tachycardia
- Lacrimation and rhinorrhoea
- Uncontrollable yawning
- Piloerection (hence the term 'cold turkey' used to describe the abstinence syndrome)
- Sweating and fever
- Insomnia

withdrawn. Renewed use after a period of abstinence may thus result in fatal respiratory depression and this mechanism is likely to be responsible for a significant percentage of heroin-associated deaths following enforced abstinence in hospital or prison.

Chronic use produces both physical and psychological dependence, with a characteristic withdrawal syndrome on abstinence, dose reduction or the administration of an opiate antagonist such as naloxone. The intensity and time scale of the withdrawal reaction are, however, dependent on the particular opiate taken. Withdrawal features do not put life at risk, but they can be prolonged and severe (Table 20.24). Threatened abstinence can thus result in manipulative drug-seeking behaviour.

Traditional detoxification is by gradual withdrawal of a substitute drug such as methadone, given orally. The rate of reduction is governed by the severity of withdrawal symptoms and the individual's desire to achieve abstinence. Alternative regimes involve the use of non-opiate drugs such as benzodiazepines or the α-adrenergic agonist clonidine. A similar drug, lofexidine, produces less hypotension and, with compliance, can help to achieve abstinence within a few weeks.

Hallucinogens

Drugs belonging to this group include lysergic acid diethylamide (LSD), dimethyltryptamine (DMT), dimethoxyamphetamine (DAM) and psilocybin, which is found in some species of fungi (magic mushrooms). They all produce hallucinations without reducing conscious level and have become established in the UK as part of the 'acid house' dance culture. They are taken to produce euphoria, visual hallucinations and other perceptual changes. Associated physical features are due to sympathomimetic activity and include tachycardia, pupillary dilation, tremor and sweating. In contrast to many other drugs of misuse, the hallucinogens do not produce physical dependence and are generally taken only in particular situations, without obvious withdrawal features on abstinence. Adverse reactions generally relate to the potentially frightening nature of the perceptual changes induced.

The 1990s have seen increasing use of a synthetic amphetamine analogue, 3,4-methylenedioxy-methylamphetamine (MDMA), commonly known as ecstasy.

Its mixed hallucinogenic and stimulant properties are associated with the development of transient paranoid psychotic features, which may become chronic, or anxiety and depressive symptoms. Adverse physical effects include cardiotoxicity, epilepsy, hyperthermia, intracerebral haemorrhage and recurrent jaundice. There is evidence that even limited use may cause lasting cerebral changes.

Volatile substance misuse

Several substances may be used, including adhesives (glue sniffing), dry-cleaning solvents, correcting fluid, cigarette lighter fuel and aerosol products. Prevalence is difficult to ascertain because of underreporting, but it occurs more commonly in boys during the early teenage years. The problem is closely linked with various conduct disorders and dysfunctional family dynamics. Deaths from butane gas aerosol use are increasing in the UK. With continued use, psychological dependence and tolerance may develop, but there are no specific withdrawal features. In one-third of cases there is transient disorientation with frightening auditory and visual hallucinations. Death may result from unconsciousness and aspiration of stomach contents.

The management of acutely disturbed behaviour

Disturbed or violent behaviour has numerous and diverse causes including psychotic illness, personality disorder, cerebral pathology, substance intoxication or withdrawal and wilful aggression. The essential element in management is identification of the underlying cause but often, before this can be investigated, rapid symptomatic control is required to prevent injury or damage. Non-pharmacological strategies such as attempts at non-confrontational negotiation, distraction or seclusion may be effective but require expertise, time and a compliant patient. Urgent necessity may render these approaches impractical and, in such cases, medication should be considered.

Irrespective of the drug group chosen, there are general safety principles that must be adhered to in rapid tranquillization:

- facilities for resuscitation should be available
- pulse, blood pressure and respiratory rate should be checked every 5–10 min
- once sedation is achieved, control should be maintained by oral drug administration
- extreme caution is required when treating the elderly, physically debilitated patients or children.

Antipsychotics

In emergency situations, antipsychotic drugs are used for their sedative, rather than their antipsychotic properties. Intramuscular antipsychotic preparations offer little advantage over drugs given orally in achieving behavioural control. For example, similar peak plasma levels of Haloperidol are reached in 20 min after both oral and intramuscular administration. Oral preparations should be used if possible, but difficulties may arise in treating extremely disturbed, non-compliant patients. In such circumstances, intramuscular administration is likely to be the favoured option. The intravenous administration of antipsychotics is hazardous: high concentrations of the drug may reach the heart suddenly, especially in struggling patients, and precipitate fatal arrhythmias.

Haloperidol may be given orally 3–5 mg two or three times daily, or 2–10 mg every 4–8 h by intramuscular injection up to a maximum of 60 mg in a 24-h period. An initial loading dose of up to 30 mg may be required in extreme situations.

Important adverse reactions may occur. Acute dystonic reactions occur in up to 20% of patients receiving antipsychotic drugs. Young men and children appear to be at particular risk. Slow, sustained muscular contraction can result in spasm or involuntary movements. This may manifest as torticollis, retrocollis, writhing movements of the entire body (opistinotonus), dysarthria, dysphagia or oculogyric crisis characterized by fixed deviation of the eyes. Onset is within hours of parenteral administration or days if the drug has been given orally. Dramatic presentations may be misidentified as tetanus, status epilepticus or hysteria. The disorder is self-limiting but it is intensely distressing. It can be relieved rapidly by intravenous procyclidine.

Neuroleptic malignant syndrome is a rare idiosyncratic response to antipsychotic medication characterized by hyperthermia, muscle rigidity, tremor, mental state changes (agitation, confusion, coma), autonomic instability, tachycardia, labile blood pressure, sweating and raised creatinine phosphokinase (CPK). Death may occur in up to 20% of cases, usually secondary to renal or cardiorespiratory failure. Treatment requires the immediate withdrawal of all antipsychotic agents and transfer to intensive care facilities for specialist treatment.

Benzodiazepines

These drugs are useful and generally safe in controlling disturbed behaviour. They have no antipsychotic effect but are potent sedative, anxiolytic, anticonvulsant and muscle-relaxant agents. Given within the normal therapeutic range, benzodiazepines have little effect on respiratory or cardiovascular function, but with high doses, especially if given intravenously, oversedation, hypotension and respiratory depression can occur. The specific benzodiazepine antagonist flumazenil, given intravenously, rapidly reverses these toxic effects. It should be noted that although the response to benzodiazepines is generally predictable, disinhibition, confusion and paradoxical aggression may be seen in some predisposed individuals with personality disorders.

Lorazepam may be used for rapid tranquillization by oral (2–4 mg repeated 6 hourly up to a maximum of six doses in 48 h) and intravenous routes (25–30 µg/kg to approximately 2 mg/70 kg, repeated 6 hourly if required). Absorption from intramuscular injection sites is slow and offers no advantage over oral administration.

Antipsychotic–benzodiazepine combinations

This is a highly effective regime and allows lower doses of both drugs to be used. Toxicity is thus reduced and repeated administration is less likely to be necessary to gain behavioural control. An example would be 5 mg haloperidol with 2 mg lorazepam given intramuscularly and repeated 6 hourly if required.

Deliberate self-harm and suicide

DSH refers to non-fatal acts of self-injury such as poisoning, cutting or mutilation. Synonyms include attempted suicide and parasuicide, but both of these terms convey a sense of failure in an act designed to be fatal, and are best avoided since many individuals who self-harm do not express a wish to die. UK rates for general hospital attendance following DSH average around 150–200 per 100 000 population and it is the most common reason for acute hospital admission in women. In men, it is second only to ischaemic heart disease. In recent years there has been a shift in the gender ratio away from a female preponderance towards parity, mainly due to an increased incidence of DSH in young men. Repetition is common, with studies identifying hospital readmission rates of around 15% within 12 months of the index presentation.

DSH is a potent risk factor for completed suicide. In the year after DSH, 1% of individuals complete suicide and 3–10% may do so eventually. As a group, DSH patients have an overall risk of suicide 100 times that of the general population. Between 30 and 40% of all suicides have a history of self-harm and in up to 25% of suicide deaths, the individual will have presented to the general hospital after self-harming in the preceding year. The severity of an individual episode of DSH does not, however, correlate well with the degree of underlying psychological distress and thus all patients presenting to hospital after self-harm should be offered psychosocial assessment aimed at identifying:

- underlying psychiatric illness
- high suicide risk
- coexisting alcohol or drug problems
- social difficulties.

In some centres this work is undertaken exclusively by psychiatric staff, but in others appropriately trained medical, nursing or social services staff may be involved. Where this occurs, it is important that there are clearly defined procedures in place to facilitate immediate access to psychiatric opinion.

Suicide risk assessment

In assessing suicide risk, four main issues should be considered: the history of any self-harm event, medical and psychiatric risk factors, present psychiatric state and social circumstances.

History of the deliberate self-harm event

Intent correlates with the perceived dangerousness of the method used, the degree of preparation in the planning of the event, the presence of associated final acts (such as a suicide note or placing financial affairs in order) and precautions against discovery or prevention of the act.

Psychiatric and medical risk factors

Risk factors include a history of previous DSH, a history of past psychiatric contact, a family history of psychiatric disorder, suicide or alcohol misuse, chronic or painful physical illness, and chronic drug or alcohol misuse.

Present psychiatric state

It is important to screen for depressive illness: psychological features of depression such as inappropriate guilt, hopelessness, pessimism and worthlessness are of particular significance. Current suicidal thinking should be explored: the patient should be asked specific questions about suicidality in a graded way from ambivalence about living to active suicide plans. There is no evidence to suggest that this type of enquiry precipitates suicidal behaviour in vulnerable individuals and it is an essential part of any thorough psychosocial assessment. It is also important to appreciate that suicidality is dynamic. An individual's mental state can change quickly and thus regular face-to-face reassessment may be necessary. Other psychiatric conditions such as schizophrenia, personality disorders or substance misuse should be considered.

Social circumstances

Social isolation and unemployment are risk factors. It is important to establish whether family support is available, and how the family views the current episode of self-injury. Enquiry should be made as to whether other forms of support are available (e.g. social services) and whether the difficulties are likely to diminish or multiply as a result of the self-harm.

In all cases, suicide risk should be assessed and considered when establishing a treatment plan. Certain patient groups, including the elderly, those with learning difficulties and young people, present particularly difficult assessment problems and referral to specialist psychiatric services should be considered.

Which patients should be referred for psychiatric opinion?

Many psychological problems are identified and treated by the surgical team, but others may require more specialized interventions. There are no immutable rules for psychiatric referral, but the following are useful guidelines:

- where there is uncertainty about the diagnosis of comorbid depression in physically unwell patients with multiple somatic features

- where the choice of psychoactive medication is complicated by polypharmacy or severe organic disease
- where a psychiatric disorder has not responded to first-line treatment
- where there is a high risk of suicide or self-harm
- where inappropriate guilt, hopelessness or worthlessness are prominent features of depression
- where there is evidence of psychotic illness (delusions or hallucinations)
- where severe behaviour disturbance compromises surgical care
- where psychiatric morbidity is identified during surgical assessment, e.g. debilitating anxiety, depressive illness or alcohol or other drug misuse
- where there is a history of psychological problems complicating previous surgery
- where there is a long history of multiple, unremitting medically unexplained symptoms and numerous contacts with a variety of different specialists
- where there is evidence of body image disturbance and a preoccupation with weight and shape
- in cases where it appears as though the patient is intentionally feigning illness.

Guide to further reading

CRAG/SCOTMEG Working Group on Mental Illness (1994). *The Management of Alcohol Withdrawal and Delirium Tremens. A Good Practice Statement.*

Eagle, K. A., Brundage, B., Chaitman, B. R. *et al.* (1996). Guidelines for perioperative cardiovascular evaluation for non cardiac surgery. Report of the ACC/AHA Task Force on Practice Guidelines. *Circulation* **93**: 1278–1317.

Grubb, N. R. (1998). The end of the heparin pump? Low molecular weight heparin has many advantages over unfractionated heparin. *BMJ* **317**: 1540–1541.

Hardaway, R. M. (1998). Traumatic and septic shock alias post-trauma critical illness. *Br J Surg* **85**: 1473–1479.

Mangano, D. T., Layug, E. L., Wallace, A. *et al.* (1996). Effect of atenolol on mortality and cardiovascular morbidity after noncardiac surgery. *N Engl J Med* **335**: 1713–1720.

Mayou, R. A. and Hawton, K. E. (1986). Psychiatric disorder in the general hospital. *Br J Psych* **149**: 172–190.

Royal College of Physicians and Royal College of Psychiatrists (1995). *The Psychological Care of Medical Patients. Recognition of Need and Service Provision (CR35).*

Royal College of Psychiatrists (June 1994). *The General Hospital Management of Adult Deliberate Self Harm. A Consensus Statement on Standards for Service Provision (CR32).*

Royal College of Surgeons of England and the Royal College of Psychiatrists (1997). *Report of the Working Party on the Psychological Care of Surgical Patients (CR55).*

Scottish Office Department of Health, National Medical Advisory Committee (1998). *The Management of Patients with Mental Disorders and/or Disturbed Behaviour who Present to Accident and Emergency Departments.*

Wareham, N. J. and O'Rahilly, S. (1998). The changing classification and diagnosis of diabetes. *BMJ* **317**: 59–60.

Minimal access therapy

1 • Definition, scope and spectrum of minimal access therapy

2 • Technology and set-up for minimal access surgery

3 • Minimal access surgery

4 • Interventional flexible endoscopy

5 • Percutaneous interventional radiology

6 • Image-guided microtherapy

'I never say of an operation that it is without danger'
– August Bier (1861–1949)

Section 21.1 • Definition, scope and spectrum of minimal access therapy

One of the significant changes in medical practice that has evolved gradually during the last two decades, but which has gathered substantial momentum more recently, is the reduction of the traumatic insult inevitable with surgical interventions. The term 'minimally invasive surgery/intervention' was coined initially to describe these surgical and interventional approaches. This terminology, although still in current usage, is inappropriate for two reasons. In the first instance, it carries connotations of increased safety, which is not the case. Secondly, it is semantically incorrect, since to invade is absolute, and indeed such interventions are as invasive in terms of reach of the various organs and tissues as is open surgery. The hallmark of the new approaches is the **reduction of the trauma of access without compromising exposure** of the anatomical region for the intended operation/intervention. Hence, a more appropriate generic term is minimal access therapy (MAT).

MAT comprises several approaches, involves various disciplines and cuts across the various specialties within these disciplines, but in essence it has three arms:

- minimal access surgery (MAS)
- interventional flexible endoscopy (IFE)
- percutaneous interventional radiology (PIR).

To a large extent, these therapeutic approaches are complementary and increasingly they are used in combination in the treatment of the individual case. Indeed, MAT has stressed the need for regrouping of existing specialists from different disciplines to form multi-disciplinary disease-related treatment (MDRT) groups,

e.g. gastrointestinal, angiological and musculoskeletal. Real progress and efficiency in management and therapy for all disease processes are likely to depend on the establishment of effective MDRT groups as distinct from the current restrictions inherent in the treatment of patients within separate specialties and disciplines. To illustrate the point, management of patients with complex gastrointestinal disorders would benefit considerably from gastrointestinal surgeons working in close co-operation with gastroenterologists and gastrointestinal radiologists. Indeed, the surgical gastroenterologist has much more in common with these colleagues than with other surgical specialties such as orthopaedics and vascular surgery. In a sense, referral of a patient from one specialty to another when both share the same system-based clinical interest and expertise illustrates the weakness and inefficiency of the current system.

The scope of MAT is to minimize the traumatic insult to the patient without compromising the safety and efficacy of the treatment compared with the traditional open surgery. If this is achieved, than the recovery of the patient is expedited with the positive gain of a reduced hospital stay and an accelerated recovery to full activity and work. Thus, aside from achieving the objective of ambulatory or short-stay hospital care, there is a real benefit to the country as a whole by the significant reduction in the period of short-term disability of the patient following discharge from the hospital.

All three major components of MAT rely on image-display systems and technology, in addition to operator skill. Thus, the endoscopic surgeon, the interventional flexible endoscopist and the interventional radiologist all operate from displayed images of the operative field rather then reality. Three considerations follow from this. The first is that these interventions and operations are technology dependent in that the procedure cannot be performed if the imaging system [computed tomographic (CT) scan, flexible videoendoscope, laparoscope-charged couple device (CCD)-monitor display] fails. Secondly, the image with the current systems is two-dimensional and thus the operator has to process the image mentally, both for identification of the target structures and for the monocular (pictorial) depth cues to perform purposeful and precise manipulations. Thirdly, and this applies particularly to MAS, the visual and the motor axis of the operator are no longer aligned, and with the current TV monitor display, the image is far removed from the actual operative site. Thus, the surgeon is confronted with a mapping problem and cannot look at his or her hands during the manipulations. These restrictions can be overcome with training, but none the less require certain innate attributes.

Section 21.2 • Technology and set-up for minimal access surgery

Some of the technology used, e.g. high-frequency electrosurgery, ultrasound scanning and ultrasonic dissection, are covered elsewhere **[see Module 2, Vol. I]**. In this section only those devices, equipment and instruments needed for the conduct of MAS operations are covered.

Image systems

Light sources and light cables
Two types of light source are in use: xenon and metal halide (halogen). Xenon has a more natural colour spectrum, i.e. whiter, and a smaller spot size than halide (4.5 mm vs > 6 mm). In practice, the yellow light of the halogen bulb is compensated for in the video-camera system by white balancing. Both types of light source have infrared filters.

The output from the light sources is ducted to the telescope by light cables that contain either glass-fibre bundles or special fluid. The glass-fibre light cables are more commonly used in MAT, largely because of their flexibility, although they are less efficient than the fluid light guides owing to fibre mismatch at the junctions. Adaptation (coupler/condenser) lenses at the junction of glass fibre cables reduce this problem with telescopes. Aside from being less flexible, fluid light cables are not autoclavable.

Telescopes
Currently, the majority of telescopes used in MAS are of the **rigid viewing** type based on the Hopkins rod–lens system. These telescopes vary in diameter and in their direction of view. In laparoscopy, the 10 mm telescopes with zero (forward viewing) or 30° and 45° forward oblique directions (view angles) are the most commonly employed (Figure 21.1). For the same

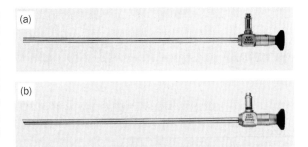

Figure 21.1 (a) Forward-viewing 0° 10 mm laparoscope; (b) oblique 30° 10 mm laparoscope.

diameter, the forward-viewing telescope transmits more light than the oblique types and is easier to use since the visual field is constant irrespective of the axis of rotation in which the telescope is held. However, the 30° telescope has considerable advantages that outweigh these limitations. It permits 'looking down' on the operative field and this facilitates dissections. Furthermore, by rotating the axis of this telescope the object can be scanned from all sides. **Operating rigid telescopes** have an insufflating port and an instrument channel (Figure 21.2). They are used in gynaecology and some endoluminal work. The Hopkins rod–lens system can be replaced by special gradient index glass rod (Selfoc, Grin) to good effect in very narrow and short, rigid telescopes.

Fibreoptic telescopes form the mainstay of diagnostic and therapeutic IFE. In essence, the flexible endoscope consists of two fibreoptic bundles: one for light transmission and the imaging bundle that relays the image of the object to the eyepiece. Fibreoptic telescopes do not provide the same resolution quality as rigid ones and usually produce a much smaller image. However, they are steerable. The main advantage of the optical glass fibre is its ability to transmit light over large distances with negligible losses by total internal reflections. The light bundles are made from multiple

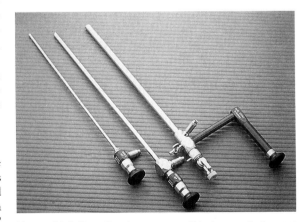

Figure 21.2 Operating laparoscope. This has an instrument channel. It is used in endoluminal laparoscopy and in operative laparoscopic gynaecology.

25 μm glass fibres without any need for specific alignment of the individual fibres, i.e. the light bundle is non-coherent. This is in sharp contrast to the image bundle responsible for the transmission of the image from the lens objective to the ocular eyepiece of the endoscope. In this instance the fibres have to be arranged coherently, i.e. the alignment of each fibre from one end of the bundle to the other must be maintained.

The objective lens at the distal end of the endoscope is used to focus the image on to the image bundle. As each imaging glass fibre (6–10 μm) admits only the light aligned with its axis, it relays only a tiny fraction of the image, called a 'picture element' or 'pixel'. Thus, several thousands of imaging fibres are needed for adequate transmission of the total image. Hence, the resolution of an endoscope is directly proportional to the number of fibres packed coherently within the image bundle ($2.5–10 \times 10^3$). When some of the constituent fibres break (with usage) the image is seen to contain 'black spots'. These represent lost pixels.

Optoelectronic telescopes have the CCD incorporated within the image plane of the objective lens at the distal end of the telescope (chip on stick technology). The advantage is that the system has fewer interfaces where image quality can be degraded and greater light sensitivity that the rigid telescope–camera assembly. In addition, the optoelectronic laparoscope has a deflecting tip.

Optical specifications of telescopes
These are the **field of view (FOV) or visual field, viewing angle, the direction of view, the magnification, the working distance, the aperture and external pupil**. The FOV or visual field is the area seen through the telescope. The corresponding angle (viewing angle) is the angle subtended on the objective lens of the telescope by the conversion of light from two opposite points on the diameter of the FOV. The viewing angle is typically 70° but telescopes with larger angles (80°) and hence FOV (fish-eye lens) are now available. The direction of view is the angle between the centre of the FOV and the longitudinal axis of the telescope (Figure 21.3). The direction of view from forward viewing (0°) of rigid telescopes is changed by use of prisms such that 30°, 45° and 70° oblique viewing telescopes are available. The working distance relates to the distance between distal end of the tele-

scope and the operative field. As this distance is increased, the FOV increases but the magnification decreases, and vice versa. Most telescopes are optimized for the best working distance, which is usually 30 mm. However, in laparoscopic surgery, the optimum working distance is between 75 and 150 mm. The objective and the ocular lenses determine the magnification of the telescope. The aperture is an iris-like opening within the telescope that limits the diameter of the optical pathway. A small aperture leads to a large depth of field, but to a low brightness. The external pupil is the diameter of the image bundle behind the ocular lens. The best imaging is achieved when the external pupil of the telescope coincides with the entrance pupil (iris) of the human eye.

Peripheral barrel distortion (fish-eye effect) is inevitable when the objective lens has a very short focal length or a wide angle. Distortion is caused by a change in the magnification from the centre of the image to the margins such that straight lines appear as curved, and objects at the periphery appear smaller or larger than the same objects in the centre. Peripheral distortion is more pronounced when the FOV and viewing angle of the lens are increased. Distortion affects the assessment of distances by the operator. Distortion-compensating 'aspheric' lenses are used to minimize peripheral distortion in wide-angle viewing telescopes.

Charged couple device cameras
All modern miniature cameras used in MAT are based on the CCD chip. The camera system has two components: (i) the head of the camera, which is attached to the ocular of the telescope; and (ii) the controller, which is usually located on the trolley along with the monitor. This separation provides a technical advantage, allowing the production of lightweight camera heads that do not hamper handling of the telescope. The camera head consists of an objective lens that focuses the image of the object on a CCD chip. The lens magnification ability is related to its focal length. Larger focal lengths produce larger images with less brightness. The use of 'zoom' lenses with variable focal lengths is thus an advantage.

The CCD chip is covered with light-sensitive photoreceptors that generate **pict**ure **el**ements (pixels) by transforming the incoming photons into electronic charges (or photoelectric charges). The electronic charges are then transferred from the pixels into a storage element on the same CCD chip. A subsequent readout (scanning) at a defined clock frequency results in a black and white image with grey tones. The number of pixels determines the resolution (the larger the pixel number, the higher the resolution). The average chip today contains 250 000–380 000 - pixels.

Cameras are classified in accordance with the number of CCDs they contain, into single-chip or three-chip types. These differ amongst other things in the way that they relay colour information to the monitor.

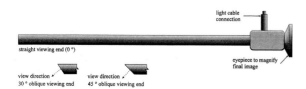

Figure 21.3 Diagrammatic representation of the direction of view of a laparoscope.

To create a coloured video image from the original black and white image a process of colour separation is used. In a single-chip camera, colour separation is achieved by adding a mosaic (stripe) filter that covers the whole chip. Each stripe accepts one of the complimentary colours (magenta, green, cyan or yellow) and each pixel is assigned to one stripe. The resolution is therefore reduced in this system. In three-chip cameras colour separation is achieved with a prism system (microlenses) that overlies the CCD chips. Each chip receives only one of the three primary colours (red, green or blue). Hence, each pixel encodes one colour dot. This technique gives a much higher resolution and a better image quality because the pixel number is tripled. The disadvantages of three-chip cameras are the larger size and increased weight (Figure 21.4).

White balance is necessary for both single and three-chip cameras to normalize the system to the spectrum of the light source used. The white balance is carried out after assembly of the system with the telescope pointing at a white surface. A button on the camera controller or the camera head itself is pressed to set the white balance. Black balance is only necessary for three-chip cameras to normalize the chips to one another. It is only performed once for a specific combination of camera head and controller.

Image-display system

Currently, the system uses one or two television monitors mounted on trolleys that also house the light source, camera control unit, insufflator, etc. The resolution of the monitor should be high and preferably not less than that of the camera. Its diagonal in inches gives the size of the monitor. The position of the monitor in relation to the surgeon is important. Aside from distance (four times the diagonal length of the monitor), the surgeon should face the monitor directly and the height should not exceed, and if possible, should be below the geometric eye point of the surgeon. Degraded performance ensues if the operator has to look up or sideways to view the operative field on the monitor.

Research has shown that the best endoscopic task performance is obtained when surgeons look down at the image in front of them. This permits 'gaze-down' viewing and restores the alignment of the visual with the motor axes of the operator. Image-display systems are now available that project the image on to a sterile screen overlying the chest of the patient. This considerably facilitates both cerebral processing of the image and endoscopic manipulations such that both task quality and task efficiency are improved (Figure 21.5). The limitations of the current gaze-down image-display systems is diminished resolution and colour balance compared with the high-resolution monitors.

Three-dimensional video systems

The requirement of stereoscopic vision is based on the need for precise and fast manipulations, particularly with the increasing complexity of endoscopic operations where perception of space is essential. In addition, enhanced perception of details and surfaces of anatomical structures and pathological processes leads to improvements in endoscopic diagnosis.

The most common systems in current usage depend on rapid time-sequential imaging with two cameras and one monitor and are based on the physiological phenomenon of retinal persistence (after-image). Both channels alternate (open and close) with sufficient speed (50–60 Hz) to avoid detection of flicker by the human eye. The monitors must therefore have double this frequency (100–120 Hz). Sequential switching between the two eyes is necessary to ensure that the correct image (left and right) falls on the corresponding retina. This is achieved by wearing special optical glasses that act (by remote signalling) as alternating shutters to each eye. The problem with these optical shutters, especially the active battery-operated liquid crystal display (LCD) types, is loss of brightness and colour degradation. To date, there is no evidence that three-dimensional (3D) systems impart any benefit to the conduct of endoscopic operations and most have adverse effects on the surgeons.

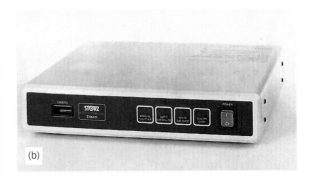

(a)   (b)

Figure 21.4 Three-chip CCD camera docked to a laparoscope.

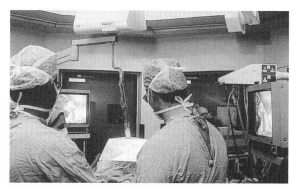

Figure 21.5 Projection of the video image on a sterile screen on top of the patient's chest, permitting gaze-down viewing.

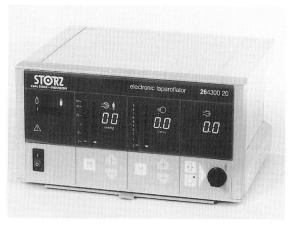

Figure 21.6 Modern laparoscopic insufflator.

Devices

Automatic insufflators

Classical laparoscopic surgery uses controlled pressure insufflation of the peritoneal cavity to achieve the necessary work space by (i) distending the anterolateral abdominal wall and (ii) depressing the hollow organs and soft tissues. For operative laparoscopy, CO_2 is the preferred gas because it does not support combustion (hence electrosurgery can be used), is very soluble (reduces but does not abolish the risk of gas embolism) and is cheap. Nitrous oxide is preferred by some for diagnostic laparoscopy performed under local anaesthesia and sedation because it is reputed to cause less pain. Several other inert gases have been tried experimentally as alternatives to CO_2 for operative laparoscopy, but none offers any haemodynamic advantages and they are potentially more hazardous by virtue of their decreased solubility in water. Automatic insufflators have the necessary sensors and circuits that enable the surgeon to preset the insufflating pressure and the device supplies gas (at a rate that is also controllable) until the preset intra-abdominal pressure selected by the surgeon is reached when gas flow ceases. The insufflator activates and delivers gas automatically when the intra-abdominal pressure falls (due to gas escape and leakage from the ports) at any stage during the operation. Modern automatic insufflators (Figure 21.6) incorporate bacteriological filters along the gas line and some can heat the gas to 37°C. This additional measure was introduced to prevent heat loss (from the cold gas), particularly during long operations.

There is no doubt that pressurized pneumoperitoneum gives the best exposure for laparoscopic surgery, but the positive pressure induces adverse effects that are pressure related. For this reason, the intra-abdominal pressure should be kept as low as is possible. In adults, a pressure of 10–12 mmHg give adequate exposure and in children the level should be kept lower, at 6–8 mmHg. A positive-pressure pneumoperitoneum has cardiovascular, neuroendocrine and metabolic consequences. The cardiovascular effects include:

■ reduction in the cardiac output/index
■ increase in the systemic vascular resistance
■ increased preload
■ increased pulmonary vascular resistance
■ diminished hepatic, splanchnic and renal flow.

The cardiac changes are similar to those of congestive cardiac failure. Although these changes are well tolerated with good anaesthesia in healthy individuals, **they impose an added risk in patients with established heart disease.** The neuroendocrine and metabolic changes induced by the positive-pressure pneumoperitoneum that have been documented in humans are:

■ release of renin and aldosterone (four-fold elevation)
■ sympathicomimetic response (vasopressin, adrenaline and noradrenaline release)
■ renal vasoconstriction: urinary sodium retention and temporary tubular renal dysfunction.

Gas embolism, although rare, is a well-documented complication that may be fatal (see below).

Abdominal wall-lift gasless systems

These systems were developed primarily to obviate the adverse cardiovascular effects of the positive-pressure pneumoperitoneum in patients with cardiac disease. They are also used in trauma patients (increased risk of gas embolism) and in cancer patients to avoid CO_2 insufflation on the pretext (unconfirmed; see below) that insufflation of this gas causes dissemination of the tumour. All may be used completely without gas insufflation (gasless laparoscopy) or with low-pressure insufflation (4–6 mmHg).

The various systems can be grouped as follows:

■ rubber tube sling abdominal wall lift
■ planar intraperitoneal abdominal wall retraction lift devices
■ extraperitoneal (subcutaneous) abdominal wall-lift devices.

None of these techniques gives as good a laparoscopic exposure as the pressurized pneumoperitoneum, for

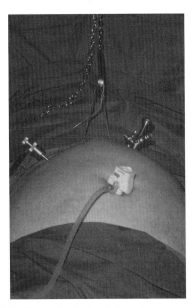

Figure 21.7 Sling abdominal wall-lift system.

two reasons: (i) they cause a tent-like elevation of the abdominal wall rather than an elevated expansion, and (ii) they do not depress the hollow organs and omentum. Exposure is, however, improved when low-pressure CO_2 insufflation is added. Randomized prospective clinical studies have demonstrated that gasless/low-pressure mechanical lifts virtually abolish the cardiovascular, hormonal and metabolic changes during surgery and significantly reduce postoperative CO_2 narcosis.

Rubber tube sling abdominal wall lift
This is the simplest, cheapest and in many ways the most versatile technique. Silicone tubes either mounted on large, curved 3.0 mm trocars or attached to short, metal, solid trocars (Figure 21.7) are inserted under vision (once the pneumoperitoneum has been created

and the laparoscope introduced) through and out of the anterior abdominal wall. The two external ends are then tied together and the abdominal wall is lifted by the sling, which is then hitched by a hook-and-chain mechanism to a cross-bar. If the sling is inserted in the upper abdomen, it encircles the falciform and round ligament. This has the added benefit of displacing the falciform ligament upwards from the operative field (extremely useful in fat patients), and also results in elevation of the liver through traction on the round ligament (Figure 21.8). Once the sling is in place, the insufflation pressure is reduced to 4–6 mmHg.

Planar intraperitoneal abdominal wall retraction lift devices
There are various systems, all based on the same principle. The retracting rod is inserted through a small wound inside the peritoneal cavity without any prior pneumoperitoneum. The retracting rod is then opened (Y or fan configuration) and attached to the lifting mechanism which, in the Laparolift system, is motorized. With the Laparolift system, an inflatable 'doughnut' (Figure 21.9) can be used instead of a metal rod.

Extraperitoneal abdominal wall-lift devices
These are the latest generation of abdominal wall-lift devices and offer significant advantages, particularly over the metal intraperitoneal systems, because they provide lift through the subcutaneous plane (completely extraperitoneal). There is some concern with the planar intraperitoneal abdominal wall systems on the extent of pressure damage and necrosis to the anterior parietal peritoneum, as the force exerted by these systems is high and sustained throughout the duration of the operations. The risks, therefore, include adhesion formation and, perhaps more importantly, the potential for tumour cell implantation in cancer cases. The extraperitoneal systems, exemplified by the Hashimoto sys-

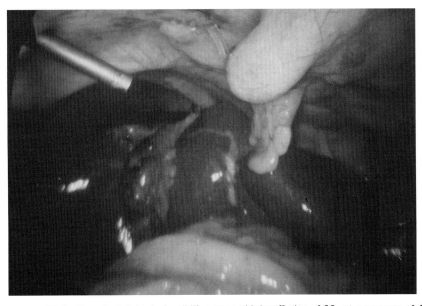

Figure 21.8 Exposure provided with a sling abdominal wall-lift system with insufflation of CO_2 at a pressure of 4.0 mmHg.

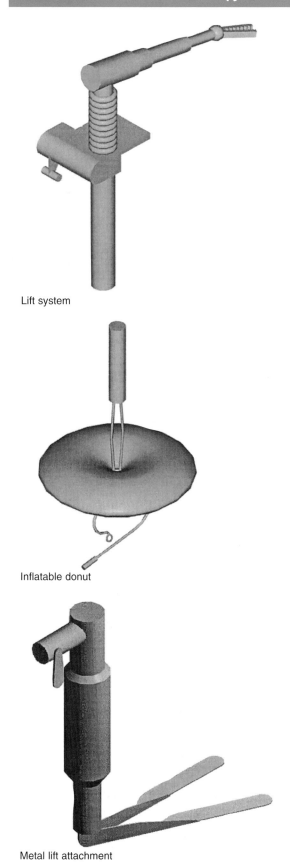

Lift system

Inflatable donut

Metal lift attachment

Figure 21.9 Inflatable donut and metal lift attachment used with the Laparolift intraperitoneal planar lift system.

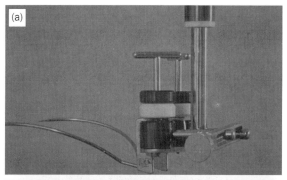

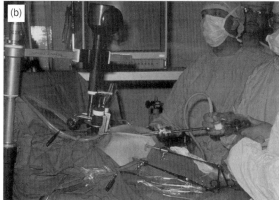

Figure 21.10 (a) Laparotensor subcutaneous lift system; (b) in use.

tem of subcutaneous Kirscher wires and pulleys system and the Laparotensor, overcome this problem. The Laparotensor (Figure 21.10) provides lift through specially shaped curvilinear needles modelled by finite element analysis to provide a more uniform lift of the anterior abdominal wall. The exposure is still, however, not as good as that obtained with insufflation, although it is improved by low-pressure CO_2 insufflation. The disadvantage of the LaparoTensor is encroachment of the operative space by the subcutaneous needles, which interferes with the optimal positioning of the ports.

Hand-assisted laparoscopic surgery

In this instance, a small wound is made within the operative field through which the hand of the surgeon or the assistant can be inserted, largely for retraction purposes. A special appliance, e.g. sleeve, seal bubble or sealing cuff (Figure 21.11), is used to prevent gas escape and thus maintain the pneumoperitoneum. Undoubtedly, hand-assisted surgery facilitates antireflux surgery, splenectomy and laparoscopic colon surgery. Careful planning is essential, in relation to both the placement of the ports and the incision for the appliance, which has to be sited in the correct position for the operation. This incision is also used for specimen extraction, e.g. spleen and colon. The disadvantage of hand-assisted laparoscopic surgery is that the operative field is encroached significantly when the hand of the surgeon or the assistant is inside the peritoneal cavity, restricting manipulations. Nonetheless, with

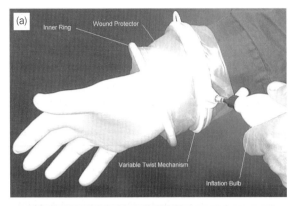

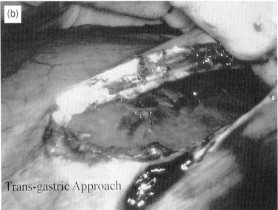

Figure 21.11 (a) Endo-cuff device for hand-assisted laparoscopic surgery; (b) hand-assisted laparoscopic transgastric removal of leiomyoma on posterior wall of stomach.

careful selection of cases and proper utilization the benefits generally outweigh the disadvantages of such an approach.

Instrumentation

Types
The current instrumentation for MAS is based on the respective instruments used in open surgery: the MAS instruments are simply longer and narrower. This basic design is, however, inappropriate for remote manipulations and is being replaced by purpose-designed instruments for endoscopic surgery that overcome the limited degrees of freedom of movement (d.o.f. = 4) available to the surgeon to varying extents. The newer generation of instruments falls into various categories:

- coaxial curved instruments that are introduced through flexible ports
- steerable instruments
- shape-memory-based instruments
- parallel occlusion and prehensile instruments.

Coaxial curved instruments
Coaxial curved instruments were developed to address some of the limitations of straight instruments. They are essentially straight instruments but have a curvature just proximal to the functional terminal segment (scissors

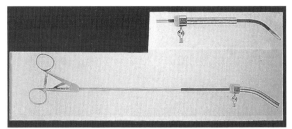

Figure 21.12 Coaxial curved instruments introduced through valveless metal flexible ports.

blades, grasping jaws, etc.) such that when the instrument is rotated along its long axis, the direction of the function tip can be changed through a circle with a diameter of 2.5 cm. They are introduced through valveless flexible metal ports (Figure 21.12). They greatly facilitate both sharp and blunt dissection and can be used to 'hook' structures for retraction purposes.

Steerable instruments
These are essentially electrically driven motorized 'endoeffector' instruments, the functional tip of which can be moved in any direction by actuator motors situated in the handle. These steerable instruments still require considerable research and development before they are introduced into routine MAS practice.

Shape-memory-based instruments
Nickel–Titanium (NiTi) alloys have unique shape-memory properties because of their unique crystalline structure. This enables the material to exist in two states: resting (martensite) or stressed (austenite). In essence, the material can be deformed or stressed by as much as 8% and return to its pristine shape when released without sustaining any structural damage or metal fatigue. This property is known as superelasticity or pseudoelasticity, and is used extensively in a variety of appliances and devices, e.g. all of the 'wall' wire stents used for palliation of obstructing cancers (bile duct, oesophageal, colonic) are made from NiTi. They are introduced in the 'stressed compressed' state and released for expansion to the unstressed (martensite) state once in position. In MAS, instruments containing shape-memory alloy components are useful for variable curvature instruments and dissectors. The principle is

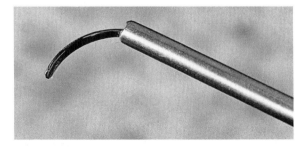

Figure 21.13 Shape-memory variable curvature dissecting spatula.

the same. The functional element of the instrument is housed within a straight tube during insertion through the port. The functional tip is extruded once the instrument is in the peritoneal cavity. The extent of extrusion of the functional element from the tube determines the curvature of the instrument as it is deployed (Figure 21.13).

The other property of NiTi alloys is known as temperature-dependent shape-memory change. As a result of special heating treatment, the alloy will change shape (martensite to austenite) when mild heat is applied to it, so that it bends to a predetermined configuration when heated to body temperature. This temperature-dependent shape-memory change underlies the novel technology of interrupted suturing with NiTi fine wire constructs that will enable efficient and easy tissue approximation in the future.

Parallel occlusion and prehensile instruments
All of the currently available laparoscopic graspers inflict a crushing injury on the tissues picked up by the jaws, even when labelled atraumatic. This is because the jaws are pivoted at one end and, therefore, the occlusive force exerted by the opposing surfaces is not uniform but varies along the length of the jaw, with the force being greatest near the fulcrum. This is very different from the situation when tissue is picked up by a dissecting forceps (pick-ups) in open surgery, where the two ends of the instrument approximate each other in a parallel fashion. Parallel occlusion graspers and bowel clamps, some based on NiTi components, are thus much less traumatic than the standard instruments.

The prehensile grasper is an even more advanced instrument. It was designed to reproduce the process of delicate 'ring grasping', enacted between the thumb and the index finger of the hand. With this segmented-jaw instrument, bowel loops including the colon can be picked up without any compression of the walls (Figure 21.14).

Reusable versus disposable instruments
The ongoing debate on the relative merits of these two categories has centred on costs. This is unfortunate in that good practice requires usage of both. Reusable instruments are precision engineered and are made of high-quality materials to ensure the rigours of repeated usage and in particular autoclaving. The lifetime of such instruments depends on the care with which they are handled during surgery and sterilization, but even under optimal conditions, these delicate instruments require frequent repair and replacement. This problem has led to the development of semidisposable or limited-use instruments. Semidisposable instruments deploy the functional component once or a limited number of times but the rest of the instrument (shaft and handle) is reusable.

Disposable instruments are mass produced of cheaper materials but have the advantage that emanates from single-use only, i.e. the instrument is in its pristine function when used. This singular advantage is lost when disposable equipment is reused. **This is a dangerous practice, because cleaning of tissue debris and blood from the insides of disposable equipment is not possible and hence carries the risk of disease transmission.** There are medicolegal implications to this since the manufacturers of such disposable instruments indicate quite clearly on the packaging 'single-use only', and thus any consequences of repeated usage are legally indefensible. Some disposable instruments have no reusable counterpart, e.g. endostaplers and multifire clip applicators. The use of disposable instruments is particularly indicated in patients with viral infections such as hepatitis B and C and acquired immunodeficiency syndrome (AIDS).

Robots and master–slave manipulators
There is an important difference between robots and master–slave manipulators. A robot is programmed to perform a task independently, whereas a master–slave manipulator is under immediate and constant control of the operator. It simply copies and translates the hand movements made by the surgeon. Thus, surgical robots are really master–slave manipulators. These are not in routine usage but existing prototypes, e.g. Mona, enable telepresence surgery, i.e. operating on the patient from a console that is at variable distance from the operating table. It seems likely that master–slave manipulators will be used in the future for delicate microvascular anastomoses, e.g. coronary revascularization, as the precision of suturing by the robotic arms through the computer interface is much more precise. The movements of the surgeon's hands are scaled down and tremor is abolished by the computer interface between the surgeon and the master–slave manipulator arms.

Operating theatres
There is no doubt that the design and configuration of the current operating theatres, including the operating table, are unsuitable for MAS. This has led to an existing situation that is ergonomically unsound and, in certain aspects, unsafe, with free-standing devices coupled to connecting floor-trailing cables to the sterile area, and

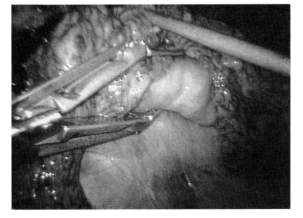

Figure 21.14 Prehensile grasper holding the transverse colon.

a variety of foot switches. The surgeon has no immediate control on the power output of energized systems used, there is no integration among the various systems components, and inadvertent activation of foot pedals is a real hazard. The pedestal configuration of the operating table and trolley-mounted TV display systems add to the difficulties such that the surgeon does not have optimal viewing and has to adopt strenuous postures during the surgical intervention. Purpose-designed operating theatres for MAS should include a bus system that incorporates all of the technologies needed with the appropriate interface, such that the surgeon can adjust the power output of all of the devices from a sterile pad in the vicinity of the operative area, adjustable image-display systems and a modular operating table that can support the patient in various positions and that enables the surgeon to sit down with sterile elbow rests. Considerable research and development is taking place to achieve such a MAS operating theatre for the next millennium. Meanwhile, with the existing set-up, it makes sense that hospitals designate certain operating theatres for MAS. This carries a number of positive advantages that help to overcome the current deficiencies. The nursing staff are familiar with the technology used and, together with the surgeons, optimize the layout for safe and efficient usage. Care and maintenance of devices and fragile equipment are ensured.

Section 21.3 • Minimal access surgery

Although this was being practised in a small number of centres as far back as the 1970s, when limited surgery was conducted by direct viewing through the laparoscope, it was only with the advent of the miniature CCD camera in the mid-1980s that MAS became established in routine surgical practice. It has undoubtedly had a significant impact (not all good) on the surgical operative management across all of the surgical specialties. It has also led to some significant positive changes in attitude to open surgery. Thus, open surgery is now practised without the recourse to unnecessary large wounds and patients are no longer starved for several days after surgery.

MAS is now established in general surgery (laparoscopic, endoluminal and retroperitoneal surgery), chest surgery (thoracoscopic surgery), orthopaedics (arthroscopic surgery), urology (laparoscopic and endoluminal urology), spinal surgery, etc. Undoubtedly, within such a relatively short period, the laparoscopic approach has largely replaced open surgery for certain operations such as cholecystectomy, sympathectomy, cardiomyotomy and antireflux surgery.

Benefits, limitations and risks of minimal access surgery

Benefits
The benefit of MAS derives primarily from the reduced traumatic insult to the patient by the surgical

intervention. The total operative trauma sustained by patients has two components: (i) the trauma of access and (ii) the procedural trauma, i.e. that of the actual operation. It is the ratio of these two components that determines the benefit from MAS. Thus, at one end (Figure 21.15) there are operations where the procedural trauma is minimal, e.g. myotomy, sympathetic denervation, meniscectomy and antireflux surgery, and the trauma of access accounts for the major portion of the operative insult. These are the disorders that benefit most when surgery is conducted by the MAS approach. At the other end, the procedural trauma accounts for most of the operative traumatic insult and the access wound contributes only a relatively minor part. These operations, e.g. pancreaticoduodenectomy and major resections with complex anastomoses, are unlikely to benefit from the MAS approach, aside from being much more difficult to execute, thus incurring a substantially increased operating time. In between these two extremes, there are several operations that benefit the patient when performed by the MAS, but a threshold is reached when the risks and disadvantages outweigh the benefit. The exact threshold has not been established and is likely to change in the future with improved technology for more efficient and safer execution of operations by the MAS approach.

Another factor that may be involved but that has been insufficiently researched is the conduct of an operation in a closed environment. In the case of abdominal MAS, this translates into absence of exposure or drying of intestinal loops and lack of contamination of the intra-abdominal contents with operating room air, which has been demonstrated to contain endotoxin. One group has suggested, on the basis of animal experimentation, that the reduced exposure to endotoxin in the operating room air accounts, in part, for the abrogated systemic stress response that has been demonstrated after closed MAS operations compared with open surgical interventions.

The inevitable non-specific depression of the immune system after surgery has been shown to be less

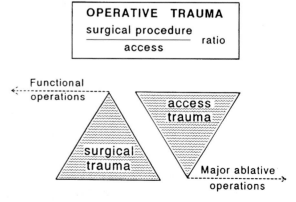

Figure 21.15 Diagrammatic representation of the concept of procedure/access trauma that determines the benefit or otherwise of using the MAS versus open surgical approach.

intense after MAS. The problem, however, has been that most human studies have been undertaken in patients undergoing surgery for benign disease, where the temporary non-specific immune suppression is of little consequence. Confirmation of this important finding requires randomized studies in patients undergoing surgery for cancer which, if confirmed, would constitute an undoubted benefit.

An important, often overlooked benefit, of MAS is the significant reduction in the wound-related complications, particularly serious wound infections and dehiscence, that incur a substantial morbidity and cost. Thus, for example, although 12 randomized trials on laparoscopic versus open appendicectomy have not shown a significant difference in the recovery of these patients, all have confirmed a significant reduction in the incidence of wound infection following laparoscopic appendicectomy. Complications may arise in laparoscopic port-site wounds, e.g. infections, bruising, haematoma and hernia formation.

MAS reduces significantly internal adhesion formation. The extent of this benefit can be judged by the reported incidence of adhesion formation after open surgery, which varies between 65 and 90%, and the documented observation that adhesions are the most common cause of acute intestinal obstruction nowadays. The vastly improved cosmetic result is of importance in young patients, especially females, although occasionally the result is far from perfect (Figure 21.16).

In general, the hospital costs of MAS operations are lower that the equivalent open operations, largely as a result of the reduced hospital stay, which more than offsets the increased operating costs. The operating costs are themselves influenced by the extent of disposable equipment used and its nature. Aside from this, the operating room charges are higher, since the determining factor here is operative time. Prospective studies in Scandinavia have shown that the cost savings (hospital + community costs including unemployment/insurance during the period of short-term disability) for such operations as antireflux surgery and cholecystectomy are very substantial (by as much as 30–60%).

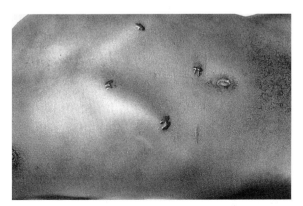

Figure 21.16 Keloid formation in port wounds after laparoscopic cardiomyotomy.

Other operations such as laparoscopic hernia repair incur a higher hospital cost but a reduced total cost because of the early return to employment.

Recovery to full activity and return to independence are especially important in the elderly. Thus, although the benefit in terms of hospital stay in this age group may not be significant, the accelerated return to the activity level enjoyed by the patient before the operation is important. Another related aspect is the ability of elderly patients to regain an independent existence. This aspect has important implications for community care and merits investigation, since many elderly patients undergoing successful open surgery for cancer lose their ability to lead independent lives and require care in nursing homes. The extent of this problem has never been quantified.

Limitations

With the current technology and image display, MAS has the following intrinsic limitations.

- **Restricted vision**: compared with normal stereoscopic vision, the display available by the best CCD-TV monitor system is inferior in terms of resolution and precise depth information, and because it provides a tunnel vision, i.e. only the small field captured by the lens objective of the telescope is seen by the surgeon at any one time. In addition, the visual axis of the surgeon is no longer aligned with his or her hands, although this restriction is likely to be overcome by the next generation of image-display systems that project the videoimage on the patient cephalad to the operating site. Even so, the surgeon has to process the image cerebrally all of the time, for accurate interpretation, which is crucial for safe execution of the operation. Thus, MAS is much more cerebrally intensive and causes mental fatigue to a greater extent than open surgery. Although never quantitated, it seems likely that the average individual becomes fatigued after operating from an image beyond 2.5–3.0 h. This is of considerable practical importance as interpretation, judgement and dexterity decline with the onset of fatigue. Two options have been suggested to overcome this problem in long MAS operations. The first is a change of surgeon half way through the operation. The second consists of strategic rest breaks by the entire surgical team, including the scrub nurse, every 2 h. During these breaks, the pneumoperitoneum is deflated, and this in itself benefits the patient.
- **Kinematic restriction**: the degrees of freedom of movement (d.o.f.) available for manipulation by the surgeon is limited to 4 by the conventional straight long instruments and to 6 by the curved coaxial instruments. This contrasts with the 23 d.o.f. of the arm–hand combination in open surgery. No doubt, this limitation will be overcome by steerable endoeffectors. However, with the current standard instrumentation, this

restriction is real and accounts for the reduced efficiency of MAS, i.e. these interventions require a longer execution time than equivalent open operations.

- **Reduced tactile and force feedback**: this is the least troublesome in the sense that most experienced surgeons in open surgery do not touch the tissues directly with the hands and have learned to process the 'tactile feedback' through the instrument–tissue interface. None the less, this feedback is reduced in MAS for two reasons: (i) much longer instruments and (ii) friction between the instrument and the ports.

The scope of research and development in MAS technology, which should now be regarded as an integral component of surgical research, is to address these limitations in conjunction with engineers, physicists and mechatronics experts.

Abdominal minimal access surgery: laparoscopic surgery

Spectrum of laparoscopic operations
Several operations can now be performed by the laparoscopic approach, but feasibility must not be equated with benefit to patient outcome. In this respect, laparoscopic operations can be classified into four groups:

- group I: operations where the laparoscopic approach provides an undoubted benefit and has replaced open intervention
- group II: operations where the laparoscopic approach appears to be beneficial and safe but more information is needed
- group III: operations that are currently under evaluation and should not be attempted outside clinical trials
- group IV: unsuitable operations: no benefit, increased risk.

Group I
This group includes cholecystectomy, cardiomyotomy, nerve sections, antireflux surgery, splenectomy, adrenalectomy for non-malignant tumours and operation for varicocele.

Group II
This group includes hernia repair (especially recurrent and bilateral), appendicectomy, adhesiolysis, surgical treatment of ductal calculi, segmental colonic resections for diverticular disease or sessile polyps, rectopexy, enucleation of insulinomas, nephrectomy for benign disease, distal pancreatic resections, oesophagectomy for oesophageal cancer and palliative bypass surgery for inoperable cancer.

Group III
This group includes resections for potentially curable invasive cancer where, because of the possibility (unproven) of dissemination, routine laparoscopic resections are not recommended and these should be confined to randomized trials or specific centres involved in research and evaluation until this issue is resolved, e.g. resection for colonic cancer, laparoscopic liver resections.

Group IV
This group is made up of major resections usually for cancer, where the trauma of access forms only a small percentage of the total operative insult. In this situation, the laparoscopic approach provides little benefit and carries increased risk, including a longer intervention, e.g. pancreaticoduodenectomy, D_2 gastrectomies for potentially curative gastric cancer.

Pneumoperitoneum
The vast majority of laparoscopic operations is currently performed after the creation of a positive-pressure CO_2 pneumoperitoneum. This can be produced by the closed technique using the Veress needle or by the open technique, i.e. insertion of the optical port through a small surgical wound in the umbilical region.

Closed pneumoperitoneum
Classically, this is produced by the insertion of a Veress needle through the immediate subumbilical area in a previously unoperated abdomen. The propensity for visceral and major vascular damage (aorta, iliac vessels and vena cava) is well documented unless the technique is flawless. **It must be remembered that the distance between the anterior abdominal wall and the aorta and its bifurcation into the iliac vessels averages only 2.0 cm.** Some surgeons have abandoned completely the creation of a closed pneumoperitoneum and use the open technique routinely whether or not the patient has had previous surgery. The need for meticulous technique even in this situation is highlighted by the reported incidence of injuries sustained during the creation of an open pneumoperitoneum, although the incidence is undoubtedly lower.

Some incisions carry a greater risk than others when the closed technique is used, e.g. central transverse and midline incisions, as opposed to peripheral ones, e.g. appendicectomy scar, Pfannenstiel and subcostal. With the correct technique, the closed method is safe for patients with peripheral scars, but the open technique is to be preferred for central incisions. If a closed peritoneum is to be created in a previously operated abdomen, the Veress needle insertion should be far removed from the scar. The most popular measure used to ensure that the Veress needle is lying in free intraperitoneal space is the saline drop test.

The problem of access is not resolved once a closed pneumoperitoneum is created successfully in a patient with a scarred abdomen, since the blind insertion of the optical port may impale adherent structures missed by the Veress needle. An optically guided cannula such as the Visiport (Figure 20.17) is highly recommended in these cases. It is good practice once the telescope is

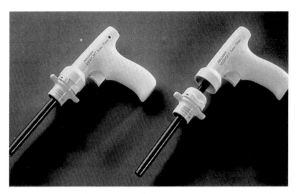

Figure 21.17 Visiport for visually guided entry of the first (optical) cannula in patients with scarred abdomens.

inserted to scan the abdomen, primarily to establish that no injury has been sustained during the creation of the pneumoperitoneum and insertion of the optical port.

Open pneumoperitoneum
This technique dispenses completely with the Veress needle and was originally introduced by Hasson for gynaecological laparoscopy. The technique entails a small subumbilical incision that is taken down behind the umbilical skin to the raphe and linea alba, which is then divided and the peritoneum opened. A sealing optical cannula of the Hasson type is then inserted and held in place by sutures (Figure 21.18). Insufflation of the peritoneal cavity is then commenced through the side port of the Hasson cannula. A modification of this technique that is favoured by the author is the transumbilical open technique. This entails grasping the edges of the umbilical ring with division of the skin of the umbilical pit. This exposes the linea alba, which is divided. A Kelly clamp or equivalent is then used to penetrate the peritoneum. This technique is simpler and easier to perform. It carries two advantages, i.e. an ordinary reusable or disposable 11.0 mm cannula can be used (inserted over a plastic rod) and the residual scar is invisible (situated in the umbilical pit).

Relative contraindications for positive-pressure pneumoperitoneum
A positive-pressure pneumoperitoneum has adverse effects on the heart. The cardiovascular, neuroendocrine and renal changes are similar to those encountered in congestive heart failure. The adverse cardiovascular changes are a 65% increase in the systemic resistance, a 90% increase in pulmonary vascular resistance and a

20–59% decrease in the cardiac index. Although these changes are well tolerated by otherwise fit patients with good general anaesthesia, patients with heart disease may not be able to cope. Although there is as yet no general consensus, positive-pressure pneumoperitoneum should be avoided in patients in the intermediate-risk category for cardiac complications during surgery [see Modules 3 and 20, Vol. I]. These patients should undergo laparoscopic surgery using gasless or low-pressure techniques. In patients in the minor risk category, the intra-abdominal pressure should be kept as low as is possible for adequate exposure.

Basic operative principles of laparoscopic surgery
In general, the same basic principles apply as in open surgery, with the necessity for meticulous technique [see Module 2, Vol. I]. MAS surgery is perhaps less forgiving than open surgery, in that mistakes in the identification of anatomical structures are more likely and control of bleeding and contamination is less easy.

Case selection
Aside from expertise, case selection is crucial to a successful outcome. It is influenced by experience of the surgeon with a particular operation, the build of the patient, previous open surgery, the nature and extent of the underlying pathology and the presence of comorbid disease. Thus, the experienced surgeon should be able to perform complicated cases, whereas the beginner should complete his or her learning curve on easy, thin and fit patients (ASA I and II) with uncomplicated disease.

Control of bleeding
Bleeding during laparoscopic surgery always appears worse on the TV monitor than it actually is. The surgeon, irrespective of experience, should keep to two rules: (i) finite time (maximum 5 min to achieve control); and (ii) immediate conversion if the patient is becoming hypotensive or the view is obscured. Otherwise, the first step consists of picking adjacent tissue (omentum, gallbladder, small intestinal loop) and placing it over the bleeding point for the assistant to hold in place. Two instruments, an atraumatic grasper and a suction/irrigator, are then introduced. As the assistant lifts the tissue over the bleeding site, this is irrigated to expose and identify the bleeding vessel, which is then picked by the atraumatic grasper. If the vessel is small, it can be electrocoagulated; otherwise, the sucker is replaced by a clip applicator, which is used to clip the vessels as it is held up by the atraumatic grasper. Sometimes, the vessel cannot be identified, as it retracts in surrounding fat. In this situation, suture ligation of the bleeding area is often successful in achieving control.

The argon gas beamer is very useful for control of surface bleeding, but care should be taken during its use to ensure against an excessive rise in the intra-abdominal pressure [see Module 2, Vol. I].

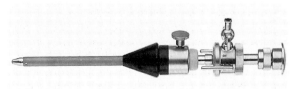

Figure 21.18 Hasson's cannula for open laparoscopy.

Conversion

This has been termed the 'Achilles heel' of laparoscopic surgery. Conversion can be **elective**, i.e. the surgeon decides for one reason or another that the operation is best conducted by the open approach, or **enforced**, when the surgeon is forced to convert to open surgery because of the onset of a major or life-threatening intraoperative complication. Evidence from the reported literature indicates that whereas the outcome of patients is not influenced adversely by elective conversion, **the morbidity is undoubtedly higher in those requiring enforced conversion.** Thus, from the practical viewpoint, the decision for conversion during the course of a laparoscopic operation reflects good judgement and common sense, and impacts on the clinical outcome of the patient.

Elective conversion is indicated:

- **when the exposure obtained is inadequate or the anatomy so disturbed by the pathology or adhesions that visual anatomical planes for safe dissection are not available to the surgeon**
- **on failure of progress of the operation for any reason.**

Exposure may be obscured by various causes, including excessive fat or enlarged left lobe of the liver (antireflux surgery), redundant colon (segmental colectomy) and gaseous distension of the small intestine. The anatomy may be disturbed by severe adhesions from previous surgery, or the lesion may be too large or complicated by fixation or fistulation to adjacent structures, etc. The diseased organ itself may be so enlarged as to preclude safe dissection and delivery, e.g. laparoscopic splenectomy is hazardous if the longitudinal axis of the organ exceeds 20 cm.

Failure of progress of the operation and misperception of the anatomy are probably the most common causes for iatrogenic injuries during laparoscopic operation and, to some extent, are linked. Failure of progress must be differentiated from a long procedure that is progressing well, i.e. the component steps of the operation are being executed and the dissection is purposeful. All that needs to be done in this situation is for the operative team to take a strategic break, during which time the CO_2 pneumoperitoneum is desufflated. Failure of progress essentially means that the surgeon is operating down a blind alley and is making little headway towards the execution of the intended operation. Some authors set a time limit and refer to this as the 'golden period'. The true picture is best reflected by the observation that a laparoscopic operation should proceed smoothly and conversion should be considered as soon as it becomes a struggle.

Tissue reduction and specimen extraction

This is an important consideration in ablative laparoscopic surgery and applies to all specimens irrespective of their perceived nature (benign or malignant). Safe practice entails (i) that the exit wound is of sufficient size and (ii) wound protection to ensure that there is no contact between the specimen and the parieties during delivery. The importance of wound protection is demonstrated in relation to laparoscopic cholecystectomy for symptomatic gallstone disease. The vast majority of these is squeezed out through an unprotected port wound. The incidence of unsuspected gallbladder cancer in these patients is variously reported in the literature between 0.5 and 1% (age dependent). There have been at least 25 reported instances of port-site tumour nodules due to tumour cell implantation after extraction of gallbladder (through an unprotected wound) containing an unsuspected carcinoma. Various devices can be used for protected extraction, including rip-proof bags, extraction sleeves, O-ring plastic drapes and the EPAB bubble (Figure 21.19). Protected extraction is mandatory for cancer specimens, even if this is through natural passages such as the rectum or vagina.

Tissue reduction enables extraction through small wounds but is applicable only to benign specimens, e.g. splenectomy for haematological disorders and uterine fibroids. Tissue reduction can be carried out by mechanical fragmentation or morcellation with electrically powered morcellators (Figure 21.20). In the case of splenectomy, tissue reduction should be carried out inside a rip-proof bag to prevent implantation of splenic fragments on the serosal surfaces, with the development of splenosis.

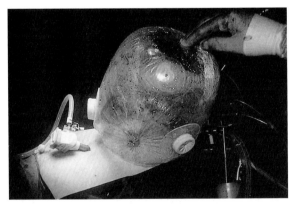

Figure 21.19 EPAB bubble used for extraction of intra-abdominal specimens.

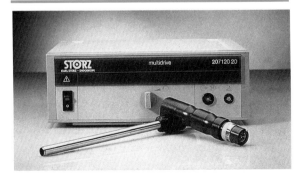

Figure 21.20 Electrically powered morcellator.

Complications of laparoscopic surgery

General

Compared with open surgery, the overall incidence of systemic complications such as pulmonary collapse and infection is low. Pneumothorax may occur, usually after laparoscopic antireflux surgery, but this is rare and easily dealt with by an intercostal underwater seal drain.

The systemic complication that is specific to laparoscopic surgery is CO_2 embolism. This can prove fatal. In most cases, it results from a technical error, e.g. insufflation through the Veress needle accidentally impaled in the uterus or liver, but there have been instances where CO_2 embolism occurred during an otherwise technically perfect operation. Presumably, the gas enters the circulation through unsealed vessels in sufficiently large amounts that exceed its solubility. One dramatic fatal case involving laparoscopic hysterectomy was found to have evidence of cerebral gas embolism in the absence of a cardiac septal defect. The explanation for this is the existence of connections between the pulmonary and systemic circulations through the bronchial blood supply. The risks of gas embolism are accentuated when the argon gas beamer is used laparoscopically. This gas is much less soluble that CO_2. Venting of the pneumoperitoneum (by opening the valves of one of the ports) is essential for the safe deployment of Argon gas plasma coagulation. The risk of CO_2 embolism is also high during laparoscopic hepatic resection unless special precautions are taken, and during retroperitoneal/extraperitoneal endoscopic procedures.

The symptoms of gas embolism include a sudden drop in the blood pressure in the absence of bleeding (outflow block of the right ventricle) and in the presence of a raised central venous pressure. A crunching precordial murmur is audible with the stethoscope. The diagnosis is readily made by echocardiography (if available at the time). The treatment includes immediate deflation of the pneumoperitoneum with cessation of the CO_2 flow and head-down posturing of the patient.

Serious synergistic narcotizing infections of the port wounds have been reported. There is little information on the relative incidence of thromboembolic disease after laparoscopic compared with open surgery, but instances of pulmonary embolism have been documented and the prophylactic measures needed to prevent DVT should not be relaxed because of the laparoscopic approach [see Modules 3 and 20, Vol. I].

Iatrogenic injuries

These have detracted from the overall benefit of laparoscopic surgery to the extent that in the UK 17% of litigation cases handled by the Medical Defence Union now relate to laparoscopic general and gynaecological surgery. Some of these iatrogenic injuries prove fatal. **The most common reason for death in the postoperative period is delay in the recognition of the intra-abdominal complication and timely surgical intervention.** The important iatrogenic injuries are:

- major retroperitoneal vascular injuries (MRVI)
- bowel injuries
- bile-duct injuries
- ureteric injuries.

Major retroperitoneal vascular injuries: these relate to injuries to the lower aorta, iliac vessels and vena cava. The majority are sustained during the creation of a closed pneumoperitoneum or blind insertion of the first (optical) cannula, with a reported incidence of 0.01–0.05%. Cases have been documented following the creation of an open pneumoperitoneum, but these are very rare occurrences. The bleeding may be immediate (iliac vessels), but if the lower aorta and vena cava are damaged, the blood loss may be initially retroperitoneal and contained by the overlying fascia and root of the mesentery. In this instance, the cardiovascular collapse may be delayed by some 10–15 min. Tachycardia is, however, always present. The immediate recognition of such injuries with prompt volume replacement and surgical intervention are the important factors in survival. In the absence of free intraperitoneal blood, a quick scan with the laparoscope with the patient in the Trendelenberg position will reveal a bluish retroperitoneal expanding and pulsatile mass. Immediate extensive midline laparotomy with proximal vascular control and repair is essential and should save the patient. The reported mortality of such injuries varies from 5 to 10%.

The iliac vessels may be damaged during laparoscopic hernia repair, anterior resection and pelvic lymphadenectomy, and the right branch of the hepatic artery may be damaged during cholecystectomy. A looped right hepatic artery is particularly prone to damage unless great care is taken during the dissection of the cystic pedicle of the anatomy obscured by adhesions, fat or inflammatory oedema. Prompt conversion with application of Pringle's manoeuvre (by fingers or a vascular clamp) will achieve immediate vascular control and enable vascular repair of the damaged artery.

Damage to the inferior epigastric vessels is usually sustained by a port inserted along the line of these vessels. Unless recognized and dealt with, this injury results in an extensive rectus sheath haematoma that requires intervention by open evacuation and ligature of the bleeding vessels.

Bowel injuries: the main problem with small and large bowel injuries during laparoscopic general and gynaecological surgery is that 60% of them are missed at operation and declare themselves in the postoperative period or after discharge from hospital with generalized peritonitis. Most of these missed injuries are caused by collateral damage following the use of energized dissection systems, particularly electrosurgery. The pathology in this instance is a full-thickness thermal lesion without immediate loss of integrity of the bowel wall. Sloughing of the necrotic area and perforation ensue over a variable period after surgery, with the development of acute bacterial peritonitis. The risk factors for a fatal outcome include perforation of the colon (as distinct from duodenum and small intestine) and delayed diagnosis. Treatment is by immediate laparotomy. These injuries are largely preventable by the adoption of the correct surgical technique and safe use of energized dissection systems [see Module 2, Vol. I].

Bowel and stomach injuries sustained by instruments such as graspers and scissors are less of a problem because they are immediately apparent during surgery. The treatment entails suture closure of the perforation laparoscopically, if the surgeon has the necessary expertise, or by conversion to open surgery, if not. A course of antibiotics against Gram-negative organisms (especially for distal ileal and large bowel injuries) is commenced at the time of surgery and continued for 5 days postoperatively.

- **Bile-duct injuries**: there is evidence that the incidence of bile-duct injuries approximates to that following open cholecystectomy, despite the undoubted temporary increase when laparoscopic cholecystectomy was introduced in surgical practice in the late 1980s. The use of routine intraoperative cholangiography during laparoscopic cholecystectomy may reduce the incidence of bile-duct injuries, although this remains unproven. There is, however, good evidence that intraoperative cholangiography identifies injuries during the intervention and thus enables timely primary repair. The majority of bile duct injuries (60–80%) are not recognised at the time of laparoscopic cholecystectomy.
- **Ureteric injuries**: the ureters are at risk during pelvic laparoscopic surgery, e.g. anterior resection, rectopexy, hysterectomy, pelvic lymphadenopathy, and during retroperitoneal surgery, e.g. lumbar sympathectomy. The best prevention is identification of the respective ureter during the procedure and preservation of its blood supply. Damage may be by inclusion in clips, sharp dissection or collateral damage from electrosurgery.

Port-site wound hernias
Herniation through port-site wounds is the result of inadequate closure of the musculoaponeurotic layers of the abdominal wall. The incidence (overall percentage) is size related, with the majority of hernias occurring in wounds larger than 10 mm. Port-site hernias are also more common in the lower abdomen below the arcuate line. Port-site hernias may present acutely with intestinal obstruction, often due to partial entrapment of a knuckle of bowel (Richter's type hernia). The diagnosis may not be immediately apparent, as often there is no superficial skin bulge. CT has been recommended for establishing the diagnosis.

Laparoscopic surgery for intra-abdominal malignancy
This has generated the greatest debate with extreme viewpoints for and against the laparoscopic approach,

especially for potentially curative cancer. The debate has been enhanced by reports of port-site deposits following laparoscopic resection of certain cancers, especially colonic. Although there were initial reports based on small retrospective series by surgeons with limited experience that indicated a significant problem, i.e. port-site deposits of 2–10% at 1–2 years of follow-up, subsequent much larger series of colorectal cancer resections have shown an incidence of 1% or less. There are no exact data on the incidence of wound deposits after open colorectal surgery, except for one large retrospective series that showed an incidence of 0.6% at 1 year, rising to 1% over subsequent years. What is now known from recent studies is that viable cancer cells can be harvested from the peritoneal cavity by saline lavage in 30% of patients undergoing open surgery for colorectal cancer. Thus, the potential for tumour implantation exists and cannot be ignored. There is no evidence from animal experiments that CO_2 pneumoperitoneum causes increased growth of tumour cells implanted within the peritoneum cavity compared with open laparotomy, but it does appear to enhance growth of subcutaneous tumour implants. The mechanisms for dissemination of viable exfoliated cells and their implantation in port wounds are not known. Several hypotheses have been suggested and investigated without any definite conclusions: CO_2 convection currents and chimney effect, trauma, effect of compounds in electrosurgical smoke produced in a closed environment and devitalization of the parieties by the port. What appears certain is the individual variation in the incidence of port-site deposits reported from different centres and surgeons, with some having no such instances in their series, and others a worrying incidence. Thus, the 'surgeon factor' as in open surgery for colorectal cancer may be very important.

Detailed analysis of the reported instances of port-site deposits after laparoscopic surgery for colonic cancer has shown that it is related to the extent of transmural spread, with all but a few of the reported cases being either Duke's B or C. One instance of a port-site deposit in a Duke's A lesion had intracorporeal anastomosis with the bowel ends open. There are some inferences from this analysis, which are backed by data from peritoneal cytology studies. The most important is that exfoliation of viable tumour cells, spontaneously or during surgery, occurs once the tumour has penetrated the entire thickness of the bowel wall. Thus, the probability of port-site deposits arises in these tumours, especially if bulky and with serosal involvement. Selection of cases based on the tumour stage is therefore prudent and advisable. On this evidence, laparoscopic resections of Duke's A colon cancer should be safe. The same applies to early gastric cancer, especially if the tumour is < 3.0 cm. The second inference relates to the special precautions that must be taken during laparoscopic surgery for cancer to minimize possible exfoliation and implantation. These are:

- the tumour must never be handled by the laparoscopic instruments
- early devascularization of the intended resection segment must be carried out
- the pneumoperitoneum must be aspirated rather than desufflated rapidly
- all port wounds must be irrigated with distilled water or povidone iodine.

Indications for laparoscopic surgery in intra-abdominal cancer
Laparoscopic surgery is established in the following:

- **staging of certain tumours:** the benefit here is considerably improved if the visual findings are supplemented by laparoscopic contact ultrasonography. Undoubted benefit has been established in the staging of patients with pancreatic, oesophageal and gastric cancer. The laparoscopic staging should be conducted in the same session as the intended operation. Some advocate that the staging laparoscopy should be performed in a prior session. This is unnecessary and exposes the patient to two interventions under general anaesthesia, and furthermore increases the costs
- **resection of T_1 tumours and large sessile polyps:** provided expertise is available and with the right precautions, these tumours can be resected laparoscopically with no added risk in terms of disease-related long-term survival. Laparoscopic D_1 gastrectomy would seem ideal for early gastric cancer > 3.0 cm with submucosal invasion detected by gastric endosonography. However, the reported data are limited and the follow-up periods too short to permit any conclusions on efficacy and safety. Laparoscopic wedge resection without lymphadenectomy may be adequate in small lesions, ≥ 3.0 cm, of certain macroscopic endoscopic type **[see Gastrointestinal Disorders, Vol. II]**
- **palliation of incurable disease** by either resection or bypass.

Currently, tumours that are advanced but still potentially curable by resection with adjuvant therapy, e.g. Duke's B and C colonic cancers, gastric cancers invading the muscularis propria (T_2, T_3), should only be resected laparoscopically in centres involved in the evaluation of these laparoscopic procedures within the confines of prospective clinical trials.

There are no restrictions on the resection of benign tumours such as leiomyomas, insulinomas or large sessile polyps by the laparoscopic approach. Indeed, these patients derive considerable benefit when treated by this approach.

Endoluminal minimal access surgery

Established examples of this approach include arthroscopic surgery, transanal endoscopic microsurgery (TEM), and the laparoendoluminal approach for benign gastric lesions or polyps and some types of early gastric cancer.

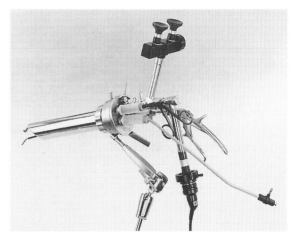

Figure 21.21 Buess' operating proctoscope used for TEM.

Transanal endoscopic microsurgery

Pioneered by Buess, TEM has opened new therapeutic possibilities for the treatment of rectal tumours up to the peritoneal reflection: large adenomas and early carcinomas **[see Gastrointestinal Disorders, Vol. II]**. The operating proctoscope has a stereoscopic telescope for the operator, and permits CO_2 insufflation and the attachment of a CCD camera for monitor display of the operative field for the assistant and scrub nurse. The proctoscope has sealed portholes for the insertion of instruments used for the resection and closure of the defect (Figure 21.21).

Laparoendoluminal gastric approach

This technique is particularly suited for lesions on the posterior wall of the stomach, fundus and oesophagogastric junction. An experienced laparoscopic surgeon and a skilled endoscopist work together. The procedure starts with a laparoscopic inspection and placement of a detachable clamp just distal to the duodenojejunal junction. Following passage of a flexible endoscope and insufflation of the stomach, this is entered from the serosal side between the lesser and greater curvatures with an Innerdyne cannula (Figure 21.22), which is then expanded to 10 mm for insertion of the laparoscope and insufflation of the stomach with CO_2. A second Innerdyne cannula is inserted as an instrument channel and stretched to 5.0 mm once in place. The second assisting instrument is brought down via the operating channel of the flexible endoscope, which for this reason must have a large instrument channel (4.2 mm).

Section 21.4 • Interventional flexible endoscopy

IFE is an established major component of therapeutic gastroenterology. It is most commonly used for:

- retrieval of swallowed or inhaled foreign bodies
- dilatation of benign strictures

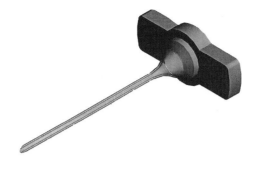

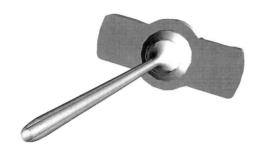

Figure 21.22 Expandable Innerdyne cannula.

- percutaneous endoscopic gastrostomy (PEG)
- control of gastrointestinal bleeding
- management of ductal stones, cholangitis and pancreatitis
- treatment of gastrointestinal polyps and some forms of early mucosal cancer
- palliation of incurable bronchial, gastrointestinal, biliary and pancreatic malignancy.

Removal of foreign bodies

Foreign bodies are either inhaled into the tracheobronchial tree or swallowed. All inhaled foreign bodies must be removed by bronchoscopy as a matter of urgency because of the inevitable serious complications, pulmonary collapse, abscess and fistula formation. By contrast, the majority of swallowed foreign bodies negotiate the gastrointestinal tract and are passed spontaneously, but 10% require intervention by flexible endoscopy. The indications for extraction of swallowed foreign bodies are:

- the foreign body has sharp edges or points that may lacerate or perforate the gastrointestinal tract, e.g. open safety pins, chicken bones
- the foreign body is toxic or corrosive, e.g. swallowed batteries, some marbles because of toxic colour coating
- the foreign body causes acute obstruction in the oesophagus, usually at the cricopharyngeal sphincter, level of the aortic arch or the lower oesophageal sphincter

- all foreign bodies that remain in the stomach for more than 72 h
- bezoars: these require debulking by endoscopic fragmentation using wire loops before piecemeal extraction.

The instruments used vary with the nature of the foreign body and include rat-tooth forceps (for coins), Dormia baskets (solid, round objects) and suction caps (soft food bolus). In some instances, extraction has to be shielded by use of an overtube, e.g. extraction of razor blades by rubber-coated forceps.

Dilatation of benign strictures

Dilatation of strictures or stenosis of surgically constructed anastomoses is performed with either solid tapered dilators, e.g. Celestin's, or balloons attached to devices that monitor the balloon pressure when inflated. The latter are more popular, can be used to dilate strictures not accessible by the solid dilators, e.g. gastroduodenal strictures, and also give better results for achalasia. However, a randomized study has shown that in the treatment of benign strictures of the oesophagus due to reflux oesophagitis, tapered solid dilators give better results than balloon dilatation in terms of the duration of the dysphagia-free period and the need for further dilatation.

Gastrointestinal bleeding

Endoscopic control of gastrointestinal bleeding is undertaken for both non-variceal and variceal bleeding. Single large-channel instruments (3.7–4.2 mm) or twin-channel endoscopes that permit suction of blood and secretions are used. The treatment modalities deployed can be grouped as thermal, injection and vascular occlusive devices (Table 21.1).

The use of the endoscopic heater probe in conjunction with adrenaline injection for the control of gastrointestinal bleeding is simple, safe, effective and one of the least expensive methods. Although electrical energy is used to heat the probe, there is no contact of electrical current with the tissues. The heater probe is as effective, more convenient to use and safer than Nd:YAG laser photocoagulation. Electrocoagulation

Table 21.1 Modalities for endoscopic control of gastrointestinal bleeding

Modality	Examples
Thermal	Monopolar coagulation, bipolar coagulation, argon plasma coagulation, heater probe coagulation, laser photocoagulation, microwave energy
Injection	Sclerosants, vasoconstrictors, fibrin/thrombin glue, etc.
Vascular occlusive devices	Bands (oesophageal varices), endoscopic metal clips for vessels

can be delivered endoscopically using either monopolar or bipolar (BICAP) electrodes. Although the efficacy in achieving haemostatic control is similar in both, the bipolar system is considerably safer [see Module 2, Vol. I]. Photocoagulation using laser energy, e.g. Nd:YAG delivered endoscopically via an optical fibre, is practised in some centres. However, randomized clinical trials have shown no specific benefit of laser photocoagulation over other thermal or injection methods.

Therapeutic endoscopy is used routinely for the following causes of non-variceal gastrointestinal bleeding:

- peptic ulcers and erosive gastritis
- Mallory–Weiss tears
- Dieulafoy lesion
- diffuse gastric antral vascular ectasia (watermelon stomach). [Gastrointestinal Disorders, Vol. II]

The surgical threshold in patients treated by therapeutic endoscopy for non-variceal gastrointestinal bleeding is an important consideration [see Module 6, Vol. I]. Attempts at endoscopic control are not effective in the following:

- chronic penetrating posterior duodenal ulcer eroding the gastroduodenal artery
- chronic deep gastric ulcer eroding the splenic or hepatic artery
- extensive colonic arteriovenous malformations.

Nowadays endoscopic control is the first-line management for control of variceal haemorrhage following resuscitation. Endoscopic sclerotherapy used to be the mainstay but is now challenged by endoscopic band ligation of varices (Figure 21.23). Randomized trials have confirmed equal efficacy of control of variceal haemorrhage by these two methods [see Hepatobiliary and Pancreatic Disorders, Vol. II].

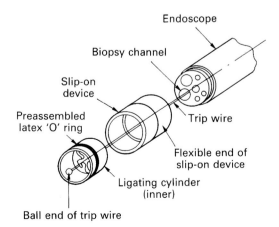

Figure 21.23 Mechanism used for rubber-band ligation of oesophageal varices.

Management of ductal stones, cholangitis and pancreatitis

Endoscopic extraction is the gold-standard management of ductal calculi and usually precedes cholecystectomy, although in centres with the necessary surgical expertise, laparoscopic stone extraction, especially via the cystic duct, is challenging the established role of endoscopic stone extraction (ESE). A preliminary sphincterotomy (papillotomy) is undertaken prior to extraction of stones by balloon catheter or Dormia basket. The morbidity of ESE is low and includes bleeding, pancreatitis, cholangitis, impaction of the Dormia basket (usually when large stones are trapped) and perforation of the duodenum. Balloon dilatation of the choledochal sphincter instead of papillotomy is practised in some centres prior to stone extraction. The reported studies with this technique are limited and it is by no means certain that the procedure is safer than endoscopic papillotomy. Failures of ESE may be due to previous gastric surgery (Roux-en-Y) or because of large or occluding stones. A pigtail stent is inserted if stones cannot be retrieved and the patient is jaundiced. Surgical treatment (open or laparoscopic) is necessary for these patients unless they are poor risks (ASA III, IV).

Endoscopic sphincterotomy with extraction of stones, if present, is the required treatment of patients admitted with bacterial cholangitis and has replaced open surgery. It is undertaken as an urgent procedure in view of the serious nature of this condition, which can prove fatal as a result of septic shock. In the severely ill patient, the endoscopic placement of a nasobiliary drain is a life-saving procedure, with stone extraction performed at a later stage.

The role of ERCP and papillotomy in severe necrotizing pancreatitis is uncertain. For some years it was advocated in these patients because of the results of a randomized trial that indicated benefit from this procedure in these seriously ill patients. However, more recent trials and prospective studies have shown that the procedure is only of benefit in patients with ampullary stone obstruction with jaundice and cholangitis. In all other cases, the consensus view is that ERCP is ill advised in the acute stage of the disease.

Endoscopic methods are well established for the treatment of pancreatic pseudocysts complicating acute pancreatitis, extraction of pancreatic calculi and stenting in some patients with chronic pancreatitis and sphincterotomy of the minor papilla in patients with pancreas divisium [see Hepatobiliary and Pancreatic Disorders, Vol. II].

Treatment of early gastrointestinal cancer

Therapeutic IFE may be used for the following:

- ablation of mucosal cancer/severe dysplasia (laser)
- excision of polyps
- ablation of premalignant mucosa, e.g. Barrett's columnar cell change (laser or argon ion plasma)
- submucosal resection of early gastric cancer.

Excision of colonic polyps is one of the most common flexible interventional procedures performed in gastroenterology and electrosurgical wire loops are used for this purpose. Retrieval of the polyp and its submission for histological examination are essential. Colonoscopic polypectomy for pedunculated polyps is safe provided it is performed with the necessary expertise. Sessile polyps are more difficult and dangerous to excise endoscopically, and if large (> 2.0 cm) should be removed surgically. Special techniques, including submucosal injection of adrenaline/saline solution, are used for the endoscopic resection of small sessile colonic polyps. Even so, the risks of bleeding and perforation of the colon are greater than following excision of pedunculated polyps.

Early gastric cancer is defined histologically when the lesion is confined to the mucosa and submucosa. It is becoming increasingly relevant in Western countries as early gastric cancer is diagnosed much more frequently with open access endoscopy. The extent of submucosal invasion (superficial or deep, sm_{1-3}) appears to determine the incidence of spread to the level 1 regional lymph nodes (N_1). Overall, some 15% of early gastric cancers have lymph-node deposits. The incidence of regional node spread increases when early gastric cancer invades the submucosa. The dilemma, therefore, in the management of patients with early gastric cancer (local endogastric ablation/removal or wedge resection versus D_1 or D_2 gastrectomy) centres on this issue. The endoscopic macroscopic type of lesion and level of submucosal involvement by gastric endosonography to define the extent of submucosal involvement (sm_1, sm_2, sm_3) can, in theory, be used in the selection of the appropriate treatment in the individual case, provided they are reliable indicators of regional node involvement [see Gastrointestinal disorders, Vol. II]. The interventional flexible endoscopic approach appears to be suitable for superficial early gastric cancer not involving the submucosa. The techniques include submucosal resection after adrenaline/saline injection in the submucosal layer and laser ablation.

Palliation of malignancy

Therapeutic endoscopy is extensively used in the palliation of obstructing inoperable cancer of the bronchus and oesophagus, biliary–pancreatic cancers and, more recently, obstructing colorectal cancer. In many of these cases, there is a choice between the endoscopic and radiological interventional approaches (see below), but in complex cases both may be needed in the individual patient.

The techniques include dilatation, stenting and recanalization with laser (either Nd:YAG, or photodynamic ablation [see Module 2, Vol. I]. Increasingly expandable metallic stents, usually made of NiTi alloy (Nitinol) are used in preference to plastic stents. In the oesophagus (Figure 21.24), these are easier to insert and do not usually require preliminary dilatation.

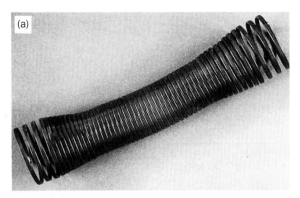
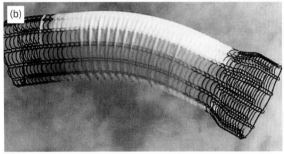

Figure 21.24 Metallic expandable stents used to palliate dysphagia in a patient with inoperable cancer of the oesophagus.

Some retrospective reports have indicated reduced morbidity and better palliation of dysphagia with expandable metallic wall stents than with plastic or reinforced silicon stents. However, there have been no randomized studies and plastic/silicon oesophageal stents (Celestin, Nottingham, etc.) are cheaper. It is not known whether adjuvant radiotherapy after stenting increases the dysphagia-free period and the quality of life. This important issue is being addressed by two randomized clinical trials.

Relief of jaundice and itching is obtained by endoscopic stenting of inoperable biliopancreatic cancer but, in time, these stents (plastic and metallic) become occluded by tumour overgrowth or ingrowth when jaundice and cholangitis supervene. The situation is remedied by restenting. There is some controversy with regard to stenting of jaundiced patients with operable biliary or pancreatic/periampullary tumours. The potential benefits are relief of jaundice and improvement in renal function if surgery is delayed. The disadvantages include the risk of infection (cholangitis) and reduced calibre of the proximally dilated bile duct, i.e. smaller and more difficult anastomosis. In general, hepatobiliary surgeons favour avoidance of stenting before surgery, if the general condition of the patient is good.

Section 21.5 • Percutaneous interventional radiology

Interventional radiology uses the imaging modalities of ultrasound, fluoroscopy, CT, magnetic resonance imaging (MRI) or a combination of techniques to provide image guidance of simple and more complex procedures. The appropriate imaging modality used depends on the relative requirement for real-time imaging, the ability of that modality to provide the necessary target or instrument visualization, the appropriate regional cross-sectional (axial, coronal or sagittal) or systems-based (vascular, biliary or urological) navigation, the safe completion of the procedure based on the patient's condition, and the procedure.

Interventional radiological techniques

Interventional radiology increasingly contributes to the management of many surgical conditions (Table 21.2). The rapid pace of technological advance in imaging modalities, image processing and instrumentation has increased the technical success rate and reduced the complication rate of many procedures. In some instances interventional radiological procedures have replaced conventional surgical methods, and in other cases they provide a useful addition to the surgical management. The close integration of an interventional radiologist and the specialized surgical team is essential to achieve the full benefit to the overall patient management and outcome. The increasing range of procedures, the instrumentation and complexity of interventional radiology emphasize the need for careful

Table 21.2 Interventional radiological techniques

- Biopsy
- Drainage
- Dilatation
- Stenting
- Formation of extra-anatomic tract
- Foreign body retrieval
- Embolization
- Line placement
- *In situ* ablation

Table 21.3 Interventional radiological procedures: general considerations

- Patient preparation
  Patient consent
  Coagulation
  Level of co-operation required
  Monitoring blood pressure, pulse oximetry
  Need for sedation, analgesia, anaesthesia: local or general
  Need for antibiotic prophylaxis
  Contraindication to imaging: X-ray, MRI
  Aftercare

- Site for intervention
  Radiology department
  Ward/intensive care unit
  Theatre

- Choice of imaging modality
  Planning imaging
  Procedural imaging: navigation
  Anatomical basis for procedure

case selection and case discussion to ensure the appropriate management plan and choice of the most beneficial method of treatment, either surgical or interventional radiological, or a combination.

For all radiological interventions, several issues require consideration by the ward staff and the surgical team. These are outlined in Table 21.3. An appropriate integration of the interventional radiologist in the surgical team allows for formulation of algorithms of management and protocols for patient preparation and aftercare to ensure appropriate patient management.

Patient preparation includes informed consent and the ability to describe the procedure to the patient. The attendant risks and benefits should be understood by the clinician obtaining the patient's consent. As the vast majority of interventional radiological procedures is performed with sedation, analgesia and local anaesthesia, the level of co-operation of the patient required for safe execution of the procedure is essential, e.g. percutaneous hepatobiliary interventions require the patient to be able to control respiration. While the majority of interventional procedures is performed in the radiology department using static imaging systems, the ability to use mobile forms of image guidance such as ultrasound extends the site for intervention to include the ward, intensive care unit or theatre.

Choice of imaging modality

The choice of the interventional imaging modality may differ from the planning imaging. For instance, whereas a lesion in the liver may be seen on CT, the appropriate biopsy or ablation may be performed percutaneously under ultrasound. The advances and developments in image modality are a continuous process and the nature of image guidance will change with further advancement. In addition, the practicality assessment, particularly in relation to availability, will depend on local circumstances and imaging resources. The particular choice rests with the interventional radiologist. An understanding of the above characteristics will assist surgeons when they discuss patients for radiological intervention. The choice of procedural imaging will depend on the accuracy of navigation of the instrument to the target and the anatomical basis for the procedure.

The characteristics of the ideal procedure of image-guidance modality are outlined in Table 21.4. Of

Table 21.4 Characteristics of the ideal procedural imaging modality

• Navigation	Real-time display
	Cross-sectional/multiplanar
	Surface information
• Therapy monitoring	
• Practicality	Safe (radiation)
	Cheap
	Available

particular importance is the requirement for accuracy for navigation. The ideal modality instantaneously refreshes the image of the orientation of the instrument to the target or adjacent structures, i.e. provides real-time display. Axial cross-sectional display of the anatomy by CT may be appropriate, but multiplanar imaging (coronal, sagittal or oblique planes) by ultrasound or MRI provides more directional information. Display of surface information is less readily available than with endoscopic surgery, but the outline of the surface may be achieved by injection of contrast agents (e.g. angiography or cholangiography).

The ability to monitor the therapeutic procedure is essential. While this may be relatively simple for dilatation or recanalization of tubular structures such as vessels, bile ducts and ureters, the ability to monitor tissue ablation is potentially available only with MRI and ultrasound.

The anatomical basis of navigation for a procedure can be separated into navigation within or around a solid organ, e.g. kidney or liver, or region, e.g. pelvis or thorax, or on the basis of a tubular structure or system such as vascular, biliary, gastrointestinal or urological conduit, e.g. ureter, urethra, uterus or fallopian tube. The requirements for each type of anatomical basis for navigation are different and are shown in Table 21.5. The ability of imaging modalities to provide these characteristics varies and an assessment of each modality on an arbitrary scale is given in Table 21.6.

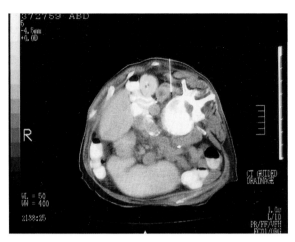

Figure 21.25 CT-guided biopsy of retroperitoneal mass/collection.

Image-guided biopsy

The specific considerations for biopsy procedures relate to:

- route of access for biopsy device
- choice of imaging modality
- choice of needle
- likely successful result
- possible morbidity.

The route of access is generally the shortest route from skin or access point to the lesion, avoiding vital structures, which would result in complications, e.g. lung, bowel or major vessels. The choice of imaging modality is usually ultrasound or CT. The multiplanar facility, real-time display, relative mobility, low cost and lack of radiation are particular advantages of ultrasound, whereas CT may be required for smaller lesions that cannot be accurately imaged or when obscured by gas, either in the pleural space or gut, or in the retroperitoneum or bone (Figure 21.25). In addition, intravenous contrast enhancement may indicate a viable part of the tumour likely to produce more histological accuracy.

The choice of biopsy device will depend on the pathological requirements. The devices available range from aspiration cytology needles and aspiration biopsy needles, to mechanical solid biopsy devices. The accuracy rates for most percutaneous biopsies exceed 80%, while the complication rates are low (< 1.5%). These are operator dependent, however, and emphasize the value of a skilled interventional radiologist performing biopsies under optimum imaging modality and conditions.

Advanced biopsy techniques

In certain situations percutaneous biopsy of lesions may not be safe. In particular, liver biopsy in patients with abnormal coagulation is a common problem. This may be overcome by using a plugged liver biopsy technique. The coagulation abnormality is corrected by adminis-

Table 21.5 Requirements for navigation

• Solid organ/regional	Real-time
	Structural anatomy: cross-sectional
	Surface view
	Tissue differentiation/lesion
	conspicuity:
	Hepatic
	Abdominal
	Thoracic
	Pelvic
• Tubular system	Real-time
	Structural anatomy: 'intensity projection'
	Lesion conspicuity:
	Vascular
	Biliary
	Gastrointestinal
	Urological
	Gynaecological

Table 21.6 Assessment of imaging modality

Modality	Real-time	Tubular	Solid	Lesions	Practicality
Fluoroscopy	5	4	1	1	4
Ultrasound	5	2	3	1	4
CT	3	3	4	3	3
MRI: closed	2	2	5	5	1
MRI: open	2	2	5	4	1

1, very poor; 5, very good.

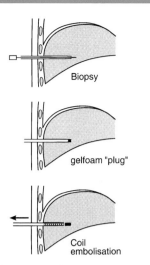

Figure 21.26 Percutaneous liver biopsy with tract embolization.

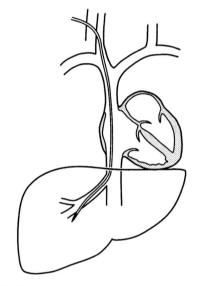

Figure 21.27 Transjugular liver biopsy.

tration of the platelets and coagulation factors. In addition, embolization of the biopsy tract with coils or particulate matter is employed to reduce the risk of haemorrhage (Figure 21.26). The alternative transvascular technique may be used through the transjugular approach. With this technique, under ultrasound guidance the right internal jugular vein is accessed and a biopsy catheter needle passed down the superior vena cava and right atrium into the right hepatic vein and thence into the liver parenchyma (Figure 21.27). A similar technique may also be employed from the transfemoral approach.

Image-guided drainage

The specific considerations for image-guided drainage of fluid collections relate to procedure planning:

- route of access for drainage.
- choice of imaging modality

- technique and choice of drainage device
- likely successful result
- possible complications.

CT- or ultrasound-guided percutaneous drainage of simple subcutaneous, intra-abdominal, pleural or pelvic fluid collections has replaced surgical intervention. Successful drainage of more complicated collections is also possible but may require multiple drainage catheters or subsequent surgical drainage. In the latter situation, the initial radiological drainage allows an improvement in the patient's general condition such that surgical intervention, if and when indicated, is carried out with less risk to the patient.

Whereas ultrasound is often used for subcutaneous or simple intra-abdominal or pelvic collections, the additional accuracy and resolution of CT reduce the risk of injuries to intra-abdominal organs. CT is therefore preferable, especially in anatomically crowded areas. Alternatively, or in the absence of CT facilities, the combination of ultrasound with fluoroscopy may provide better visual guidance than ultrasound alone in more difficult cases. This requires transfer of the patient to the fluoroscopy room.

An initial diagnostic fine needle aspiration may be performed prior to drainage. One of two techniques may be employed for draining the fluid collection or pus:

- over-the-wire technique
- trocar-mounted catheter.

The trocar technique is appropriate for large superficial collections, while the over-the-wire technique has the advantages of a greater degree of accuracy and fewer traumatic preliminary steps (Figure 21.28a, b). In either case, the catheter used should be large enough for adequate drainage, usually 8–12 French. Larger, 12–18 Fr catheters may be required for more particulate or thick material (Figure 21.28c). Isotonic saline irrigation of the cavity is performed concomitantly during the procedure. Aftercare includes further irrigation with continuous drainage with or without suction. The patient's condition usually improves within 24–48 h. Failure

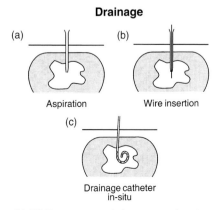

Figure 21.28 Percutaneous drainage: over-the-wire technique.

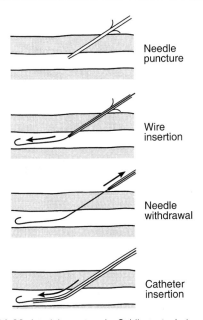

Figure 21.29 Arterial puncture by Seldinger technique.

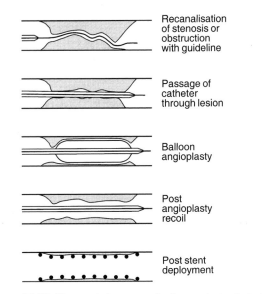

Figure 21.30 Phases during recanalization and stenting of arterial stenosis.

may imply inadequate drainage, misplacement of the tube or insufficient irrigation and suction. Careful repositioning of the catheter may be required. Continuous drainage over several days may signify the presence of a fistula. When suspected, a contrast study performed through the drainage catheter will identify the site and type of the fistulous communication. Successful percutaneous drainage of simple collections is achieved in 80–100% of cases. **Major complications include septicaemia, haemorrhage and damage to adjacent structures.**

Recanalization, dilatation and stenting

The specific considerations for recanalization, dilatation and stenting procedures relate to planning of the procedure:

- route of access for procedure
- choice of imaging modality
- technique and choice of recanalization and dilatation devices
- requirements for stenting
- likely successful result
- possible complications.

The route of access varies, depending on the anatomical site of the obstruction, the system involved (vascular, biliary, gastrointestinal, urological, etc.), and the safest and technically most feasible approach.

Recanalization, dilatation and stenting procedures are usually performed under fluoroscopy. A vascular procedure is performed by accessing the vessel using the Seldinger technique (Figure 21.29).

Balloon dilatation has replaced use of solid dilators in the dilatation of strictures or occlusions within the majority of anatomical tubes above 3 mm in size. An initial contrast study is required to confirm the site and

extent of the stenosis or obstruction. The technique usually involves manipulation of the catheter and guide wire under fluoroscopy across the stenosis or occlusion, followed by confirmation of position and subsequent dilatation with a balloon catheter to an appropriate size consistent with the original diameter of the tube (Figure 21.30). Confirmation of patency is achieved by contrast injection. This technique is generally applied to the systems outlined in Table 21.7.

Following recanalization and dilatation, certain strictures or obstruction are prone to recoil, early or late restenosis. In this situation, particularly when the underlying cause is the result of malignancy in the gastrointestinal, biliary or urological tract, or due to severe atherosclerosis, the placement of a mechanical stent is often indicated (Figure 21.31). The type and material of the stent vary widely and are dependent on the site, structure and pathology of the obstruction, the delivery system requirements, the accuracy of placement

Table 21.7 Interventional radiological dilatation/recanalization

System	Target
Vascular	Arterial
	Venous
Gastrointestinal	Oesophagus
	Duodenum
	Rectum
Biliary tract	Left and right hepatic ducts
	Common hepatic duct
	Common bile duct
Urinary tract	Ureter
	Urethra
Gynaecology	Fallopian tube
Ophthalmology	Lachrymal duct

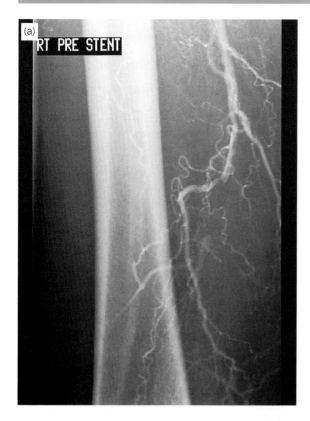

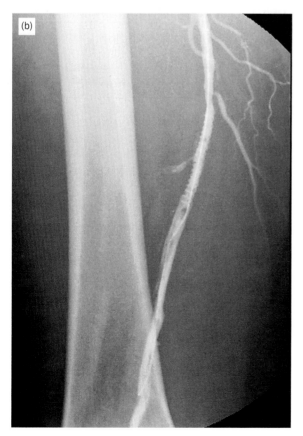

required, the compliance of the obstruction and the risk of stent migration. In the vascular system these are customized to the vessel and to the area of interest and are usually of metallic construction (stainless steel or Nitinol). In both gastrointestinal and biliary tracts, the stents used are either plastic or expanding metal wall stents of similar construction. Most percutaneous biliary stents used nowadays are metallic, owing to their self-expanding designs. Expanding metallic stents are also increasingly preferred to plastic types for obstructions in the gastrointestinal tract. Urological stents are most commonly plastic.

The results of recanalization, dilatation and stenting are variable, the major factors determining outcome being the site, the geometry of the lesion (diameter and length of obstruction) and the underlying pathology.

Formation of an extra-anatomic tract

This is best exemplified by the transjugular intrahepatic portasystemic shunt (TIPSS), which is a radiologically performed shunt between the right hepatic vein and the portal vein through the liver parenchyma. The procedure decompresses the portal hypertension in patients with variceal haemorrhage due to cirrhosis and can be used as an alternative to endoscopic sclerotherapy. The long-term patency beyond 6 months is, however, low. Its most useful indication is in patients with Child's C cirrhosis and bleeding varices awaiting hepatic transplantation.

The procedure is performed under fluoroscopy, intravenous sedation, analgesia and patient monitoring. The internal jugular vein is punctured under ultrasound guidance and a standard Seldinger technique is used. Similarly to a transjugular liver biopsy, a catheter is passed down the superior vena cava across the right atrium into the right hepatic vein. A modified needle is introduced through the catheter. This needle is passed across the liver and a portal vein accessed. Initial portal vein pressure is then recorded, and using standard catheter guide-wire angioplasty techniques the tract in the liver parenchyma between the hepatic and portal vein is dilated and then stented (Figure 21.32).

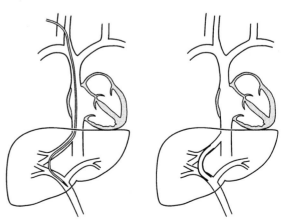

Figure 21.31 Femoral artery recanalization and stenting: (a) before and (b) after procedure.

Figure 21.32 Transjugular intrahepatic portosystemic shunt.

Foreign body retrieval

Inadvertent misplacement or fracture of a venous vascular device may embolize to the great veins, heart or pulmonary artery. In this situation, there is an urgent clinical requirement to retrieve the foreign body as it may cause thrombosis, infection or a functional complication, e.g. cardiac arrhythmia. If misplaced or lost in the arterial system, distal embolism may result in thrombosis, occlusion and ischaemia. Similar problems may be encountered in the biliary, gastrointestinal or urological tract.

Radiological retrieval is a better alternative to surgery if the site is difficult to access surgically or requires a major operation. The imaging modality used for retrieval of foreign bodies is usually fluoroscopy. A combination of catheter and guide-wire techniques is used to approximate a snare device to the foreign body. Once grasped, the foreign body may be retrieved percutaneously if small, or using a more accessible surgical site if larger.

Embolization

Blockage of the arterial supply is employed to reduce vascular inflow to a tumour, arterial venous malformation, aneurysm or abnormal vasculature (Figure 21.33). Embolization of bleeding vessels due to trauma, severe pancreatitis or iatrogenic injuries may also be employed. The emerging field of specific drug delivery by chemoembolization of the tumour has been employed, particularly in the liver and breast, and is likely to be utilized extensively for gene cancer therapy, e.g. infection of tumours with p53-adenovirus products. The types of embolization agent are outlined in Table 21.8. Temporary embolization agents are used

Table 21.8 Embolization agents

Nature	Agent
Temporary	Gelatin sponge, thrombin, etc.
Permanent	Polyvinyl alcohol, ethanol, cyanomethacrylate, coils, balloons
Chemoembolization	Cytotoxic drug + lipiodol, etc.

where the blockage of the vasculature is required only temporarily, with subsequent restoration of blood flow to the area. Permanent blockage of blood supply is intended to produce lasting devascularization. The type of agent used will depend on the size of vessels targeted. Ethanol injection is used for capillary embolization. For arteriolar obstruction, e.g. treatment of arteriovenous malformations, polyvinyl alcohol particles of an appropriate size are used. If larger vessel occlusion is required cyanomethacrylate, coils or balloons are employed. In chemoembolizaton a combination of a cytotoxic drug with a temporary or permanent embolization agent is used.

Embolization is a technically demanding and potentially dangerous procedure. It should only be undertaken by interventional radiologists with experience in the agents used and under appropriate imaging facilities of a vascular suite with appropriately trained staff.

Line placement

Increasingly, the benefits of image-guided placement of central vein catheters has been shown to be preferable to standard surgical placement. The placement of central line catheters for renal dialysis, chemotherapy, nutritional support, etc., is performed most commonly in the axillary, subclavian and internal jugular veins. Ultrasound or fluoroscopic guidance and standard Seldinger techniques are used for radiological placement. Image guidance is used both for the initial puncture and for successful placement of the catheter within the superior vena cava, allowing appropriate length and position of catheter to reduce long-term complications. In problem cases of long-term central access, alternative routes, e.g. azygos vein, inferior vena cava or hepatic vein, may be employed.

In situ ablation

The development of ablation devices into smaller delivery systems has opened the potential for percutaneous image-guided ablation of tumours in solid organs, particularly the liver. The image-guided system used may be ultrasound, CT or potentially MRI. The ablation modality deployed can be cryotherapy or extreme heating by radiofrequency current, microwave, laser fibres and high-intensity focused ultrasound. The last method requires only accurate imaging of the lesion and targeting of the focused ultrasound beam for ablation of the lesion; it is thus a tractless ablation technique.

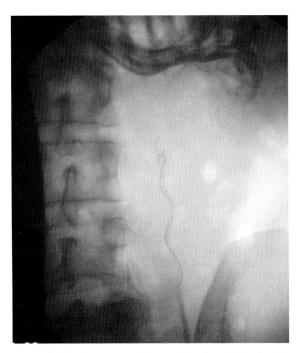

Figure 21.33 Transjugular left gonadal vein embolization for varicocele.

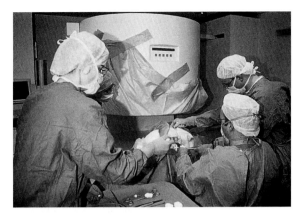

Figure 21.34 Open (operating) magnetic resonance imaging system (Siemens Magnetom Open System) used for image-guided microtherapy.

Section 21.6 • Image-guided microtherapy

This approach is still in its infancy, with the necessary facilities being available in only a few centres, but it represents the greatest growth area of MAT. Image-guided microtherapy (minimally invasive microtherapy, image-guided tomographic microtherapy) combines real-time tomographic imaging, interventional radiology, frameless stereotactic navigation and endoscopic surface viewing. The essence of this new approach is the combination of surface viewing of the operative field or target organ with real-time tomographic imaging of the operative tissue volume, e.g. the liver during *in situ* ablation of a tumour by cryosurgery or thermal ablation, when the destruction of the lesion is witnessed as it is being inflicted. The benefit of this dual-imaging approach is the increased precision of the therapeutic effect, especially when frameless stereotaxis is used. As a result, the instruments, probes and endoscopes are scaled down to 1.0 mm or less. Because of the small instruments, the majority of these interventions are performed under local anaesthesia and sedation, largely as outpatient cases.

The real-time imaging techniques used are CT–fluoroscopy hybrid systems and open MRI magnets (for parenchymal imaging), together with microendoscopes for surface viewing. Thus, the operator has two images: the endoscopic colour surface view and tomograms of the tissues and organs. With open magnet systems (Figure 21.34), the patient is housed in the imaging machine during the intervention. In this instance, because of the strong magnetic field, all of the instru-ments, monitors, endoscopes and devices must be made of non-ferromagnetic materials. With the spiral CT–fluoroscopy hybrid systems, the patient is placed on a moving operating table, which shuttles between fluoroscopy and advanced real-time spiral CT scanning (as needed) during the procedure.

The established usage of image-guided microtherapy comprises:

- biopsy including subclinical lesions of the breast detected by screening
- *in situ* tumour ablation of solid organs, especially the liver, and bone
- various sympathectomies
- spinal periradicular and disc surgery.

Image-guided microtherapy is likely to play a significant role in cancer treatment, especially with the increasing use of *in situ* ablation techniques and the introduction of gene therapy based on various forms of p53, since it should enable precise targeting. These two treatment modalities are likely to be complementary, with *in situ* ablation being used to debulk the lesion and gene therapy to eradicate residual disease.

Guide to further reading

Cuschieri, A. (1995). Wither minimal access surgery: tribulations and expectations. *Am J Surg* **169**: 9–19.

Hashimoto, D., Nayeem, A. S., Kajiwara, S. *et al.* (1993). Laparoscopic cholecystectomy: an approach without pneumoperitoneum. *Surg Endosc* **7**: 54–56.

Joris, J. L., Noirot, D. P., Legrand, M. J., Jacquet, N. J. and Lamy, M. L. (1996). Haemodynamic changes during laparoscopic cholecystectomy. *Anaesth Analg* **76**: 1067–1071.

Koivusalo, A.-M., Kellokumpu, I. and Lindgren, L. (1996). Gasless laparoscopic cholecystectomy: comparison of postoperative recovery with conventional technique. *Br J Anaesth* **77**: 576–580.

Koivasulo, A.-M., Kellokumpu, I., Scheinin, M. *et al.* (1996). Randomized comparison of the neuroendocrine response to laparoscopic cholecystectomy using either conventional or abdominal wall lift techniques. *Br J Surg* **83**: 1532–1536.

Seibel, R. M. M. (1997). Image-guided minimally invasive therapy. *Surg Endosc* **11**: 154–162.

Soehendra, N., Binmoeller, K. F., Seifert, H. and Schreiber, H. W. (1998). *Therapeutic Endoscopy: Color Atlas of Operative Techniques for the Gastrointestinal Tract*, Thieme, Stuttgart.

Struthers, A. D. and Cuschieri, A. (1998). Cardiovascular consequences of laparoscopic surgery. *Lancet* **352**: 568–570.

Van Laetham, J.-L., Cremer, M., Peny, M. O., Delhaye, M. and Deviere, J. (1998). Eradication of Barrett's mucosa with argon plasma coagulation and acid suppression: immediate and mid-term results. *Gut* **43**: 747–751.

Quality of life and rehabilitation in the surgical patient

1 • Quality-of-life measurements in surgery

2 • Influence of surgery on quality of life

3 • Rehabilitation

'Here, at whatever hour you come, you will find light and help and human kindness' – Albert Schweitzer (1875–1965), inscribed on the lamp outside his jungle hospital at Lambaréné

Section 22.1 • Quality-of-life measurements in surgery

The concept of quality of life

The effects of disease and its treatment on patients have traditionally been assessed by studying clinical outcome, e.g. disease-specific or corrected survival, disease-free survival, recurrence-free survival and length of hospital stay. These end-points, as well as socio-economic factors such as time spent off work and treatment costs, are incorporated into clinical trials in order to determine the 'best' form of treatment of the disease being studied. However, the disease and its treatment may have an impact not only on survival (quantity of life), but also on the well-being of the individual. The concept of 'quality of life' was thus introduced in order to measure the effect of illness, disease and its treatment on the patient's welfare by going beyond the physician-dominated indicators of the patient's progress.

Unfortunately, there is no universal agreement or conceptual definition of quality of life. Various definitions have been proposed, depending on the context and type of study in which the term is being used (Table 22.1). In the medical context, the term 'health-related quality of life' (also known as subjective health status) is increasingly being used to specify the impact of health and disease on quality of life.

Despite the differences in definition, there has been agreement amongst researchers that quality of life displays of three fundamental characteristics:

- multidimensional
- subjective
- dynamic.

Multidimensional

The quality-of-life construct is made up of a number of domains or dimensions that are intimately related. The three main domains, which are commonly referred to in the literature, are:

- **physical**: refers to the patient's perceived ability to carry out daily activities and tasks which require energy expenditure

Table 22.1 Quality-of-life definitions

Cella and Cherin	'Patient's appraisal of and satisfaction with their current level of functioning as compared to what they perceive to be possible or ideal'
Schumacher et al.	'Individual's overall satisfaction with life and their general sense of personal well-being'
Schipper	'a pragmatic, day to day, functional representation of a patient's physical, psychological, and social response to a disease and its treatment'
Calman	'the extent to which hopes and ambitions are matched by experience'
World Health Organization Quality of Life Group	'an individual's perception of their position in life in the context of the culture and value systems in which they live and in relation to their goals, expectations, standards and concerns. It is a broad ranging concept affected in a complex way by the person's physical health, psychological state, level of independence, social relationships and their relationships to salient features of the environment'
Grant et al.	'a personal statement of the positivity or negativity of attributes that characterises one's life'
Ferrans and Powers	'an individual's perceptions of well-being that stem from satisfaction or dissatisfaction with dimensions of life that are important to the individual'

■ **social**: refers to the patient's relationship with and the ability to integrate with members of the family, neighbourhood, place of work and other communities

■ **psychological**: refers to aspects such as depression, anxiety, fear, anger, happiness and peacefulness.

Other areas are also used in quality-of-life studies, e.g. spirituality, culture and freedom.

Subjective

Quality of life is dependent on the patient's perceptions, beliefs, feelings and expectations and it follows that quality-of-life data should be derived from the patient's own appraisal of his or her health and well-being. Information obtained from assessing the level of patients' behaviour or level of functioning, e.g. 'I can walk a hundred metres' or 'I am sleeping for three hours', should be distinguished from assessments of subjective well-being, e.g. 'My mobility is moderately impaired' or 'My sleep is greatly disturbed'. It is recommended that quality of life is assessed by the patient as far as possible, rather than by external observers or proxies. Studies have shown a lack of agreement between quality-of-life information reported by the patient and by relatives or health-care professionals.

Dynamic

Quality of life is dynamic since it varies over time, and depends on changes within the patient and in his or her surroundings. Thus, an initial assessment should be made before treatment commences (baseline assessment) and further assessments made at regular time intervals thereafter. In this way, the clinician is able to monitor changes in a patient's quality of life brought about by disease progression or regression, and by the short-term and long-term effects of treatment.

The uses of quality-of-life assessments

There are several potential uses of quality-of-life assessments in surgical practice. One is to monitor the health and quality of life of individual patients, but this is rarely done at present as part of routine clinical practice. In contrast, quality-of-life assessments are being increasingly used in a research context when comparing various treatment options. These assessments may be incorporated into cross-sectional or case-controlled studies, or in prospective randomized controlled clinical trials (phase III studies). Examples of the former include comparisons of quality of life between restorative rectal resection and permanent stoma formation for rectal cancer, and comparison of mastectomy and lumpectomy for breast cancer. In phase III trials, quality of life may be either a primary or a secondary end-point. Quality of life is considered to be the main study end-point when the effects of the treatments being studied on survival are similar, e.g. chemotherapy regimens employed in the palliation of advanced cancer. More commonly, quality of life is used as a secondary end-point, especially if the effects of the treatments on

survival and/or tumour recurrence are unknown. Quality-of-life assessments are also used by economists and health-care providers to determine the cost-effectiveness of various forms of treatment and, for this purpose, the quality-adjusted life year (QALY) represents 1 year of healthy life expectancy.

Measurement of quality of life

Detailed information on quality of life can be obtained by means of an open-ended interview, but unless this information can be quantified in some way, its value for research purposes is limited. Quality-of-life data are thus collected using structured questionnaires consisting of a number of items (questions or statements), which tap various dimensions of quality of life. The answers to these items are then given a score.

The questionnaire may be administered in various ways, e.g. by an interviewer, with the advantage that any errors of misunderstanding are kept to a minimum and the number of missing answers is kept low. However, most questionnaires are now constructed in simple and straightforward language and may be completed in less than 10 min. These questionnaires may be self-administered; the patient completes the questionnaire in hospital or at home with the least external interference. This approach is usually recommended as being less open to bias introduced by the interviewer.

In some cases, the patient is too ill to complete a questionnaire. In an attempt not to lose any quality-of-life data, some researchers have employed a proxy or surrogate respondent to answer the questionnaire instead of the patient. This approach also ensures that there is no stress on the patient. However, studies have shown that although proxy respondents who are very close to the patient, for example, carers and spouses, agree closely with the patient on answers to questions on physical function, agreement on other items is poor.

Classification of quality-of-life instruments

Quality-of-life instruments may be generic or specific.

Generic

These are based on a broad and global concept of quality of life, and are designed to assess many dimensions of health-related quality of life. There are two types of generic questionnaires: health profiles and health indices.

■ **Health profiles** contain a number of items (questions) that are related to various aspects of quality of life. The questions usually tap a wide range of domains and a separate score is given for each domain. A well-known generic quality-of-life questionnaire is the SF-36. This consists of 36 items, measuring eight dimensions of health on multi-item scales, plus a further dimension on a single-item scale, which measures any change in health occurring over the previous year. The eight dimensions measure physical functioning, social functioning, role limitations because of physical and emotional problems, mental health energy and vitality, and also pain and general health perception. The scoring scale ranges from 0 to 100, with lower scores indicating worse health. An improved version, the SF-36 version 2.0, is in widespread use, and is currently the generic questionnaire of choice.

The main advantage of health profiles is not only that they allow comparison of various domains of quality of life for the condition being studied, but also that a comparison can be made across population and disease states. However, these instruments may lack responsiveness (sensitivity), and changes brought about by treatment of a particular condition may not always be identified.

■ **Health indices**: in this instance, the questions are designed so that the scores generated from all of the answers are added up to give a single number or index. There is a range of possible scores from a minimum of 0, representing death, to a maximum of 1.0. The maximum value represents quality of life achieved with perfect health. This approach is preferred by health economists who use health indices to carry out cost–benefit analysis, and health indices may be used to derive QALYs. A QALY is 1 year spent in good health; the quality of the year is low if health is poor. QALYs are derived by multiplying life expectancy with an index of health or disease, e.g. Rosser Index. They do not measure quality of life as such, but rather give a value to the outcome of treatment in terms of years spent in an improved health state. QALYs may be combined with treatment costs, and cost that is incurred by a particular form of treatment is calculated per QALY gained. QALYs have been criticised on the grounds that they are often based on unvalidated and unreliable data.

Specific
These questionnaires, although similar in format to the health profiles, are designed for use for a particular condition only. There are various types:

■ **domain-specific** questionnaires focus in detail on one dimension only, e.g. 'Hospital Anxiety and Depression Scales' to assess the psychological domain
■ **disease-specific** instruments measure quality of life in patients who suffer from a particular disease, such as cancer, e.g. the EORTC QLQ-C30, which consists of questions on the domains of quality of life that may be affected in cancer patients. More specific modules have also been developed to focus on one cancer, e.g. the colorectal cancer module (EORTC QLQ-CR38) containing questions that are of relevance only to patients who are suffering from or being treated for this cancer
■ **population-specific** instruments, for use in subgroups of people such as the elderly and children, are designed to assess the relevant aspects of quality of life in the population being studied

■ **symptom-specific** questionnaires, e.g. the McGill pain questionnaire, deal in detail with only one symptom.

The advantage of these questionnaires is that emphasis is made on a specific area of quality of life, rather than assessing quality of life globally. Such instruments are more responsive to changes brought about by the disease being studied and its treatment. Another advantage is that these questionnaires are clearly related to the condition or population being treated by the clinician.

Testing the psychometric properties of an instrument

Psychometry (Greek: *psyche* = mind, *metron* = measure) is the science of measuring mental functions. This science is applied to the construction and development of quality-of-life instruments. The psychometric properties of a good quality-of-life tool are validity, reliability and responsiveness.

Validity
This examines whether a questionnaire is measuring what it intends to measure rather than something else. There is a number of approaches to the process of validation.

Face validation determines whether the questionnaire measures the intended dimension and also that the items are worded clearly and in a style that is easily understood. **Content validity** is the degree to which the questions tap the main aspects of the dimension being measured. **Criterion validity** is the extent to which a questionnaire correlates with a gold standard. In quality-of-life research, no true gold-standard instrument exists, so the best instrument available is used instead. The new instrument and the well-established one are administered to patients concurrently, and the two are correlated (**concurrent validity**). The predictive power of each instrument may also be compared (**predictive validity**). The items that measure levels of physical functioning, (**functional or performance status**) are sometimes validated against objective scales of performance.

Construct validity is an approach whereby a questionnaire is tested against a hypothesis. Thus, validation is strengthened or weakened when the hypothesis being tested is confirmed or refuted. **Convergent validity** is the degree to which instruments measuring the same dimension correlate with one another. **Discriminant validity** is the lack of correlation between instruments that are measuring unrelated dimensions.

Reliability
A questionnaire is reliable if it produces consistent and similar results from the same individual person after repeated administration, with no evidence of change occurring in that person. **Test–retest reliability** is administered to the same population sample on two or more different occasions and the answers are then

correlated. Test–retest reliability may be affected by the conditions of administration, changes in the health status of the population being assessed, and the period between one test and another. **Internal consistency reliability** is assessed by determining the extent to which a number of items measuring a particular dimension is actually doing so. **Inter-rater reliability** refers to a comparison of the results generated when the questionnaire is administered to the same population by different interviewers.

Responsiveness
The questionnaire should be able to detect any changes in quality of life resulting from disease or treatment. Responsiveness can only be assessed in a longitudinal study.

Conducting a quality-of-life study
A quality-of-life study may be either longitudinal (this includes clinical trials), in which quality-of-life changes are assessed before and after an intervention, or cross-sectional, where quality of life is assessed at one point in time. The choice of questionnaire depends on the type of study being conducted. In a cross-sectional study, useful information is obtained from a generic questionnaire, while in a longitudinal study a disease-specific questionnaire is more responsive to change. In practice, however, both types of questionnaire may be used.

In general, quality of life in cancer trials is assessed by a modular approach, using a generic and a cancer-specific questionnaire (core questionnaire) as well as a questionnaire specific to the cancer being studied. The psychometric properties of the questionnaire must be well proven, but if an untested instrument is used, it should be administered concurrently with the well-established one. The instruments used must be sufficiently detailed in order to carry out an adequate measurement of the specified dimensions. However, a lengthy instrument may induce fatigue in the responders and may lead to poor compliance.

The method of administration (self, interview, proxy) has an important bearing on the results obtained. The frequency of administration depends on the type of study and the treatment being assessed; in a longitudinal study, a baseline assessment is conducted before the commencement of treatment, and in randomized studies this is done on randomization. A further assessment is carried out during treatment and follow-up assessments are carried out at regular intervals thereafter. Follow-ups are evenly spaced, usually every 2–3 months. More frequent assessments may not be acceptable to patients.

The recall period of the questionnaire is determined by the type of study being carried out. In a cross-sectional study, the recall periods may be between 2 and 4 weeks. Longer recall periods are not recommended. In a longitudinal study, the recall period is usually shorter, preferably 1 week or less, since frequent assessments are being made.

Section 22.2 • Influence of surgery on quality of life

Cancer
Cancer is a leading cause of death in Western countries, second only to cardiovascular disease, and its treatment is associated with a significant degree of morbidity. It is therefore understandable that quality-of-life assessments had their origin in this area. The Karnofsky Performance Status Index was introduced in 1948 in an attempt to measure the functional status of patients with advanced cancer. The scale ranges from 0 (death) to 100 (no complaints). It is still being used nowadays despite its limitations. Although it is simple to score, it is physician administered, possibly resulting in external bias and interobserver variation, and evidence of its reliability is poor. The World Health Organization (WHO) produced the WHO Functional Scale, which is similar to the Karnofsky but simpler to use, although there has been no confirmation of its reliability and validity.

Further advances in the field of quality of life led to the development of cancer-specific instruments. One of these, the QLQ-C30 has been developed by the European Organization for the Research and Treatment of Cancer (EORTC). It is used both in clinical trials and other prospective and retrospective studies. It is a multidimensional questionnaire consisting of nine scales: five are functional scales (physical, role, cognitive, emotional and social), three are symptom scales (fatigue, pain and nausea, and vomiting) and one is a global health status and quality-of-life scale. There are also six single-item measures (dyspnoea, insomnia, appetite loss, constipation, diarrhoea and financial difficulties).

The QLQ-C30 is the core questionnaire, as it is suitable for all cancer patients, but there are also supplementary questionnaires (modules) specific to the cancer being studied. The combination of the core questionnaire and the module yields detailed information on many quality-of-life dimensions that are affected by cancer and its treatment. Examples of these modules are QLQ-BR23 (breast cancer), QLQ-LC13 (lung cancer) and QLQ-CR38 (colorectal cancer).

Another quality-of-life questionnaire developed for cancer clinical trials is the Rotterdam Symptom Checklist. It consists of 30 questions on various aspects of the physical and psychological dimensions of quality of life. It is used less nowadays owing to the greater acceptability of the QLQ-C30. Other quality-of-life instruments are used in oncology studies. Most of them are study specific, with little evidence available on their validity and reliability. A list of quality-of-life instruments is given in Table 22.2.

Oesophageal cancer
Quality-of-life studies on oesophageal cancer have dealt with both curative and palliative treatment of this dis-

Table 22.2 Quality-of-life instruments in oncology

- Activities of Daily Living (ADL)
- Breast Cancer Chemotherapy Questionnaire (BCCQ)
- Bowel Symptom Questionnaire (BSQ)
- Cancer Rehabilitation Evaluation System (CARES)
- Comfort Index
- Daily Diary Card
- Disease Activity Index (DAI)
- Eastern Cooperative Oncology Group Scale (ECOG)
- European Organization for Research and Treatment of Cancer Quality of Life Core Questionnaire (EORTC QLQ-C30)
- European Organization for Research and Treatment of Cancer Quality of Life Questionnaire Modules: Lung Cancer (QLQ-LC13), Colorectal Cancer (QLQ-CR38), Breast Cancer (QLQ-BR23), Head and Neck Cancer (QLQ-H&N35), Oesophageal Cancer (QLQ-OES24), Pancreatic Cancer (QLQ-PAN26)
- Fatigue Symptom Inventory (FSI)
- Ferrans and Powers Quality of Life Questionnaire – Cancer version
- Functional Assessment of Cancer Therapy (FACT)
- Functional Living Index for Cancer (FLIC)
- General Health Questionnaire (GHQ)
- Gastrointestinal Quality of Life Index (GIQLI)
- General Satisfaction Questionnaire (GSQ)
- Hospital Anxiety and Depression Scale (HAD)
- International Breast Cancer Study Group – Quality of Life Questionnaire (IBCSG-QL)
- Karnofsky Performance Status (KPS)
- Linear Analogue Self-Assessment Scale (LASA)
- Lung Cancer Symptom Scale (LCSS)
- Medical Outcomes Study – Short Form 36 (SF-36) and Short Form 12 (SF-12)
- Nottingham Health Profile (NHP)
- Ostomy Adjustment Scale (OAS)
- Patient Generated Index (PGI)
- Psychological General Well-Being Index (PGWB)
- Quality of Life Index – Cancer (QLI-C)
- Quality of Life Index for Colostomy Patients (QLI-CP)
- Quality of Life Index (Padilla)
- Quality of Life Index (Spitzer)
- Quality of Life Index – Radiotherapy (QLI-RT)
- Quality Adjusted Time Without Symptoms or Toxicity (Q-TWiST)
- Rotterdam Symptom Checklist (RSC)
- Sickness Impact Profile (SIP)
- State–Trait Anxiety Inventory (STAI)
- Summary Satisfaction Index (SSI)
- WHO Functional Scale

ease. Studies have shown that palliation of malignant dysphagia improves quality of life, and treatments that show an improvement in quality of life in the short term include laser photoablation and endoscopic intubation. However, quality of life worsens as a patient's general condition deteriorates during the terminal phase of the illness. Total oesophagectomy also improves quality of life; although the performance status in cured patients is similar to that in those operated on for palliation, pain status and global quality of life is better in the curative group. In the long term, survivors of oesophageal carcinoma enjoy satisfactory quality of life.

Gastric cancer

Most studies have compared the types of gastric surgery for cancer. Symptomatic outcome is much better after partial gastrectomy than after total gastrectomy, and those patients who had a pouch reconstruction following total gastrectomy score better on quality-of-life questionnaires than those without a pouch.

Pancreatic cancer

A Comfort Index, or the ratio of good palliation to duration of survival, has been devised for pancreatic cancer. The Comfort Index in patients who have limited regional or systemic metastases and who undergo a stomach-preserving gastric bypass exceeds 50%, while in those whose cancer is not bypassed the Comfort Index is less then 40%. In patients with extensive systemic metastases, the Comfort Index is less than 30%, irrespective of treatment. For patients suffering from localized cancer of the pancreatic head, a pylorus-preserving pancreaticoduodenectomy offers a better resumption of social activity than a Whipple's operation, although the survival rates after both operations are similar.

Colorectal cancer

Physical problems after rectal cancer surgery are mainly sexual, urological or defecatory. Male sexual problems are erectile and ejaculatory dysfunction, as well as loss of desire and anorgasmia. Sexual problems in females have not been as extensively researched. The problems described are fewer, and include cessation of intercourse, anorgasmia and dyspareunia. There is a higher prevalence of sexual problems in patients treated by a low anterior resection and abdominoperineal resection than those who have a high anterior resection. Abdominoperineal resection is associated with more urological problems than anterior resection, but the results in some studies are not statistically significant. Operative techniques such as total mesorectal excision with autonomic nerve preservation, in which the pelvic nerves are carefully identified during surgery, may result in less sexual and urinary dysfunction.

A number of studies has been carried out assessing defecatory function following surgery for rectal cancer. The common symptoms assessed are frequency of bowel motion, urgency and faecal leakage or incontinence. Other studies also report on the prevalence of diarrhoea, constipation and flatus.

Many relevant issues emerge from these studies. Bowel function, which may be erratic preoperatively owing to the tumour, may not improve postoperatively. Social problems have also been described after rectal cancer surgery. Patients may be embarrassed about the presence of a colostomy or because of foul odours produced from the stoma, resulting in decreased social activities with family and friends. Similar problems beset those who are incontinent of flatus and/or faeces following a restorative rectal resection. Psychological problems also occur, mainly in colostomy patients. Some authors report a high incidence of depression and low self-esteem in these patients when compared with patients who have undergone restorative surgery. To date, however, formal quality-of-life studies in colorectal cancer surgery are few.

Lung cancer

Lung cancer patients have a higher prevalence of dyspnoea but similar overall quality of life compared with those with benign lung disease. Following surgery, quality of life in cancer patients decreases, but then improves and reaches preoperative levels by 6–9 months.

Breast cancer

Quality of life has been assessed in patients with early breast cancer participating in a randomized trial comparing mastectomy to tumorectomy and radiotherapy. There is a more severe impairment of body image in the mastectomy group than in the breast-conserving group but there is an improvement in overall quality of life in both groups with the passage of time.

Comparative studies between operated breast cancer patients with those suffering from benign disease have shown that patients with breast cancer have poorer levels of physical functioning but greater positive psychosocial adaptation, such as improved life outlook, enhanced interpersonal relationships, and deeper spiritual and religious satisfaction. Comparison of healthy 8-year survivors of breast cancer with normal controls reveals no differences in quality-of-life scores apart from impaired sexuality. However, patients who develop tumour recurrence or a new primary breast cancer experience worse quality of life in all domains except for social functioning.

Benign disease

Chronic pancreatitis

Pain is a major symptom in chronic pancreatitis, and surgery should be considered when conservative measures fail to relieve pain, and when pain interferes with the patient's quality of life. After duodenum-preserving resection of the head of pancreas, pain scores decrease by 95% and quality of life is significantly improved.

Gastro-oesophageal reflux disease

Medical treatment is the initial treatment of choice for gastro-oesophageal reflux disease. In a multicentre European clinical trial comparing ranitidine with omeprazole, patients who were treated with either drug had an improvement in symptoms and quality of life, although the improvement was better in the omeprazole-treated group. Surgery is reserved for those who relapse with medical treatment, and after laparoscopic fundoplication, patients have good quality-of-life scores on a specific questionnaire, better than untreated patients and as good as or better than those on optimal medical treatment.

Inflammatory bowel disease

Patients suffering from Crohn's disease have been shown to have a poorer quality of life than those with ulcerative colitis. Patients whose disease is in the quiescent phase have better quality-of-life scores than those with active disease and, in general, quality of life in patients suffering from either ulcerative colitis or Crohn's disease and awaiting surgery is poor. Surgery usually improves quality of life, and there is a perception that restorative proctocolectomy with ileoanal pouch for ulcerative colitis is preferable to panproctocolectomy with ileostomy. This has not been documented by formal quality-of-life studies, however.

Abdominal aortic aneurysm

Repair of an abdominal aortic aneurysm carries significant morbidity and mortality, but few studies have assessed quality of life following this procedure. It has been reported that a good quality of life is achieved in octogenarians who survived either elective or emergency abdominal aortic aneurysm repair.

Conclusions

Quality-of-life studies highlight various important issues in surgical practice. There are, however, methodological deficiencies that need to be rectified so that better quality data are obtained from future studies. Currently, the best way to assess quality of life is in the context of a randomized controlled clinical trial, although case-controlled and cross-sectional studies have their merits. The dynamic nature of a person's quality of life in cancer can only be assessed in a prospective study, where measurements are made at various times before, during and after treatment. The correct choice of questionnaire is very important. It should be psychometrically sound, with firm evidence of validity, reliability and responsiveness. The instrument should be self-administered. The type of study determines whether a generic or a condition-specific questionnaire, or both, is used. Further refinement of existing questionnaires (Tables 22.2 and 22.3), rather than developing new ones, may help in improving the quality of research.

Section 22.3 • Rehabilitation

Rehabilitation is an important aspect of surgical treatment and applies to all surgical specialties, but is particularly relevant to trauma and orthopaedic surgery. It necessitates the co-ordinated activity of the rehabilitation team that operates within the hospital (medical and nursing team, physiotherapists, occupational therapists, dieticians, psychologists, stoma therapists, etc.) and the community (social workers, district nurses and general practitioners). **The objective is the achievement of the optimum mental and physical state necessary to overcome a disability incurred by trauma or ablative surgery for disease, thereby enabling independence and active involvement in family life and society, and return to gainful employment.**

Rehabilitation in musculoskeletal disorders

Rehabilitation may be viewed from a point of view of the musculoskeletal system in terms of the recovery

Table 22.3 Quality-of-life instruments in surgery (excluding oncology)

- Activities of Daily Living (ADL)
- Aberdeen Dyspepsia Questionnaire (ADQ)
- Bowel Symptom Questionnaire (BSQ)
- Crohn's Disease Activity Index (CDAI)
- Constipation Score (CS)
- Daily Diary Card
- Disease Activity Index (DAI)
- Dyspepsia Questionnaire (DQ)
- General Health Questionnaire (GHQ)
- Gastrointestinal Quality of Life Index (GIQLI)
- General Satisfaction Questionnaire (GSQ)
- Hospital Anxiety and Depression Scale (HAD)
- Inflammatory Bowel Disease Questionnaire (IBDQ)
- Karnofsky Performance Status (KPS)
- Medical Outcomes Study – Short Form 36 (SF-36) and Short Form 12 (SF-12)
- Nottingham Health Profile (NHP)
- Ostomy Adjustment Scale (OAS)
- Patient Generated Index (PGI)
- Psychological General Well-Being Index (PGWB)
- Psychological Adjustment to Illness Scale (PAIS)
- Quality of Life in Duodenal Ulcer Patients (QLDUP)
- Quality of Life Index for Colostomy Patients (QLI-CP)
- Quality of Life Index (Padilla)
- Quality of Life Index (Spitzer)
- Sickness Impact Profile (SIP)
- State–Trait Anxiety Inventory (STAI)
- Rosser Index
- WHO Functional Scale

from unplanned trauma caused by chance accident and recovery from surgical trauma that may include amputation following vascular disease. In both cases the needs of the whole patient and his or her family must be catered for and must, if possible, span the whole of the subject's lifestyle, including pastimes as well as work.

Rehabilitation following generalized trauma

Following simple injuries patients may be taught simple exercises that they can carry out at home, supervised at outpatient follow-up. While in hospital an attitude of progress towards recovery must be engendered from the first day as otherwise a state of regression to a dependent state rapidly becomes established. The role of physical rehabilitation after simple injuries is often taken for granted, although in times of scant resources it would be better if its use were confined to those accurately assessed as gaining useful benefit. For example, therapy following even quite minor hand injury may be essential to ensure early return to work, although commonly provided mass rehabilitation classes such as back or knee groups have not been proved to be a valuable use of resources.

After multiple injuries affecting many limb segments, often associated with head injuries, the role of rehabilitation needs to be carefully considered as early as possible once medical and surgical management permits. In these cases, which are less common, disproportionately large resources may be required to ensure that recovery is optimal in the multiply injured. Here, the professionals allied to medicine, including physiotherapists, occupational therapists and others should be asked to make an early assessment. For example, following a head injury, which may have involved many months in bed, besides the related motor recovery, aid may be required in speech, and the effects of psychological disturbance are often underrated unless fully assessed by careful psychological examination.

The role of the surgeon is to act as a first among equals in assembling a team, or ideally the surgeon may seek the co-operation of a specialist in rehabilitation. Following assessments the team must collate a plan of action culminating not in discharge from hospital but in restoration to as normal a preinjury lifestyle as is practical. However, rehabilitation should not be overambitious and limitations set by disability must be appreciated. The setting of unrealistic and overoptimistic goals is as counterproductive as setting no goals at all.

Rehabilitation after amputation

The amputee, whether as a result of trauma or vascular diseases, has very specific problems to cope with in the aftermath of surgery. The rehabilitation of this specific group of patients is, however, an ideal model for discussion since the care highlights all aspects of rehabilitation. The trauma of the surgery has a profound psychological effect on the individual concerned. For the traumatic amputee there has been no warning or preparation. The majority of these patients are young and following the accident there may be considerable anguish, disbelief and despair at the amputation and the perceived problems that may follow. The initial postoperative period requires considerable care and understanding and should be handled by experienced staff. Full explanation must include realistic consideration of likely outcome and description of the rehabilitation process that is to follow.

The elderly, for example the vascular amputee, however, have usually had a period of pain and suffering prior to the surgery. The patient will have often chosen amputation as a means of relieving the severe pain of a gangrenous limb. Counselling preoperative patients is extremely valuable and should, wherever possible, be undertaken by experienced staff. In addition, relatives need to be included in these discussions as their understanding and reassurance can help the patient to overcome the natural fear of the future.

The rehabilitation of the amputee and consequent independence is influenced by several factors. In the first instance, the level of lower limb amputation can profoundly affect the ability of the patient to walk with a prosthesis and gain the fullest mobility possible. The bigger the amputation the greater the psychological effect on the patient, and secondly the greater the effort required to walk. The expertise of the rehabilitation team and the facilities at their disposal can similarly affect the ultimate success of the rehabilitation process. The levels of amputation are shown in Figure 22.1.

The hindquarter and hip disarticulation are unusual levels (1% of all amputations) and usually undertaken for neoplasm in the femur or at or near the knee; walking is difficult with the prosthesis, which requires hip joints, knee joints and an ankle prosthetic replacement.

The above-knee amputation (45% of English lower limb amputees, although in some centres as low as 20%) is the second most common level and the patient who has amputation at this level will benefit from a long stump; walking requires about 75% more energy than that of a normal person. In an elderly person walking with a locked-knee prosthesis is safer, although this incurs more energy expenditure than that of a young amputee with a free or stabilized knee. However, the stability provided by the lock is often essential in the elderly person in whom balance and strength are often reduced. The GrittiStokes amputation is advocated by some surgeons but has no end bearing, tends to have difficult prosthesis suspension and does not normally allow the use of a modern prosthetic knee. Its use is very limited and is not considered as an amputation of choice.

The below-knee amputation is the amputation of choice, especially in the elderly (45% of English prim-

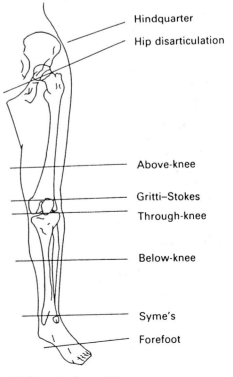

Figure 22.1 Levels of amputation.

ary amputees, in some centres up to 80%). The preservation of the knee joint allows easier walking (25% more energy than normal walking), good proprioception, a lighter, more cosmetic prosthesis and significantly less psychological trauma than higher amputations. The Symes amputation (12% of amputations) is a transmalleolar amputation, with the heel pad forming the distal end. This allows the amputee to bear weight on the end. The level is possible in diabetic patients with reasonable patent blood vessels but not usually possible in atherosclerotic patients. Walking is usually successful (15–20% more energy than not walking) but the cosmetics of the prosthesis is poor, owing to the inevitable bulbous distal end, and as a consequence it is not so popular for female patients.

Phantom pain
The patients nearly all have a phantom sensation, or the feeling of the presence of a limb that has been removed. This can be a frightening and bewildering experience and counselling is needed, ideally preoperatively as well as postoperatively, to allay the fear of the unexpected feeling. It can appear soon after surgery and may last a lifetime. The sensation can take many forms, from a tingling to a feeling of hotness. The phantom limb can also truncate up, so that the foot may feel as if it is sited at the knee joint area. The phantom can also manifest as pain in the absent limb. The pain is often quite distant and may be in a joint that caused problems years before (e.g. bunion). The incidence of pain is in the order of 30–40% of the amputee population and is more common in the young traumatic amputee.

Phantom sensation requires no medical intervention apart from reassurance. Phantom pain is, however, very problematical to control. There is some evidence that the pain settles in some patients but in many it recurs in some cases years after the amputation. Normally, however, it is not present continuously and only occurs from time to time. Some specific activities may induce the pain, for example a weather change or micturition. The 41 different treatments described in one study suggest that it is difficult to treat with any one specific treatment available. The mainstay of therapy remains analgesics, transcutaneous nerve stimulation (TNS), antidepressants and counselling.

The rehabilitation team
The rehabilitation team (Figure 22.2) that cares for the amputee of whatever age must be a closely integrated group of professionals who work together. This ensures the amputee is given total care in a constructive, coordinated environment. The environment for care should be cheerful and encouraging. The medical team should include the operating surgeon and the rehabilitation specialist. In some areas the medical team will vary but in all there must be a specialist responsible for prosthesis prescription. The responsibility for the overall medical care rests with the medical staff and, as in any major trauma whatever the cause, the patient may require specialized rehabilitation. The nursing staff pro-

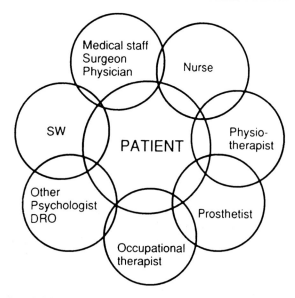

Figure 22.2 Schematic representation of the integrated nature of the rehabilitation team. SW, social worker; DRO, Disablement Resettlement Officer.

vide day-to-day care of the patient, with particular attention to pressure areas and to the care of the stump. Adequate nutrition is essential and good hygiene is important, as is effective dentition.

Physiotherapy provides assessment of early mobilization of the patient. The patient needs to be mobilized 24 h after surgery, if possible. Chest physiotherapy is used to avoid chest infections and early mobility to avoid deep venous thrombosis. The use of early walking aids has greatly enhanced the ability of the patient to mobilize. The postpneumatic ambulatory mobility (PPAM) aid (Figure 22.3) can be of help for below-knee amputations, and on some occasions for Syme's and through-knee cases; the Femurett may be used for the patient with an above-knee amputation. Once the stump is healed, mobility with a prosthesis is undertaken with the supervision of a physiotherapist and the prosthetist. The prosthetist, who is the specialist responsible for the manufacture, fitting and maintenance of the artificial leg, works closely with the therapists.

Prostheses
A wide range of prostheses is available for the amputee. For the below-knee, the standard prosthesis is the patellar tendon bearing (PTB), which has a socket to allow full weight-bearing on the stump, partly over the patellar tendon, on either side of the tibial crest and, in particular, the calf area (Figure 22.4). The prosthesis is often self-suspending, reasonably lightweight and cosmetic in appearance.

The above-knee prosthesis requires a mechanical knee. These are now endoskeletal with modular components covered in a foam faring to look cosmetically acceptable (Figure 22.5). The knee can be self-locking (locked in extension for walking, normally unlocked to sit and usually provided for the older patient), or free

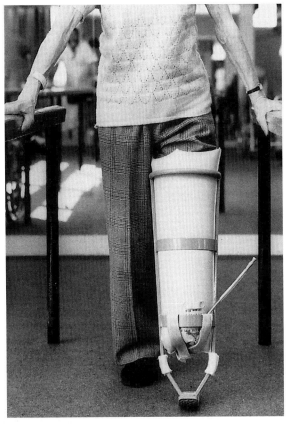

Figure 22.3 PPAM (postpneumatic ambulatory mobility) early walking aid for patients after below-knee, Syme's and through-knee amputation.

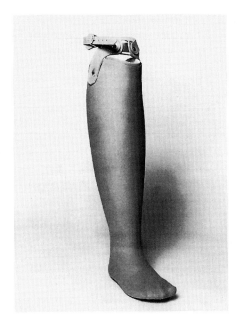

Figure 22.4 Patellar tendon-bearing (PTB) standard prosthesis for below-knee amputations.

swinging with the added options of various swing phase devices to provide smooth swing-through for the younger patient.

Since the late 1940s the use of a quadrilateral shaped socket has been popular. A recent American socket, the ischial containment socket, which is made more intimate in its fit, has been introduced. These, with the Icelandic fenestrated frame, which is much cooler and dynamic, have made the fit of prostheses more comfortable for the majority of patients. Suspension can be by way of a leather belt or an elastic belt [total elasticated support (TES) belt]. For the younger amputee a suction socket can be very successful. The latter socket is very close-fitting and the stump is in total contact; there is a valve sited at the bottom of the socket. The patient puts the stump in by way of a light bandage wrapped round the stump and then pulled out through the valve hole. A one-way valve is placed in the hole and air can leak out but not in, providing a vacuum that holds the socket on to the stump.

The choice of prosthesis naturally depends on the level of amputation but also on the projected activity of the amputee, and is usually decided by discussion with the team. Fitting of a prosthesis can begin as early as 25 days postoperatively if the stump has healed and is mature enough. However, in some circumstances a delay may be incurred in waiting for the stump to lose the postopera-

tive oedema, since too early fitting may result in a rapidly ill-fitting socket which requires early replacement. This is not ideal for the patient who is being encouraged to walk as much as possible, nor is it very cost-effective.

The occupational therapist is specially trained to teach aids to daily living skills and to assess home circumstances. The latter assessment involves domiciliary visits with patients. The advice provided ensures that services are altered to the needs of the individual once they are discharged. The training of activities of daily living (ADL) is undertaken in the hospital and concentrates on self-hygiene, personal independence and domestic skills in a kitchen.

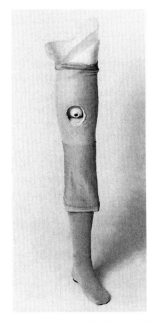

Figure 22.5 Above-knee prothesis with a mechanical knee.

Close liaison with outside groups is essential. All team members may need to discuss patient care with them; in particular, the occupational therapist and nursing staff may need to liaise with the social worker. Social workers are often attached to hospitals and wherever possible should be part of the rehabilitation team. The social worker can arrange domiciliary services, e.g. home help and meals-on-wheels, and may help with financial matters. In addition to the social worker, the general practitioner who will provide the care once discharge has occurred should be informed as to the progress and likely prognosis of the patient. District nurses are essential to ensure that nursing skills are available in a domiciliary situation.

The whole team should meet regularly to discuss the patient's progress and decide on realistic goals that the patient can achieve. The patient should be involved in the discussion so that he or she is aware of what is to be achieved. Family members also need to be kept aware of progress and of problems as they arise. Goals may need to be modified as the rehabilitation process proceeds in the light of progress.

In the case of a young amputee the return to work can be an important issue. The social worker and occupational therapist can give initial guidance and hold discussions with employers, which can be helpful. In a situation where a return to the patient's former work is not possible the patient is referred to the Disablement Resettlement Officer, who has a statutory responsibility to advise on retraining programmes and potential employers. Local charitable organizations may also offer employment advice and these services are often worth considering.

Social reintegration is important. The amputee may feel initially isolated and handicapped by his surgery. Family and friends play a vital role in encouraging the patient to get back into society. The rehabilitation team should be aware of this isolation and encourage the patient to get out. The use of clubs and societies, e.g. the British Limbless ExServicemen's Association (BLESMA) or the National Association for Limbless Disabled, can be extremely valuable. To encourage this reintegration rapid discharge to home is important, but this should be undertaken once prosthetic fitting has been completed and the occupational therapist has assessed the house. If discharged too early, demoralization of the patient and relatives can reduce the ability to achieve full potential.

The patient will need to remain in contact with a limb-fitting centre for the rest of his or her life for the maintenance and provision of prostheses. Regular reviews are initially necessary as the stump matures and the patient adapts to the new situation. The review clinics act as both a stump and prosthetic review, but also as an opportunity for open discussion on how the patient has managed at home. In this way, shortfalls in service provision and the identification of areas in which help can be provided are assessed.

Amputees can be seen to be a very specific group of patients in whom a rehabilitation team can work clearly. All patients may require varying degrees of rehabilitation, but the most important factor in achieving the optimum recovery is the close co-operation between all members of the team, with full and frank discussion of the patient's needs.

Rehabilitation in general surgical practice

After major abdominal surgery, irrespective of any physical or visceral deficit, patients experience a varying period of asthenia reflected in tiredness, diminished energy and inability to concentrate. In addition to the well-documented catabolic response to trauma, which is reversed by adequate nutrition, there are poorly understood psychological changes that often delay full recovery. These psychological changes, which are influenced by individual psychometric traits, are especially marked in patients with an external focus of control (i.e. patients who believe that they have no control over their health, this being determined by external influences). Awareness by the patient of this convalescent state and its temporary nature, together with constant encouragement, is beneficial.

Although a wide spectrum of patients require varying rehabilitation measures after general surgical treatment, in view of the limited resources, emphasis is placed on certain disease categories. The groups in need are cancer patients, patients with stomas, gastric cripples, patients with small intestinal failure (short gut syndrome) and transplant patients. The principles employed are identical to those outlined in the 'Musculoskeletal' section, and both hospital and community support is needed.

Cancer patients

These patients are especially disadvantaged. They may need major ablative surgery, which at times alters drastically their own perception of body image and may be actually disfiguring (mastectomy), or restrictive of either visceral function (total gastrectomy, colostomy), physical function (pneumonectomy) or sexual function (orchidectomy, rectal cancer surgery causing impotence). Side-effects of chemotherapy and radiotherapy may also have a negative influence on the patient's quality of life in the recovery period. In addition, patients have fears and concerns about tumour recurrence and death. This may lead to mental disorders, the most common of which is reactive depression, which may need treatment by a psychiatrist.

Perhaps more than in any other group, psychological support from the surgical and nursing team during convalescence and the early phase of rehabilitation is of paramount importance. Organizations and charities, such as CancerBACUP, Cancerlink, Macmillan Cancer Relief, Marie Curie Cancer Care and the Cancer Care Society provide, through professionals such as Macmillan and Marie Curie doctors and nurses and Linda McCartney breast cancer nurses, invaluable counselling and support to patients and their families. Not only is their service provided at hospital during the postoperative phase, but patients are also followed up in the community and given further psychological help. Cancer patients can meet and share their experiences in hospice centres, as well as benefit from further therapy.

The management of the physical sequelae of cancer treatment is part of the process of rehabilitation. Reconstructive surgery following mastectomy (use of TRAM or latissimus dorsi flaps) or the use of external breast prostheses improves the woman's perception of body image. Similarly, testicular prostheses restore a male's body image to normal following an orchidectomy for testicular or prostatic cancer. Impotence, commonly observed after an abdominoperineal resection or a low anterior resection for rectal cancer, may be treated by prostaglandin intracavernosal injections (Caverject). Incontinence of urine, also present following surgery for prostatic or rectal cancer surgery, may be improved by physiotherapy. An artificial urinary sphincter may be inserted if physiotherapy fails. Speech can be relearned after a total laryngectomy with the help of an artificial voice-box and expert speech therapy.

Stoma patients

Stoma therapy is needed for all patients with ileostomy, colostomy and urinary conduits. The success of the service provided by the stoma therapist is reflected by the infrequent problems experienced by stoma patients nowadays. In elective cases stoma therapy is started before the operation. It includes detailed explanation by the stoma therapist and the surgeon of the intended operation, the function of the stoma, the nature of the appliance, its social acceptability and details of the training period before the patient becomes fully proficient in its use. Postoperatively, the stoma therapist provides help and advice to patients, both at the hospital and in the community, and ensures that patients can manage the stoma well. Stoma care is easier nowadays, with the availability of a new generation of stoma appliances. These are designed to ensure optimal fitting and thus prevent leakages and peristomal skin excoriation. Special filters minimize foul odours.

The idea of a stoma is naturally abhorrent to most normal individuals. It is remarkable how, with adequate help from the stoma therapist and psychological support from the entire team, as well as from organizations such as the British Colostomy Association, the majority of patients cope with the situation and lead an otherwise normal social and family life.

Patients following gastric and small bowel surgery

These patients need specific therapy. This includes dietary advice and management in patients with postgastric surgery and alimentary symptoms, and nutritional treatment of patients with the small bowel syndrome. The latter entails training of the patient in the self-administration of enteral or parenteral nutri-

tion by the home hyperalimentation team. Aside from the training, which is initiated in the hospital, this process involves frequent visits to the patient's home by the nurse concerned, especially during the early phase of the home nutritional programme.

The need for long-term review is dictated by the severity of the disability and the nature of the disease that necessitated the surgical treatment. Although there are set guidelines, each patient has to be reviewed in accordance with individual needs and the home background. Voluntary societies and associations play a crucial role in accelerating the return of these patients to a full social life.

Rehabilitation of transplant patients

A successful organ transplant so dramatically improves the well-being, physical activity and independence of the recipient, that the rehabilitation process following the operation is seldom accompanied by significant physical or psychological hurdles in these patients. The change from a chronic invalid state consequent on the organ failure and its effects on the other systems, to an increasingly active normal lifestyle, is so real and has such an impact on these patients that they are prepared to put up with all that is required in terms of follow-up requirements and immunosuppressive therapy. By contrast, emotional and psychopsychiatric problems are very common in relatives of the deceased donor. Counselling and support of these bereaved relatives is essential. The knowledge that the donation was successful in restoring health to a chronically sick patient helps these unfortunate individuals in the acceptance and resolution of the bereavement process. None the less, although often asked for, the identity of the recipient must never be divulged to the donor relatives. Likewise, patients receiving allogeneic organ grafting should not know the source of their successful transplant. The problems faced by all transplant patients following a successful operation are shown in Table 22.4.

The need for indefinite immunosuppressive therapy carries a number of adverse consequences: organ toxicity, infective complications (bacterial, viral and fungal) and an increased incidence of lymphomas and other tumours. Most current immunosuppressive regimens are based on cyclosporin A and this has resulted in a significant improvement in graft survival compared with the precyclosporin era. None the less, cyclosporin

---

Table 22.4 Problems specific to transplant recipients

- Immunosuppressive therapy and its complications
- Infective risks
- Development of tumours
- Recurrence of original disease
- Late surgical complications
- Chronic rejection
- Osteoporosis

is both nephrotoxic and hepatotoxic. Viral infections may be transmitted to the recipient during the perioperative period. These include cytomegalovirus (CMV) and hepatitis (particularly hepatitis C and other non-A non-B). Instances of acquired immunodeficiency syndrome (AIDS) have now been reported, although mercifully they have been rare. Aside from these infections associated with the operation, the resistance to invasion by pathogens is compromised by the immunosuppressive therapy, and for this reason these patients have to be counselled accordingly. Any infection requires active intervention using the appropriate antibiotic.

Another problem relates to recurrence of the original disease for which the transplant operation was carried out. This applies to tumour recurrence and recurrence of specific hepatic disease after liver transplantation. Recurrence of tumour after hepatic transplantation for primary hepatic malignancy (hepatomas and cholangiocarcinomas) is almost universal and is the reason why hepatic transplantation for these tumours is no longer practised except for small fibrolamellar variants of hepatocellular carcinoma. The same dismal outcome from early recurrence has been observed in patients undergoing 'cluster transplantation' for advanced malignancy in the supracolic compartment, and these heroic procedures are no longer practised.

Recurrence of hepatic disease may be encountered in patients undergoing transplantation for primary biliary cirrhosis or Budd–Chiari syndrome and in chronic carriers of hepatitis B and C. Currently, primary biliary cirrhosis is considered to be a form of chronic graft-versus-host disease and is associated with various immunological abnormalities. It is not surprising, therefore, that recurrence of the disease in the transplanted liver can occur and is, indeed, well documented. It is accompanied by the same serological findings (circulating immune complexes and elevated immunoglobulin M) despite the continued immunosuppressive therapy.

However, transplantation is still worthwhile in these patients, as the majority have minimal disease and lead active lives despite abnormal liver function tests and subclinical or mild icterus. The experience at Denver Pittsburgh has shown that recurrence of the Budd–Chiari syndrome is encountered if the patients are not kept on anticoagulant therapy indefinitely. Chronic carriage of the hepatitis B or C virus is associated with the development of both cirrhosis of the liver and hepatocellular carcinoma. Thus, in chronic carriers the transplanted liver becomes infected with the virus, with the development of hepatitis B-related disease in the transplanted organ unless specific mea-sures are employed at the time of surgery (human antiHBs hyperimmune globulin during the anhepatic phase of the operation) and specific anti-viral therapy **[see Disorder of the Liver, Vol. II]** although the transplanted liver may become infected subsequently from virus present in extrahepatic tissue such as the pancreas.

The specific surgical problems that may impair or jeopardize the function of an otherwise successful transplant include biliary obstruction after orthotopic liver transplantation and vesicoureteric reflux or obstruction after renal transplantation, although chronic rejection remains the most frequent cause for graft failure and the need for retransplantation in the long term.

The most common metabolic problem is osteoporosis. This is usually encountered in patients after liver transplantation, especially when the procedure is performed for primary biliary cirrhosis. Osteoporosis in transplant patients is also associated with the requirement for large doses of corticosteroids soon after the operation, reduced physical activity and prolonged recumbency. The incidence and severity of osteoporosis have been reduced with the new cyclosporin-based regimens and with the routine administration of microcrystalline calcium hydroxyapatite.

Guide to further reading

Bowling, A. (1997). *Measuring Health: A Review of Quality of Life Measurement Scales*, Open University Press, Buckingham.

Bowling, A. (1995). *Measuring Disease: A Review of Disease-Specific Quality of Life Scales*, Open University Press, Buckingham.

Camilleri-Brennan, J. and Steele, R. J. C. (1998). Quality of life after treatment for rectal cancer. *Br J Surg* **85**: 1036–1043.

McLeod, R. S. and Baxter, N. (1998). Quality of life of patients with inflammatory bowel disease after surgery. *World J Surg* **22**: 375–381.

Montazeri, A., Gillis, C. R. and McEwen J. (1998). Quality of life in patients with lung cancer: a review of the literature from 1970 to 1995. *Chest* **113**: 467–481.

Murdoch, G. and Donovan, R. B. (1988). *Amputation Surgery and Lower Limb Prosthetics*, Blackwell Scientific Publications, Oxford.

Streiner, D. L. and Norman, G. R. (1995). *Health Measurement Scales: A Practical Guide to their Development and Use*, Oxford University Press, Oxford.

Troup, I. M. and Wood, M. (1982). *Total Care of the Lower Limb Amputee*, Pitman, London.

Walker, S. R. and Rosser, R. M. (1993). *Quality of Life Assessment: Key Issues in the 1990s*, Kluwer Academic Publishers, Dordrecht.

MODULE 23

Assessment and professional development

1 • Principles of clinical studies

2 • Nature and principles of surgical audit

3 • Human reliability assessment

4 • Principles of cost-effectiveness analysis in surgery

5 • Legal aspects of surgical practice

6 • The Internet

7 • Computers, medicine and the twenty-first century

'Don't wait till the last judgement. It happens every day' – Albert Camus (1913–1960)

Section 23.1 • Principles of clinical studies

Clinical research can be divided into two broad areas, observational and experimental. In the former, the research involves observing a population or group of patients either prospectively or by examining data concerning the subjects. These data may be already available or they may be collected prospectively. Techniques of observational research include qualitative research, surveys, case–control studies and some forms of cohort study. In experimental research, in contrast, a specific intervention is involved. Clinical experimental research can include some types of cohort studies and randomized, controlled trials. In the development of new drugs, particularly for cancer treatment, phase I and phase II cohort studies are followed by a phase III randomized trial, where the drug is compared either with placebo or with standard treatment [see Module 15, Vol. I].

Another important aspect of clinical research is the systematic review, and the meta-analysis in particular. Systematic reviews and meta-analyses are used in the development of evidence-based clinical guidelines and today all guidelines should be accompanied by grading of recommendations based on the strength of evidence. The definitions of the types of evidence and how these relate to the grading of recommendations vary but the most widely used system originates from the US Agency for Health Care Policy and Research (Table 23.1).

Qualitative research

Certain areas of health service research are not amenable to quantitative analysis. Examples would be examining techniques of training, trying to find out why individuals prefer certain sorts of diet and exploring why patients delay before seeking medical advice after the onset of symptoms. Qualitative research is

---

Table 23.1 Definitions of the types of evidence and the grading of recommendations used by the US Agency for Health Care Policy and Research.

Statement of evidence

Ia Evidence obtained from meta-analysis of randomized, controlled trials

Ib Evidence obtained from at least one randomized, controlled trial

IIa Evidence obtained from at least one well-designed controlled study without randomization

IIb Evidence obtained from at least one other type of well-designed quasi-experimental study

III Evidence obtained from well-designed non-experimental descriptive studies, such as comparative studies, correlation studies and case studies

IV Evidence obtained from expert committee reports or opinions and/or clinical experiences of respected authorities

Grades of recommendations

A Requires at least one randomized, controlled trial as part of a body of literature of overall good quality and consistency addressing the specific recommendations (evidence levels Ia, Ib)

B Requires the availability of well-conducted clinical studies but no randomized clinical trials on the topic of recommendation (evidence levels IIa, IIb, III)

C Requires evidence obtained from expert committee reports or opinions and/or clinical experiences of respected authorities. Indicates an absence of directly applicable clinical studies of good quality (evidence level IV)

often used in combination with quantitative research, although both can exist independently.

Surveys

Surveys are used to investigate what is happening at a given point in time or during a given period. This is a useful technique for studying complicated situations and opinions. It is, however, very dependent on careful data collection. Surveys are frequently carried out by distributing questionnaires by post, but frequently the response rate is poor. Unless the response rate is close to 100%, useful conclusions about the population being studied cannot be drawn. Techniques for improving response rate include reminder letters and telephone calls. The most effective technique, however, is to carry out the survey by personal contact between the researcher and the members of the population being studied.

Case–control studies

A case–control study is a technique whereby a control group is compared with a study group in a non-randomized fashion. However, the individuals in the control group are carefully selected so that they have the same characteristics as the subject of the study except for the characteristics that are under investigation. Case–control studies can be used to investigate the aetiology of disease. If there is a hypothesis that a certain disease may be caused by a certain variable then individuals with the disease (cases) can be matched with individuals without the disease (controls) who are identical with the cases in all respects other than the variable under study. Case–control studies may also be used to study adverse effects of treatment, although this is probably best done by a randomized, controlled trial.

Under certain circumstances it may not be appropriate to have the same number of cases and controls and each case may be matched with more than one control. The disadvantage of case–control studies is that they are more open to bias than randomized, controlled trials and in a good case–control study the selection of the cases must be performed in such a way that bias is minimized.

Cohort studies

In cohort studies groups are investigated over a certain period and changes occurring during that period are recorded. This can be done either retrospectively or prospectively and the data may be collected routinely or specifically. Cohort studies can be used to investigate the outcome of treatment when a randomized, controlled trial is impossible for ethical reasons. They may also be used to look at different methods of delivering a service, e.g. the relationship between specialization or case volume and outcome. Clearly, cohort studies can either be observational or, when an intervention is introduced, experimental.

Randomized, controlled trial

The randomized, controlled trial is perhaps the gold standard in terms of evaluating a new treatment or comparing two established forms of treatment. It is essential, however, that there is genuine doubt as to the effectiveness of a new treatment or the choice between two treatments before a randomized trial can be considered ethically justifiable. It is also essential, as with all research, that patients entered into randomized control trials do so after giving fully informed consent and this can sometimes be difficult to achieve, especially when treatment is being compared with no treatment or placebo. This is particularly true when a surgical intervention is being compared with no treatment or a nonsurgical intervention.

The ideal design of a randomized trial is the double-blind structure, where neither the patient nor the assessing doctor is aware of the treatment option. This is extremely difficult to achieve in surgical trials and often impossible. For a randomized trial to be effective, it is essential that the randomization process is truly random and that the decision to enter the patient into the trial is made before randomization takes place. Any deviation from this principle is likely to allow the introduction of unacceptable bias.

Another common type of error (sometimes referred to as a type II error) is making assumptions about a negative result of a randomized, controlled trial based on too few numbers. While designing a trial it is important to ensure that it has sufficient power to detect the difference between the treatment and control groups or between the two treatment groups. It follows that the smaller the expected effect of the treatment, the larger the trial will have to be to detect the effect.

Systematic reviews and meta-analysis

Increasingly, it is being recognized that evidence-based care should be based on a systematic review of the available evidence. For a systematic review to be valuable it must be based on a complete database derived from a clearly defined search of the literature. The criteria used to assess the quality of the evidence reviewed must be stated (see Table 23.1) and it is important that the abstracted data are analysed using accepted and well-validated methods.

The most powerful type of systematic review is the meta-analysis, in which data from individual randomized, controlled trials are pooled and reanalysed. This is particularly helpful when there has been a number of small trials or where there have been trials with contradictory results. There are two types of meta-analysis, which depend on the source of the data. The MAL meta-analysis involves abstracting data from published papers, whereas in a MAP meta-analysis, original single-patient data are obtained from the authors of the published papers. Although more difficult to perform, MAP analysis is more reliable.

While meta-analysis is powerful, there are some problems and two main disadvantages. Firstly, meta-analyses are often based only on trials that have been published and thus are usually biased towards a positive result. Secondly, data from trials included in a meta-analysis often refer to heterogeneous groups of patients and are not therefore strictly comparable. The effects of this can be minimized using specific statistical techniques, but it still represents a significant problem in the interpretation of meta-analysis.

Section 23.2 • Nature and principles of surgical audit

This section covers the principles and application of audit to the practice of surgery. Surgical audit is a tool that uses a peer-review process to enable change based on need. It can evaluate structure, process or outcome. The audit cycle and critical event analysis can be used to change many aspects of surgical practice, including training, quality assurance, morbidity, mortality and resource allocation.

Background

Stories abound that audit is as old as history; certainly in surgical circles simple registration of operative results and morbidity and mortality meetings have been commonplace for many years. However, for most doctors, audit appeared more formally in the UK as part of the 1989 Government White Paper 'Working for Patients'. In this paper, audit was defined as 'the systematic, critical analysis of the quality of medical care including the procedures used for diagnosis and treatment, the use of resources, and the resulting outcome and quality of life for the patient'. Networks to support medical teams were established: the Clinical Resource and Audit Group (CRAG) in Scotland and Medical Audit Advisory Groups (MAAGs) in England and Wales. This has been a costly exercise, with an estimated £800 000 000 being spent on audit in the UK between 1990 and 2000. Despite this massive input of financial resource, evidence for a change in the culture of evaluating change is patchy, even though attitudes to audit, in theory at least, are positive.

The General Medical Council (GMC), however, is uncompromising. The wording in their most recent pamphlets unequivocally states that doctors must monitor and evaluate the quality of care that they are providing to their patients. This suggests that failure to measure the quality of care provided is a possible breach of professional responsibility and could, in theory, lead to referral to the GMC. Some recent high-profile cases have served to stiffen rather than soften government resolve and the 1998 White Papers 'Designed to Care' and 'The New NHS' have put quality at the centre of reforms in the UK. In Scotland a report entitled the 'Acute Services Review' is clear about the link between quality and explicit standards and the need for more information to be in the public domain.

The need for an understanding of basic audit methods and their practical application has therefore never been greater. However, knowledge of audit cannot be assumed, as undergraduate and postgraduate teaching on the subject is often deficient.

Principles of audit: theoretical issues

To paraphrase the Mad Hatter in Lewis Carroll's 'Alice in Wonderland': 'there is so much to do, and so little time to do it'. A convenient method for describing the broad nature of the work of a doctor is to look at the structure, process and outcome of care. In simple terms this describes the tools of the trade (structure), what we do with these tools (process) and how effective we are with the tools (outcome). Measurement of each of these variables will demand qualitative as well as quantitative techniques, with comparison of outcomes being most related to a measurement of the quality of care being delivered. There is some evidence, however, that adequate processes can be as effective in measuring quality as outcomes, but neither process nor outcome will reflect adequate quality if the basic structure for care is not in place. An example, using colonic polyps and cancer, will illustrate this point.

(i) A register of patients with colonic polyps is an example of a basic structure of care. Knowing that the prevalence of these polyps is 0.1% of the population allows a clinician to determine whether all patients with polyps are known about in the area. Without this essential knowledge, data on processes and outcomes will be unreliable.

(ii) The monitoring of patients with a history of colonic polyps is an example of the process of care. It is becoming a medical–legal issue that such patients should have their colon checked every 3–5 years and the recording and monitoring of this process will protect both professional and patient alike.

(iii) The incidence of colon cancer in patients with colonic polyps is an example of outcome of care, as this is a potentially treatable precursor of colon cancer in the population. If the register of patients known to have had polyps is inadequate or if the process is not being implemented, outcomes will be poorer. In other words, structure, process and outcome are dependent on each other but independently measurable.

To begin to measure the structure, process or outcome of care two important definitions need to be considered:

▪ a criterion is that element of care that has to be present as defined by best practice
▪ the standard of care is the percentage of times that the criterion is present in the 'real world'.

An example will illustrate this. Patients under the age of 70 years with a history of colonic polyps should have their colon examined every 3 years. This is a criterion for good care of these patients and describes the disease, the process and the time-scale. These three variables combine to give one measure of quality of care for patients with colonic polyps. It is, however, impossible to examine the colon of every patient known to have had colonic polyps. This is because some individuals may refuse to undergo colonoscopy or may persistently default, failing to take the bowel preparation or even failing to turn up for their appointment. In such circumstances, it is reasonable to assume a standard that 90% of patients with a history of colonic polyps will have their colon checked every 3 years, with the remaining 10% representing those who refuse or default from colonoscopy.

There are two main mechanisms for evaluating the quality of care being delivered by doctors and their teams. The first is the audit cycle and the second is critical event analysis (also known as significant event analysis). The former is more quantitative in nature and the latter is more qualitative. Any quality-assurance programme should include both.

The audit cycle

Evaluation of change through a completed audit cycle is described in the following stages (Figure 23.1).

Reason for choice of subject

The choice of audit subject should have the potential for change and the subject should be relevant to the quality of care being determined. As mentioned earlier (by the Mad Hatter), there are so many potential areas to audit and thus priorities should determine that the most important areas, as determined by the team, should be audited early. The key to successful audit is to keep the audit focused.

Criterion/criteria chosen

The criterion or criteria selected should be based on the best evidence available, such as published guidelines and a literature search, and should be relevant to the subject of the audit. These criteria form the basis by which the quality of care being delivered will be measured.

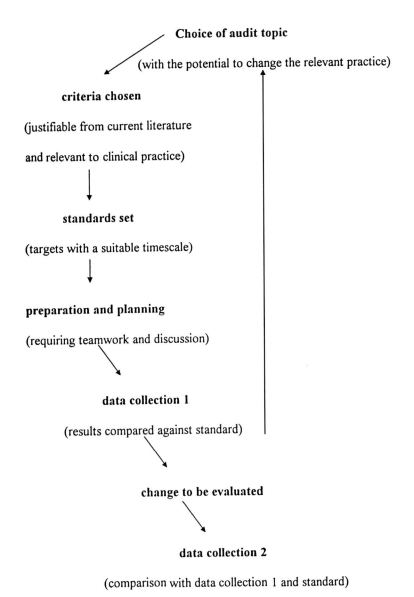

Figure 23.1 The audit cycle.

Standards set

Standard setting is often controversial because it is an explicit statement of the quality of care that **should** be delivered and is a recognition that **actual** quality of care often falls short of this. A realistic time-scale to achieve a standard should be determined, for example over a period of years, with targets set to provide a framework against which progress towards the standard can be measured. For example, patients with a history of polyps will have their colon examined every 3 years (criterion), 90% of such patients will have their colon examined within 5 years (standard), 50% of polyp patients will have their colon examined in the third year and 70% by the fourth year (targets) towards the standard of 90%.

Planning and preparation

Lack of planning and preparation are the reasons that most audit cycles fail. It is vital that the whole team (including clerical, nursing and medical staff in the example given) is aware of any audit being carried out for ethical as well as practical reasons. Delegated responsibility and an appropriate time-scale should be determined and full agreement achieved to evaluate change.

Data collection

To evaluate change, two collections of data will be required: one to measure the current care being delivered and the second to evaluate whether change has improved the situation (or not). A glance through the surgical literature will demonstrate that many 'audits' cited in surgical papers are merely data collections with suggestions for change. Adequate preparation and planning should ensure that any change is evaluated and thus will justify the time and effort involved in carrying out the audit. The collections of data should be compared against the targets or standard, with the whole team being informed of progress.

Critical event analysis

The second example of an audit mechanism is the significant or critical event analysis, sometimes called a confidential enquiry. This is a qualitative or descriptive technique for describing events that happen unexpectedly in the delivery of care, either to an individual or to the department. The event should be significant in how it affects the individual or the team, and should be carried out in an atmosphere of trust rather than threat. This process will encourage the culture required to promote audit to change in a positive manner. A suggested format for a description of significant event analysis is as outlined below.

- Describe the significant event.
- Why did it occur?
- What has been changed?
- What has been learned?
- Has the change been continued?

An example of critical event analysis could come from the colonic surveillance programme outlined above. A man of 50 years who had three 1 cm polyps removed from the ascending, transverse and sigmoid colon 3 years earlier returns for colonoscopy. Bowel preparation is good, but an inexperienced and unsupervised junior fails to get beyond the sigmoid colon. Having seen no abnormality to that point, the junior arranges a colonoscopy for 3 years hence. However, within 18 months, the patient returns with an altered bowel habit and investigations reveal a colonic carcinoma in the transverse colon. Critical event analysis highlights that the colonoscopy carried out by the junior was inadequate. The unit decides that all surveillance colonoscopy should be performed by an experienced and appropriately trained member of staff, unless the colonoscopy clearly views the full colon and total colonoscopy is confirmed by ileal biopsy, repeat colonoscopy or radiological review by double-contrast enema is required. Subsequent review of the endoscopy lists 6 months later confirms that this change in personnel conducting colonoscopy has been implemented; 70% of colonoscopy now views the whole colon at the first attempt.

Finally, for either of the above mechanisms to continue it will be necessary to implement a system whereby future change can be measured periodically with the minimum of effort. It is the lack of system development that makes the audit process more arduous and time consuming than it should be.

Principles of audit: practical issues

In practical terms there are two main issues to be addressed: (i) an adequate infrastructure within the organization, and (ii) the appropriate application of information management and technology. To provide an adequate infrastructure for supporting audit for quality assurance will require:

- a lead person with responsibility for audit
- planning of the audit
- system development dictated by best practice, e.g. based on guidelines
- a series of audit mechanisms required to be in place to check that the systems are performing adequately
- a peer review process to allow comparison between individuals or groups to identify and disseminate examples of good practice and identify and correct examples of poor practice.

To make the most of good organization and a tight infrastructure the potential for and use of IT will need to be maximized. In practice, the audit systems that have become successfully established, have usually been developed by clinicians with a particular interest in audit and with skills in information technology (IT). This has allowed the development, often over several years, of systems from the 'bottom up' (i.e. from the surgical workforce) rather than those imposed by middle or senior management ('top down') sometimes generated by computer software engineers with little knowledge of surgical life. The administrative structure for surgical audit is usually conducted through a hospital, regional or national committee, often comprising representatives of all interested parties. For larger ongoing audits, there may be full-time facilitators of the audit, although most members of audit committees are involved on a voluntary basis through interest in the concepts and development of audit. The collection of valid and reliable data needs to be as simple and straightforward as possible, and has evolved from punch cards through stand-alone personal computers to systematically collated data with customized software on intranet systems.

Collection and analysis of information

The choice of which audit software or tool to use in a given surgical setting may require detailed evaluation as to the local applications before a system is chosen and put into action. The ideal system should:

- be designed for use in a hospital environment with multiple users
- allow simple and rapid data collection (this may include the use of an optical reader or scanner to input data into a computer)
- have a logical and well-structured data entry
- be user friendly by clerical, nursing and medical staff
- generate appropriate documents such as discharge summaries
- talk to other departments (e.g. pharmacy) and other management systems
- allow derivation of and access to mortality and morbidity data

Two such audit systems are the Lothian Surgical Audit (LSA) System and the British Association of Surgical Oncologists breast database. The LSA software was developed for installation on personal computers or networked terminals at minimum cost, linked to the hospitals in the region and more recently to other hospitals and regions in the UK. Although the LSA system applies to most surgical specialties (ranging from vascular surgery through general and specialist surgical practices to gynaecology) and the British Association of Surgical Oncology breast database is confined to breast conditions alone, both systems aim to integrate audit with routine data gathering using intranet technology and allow the generation of documents such as letters to general medical practitioners and discharge summaries and the mapping of codes to other data systems (such as the Read code system of diseases).

    The funding of these committee structures and the financial support for the hardware (computers) and software (although some of the best audit packages are almost free) may be through local (e.g. hospital), regional or national structures, either by top slicing or ring fencing part of the general budget or through specifically funded audits. In addition to these resource implications there are training issues for users of the system. The dissemination of information locally may be through weekly or monthly meetings using time set aside specifically for the activity; indeed, some centres suspend all elective surgery for half a day each month

and hold interspecialty or single-specialty nursing, anaesthetic and surgical audit meetings. Wider dissemination of audit findings may be through college, governmental or specialty association meetings and through peer-reviewed journals. Individual audits may be developed into a full quality-assurance programme. The structure for providing such a quality assurance programme should therefore include:

- a defined clinical programme
- a lead person with full responsibility for feeding back performance periodically
- evidence-based criteria
- agreed standards
- customized software to run systems
- agreed methods for consistent and rigorous data collection
- an agreed timetable to review changes.

Audit in practice

Many published surgical papers with the term audit in the title do not actually follow the audit process and are simply collections of data. A simple framework to apply to any audit is to ask the following questions.

- Why was it done?
- How was it done?
- What did it find?

Audit has been used to good effect to change practice in training, surgical practice, the development of risk assessment **[see Module 3, Vol. I]**, quality assurance, morbidity and mortality audit and issues relating to surgical resources. Examples in each of these fields are given below.

Training

While audit is not yet compulsory for surgical trainees, general medical practitioner registrars have to conduct and submit an audit project as part of their summative assessment for Membership of the Royal College of General Practitioners (MRCGP). This demonstrates that it is possible for trainees, even in a 6-month period, to conduct a worthwhile audit. Some surgical trainees also undertake and complete an audit project. In addition, audit has been used to examine the training of trainees themselves. The Lothian Surgical Audit System was used to compare the training received and the time required in theatre against actual operations performed by surgical trainees to ascertain the need for an additional 270 operating days and £1.3 million required per annum to achieve an adequate level of training.

Surgical practice

Since 1982 surgeons in Lothian Region, Scotland, have driven the development of computerized audit in everyday practice as an educational tool (a weekly meeting and annual report) and as an accurate record of surgical activity. The establishment of specialist surgical units, improved results after colonic surgery and the demise of outmoded techniques have all been attributed to this regional audit. While changes in surgical practice require repeated education and typically occur over 3–4 years, audit has significantly influenced and improved surgical practice. However, even large audits may not be able to demonstrate that changes in surgical practice are directly attributable to the audit alone, owing to clinical developments over the period of the audit.

Quality assurance

The National Health Service Breast Screening Programme (NHSBSP) has a quality-assurance programme for the maintenance of minimum standards and the continuous improvement in the performance of all aspects of breast screening to ensure that all women have access to a uniformly high service. The breast screening programme seeks to review performance and outcomes of individual breast screening units. By examining a range of performance indicators including radiological, pathological and surgical data against set criteria and standards, the quality-assurance programme audits the provision of breast screening services throughout the UK. Where the service differs from set standards detailed examination of the data can suggest reasons why and courses for improvement; re-audit of the next year's data demonstrates whether improvements towards the required standards have been achieved.

Morbidity and mortality

One of the most useful risk assessment and scoring systems to arise from surgical audit is POSSUM (Physiological and Operative Severity Score for the enUmeration of Mortality and morbidity) **[see Module 3, Vol. I]**. POSSUM has now been widely validated and comprises 18 factors giving a numerical assessment. It comprises two parts: 12 physiological factors of four grades, plus six operative factors of four grades. The resulting score can be entered into logistical regression analysis equations to yield numerical values for both morbidity and mortality. Alternatively, the risk may be displayed graphically. Used in gastrointestinal, vascular and urological surgery, it provides excellent matching of predicted and observed values and can be used as a practical means of morbidity audit as well as mortality audit. The POSSUM system thus allows comparisons between surgical units and hospitals by taking into account medical conditions, case mix and some non-surgical factors (but not others such as the lack of high dependency or intensive care).

Multidisciplinary national audit of surgical mortality in the UK is now well established. The Scottish Audit of Surgical Mortality (SASM) evolved from regional audits and examines all deaths on surgical wards or within 30 days of an operative procedure (including endoscopy). Compliance by surgeons of all specialties and anaesthetists is extremely high (95%), with all deaths peer reviewed by independent anaesthetists and surgeons; 10% of deaths go on to a further, more detailed case note assessment by a surgeon or anaesthetist with a specialist interest in the field in question.

For the 4500 deaths examined each year, the resource implications at £40 per death analysed are relatively small. The feedback to clinicians is through individual feedback for each death, the circulation of detailed case note assessments amongst the surgical community and by the publication of an annual report. Using multiple audit cycles, SASM has led to a progressive improvement in several areas of surgical and anaesthetic practice.

A further contrasting audit, the National Confidential Enquiry into Perioperative Deaths (NCE-POD), examines just 10% of patients but targets specific areas of surgical practice. Despite the differences in approach, both large-scale audits have highlighted deficits in the provision of high-dependency and intensive care facilities, deficits in communication between grades and specialties, and poor clinical record keeping, and have identified problems with the seniority of surgeons and anaesthetists operating and the timing of surgery. The issue of who operates, and when, led to the recognition that senior staff need to become more involved in surgical emergencies and the need to provide adequate daytime emergency theatre provision.

Resource

Audit can also be used to demonstrate changes and influence resource allocation. In an audit of 180 466 procedures prospectively recorded over a 10-year period in a single UK health board, the operations were weighted to reflect workload. While the annual case load (case counting) fell by 12% over the 10-year period, this was due to the decrease in minor operations. However, the equivalent workload rose by 2.7% owing to an increase in complex major operations. Thus, surgical audit can be used to demonstrate qualitative changes in clinical practice with time.

Implications

The importance of audit as a mechanism for measuring change in the delivery of quality of care is emphasized in the impending introduction of clinical governance in the UK (MEL 1998–75). Standards of care show enormous variation and the dissemination of best practice is vital if these variations are to be reduced. An understanding of the basic audit process is therefore fundamental to ensuring that improving the quality of care being provided is a lifelong professional commitment with professionals, patients and the government all satisfied that checks and balances are in place to ensure that everyone gets a fair deal.

Section 23.3 • Human reliability assessment

Human reliability assessment (HRA) has been used in high-risk industry (e.g. nuclear industry) as a measure of prevention of accidents, the consequences of which would be catastrophic. The techniques used borrow from expertise in three fields: engineering, psychology and ergonomics, the ultimate aim being to reduce errors, such that the risk of the task or activity is as low as is reasonably possible (ALARP). HRA differs from audit used in surgical practice in that it is both prospective and prescriptive from the start, i.e. the methodology identifies:

- what may go wrong
- the probability of this happening
- the consequence were it to happen
- the necessary defence systems that need to be incorporated to ensure that the risk is in the ALARP region.

The techniques of HRA are being adapted to surgical practice, and should considerably enhance the safety and improve the outcome of surgical intervention, although it is important to stress that clinical HRA is still in its infancy, despite its undoubted potential in this direction.

Human errors

Before discussing HRA, it is important to outline the nature and consequence of errors. There are several classifications of errors, but the model proposed by Rasmussen is applicable with modifications to surgery:

- **skill-based level**: relating to faulty execution of a task
- **rule-based level**: misclassification or misdiagnosis leading to the application of the wrong rule
- **knowledge-based level**: arising from incomplete or incorrect knowledge.

In addition, errors as stressed by Reason fall into two broad categories: active and latent. In general, **active errors** are enacted by front-line operators and have an immediate effect, e.g. a driver crashes a car, or a surgeon inflicts an injury to the aorta during the creation of a closed pneumoperitoneum for laparoscopic surgery. By contrast, **latent** errors (hidden within the system) may lie dormant and undetected, causing no adverse effect until they summate to create the necessary trajectory for a major catastrophe. Many of the major disasters that could not conceivably happen, but did, e.g. Three Mile Island, Chernobyl, Zeebrugge ferry, were the outcome of latent errors related to bad decision making, bad management, faulty practice, inadequate maintenance, etc. In his seminal monograph on human error, J. Reason states: 'Rather than being the main instigators of an accident, operators tend to be the inheritors of system defects caused by poor design, incorrect installation, faulty maintenance and bad management decisions.' There is an exact parallel in surgical practice, where a combination of latent errors is more often responsible for a fatal disaster than front-line errors enacted by a surgeon during the course of an operation. The following case illustrates this combination of latent errors.

- The patient was scheduled for laparoscopic endogastric removal of a localized sessile lesion in the posterior wall of the stomach.

- Before the operation, the surgeon was informed by the theatre sister that the 'new' flexible endoscope was away for repair and only the 'old spare' endoscope was available.
- This endoscope was inserted after induction of anaesthesia to locate the lesion. The endoscope was left *in situ* as is required by the procedure.
- The surgeon and assistant left the operating theatre to scrub and gown.
- The anaesthetist left the operating room, leaving an anaesthetic nurse.
- The surgeon, on returning to the operating room, notices gross distension of the patient's abdomen: the insufflating valve of the 'old endoscope' had jammed, with resulting continuous insufflation over a period of 5 min.
- Remedial action was taken: immediate aspiration of air via the endoscope followed by open laparoscopy. This showed serosal splits in the stomach but no complete breach. Nasogastric suction was instituted and the operation postponed. The patient recovered from this ordeal without any complication and had the operation 6 weeks later with the 'new flexible endoscope' without any mishaps: the pathology of the excised lesion was 'ectopic pancreatic tissue'.
- The outcome was thus two hospital admissions, two exposures to general anaesthesia, and fortunately no serious complication.

On review of this potentially disastrous incident, the following latent errors can be identified.

- The hospital was not equipped with all necessary instruments and devices needed for the operative work done.
- The equipment was not maintained and checked regularly for malfunction.
- The surgeon accepted use of the 'old spare' endoscope and did not test it before use.
- The anaesthetist left the operating theatre when the surgeons were scrubbing up.

There is evidence that the risk of latent errors increases with the complexity of the activity, especially if it entails the use of advanced high technology.

Consequence of errors

The consequence of an error is of crucial importance and the spectrum varies from no consequence to serious or fatal. Thus, some errors are intrinsically more important than others, although the effect (consequence) of an error varies with extraneous circumstances. Thus, for example, a car driver who skids on a patch of black ice may crash into a wall and sustain serious or fatal injuries or kill an innocent pedestrian, or he may be 'lucky' and hit neither wall nor pedestrian and escape unhurt, i.e. the same error can result in quite different consequences. In the case referred to above, gastrointestinal perforation could have easily occurred and it was fortuitous for the surgeon and the patient that it did not. Likewise, in endoscopic surgery, a surgeon may exert too much tenting force during the use of electrosurgical knife, with inevitable follow-through of the hook knife once the tissue is cut. It is a matter of luck whether the hook knife stops in mid-air (no consequence), or impinges into bowel or large vessel (serious consequence). **Thus avoidance of all errors underlies safe execution, and in this respect there is no such thing as an inconsequential error in surgical practice, but some are more important than others.**

Generic methodology of human reliability assessment

As outlined by Kirwin, HRA as developed for use in high-risk industries entails 10 steps:

- problem definition
- task analysis
- human error analysis
- representation
- screening
- quantification
- impact assessment
- error reduction
- quality assurance
- documentation.

Human reliability assessment steps

(i)   **Problem definition** entails precise objective of the system/activity and the problem(s) that can occur and that must be avoided. In the context of a surgical operation, this may be 'local recurrence' after resection for cancer, anastomotic dehiscence, infection after hip replacement surgery, etc.

(ii) **Task analysis** involves identification of the nature of all the component steps of the activity or operation, including the use of specific equipment. There are several types of task analysis used by industry but the one that is most applicable to surgery is **sequential task analysis**. This looks at the task in terms of the actions of the operator in a chronological sequence. Task analysis in the case of a surgical operation includes the selection criteria (indications), all the component steps of the operation, all the equipment used and the experience of the surgeon with the procedure.

(iii) **Human error identification** (HEI) is a crucial component of the process. All conceivable errors that may occur during the steps of the procedure, their nature and consequence have to be identified and categorized. There are various methods of error categorization but the one that is most applicable to surgery is that based on external error modes (EEMs), outlined in the systematic human error reduction predictive approach (SHERPA) proposed by Embrey. HEI also includes identification of factors that influence human performance (performance-shaping factors). These are very important in surgical practice.

(iv) **Representation**: this step consists of modelling the human errors and the recovery paths in order to quantitate their effect on the system or outcome. This process involves the integration of human errors with hardware (devices/equipment) failures in a fault/event tree.

(v)   **Screening**: during this step all identified errors are screened such that inconsequential and insignificant errors are excluded from the study. Screening does not apply to surgical HRA as all errors enacted during surgery may be consequential, some more than others.

(vi) **Quantification**: in this step the probability of any given error occurring is estimated (human error probability or HEP) as well as human error recovery probability by a variety of human reliability quantitation techniques. HEP is simply derived from the number of errors encountered/number of opportunities for the error to occur. In the high-risk industry this is simply an estimate based on a predictive analysis. In surgery, HEPs can be quantitated accurately by using an observational data capture based on videorecording of the operations. The material is then analysed for the error rates by an expert in conjunction with an ergonomist. This technique provides a very accurate estimate of both procedural (interstep) and execution (intrastep) errors enacted by a surgeon during a specific operation.

(vii) **Impact assessment**: at this stage, decisions are made on whether improvements in human reliability are needed with respect to the activity/system/operation.

(viii) **Error reduction**: this is the remedial step when defence systems are introduced to prevent the errors and thus achieve a safe and consistent performance. In surgery, this should translate to achieving the lowest possible morbidity and best possible outcome. Taking surgery for colorectal cancer as an example, this would mean low immediate morbidity including anastomotic dehiscence and abolition of local recurrence of the disease.

(ix) **Quality assurance**: essentially, this is an ongoing audit to ensure that the improved system/execution/performance is maintained.

(x)   **Documentation** is necessary to stipulate the conditions or measures necessary to achieve the goals, i.e. safe and optimal execution of an operation. In the case of surgery, this should form the basis of guidelines for operative treatment of various disorders.

Adaptation of human reliability assessment to surgical practice

The generic HRA described is readily adaptable to operative surgery but certain modifications are needed. In the first instance, the errors and their HEPs are obtained by observational data capture and the relative importance of the errors has to be decided by a group of experts on the subject. Secondly, the system has to be simplified to render it feasible in clinical practice. In this respect, all operations have crucial steps that determine success or failure. These steps are not easily separated. For example, in the creation of an anastomosis, the outcome (healing or dehiscence of the anastomosis) is not dependent only on a single task (suturing or stapling) but also on preparation of the bowel ends, ensuring a good blood supply, anastomosis without any tension, etc. Thus, rather then tasks, one has to consider **hazard zones** that consist of a series of interrelated tasks. For each operation, the hazard zones are identified, rather than individual steps.

HRA has been used to improve outcome, especially reduction of infection following hip-joint replacement surgery and in laparoscopic surgery. In one study on 20 laparoscopic cholecystectomies undertaken by specialist registrars 189 errors were recorded using a video-based observational data capture, 16 of which required corrective action during the procedure.

Section 23.4 • Principles of cost-effectiveness analysis in surgery

Decision makers are increasingly faced with the challenge of reconciling growing demand for health-care services with available resources. Out of this economic fact of life arises the key concept of 'opportunity cost' (i.e. the benefits to patients that are forgone by using a resource in one way rather than its next best alternative). Those responsible for allocating resources need to prioritize between competing uses so that maximum benefit (health gain) can be obtained from any given budget. Hence, choices have to be made about which services to provide in order to maximize patient benefit and to minimize opportunity cost; in other words, decisions about how to maximize the efficiency of the health-care system.

The role of cost-effectiveness analysis (CEA) is to provide a framework for decision making regarding the relative value of health-care interventions and programmes. For example, at the level of the health service, commissioners may have to decide on the appropriate specialty mix that they wish to purchase for their population. In this broad context, CEA can be used to determine whether the resources available should be spent on general surgery or medical oncology or some other area of health care. Choices may also have to be made at the disease level, where CEA can be used to determine, for example, whether extraperitoneal laparoscopic inguinal hernia repair is a more efficient treatment than open herniorrhaphy.

CEA has become an integral component of decision making in some areas of health care. For example, in Australia and Canada, economic evaluation is now a mandatory requirement in applications for public reimbursement of new drugs. The growing requirement to demonstrate the efficiency of new technologies means that CEA is increasingly becoming required

- LF is more effective than OF and no more costly

- LF is less costly than OF and no less effective

- LF is more effective than OF and more costly, but the incremental resources necessary to provide LF could not be used to generate a greater number of benefits elsewhere

- LF is less effective than OF and less costly, and the incremental resources necessary to provide OF could be used to generate a greater number of benefits elsewhere

Figure 23.2 Four possible conditions that would ensure that laparoscopic fundoplication (LF) is more efficient than open fundoplication (OF) in the treatment of gastro-oesophageal reflux disease.

as a part of health service research proposal grants to both the NHS Research and Development (R&D) programme and the Medical Research Council.

Although CEA is not, as yet, a formal requirement for the evaluation of surgical interventions prior to use in the NHS, cost-effectiveness studies are appearing more frequently in the medical literature, including surgery journals. Surgery is not immune from external pressures to set priorities based on the costs and benefits of surgical interventions and, increasingly, clinicians and other health service staff will have to contribute to this sort of decision making. It is important, therefore, that they are able to understand the key concepts and critically to appraise published cost-effectiveness studies. Using examples of published studies in the field of surgery, this section describes the key elements of a study, the different approaches to CEA and the usefulness of the information that they provide.

Defining cost-effectiveness analysis

CEA can be defined as the 'comparative analysis of alternative courses of action in terms of both their costs and consequences' (Drummond *et al.*). There are two key elements contained within this definition. The first of these is the term 'comparative'; in the same way that clinical evaluation requires a comparison of two or more interventions, so too does any economic analysis aimed at generating information to assist with resource allocation. It is not possible to assess the cost-effectiveness of a new intervention in isolation; there would have to be an assessment of the costs and outcomes of the technology compared with usual practice. The second key element in the definition is that CEA is concerned not only with costs, but also with the consequences for health and other things that are valued.

During the 1990s there has been a rapid expansion in the cost-effectiveness literature in all areas of health technology, including surgery. In a comparison of studies conducted from 1979 to 1990 with studies conducted from 1991 to 1996, Elixhauser *et al.* identified a total of 133 studies published during 1979–1990 and 185 studies published during 1991–1996 evaluating the cost-effectiveness of surgical interventions. This represents an annual average of 11 and 31 articles, respectively, for each of these periods.

Despite the increased trend towards CEA, the meaning of the term 'cost-effective' used in the literature varies considerably and the term is often used inappropriately. Incorrect interpretations often include equating 'cost-effective' with 'cost-savings'. The correct interpretation of a cost-effective intervention is one that has a differential outcome relative to a competing alternative, which is worth its differential cost. By way of illustration, consider the comparison of open and laparoscopic fundoplication in the treatment of gastro-oesophageal reflux disease. Although there have been some randomized, controlled trials comparing the two procedures, no study has yet explored their relative cost-effectiveness. Figure 23.2 describes the conditions required for cost-effectiveness using the example of gastro-oesophageal reflux disease.

Key concepts in economic evaluation

This section introduces some of the important concepts in CEA.

Measuring outcomes

A range of outcome measures is now used to evaluate health-care technologies. These can be broadly divided into:

- clinical measures
- patient-based measures.

Clinical measures are based on the physiological or pathological measurements made by clinicians and may have little relationship to patients' feeling of well-being (e.g. measuring the size of a patient's gallstones). Patient-based outcome measures are more closely related to patients' perceptions of illness and, in terms of a spectrum of sophistication, run from the measurement of patients' symptoms to a detailed assessment of the impact of a condition and its treatment on patients' functioning and general well-being. The latter is often described as a measure of **health-related quality of life** (HRQL); for example, an instrument has been developed by Eyspach *et al.* to assess the impact of gastrointestinal surgery on various aspects of a patient's life, including physical, psychological, sexual and social domains. Of course, some measures of outcome are of great interest to clinicians and patients alike, mortality and survival rates being the most obvious examples.

Various outcome measures used in clinical evaluation are used in economic appraisal, but they differ in the information value they offer for resource allocation. In judging the potential value of an outcome measure for CEA, the following issues are relevant.

- **Is the measure unidimensional or multidimensional?** Assessing the relative value for money of health-care interventions is more straightforward when outcomes can be expressed on a unidimensional scale, e.g. percentage risk of cancer recurrence or life-years gained. When outcomes are inherently multidimensional, however, methods are required to express them on a single scale.
- **Does the measure fully or partially reflect the effectiveness of the interventions?** It makes little sense to select an outcome measure for

a CEA because it is unidimensional if it only partly reflects the differences between interventions, e.g. the use of surgical complications in isolation from recurrence rates and time to recovery in a CEA of open versus laparoscopic hernia repair.

- **Is the measure condition specific or generic?** Decisions about resource allocation often need to be taken across specialties and disease areas. If these decisions are to be informed by CEA in this context, it is crucial that the outcome measure adopted is generic, i.e. that it has meaning outside the clinical area within which it is used. For example, Kald *et al.* expressed outcomes in an evaluation of laparoscopic and open hernia repair in terms of time off work and time to complete recovery. However, this condition-specific measure would be of little use to a decision maker faced with the choice of allocating additional resources to that programme versus, for example, a new drug for hypertension, because there would be no basis for comparison between them.

Generic measures of outcome: the quality-adjusted life year

Faced with the demands of cross-programme comparison of the results of CEA, there have been attempts to develop generic measures of benefit. The most popular example of this is quality-adjusted life year (QALY). The premise of the QALY is that health care seeks to generate two general forms of outcome, increased life expectancy and improved HRQL, and the measure embodies both elements. Figure 23.3 provides an illustration of how QALYs are calculated. For a given condition, length of life is measured along the horizontal axis in terms of life-years. The vertical axis shows how each life-year is weighted, to represent the HRQL typically associated with it, using a scale running from 0 (equivalent to death) to 1 (equivalent to good health). The area under these 'QALY profiles' represents the expected QALYs associated with the prognosis following a specific intervention, and the difference between the areas under the two profiles represents the additional QALYs generated by one intervention over

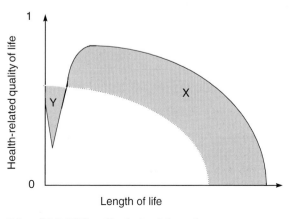

Figure 23.3 QALY profiles for two interventions.

another (in this case the shaded area X minus the shaded area Y). In addition to being a generic measure of benefit in health care, the weighting system in the QALY is used as a means of combining the various domains of HRQL such as pain and social function.

To estimate QALYs in any specific study, two types of data are required. Life expectancy is usually taken from available clinical studies, although these may only report mortality or survival rates requiring assumptions if these are to be translated into estimates of life expectancy. The more difficult data for QALY estimation are the weights (often referred to as utilities, preferences or values) to quality adjust the life-years. Various methods exist to elicit these weights which, in terms of sophistication, range from the use of plausible ad hoc values posited by the authors of studies, to the use of preference-based instruments to elicit from individuals the weights that they would attach to particular states of health.

In CEA, one of three methods is typically used to elicit these weights directly: standard gamble, visual analogue and time trade-off. Although each method uses a different technique, they share the common intention of establishing the relative value of a particular health state in relation to the states of perfect health and death. In estimating weights for states of health, a decision needs to be taken regarding from whom these should be elicited. One approach is to use the methods directly on patients in a prospective study to value their actual state of health over time. Another approach is for the weights to be elicited from a group of patients, clinicians or members of the public based on descriptive scenarios. In their evaluation of laser-assisted angioplasty for peripheral arterial occlusions, Sculpher *et al.* generated descriptive scenarios based on a sample of patients with claudication or critical ischaemia and then elicited values for health states from a sample of health professionals and the general public using both the time trade-off technique and visual analogue rating scale.

In recent years, the effort of having to elicit a set of weights for each and every QALY-based evaluation has been avoided by the development of standardized generic classifications of states of health that, in principle, can be applied to all clinical areas. These systems also provide a predetermined weight for each state of health. An example of this sort of system is the EuroQol (EQ-5D), which defines states of health in terms of five dimensions: mobility, self-care, usual activities, pain and depression/anxiety. Each dimension has three levels that can be used to classify a patient at a given point of time into one of 245 states of health. On the basis of interviews undertaken with 3395 randomly selected members of the public, weights have been estimated for each of these states of health. Therefore, if prognoses can be described in terms of these various EQ-5D states of health, QALY profiles can be defined for various interventions without specially having to elicit weights.

Estimating costs

Costing exercises can be seen as a two-stage process. The first stage involves estimating the type and number of physical resources used as part of an intervention or programme or as a result of a clinical condition (e.g. the number of days in hospital, the type and grade of staff during a therapeutic procedure, and the dose and type of prophylactic antibiotics used prior to surgery). The second stage involves attaching monetary values to these measures of resource use by multiplying the resource use counts by their appropriate unit costs. For any intervention, the assessment of resource costs should not be limited to those directly associated with providing the technology, but should also consider the stream of costs associated with the course of a disease and its management.

Establishing which measures of resource to use and costs to include is determined by the perspective of the analysis. While a variety of perspectives are possible, of

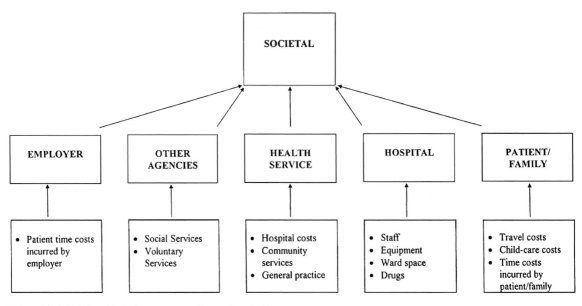

Figure 23.4 Relationship between perspective and costing.

particular importance are those based on one or more of the following: the hospital or other provider, the health service, the government, or society in general. The societal perspective represents the broadest viewpoint for an analysis, as this will include all costs regardless of who incurs them.

For example, from a societal perspective, cost is represented by the monetary value of the total resources used regardless of who incurred them; from a hospital perspective, it is the monetary value of resources used in providing treatment; and from the patient's point of view, it is the out-of-pocket expenses and impact on work and leisure time attributable to the intervention under investigation. As a result, costs are usually divided into a number of categories:

- direct health-care costs
- direct non-health-care costs
- productivity costs.

The relationship between study perspective and the categorization of costs is illustrated in Figure 23.4.

It is rapidly becoming recognized that if the objective of CEA is to identify the efficient uses of social resources for health care then the most relevant perspective for economic evaluations is the societal perspective. From the societal perspective there is no difference between health-care costs and costs outside the health-care sector, and hence no theoretical reason exists for their exclusion. For this reason, it is considered the preferred approach.

Adopting the societal perspective has several main implications that distinguish it from approaches with more limited perspectives. Firstly, it usually involves measuring and valuing resource use that do not have market prices attached to them, such as the time costs that patients incur when undergoing treatment and recuperating. Secondly, it means that certain costs should not be included in the evaluation because they represent transfers from one sector to another, rather than imposing a net cost on society (e.g. social security payments).

Although adopting an overall societal perspective in evaluating alternative allocations of health resources is important, it may also be important that particular implications to both the relevant decision makers and other parties are considered in an evaluation. While society as a whole bears all the costs, it will be the relevant organizations who actually make resource allocation decisions and who may have varying objectives that should be recognized in a CEA. Potential cost shifts between sectors may have important implications for decision makers. Full enumeration of all relevant costs and benefits in a societal evaluation, however, will enable the results to be examined from narrower perspectives.

Whether the results of analyses from alternative perspectives will differ from the social perspective will depend on the impact the intervention has on shifting costs into or out of the financial responsibility of the selected decision maker. Hence, if a more restrictive perspective is taken (e.g. hospital), the results may not hold for society as a whole and decision makers must

therefore be careful in basing policy decisions on the results of studies that take a narrower perspective. For example, assuming similar clinical outcomes, Begren *et al.* reported cost savings of 2400 SEK from laparoscopic cholecystectomy, compared with open cholecystectomy, from a societal perspective. However, the laparoscopic technique was 2000 SEK more costly from a narrower hospital perspective. In this case, the relative efficiency of laparoscopy was clearly dependent on the perspective adopted in the study.

Direct costs

Direct costs include the value of resources that are used in both the provision of an intervention and those associated with current and future consequences, which can be directly attributed to the intervention (e.g. side-effects). Typically, direct costs are separated into direct health-care costs and direct non-health-care costs.

Direct health-care costs include the costs of medications (prescription and non-prescription), devices, diagnostic tests, treatment services, prevention services, rehabilitation and training and education programmes. For example, in an evaluation of the cost-effectiveness of revascularization for femoropopliteal disease, Hunicnk *et al.* included the initial costs of inpatient and outpatient visits, the costs of amputation and rehabilitation, together with the annual costs of treatment after an amputation or with major morbidity. This category of cost is usually the dominant one in most CEAs and is often the only one considered, particularly when a narrow perspective is adopted (e.g. hospital).

When evaluating direct health-care costs it may also be important to distinguish between fixed and variable costs. Fixed costs represent the part of total cost that remains constant across the number of interventions performed (e.g. the cost of buildings, related overheads), while variable costs vary directly with the volume of services produced (e.g. consumables). This distinction is particularly important when the level of volume may have a significant impact on the relative value for money of an intervention. For example, a study of disposable versus reusable laparoscopic instruments showed that disposables generated high variable costs and zero fixed costs, while reusables generated high fixed costs and low variable costs.

In addition to direct health-care costs, other non-health-care resources may be incurred due to the intervention or its follow-up. For example, a patient may incur out-of-pocket expenses (e.g. travel costs) to attend a particular service or additional household expenditure (e.g. child care) as a direct result of an intervention. These are categorized as **direct non-health-care costs**. In a randomized trial of immediate discharge of surgical patients to general practice versus outpatient follow-up, Florey *et al.* evaluated the time taken for visits and the cost of travel incurred by the patient, as well as direct health service costs.

Valuing direct costs

The methodology of costing in a CEA should also be based on the theory of opportunity cost. Although it is generally accepted that market prices can be used as sufficiently close approximation of the opportunity cost of a resource, significant biases should be identified, and appropriate adjustments made, where prices are likely to diverge significantly from opportunity costs.

Market imperfections mean that some prices will clearly not reflect their opportunity cost. For example, a cost-to-charge ratio is often applied to US hospital charges to obtain a more accurate estimation of cost. An adjustment is necessary because the charges include an element of profit in excess of a reasonable rate of return on capital. The charge will exceed the opportunity cost to society of the resources used.

Finally, in the case of non-marketed resources (e.g. patient time, informal care), alternative methods must be used to derive 'shadow prices'. Although shadow prices do not actually exist in the market place, they represent the true social value of non-marketed resources. One of the most significant non-marketed resources is time. Attending any service requires the patient (and occasionally friends, relatives or carers) to sacrifice time (e.g. travelling to and from the service, waiting time and treatment and recovery time). This time is not a free resource; time spent receiving treatment means that time doing something else has to be given up (i.e. enjoying leisure pursuits or work time). For similar reasons, the use of unpaid resources (e.g. volunteers) also involves an opportunity cost.

As yet there is no firm consensus regarding the most appropriate technique for measuring the opportunity cost of time. The best approximation of the opportunity cost of time for working-age adults is usually seen as the wage they are or could be making, in paid work; however, this may vary according to whether the time lost involves work or leisure time and whether unemployment in the workforce exists. Alternatively, the unit cost of unpaid resources may be inferred from the market prices of related resources. For example, the unit cost of an informal carer might be based on the hourly wage rate of a care assistant.

Productivity costs

Productivity costs result from the time lost from usual activities due to both morbidity and premature mortality and are distinct from patients' (and others') time inputs into the process of health care. Costs associated with morbidity include the value of lost productivity resulting from impaired ability to work during recuperation and convalescence, and the value of lost leisure time resulting from impaired ability to participate in usual leisure activities. In contrast to morbidity costs, mortality costs result from changes to life expectancy resulting from an intervention.

The impact of productivity costs may be particularly relevant in an evaluation of surgical interventions. In an evaluation of treatment of gallstone disease by open and laparoscopic cholecystectomy and by extracorporeal shockwave lithotripsy (ESWL), Cook *et al.* reported that the results were dependent on the inclusion of productivity costs. Although laparoscopy was deemed more cost-effective than either open or ESWL with or without the inclusion of morbidity costs, by contrast, comparisons between open and ESWL were highly sensitive to the inclusion or exclusion of morbidity costs.

Valuing productivity costs

Traditionally, the human capital method, based on the individual's gross wage rate, has been used to assign a monetary value to the potential lost production as a consequence of the disease and treatment. However, the validity of this method has come under increasing scrutiny. For instance, the use of this method of valuation could discriminate against people outside the labour force (e.g. students, homemakers, the elderly). Furthermore, it has been suggested that there may be different productivity losses associated with short-term and long-term absences than suggested by the human capital approach. Productivity losses incurred as a result of short-term absences may be overestimated using the human capital approach, if either the individual makes up the lost time on return to work, or there is sufficient spare capacity within a company for workers to cover for a sick colleague. For long-term absences, the presence of unemployment may result in an individual on sick leave being replaced by someone currently unemployed, resulting in significantly lower estimates of productivity costs than implied using the human capital approach.

Another problem with valuing productivity costs is the risk of double-counting. It can be argued that generic measures of benefit already include some measure of 'productivity costs' within them. For example, individuals' valuation of lost leisure time due to morbidity is typically reflected in the quality-adjustment weight they provide for health states with a decrement in social function. Therefore, the valuation of changes in productivity in monetary terms using human capital methods within studies using QALYs risks double counting.

In critically appraising a cost analysis, it is important to be confident that all the relevant costs have been included, or adequate justification has been provided supporting their omission, given the perspective of the study.

Sources of evidence

The quality of a CEA will in part be determined by the quality of its data sources. The debate that exists in clinical evaluation about the value and feasibility of randomized, controlled trials (RCTs), relative to observational studies, also takes place in relation to economic analysis. Increasingly, RCTs are being used as a vehicle for the collection of resource use and outcome data for economic evaluation. For example, the economic analysis of laparoscopic versus open repair for inguinal hernia by Wellwood *et al.* involved the prospective collection of a range of outcome and resource use data on 400 patients randomized to either laparoscopic or open repair. In the field of surgery, RCTs are used less frequently than in other clinical areas, with practical problems relating to patient recruitment, blinding, differences in skills due to a learning curve and the length of follow-up required. It has been argued that, despite these problems, the RCT remains the design of choice for evaluating surgical procedures, and the challenge is to find solutions to the potential problems, e.g. patient preference trials.

Although the inclusion of economic evaluations alongside randomized trials has been growing in recent years, economists' input into trial design tends to be limited to advice on the type of cost data to collect and the method of its collection. There is, however, a number of important design issues, which may need to be addressed in addition to the selection of outcome measures discussed previously. An example is the sample size of a trial. As well as estimating effectiveness differences of economic importance, trialists may consider designing a study to detect important cost differences. In fields outside surgery, where trials have been primarily designed to detect differences in effectiveness, sample sizes have been shown to be too small to detect relatively large differences in costs. It would seem important, therefore, for sample size calculations to incorporate issues of cost-effectiveness, not just clinical effectiveness. To do this, it is necessary to define an economically important difference in costs and outcomes.

Modelling

Although many consider the RCT to be the ideal design to measure key parameters in an evaluation (e.g. clinical effectiveness), decision making may require these data to be augmented by information from other sources and plausible assumptions about things that are hard to measure. Decision analytic models offer a framework to synthesize data from a range of sources and assumptions regarding unmeasured (or unmeasurable) parameters. For example, although an economic evaluation may demonstrate that a given technology is cost-effective in a particular context, or cost-effective based on an intermediate outcome, uncertainty about either the generalizability of the results or the link between intermediate outcomes and final health outcomes may affect the usefulness of the findings. In these cases there is a clear role for modelling in linking intermediate clinical end-points to final outcomes (e.g. life-years saved) or generalizing results to other settings. For example, Lawrence et al., in an RCT of laparoscopic and open hernia repair, explored the impact of extrapolating short-term recurrence rates derived from the RCT to long-term recurrence rates at 2 years and 10 years and reported that the direction of cost-effectiveness was not sensitive to these assumptions.

The use of decision analysis to estimate the relative cost-effectiveness of an intervention may also be valuable in the absence of direct head-to-head RCTs involving comparisons of the intervention and comparator under investigation, or in the absence of data for certain parameters. For example, in the absence of head-to-head comparisons of proton pump inhibitors (PPIs) with surgical fundoplication for the management of patients with severe oesophagitis, Huedebert et

al. used a decision analytic model to compare the two strategies. The authors used a model to estimate the cost-utility of the two interventions using probabilities derived from the literature and a modified Delphi panel to obtain estimates of utilities and probabilities that were not available in the literature.

Time horizon

For many conditions, particularly chronic ones, the resource implications and effects on patients' health take place over many years. It is, therefore, important that an economic assessment has a time horizon that is consistent with the duration of these effects. For example, in an evaluation of medical costs following coronary angioplasty or bypass surgery for angina, the initial direct health-care cost of angioplasty was 65% that of surgery; however, after 5 years this figure had risen to 95% that of surgery. In these circumstances, it may be inappropriate to reach definite conclusions about the relative cost-effectiveness prior to adequate follow-up.

The time dimension of costs and outcomes gives rise to another key concept in economic analysis, that of the process of discounting costs and benefits. Discounting involves adjusting future costs and benefits downwards to express them in terms of their present value. The rationale for discounting can be explained in two ways. The first of these is positive time preference, which suggests that as individuals and as society we prefer good things (such as improvements in our health) earlier and bad things (such as resource costs) later. Therefore, costs and outcomes that occur in the future are valued less than those that occur in the present. Discounting is an attempt to reflect this preference in the calculus of economic evaluation. Evidence indicates that individuals' intertemporal preferences are rather more complex than discounting assumes.

The second interpretation of discounting is the concept of opportunity cost introduced earlier. The clearest illustration of this is that if £50 000 is used to buy a piece of surgical equipment today, the interest that could have been earned had the money been placed in a bank deposit is lost. Hence, the cost of employing a resource today can be considered greater than that in 10 years' time because of the opportunity costs that are incurred over the 10-year period. The opportunity cost rationale is firmer when discounting relates to costs rather than to outcomes, and this is one reason why the discounting of outcomes at the same rate as costs in an economic evaluation has been questioned. In practice, existing guidelines in the UK recommend discounting costs at 6% and health outcomes at 1.5–2%.

Dealing with uncertainty

All cost-effectiveness analyses produce estimates of the costs and outcomes of interventions in conditions of uncertainty. This will be associated with the data inputs, such as estimates of resource use, the probability of particular clinical events and the unit costs of resources; the methods of analysis used, such as the discount rate employed; and the extent to which the analysis can be

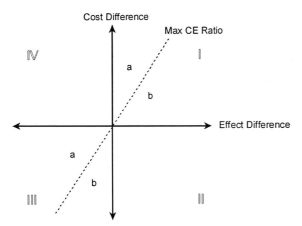

Figure 23.5 The cost-effectiveness plane: a diagrammatic representation of the costs and outcomes of two interventions.

generalized to routine clinical practice. For particular inputs, the analyst may have a very good knowledge of what the true values are based on clinical trials and observational studies. For other aspects of the study, however, the current level of certainty concerning the correct value may be extremely limited.

In a sensitivity analysis, some integral inputs in the analysis are changed by a meaningful amount or varied from worst case to best case, and the impact on the cost-effectiveness of an intervention is recalculated. The resulting difference provides the decision maker with an indication of how sensitive the results are to a substantial but not implausible change in that parameter. If the major results are insensitive to a reasonable variation in a parameter, then the decision maker can be relatively sure that the conclusions are robust to the assumptions made about that parameter. In cases where variations in parameters cause wide divergences in the results, threshold analysis can be performed to identify critical values of particular inputs, which cause the results to change. The decision maker can then make assessments of the relative likelihood of each scenario before deciding whether to implement the programme.

Decision rules in economic evaluation

Comparing costs and outcomes

The assessment of relative cost-effectiveness requires a formal comparison of costs and outcomes to ascertain whether any of the conditions detailed in Figure 23.2 exist, based on some clear decision rules.

This process is illustrated in Figure 23.5, which is often referred to as the cost-effectiveness plane. To explain this diagram, assume that the costs and outcomes of two treatment options, A and B, are being compared. The vertical axis of the graph shows the differential cost of the two interventions ($Cost_A$ minus $Cost_B$): A is more costly than B above the origin, and B is more costly below the origin. The horizontal axis relates to the differential outcomes achieved by the two options ($Outcome_A$ minus $Outcome_B$): A is more effective to the right of the origin and B is more effective to the left of the origin. On this basis, it is possible to define four

quadrants. In quadrant I, A is more costly and more effective; in quadrant II, A is less costly and more effective; in quadrant III, A is less effective and less costly; and in quadrant IV, A is more costly and less effective.

Establishing the presence of dominance

The most straightforward decision rule concerning relative cost-effectiveness states that if an intervention, say A, falls into quadrant II, and A is less costly and more effective, it is said to 'dominate' B. Similarly, if the comparison fell into quadrant IV, A would be more costly and less effective, and would be dominated by B. Under either of these conditions, the decision maker would feel safe in concluding that the dominant option was the more cost-effective.

Assessing relative efficiency when dominance is not established

In practice, it is rare that the costs and outcomes in an economic study lend themselves to the dominance rule, and it is usually the case that one option is more effective than the other, but also more costly (quadrants I and II in Figure 23.5). The critical issue here is whether the additional cost (referred to as the incremental cost) is worth paying for the additional benefits (incremental benefits). The decision rules developed to address this issue focus on the incremental cost per additional unit of outcome of A relative to B. This is calculated as ($Cost_A$ minus $Cost_B$)/($Outcome_A$ minus $Outcome_B$), and is represented by the gradient of the dotted line in quadrant 1.

When non-dominance exists, the characteristics of outcome measures described earlier become all-important. The first important characteristic is that the outcome measure used in a study should be unidimensional in order that it is unequivocal that one intervention is more effective and that it is possible to express additional costs and effects in the form of an incremental ratio.

The second important characteristic of an outcome measure when there is no dominance is the level of efficiency in which the decision maker is interested. If the decision maker is a team of clinicians concerned with maximizing the outcomes achieved in the management of a specific condition, the outcome measure they use can simply be relevant to that condition. If, however, the decision maker is a purchaser responsible for maximizing the benefits from health care in a range of specialties and disease areas, the outcome measure required should be generic, i.e. it should have meaning across the whole health-care system. Although it is helpful to think of CEA being used to inform decision making at these two different levels, it is important to recognize that while a generic measure can address efficiency at both levels, condition-specific measures will be restricted to decisions at the disease level only.

Level of decision making: disease area

If the decision maker is concerned with maximizing the outcomes that can be achieved from a fixed budget in a specific clinical area, the requirements are that the outcome measure adopted in an economic appraisal should be relevant to the clinical area, an adequate representation of the differential effectiveness to the options under consideration, unidimensional and widely used in studies undertaken to inform resource allocation in that area. There are several of examples in the surgical field of studies to inform decision making at this level. For example, in evaluating laparoscopic versus inguinal hernia repair, Lawrence et al. reported the incremental cost of laparoscopic repair per pain-free day and Liem et al. reported the incremental cost per recurrence avoided.

In order to maximize the outcomes achieved in a clinical area, the decision maker would need to compare the ratios reported in all relevant studies and allocate additional resources to those programmes with the lower incremental ratios, or fund these interventions by removing funding from the programmes with relatively high ratios. In practice, there are enormous difficulties in obtaining sufficient information to facilitate such a ranking process. Information on the costs and benefits are required for all possible interventions in a given disease area. Such data are neither routinely collected nor easy to generate.

Level of decision making: health-care system

Although the choice of a unidimensional, condition-specific measure of outcome may be deemed sufficient for decisions within a disease area, health-care purchasers are likely to take a broader perspective in terms of the outcomes they are trying to maximize. In principle, their focus is on decisions at the level of the whole health-care system. This involves judgements about the relative value of outcomes achieved in clinical areas as diverse as surgery and gerontology, which means that condition-specific outcomes need to be translated into a generic measure of benefit (e.g. QALYs) that has meaning in all of these areas. Hence, it is recommended that studies incorporate a generic measure of HRQL that generates weights for QALYs alongside any condition-specific measures. Lawrence et al., in a study comparing laparoscopic with open inguinal hernia, assessed HRQL using EuroQol (EQ-5D) and measured pain using a linear analogue scale, allowing decision makers to address the relative cost-effectiveness of the intervention at both levels.

In a similar manner to decisions performed at the level of disease area, economic evaluations using QALYs also relate costs and outcomes in the form of a ratio: the incremental cost per additional QALY. Although this form of analysis is essentially a special case of CEA, it is usually referred to as a cost–utility analysis. For example, in a cost–utility analysis of laser-assisted angioplasty for patients with peripheral arterial occlusions, Sculpher et al. estimated that the incremental cost per QALY generated by the use of a laser, over standard angiography, was £3040 for patients with claudication and £1810 for patients with rest pain or ulceration.

In contrast to CEAs using condition-specific measures of outcome, if a new intervention is both more expensive and generates greater effectiveness, then the use of a single index measure of health benefit enables diverse programmes or interventions, producing different types of health outcomes, to be compared. Consequently, the impact of reducing other programmes to fund the new intervention can be addressed because the additional benefits derived from adopting the new intervention can be compared to the lost benefits from reducing alternative interventions or programmes. QALY-based analyses have the potential advantage of moving beyond questions relating to the relative efficiency within a specific disease area to issues relating to the relative cost-effectiveness of different interventions across a variety of clinical areas.

In practice, there are enormous difficulties in obtaining sufficient information to facilitate such a ranking process. Information on the costs and benefits is required for all possible health problems and for all alternative interventions. The paucity of available data on the cost-effectiveness of interventions across the entire health sector was widely recognized as a major deficiency in the Oregon priority setting process. Similarly, the use of cost-effectiveness league tables has been criticized because of the methodological differences between many of the studies and the limited programmes included.

It is evident that CEA is unlikely to provide a complete technical solution to the problem of allocating resources in the health-care sector. However, adopting an economic way of thinking (i.e. considering a broad range of alternatives and assessing their relative costs and benefits) is vital if the evaluation of interventions is to be based on explicit and accountable criteria.

Conclusions

CEA is increasingly used in health-care decision making. It is important to be aware of the various components of a study and to be able to judge its quality.

Section 23.5 • Legal aspects of surgical practice

In relation to personal injuries litigation, the practice of surgery is governed by the law of torts (civil wrongs) and contract law. This section will consider the law from a UK perspective, but reference will also be made to case law from other Anglo-American legal systems, such as the USA, Canada and Australia, since the law in these countries is similar to that of the UK. There are several separate legal systems in the UK, but the law in each of these jurisdictions is broadly similar, hence this chapter will refer to 'UK law', for simplicity.

Torts (civil wrongs)

In the UK, it is generally accepted that no contract exists between a doctor and a patient who is receiving treatment under the NHS. In such cases, the law of torts, rather than contract law, applies. An NHS Trust or Health Board is responsible for the acts or omission of each of its employees, and that body will generally be sued, rather than the surgeon, personally. Surgeons should, however, ensure that they subscribe to a medical defence society, to cover legal expenses arising from coroners' inquests and fatal accident inquiries, appearances before disciplinary bodies such as the General Medical Council, and claims arising from work performed outside the NHS, such as the treatment of private clients.

Consent: the tort of 'battery'

Any touching of a patient without his or her agreement is generally regarded by the law as an 'assault' or 'battery'. This entitles the aggrieved patient to sue the surgeon for financial recompense. The importance that the law places on the requirement for consent arises from a recognition of a patient's moral right to self-determination and bodily autonomy. In 1914, in the American case of *Schloendorff v Society of New York Hospital*, this was expressed as follows.

> **Every human being of adult years and sound mind has a right to determine what shall be done with his own body; and a surgeon who performs an operation without his patient's consent commits an assault.**

Despite the use of the emotive terms 'battery' and 'assault', the courts have made clear that no overtly hostile intention or motive on the part of the person doing the 'touching' needs to be established. This is illustrated by the Canadian case of *Malette v Shulman* (1988), in which a Jehovah's Witness was given a blood transfusion without her consent. The surgeon acted from the best of motives – to save the patient's life – but was nonetheless successfully sued.

Capacity to consent

The reference in *Schloendorff* to the patient being 'of adult years and sound mind' serves to remind us that not all patients have the capacity to consent to treatment. In the UK, a person is 'of adult years' for the purposes of medical treatment once he or she has attained the age of 16. Following the case of *Gillick v West Norfolk and Wisbech Area Health Authority* in 1986, children who are younger than this may also be competent to give consent if their doctors judge that they are sufficiently mature to understand a procedure and its consequences.

In the case of younger children, parental consent must be sought. Dr James Taylor, an eminent cardiologist, was recently found guilty of serious professional misconduct by the UK General Medical Council when he undertook a high-risk operation on a child without her parents' consent. Indeed, the parents had expressly refused to consent to the procedure. The child died the day after the operation and Dr Taylor may now face a suit for battery.

A patient who is unconscious is, of course, unable to give consent. In such circumstances a surgeon may undertake essential, emergency surgery without consent, so long as there is no reason to suppose that the patient, if competent, would have withheld consent. This is based on the idea that the doctor is acting out of necessity to save the patient's life or to safeguard his or her health. In the case of *Re R (a minor) (wardship: consent to treatment)* in 1992, Lord Donaldson MR stated:

> **... in cases of an emergency a doctor may treat the patient notwithstanding the absence of consent, if the patient is unconscious or otherwise incapable of giving or refusing consent and there is no one else sufficiently immediately available with authority to consent on behalf of the patient.**

It should be noted, however, that third parties cannot generally give consent even where an adult patient is incompetent. The common medical practice of obtaining consent from relatives when a patient is unable to consent for him or herself is a matter of good medical practice and courtesy only. In the case of *Re F (mental patient: sterilization)* in 1990 Lord Goff stated:

> **Where ... a surgeon performs an operation without his consent on a patient temporarily rendered unconscious in an accident, he should do no more than is reasonably required, in the best interests of the patient, before he recovers consciousness.**
>
> **... The point has however arisen in a more acute form where a surgeon, in the course of an operation, discovers some other condition which, in his opinion, requires operative treatment for which he has not received the patient's consent. In what circumstances he should operate forthwith, and in what circumstances he should postpone the further treatment until he has received the patient's consent, is a difficult matter ...**

In the unreported case of *Bartley v Studd* the patient had consented to a hysterectomy operation. During the procedure, the surgeon removed the patient's ovaries. He did not have consent for this, and this part of the procedure was not urgently medically necessary. The patient successfully sued the surgeon for battery. Similarly, in *Murray v McMurchy* a surgeon who sterilized a patient during a caesarean operation was successfully sued. The sterilization was not immediately medically necessary, and it would not have been unreasonable to have postponed the operation to allow the patient's own views to be determined. In contrast to this, in *Marshall v Curry* the surgeon removed a diseased testicle during a hernia operation. The suit failed since the surgeon was able to show that removal was necessary 'in the interest of his patient and for the protection of his health'. *Marshall v Curry* was decided in 1933, when the risks posed by anaesthetics were greater, and it is questionable whether a similar case would be decided the same way today.

It is important to note that a patient can succeed in a battery action even where no actual physical injury has been caused – the fact that the patient did not consent is sufficient.

'Informed' consent

In the majority of cases, a patient's complaint is not that he or she gave no consent whatever to the operation, but rather that the consent was not a 'true' or 'fully informed' one, since the surgeon did not reveal all of the risks inherent in the operation. It must be emphasized that consent is a process – it is more than a signature on a piece of paper. Some of the discussions following the recent outcry over the Bristol intensive care trial suggest that not all doctors appreciate this. It has been alleged that 43 babies died as a result of an experimental treatment, and the parents of some of these children are claiming that they did not give fully informed consent. A representative from North Staffordshire NHS Trust has attempted to counter this by stating that the Trust holds consent forms signed by all the parents.

In the case of *Chatterton v Gerson* it was stated that 'once the patient is informed in broad terms of the nature of the procedure which is intended, and gives her consent, that consent is real'. This suggests that a surgeon need not describe the operation in minute detail to a patient before it can be said that the patient is capable of giving valid consent. However, a consent can only be considered to be meaningful if the patient understands the necessity for the operation, and the likely prognosis should the patient decline to consent to it. The potential benefits likely to flow from a successful operation and alternative treatments should also be discussed with patients. Any material risks or side-effects associated with the procedure ought to be explained. This begs the question as to what is considered to be a 'material' risk.

The courts have tended to restrict the operation of the 'battery' action to cases in which the patient alleges that he or she did not give any consent whatever to the operation that was actually performed. Where a patient concedes that consent was given, but claims that this was not based on adequate information about the risks associated with the operation, the courts have held that an action for negligence is the more appropriate remedy. This will be discussed further below.

The tort of negligence

A patient who alleges that he or she has been harmed by a surgeon will not succeed in obtaining compensation unless it can be proved, on the balance of probabilities, that:

- the surgeon in question owed the patient a duty of care
- the surgeon breached that duty of care (i.e. that the surgeon was 'negligent') and
- the breach has caused, or materially contributed to, loss or damage to the patient.

The 'balance of probabilities' means that a patient must satisfy a court that his or her allegations are more likely to be true than not.

That a duty of care is owed by a surgeon to a patient is rarely in dispute; once a surgeon agrees to operate on a patient, the former owes the latter a duty to act with reasonable care. This duty was described in the 1925 case of *R. v Bateman*, in relation to doctors in general, as follows:

> **If [the doctor] accepts the responsibility and undertakes the treatment and the patient submits to his discretion and treatment accordingly, he owes a duty to the patient to use diligence, care, knowledge, skill and caution in administering the treatment.**

In the important case of *Bolam v Friern Hospital Management Committee* in 1957, McNair J. directed the jury that a doctor

> **… is not guilty of negligence if he has acted in accordance with a practice accepted as proper by a responsible body of medical men skilled in that particular art.**
> **… Putting it the other way round, a [doctor] is not negligent, if he is acting in accordance with such a practice, merely because there is a body of opinion who would take a contrary view.**

What amounts to 'reasonable care' is judged in the light of procedures common at the time of the alleged negligence – that is, the standards prevalent at the time of the operation – a surgeon is not judged by the application of hindsight.

As McNair J. stated in *Bolam*, if there are differing bodies of opinion as to the preferred treatment, a judge is not at liberty simply to pick the one that he or she prefers. Hence, in *Maynard v West Midlands Regional Health Authority* it was stated that:

> **It is not enough to show that there is a body of competent professional opinion which considers that [the surgeon's decision] was a wrong decision, if there also exists a body of professional opinion, equally competent, which supports the decision as reasonable in the circumstances.**

Furthermore, differences of opinion and practice exist and will always exist, in the medical as in other professions. There is seldom any one answer exclusive of all others to problems of professional judgement. A court may prefer one body of opinion to the other, but that is no basis for a conclusion of negligence. The court in *Bolam* approved the Scottish case of *Hunter v Hanley* (1955) in which it was stated:

> **In the realm of diagnosis and treatment there is ample scope for genuine differences of opinion and one man is clearly not negligent merely because his conclusion differs from that of other professional men, nor because he has displayed less skill or knowledge than others would have shown. The true test for establishing negligence in diagnosis or treatment on the part of a doctor is whether he has been proved to be guilty of such failure as no doctor or ordinary skill would be guilty of if acting with ordinary care.**

A surgeon has a duty to be aware of important medical advances: he or she is not expected to have read every article in every medical journal, however obscure, but ought to be familiar with seminal papers, in mainstream journals. The fact that a junior surgeon has less experience than others is no defence to a negligence suit, but it may be relevant to the issue of whether supervision of the less experienced surgeon should have been provided by his or her mentors, or the hospital.

Res ipsa loquitur

This Latin tag means literally 'the facts of the case speak for themselves'. In some cases the very fact that a person has been injured raises an inference that someone has been negligent. The courts are reluctant to apply this principle to cases of alleged medical negligence, and it will generally only operate where the injury to the patient is one that manifestly ought not to have occurred had due care been exercised. The fact that a patient has suffered a catastrophic injury will not of itself allow the patient to rely on this principle. This point is illustrated by the case of *Howard v Wessex Regional Health Authority* (1994) in relation to a patient who had been rendered tetraplegic.

The principle was successfully applied in the case of *Clark v MacLellan* (1983). The surgeon was negligent in performing an anterior colporrhaphy at an inappropriate time, within 4 weeks from the patient having given birth. This should not have been performed until 3 months after birth. According to Peter Pain J.:

> **Where ... there is but one orthodox course of treatment and [the surgeon] chooses to depart from that, his position is different. It is not enough for him to say as to his decision simply that it was based on his clinical judgment. One has to inquire whether he took all proper factors into account, which he knew or should have known, and whether his departure from the orthodox course can be justified on the basis of these factors.**

A common situation in which the principle of *res ipsa loquitur* is applied is in relation to the 'swab cases'. While a surgeon is not responsible for the negligence of other members of the medical team, such as theatre nurses, merely because the surgeon is in charge of the operation, the responsibility for ensuring that all extraneous objects are ultimately removed from the patient's body lies with the surgeon. In the case of *Mahon v Osborne* in 1939, Lord Justice Goddard stated:

> **If ... a swab is left in the patient's body, it seems to me clear that the surgeon is called on for an explanation, that is, he is called on to show not necessarily why he missed it but that he exercised due care to prevent it being left there.**

In the American case of *Ravi v Coates* it was held that a surgeon could not shift his liability for the leaving of a sponge in a body cavity by explaining that he had delegated the task of counting the sponges. In *Frandle v MacKenzie*, a Canadian case, a surgical sponge had been left in the patient following a hip operation. The surgeon had failed to order a final count of the sponges and was held to be 80% to blame, with the nurses 20% liable.

Causation

A patient must show that the surgeon breached his or her duty of care to the patient (in other words, that the surgeon was negligent) but also that this breach caused the patient's injury. Failure to establish this causal link between the surgeon's behaviour and the injury will result in failure of the patient's claim for compensation. This is illustrated by the case of *Barnett v Chelsea and Kensington Hospital Management Committee* (1969). The patient attended his local casualty department, complaining of acute stomach pains, but the doctor advised the patient to go home, without having examined him. The patient died of arsenic poisoning, and it was accepted that the doctor had been negligent in not attending to him. However, it transpired that there was no cure for the patient's condition; had he been seen by the doctor, the patient would still have died. His widow was accordingly unable to show that the doctor's negligence had caused the patient's death, hence her suit for compensation did not succeed.

Negligence and consent

As already noted, where a patient alleges that his or her consent to an operation was not based on adequate information about the risks associated with that operation, then an action based on negligence is more appropriate than one based on battery. It is part of a surgeon's duty to act with reasonable care towards a patient that the patient should be given appropriate information about an operation before being asked to consent to it.

The leading case is that of *Sidaway v Board of Governors of the Bethlem Royal Hospital and the Maudsley Hospital* (1985). The patient had suffered from pain in her shoulder and neck for a number of years. Her consultant neurosurgeon recommended that she have an operation to her spinal column to alleviate the pain. Mrs Sidaway was warned that the nerve root might be disturbed as a result of the operation but she was not told that there was a risk of spinal cord damage, which could render her paraplegic. The former risk was assessed at a 2% chance, and the latter represented a less than 1% risk. Unfortunately, the latter risk materialized and she became severely disabled as a result. The House of Lords, the supreme court in the UK in cases of personal injury, decided that the risk that in fact materialized was too remote, and that Mrs Sidaway's surgeon was under no duty to warn her about such a risk, in order for her consent to be valid.

The test for determining whether a risk was to be regarded as material or not was based on the *Bolam* standard, as previously described; in other words, the surgeon would not be considered to have been negligent in failing to advise Mrs Sidaway of this risk if there was evidence that a responsible body of surgeons would have acted similarly, in the circumstances. In the Scottish case of *Moyes v Lothian Health Board* (1990) Lord Caplan stated:

> **As I see it the law in both Scotland and England has come down firmly against the view that the**

doctor's duty to the patient involves at all costs obtaining the informed consent of the patient to specific medical treatments. When the patient entrusts himself to the doctor he expects, and is entitled, to be kept fully informed about decisions which have to be taken and which may concern his welfare but the paramount expectation is that the doctor will do what is best to care for the patient's health. In general it will be consistent with that primary responsibility that the doctor should acquaint the patient with the risks facing him and that becomes particularly critical when the risk is a severe risk for, as Lord Bridge observes in *Sidaway*, in such a case the patient may want to be able to decide whether he should submit himself to a significant risk or even secure a second opinion.

How 'significant' does a risk have to be before a surgeon is required to mention it to a patient? The risk associated with the procedure in the case of *Moyes* was 0.2–0.3%. This was described by the court as a 'slight risk', not a material one. In the American case of *Canterbury v Spence* it was held that a 1% risk of paralysis resulting from a laminectomy was of sufficient magnitude to warrant being disclosed to the patient. In the *Sidaway* case Lord Bridge referred to a 'substantial' risk of a grave adverse consequence as being a 10% risk of a stroke. He stated that a patient ought to be appraised of this magnitude of risk. As we have seen, the injury that ultimately became manifest in the *Sidaway* case was based on a risk of less than 1%, and it was held that this risk was too remote to be mentioned. In contrast to this, in the case of *Newell v Goldenberg* it was held that a surgeon was negligent in failing to warn the patient of a 1: 2300 risk of failure in a sterilization operation. Which risks need to be communicated to a patient very much depend on the usual practice of surgeons who commonly undertake such operations. In the *Moyes* case, Lord Caplan referred to the decision in *Sidaway*, and concluded:

> … I can read nothing in the majority view in *Sidaway* which suggests that the extent and quality of warning to be given by a doctor to his patient should not in the last resort be governed by medical criteria.

In the more recent case of *Bolitho v City and Hackney Health Authority* (1997) it was stated by Lord Browne-Wilkinson in the House of Lords that:

> … the court is not bound to hold that a defendant doctor escapes liability for negligent treatment or diagnosis just because he leads evidence from a number of medical experts who are genuinely of opinion that the defendant's treatment or diagnosis accorded with sound medical practice.

Here, the courts are stressing that it is a matter of law whether the doctor in question has fallen below the standard of reasonable care, i.e. it is not the case that the medical profession sets its own standard. Despite the fact that lip-service is paid to this principle, the courts rely on the testimony of other doctors to provide evidence of what can be expected from a doctor in partic-

ular circumstances, and the courts are very reluctant to hold that a practice accepted by medical practitioners themselves is nonetheless a negligent one.

The Australian case of *Roger v Whitaker* provides a rare example of a court being prepared to criticize a standard set by a medical professional body. The case involved an opthalmologist who had not warned a patient of a 1:14 000 risk of blindness associated with a procedure. Despite the fact that it was accepted medical practice not to warn patients of this remote risk, the doctor was found to have been negligent in failing to do so.

Explanations given to patients about surgical procedures should not be couched in complex medical terminology; patients need to be given information that they can understand. It should be borne in mind that patients appear to remember little of the information that is given to them prior to surgery. Ideally, the surgeon who is to perform an operation ought to be responsible for obtaining the informed consent of the patient. It is advisable for a separate member of the medical team to discuss the procedure with the patient, also. Patients generally find it easier to talk to nurses than surgeons and may be more able to ask questions of the nurse.

It has been suggested that following any skin incision, numbness may result in the area surrounding the wound. This is unavoidable, but may cause patients some distress if they have not been warned in advance. All surgical procedures are associated with some bleeding, and wound haematomas may occur. A patient properly prepared is more likely accept these problems than a patient who has been given no preoperative information (Hobsley and Scurr).

The authors also suggested that almost one-third of patients over the age of 40 years who undergo major surgery may develop an isotopically detectable deep vein thrombosis. They recommend that all patients be assessed to determine the risk of this, and suitable precautions taken. This may include giving such patients heparin after surgery.

What else ought a surgeon to tell his or her patient? In the Canadian case of *Casey v Provan* it was held that the surgeon was not under a duty to inform a patient that a major part of the surgery would be carried out by a senior resident surgeon rather than by a vascular surgeon, and according to *Hopp v Lepp* a surgeon is under no duty to tell a patient that the operation is the first of its kind that the surgeon will have performed.

Recording consent

Consent need not be in writing: it may be oral or implicit. The importance of obtaining written consent lies in the fact that it is much easier to establish that a patient did in fact consent to a procedure if there is a signature from the patient. An injured party generally has 3 years within which to commence litigation for personal injury, but this period may be extended by the court, hence there may be a considerable time gap between a patient undergoing an operation and the surgeon being required to demonstrate that consent was in fact obtained. Written consent to all but the most minor procedures is therefore recommended. In *Chatterton v Gerson* reference was made to consent forms:

> **… getting the patient to sign a pro forma expressing consent to undergo the operation 'the effect and nature of which have been explained to me,' as was done here in each case, should be a valuable reminder to everyone of the need for explanation and consent. But it would be no defence to an action … if no explanation had in fact been given. The consent would have been expressed in form only, not in reality.**

In the Canadian case of *Ferguson v Hamilton Civic Hospitals* the surgeon explained the procedure and risks of an angiography to a patient after the patient had been given tranquillizers and while the patient was outside the operating theatre. It was held that this was negligent. It should be noted that the patient's case failed, nonetheless, since the surgeon's negligence had not **caused** the patient's injury; the patient would have undertaken the medical treatment even if he had been fully informed of the risks involved. This case reminds us of the third hurdle facing patients in a negligence suit: the requirement to prove that the surgeon's negligence actually caused the patient's injury.

Examples of negligence

Diagnosis

In *Taylor v West Kent Health Authority* failure to follow up a cytology report with a biopsy in a case of suspected breast cancer was held to be negligent. Negligence was also established in the case of *Judge v Huntington Health Authority*, in which the surgeon had failed to detect a 5-mm breast lump.

The diagnosis of gastroenteritis in a patient with appendicitis was negligent in the case of *Daniels v Kay*. The patient was advised that it was safe for her to travel to Singapore. Her appendix burst on arrival in that country and the patient was awarded £23 750 in compensation.

During surgery

Harpwood cites figures from the Medical Defence Union to the effect that allegations of medical negligence arising from keyhole surgery have increased by 50% in the past 7 years. A quarter of cases involves the perforation of intestines or blood vessels. In *Myles v West Kent Health Authority* the surgeon was negligent in cutting a patient's bile duct during keyhole surgery to removal her gallbladder and the patient was awarded £60 000 compensation.

In *Carter v City and Hackney Health Authority* a surgeon who punctured a patient's gallbladder while making three attempts to carry out a liver biopsy was held to have been negligent. In the Canadian case of *Andree v Pierce* the surgeon attempted to complete within 10 min a laryngotomy, that generally required between 30 and 45 min of surgery. He caused a haemorrhage and the court determined that his haste was

evidence of negligence. In *Chaunt v Hertfordshire Area Health Authority* a woman who became pregnant after a negligently performed sterilization operation was awarded compensation. She had been required to undergo two further operations.

Postoperatively

Patients need to be monitored following surgical operations and failure to monitor is common grounds for a medical negligence suit. In *Newbury v Bath District Health Authority* a patient who suffered a loss of sensation succeeded in establishing that this was due to a lack of proper postoperative care. She was left severely disabled and was awarded £200 000 in compensation.

Contract law

Where a patient is treated privately, rather than under the auspices of the NHS, there may be a contract between the patient and his or her surgeon, and a surgeon who breaches that contract may be sued for damages. In general, a surgeon owes similar duties of care as a result of contract law as previously described in relation to tort law. However, a surgeon who guarantees certain results may be liable to compensate a patient if these results do not materialize. This is illustrated by the case of *Thake v Maurice*, in which the patient alleged that his surgeon had guaranteed the success of a sterilization operation. It was decided by the court that the surgeon would only be taken to have offered such a guarantee of success if he had expressly stated so, in clear terms. The surgeon was, however, found liable for failing to warn the patient of the possibility of natural reversal. In the Canadian case of *La Fleur v Cornelis* a surgeon promised his patient that she would be happy with the results of an operation to reduce the size of her nose. He did not, however, warn her of the risks of deformity inherent in the operation, and was liable to compensate the patient for scarring and deformity.

Conclusions

The law recognizes that medicine is not an exact science, and accepts that the mere fact that a patient's operation has not been entirely successful is not necessarily evidence that the surgeon has been negligent. In *Thake v Maurice* the judge stated:

> **It is the common experience of mankind that the results of medical treatment are to some extent unpredictable and that any treatment may be affected by the special characteristics of the particular patient. It has been well said that 'the dynamics of the human body of each individual are themselves individual'.**

Communication with the patient is of paramount importance. Patients who have been advised in advance about the possibility of a less than satisfactory outcome are much less inclined to seek legal redress when such risks materialize. Where negligence is involved, an honest explanation given to the patient at an early stage may also help to lessen the likelihood of suit; many patients resort to the legal process in an attempt to find out what went wrong, rather than for financial recompense.

Section 23.6 • The Internet

This section contains an introduction to the facilities offered via the global communications system known as the Internet. The approach is to provide a guided tour of the services available for accessing and exchanging electronic information. It is hoped that by removing some of the mystique and exposing the underlying technology, surgeons will be placed in a better position to access and use the Internet as a valuable means of continued professional development during their careers.

Nature and resources offered by the Internet

One view of the Internet is that of a communications network than spans the globe, rather like the telephone network with which we are all familiar. The major differences are that the telephone network requires a telephone at both ends of the link with information transferred using speech, whereas the Internet requires a computer at either end of the link and the information is transferred in a form that humans cannot readily interpret. Another significant difference is that while the cost of a telephone call depends on the distance to the destination, the cost of transferring information over the Internet is independent of the distance involved and is normally charged at a rate equivalent to the cost of a local telephone call. This has led to a flourishing growth in the use of the Internet as a low-cost substitute for long-distance telephone calls, but this is just one of many potential benefits.

Telephones have a unique identifying number that is dialled in order to establish a link with their owner. Similarly, every computer connected to the Internet has a unique identifying number by which it can be contacted. However, with a telephone one may have to carry a telephone directory of contact names and associated numbers, whereas to access a user via the Internet they can be referred to by name, e.g. ricketts computing.dundee.ac.uk, and the translation to their unique Internet identifying number will be automatically handled by the computer.

Individual computers are capable of storing and retrieving considerable amounts of information without appreciable delay. When connected together, this potential resource is multiplied. Estimates vary as to the number of computers connected to the Internet, but in the UK it is in excess of 5 million (ref: http://www.headcount.com/), with potentially 100 million world-wide and growing rapidly.

Let us assume that your particular interests make you 1:1000, i.e. in a random sample of 1000 people there will be one who will share your interest in a particular topic. Then, given the 100 million users of the Internet there could be 100 000 users who share that particular interest. Let us further assume that only one in 100 of those users will speak your language and share your culture. This would mean that there are 1000 people accessible via the Internet, for the cost of a local telephone call, who share your interest and with whom you can communicate. The potential opportunity therefore exists to exchange knowledge with these 1000 users to your mutual benefit.

The potential for sharing information is one of the factors that fuels the expansion in the use of the Internet. The following sections aim to outline some of the facilities offered by the Internet that may benefit readers.

Electronic mail

Electronic mail (e-mail) is a facility for exchanging via the Internet much of what can currently be exchanged via the normal postal services. Letters, memos, charts and pictures can be sent just as readily as faxes are currently sent. In addition, attachments can be included such as sound extracts, video recordings, computer software, previously written reports and animations. Anything that can be stored on a computer can be transmitted (and received) using e-mail to anyone connected to the Internet anywhere in the world. Particularly noteworthy is that the e-mail message will normally arrive at its destination computer within minutes of being sent and will cost the equivalent of a local telephone call.

Rapid access to research reports

A significant proportion of every researcher's effort is applied to maintaining contact with the frontiers of development within their speciality. This used to be achieved via frequent trips to the local libraries and/or significant investment in journals. Despite the best endeavours of journal editors the delays associated with paper publications meant that findings would typically between 6 months and 2 years behind the time when the information was first made available. Now publication via the Internet offers the potential to reduce significantly and possibly to remove this delay altogether.

A further problem facing the active researcher is the task of locating articles containing relevant information within the large volume of publications available. This previously depended on careful searching of likely journals and the associated citation indices and various published abstracts. Now, with electronic indexing of journal articles, the search process can be handled rapidly using computers and the abstracts can be inspected via the Internet without even moving from the desktop computer.

The Internet is quickly becoming the first-choice medium because it offers a low-cost channel for the speedy communication of research findings to a world-wide audience. This move is supported and encouraged in the UK by several of the research funding bodies who request that research findings are made available via the Internet as well as by the more traditional routes to publication of non-electronic journals and conferences.

Libraries of software, images and videos

The software industry has long promoted the concept of reuse, although with limited mechanisms for rapid and low-cost distribution the implementation of the concept was constrained. The advent of the Internet providing rapid access to remote sites has revolutionized distribution in this as in many other areas. There was a significant volume of very good material available either free or at replication costs via the Public Domain and Shareware suppliers using postal services. However, the problems of locating appropriate material are similar to those associated with locating appropriate research publications, and were only overcome with the availability of software libraries accessible via the Internet.

Teaching and learning materials

The preparation of material for teaching and learning is extremely time-consuming. Estimates for the time spent producing such materials vary considerably, according to an author's familiarity with the topic, the extent of supporting material required, ease of access to means of production, experience, etc. Estimates for the time taken to prepare a 1-h lecture vary from 10 to 100 h. There is therefore considerable benefit to be gained from reusing materials created by other authors in return for due credit. The Internet is a particularly rich source of teaching and learning material. This is due in part to academic staff granting access to the material that they produce. Another rich source of material is the many companies who provide information to support their users and to attract new customers.

Special-interest groups

As their name suggests, special-interest groups (SIGs) are formed by Internet users who have a common interest, e.g. 3D graphics, orthopaedics or model aircraft. A group offers a forum where members can send, via e-mail, details of technical problems that they may have and that other members of the group can then read and respond to. The questions and any replies are collected together so that in time the group creates a corporate memory, which is available to all. Members also post details of book reviews and forthcoming conferences or any information that may be of interest to the group. Often, a subgroup of the more experienced members will assemble a set of frequently asked questions (FAQs) and their answers. New members are encouraged to consult the FAQs before posting questions to the group. FAQs can significantly reduce the volume of e-mail traffic within SIGs.

Gaining access to the Internet

Selecting a suitable personal computer

Let us assume that you have no access to computer equipment and little or no knowledge of what you require. Approach the problem in the same way as you would buying a new car. You would first decide what type of role you envisaged for the car, e.g. a large-capacity vehicle for family holidays or a compact vehicle for commuting. You would probably purchase a couple of car magazines, read the latest reviews and familiarize yourself with current prices. You would talk to colleagues and ask what recommendations they would make. You might talk to the Automobile Association or the Royal Automobile Club and ask what they would recommend. You might even visit some showrooms, but you would be wary of the salespeople and never commit to buying on a first visit. Eventually, based on necessarily incomplete information, you would make a decision in the full knowledge that in a month or two a better offer would present itself.

Buying a computer for Internet access follows a similar procedure. The optimum route to success is to find a colleague who already has access to the Internet and ask them to show you what equipment they have, how they use it and which supplier they would recommend. The next step would then be to leave your money at home, visit the supplier and ask them which models they would suggest you purchase. Take all of the information they offer, resisting the temptation to buy, and leave. Back in the comfort of home or the office, take the time to consult a range of sources of information including any IT advisers at work, read some of the magazines and talk to contacts.

Eventually, assuming you still wish to proceed, you will probably select a personal computer that runs an operating system such as Microsoft Windows (Windows 98 or Windows NT). The computer will comprise a screen, a keyboard, a pointing device called a mouse, the main box holding the processor (minimum 400 MHz), memory (64 MB) for holding the programs and associated data, and disk drives (minimum 4 GB and 1.4 MB 3.5″ floppy drive) for storing programs and data when not in use, and a modem (56 Kbaud) to connect the computer to the Internet via the telephone system. You should also consider including, as preferred but optional extras, a CD-ROM (minimum 32 times normal speed) to enable you to install new software and an inkjet printer to provide hard copy. Other non-essential extras for your computer system include a scanner with optical character recognition (OCR) software to enable you to capture information directly from paper documents, and a Zip drive for making safe copies of your work.

You should expect to pay between £600 and £1500 for your computer system. The cheaper systems tend to be produced by the less well-known manufacturers. They offer better value for money but the risk of disappointment is higher. Some of that risk can be offset by only purchasing equipment that has a 3-year warranty. This length of warranty is sufficient, since you will probably replace the complete system after 3 years, assuming that it has been useful, since by then it will be very old technology. At that stage the resale value of the computer will be negligible, so during its life the computer will cost £4–10/week plus running costs, which will mainly be telephone charges.

Choosing an Internet service provider

Access to the Internet is via an Internet service provider (ISP). This provides software which, when installed on the computer, will automatically dial and connect the user to the Internet, via his or her own telephone line, for the cost of a local call. The ISP will normally also provide a range of facilities including an e-mail address (or addresses) for the user, access to SIGs, also known as news groups, and space to create a personal site on the Internet, known as a web site. Each of these facilities will be examined in detail later.

Until recently, most ISPs charged subscribers for access to the Internet. Typical rates were £10 per month. However, several companies now offer Internet access free of charge to subscribers and currently there are reported to be over 40 free providers. It seems likely that those ISPs who continue to charge their subscribers will need to offer additional and unique services to maintain their current customers. The 'free' ISPs generate their revenue in a variety of ways including levies on advertisers for access to subscribers and agreements with telephone-line providers based on the additional use by their subscribers.

Information technology training
Operating a computer is similar in many respects to driving a car. Once you have developed the techniques it is a straightforward process. Now cast your mind back to those early days of learning to drive. Remember the difficulty you had just starting the engine and when selecting a gear seemed impossible without stalling? Can you recall the nightmare of trying to reverse a vehicle into a small parking place? The transition from learner to competent driver was made possible by the presence of an experienced instructor plus time set aside to learn and practise.

The same strategy will serve you well should you decide to embrace IT. You can learn without an instructor, but if you want to achieve the competent driver stage with minimum overall effort then the author recommends enrolment on an introductory IT course at your place of work or local college. This will provide the basic knowledge and skills to operate a computer, providing a foundation on which to build the additional skills appropriate for your particular needs.

Sending and receiving electronic mail

What is e-mail?
Electronic mail (e-mail) is one of several facilities available via the Internet. It enables the exchange of electronic information, via the computer, with any other Internet user. Electronic information is anything that

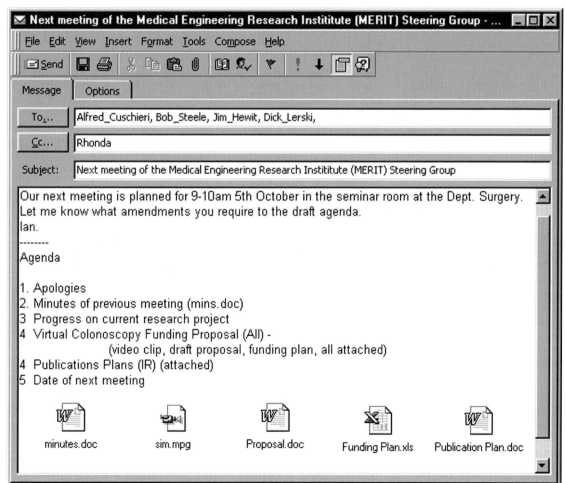

Figure 23.6 Microsoft Outlook e-mail tool.

can be stored as a file on the computer and includes letters, memos, reports, pictures, cartoons, videos, audio recordings, and any combination of these.

How to send and receive e-mail

In the following example, Microsoft Outlook, a widely used e-mail software tool, was used to create an e-mail, as shown in Figure 23.6. There are four components to the e-mail:

- a circulation list
- a subject title
- the body of the message
- several attached documents.

The complete message is to be sent to each of the people whose names are listed. In the author's electronic address book, also held on the computer, he maintains contact details for most people with whom he exchanges information. The contact details include name, postal address, e-mail address, and telephone and fax numbers. The e-mail software will substitute each recipient's unique e-mail address once it is given the command to 'send' the message.

How to incorporate electronic attachments

The body of the message, e.g. 'Our next meeting ...', is entered via the keyboard and then copies of previously prepared material, e.g. minutes.doc, sim.mpg, were attached by selecting those files by name from a list of all the files available on the computer. The small annotated pictures, known as icons, were automatically provided by the e-mail software.

Once the 'send' button is selected the e-mail software establishes a link with the ISP by automatically dialling the appropriate telephone number using the modem attached to the computer. Once the call is answered the sender's e-mail software will confirm with the ISP's computer that he is a registered user of the ISP's resources and then copy the e-mail to the ISP before disconnecting the telephone call. The entire communication with the ISP typically takes no more than a couple of minutes and would be charged, along with any other local telephone calls, to the sender's telephone account.

Meanwhile, the ISP computer will send the e-mail on to its multiple destinations. When the e-mail recipients next connect to their ISP they will be notified of the arrival of a new e-mail message and they will then be able to use their own e-mail software to transfer a copy of the message, with all of its attachments, from their ISP to their computer. Once the message is on their computer they will be able to read it, open each of the attached files and, if required, prepare an e-mail response.

Thus, e-mail messages can be transmitted to any destination around the globe in minutes and at the cost of a local telephone call.

The World Wide Web

What is the World Wide Web?

The Internet provides a world-wide communication network to which almost all computers in universities and an increasingly large proportion of company computers are connected. However, being interconnected does not guarantee that information can be exchanged.

Consider the analogy of using the telephone network and what happens if, from a telephone, one erroneously dials the number for a fax machine. The connection will be made, so you will be charged for occupying the line, but no useful information will be exchanged. The problem is that the format of information used by fax machines (tones) is not compatible with the format used by humans (voice).

To exchange information successfully over any link requires that the information be in a compatible format and often requires the use of devices at each end to encode and decode the information to and from the format required by the link.

The World Wide Web (www) is that section of the Internet in which the connected computers provide their information in a compatible format and for which there is readily available software to translate that format to a human readable form. The basic format is called HyperText Markup Language (HTML) and the translation software is termed a www browser. Microsoft's Internet Explorer and Netscape are examples of commonly used HTML browsers.

The www is sometimes described as a virtual network because, although it may be helpful to think of it as a separate network, it is not physically separated from the non-www parts of the Internet. The www is a virtual network in much the same way as the telephone network is a virtual network, since the telephone network is not physically separated from the network of fax machines.

Using browser software

Figure 23.7 shows a view of Microsoft Internet Explorer, which the author uses as his www browser. It is configured so that immediately after being launched it will connect via the ISP to the author's www site at the University of Dundee (http://plough.mic.dundee.ac.uk/index.html). To browse any other www site either:

- enter the site's unique www address into the Internet Explorer's address box (e.g. http://www.rcsed.ed.ac.uk/)
- use the mouse pointer to select a www site address that has been previously stored as a **favourite** link and assigned a suitable name, e.g. RCSEd Surgical Gateway, or
- use the mouse pointer to select any of the www site links on the currently displayed www page. www site links are underlined, e.g. summary CV.

The www browser software will be supplied free of charge upon registering with an ISP.

Searching for relevant information

We have seen how to connect to the Internet and how to link to a known address on the www. How do we cope when we lose the address of a www site or we do not know the address and only have a vague idea of the type of information we are seeking? Where do we find help when we come to searching for a hitherto

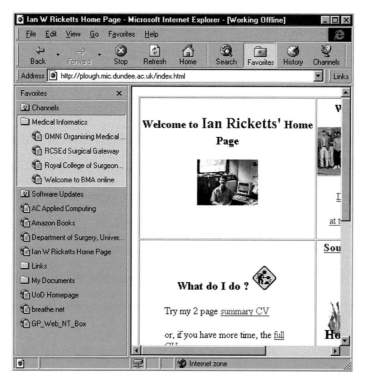

Figure 23.7 Microsoft Internet Explorer www browser.

unknown www site? This is when to call on the services of a www search engine. This offers a similar service to that offered to telephone users by Directory Enquiries, but with two major differences.

■ The www directory entries are compiled automatically and are updated frequently, removing any worries about 'late entries'.

■ The user is not constrained in the choice of search topic(s) when using a www search engine. A search engine will look for several words or search terms that summarize the topic on which further information is required and it will respond with a list of addresses for www sites that contain references to those search terms.

Figure 23.8 shows the Alta Vista www search engine (www.altavista.com) and its response when asked to search for www links to '3rd molar'. The response to this enquiry took less than 2 s and the search engine located 1 729 345 potentially relevant www links. It also recommended that the search be refined (shortened) by adding further items to the search list.

To follow the '3rd Molar Project Web' link one of the highlighted links, e.g. 3rd Molar Project www, is selected using the mouse cursor. To enable a link to be revisited at a later time the address should be saved to a list of favourite links.

Alta Vista is just one of many search engines. To find the www addresses of other search engines one could ask Alta Vista to search for 'Search Engines'. Equally effective approaches include talking to colleagues and asking for their recommendations, consulting professional journals and visiting one of the many news groups.

Accessing news groups

Using a news reader

As mentioned earlier, news groups (or SIGs) are formed by Internet users with common interests. To access the news group material one needs a **news**

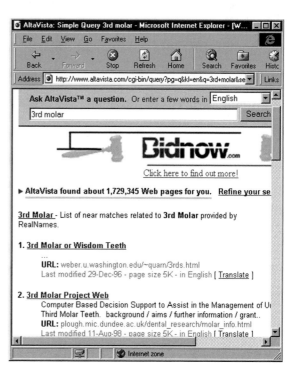

Figure 23.8 Searching for a www site.

reader. Microsoft includes a news reader within their Outlook Express software and this is shown in Figure 23.9. Once a user is registered with your ISP he or she will be given access to that ISP's news server (e.g. news.sol.co.uk), which can be regarded as the news vendor. To see what news groups are available to be consulted the user then selects 'News Groups' and will be presented with a list of the several thousand available groups. The news group in Figure 23.9 was located by extracting from the full list of news groups only those that had 'health' in their title and then choosing 'uk.people.health' from that shortlist.

Individual items of news in the list can be read by selecting them from the list of subjects and then their content will be displayed. A response can be posted to an individual author or to the entire group by selecting the appropriate menu item, e.g. 'Reply to Group', and inserting the text of the reply together with any file attachments. Experienced news group users tend to exchange information with individual members and only post to the entire group the summarized 'question and answer'.

Finding the news groups relevant to you

The efficient method of finding the most relevant news groups is to use a search engine, e.g. www.altavista.com. Unfortunately, the searches are dependent on the target words supplied by the user and they may ignore relevant articles that do not contain these target words. It is wise, therefore, to use a combination of regular visits to those news groups that overlap with your interests as well as regular visits to your favourite search engine.

Restricting membership and access to news group

A potentially useful extension of news groups is to restrict the membership of the group and thereby access to the information held by it. For example, restricting membership to the employees of a particular company makes it feasible to post company-confidential information to the group, e.g. the latest sales figures.

This raises the question of the security of the information exchanged via a computer network. This is a rather large topic to address but there is a wide range of mechanisms available to protect against access by non-approved persons. As a proof by demonstration, the electronic transfer of highly sensitive and commercially valuable information is conducted over electronic networks on a daily basis and breakdowns in security are rare.

Keeping informed via a list server

What is a list server?

A list server is best thought of as a combination of news group and e-mail. List servers are established by groups of users with common interests and can be consulted in the same way as any other user group. The unique feature of a list server is that whenever any member posts a message to it a copy of their message will be automatically e-mailed to each of the list's registered members.

The advantage of list servers is that they remove from the user the requirement to be proactive. As soon as a member posts any item you will receive it and thereby be kept fully informed of developments. The disadvantage is that if the group is active then a large amount of time may be spent dealing with e-mails from the list server; while you may at times wish to be kept up to date with developments, there may be other times where there are more pressing duties to attend to.

A refinement used with some list servers is the intervention of a human 'moderator' or 'gate keeper', whose role is to approve the content of all e-mails before they are included on the list and therefore before they are copied to the individual members. The presence of a moderator tends both to reduce the volume of traffic and to improve the quality of the content.

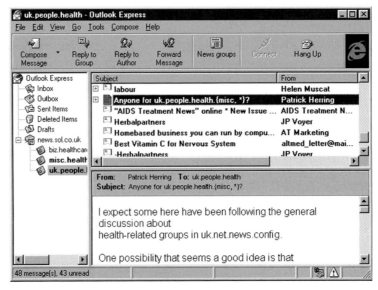

Figure 23.9 Reading the news.

Locating a relevant list server

The AltaVista search engine provided a number of potentially useful www addresses when asked to search for links to 'list servers UK', including a link to the United Kingdom Medical List Servers (Figure 23.10).

Registering with a list server

Once a relevant list server has been located, then joining it is usually a simple matter of sending an e-mail to its registration address and inserting in the e-mail the instructions to join (or subscribe). Most list servers have a www site, which includes instructions on the particular format of message that they expect to receive. As an example, Figure 23.11 shows the e-mail message that one would send to enrol with the Focal Institute for Scottish Health Informatics (FISHI), which is hosted by the UK Mailbase server.

All you would need to do is to substitute your **first name** and **surname** in this message. Your e-mail address would be attached automatically when you sent the message so the list server would know where to send its postings.

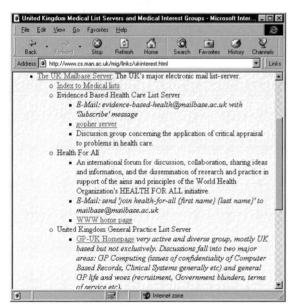

Figure 23.10 Locating relevant list servers.

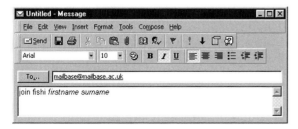

Figure 23.11 How to join the Focal Institute for Scottish Health Informatics.

Maintaining the integrity of the information on your computer

Guarding against loss of data

Loss of data is not inevitable but it is wise to assume that it will occur and to establish a procedure to minimize the time taken to recover. The causes of loss of data are many and varied, with the more exotic generally getting the greatest publicity, e.g. computer viruses; however, the more mundane, e.g. accidental file deletion, should not be overlooked.

Whenever data are lost it will cost some effort to recover, but if a few simple procedures are put in place it is likely that most of the original information will be recoverable, whatever the cause of its loss. The challenge is to identify a procedure that is not so onerous that you do not follow it.

Almost all current computers are equipped with both a large-capacity but non-removable disk and a smaller capacity removable disk drive. When creating any computer files you should make regular and frequent copies of your latest work on to a removable disk. While writing this article, the author kept the master copy of the article on the large-capacity non-removable disk and transferred a copy of the article on to a removable disk every 15–20 min to limit the impact of any failure. Making the safe or backup copy took a matter of seconds.

As the article grew in size, especially with the inclusion of figures, it became too large to save on a single removable disk. At that stage the author used a utility program called Winzip (available over the Internet) to compress the file by a factor of 10 times so that again it fitted on to a single removable disk. The compress and copy operation still took less than 1 min and if anything had gone wrong with the master copy, the work could have been recovered up to the point of making the last backup copy, so that at worst 15–20 min of work would have been lost. A computer is a potential target for theft or fire, so upon leaving the machine it is advisable to take the removable disk with the latest copy of the article away.

On occasion the author also used the Internet to mail a copy of his work to a remote site as an attachment to an e-mail message. He then had the option to retrieve the message subsequently.

To keep information confidential, an encryption program can be used. This translates an otherwise readable document in to a form that is unreadable without access to the associated password or keyword. For instance, Microsoft's Word processor includes the option of storing files in an encrypted format. Then, if the disks or the computer are accidentally misplaced the encrypted files will be inaccessible to all but the most determined of readers.

More robust encryption mechanisms are available and a search of the www will provide a range of both software and hardware tools with which to protect information from any reader who does not have the keywords. However, as with most things, the better versions will cost more.

Data corruption from software viruses

A software virus is a program that arrives uninvited on the computer and the purpose of which is to corrupt the files on the disk. The virus can arrive by a variety of routes, including your use of an already infected disk in the computer and the receipt of a document or program over the Internet. Software viruses are endemic and it is therefore recommended to purchase an antivirus program to guard the computer against infection. Once installed, the antivirus will detect the arrival of a virus, notify the user, and enable its removal before it can damage any files. The antivirus software should include an update service, available over the Internet, so that your work is protected against any new viruses.

All of the computers used by the author have antivirus software installed and he has not lost any information because of virus attack subsequent to that installation.

Ensuring that data sources are reliable

The Internet provides access to vast stores of information but very few of the providers offer any guarantees as to the quality of the information. In common with software suppliers, none of the 'information providers' offers to accept responsibility for consequential damage caused by its use. That responsibility, as always, rests with the user.

To counteract the widespread lack of quality controls, a number of mechanisms is now being established. Some groups have established 'seals of approval', which are issued to Internet sites whose information meets the group's standards. Other groups have created Internet sites from which they will only link to other sites of which they approve. Given the highly dynamic nature of Internet links, both solutions require a considerable and continuing investment to maintain, but the benefits are also considerable.

To find good-quality information on the Internet one should use the same approach as when looking for it in other forms, i.e. seeking the recommendations of professional bodies and the views of trusted colleagues and, perhaps most importantly, being sceptical.

Internet sources of information

This following list is supplied as a starting point for an exploration of the Internet.

Free Internet service providers
- BT
- Freeserve
- Free-Online
- Martin Dawes
- Tesco
- Virgin
- Yahoo.

Sources of information on medical topics
- American Medical Association
- British Medical Association
- British Medical Journal
- Focal Institute for Scottish Health Informatics

- Gateway to the Orthopaedic Internet
- NHS Executive
- OMNI: Organising Medical Networked Information
- PubMed National Library Medicine search service
- Royal College of Surgeons (Edinburgh): Surgical Internet Information Gateway
- Royal College Surgeons (England)
- Scottish Intercollegiate Guidelines Network
- Scottish Respiratory Site
- SHOW – Scottish Health on the Web.

Search engines
- Alta Vista
- Hotbot
- Infoseek
- Lycos
- Yahoo.

Others
- HENSA: Higher Education National Software Archive
- Mailbase: electronic discussion lists for the UK higher education community.

As a professor in applied computing the author admits to a slight bias, but believes that computers in combination with the Internet offer significant benefits to the majority of users.

Access to remote sources of information and the ability to share experiences with colleagues and co-workers are potential benefits, but we must also consider the costs, i.e. the computer equipment and human resource, which will need to be transferred from other activities to realize the potential. As with any other activity the costs and the benefits should be examined and those activities that offer the largest gains should be pursued.

The author hopes that he has provided some useful insights into the potential uses of the Internet and that the reader feels encouraged to explore further.

Section 23.7 • Computers, medicine and the twenty-first century

'Messers Hubbard and Bell want to install one of their "telephone devices" in every city. The idea is idiotic on the face of it. Furthermore, why would any person want to use this ungainly and impractical device when he can send a messenger to the telegraph office and have a clear written message sent to any large city in the United States?' – 1876 committee report from The Telegraph Company

Introduction

Recent technical improvements in personal computers and the widespread growth of the Internet have created an environment where superfast data propagation is commonplace. Healthcare is one of the many facets of this information explosion. Patients who visit the doctor's office today are likely to already have visited a world-wide web (WWW) page about their provisional diagnosis. The physician or surgeon of the twenty-first century must keep abreast of rapidly evolving computer technologies. This section will cover the common uses of computers and the Internet that are currently employed by healthcare providers and consumers. A glimpse into future applications and potential shortcomings will be discussed.

Internet

History

The Internet was not born on any single day. Its beginnings were in the USA with the Advanced Research Project Agencies (ARPA), a federal organization created in response to the 1954 launch of the Soviet *Sputnik*. ARPA researchers investigated packet-switching technology, which de-emphasized hub systems and allowed for multiple routes of information travel. This was particularly applicable in the existing political climate because there was fear of a central, devastating nuclear strike on the USA by the Soviet Union. A decentralized system would continue to function even though key military and intelligence locations had been completely destroyed.

In 1972, ARPA was renamed The Defense Advanced Research Projects Agency (DARPA) and a Network Control Protocol was created to transfer data between hosts running on the same network. Shortly afterwards, a protocol called Transmission Control Protocol/Internet Protocol (TCP/IP) was developed by DARPA scientists that allowed diverse computer networks to interconnect with each other.

In 1983 programmers at The University of Wisconsin created the Domain Name System, which allowed information packets to be directed to a domain name, and the foundation for the modern Internet was laid. That same year Microsoft® unveiled Windows©, which allowed users of the software to view and interact with multiple application programs simultaneously. The last two decades have been characterized by a massive increase in personal computer sales. The newer machines are relatively inexpensive and much more user-friendly than previously released models. Most are equipped with modems, devices allowing computer-to-computer communication over a telephone line.

On 24 October 1995, the United States Federal Networking Council unanimously passed a resolution defining the term Internet.

The Federal Networking Council agrees that the following language reflects our definition of the term 'Internet'.

'Internet' refers to the global information system that

   (i)   is logically linked together by a globally unique address space based on the Internet Protocol (IP) or its subsequent extensions/follow-ons;

   (ii) is able to support communications using the TCP/IP suite or its subsequent extensions/follow-ons, and/or other IP-compatible protocols; and

   (iii) provides, uses or makes accessible, either publicly or privately, high-level services layered on the communications and related infrastructure described herein.

                                 (http://www.fnc.gov/)

Catalysed by the strong personal computer market, use of the Internet increased dramatically. The number of people with access to the Internet has grown from thousands in the mid-1980s to millions in the late 1990s. In 1991, the National Science Foundation lifted the restriction on commercial utilization of the Internet. Shortly thereafter, the phrase 'world-wide web' was coined in Switzerland, representing the portion of the Internet allowing text and graphics to be shown simultaneously. Programs, called browsers, are created to fetch and display the documents containing text and graphics, which are now known as WWW pages, or webpages for short.

At present, the number of people who potentially have access to the Internet is difficult to measure. Most public libraries offer an Internet station, as do nearly all universities. Soon the number of people world-wide who have the ability to get online will outnumber the people who do not. More and more patients obtain their supplemental health-related knowledge through information obtained from webpages. In fact, the number of people in America who use the Internet for medical information has climbed from 7.8 million in 1996 to over 30 million in 1999.

Patient-oriented webpages

Modern patients are very different from those of earlier centuries or even decades. They demand, and deserve, a right to informed consent about procedures or operations performed upon them. In addition to personal one-on-one counselling by the surgeon and his or her staff, patients seek other sources of information about their disease process. An obvious turning point is the WWW, initially known as the 'Information Super Highway.' However, not all of the information on a webpage that a patient might visit is true, applicable, or even useful. At present there is no quality assurance system to ensure that medical webpages contain information universally accepted as fact. In a recent review of representation of common vascular surgical problems on the WWW, Soot and colleagues found that 96/150 sites (66%) had virtually no useful patient-oriented information. Of the vascular websites that contained information felt to be relevant to patient education, 33% had areas that were classified by the authors as misleading or unconventional. A publication on laparoscopy and the WWW contains similar findings.

Until the problems of verifying the accuracy and integrity of the content presented in medical webpages are solved, it is up to healthcare professionals to guide patients to reliable online information. One way to do this is to produce a 'selected links section', to recommend to patients who seek additional medical information on the WWW. A program to do this was established at the Family Practice Department of Medical College of Wisconsin, Milwaukee, USA. Patients were given access to webpages that had been previously peer reviewed. In this study 94% of patients found this group of webpages useful and 77% said that they would modify an unhealthy behaviour because of information that they had read on the webpages.

The most popular starting point for patients seeking information online is a 'search engine'. Search engines are specialized webpages that function as a topic index for the rest of the WWW. However, no one engine is a complete reference and, as a whole, they are frequently inefficient when searching for medical content, often containing irrelevant information. Many corporate health webpages, or infomediaries, also attempt to guide web visitors to relevant medical webpages within their system. Often these are heavily sprinkled with advertising banners and do not contain peer-reviewed material.

Despite the drawbacks of certain sites, there are many webpages that are useful for patients and contain information that cannot be easily found using another medium. For example, in small towns there may be difficulties in obtaining prosthetic devices for women after mastectomy. In cyberspace, however, there are a variety of mail order shops available, including Reflections Post-Mastectomy Boutique (http://www. reflections-boutique.com/), Comfortably Yours (http:// bizserve.com/mastectomy/index.html), and Ladies First, Inc. (http://www.wvi.com/~ladies1/). Each of these offer mail order purchase and delivery of apparel specially designed especially for women who have previously undergone mastectomy. Other product information may be found at http://www.oandp.com, a resource for Orthotics & Prosthetics information, http://www. fashfirst.com, a nursing home apparel company, and http://www.ktv-i.com/news/nf05_07_97.html, a wheelchair maintenance webpage. Countless disease-specific product webpages exist and it is up to healthcare professionals to recommend proper sites to their patients.

Chat rooms are locations on the Internet where simultaneous communication between two or more people is possible. This may be in the form of typing messages back and forth, or in some cases, actually speaking into a microphone and hearing others through the computer's speakers. These chat rooms are usually segregated by topic. The medical application here is in the form of online support groups, especially useful in uncommon diseases. Through discussion with others who share their diagnosis and have experienced treatment, practical tips on coping and emotional support may be obtained. At the cancer information and support international webpage (http://www.cancer-info.com) there are chatrooms available for a variety of cancers. Specific chatrooms include those for Ewing's Sarcoma, multiple myeloma, glioblastoma, gall bladder cancer and pancreas cancer, as well as more common malignancies.

Chatrooms are not immune from the hazards of Internet usage. People feigning illnesses have been reported to reside in chat rooms. Exhibiting a form of Munchausen syndrome, these people appear to thrive on the attention and support afforded to them in these online support groups. The abundance of disease-specific information available on the WWW unfortunately gives people with factitious disorders details to support their claim and make their story believable.

Similar to chat rooms, e-mailing lists are gaining popularity as avenues in which healthcare professionals can share practice parameters and discuss interesting or problematic cases. These function as discussion groups but not in 'real time'. Instead, messages written by members of the list are distributed on a regular basis, via e-mail, to people who are subscribers. The requirement of a working e-mail address may discourage impostors in this type of forum.

Public health

Application of Internet technologies in the public health system has potential to markedly improve global healthcare through better surveillance and information systems. Flu Net (http://oms.b3e.jussieu.fr/flunet/) has been developed to study the global characteristics of influenza and provide an alert system for epidemic outbreaks. Other similar co-operative efforts include the World Health Organization's Communicable Disease Surveillance and Response effort (http://www.who. int/emc/). As world-wide access to the Internet grows, public health applications will follow.

Physician webpages

Until recently, physicians who advertised were immediately discredited or arrested. However, there seems to be some relaxation of these notions with respect to physician webpages, certainly one form of advertising. Many of the corporate medical webpages, such as Medscape, offer member physicians the opportunity to easily create and publish a webpage. Credentials, special interests or experiences, and the *curriculum vitae* are often included. However, a physician's webpage has the potential to be more than an inexpensive and accepted form of personal advertising. A frequently asked questions section (FAQ) can pre-emptively answer common patient questions about the illnesses the doctor treats. Also, non-medical FAQs would include directions to the facility, office hours, and policies on prescription refills. 'What to watch for' sections describing postoperative problems and clues to early diagnosis may prompt patients to seek medical advice early rather than late.

Continuing medical education

Depending on location, most healthcare professionals are required to obtain some form of continuing medical education (CME). Credits for this may include attending lectures, taking self-assessment quizzes, watching videos or teaching courses. Frequently this requires travel and time away from practice. Obtaining

CME credit online will be an important application of the WWW because the doctor need not leave home, performing these requirements at leisure. He or she can study the online syllabus and images and, given the anonymity afforded by the web, can honestly answer the self-assessment questions.

There are a number of webpages offering some form of access to CME credits, including Helix (http://www.helix.com), Medconnect (http://www.medconnect.com), and Medivision (http://www.medivision-volt.com/listings.htm) among many. Some of these are commercial webpages, which require a membership and charge a fee for the credit obtained. The fees will generally pale in comparison to travel costs incurred during a trip to obtain CME.

Like most Internet venues, obtaining online CME credit is not without imperfections. Potentially, healthcare professionals may neither study the material nor honestly assess their knowledge by the self-test, but still obtain the required credit. This abuse defeats the very philosophy of CME.

Clinical trials

Current treatment practices in nearly all fields of medicine are based on previous clinical trials. Often these trials are fraught with labour-intensive paper work and discarded data due to non-adherence to strict protocols. Specific portions of clinical trials that the Internet can facilitate include randomization, patient and physician recruitment, data entry, and the widespread distribution of trial progress. International trials are more feasible using this technology, eliminating lag times associated with overseas correspondence. A clinical trials resource centre (http://pharminfo.com/conference/clintrial/ct_rsc.html) is available, which includes an international listing of more than 5200 clinical trials that are actively recruiting patients.

Literature searches

Even the staunchest opponent of the Internet movement must admit that this technology allows a near effortless search of the medical literature. Numerous educational organizations and private companies operate webpages offering free searches of the Medline' database. At present, these include PubMed (http://www.ncbi.nlm.nih.gov/PubMed/), MedPortal (http://www.medportal.com/), Healthgate (http://www.healthgate.com/medline/search-medline.shtml), and Medscape (http://www.medscape.com), to name only a few. The available searches include articles written in languages other than English and are current to within 10 years. Mostly, abstracts can be obtained from these queries but often entire articles can be ordered and purchased. This is especially helpful in articles published in hard-to-find journals where inter-department library loan is often slow.

E-mail

Electronic mail (e-mail) has been one of the real triumphs of the Internet. Using e-mail, a person can correspond, almost instantaneously, with anyone else in the world with an e-mail account. Although a large portion of the e-mail sent today is clearly social in nature, this exciting but simple technology has tremendous medical application. The physician of the next decade will communicate by e-mail with patients, families, colleagues, therapists, and hospital administrators. It is not far-fetched to assume that even non-urgent ward calls and 'beeps' will be replaced by electronic messages.

Current e-mail use has been tempered mainly by physicians who fear that easier personal access will cause a bombardment of messages requiring return. Ellis *et al.* use e-mail for postoperative follow-up after ambulatory surgery and feel that potential benefits include cost savings, ease in collecting quality improvement data, and the potential for increased reporting of unpleasant events. Potential pitfalls of e-mail follow-up include lack of universal home Internet access, privacy and security concerns, and possible delay in response to messages that require emergent responses or actions.

Certain guidelines should be employed when corresponding by e-mail with colleagues, patients and families. First, e-mail may be included in the patient's medical record. As such, the same discretion should be used when communicating in this fashion as would be used when writing in the chart. Second, the exact identity of the recipient must be guaranteed prior to sending information, which may be linked to that patient's private medical records. Finally, potential for misunderstandings may be magnified given the lack of 'real-time' communication nuances including word inflection and emotion. Clearly expressed thoughts with specific words and phrases should be used.

Telemedicine

The availability of 'store and forward' transfer of text and images has made telemedicine possible. Telemedicine is the delivery of healthcare and sharing of medical knowledge using telecommunication systems. Some, but not all telemedicine is performed over conventional telephone lines via the Internet.

This technology has been used to deliver healthcare to underprivileged areas of the world. In isolated areas hospitals have integrated telemedicine systems into the fields of dermatology, cardiology, pathology, endoscopy and radiology. Norway was the first country to implement a fee schedule for teleconsultations, opinions rendered by a consulting physician at a distance from the patient. Telemedicine systems have also been shown to be helpful in assisting in the selection of patients for triage to tertiary care centres. In the traumatic neurosurgery realm, this system has been shown to be safe and cost-effective by Bailes and co-workers .

Patient follow-up, especially in areas where transport to the nearest physician or operating surgeon is difficult, has be shown to be feasible online. DeBakey and colleagues have shown the Internet to be useful in follow-up of a patient who underwent mitral valve replacement in America and is now residing in the former Soviet Union. The patient's medications, electrocardiographs, and activity status were reviewed in America via the Internet and specific clinical recommendations were made, all while the patient remained in the former Soviet Union.

Teleconsulting

Using telemedicine for medical consultation is 'teleconsulting'. Teleconsultations will ensure that no area in the world equipped with an Internet connection will be without specialists to render opinions. Beginning in 1999, USA physicians performing teleconsultations will be financially compensated for their services. Initially, this will be limited to patients residing in a rural, underprivileged area with the referring physician physically present. As patients and doctors become more comfortable with this set-up, this field of medicine is sure to grow.

Telesurgery

Telesurgery is the use of telecommunications technologies to facilitate performance of an operation. Telesurgery is most applicable in the fields of laparoscopy, endoscopy, and arthroscopy because all rely heavily on images and optics. During a conventional laparoscopic procedure, the operating surgeon looks at a video monitor and manipulates his or her hands on instruments that traverse the abdominal cavity. Although some tactile sense is used, the surgeon relies heavily on depth perception as a two-dimensional video image is converted within the operator's mind into the three-dimensional anatomy.

On 29 August, 1996 a laparoscopic procedure was first broadcast in interactive fashion over the Internet. Surgeons in the USA and Argentina actively discussed portions of the operation while the case was underway. This interactive broadcast brought up many questions concerning the new combination of technologies; namely, is it ethical, appropriate, and safe to actually perform surgery over the Internet?

Already, however, the envelope is being pushed. A laparoscopic procedure has been performed by a surgeon at a distance from a patient.

By manipulating handles connected to a computer in command of instruments inside a patient's abdominal cavity, Dr Favretti performed a laparoscopic gastric banding in 1999 while being a distance of 6 feet from the patient.

Telementoring

Perhaps more practical than performing an entire operation at a distance, is the idea of surgical telementoring. In this scenario, an experienced surgeon (mentor) located at a central hub, guides less experienced surgeons through selected difficult portions of a procedure using voice and visual cues while watching their progress on a computer monitor. The telementoring concept has been shown to be a safe, potentially cost-saving system for training surgeons in advanced laparoscopy.

One of the most interesting examples of telementoring has come aboard the USS *Abraham Lincoln* aircraft carrier. While cruising in the Pacific Ocean, five laparoscopic inguinal hernia repairs have been performed on seamen under shore-based telementor guidance. Laparoscopic surgery is but one of the many specialties that have an application in this field of telemedicine. Real-time telementoring has been reported to be useful in complex ophthalmologic, urologic, and neurologic clinical situations.

Electronic medical record

At present, most hospitals use analogue medical records. Doctors write progress notes and orders and nurses write patient status and medication delivered notes. Often dictated operative notes, history and physicals, and discharge summaries, as well as ancillary notes, are transcribed and the typed pages placed in the chart. Lab values are printed, but require frequent updates and cumulative results have to be reprinted and delivered daily to the 'chart'. After patient discharge, the chart is stored in a medical records area. Often after a certain time period it is moved to an off-site storage facility, or even discarded.

What makes this whole process even more inefficient is the fact that these processes are generally unique to each hospital complex. When a patient changes hospitals or geographic areas, there is poor immediate access to the medical record available for a new physician. These shortcomings have been improved by fax technology; however, it is still a cumbersome, time-consuming process with several rate-limiting steps.

Digitalizing the medical record will be a remarkable and welcome change. Computer-based medical records will be more than mere electronic versions of the analogue record. They will be a globally accepted way to examine a patient's past medical history. Even more helpful will be the use of a universal language, like web-based hypertext mark-up language (HTML), that allows simultaneous examination of text and graphics. Not only will a previous radiograph report be available for the new physician, but also an online view of the test itself. The Internet will permit confidential transfer of the entire digital medical record between healthcare providers.

There are unlimited improvements in patient care that this system will provide. Drug addicts who rotate from hospital to hospital in search of narcotics will have a tell-tale digital medical record, which will be immediately accessible by any hospital in the world. Also, the involvement of the Internet will make additional data available to the clinician. Constantly updated databases will provide reminders of ongoing clinical trials concerning a patient's diagnosis. A reference library of journal articles will be available, and will be cued by the diagnosis, symptoms, or physical findings. Substantial financial benefits also await a hospital system that will eliminate the cost of manufacturing, storing, filing and retrieving analogue charts

At present, the digital medical record is not common in clinical practice. The transition between hospital platforms is not yet seamless and software is being created to allow this to happen. One unifying project is the CareWeb, which attempts to provide architecture for retrieval of electronic medical records from heterogeneous data sources on the WWW.

Uniform usage by doctors of the electronic medical record will require significant improvements in hardware as well as software. This must mean smaller computers (palm-sized) that are cordless, have a long battery life and have built-in, reliable operating systems. Scanners, or the devices that produce the recorded images, will need to have higher resolution and produce an image able to be compressed for smaller storage size. The 'connection', or the way the information is transferred, must be fast, to limit wait time.

Conclusion

The practice of medicine is ever changing. Computers and the Internet will markedly improve healthcare. There will be better informed patients, doctors with a world of medical literature at their fingertips, and easier communication between the two. There will be fewer areas which have no specialists available for consultation. During difficult laparoscopic procedures a telementor will be called upon for assistance by an inexperienced surgeon. The electronic medical record will be a cost-effective and more efficient way to follow patients. Doctors must keep abreast with these changes and play a role in their development.

Table 23.2 Referenced webpages and URL

Webpage title	URL
Cancer Information Chat	http://www.cancer-info.com/chat/
Careweb	http://clinquery.bidmc.harvard.edu/people/jhalamka/lookup.htm
Clinical Trials Center	http://pharminfo.com/conference/clintrial/ct_rsc.html
Fashion First	http://www.fashfirst.com/
Flu Net	http://oms.b3e.jussieu.fr/flunet/
Healthgate	http://www.healthgate.com/medline/search-medline.shtml
Helix	http://www.helix.com
Keep-em rolling	http://www.ktv-i.com/news/nf05_07_97.html
Medconnect	http://www.medconnect.com
Medivision	http://www.medivision-volt.com/listings.htm
Medportal	http://www.medportal.com/
Medscape	http://www.medscape.com
Orthotics/Prosthetics	http://www.oandp.com
Physicians Online	http://www.po.com/
PubMed	http://www.ncbi.nlm.nih.gov/PubMed/
Reflections Boutique	http://www.reflections-boutique.com/
World Health Organization	http://www.who.int/

Table 23.3 Glossary

Browser	Program that displays WWW pages.
Chat room	Webpage that allows typed messages to be circulated among visitors, usually about a specific subject
.com	.commercial, representing the suffix for a commercial webpage
E-mail	Electronic mail, the system of sending instantaneous typed messages to another person using the Internet
FAQ	Frequently asked questions
Hardware	Physical computer equipment such as a monitor, modem, printer, etc.
Homepage	Interchangeable with webpage, perhaps representing the opening page of a larger site
HTML	Hypertext markup language, the flexible, powerful programming language in which webpages are written
HTTP	Hypertext Transfer Protocol, the underlying system for information transfer on the Internet
Internet	A system of interconnections of computers allowing data transfer
Modem	Modulator-demodulator, a device enabling computers to transmit information over telephone lines
Search engine	Specialized webpage that functions as a topic index for a portion of the WWW
Software	Programs, or applications, used by computers to accomplish specific tasks
Telemedicine	Delivery of healthcare and sharing of medical knowledge using telecommunication systems
Webpage	A document, displayed by a browser, that contains text and images and is transferable on the WWW
WWW	World-wide-web, that portion of the Internet where text, graphics, and sounds are displayed simultaneously with a high degree of user friendliness

Guide to further reading

Section 23.1

Black, N. (1994). Experimental and observational methods of evaluation. *BMJ* **309**: 540

Mays, N. and Pope, C. (1996). *Qualitative Research in Health Care*, BMA Publications, London.

Thompson, S. G. and Pocock, S. J. (1991). Can meta-analysis be trusted? *Lancet* **338**: 1127–1130.

Yusuf, S., Collins, R. and Peto, R. I. (1984). Why do we need some large sample randomised trials? *Statist Med* **3**: 409–420.

Section 23.2

Aitken, R. J., Nixon, S. J. and Ruckley, C. V. (1997). Lothian Surgical Audit: a 15 year experience of improvement in surgical practice through regional computerised audit. *Lancet* **350**: 800–804.

Campling, E. A., Devlin, H. B., Hoile, R. W. and Lunn, G. S. (1997). *Who Operates When?* A report by the National Confidential Enquiry into perioperative deaths, Lincoln's Inn Fields, London, pp. 35–43.

Copeland, G. P., Jones, D. and Walters, M. (1991). POSSUM: a scoring system for surgical audit. *Br J Surg* **78**: 356–360.

Crofts, T. J., Griffiths, J. M., Sharma, S., Wygrala, J. and Aitken, R. J. (1997). Surgical training: an objective assessment of recent changes for a single health board. *BMJ* **314**: 891–895.

Donabedian, A. (1992). Quality assurance. Structure, process and outcome. *Qual Stand* **7**(11 Suppl QA): 4–5.

Flanagan, J. C. (1954). The critical incident technique. *Psychol Bull* **51**: 327–358.

Grol, R. and Wensing, M. (1995). Implementation of quality assurance and medical audit: general practitioners' perceived obstacles and requirements. *Br J Gen Pract* **45**: 548–552.

Lough, J. R. M., McKay, J. and Murray, T. S. (1995). Audit: trainers' and trainees' attitudes and experiences. *Med Educ* **29**: 85–90.

Mant, J. and Hicks, N. (1995). Detecting differences in quality of care: the sensitivity of measures of process and outcome in treating acute myocardial infarction. *BMJ* **311**: 793–796.

Marinker, M. Standards, in *Medical Audit In General Practice* (M. Marinker, ed.), MSD Foundation, London, pp. 22–23.

Potter, M. A., Nixon, S. J. and Aitken, R. J. (1996). A 10 year analysis of case load and weighted workload in a single health board. *Ann R Coll Surg Engl* **78**(1 Suppl.): 11–13.

Section 23.3

Joice, P., Hanna, G. B. and Cuschieri, A. (1998). Errors enacted during endoscopic surgery – a human reliability analysis. *Appl Ergon* **29**: 409–414.

Kirwin, B. (1998). Human reliability assessment, in *Evaluation of Human Work. A Practical Methodology*, 2nd edn (J. R. Wilson and E. N. Corlett, eds), Taylor & Francis, London, pp. 921–968.

Reason, J. (1994). *Human Error*, Cambridge University Press, Cambridge.

Section 23.4

Begren, U., Zethraeus, N., Arvidsson, D. *et al.* (1996). A cost-minimization analysis of laparoscopic cholecystectomy versus open cholecystectomy. *Am J Surg* **172**: 305–310.

Black, N. (1996). Why we need observational studies to evaluate the effectiveness of health care. *BMJ* **312**: 1215–1218.

Brooks, R. (1996). EuroQol: the current state of play. *Health Policy* **31**: 53–72.

Drummond, M. F., O'Brien, B. J., Stoddardt, G. L. and Torrance, G. W. (1997). *Methods for the Economic Evaluation of Health Care Programmes*, 2nd edn, Oxford University Press, Oxford.

Elixhauser, A., Halpern, M., Schmier, J. and Luce, B. (1998). Health care CBA and CEA from 1991 to 1996: an updated bibliography. *Med Care* **36**(Suppl.): S1–9.

Eyspach, E., Williams, J. I., Wood-Dauphinee, S. *et al.* (1993). The gastrointestinal quality of life index (GIQLI) development and validation of a new instrument. *Chirugia* **64**: 264–274.

Florey, C. du V., Yule, B., Fogg, A. *et al.* (1994). A randomized trial of immediate discharge of surgical patients to general practice. *J Public Health Med* **16**: 455–464.

Lawrence, K., McWhinnie, D., Goodwin, A. *et al.* (1996). An economic evaluation of laparoscopic versus open inguinal hernia repair. *J Public Health Med* **18**: 41–48.

Liem, M. S., Halsema, J. A., van-der-Graaf, Y. *et al.* (1997). Cost-effectiveness of extraperitoneal laparoscopic inguinal hernia repair: a randomized comparison with conventional herniorrhaphy. Coal trial group. *Ann Surg* **22**: 668–675.

Sculpher, M., Michaels, J., McKenna, M. and Minor, J. (1996). A cost–utility analysis of laser assisted angioplasty for peripheral arterial occlusions. *Int J Technol Assess Health Care* **12**: 104–125.

Wellwood, J., Sculpher M. J., Stoker, D. *et al.* (1998). Randomised controlled trial of laparoscopic versus open mesh repair for inguinal hernia: outcome and cost. *BMJ* **317**: 103–110.

Section 23.5

Brazier, M. (1992). *Medicine, Patients and the Law*, 2nd edn, Penguin, London.

Dickson, R. H. (1997). *Medical and Dental Negligence*, 1st edn, T & T Clark, Edinburgh.

Harpwood, V. (1998). *Medical Negligence and Clinical Risk: Trends and Developments 1998*, 1st edn, Monitor Press, Suffolk.

Hobsley, M. and Scurr, J. (1994). General surgery, in *Medical Negligence*, 2nd edn (M. Powers and N. Harris, eds), Butterworth, London, Chap. 33.

Mason, K. and McCall Smith, R. A. A. (1994). *Law and Medical Ethics*, 4th edn, Butterworth, London.

Section 23.7

Aucar, J. A., Doarn, C. R., Sargsyan, A., Samuelson, D. A., Odonnell, M. J. and DeBakey, M. E. (1998). Use of the Internet for long-term clinical follow-up. *Telemed J* **4**: 371–374.

Bailes, J. E., Poole, C. C., Hutchison, W., Maroon, J. C. and Fukushima, T. (1997). Utilization and cost savings of a wide-area computer network for neurosurgical consultation. *Telemed J* 1997; **3**: 135–139.

Bell, J. D. and Fay, M. T. (1997). A longitudinal study of the attitudes of the medical profession towards competition and advertising. *NZ Med J* **110**: 410–412.

Brailer, D. J. and Hackett, T. S. (1997). Points [and clicks] on quality. *Hosp Health Networks* **71**(22): 32.

Cadiere, G. B., Himpens, J., Vertruyen, M. and Favretti, F. (1999). The world's first obesity surgery performed by a surgeon at a distance. *Obes Surg* **9**: 206–209.

Camara J. G, Rodriguez R. E. (1998). Real-time telementoring in ophthalmology. *Telemed J* 1998; **4**: 375–377.

Cubano, M., Poulose, B. K., Talamini, M. A., *et al.* (1999). Long distance telementoring. A novel tool for laparoscopy aboard the USS Abraham Lincoln. *Surg Endosc* **13**: 673–678.

Ellis, J. E., Klock, P.A., Mingay, D. J. and Roizen, M. F. (1999). Use of electronic mail for postoperative follow-up after ambulatory surgery. *J Clin Anesth* **11**: 136–139.

Flahault, A., Dias-Ferrao, V., Chaberty, P., Esteves, K., Valleron, A. J. and Lavanchy, D. (1998). FluNet as a tool for global monitoring of influenza on the Web. *JAMA* **280**: 1293.

Gandsas, A., Altrudi, R., Pleatman, M. and Silva, Y. (1998). Live interactive broadcast of laparoscopic surgery via the Internet. *Surg Endosc* **12**: 252–255.

Gilas, T., Schein, M. and Frykberg, E. (1998). A surgical Internet discussion list (Surginet): a novel venue for international communication among surgeons. *Arch Surg* **133**: 1126–1130.

Halamka, J. D. and Safran, C. (1998). CareWeb, a web-based medical record for an integrated healthcare delivery system. *Medinfo* **9**(Part 1): 36–39.

Helwig, A. L., Lovelle, A., Guse, C.E. and Gottlieb, M. S. (1999). An office-based Internet patient education system: a pilot study. *J Fam Pract* **48**: 123-127.

Kane, B. and Sands, D. Z. (1998). Guidelines for the clinical use of electronic mail with patients. The AMIA Internet Working Group, Task Force on Guidelines for the Use of Clinic–Patient Electronic Mail. *J Am Med Inform Assoc* **5**: 104–111.

Lee, B. R., Caddedu, J. A., Janetschek, G. *et al.* (1998). International surgical telementoring: our initial experience. *Stud Health Technol Inform* **50**: 41–47.

Levine, S. R. and Gorman, M. (1999). 'Telestroke': the application of telemedicine for stroke. *Stroke* **30**: 464–469.

McLauchlan, G. J., Cadogan, M. and Oliver, C. W. (1999). Assessment of an electronic mailing list for orthopaedic and trauma surgery. *J R Coll Surg Edin* **44**: 36–39.

Peterson, M. W., Galvin, J. R., Dayton, C. and D'Alessandro, M. P. (1999). Realizing the promise: delivering pulmonary continuing medical education over the Internet. *Chest* **115**:1429-1436.

Rosser, J. C., Wood, M., Payne, J. H. *et al.* (1997). Telementoring. A practical option in surgical training. *Surg Endosc* **11**: 852–855.

Sacchetti, P., Zvara, P. and Plante, M. K. (1999). The Internet and patient education–resources and their reliability: focus on a select urologic topic. *Urology* **53**: 1117–1120.

Satoh, T., Takahashi, K., Yahata, K. *et al.* (1997). Application of Internet technology in public health. *Nippon Koshu Eisei Zasshi* **44**: 518–522.

Schulam, P. G., Docimo, S. G., Saleh, W., Breitenbach, C., Moore, R. G. and Kavoussi, L. (1997). Telesurgical mentoring. Initial clinical experience. *Surg Endosc* **11**: 1001–1005.

Shortliffe, E. H. (1998). The evolution of health-care records in the era of the Internet. *Medinfo* **9**(Part 1): 8–14.

Soot, L. C., Moneta, G. L. and Edwards, J. M. (1999). Vascular surgery and the Internet: a poor source of patient-oriented information. *J Vasc Surg* **30**: 84–91.

Spielberg, A. R.(1998). On Call and Online. *JAMA* **280**: 1353–1359.

Stephenson, J. (1998a). Patient pretenders weave tangled 'Web' of deceit. *JAMA* **280**:1297.

Stephenson, J. (1998b). Physicians find teleactivity hot near the North Pole. *JAMA* **280**: 1296.

Strode, S. W., Gustke, S. and Allen, A.(1999). Technical and clinical progress in telemedicine. *JAMA* **281**: 1066–1068.

Index